# Guidelines for drinking-water quality

## SECOND EDITION

### Volume 2
### *Health criteria and*
### *other supporting information*

World Health Organization
Geneva
1996

WHO Library Cataloguing in Publication Data

Guidelines for drinking-water quality. - 2nd ed.
    Contents: v.2. Health criteria and other supporting information
    1. Drinking water – standards
    ISBN 92 4 154480 5 (v. 2) (NLM Classification: WA 675)

The World Health Organization welcomes requests for permission to reproduce or translate its publications, in part or in full. Applications and enquiries should be addressed to the Office of Publications, World Health Organization, Geneva, Switzerland, which will be glad to provide the latest information on any changes made to the text, plans for new editions, and reprints and translations already available.

The designations employed and the presentation of the material in this publication do not imply the expression of any opinion whatsoever on the part of the Secretariat of the World Health Organization concerning the legal status of any country, territory, city or area or of its authorities, or concerning the delimitation of its frontiers or boundaries.

The mention of specific companies or of certain manufacturers' products does not imply that they are endorsed or recommended by the World Health Organization in preference to others of a similar nature that are not mentioned. Errors and omissions excepted, the names of proprietary products are distinguished by initial capital letters.

TYPESET IN THE NETHERLANDS
PRINTED IN AUSTRIA
94/9960 – Mastercom/Wiener Verlag – 8000

# Contents

# Preface

In 1984 and 1985, the World Health Organization (WHO) published the first edition of *Guidelines for drinking-water quality* in three volumes. The development of these guidelines was organized and carried out jointly by WHO headquarters and the WHO Regional Office for Europe (EURO).

In 1988, the decision was made within WHO to initiate the revision of the guidelines. The work was again shared between WHO headquarters and EURO. Within headquarters, both the unit for the Prevention of Environmental Pollution (PEP) and the ILO/UNEP/WHO International Programme on Chemical Safety (IPCS) were involved, IPCS providing a major input to the health risk assessments of chemicals in drinking-water.

The revised guidelines are being published in three volumes. Guideline values for various constituents of drinking-water are given in Volume 1, *Recommendations,* together with essential information required to understand the basis for the values. Volume 2, *Health criteria and other supporting information,* contains the criteria monographs prepared for each substance or contaminant; the guideline values are based on these. Volume 3, *Surveillance and control of community supplies,* is intended to serve a very different purpose; it contains recommendations and information concerning what needs to be done in small communities, particularly in developing countries, to safeguard their water supplies.

The preparation of the current edition of the *Guidelines for drinking-water quality* covered a period of four years and involved the participation of numerous institutions, over 200 experts from nearly 40 different developing and developed countries and 18 meetings of the various coordination and review groups. The work of these institutions and scientists, whose names appear in Annex 1, was central to the completion of the guidelines and is much appreciated.

For each contaminant or substance considered, a lead country prepared a draft document evaluating the risks for human health from exposure to the contaminant in drinking-water. The following countries prepared such evaluation documents: Canada, Denmark, Finland, Germany, Italy, Japan, Netherlands, Norway, Poland, Sweden, United Kingdom of Great Britain and Northern Ireland and United States of America.

Under the responsibility of a coordinator for each major aspect of the guidelines, these draft evaluation documents were reviewed by several scientific institutions and selected experts, and comments were incorporated by the coordinator and author prior to submission for final evaluation by a review group. The review group then took a decision as to the health risk assessment and proposed a guideline value.

During the preparation of draft evaluation documents and at the review group meetings, careful consideration was always given to previous risk assessments carried out by IPCS, in its Environmental Health Criteria monographs, the International Agency for Research on Cancer, the Joint FAO/WHO Meetings on Pesticide Residues, and the Joint FAO/WHO Expert Committee on Food Additives, which evaluates contaminants such as lead and cadmium in addition to food additives.

It is clear that not all the chemicals that may be found in drinking-water were evaluated in developing these guidelines. Chemicals of importance to Member States which have not been evaluated should be brought to the attention of WHO for inclusion in any future revision.

It is planned to establish a continuing process of revision of the *Guidelines for drinking-water quality* with a number of substances or agents subject to evaluation each year. Where appropriate, addenda will be issued, containing evaluations of new substances or substances already evaluated for which new scientific information has become available. Substances for which provisional guideline values have been established will receive high priority for re-evaluation.

# Acknowledgements

The work of the following coordinators was crucial in the development of Volumes 1 and 2 of the *Guidelines*:

J. K. Fawell, Water Research Centre, England (inorganic constituents)
J. R. Hickman, Department of National Health and Welfare, Canada (radioactive materials)
U. Lund, Water Quality Institute, Denmark (organic constituents and pesticides)
B. Mintz, Environmental Protection Agency, United States of America (disinfectants and disinfectant by-products)
E. B. Pike, Water Research Centre, England (microbiology)

The coordinator for Volume 3 of the *Guidelines* was J. Bartram of the Robens Institute of Health and Safety, England.

The WHO coordinators were as follows:

*Headquarters*: H. Galal-Gorchev, International Programme on Chemical Safety; R. Helmer, Division of Environmental Health.
*Regional Office for Europe*: X. Bonnefoy, Environment and Health; O. Espinoza, Environment and Health.

Ms Marla Sheffer of Ottawa, Canada, was responsible for the scientific editing of the guidelines.

The convening of the coordination and review group meetings was made possible by the financial support afforded to WHO by the Danish International Development Agency (DANIDA) and the following sponsoring countries: Belgium, Canada, France, Italy, Netherlands, United Kingdom of Great Britain and Northern Ireland and United States of America.

In addition, financial contributions for the convening of the final task group meeting were received from the Norwegian Agency for Development Cooperation (NORAD), the United Kingdom Overseas Development Administration (ODA) and the Water Services Association in the United Kingdom, the Swedish International Development Authority (SIDA), and the Government of Japan.

The efforts of all who helped in the preparations and finalization of the *Guidelines for drinking-water quality* are gratefully acknowledged.

# Acronyms and abbreviations used in the text

| | |
|---|---|
| AAS | atomic absorption spectrometry |
| A/C | asbestos-cement |
| ADA | ampicillin-dextrin agar |
| ADI | acceptable daily intake |
| a.i. | active ingredient |
| AIDS | acquired immunodeficiency syndrome |
| ALAD | aminolaevulinic acid dehydratase |
| ALAT | alanine aminotransferase |
| AOC | assimilable organic carbon |
| APHA | American Public Health Association |
| | |
| BOD | biochemical oxygen demand |
| Bq | Becquerel |
| BSP | bromosulfophthalein |
| BUN | blood urea nitrogen |
| bw | body weight |
| | |
| CAS | Chemical Abstracts Service |
| cfu | colony-forming units |
| CHO | Chinese hamster ovary |
| CMC | carboxymethyl cellulose |
| | |
| DENA | diethylnitrosamine |
| DMAA | dimethylarsinic acid |
| DNA | deoxyribonucleic acid |
| DOPA | 3,4-dihydroxyphenylalanine |
| | |
| ECG | electrocardiogram |
| EDTA | edetic acid |
| EEG | electroencephalogram |
| EIEC | enteroinvasive *E. coli* |
| EP | erythrocyte protoporphyrin |
| EPA | Environmental Protection Agency (USA) |
| ETEC | enterotoxigenic *E. coli* |

| | |
|---|---|
| FAO | Food and Agriculture Organization of the United Nations |
| FPD | flame photometric detection |
| | |
| GC | gas chromatography |
| GCI | general cognitive index |
| GEMS | Global Environment Monitoring System |
| GOT | glutamic-oxaloacetic transaminase |
| GPT | glutamic-pyruvic transaminase |
| | |
| h | hour |
| HD | Hodgkin disease |
| HDL | high-density lipoprotein |
| HPLC | high-performance liquid chromatography |
| | |
| IARC | International Agency for Research on Cancer |
| ICRP | International Commission on Radiological Protection |
| ID | infective dose |
| Ig | immunoglobulin |
| IgG | immunoglobulin G |
| IgM | immunoglobulin M |
| ILO | International Labour Organisation |
| IPCS | International Programme on Chemical Safety |
| IQ | intelligence quotient |
| ISO | International Organization for Standardization |
| | |
| JECFA | Joint FAO/WHO Expert Committee on Food Additives |
| JMPR | Joint FAO/WHO Meeting on Pesticide Residues |
| | |
| $LC_{50}$ | lethal concentration, median |
| $LD_{50}$ | lethal dose, median |
| LH | luteinizing hormone |
| LOAEL | lowest-observed-adverse-effect level |
| LT | heat-labile enterotoxin |
| | |
| MAC | *Mycobacterium avium* complex |
| MAIS | *Mycobacterium avium, M. intracellulare, M. scrofulaceum* complex |
| MDI | mental development index |
| MFL | million fibres per litre |
| MIB | 2-methylisoborneol |
| MMAA | monomethylarsonic acid |
| MNCV | motor nerve conduction velocity |
| MS | mass spectrometry |
| MSCA | McCarthy Scales of Children's Abilities |
| MTD | maximum tolerated dose |

| | |
|---|---|
| NADPH | nicotinamide adenine dinucleotide phosphate (reduced) |
| NAG | non-agglutinable |
| NCI | National Cancer Institute (USA) |
| NCV | non-cholera vibrios |
| NEU | nitrosoethylurea |
| NHANES | US National Health and Nutrition Examination Survey |
| NHL | non-Hodgkin lymphoma |
| NOAEL | no-observed-adverse-effect level |
| NTA | nitrilotriacetic acid |
| NTP | National Toxicology Program (USA) |
| NTU | nephelometric turbidity unit |
| | |
| Pa | Pascal |
| PDI | psychomotor development index |
| $pK_a$ | log acid dissociation constant |
| PMTDI | provisional maximum tolerable daily intake |
| PTWI | provisional tolerable weekly intake |
| PVC | polyvinyl chloride |
| | |
| RNA | ribonucleic acid |
| | |
| SAED | selected-area electron diffraction |
| SAP | serum alkaline phosphatase |
| SGOT | serum glutamic-oxaloacetic transaminase |
| SGPT | serum glutamic-pyruvic transaminase |
| SMR | standardized mortality ratio |
| ST | heat-stable enterotoxin |
| STS | soft tissue sarcoma |
| | |
| $T_3$ | triiodothyronine |
| $T_4$ | thyroxine |
| TCU | true colour unit |
| TDI | tolerable daily intake |
| TDS | total dissolved solids |
| TEM | transmission electron microscopy |
| TOC | total organic carbon |
| TPA | tetradecanoyl-phorbol-acetate |
| | |
| UNEP | United Nations Environment Programme |
| UV | ultraviolet |
| WHA | World Health Assembly |
| WHO | World Health Organization |

# 1.
# Introduction

This volume of the *Guidelines for drinking-water quality* explains how guideline values for drinking-water contaminants are to be used, defines the criteria used to select the various chemical, physical, microbiological, and radiological contaminants included in the report, describes the approaches used in deriving guideline values, and presents, in the form of brief monographs, critical reviews and evaluations of the effects on human health of the substances or contaminants examined.

This edition of the *Guidelines* considers many drinking-water contaminants not included in the first edition. It also contains revised guideline values for many of the contaminants included in the first edition, which have been changed as a result of new scientific information. The guideline values given here supersede those in the 1984 edition.

Although the number of chemical contaminants for which guideline values are recommended is greater than in the first edition, it is unlikely that all of these chemical contaminants will occur in all water supplies or even in all countries. Care should therefore be taken in selecting substances for which national standards will be developed. A number of factors should be considered, including the geology of the region and the types of human activities that take place there. For example, if a particular pesticide is not used in the region, it is unlikely to occur in the drinking-water.

In other cases, such as the disinfection by-products, it may not be necessary to set standards for all of the substances for which guideline values have been proposed. If chlorination is practised, the trihalomethanes, of which chloroform is the major component, are likely to be the main disinfection by-products, together with the chlorinated acetic acids in some instances. In many cases, control of chloroform levels and, where appropriate, trichloroacetic acid will also provide an adequate measure of control over other chlorination by-products.

In developing national standards, care should also be taken to ensure that scarce resources are not unnecessarily diverted to the development of standards and the monitoring of substances of relatively minor importance.

Several of the inorganic elements for which guideline values have been recommended are recognized to be essential elements in human nutrition. No attempt has been made here to define a minimum desirable concentration of such substances in drinking-water.

## 1.1 General considerations

The primary aim of the *Guidelines for drinking-water quality* is the protection of public health. The guidelines are intended to be used as a basis for the development of national standards that, if properly implemented, will ensure the safety of drinking-water supplies through the elimination, or reduction to a minimum concentration, of constituents of water that are known to be hazardous to health. It must be emphasized that the guideline values recommended are not mandatory limits. In order to define such limits, it is necessary to consider the guideline values in the context of local or national environmental, social, economic, and cultural conditions.

The main reason for not promoting the adoption of international standards for drinking-water quality is the advantage provided by the use of a risk-benefit approach (qualitative or quantitative) to the establishment of national standards and regulations. This approach should lead to standards and regulations that can be readily implemented and enforced. For example, the adoption of drinking-water standards that are too stringent could limit the availability of water supplies that meet those standards—a significant consideration in regions of water shortage. The standards that individual countries will develop can thus be influenced by national priorities and economic factors. However, considerations of policy and convenience must never be allowed to endanger public health, and the implementation of standards and regulations will require suitable facilities and expertise as well as the appropriate legislative framework.

The judgement of safety—or what is an acceptable level of risk in particular circumstances—is a matter in which society as a whole has a role to play. The final judgement as to whether the benefit resulting from the adoption of any of the guideline values given here as standards justifies the cost is for each country to decide. What must be emphasized is that the guideline values have a degree of flexibility and enable a judgement to be made regarding the provision of drinking-water of acceptable quality.

Water is essential to sustain life, and a satisfactory supply must be made available to consumers. Every effort should be made to achieve a drinking-water quality as high as practicable. Protection of water supplies from contamination is the first line of defence. Source protection is almost invariably the best method of ensuring safe drinking-water and is to be preferred to treating a contaminated water supply to render it suitable for consumption. Once a potentially hazardous situation has been recognized, however, the risk to health, the availability of alternative sources, and the availability of suitable remedial measures must be considered so that a decision can be made about the acceptability of the supply.

As far as possible, water sources must be protected from contamination by human and animal waste, which can contain a variety of bacterial, viral, and protozoan pathogens and helminth parasites. Failure to provide adequate protection and effective treatment will expose the community to the risk of outbreaks of intestinal and other infectious diseases. Those at greatest risk of waterborne disease are infants and young children, people who are debilitated or living under unsanitary conditions, the sick, and the elderly. For these people, infective doses are significantly lower than for the general adult population.

The potential consequences of microbial contamination are such that its control must always be of paramount importance and must never be compromised.

The assessment of the risks associated with variations in microbial quality is difficult and controversial because of insufficient epidemiological evidence, the number of factors involved, and the changing interrelationships between these factors. In general terms, the greatest microbial risks are associated with ingestion of water that is contaminated with human and animal excreta. Microbial risk can never be entirely eliminated, because the diseases that are waterborne may also be transmitted by person-to-person contact, aerosols, and food intake; thus, a reservoir of cases and carriers is maintained. Provision of a safe water supply in these circumstances will reduce the chances of spread by these other routes. Waterborne outbreaks are particularly to be avoided because of their capacity to result in the simultaneous infection of a high proportion of the community.

The health risk due to toxic chemicals in drinking-water differs from that caused by microbiological contaminants. There are few chemical constituents of water that can lead to acute health problems except through massive accidental contamination of supply. Moreover, experience shows that, in such incidents the water usually becomes undrinkable owing to unacceptable taste, odour, and appearance.

The fact that chemical contaminants are not normally associated with acute effects places them in a lower priority category than microbial contaminants, the effects of which are usually acute and widespread. Indeed, it can be argued that chemical standards for drinking-water are of secondary consideration in a supply subject to severe bacterial contamination.

The problems associated with chemical constituents of drinking-water arise primarily from their ability to cause adverse health effects after prolonged periods of exposure; of particular concern are contaminants that have cumulative toxic properties, such as heavy metals, and substances that are carcinogenic.

It should be noted that the use of chemical disinfectants in water treatment usually results in the formation of chemical by-products, some of which are potentially hazardous. However, the risks to health from these by-products are extremely small in comparison with the risks associated with inadequate disinfection, and it is important that disinfection should not be compromised in attempting to control such by-products.

The radiological health risk associated with the presence of naturally occurring radionuclides in drinking-water should also be taken into consideration, although the contribution of drinking-water to total ambient exposure to these radionuclides is very small under normal circumstances. The guideline values recommended in this volume do not apply to water supplies contaminated during emergencies arising from accidental releases of radioactive substances to the environment.

In assessing the quality of drinking-water, the consumer relies principally upon his or her senses. Water constituents may affect the appearance, odour, or taste of the water, and the consumer will evaluate the quality and acceptability of the water on the basis of these criteria. Water that is highly turbid, is highly coloured, or has an objectionable taste or odour may be regarded by consumers as unsafe and may be rejected for drinking purposes. It is therefore vital to maintain a quality of water that is acceptable to the consumer, although the absence of any adverse sensory effects does not guarantee the safety of the water.

Countries developing national drinking-water limits or standards should carefully evaluate the costs and benefits associated with the control of aesthetic and organoleptic quality. Enforceable standards are sometimes set for contaminants directly related to health, whereas recommendations only are made for aesthetic and organoleptic characteristics. For countries with severely limited resources, it is even more important to establish priorities, and this should be done by considering the impact on health in each case. This approach does not underestimate the importance of the aesthetic quality of drinking-water. Source water that is aesthetically unsatisfactory may discourage the consumer from using an otherwise safe supply. Furthermore, taste, odour, and colour may be the first indication of potential health hazards.

Many parameters must be taken into consideration in the assessment of water quality, such as source protection, treatment efficiency and reliability, and protection of the distribution network (e.g., corrosion control). The costs associated with water quality surveillance and control must also be carefully evaluated before developing national standards.

## 1.2 The nature of the guideline values

Guideline values have been set for potentially hazardous water constituents and provide a basis for assessing drinking-water quality.

(a) A guideline value represents the concentration of a constituent that does not result in any significant risk to the health of the consumer over a lifetime of consumption.

(b) The quality of water defined by the *Guidelines for drinking-water quality* is such that it is suitable for human consumption and for all domestic purposes, including personal hygiene. However, water of a higher quality may be required for some special purposes, such as renal dialysis.

(c) When a guideline value is exceeded, this should be a signal: (i) to investigate the cause with a view to taking remedial action; (ii) to consult with, and seek advice from, the authority responsible for public health.

(d) Although the guideline values describe a quality of water that is acceptable for lifelong consumption, the establishment of these guideline values should not be regarded as implying that the quality of drinking-water may be degraded to the recommended level. Indeed, a continuous effort should be made to maintain drinking-water quality at the highest possible level.

(e) Short-term deviations above the guideline values do not necessarily mean that the water is unsuitable for consumption. The amount by which, and the period for which, any guideline value can be exceeded without affecting public health depends upon the specific substance involved.

It is recommended that when a guideline value is exceeded, the surveillance agency (usually the authority responsible for public health) should be consulted for advice on suitable action, taking into account the intake of the substance from sources other than drinking-water (for chemical constituents), the toxicity of the substance, the likelihood and nature of any adverse effects, the practicability of remedial measures, and similar factors.

(f) In developing national drinking-water standards based on these guideline values, it will be necessary to take account of a variety of geographical, socioeconomic, dietary, and other conditions affecting potential exposure. This may lead to national standards that differ appreciably from the guideline values.

(g) In the case of radioactive substances, screening values for gross alpha and gross beta activity are given, based on a reference level of dose.

It is important that recommended guideline values are both practical and feasible to implement as well as protective of public health. Guideline values are not set at concentrations lower than the detection limits achievable under routine laboratory operating conditions. Moreover, guideline values are recommended only when control techniques are available to remove or reduce the concentration of the contaminant to the desired level.

In some instances, *provisional* guideline values have been set for constituents for which there is some evidence of a potential hazard but where the available information on health effects is limited. Provisional guideline values have also been set for substances for which the calculated guideline value would be (i) below the practical quantification level, or (ii) below the level that can be achieved through practical treatment methods. Finally, provisional guideline values have been set for certain substances when it is likely that guideline values will be exceeded as a result of disinfection procedures.

Aesthetic and organoleptic characteristics are subject to individual preference as well as social, economic, and cultural considerations. For this reason, although guidance can be given on the levels of substances that may be aesthetically unacceptable, no guideline values have been set for such substances where they do not represent a potential hazard to health.

The recommended guideline values are set at a level to protect human health; they may not be suitable for the protection of aquatic life. The guidelines apply to bottled water and ice intended for human consumption but do not apply to natural mineral waters, which should be regarded as beverages rather than drinking-water in the usual sense of the word. The Codex Alimentarius Commission has developed Codex standards for such mineral waters.[1]

## 1.3 Criteria for the selection of health-related drinking-water contaminants

The recognition that faecally polluted water can lead to the spread of microbial infections has led to the development of sensitive methods for routine examination to ensure that water intended for human consumption is free from faecal contamination. Although it is now possible to detect the presence of many pathogens in water, the methods of isolation and enumeration are often complex and time-consuming. It is therefore impracticable to monitor drinking-water for every possible microbial pathogen. A more logical approach is the detection of organisms normally present in the faeces of humans and other warm-blooded animals as indicators of faecal pollution, as well as of the efficacy of water treatment and disinfection. The various bacterial indicators used for this purpose are described in Chapter 9. The presence of such organisms indicates the presence of faecal material and, hence, that intestinal pathogens could be present. Conversely, their absence indicates that pathogens are probably also absent.

Thousands of organic and inorganic chemicals have been identified in drinking-water supplies around the world, many in extremely low concentrations. The chemicals selected for the development of guideline values include those considered potentially hazardous to human health, those detected relatively frequently in drinking-water, and those detected in relatively high concentrations.

Some potentially hazardous chemicals in drinking-water are derived directly from treatment chemicals or construction materials used in water supply systems. Such chemicals are best controlled by appropriate specifications for the chemicals and materials used. For example, a wide range of polyelectrolytes are now used as coagulant aids in water treatment, and the presence of residues of the unreacted monomer may cause concern. Many polyelectrolytes are based on acrylamide polymers and co-polymers, in both of which the acrylamide monomer is present as a trace impurity. Chlorine used for disinfection has sometimes been found to contain carbon tetrachloride. This type of drinking-water contamination is best controlled by the application of regulations governing the quality of the products themselves rather than the quality of the water. Similarly, strict national regulations on the quality of pipe material should avoid the possible contamination of drinking-water by trace constituents of plastic pipes. The control of contamination of water supplies by *in situ* polymerized coatings and coatings applied in a solvent requires the development of suitable codes of practice, in addition to controls on the quality of the materials used.

---

[1] Codex Alimentarius Commission. *Codex standards for natural mineral waters.* Rome, Food and Agriculture Organization of the United Nations, 1994 (Codex Alimentarius Vol. XI, Part III).

# PART 1
## Microbiological aspects

# 2.

# Microbiological aspects: introduction

The most common and widespread health risk associated with drinking-water is contamination, either directly or indirectly, by human or animal excreta, particularly faeces. If such contamination is recent, and if those responsible for it include carriers of communicable enteric diseases, some of the pathogenic microorganisms that cause these diseases may be present in the water. Drinking the water, or using it in food preparation, may then result in new cases of infection.

The pathogenic agents involved include bacteria, viruses, and protozoa, which may cause diseases that vary in severity from mild gastroenteritis to severe and sometimes fatal diarrhoea, dysentery, hepatitis, or typhoid fever. Most of them are widely distributed throughout the world. Faecal contamination of drinking-water is only one of several faeco-oral mechanisms by which they can be transmitted from one person to another or, in some cases, from animals to people.

One ingested waterborne pathogen, namely guinea worm (*Dracunculus medinensis*), is not faecal in origin and deserves special mention. Although it is of limited geographical distribution, this helminth is of major public health importance in endemic areas. It is the only human infection that is solely transmitted by the waterborne route, and the World Health Assembly has committed itself to the eradication of dracunculiasis by the end of 1995 (resolution WHA 44.5, 1991).

Other pathogens cause infection when water containing them is used for bathing or for recreation involving water contact, rather than by the oral route. Some may also cause infection by inhalation when they are present in large numbers in water droplets, such as those produced by showers and some air-conditioning systems or in the irrigation of agricultural land.

It is not only by causing infection that microorganisms in drinking-water can affect human health. In some circumstances, cyanobacteria can produce toxins that may remain in the water even when the cyanobacteria themselves have been removed. Finally, there are some organisms whose presence in water is a nuisance, but which are of no significance for public health.

## 2.1 Agents of significance

The human pathogens potentially transmitted in drinking-water are listed in Table 2.1. Some general information on those included in the table is given below.

### Table 2.1 Waterborne pathogens and their significance in water supplies

| Pathogen | Health significance | Main route of exposure[a] | Persistence in water supplies[b] | Resistance to chlorine[c] | Relative infective dose[d] | Important animal reservoir |
|---|---|---|---|---|---|---|
| **Bacteria** | | | | | | |
| *Campylobacter jejuni, C.coli* | High | O | Moderate | Low | Moderate | Yes |
| Pathogenic *Escherichia coli* | High | O | Moderate | Low | High | Yes |
| *Salmonella typhi* | High | O | Moderate | Low | High | No |
| Other salmonellae | High | O | Long | Low | High | Yes |
| *Shigella* spp. | High | O | Short | Low | Moderate | No |
| *Vibrio cholerae* | High | O | Short | Low | High | No |
| *Yersinia enterocolitica* | High | O | Long | Low | High(?) | Yes |
| *Legionella* | Moderate | I | May multiply | Moderate | High | No |
| *Pseudomonas aeruginosa* | Moderate | C,IN | May multiply | Moderate | High(?) | No |
| *Aeromonas* spp. | Moderate | O,C | May multiply | Low | High(?) | No |
| *Mycobacterium,* atypical | Moderate | I,C | May multiply | High | ? | No |
| **Viruses** | | | | | | |
| Adenoviruses | High | O,I,C | ? | Moderate | Low | No |
| Enteroviruses | High | O | Long | Moderate | Low | No |
| Hepatitis A | High | O | Long | Moderate | Low | No |
| Hepatitis E | High | O | ? | ? | Low | Probable |
| Norwalk virus | High | O | ? | ? | Low | No |
| Rotavirus | High | O | ? | ? | Moderate | No(?) |
| Small round viruses (other than Norwalk virus) | Moderate | O | ? | ? | Low(?) | No |
| **Protozoa** | | | | | | |
| *Entamoeba histolytica* | High | O | Moderate | High | Low | No |
| *Giardia intestinalis* | High | O | Moderate | High | Low | Yes |
| *Cryptosporidium parvum* | High | O | Long | High | Low | Yes |
| *Acanthamoeba* spp. | Moderate | C,I | May multiply | High | ? | No |
| *Naegleria fowleri* | Moderate | C | May multiply | Moderate | Low | No |
| *Balantidium coli* | Moderate | O | ? | Moderate | Low | Yes |

**Table 2.1** (continued)

| Pathogen | Health significance | Main route of exposure[a] | Persistence in water supplies[b] | Resistance to chlorine[c] | Relative infective dose[d] | Important animal reservoir |
|---|---|---|---|---|---|---|
| **Helminths** | | | | | | |
| *Dracunculus medinensis* | High | O | Moderate | Moderate | Low | Yes |
| *Schistosoma* spp. | Moderate | C | Short | Low | Low | Yes |

? = Not known or uncertain
[a] O = oral (ingestion); I = inhalation in aerosol; C= contact with skin; IN - ingestion in immunosuppressed patients.
[b] Detection period for infective stage in water at 20 °C: short = up to 1 week; moderate = 1 week to 1 month; long = over 1 month.
[c] When the infective stage is freely suspended in water treated at conventional doses and contact times: resistance moderate, agent may not be completely destroyed; resistance low, agent completely destroyed.
[d] Dose required to cause infection in 50% of healthy adult volunteers.

## 2.1.1 Agents of high health significance

Not all potentially waterborne human pathogens are of equal public health significance (Table 2.1). Some of them, including most of the ingested pathogens, present a serious risk of disease whenever they are present in drinking-water, and their elimination from it should be given high priority. Examples include strains of *Escherichia coli*, *Salmonella*, *Shigella*, *Vibrio cholerae*, *Yersinia enterocolitica*, and *Campylobacter jejuni*, the viruses described in Chapter 4, and the parasites *Giardia*, *Cryptosporidium*, *Entamoeba histolytica*, and *Dracunculus*.

While most of the pathogens of high significance in Table 2.1 are found worldwide, others are a public health problem only in limited regions of the world, e.g. guinea worm is found only in certain countries of Africa and Asia. Historically, pandemics of cholera have spread from well-defined regions where the outbreaks first occurred. Although high priority should be given to control of these pathogens in drinking-water, this is of regional significance only.

## 2.1.2 Opportunistic pathogens

Some organisms, naturally present in the environment and not normally regarded as pathogens, may cause disease opportunistically. When such organisms are present in drinking-water, they cause infection predominantly among people whose local or general natural defence mechanisms are impaired. Those most likely to be at risk include the very old, the very young, and patients in hospitals, e.g. those with burns or undergoing immunosuppressive therapy, and those suffering from acquired immunodeficiency syndrome (AIDS). Water used by such patients for drinking or bathing, if it contains excessive numbers of these agents, may produce a variety of infections involving the skin and mucous membranes of the eye, ear, nose, and throat. *Pseudomonas, Flavobacterium, Acineto-*

*bacter, Klebsiella,* and *Serratia* are examples of such opportunistic pathogens, as is *Legionella,* which can infect the lungs if inhaled in droplets. Some of these, such as *Legionella* and *Aeromonas,* can also cause disease in otherwise healthy individuals when the specific conditions prevailing within a water-supply system have enabled them to multiply to unusually high concentrations. These organisms, while clearly of medical importance, only acquire public health significance under certain conditions. Their removal from drinking-water may therefore be given moderate priority.

## 2.1.3 Nuisance organisms

Nuisance organisms, by definition, have no public health significance. However, they produce problems of turbidity, taste and odour or appear as visible animal life in the water. As well as being aesthetically objectionable, they indicate that both water treatment and the maintenance and repair of the distribution system are defective.

# 2.2 Routes of exposure

For the faeco-oral pathogens, drinking-water is only one vehicle of transmission. Contamination of food, hands, utensils, and clothing can also play a role, particularly when domestic hygiene is poor. Because of this multiplicity of transmission routes, improvements in the quality and availability of water, in excreta disposal, and in general hygiene education are all important factors in achieving reductions in diarrhoea morbidity and mortality rates ( *1* )

While many faeco-oral pathogens have been shown to cause waterborne epidemics, none of them causes epidemics exclusively by this means. Neither the identification of a specific pathogen in drinking-water nor the occurrence of a common-source epidemic can therefore be taken as proof of waterborne disease transmission. To obtain confirmatory evidence, an epidemiological investigation is required. Those infections for which there is epidemiological evidence of waterborne transmission are listed in Table 2.1

The significance of the water route varies considerably both with the disease and with local conditions. Thus, waterborne transmission of poliomyelitis has not been conclusively demonstrated, while waterborne epidemics of giardiasis, typhoid fever, and cholera have frequently been documented. One reason for this is that there are important differences between the pathogens in terms of their persistence in water, their removal by conventional water-treatment processes, and the minimum infective dose, i.e. the number of organisms needed to cause infection when taken by mouth.

## 2.3 Persistence in water

The persistence of a pathogen in water is a measure of how quickly it dies after leaving the body. In practice, the numbers of a pathogen introduced on a given occasion will tend to decline exponentially with time, reaching insignificant and undetectable levels after a certain period (Table 2.1).

A pathogen that persists outside the body only for a short time must rapidly find a new susceptible host. It is therefore less likely to be transmitted through a water-supply system than within a family or some other group living closely together, where lax personal cleanliness will allow the infection to be transferred from one person to another.

The persistence of most pathogens in water is affected by various factors, of which sunlight and temperature are among the most important. Lifetimes are shorter, sometimes much shorter, at warmer temperatures. For example, whereas enteric viruses may be detected for up to 9 months at around 10 °C, their maximum period of detection at 20 °C is nearer to 2 months (2).

Some pathogens are more resistant than others to conventional water-treatment processes, particularly chlorination at the doses and contact times usually employed. This is also indicated in Table 2.1 and discussed in further detail in Chapter 11.

## 2.4 Infective dose

For several intestinal pathogens, attempts have been made to determine the number of organisms needed to produce either a clinically apparent infection or intestinal colonization in human subjects (see Table 2.2). The significance of the results of these studies is obscure. While they undoubtedly provide an order of relative infectivity, it is doubtful whether the actual infective doses obtained are relevant to natural infections. The number of subjects exposed to infection in experimental studies is necessarily small and the experiments are designed to ensure that many of them become infected. During an outbreak, the number of subjects exposed may be very large, but only a small proportion become infected. Thus the minimum infective dose in an outbreak, and the attack rate, are probably much lower than in an experimental study. In many outbreaks of typhoid fever, the case rate can be explained only by assuming that the infective dose was low.

The likelihood of ingesting very large numbers of a pathogen on a single occasion from drinking-water is relatively small, both because enteric pathogens cannot normally multiply in water and because the water tends to disperse them. On the other hand, if polluted water is permitted to contaminate food, bacterial pathogens, initially present in small numbers, can multiply to produce very large doses.

### Table 2.2 Studies on the infectivity of various pathogens in human volunteers

| Pathogen | Reference no. |
|---|---|
| Salmonella typhi | 3, 4 |
| Other Salmonella spp. | 3 |
| Escherichia coli | 5–12 |
| Shigella spp. | 13 |
| Campylobacter jejuni | 14 |
| Vibrio cholerae | 15–17 |
| Giardia intestinalis | 18,19 |
| Echovirus 12 | 20 |
| Poliovirus type 1 (attenuated vaccine strains) | 21, 22 |
| Rotavirus strain CJN | 23 |
| General methodologies | 24 |

Bacteria that cause intestinal infections are able to invade and grow in the intestine. It is convenient, therefore, to develop a model of infection that states that, under the correct circumstances, a single infective organism must be able to initiate a clinically significant infection. The infective dose (ID) required to ensure that infection occurs in a specified proportion of subjects—for example, half the subjects ($ID_{50}$)—may be considered to represent, for a particular bacterial species, the probability that the single organism will reach the correct portion of intestine under the right circumstances to initiate a clinically apparent infection.

In a natural infection, the variables affecting this probability may be numerous and varied, as shown in Table 2.3. The transfer of the pathogen from one case to the next may appear simple, but numerous factors, including the ability to survive in the environment and the nature of the environment available to the host, play an important role. Socioeconomic factors, such as the practice of food hygiene, the availability of pure water, and the adequacy of excreta disposal, further complicate the picture.

After ingestion of the pathogen, the development of an infection depends on the balance between host factors, such as gastric acidity and intestinal immunity, tending to remove it, and factors aiding the bacteria in their attempt to colonize the intestine, such as the possession of colonization factors and adhesions. Studies in animals suggest that the growth phase and growth rate may be crucial.

After an infection has been initiated, its clinical expression is still not certain. The bacterial virulence factors, such as enterotoxin production and invasiveness, produce pathological changes, but their overt expression is countered by homoeostatic mechanisms in the gut. The multiplication of the bacteria extends the area of pathological changes, while the development of immunity inhibits the expression of bacterial virulence and results in the elimination of the pathogen. The infective dose, as determined in experimental situations, must, in part, represent the number of bacteria needed to produce disease before being overcome by the host defences. The effect of infective dose on incubation period has been demonstrated in a study on typhoid fever, which showed that the larger the adminis-

**Table 2.3 Factors determining the probability of developing clinically significant intestinal infections**

| Host | Stage of infection | Pathogen |
|------|-------------------|----------|
| Socioeconomic factors (food hygiene, availability of potable water, excreta disposal, public health measures) | Ingestion | Environmental survival |
| Antimicrobial defences, gastric acidity, etc. | Infection | Growth phase, adhesins and colonization factors |
| Immune system, antitoxic immunity | Water loss | Enterotoxin production, mucosal invasion |
| Homoeostatic mechanisms of water absorption in the gut | Diarrhoea | |

tered dose, the shorter the incubation period (4), a finding that may constitute evidence in support of that conclusion.

The physiological state of the host is another important factor. Undoubtedly the response to infection of the healthy north American adults, in whom most studies on infective dose have been performed (Table 2.2), is different from that of malnourished infants in Africa, Asia, or South America. Factors such as gastric acid production and the immune response are both influenced by nutritional status. Caution is therefore necessary in extrapolating from infective dose to epidemiological mechanism.

## References

1. Esrey SA, Feachem RG, Hughes JM. Interventions for the control of diarrhoeal diseases among young children: improving water supplies and excreta disposal facilities. *Bulletin of the World Health Organization*, 1985, 63:757-772.

2. Feachem RG et al. *Sanitation and disease: health aspects of excreta and wastewater management.* Chichester, John Wiley & Sons, 1983 (World Bank Studies in Water Supply and Sanitation, No. 3)

3. Blaser MJ, Newman LS. A review of human salmonellosis: 1. Infective dose. *Review of infectious diseases*, 1982, 4:1096-1106.

4. Hornick RB et al. Typhoid fever: pathogenesis and immunologic control. Part 1. *New England journal of medicine*, 1970, 283:686-691.

5.  Evans DG et al. Differences in serological responses and excretion patterns of volunteers challenged with enterotoxigenic *Escherichia coli* with and without the colonization factor antigen. *Infection and immunology*, 1978, 19:883-888.

6.  Evans DG et al. Administration of purified colonization factor antigens (CFA/I, CFA/II) of enterotoxigenic *Escherichia coli* to volunteers. Response to challenge with virulent enterotoxigenic *Escherichia coli*. *Gastroenterology*, 1984, 87:934-940.

7.  Levine MM et al. Diarrhea caused by *Escherichia coli* that produce only heat-stable enterotoxin. *Infection and immunology*, 1977, 17:78-82.

8.  Levine MM et al. Immunity to enterotoxigenic *Escherichia coli*. *Infection and immunology*, 1979, 23:729-736.

9.  Levine MM et al. Coli surface antigens 1 and 3 of Colonization Factor Antigen II-positive enterotoxigenic *Escherichia coli*: morphology, purification, and immune responses in humans. *Infection and immunology*, 1984, 44:409-420.

10. Levine MM et al. The diarrheal response of humans to some classic serotypes of enteropathogenic *Escherichia coli* is dependent on a plasmid encoding an entero-adhesiveness factor. *Journal of infectious diseases*, 1985, 152:550-559.

11. Mathewson JJ et al. Pathogenicity of enteroadherent *Escherichia coli* in adult volunteers. *Journal of infectious diseases*, 1986, 154:524-527.

12. Tacket CO et al. Protection by milk immunoglobulin concentrate against oral challenge with enterotoxigenic *Escherichia coli*. *New England journal of medicine*, 1988, 318:1240-1243.

13. Dupont HL et al. Inoculum size in shigellosis and implications for expected mode of transmission. *Journal of infectious diseases*, 1989, 159:1126-1128.

14. Black RE et al. Experimental *Campylobacter jejuni* infection in humans. *Journal of infectious diseases*, 1988, 157:472-479.

15. Cash RA et al. Response of man to infection with *Vibrio cholerae*. Clinical, serologic, and bacteriologic responses to a known inoculum. *Journal of infectious diseases*, 1974, 129:45-52.

16. Levine MM et al. Volunteer studies of deletion mutants of *Vibrio cholerae* 01 prepared by recombinant techniques. *Infection and immunology*, 1988, 56:161-167.

17. Levine MM et al. Safety, immunogenicity, and efficacy of recombinant live oral cholera vaccines, CVD 103 and CVD 103-HgR. *Lancet*, 1988, ii:467-470.

18. Nash TE et al. Experimental human infections with *Giardia lamblia*. *Journal of infectious diseases*, 1987, 156: 974-984.

19. Rose JB, Haas CN, Regli S. Risk assessment and control of waterborne giardiasis. *American journal of public health*, 1991, 81:701-713.

20. Schiff GM et al. Studies of Echovirus-12 in volunteers: determination of minimal infectious dose and the effect of previous infection on infectious dose. *Journal of infectious diseases*, 1984, 150:858-866.

21. Katz M, Plotkin SA. Minimal infective dose of attenuated poliovirus for man. *American journal of public health*, 1967, 57:1838-1840.

22. Minor TE et al. Human infective dose determinations for oral poliovirus type 1 vaccine in infants. *Journal of clinical microbiology*, 1981, 13:388-389.

23. Ward RL et al. Human rotavirus studies in volunteers: determination of infectious dose and serological response to infection. *Journal of infectious diseases*, 1986, 154:871-880.

24. Haas CN. Estimation of risk due to low doses of microorganisms: a comparison of alternative methodologies. *American journal of epidemiology*, 1983, 118:573-582.

# 3.
# Bacteria [1]

## 3.1 Pathogens excreted

### 3.1.1 *Salmonella*

#### General description

The genus *Salmonella* is a member of the family Enterobacteriaceae. The genus is currently subdivided into the subgenera I–IV, on the basis of biochemical characteristics. Most salmonella strains isolated from humans and warm-blooded vertebrates belong to subgenus I, while subgenera II, III (also called Arizona) and IV are more frequently associated with reptiles, in which they reside commensally. Currently more than 2000 serotypes are named. There are considerable regional variations in the prevalence of serotypes (*1*).

The virulence of *Salmonella* spp. depends on serotype and strain specificity in host range and infective dose and on host status. *S. typhi* is a specific human pathogen. In particular, *S. typhi*, *S. paratyphi* A, and *S. paratyphi* B are able to invade tissues and cause septicaemia with high temperature rather than diarrhoea. This is known as enteric fever. In humans, the majority of the other serotypes give rise to a transient intestinal infection manifesting itself as acute gastroenteritis with diarrhoea. Certain serotypes are highly pathogenic for humans, while others are devoid of any pathogenic action. Many salmonella infections are asymptomatic (*2*).

#### Routes of exposure

In the case of *S. typhi* and *S. paratyphi* A, human carriers are the source of infection, whereas milk-borne transmission can also occur with *S. paratyphi* B. The incidence of enteric fever decreases as a country becomes more highly developed in terms of controlled sewerage systems and drinking-water supplies, and the supply of pasteurized milk and dairy products. Most salmonellae are primarily pathogens of animals, which constitute important reservoirs for those infections (*2*).

---

[1] The valuable contribution made by Dr N.F. Pierce, Division of Diarrhoeal and Acute Respiratory Disease Control, WHO, Geneva, in the preparation of this chapter is gratefully acknowledged.

Salmonellae may be present in all kinds of food grown in faecally polluted environments, and are commonly isolated from poultry and livestock and foods prepared from them. Furthermore, animal feedstuffs and fertilizers prepared from animal products may be highly contaminated with salmonellae, and they are also widely distributed in the environment. The contamination of food and animal feedstuffs by water contaminated with salmonellae is considered to be an additional risk factor (*3*, *4*). Dumping of unprocessed slaughterhouse wastes into rivers has been found to be a cause of salmonellae infections. Contamination by salmonellae and conditions favouring their regrowth should be avoided at all stages of the production, transport, storage, and preparation of food, feedstuffs, and drinking-water. Sludge disposal and irrigation must always be accompanied by appropriate hygienic precautions.

The transmission routes of salmonellae are highly complex. Person-to-person transmission may occur, but the relative importance of the human and non-human reservoirs depends on the dietary, agricultural, and sanitary situation in a particular community (*2*).

### *Significance in drinking-water*

Waterborne outbreaks have been chiefly associated with *S. typhi* and much less frequently with *S. paratyphi* B or other *Salmonella* serotypes (*2*). Epidemiological studies of outbreaks suggest that the ingestion of relatively few cells of *S. typhi* may cause typhoid fever, whereas studies in volunteers (Table 2.2, p. 14) indicate that, for other *Salmonella* serotypes, millions of cells are usually required to cause gastroenteritis.

Salmonellae are excreted in the faeces of infected humans or animals. Faecal contamination of groundwater or surface waters, as well as insufficiently treated and inadequately disinfected drinking-water, are the main causes of epidemic waterborne outbreaks caused by *Salmonella* spp.

Waterborne outbreaks due to heavy contamination are usually characterized by an explosive onset. The majority of cases develop over a period of a few days, and may be followed by a secondary crop of contact cases (*2*). The geographical distribution of infections in major outbreaks is often strongly correlated with the pattern of a waterworks pipeline network.

Salmonellae can be found in open wells as a result of the drainage or flooding of contaminated surface water into unprotected well shafts. It is uncommon for salmonellae to be isolated from piped water supplies, whether treated or untreated, and their presence suggests a serious fault in the design or management of the system (*2*).

Penetration of pathogens into water sources must be avoided by the protection of groundwater and surface water catchment areas. A review of the literature has shown that, in general, pathogens will not travel further than the distance that the groundwater flows in 10 days, except in fissured rocks such as limestone and heavily fissured soils (*5*).

Drinking-water must be of low turbidity after treatment if adequate chlorination is to be achieved. Furthermore, a low load of assimilable organic carbon (AOC) in the treated water is considered to be an important factor in reducing survival time and preventing the regrowth of salmonellae within the distribution system. Reported survival times for salmonellae in drinking-water range from a few days to over 100 days.

Several outbreaks have been caused by the deposition of contaminated sediments in the distribution system for drinking-water, especially in water basins and pipes. Sediments may be shifted to new positions in the system by water pressure oscillations or temporary scarcity of water. Regular flushing of the distribution system is therefore recommended.

### 3.1.2 Yersinia

#### General description

The genus *Yersinia* is currently placed in the family Enterobacteriaceae and comprises seven species. *Y. pestis*, *Y. pseudotuberculosis*, and certain serotypes of *Y. enterocolitica* are pathogens for humans. Atypical strains within *Y. enterocolitica*, isolated most frequently from environmental samples, are grouped together as *Y. enterocolitica*-like organisms. They are nonpathogenic for humans and can be subdivided by biochemical means into *Y. intermedia*, *Y. frederiksenii*, *Y. kristensenii*, and *Y. aldovae*.

The cells of *Y. enterocolitica* are Gram-negative rods, motile at 25 °C but nonmotile in cultures grown at 37 °C. Certain strains of *Y. enterocolitica* cause acute gastroenteritis with diarrhoea, but other human diseases caused by *Y. enterocolitica* are also known. Biochemical and serological typing of enteric *Y. enterocolitica* strains show that serotypes O:3 and O:9 are commonly found in Africa, Asia, Canada and Europe, whereas serotype O:8 is exclusively isolated in the United States (6-8).

There is some evidence that *Y. enterocolitica* infection may be waterborne. The following discussion is confined to this species.

#### Routes of exposure

The transmission of *Y. enterocolitica* from the natural reservoirs to humans has been the subject of much debate. Many domestic and wild animals are considered to be possible reservoirs of *Y. enterocolitica* because of the high isolation rates of the organism from such sources. It is likely that wild animals, particularly shrews, hares, foxes, and beavers, form a natural reservoir of *Y. enterocolitica*. Swine have been implicated as a major reservoir of *Y. enterocolitica* serotypes involved in human infections.

Available evidence indicates that foods, especially meat and meat products, milk and dairy products, are the major vehicles for the transmission of *Y. enterocolitica*. Furthermore, *Y. enterocolitica* has been isolated from a variety of environmental samples, especially from water, but the serotypes isolated differ from those associated with human disease.

A number of different transmission routes have been suggested for *Y. enterocolitica*, but the ingestion of contaminated food and water is probably the most likely one (*8*). Direct transmission from person to person and from animals to humans also occurs, but its relative importance has not been clarified. Further research is needed to define the epidemiological importance of "environmental" strains of *Y. enterocolitica*.

### Significance in drinking-water

The apparent waterborne spread of *Y. enterocolitica* infection has been described in a number of reports. There is some evidence that pathogenic strains of *Y. enterocolitica* enter drinking-water via contaminated surface water or as a result of pollution with sewage (*9*). Recent studies have shown that human pathogenic serotypes of *Y. enterocolitica* are present in sewage and polluted surface water (*10, 11*).

In general, pathogenic types of *Y. enterocolitica* are not isolated from untreated or treated drinking-water unless faecal pollution has occurred. Occasionally, nonpathogenic serotypes of *Y. enterocolitica* and nonpathogenic *Y. enterocolitica*-like organisms (*Y. intermedia, Y. frederiksenii, Y. kristensenii*) may also be isolated from drinking-water. However, none of these isolates exhibit the typical virulence markers. Such isolates are probably of environmental origin without public health importance (*12*).

Water samples yielding *Y. enterocolitica* often show only slight coliform contamination. One study indicated that 25% of *Y. enterocolitica*-positive samples were negative for both total and faecal coliforms (*9*). Intensive methods of treatment are not needed in such cases. Other studies have shown a close relationship between faecal pollution and *Y. enterocolitica* isolation rates (*13*).

Standard chlorination procedures are sufficient to avoid the transmission of *Yersinia* if the treated water is of low turbidity. Free chlorine in the range required for water disinfection (0.2–0.5 mg/litre) for 10 minutes at pH 7.0 completely eradicates the bacteria; 0.05 mg/litre of ozone eradicates the organism after contact for 1 minute regardless of pH (*14*).

A special feature of *Y. enterocolitica* and *Y. enterocolitica*-like organisms is their ability to grow at low temperatures, even at 4 °C. Accordingly, these organisms can survive for long periods in water habitats. For example, *Y. enterocolitica* was detected in previously sterilized distilled water after over 18 months at 4 °C (*15*). Such long survival periods make it difficult to determine the origin of contamination when *Yersinia* are detected.

### 3.1.3 Campylobacter

**General description**

In recent years, considerable attention has been given to *Campylobacter* spp. as important agents of enteritis, gastritis, and other human diseases.

Campylobacters are Gram-negative, slender, comma-shaped rods. They also appear S-shaped and gull-winged when in pairs (*7, 16*). The organisms show a characteristic corkscrew-like motion, which can be easily seen by phase-contrast microscopy. Campylobacters are microaerophilic organisms, requiring a low oxygen tension (3–6%) for growth. Under unfavourable growth conditions, cells may form coccoid bodies.

A recent review discusses 14 *Campylobacter* species (*17*). Some are pathogens for humans and animals (e.g. *C. jejuni, C. coli, C. fetus*), while others are considered to be nonpathogenic (e.g. *C. sputorum, C. concisus*) (*16, 17*). Most of the members of the thermophilic group (growing at 42 °C) of campylobacters cause enteritis in humans. Worldwide, campylobacters are much more important than salmonellae as causes of acute gastroenteritis, but not as important as shigellas. Several major outbreaks of campylobacter enteritis were linked to the ingestion of contaminated food, milk, or water.

From the point of view of water hygiene, the thermophilic campylobacters are of greatest significance; the following discussion is therefore confined to these organisms.

**Routes of exposure**

Thermophilic campylobacters are transmitted by the oral route. The reservoirs for campylobacters include wild birds and poultry which are the most important, and other domesticated animals, such as pigs, cattle, dogs, and cats. Meat, in particular poultry products, and unpasteurized milk are therefore important sources of campylobacter infections (*16*). Milk may be contaminated with faeces or by the secretion of organisms into milk by cows with mastitis (*18*). In developing countries, the faeces of infected animals are important reservoirs. The infective dose is low (*19*).

Recent studies have shown that raw sewage frequently contains $10–10^5$ thermophilic campylobacters per 100 ml (*20, 21*). However, *Campylobacter* counts in heavily contaminated sewage can be reduced considerably by wastewater treatment processes. Thermophilic campylobacters were found in crude sludge, but were not detectable in digested conditioned sludge of filter effluent (*21*). The occurrence of campylobacters in surface waters has proved to be strongly dependent on rainfall, water temperature, and the presence of waterfowl.

## Significance in drinking-water

Several waterborne outbreaks of campylobacteriosis have been reported in the past decade. The numbers of persons involved ranged from a few to several thousands. In only two of these outbreaks were campylobacters isolated both from patients and from water samples. Unchlorinated surface water and faecal contamination of water storage reservoirs by wild birds were found to be the main causes. The consumption of unchlorinated or inadequately chlorinated surface waters is associated with a considerable risk of outbreaks of campylobacteriosis. Any contamination of drinking-water reservoirs by the excrement of waterfowl must be controlled. Consideration should be given to imposing stricter hygienic requirements for drinking-water, even if obtained from high-quality surface water, since it may be distributed without chlorination.

Campylobacters, like other bacterial pathogens, survive well at low temperatures, suggesting that cold water may be an effective vehicle of transmission. They are able to survive for several weeks (22) in cold groundwater or unchlorinated tapwater. The standard chlorination procedures are sufficient to prevent the spread of campylobacters along water mains if the water is of low turbidity.

### 3.1.4 Escherichia coli

E. coli is found in large numbers in the faeces of humans and of nearly all warm-blooded animals; as such it serves as a reliable index of recent faecal contamination of water. This topic is fully covered in Chapters 9–11. Certain strains are pathogenic for humans and it is these that are described below.

## General description

E. coli is a Gram-negative, non-spore-forming, rod-shaped bacterium which can be either motile or nonmotile (motile cells are peritrichous); growth is aerobic or facultatively anaerobic. Metabolism is both respiratory and fermentative; acid is produced by the fermentation of glucose and lactose. Catalase is produced but not oxidase, and nitrates are reduced to nitrites. In the microbiological examination of water, a biochemical description is used (see sections 9.2.1–9.2.3).

Serological typing is based on the somatic O antigens, the capsular K antigens, and the flagellar H antigens. In practice, serogrouping by O antigen is often used alone and, within a particular epidemiological context, may be satisfactory. Biochemical tests do not reliably distinguish pathogenic strains of E. coli.

## Health effects

E. coli is a normal inhabitant of the intestine, and most strains are nonpathogenic. However, subtypes able to cause gastrointestinal disease are also known. Such pathogenic E. coli strains cause intestinal disease by a variety of mechanisms. Infections may resemble cholera, dysentery, or gastroenteritis due to salmonellae. Four classes of pathogenic *E. coli* responsible for diarrhoea are recognized: enteropathogenic, enteroinvasive, enterotoxigenic, and verocytotoxin-producing (*23*).

Enteropathogenic subtypes of *E. coli* were first recognized as a result of the serological examination of strains isolated from outbreaks of diarrhoea among infants. Associations of particular serotypes with disease were observed, but the corresponding pathogenic mechanisms are not fully understood for most of these organisms. These strains have been particularly associated with outbreaks of infantile gastroenteritis (*24*).

Enteroinvasive strains of *E. coli* (EIEC) produce dysentery by a mechanism similar to that found with *Shigella* spp. These organisms invade the colonic mucosa and cause bloody diarrhoea. The property seems to be restricted to a few O groups. It must be remembered that *Shigella* and *E. coli* are closely related and that genetic material is readily exchanged between them.

Although enteropathogenic or enteroinvasive strains may cause serious illness, such epidemiological evidence as is available suggests that enterotoxigenic strains are responsible for most episodes of *E. coli* diarrhoea, particularly in developing countries. Enterotoxigenic *E. coli* (ETEC) can cause a cholera-like syndrome in infants, children, and adults.

ETEC produce either a heat-labile enterotoxin (LT), related to cholera enterotoxin, or a heat-stable enterotoxin (ST); some strains produce both toxins. The action of LT is the same as that of cholera toxin. The production of enterotoxin is controlled by plasmids.

The ability of ETEC to cause disease depends not only on the production of enterotoxin but also on their ability to colonize the small intestine. Various colonization factors, or adhesins, have been described, which enable the bacteria to attach themselves to the intestinal mucosa.

The fourth class, verocytotoxic *E. coli*, was first recognized by their production of a cytotoxin active against Vero cells in culture. The organisms commonly belong to the serogroup O157 and cause disease ranging from mild diarrhoea to haemorrhagic colitis characterized by blood-stained diarrhoea, usually without fever, but accompanied by abdominal pain. It is also a cause of the haemolytic uraemic syndrome, commonest in infants and young children, and characterized by acute renal failure and haemolytic anaemia.

### Significance in drinking-water

Isolation of *E. coli* from a water supply indicates faecal contamination. However, *E. coli* is only one species among many in the family Enterobacteriaceae. Members of the lactose-fermenting species of this group, which may be referred to colloquially as "coliforms", occur in a variety of ecological niches, not all of which are intestinal. Thus, for example, some species are associated with aquatic slimes and vegetation. The picture is further complicated by the fact that other members of the coliform group are also found in the intestine. Thus, the definitive identification of *E. coli* may be needed to determine the significance of "coliforms" in a water supply.

Conventionally, thermotolerant coliforms are identified by growth at 44–45 °C, but some isolates of *Klebsiella*, *Citrobacter*, and *Enterobacter* will also grow and ferment lactose under these conditions. The term "faecal coliforms" is often used for this group, but the term "faecal" is to be deprecated, since not all prove to be of faecal origin.

The detection of the pathogenic subtypes of *E. coli* in water supplies has seldom been attempted. Although this may be necessary in epidemiological research, the available methods are not suitable for the routine examination of water samples.

## 3.1.5 *Vibrio cholerae*
### General description

*Vibrio* species are motile, non-spore-forming, slightly curved Gram-negative rods with a single polar flagellum; they are both aerobic and facultatively anaerobic. Their metabolism is both respiratory and fermentative without the production of gas. Both catalase and oxidase are formed, and nitrates are reduced to nitrites.

Among the vibrios, special attention has focused on the identity of those causing cholera. It was for a long time believed that *Vibrio cholerae* was a unique and distinct species associated with human disease, and recognized by possession of the O1 antigens. This species was further divided into "classical" and "El Tor" biotypes, the latter distinguished by the ability to produce a dialysable, heat-labile haemolysin, active against sheep and goat red cells (*25*).

A broader definition of *V. cholerae* has now been adopted. It has been known for many years that vibrios biochemically identical to *Vibrio cholerae* O1, but lacking the O1 antigen, could be found in the aquatic environment. These were termed non-cholera vibrios (NCV) or non-agglutinable (NAG) vibrios. The term "non-O1 *V. cholerae*" is now preferred, since some may produce cholera toxin, while investigation of DNA/DNA homology between *Vibrio cholerae*, NCVs, and NAG vibrios has conclusively demonstrated that they are all very closely related. Currently, all are considered to be a single species, *Vibrio cholerae*, divided into more than 80 serological types on the basis of the O or somatic antigens. The H or flagella antigen is common to all the O groups of *V. cholerae*, and H agglutination has been used as a diagnostic test.

Only *V. cholerae* serogroup O1 causes cholera. The O1 group contains two serotypes based on variations in the O antigen factors, namely Ogawa (factors A and B) and Inaba (factors A and C). These serotypes may exist in either the classical or El Tor biotype.

## Routes of exposure

Cholera has historically been one of the major pandemic diseases. The present pandemic, unlike previous ones, is caused by *V. cholerae* O1 biotype El Tor.

Cholera is usually a waterborne disease, and numerous waterborne outbreaks have been documented. However, foodborne and nosocomial outbreaks are also important, and person-to-person transmission may occur under conditions of extreme crowding and poor hygiene. The problems of the transmission of cholera have been extensively reviewed, and although waterborne transmission is undoubtedly important, many aspects of the epidemiology of cholera are a matter for debate. Evidence has accumulated to suggest that, in some circumstances, *V. cholerae*, including serotype O1, may be part of the autochthonous microbiota of natural waters (*25, 26*).

## Health effects

Infection with *V. cholerae* O1 involves the small and large intestine. In the small intestine, the vibrios attach themselves to the mucous layer covering the villous epithelium, chemotactic processes apparently playing a role in their migration to the epithelium. After attachment, vibrios penetrate the layer of mucus and adhere to the surface of the epithelial cells. Motility seems to be essential for mucus penetration to occur. Adherence to the mucosal surface is specific, involving a receptor–adhesion interaction analogous to a lectin–ligand reaction. When present in large numbers, *V. cholerae* O1 produce an enterotoxin (cholera toxin) that causes alterations in the ionic fluxes across the mucosa with the resulting catastrophic loss of water and electrolytes in liquid stools. Cholera toxin is very similar to the heat-labile toxin produced by enterotoxigenic *E. coli*.

It seems likely that other accessory virulence factors, such as mucinase and protease, are also important in the pathogenesis of cholera. Other toxins may also be involved. Enterotoxins similar to the heat-stable toxins of *E. coli* are known to be formed by *V. cholerae* of O groups 2–84, and *V. cholerae* O1 may also produce several toxins. Cholera toxin is not produced by all strains of *V. cholerae* O1, and nontoxigenic strains are considered to be nonpathogenic.

## Significance in drinking-water

The isolation of *V. cholerae* O1 from water used for drinking is of major public health importance and is evidence of faecal contamination. However, other serogroups of *V. cholerae* may be part of the normal flora of some waters.

### 3.1.6 *Shigella*

#### General description

Shigellae are Gram-negative, non-spore-forming, non-motile rods, capable of growth under both aerobic and anaerobic conditions. Metabolism is both respiratory and fermentative; acid, but not usually gas, is produced from glucose. Lactose is seldom fermented. Catalase is usually produced, except by *Shigella dysenteriae* type 1, but oxidase is produced by one serotype only. Nitrates are reduced to nitrites.

Shigellae are serotyped on the basis of their somatic O antigens. Both group and type antigens are distinguished, group antigenic determinants being common to a number of related types. There is evidence that type antigen specificities among *Shigella flexneri* are determined by the presence of lysogenic bacteriophages. It seems likely that biotypic and serological variants are determined by the presence of phage or the carriage of plasmids. Plasmids (transferable, extrachromosomal genetic elements) were first described in this genus. Phage-typing systems exist for all groups, though they have not been widely applied, serological typing being adequate for all species except *Shigella sonnei*.

#### Health effects and routes of infection

Though shigella infection is not often spread by waterborne transmission, major outbreaks resulting from such transmission have been described. The characteristic bloody diarrhoea results from the invasion of the colonic mucosa by the bacteria. There is good reason to believe that the process is highly species-specific. Shigellae have no natural hosts other than the higher primates, and humans are the only effective source of infection. Of the enteric bacterial pathogens, shigellae seem to be the best adapted to cause human disease. Direct transmission between susceptible individuals is the usual route of infection, and the infective dose is lower than for other bacteria.

#### Significance in drinking-water

The isolation of shigellae from drinking-water indicates recent human faecal contamination and, in view of the extreme pathogenicity of the organisms, is of crucial public health significance. However, this is a rare event, possibly explained in part by the absence of a useful enrichment or selective medium for the isolation of these bacteria. Those generally used have been designed for the isolation of salmonellae and are not optimal for that of shigellae. Furthermore, without confirmatory testing, some anaerogenic strains of *E. coli* may be wrongly identified as shigellae.

# 3.2 Pathogens that grow in supply systems

All drinking-water contains assimilable organic compounds that will allow a certain degree of bacterial growth. The density of bacteria in drinking-water can and should be controlled for the reasons given in Chapter 8.

Certain bacteria in drinking-water deserve particular attention because they are opportunistic pathogens to humans, i.e. they are able to cause infections in susceptible persons. The most important organisms of this type, namely *Legionella* and *Aeromonas*, will be considered here. Other organisms, such as *Pseudomonas aeruginosa* and opportunistically pathogenic mycobacteria, have been detected in drinking-water supplies.

## 3.2.1 Legionella

### General description

The genus *Legionella*, a member of the family Legionellaceae, has 22 currently known species, of which *L. pneumophila* serogroup 1 is most frequently associated with human disease. Other serogroups of *L. pneumophila* and occasionally other legionellae have also been reported to cause disease. Legionellae are Gram-negative, rod-shaped, non-spore-forming bacteria that require L-cysteine for growth and primary isolation. The cellular fatty acids in legionellae are unique among those found in Gram-negative bacilli in that they consist essentially of branched chains. Preconcentration of legionellae from environmental samples may be required if low levels are to be detected. Immunofluorescence techniques may also be used to detect legionellae in the environment.

### Health effects

*Legionella* infections can lead to two types of disease, namely Legionnaires' disease (legionellosis) and non-pneumonic Legionnaires' disease (Pontiac fever). Legionnaires' disease is a form of pneumonia with an incubation period usually of 3–6 days. Males are more frequently affected than females, and most cases occur in the 40–70 year age group. Risk factors include smoking, alcohol abuse, cancer, diabetes, chronic respiratory or kidney disease, and severe immunosuppression, as in transplant recipients. The fatality rate in untreated cases may be 10% or higher, but the disease can be treated effectively with antibiotics such as erythromycin and rifampicin.

Legionnaires' disease is uncommon, but common-source outbreaks attract much attention. Between 100 and 200 cases are reported each year in England and Wales, and in Germany; in France, the incidence is somewhat higher, with over 400 cases per year (27). For people living in temperate climates, travelling to subtropical areas appears to be a significant risk factor, outbreaks being related to air-conditioning and hot-water systems in hotels. Hospital-associated Legionnaires' disease is the most serious form, because it usually affects debilitated persons and has a high mortality rate. The non-pneumonic form of the disease is milder, with a high attack rate, an acute onset (5 hours to 3 days) and symptoms similar to those of influenza: fever, headache, nausea, vomiting, aching muscles, and coughing. No fatal cases have been reported and few outbreaks have been recognized, possibly because the non-specific symptoms of the disease hinder its diagnosis.

## Routes of exposure

Legionellae are widespread in natural sources of water and may also be found in soils. They occur commonly in man-made water systems, particularly in hot-water and cooling-water systems. Infection is the result of the inhalation of aerosols that are small enough to penetrate the lungs and be retained by the alveoli. The degree of risk depends on four key factors: (i) the density of the bacteria in the source; (ii) the extent of aerosol generation; (iii) the number of inhaled bacteria; and (iv) the susceptibility of the exposed individual.

Legionellae multiply in the laboratory at temperatures between 20 and 46 °C. At temperatures higher than 46 °C, the bacteria will survive, but at 60 °C only for a few minutes (28). Temperatures favourable for growth may be found in cooling towers, spas, cold-water systems in buildings, hot-water systems operated below 60 °C or "dead legs" of such systems operated at higher temperatures. Aerosols may be created by the spraying of water in cooling towers or its agitation in spas. Hot-water systems are also likely to create aerosols in showers, through nozzle heads or by splashing in sinks, baths, etc. The number of inhaled bacteria depends on the size of the aerosol generated (<5 µm being most dangerous), the dispersal of the aerosol in the air, and the duration of the exposure. Host defence is an important factor that determines whether exposure to legionellae will lead to clinical disease. It is primarily for this reason that high counts of *L. pneumophila* in water systems have been reported in the absence of disease, whereas similar or lower counts have been associated with epidemics. It is also likely, although not yet adequately proven, that differences in virulence between strains partly account for these observations.

It is now apparent that legionellae can be ingested by the trophozoites of certain amoebae (*Acanthamoeba*, *Hartmanella*, *Valkampfia*, and *Naegleria*) and even grow intracellularly and become incorporated in their cysts (29). This may explain the difficulty of eradicating legionellae from water systems and may be a factor in the etiology of the non-pneumonic disease (30).

The following are generally accepted as requiring disinfection:
- sites implicated in an outbreak of Legionnaires' disease or Pontiac fever;
- hospital wards housing high-risk patients, such as an organ transplant unit;
- buildings in which the water system has not been used for some time and where large numbers of legionellae are likely to be found.

Nevertheless, it is generally advisable to design and maintain systems in such a way that colonization by *Legionella* is prevented as much as possible. Detailed instructions for achieving this have been given in several publications (*31–34*) and focus on the following aspects:

- preventing the accumulation of sludge, scale, rust, algae and slime, and removing such deposits regularly;
- maintaining hot-water temperatures permanently above 60 °C or increasing them periodically to above 70 °C, and keeping cold-water supplies below 20 °C;
- selecting materials for contact with water that do not release nutrients that support the growth of *Legionella*.

The use of biocides is generally regarded as a less effective and less desirable means of controlling legionellae in water supplies in buildings. However, their use is essential to prevent the build-up of microbial slimes in air-conditioning systems in which wet, evaporative cooling towers are used. Such systems should be kept clean and well maintained, and should be inspected weekly for fouling, accumulations of slime and scale, and corrosion; they should be thoroughly cleaned and disinfected twice yearly. Biocides are best used intermittently in clean systems (*33, 34*).

## 3.2.2 Aeromonas

### General description

*Aeromonas* spp. are Gram-negative, rod-shaped, non-spore-forming bacteria that are currently assigned to the family Vibrionaceae, although they also bear many similarities to the Enterobacteriaceae. MacDonnell et al. (*35*) have suggested the creation of a new family Aeromonadaceae. The genus *Aeromonas* is divided into two groups of which the first, the group of psychrophilic non-motile aeromonads, consists of only one species, *A. salmonicida*, an obligate fish pathogen that will not be considered further here. The group of mesophilic motile aeromonads has been divided by Popoff into three biochemically distinguishable groups (*36*), namely *A. hydrophila*, *A. sobria* and *A. caviae*. Each of these three species consists of at least three different DNA-hybridization groups, and later workers have described new species such as *A. veronii*, *A. media*, *A. schubertii*, and *A. eucreno-phila*. It may be expected that in the near future the taxonomy of the group of mesophilic aeromonads will be changed still further, but at present the classification of Popoff is that most widely accepted internationally.

### Health effects

Mesophilic aeromonads have long been known to be pathogenic for cold-blooded animals such as fish and amphibians, but in the last few decades greater attention has been given to their pathogenic significance for humans. Three major types of infection are described (*37*): (i) systemic infections, usually in seriously immunocompromised persons; (ii) wound infections (mainly after contact with surface water); and (iii) diarrhoea. In particular, the significance of *Aeromonas* as an enteropathogenic organism is the subject of much discussion. In animal test models, such as the suckling mouse test and the rabbit ileal loop test, pure cultures of *Aeromonas* have been found to cause strong fluid accumulation which can partially be ascribed to the production of extracelluar cytotoxins. However, there have been reports that, while the culture filtrate of some *Aeromonas* strains is not enteropathogenic in an animal test model, a suspension of living cells does have this property. Cell-bound factors are apparently also of importance (*38*). Asao et al. (*39*) have purified and characterized an *Aeromonas* haemolysin, which was found to be a protein with a relative molecular mass of about 50 000 that was strongly enterotoxic and cytotoxic. It has not yet been possible to purify and characterize other toxins because the toxic activity disappears rapidly when culture filtrates are manipulated. Despite the marked toxin production by *Aeromonas* strains *in vitro*, diarrhoea has not yet been induced in test animals or human volunteers, and it is assumed that such strains are only poorly able to colonize the gastrointestinal tract (*40*). Little is known about the adhesion factors of *Aeromonas* or their interaction with receptors in the gastrointestinal tract.

Epidemiological investigations have also resulted in contradictory findings on the significance of *Aeromonas* as an enteropathogenic organism. In some studies, the numbers of *Aeromonas* in the faeces of patients with diarrhoea were greater than those in control groups, whereas in other studies there was no difference, or the bacteria were found in even greater numbers in the latter. In general, it can be said that the significance of *Aeromonas* as an enteropathogenic organism is greater in tropical areas than in the temperate zone. However, infections do occur in the temperate zone as well, albeit less frequently. *Aeromonas*-associated diarrhoea usually causes an acute but self-limiting gastroenteritis but chronic disease with serious complications may also occur. The incidence of *Aeromonas* in human diarrhoeal faeces in the Netherlands was found to vary between 0.5% in winter and 3% in summer. Most isolations were made in children under five years of age or in adults above 70 years of age. Young children yielded mainly *A. caviae*, whereas *A. sobria* was usually isolated from the elderly (*41*).

### Routes of exposure

*Aeromonas* occurs in water, soil, and food, particularly meat, fish, and milk. The occurrence of *Aeromonas* in drinking-water can be studied by a variety of methods. A membrane filtration method has been described in which a selective ampicillin-dextrin agar (ADA) is used (*42*). If water samples from house installations are being examined, the addition to the sample of a complexing agent such as the disodium salt of edetic acid ($Na_2EDTA$) at a concentration of 50 mg/litre is necessary. *Aeromonas* is extremely sensitive to the traces of copper that may be present in water in domestic installations in which copper piping is used. Complexing of copper was also found to improve the survival of coliform bacteria and heterotrophic bacteria (*43*).

The number of *Aeromonas* in surface waters can vary between 0.01 and 1000 cfu/ml. Small numbers are found in springs and in seawater that is not contaminated by sewage discharges. If such discharges are present, the number of *Aeromonas* can rise to 100 cfu/ml in seawater, and more than 1000 cfu/ml in fresh water, the species *A. caviae* then being dominant. In fresh waters not subject to sewage pollution, the numbers of *Aeromonas* are usually between 10 and 100 cfu/ml. In these waters, the numbers are higher in summer than in winter, and there is a relation between the eutrophication of the water and the summer density of *Aeromonas*. In stagnant fresh water, *A. sobria* is usually the dominant species. When river water is stored in reservoirs, the number of *Aeromonas* decreases, but there is also a shift in species composition from *A. caviae* to *A. sobria*. *Aeromonas* is not usually found in groundwater or is found only in very small numbers (*44*).

Irrespective of the contamination level of the raw water, most drinking-water treatment processes appear to be able to reduce the numbers of *Aeromonas* to below 1 cfu/100 ml. However, treated water can contain larger numbers, with maxima of about 1000 cfu/100 ml as a result of regrowth in storage reservoirs with long retention times, polluted filter sand, or sudden changes in the quantities of water to be produced. Regrowth of *Aeromonas* occurs in the distribution network of most drinking-water treatment plants. The size of the *Aeromonas* population will depend on many factors but primarily on the organic content of the water and its temperature, the residence time in the distribution network, and the presence of residual chlorine.

Little is known about the type and concentrations of nutrients for *Aeromonas* in drinking-water. Van der Kooij (*45*) has suggested that *Aeromonas* prefers to grow on organic matter, e.g. from decaying nitrifying and methane-oxidizing bacteria that develop in drinking-water treatment plants or from biofilm material in distribution networks.

Control of aeromonads in drinking-water requires a multiple approach, which is similar to the general approach to limiting the regrowth of bacteria (see Chapters 8 and 9). The treatment process should effectively remove organic compounds serving as sources of carbon and energy for the growth of bacteria. Furthermore, the amount of biomass produced and subsequently released during the treatment process should be as small as possible. The distribution system should be designed in such a way that residence times are short, and it should be flushed regularly to prevent the accumulation of sediments in stretches with low water velocities. Materials in contact with drinking-water should not be a source of biodegradable compounds. These factors are of greatest importance in supplies that are not disinfected, or where the maintenance of a chlorine residual is not considered desirable for various reasons. Free available chlorine residuals of 0.2–0.5 mg/litre will generally be sufficient to control *Aeromonas* densities in water in the distribution network (*46, 47*). Chlorine or other disinfectants should not be used to control occasional increases in *Aeromonas* densities in supplies that are normally not chlorinated because biofilms on pipe walls will be disturbed, and this will result initially in increases rather than decreases in bacterial concentrations. Also, in such systems the chlorine consumption will be rather high and residuals cannot be properly maintained, thus allowing regrowth in remote stretches of the network.

The question whether the presence of *Aeromonas* in drinking-water is a risk to human health cannot be answered with certainty; however, if there is a risk, it must be small because in many countries the bacterium is not important as a causative agent of diarrhoea and is not often able to colonize the gastrointestinal tract of humans. Also, the numbers present in drinking-water are small as compared with those in other sources. In food, for instance, the numbers usually found are of the order of $10^3$–$10^5$ cfu/g. However, drinking-water is a product that is consumed daily by everyone, including groups with a reduced resistance to infectious diseases. Some of this water is consumed without previous heating, in contrast to most foods contaminated with *Aeromonas*. A cautious approach therefore appears to be justified. Numbers of *Aeromonas* in drinking-water must be controlled as far as possible. Apart from the public health reasons for the control of *Aeromonas* levels in drinking-water, experience has shown that it is a useful and sensitive indicator of general hygiene within the drinking-water production and distribution process. Currently, no guideline value can be given because local conditions (temperature, raw water source) may greatly influence *Aeromonas* counts in drinking-water.

### 3.2.3 *Pseudomonas aeruginosa*

#### General description

*P. aeruginosa* is a member of the family Pseudomonadaceae and is a mono-trichate, Gram-negative rod. It can be recognized by its production of a blue-green fluorescent pigment (pyocyanin), which, in agar cultures, will diffuse into the medium. Pigment may not be produced by strains of *P. aeruginosa* recovered from clinical specimens, and the ability to produce it may be lost on subculture. Like other fluorescent pseudomonads that occur in natural waters, *P. aeruginosa* strains produce catalase and oxidase, and ammonia from arginine, grow with citrate as the sole source of carbon, and are aerobic. *P. aeruginosa*, however, is capable of growth at 41–42 °C, and the blue-green pigment that it produces differs from the fluorescent pale green pigment (fluorescein) produced by other species of fluorescent pseudomonads found in water. It is also capable of growing anaerobically in stab cultures of nitrate agar.

*P. aeruginosa* is commonly found in faeces, soil, water, and sewage but cannot be used as an indicator of faecal contamination, since it is not invariably present in faeces and sewage, and may also multiply in the enriched aquatic environment and on the surface of unsuitable organic materials in contact with water. However, its presence may be one of the factors taken into account in assessing the general cleanliness of water distribution systems and the quality of bottled waters (see section 9.3.2).

### Routes of exposure

*P. aeruginosa* is an opportunistic pathogen. Most of the illnesses in humans for which it is responsible are caused, not by drinking water, but by contact with it. Water containing these bacteria may also contaminate food, drinks, and pharmaceutical products, causing them to deteriorate and to act as secondary vehicles for transmission. Fixtures in contact with water, such as sinks and sink drains, tap fittings and showerheads, can also be contaminated by *P. aeruginosa* and can serve as reservoirs of infection in hospitals.

### Health effects and significance in drinking-water

In healthy persons, the illnesses caused by *P. aeruginosa* are usually mild and trivial. Waterborne infections are usually associated with warm, moist environments; they include the skin rashes and pustules or outer ear canal infections (otitis externa) reported in users of indoor swimming-pools and whirlpools, where bacterial counts are high and disinfection is deficient (*48, 49*). The presence of this organism in water supplied to hospitals and for the manufacture of pharmaceutical preparations and dressings is a matter of concern because *P. aeruginosa* is a common pathogen in infections of wounds and burns and has caused serious eye infections after the use of contaminated eye drops (*50*). Hospital strains of *P. aeruginosa* can first colonize and then infect patients receiving cancer chemotherapy (*51*).

The presence of this organism in potable water also indicates a serious deterioration in bacteriological quality, and is often associated with complaints about taste, odour, and turbidity linked to low rates of flow in the distribution system and a rise in water temperature (see section 9.3.2).

## 3.2.4 Mycobacterium
### General description

*Mycobacterium* spp. are rod-shaped bacteria with cell walls having a high lipid content; this enables them to retain certain dyes in staining procedures that employ an acid wash, and they are therefore often referred to as acid-fast bacteria. The characteristics of the cell wall structure also result in a relatively high resistance to disinfectants. All mycobacteria are characterized by slow growth (generation times under optimal circumstances 2–20 hours), but within this range they are divided into "slow" and "rapid" growers. Most pathogenic species are found among the slow growers, which include the strictly pathogenic species *M. tuberculosis*, *M. bovis*, *M. africanum*, and *M. leprae*; these are not transmitted by water and have only human or animal reservoirs. Other mycobacterial species, often referred to as "atypical", have environmental reservoirs. Although many are considered to be nonpathogenic, several species are opportunistic pathogens for humans, the most important being the slow growers *M. kansasii*, *M. marinum*, *M. avium*, *M. intracellulare*, *M. scrofulaceum*, and *M. xenopi*, and the rapid growers *M. chelonae* and *M. fortuitum*. Some of these species are closely related, and the literature often describes a number of complexes rather than individual species. Examples are the "*M. bovis* complex" (which includes *M. africanum*), the "*M. avium* complex" (or MAC, which includes *M. intracellulare*), or the "*M. avium*, *M. intracellulare*, *M. scrofulaceum* complex" (or MAIS) and the "*M. fortuitum-chelonae* complex."

### Health effects

The strictly pathogenic mycobacteria are associated with classical infectious diseases such as tuberculosis and leprosy. The environmental mycobacteria may cause a range of diseases including tuberculous lung disease and disseminated infections which may also involve the skeleton (*M. kansasii*, *M. avium* complex), infections of the lymph nodes (MAIS complex), and infections of the skin and soft tissues (*M. marinum*, *M. fortuitum-chelonae* complex) (*52*, *53*). Diseases caused by opportunistic pathogenic mycobacteria are not normally transmitted from person to person but are usually the result of environmental exposure in combination with predisposing factors, such as dust retained in the lungs, surgical wounds, or immunosuppression produced by medication (transplant patients) or by underlying disease (AIDS, malignancies). Mycobacteria are generally resistant to many antimicrobial agents, hence effective treatment may be difficult.

### Routes of exposure

An extensive review of the occurrence of mycobacteria in environmental sources has been published (*54*). Tapwater has long been known to harbour saprophytic mycobacteria; in fact, one of the most commonly occurring species, *M. gordonae*, is known as the tapwater bacillus. The occurrence of opportunistic pathogenic species in tapwater has also been demonstrated by various authors (*55*, *56*). These organisms may accidentally contaminate clinical specimens during and after collection, or during processing in the laboratory; this may falsely suggest that the patients concerned are suffering from a mycobacterial infection (*57*, *58*). A link between the occurrence of mycobacteria in drinking-water and disease has sometimes been suggested. Endemic *M. kansasii* infections in Czechoslovakia were studied from 1968 onwards, the peak incidence being found in a small, densely populated district in which workers were engaged in mining, heavy industry, and power generation. *M. kansasii* could also be isolated from shower outlets in collieries, and it was later shown that the drinking-water system in the entire region was widely contaminated. It was suggested that mycobacteria from drinking-water were spread via aerosols (*59*). The high isolation frequency of *M. kansasii* from clinical specimens in Rotterdam, the Netherlands, led to an investigation of the water supply system. The organisms were frequently isolated from tapwater, and were of the same phage type and showed the same weak nitratase activity as clinical strains (*60*). The increase in the isolation frequency of the *M. avium* complex in Massachusetts, USA, has also been attributed to their presence in drinking-water (*61*). It should be noted that in all these cases there is only circumstantial evidence of a causal relationship between the occurrence of mycobacteria in drinking-water and human disease. Certainly, the low infectivity of environmental mycobacteria does not warrant the setting of standards or the institution of eradication programmes.

The ecology of opportunistic mycobacteria in water supplies is poorly understood. The bacteria have been isolated infrequently from treated water or mains water (*52, 57*) but appear to multiply within the plumbing systems in buildings as well as in taps. Increased isolation frequencies have been associated with higher temperatures (hot-water systems or cold-water pipes in the vicinity of central heating). Older buildings appear to be more frequently colonized than new ones (*61*), and transport of drinking-water over long distances also seems to increase the content of mycobacteria (*58*). Haas et al. (*62*) attempted to correlate total microscopic counts of acid-fast bacteria (hence including both pathogenic and saprophytic species) with a range of physicochemical parameters. A negative correlation with total chlorine residual and a positive correlation with turbidity and total organic carbon (TOC) was established, but these variables only accounted for a small proportion of the overall variance of counts. It might also be expected that materials used for plumbing would have an effect on mycobacterial densities, but no experimental evidence of such an effect has yet been presented.

# References

1. Leminor L. The genus *Salmonella*. In: Starr MP et al., eds. *The prokaryotes*, Vol. II. Berlin and Heidelberg, Springer-Verlag, 1981:1148-1159.

2. Lloyd B. *Salmonella*, enteric fevers and salmonelloses. In: Feacham RG et al., eds. *Sanitation and disease. Health aspects of excreta and wastewater management.* Chichester, John Wiley & Sons, 1983:251-286 (World Bank Studies in Water Supply and Sanitation, No.3).

3. Kampelmacher EH. Spread and significance of salmonellae in surface waters in the Netherlands. In: Hoadley AW, Dutka BJ, eds. *Bacterial indicators of potential health hazards associated with water.* Philadelphia, American Society for Testing and Materials, 1977:148-158.

4. Mersch-Sundermann V, Wundt W. Die bakteriologische Beschaffenheit des Wassers vom Rhein und seinen Zuflussen im Rhein-Neckar-Raum. II. Mitteilung. Salmonellen—Hygienische Bedeutung und gesundheitliche Gefahren. [Bacteriological quality

of water from the Rhine and its tributaries in the Rhine-Neckar area. Part II. Salmonellae—public health significance and health risks.] *Zentralblatt für Bakteriologie, Mikrobiologie und Hygiene*, Reihe B, 1987, 184:470-482.

5. Lewis WJ, Foster SSD, Dragar BS. *The risk of groundwater pollution by on-site sanitation in developing countries; a literature review.* Dubendorf, Switzerland, International Centre for Wastes Disposal, 1982 (Report No. 01/82).

6. Swaminathan B, Harmon MC, Mehlman JJ. *Yersinia enterocolitica. Journal of applied bacteriology*, 1982, 52:151-183.

7. Bercovier H, Mollaret HH. *Yersinia.* In: Krieg NR, Holt JG, eds. *Bergey's manual of systematic bacteriology*, Vol. 1. Baltimore, Williams & Wilkins, 1984:498-506.

8. Lloyd B. *Yersinia and yersiniosis.* In: Feacham RG, eds. *Sanitation and disease. Health aspects of excreta and wastewater management.* Chichester, John Wiley & Sons, 1983:327-330 (World Bank Studies in Water Supply and Sanitation, No. 3).

9. Schiemann DA. Isolation of *Yersinia enterocolitica* from surface and well waters in Ontario. *Canadian journal of microbiology*, 1978, 24:1048-1052.

10. Ziegert E, Diesterweg I. The occurrence of *Yersinia enterocolitica* in sewage, *Zentralblatt für Mikrobiologie*, 1990, 145(5):367-375.

11. Fukushima H et al. *Yersinia* spp. in surface waters in Matsue, Japan. *Zentralblatt für Bakteriologie, Mikrobiologie und Hygiene*, Reihe B, 1984, 179:235-247.

12. Aleksic S, Bockem HLJ. Serological and biochemical characteristics of 416 *Yersinia* strains from well water and drinking water plants in the Federal Republic of Germany: lack of evidence that these strains are of public health importance. *Zentralblatt für Bakteriologie, Mikrobiologie und Hygiene*, Reihe B, 1988, 185:527-533.

13. Weber G, Manafi M, Reisinger H. Die bedeutung von *Yersinia enterocolitica* und thermophilen campylobactern für die Wasserhygiene. [Significance of *Yersinia enterolitica* and thermophilic campylobacter for water hygiene.] *Zentralblatt für Bakteriologie, Mikrobiologie und Hygiene*, Reihe B, 1987, 184:504-514.

14. Krogulska B, Maleszewska J, Wichrowska B. [Sensitivity of *Yersinia enterocolitica* to agents used in water disinfection.] *Rocznik panstwowego zakladu higieny*, 1986, 37: 434-440 (in Polish).

15. Highsmith AK et al. Isolation of *Yersinia enterocolitica* from well water and growth in distilled water. *Applied and environmental microbiology*, 1977, 34:745-750.

16. Smibert RM. The genus *Campylobacter.* In: Starr MP et al., eds. *The prokaryotes*, Vol.I. Berlin and Heidelberg, Springer-Verlag, 1981:609-617.

17. Penner JL. The genus *Campylobacter*: a decade of progress. *Clinical reviews in microbiology*, 1988, 1:157-172.

18. Birkhead G et al. A multiple-strain outbreak of campylobacter enteritis due to consumption of inadequately pasteurized milk. *Journal of infectious diseases*, 1988, 157:1095-1097.

19. Robinson DA. Infective dose of *Campylobacter jejuni* in milk. *British medical journal*, 1981, 282:1584.

20. Steltzer W et al. Characterisation of *Campylobacter jejuni* and *Campylobacter coli* isolated from wastewater. *Zentralblatt für Bakteriologie, Mikrobiologie und Hygiene, Reihe A*, 1988, 269:188-196.

21. Holler C. Quantitative and qualitative studies of *Campylobacter* in the sewage of a large city. *Zentralblatt für Bakteriologie, Mikrobiologie und Hygiene, Reihe B*, 1988, 185:307-325.

22. Gondrosen B. Survival of thermotolerant campylobacters in water. *Acta veterinaria scandinavica*, 1986, 27:1-10.

23. Feachem RG. Environmental aspects of cholera epidemiology. III. Transmission and control. *Tropical disease bulletin*, 1982, 79:1-47.

24. Scotland SM et al. Adhesion to cells in culture and plasmid profiles of enteropathogenic *Escherichia coli* isolated from outbreaks and sporadic cases of infant diarrhoea. *Journal of infection*, 1989, 19(3):237-249.

25. Attridge SR, Rowley D. Cholera. In: Smith GR, Easmon CSF, eds. *Topley and Wilson's principles of bacteriology, virology and immunity*, 8th ed., Vol. 3. London, Edward Arnold, 1990:459-468.

26. Miller CJ, Drasar BS, Feachem RG. Cholera epidemiology in developed and developing countries: new thoughts on transmission, seasonality and control. *Lancet*, 1985:261-262.

27. Guerin JC. Epidemiology of Legionnaires' disease. From myth to reality. *Revues des maladies respiratoires*, 1992, 9 (Suppl. 1):R53-R56.

28. Brenner DJ et al. Legionella. In: Krieg NR, Holt JG, eds. *Bergey's manual of systematic bacteriology*. Vol. 1. Baltimore, Williams & Wilkins, 1984:279-288.

29. Lee JV, West AA. Survival and growth of *Legionella* species in the environment. *Society of Applied Bacteriology symposium series*, 1991, 20:121S-129S.

30. Rowbotham TJ. Pontiac fever explained? *Lancet*, 1980, ii: 969.

31. *Prevention of legionellosis*. The Hague, Gezondheidsraad, 1986.

32. *The control of legionellae in health care premises. A code of practice.* London, Her Majesty's Stationery Office, 1989.

33. Department of Health and Social Security. *Health services management. Legionnaires' disease. Cooling towers and evaporative condensers.* London, 1987 (Engineering Guidance Note 4).

34. *Report of the Expert Advisory Committee on Biocides.* London, Her Majesty's Stationery Office, 1989.

35. MacDonnell MT et al. Ribosomal RNA phylogenies for the vibrio enteric group of eubacteria. *Microbiological science,* 1986, 3(6):172-175, 178.

36. Popoff M. Aeromonas. In: Krieg NR, Holt JG, eds. *Bergey's manual of systematic bacteriology,* Vol. 1. Baltimore, Williams & Wilkins, 1984:545-548.

37. Janda JM, Duffey PS. Mesophilic aeromonads in human disease: current taxonomy, laboratory identification, and infectious disease spectrum. *Reviews of infectious diseases,* 1988, 10:980-997.

38. Stelma GN, Johnson CH, Spaulding PL. Experimental evidence for enteropathogenicity in *Aeromonas veronii. Canadian journal of microbiology,* 1988, 34:877-880.

39. Asao T et al. Purification and some properties of *Aeromonas hydrophila* hemolysin. *Infection and immunity,* 1984, 46:122-127.

40. Kuijper EJ. *Aeromonas associated diarrhoea in the Netherlands.* Amsterdam, University of Amsterdam, 1989 (thesis).

41. Havelaar AH et al. *Aeromonas* species als verwekker van diarree en infecties buiten het maag-darmkanaal in Nederland. [*Aeromonas* as the cause of diarrhoea and of infections outside the gastrointestinal tract in the Netherlands.] *Nederlands tijdschrift voor geneeskunde,* 1990, 134:1053-1057.

42. Havelaar AH, During M, Versteegh JF. Ampicillin-dextrin agar medium for the enumeration of *Aeromonas* species in water by membrane filtration. *Journal of applied bacteriology,* 1987, 62:279-287.

43. Versteegh JF et al. Complexing of copper in drinking water samples to enhance recovery of *Aeromonas* and other bacteria. *Journal of applied bacteriology,* 1989, 67:561-566.

44. Schubert RHW. Der Nachweis von Aeromonaden der "Hydrophila-Punctata-Gruppe" im Rahmen der hygienischen Trinkwasserbeurteilung. [Detection of aeromonads of the "hydrophila punctata group" in the hygienic assessment of drinking-water.] *Zentralblatt für Bakteriologie und Hygiene, I Abteilung, Originale, Reihe B,* 1976, 161:482-497.

45. Van der Kooij D. Properties of aeromonads and their occurrence and hygienic signif-icance in drinking-water. *Zentralblatt für Bakteriologie, Mikrobiologie und Hygiene, Reihe B*, 1988, 187:1-17.

46. Burke V et al. Isolation of *Aeromonas hydrophila* from a metropolitan water supply: seasonal correlation with clinical isolates. *Applied and environmental microbiology*, 1984, 48:361-366.

47. Lechevallier MW, Cawthorn CD, Lee RG. Factors promoting survival of bacteria in chlorinated water supplies. *Applied and environmental microbiology*, 1988, 54:649-654.

48. Jones F, Bartlett CLR. Infections associated with whirlpools and spas. *Society of Applied Bacteriology symposium series*, 1985, 14:61S-66S.

49. Calderon R, Mood EW. An epidemiological assessment of water quality and "swim-mer's ear". *Archives of environmental health*, 1982, 73:300-305.

50. Parker MT. Septic infections due to Gram-negative aerobic bacilli. In: Smith GR, ed. *Topley and Wilson's principles of bacteriology, virology and immunity*, 7th ed., Vol. 3. London, Edward Arnold, 1984:280-310.

51. Wade JC et al. Potential of imipenem as single-agent empiric antibiotic therapy of febrile neutropenic patients with cancer. *American journal of medicine*, 1985, 78 (6A):62-72.

52. Good RC. Opportunistic pathogens in the genus *Mycobacterium*. *Annual reviews of microbiology*, 1985, 39:347-369.

53. Wallace RJ et al. Spectrum of disease due to rapidly growing mycobacteria. *Reviews of infectious diseases* 1983, 5:657-679.

54. Collins CH, Grange JM, Yates MD. Mycobacteria in water. *Journal of applied bac-teriology*, 1984, 57:193-211.

55. McSwiggan DA, Collins CH. The isolation of *M. kansasii* and *M. xenopii* from water systems. *Tubercle*, 1974, 55:291-297.

56. Stine TM et al. A pseudoepidemic due to atypical mycobacteria in a hospital water supply. *Journal of the American Medical Association*, 1987, 258:809-811.

57. Mankiewicz E, Majdaniw O. Atypical mycobacteria in tapwater. *Canadian journal of public health*, 1982, 73:358-360.

58. Wright EP, Collins CH, Yates MD. *Mycobacterium xenopi* and *Mycobacterium kan-sasii* in a hospital water supply. *Journal of hospital infection*, 1985, 6:175-178.

59. Kaustova J et al. Endemic occurrence of *Mycobacterium kansasii* in water supply systems. *Journal of hygiene, epidemiology, microbiology and immunology*, 1981, 25:24-30.

60. Engel HWB, Berwald LG, Havelaar AH. The occurrence of *Mycobacterium kansasii* in tapwater. *Tubercle*, 1980, 61:21-26.

61. du Moulin GC et al. *Mycobacterium avium* complex, an emerging pathogen in Massachusetts. *Journal of clinical microbiology*, 1985, 22:9-12.

62. Haas CH, Meyer MA, Paller MS. The ecology of acid-fast organisms in water supply, treatment, and distribution systems. *Journal of the American Water Works Association*, 1983, 75:139-144.

# 4.
# Viruses [1]

## 4.1 General description

The viruses of greatest significance in the waterborne transmission of infectious disease are essentially those that multiply in the intestine of humans and are excreted in large numbers in the faeces of infected individuals. Although viruses cannot multiply outside the tissues of infected hosts, some enteric viruses appear to have a considerable ability to survive in the environment and remain infective. Discharges of sewage and human excreta constitute the main source of human enteric viruses in the aquatic environment. With the various analytical methods currently available, wide variations are found in the numbers of viruses present in sewage. These belong to the families shown in Table 4.1. The numbers of viruses and the species distribution will reflect the extent to which they are being carried by the population. Sewage treatment may reduce the numbers of viruses 10–1000-fold, depending on the nature and extent of the treatment given. However, it will not eliminate them entirely, and the sludge produced during sewage treatment will often contain large numbers. As sewage mixes with receiving water, viruses are carried downstream, remaining detectable for varying periods of time, depending on the temperature, the degree to which they are adsorbed on to sediments, the depth to which sunlight penetrates into the water, and other factors. Consequently, enteric viruses can be found in sewage-polluted water at the intakes to water-treatment plants.

The relationship between the occurrence of viruses in water and risks to health is not a simple one; the factors involved are discussed in section 4.3. Table 4.1 lists those viruses, infective for humans, which have been found in sewage-polluted water and the illnesses with which they have been associated.

### 4.1.1 The nature of viruses

Viruses are replicating infectious agents that are among the smallest of all microorganisms. In essence, they are nucleic acid molecules that can enter cells and replicate in them, and code for proteins capable of forming protective shells around them. The following characteristics are shared by all viruses:

---

[1]  The valuable contribution made by Dr N.F. Pierce, Division of Diarrhoeal and Acute Respiratory Disease Control, WHO, Geneva, in the preparation of this chapter is gratefully acknowledged.

**Table 4.1 Viruses pathogenic to humans which can occur in polluted water and diseases attributed to them**

| Virus family | Members | No. of serotypes | Diseases caused |
|---|---|---|---|
| Picornaviridae | Human polioviruses | 3 | Paralysis, meningitis, fever |
| | Human echoviruses | 32 | Meningitis, respiratory disease, rash, fever, gastroenteritis |
| | Human coxsackie-viruses A1–22,24 | 23 | Enteroviral vesicular pharyngitis, respiratory disease, meningitis, enteroviral vesicular stomatitis with exanthem (hand, foot and mouth disease) |
| | Human coxsackie-viruses B1–6 | 6 | Myocarditis, congenital heart anomalies, rash, fever, meningitis, respiratory disease, epidemic myalgia (pleurodynia) |
| | Human enteroviruses 68–71 | 4 | Meningitis, encephalitis, respiratory disease, rash, acute enteroviral haemorrhagic conjunctivitis, fever |
| | Hepatitis A virus | 1 | Hepatitis A |
| Reoviridae | Human reoviruses | 3 | Unknown |
| | Human rotaviruses | 5 | Gastroenteritis, diarrhoea |
| Adenoviridae | Human adenoviruses | 41 | Respiratory disease, conjunctivitis, gastroenteritis |
| Parvoviridae | Adeno-associated viruses | 4 | Latent infection following integration of DNA into the cellular genome |
| Caliciviridae | Human caliciviruses | 5 | Gastroenteritis in infants and young children |
| | Small round structured viruses (including Norwalk virus) | 14 | Gastroenteritis, acute viral gastroenteropathy (Winter vomiting disease) |
| Caliciviridae (?) | Hepatitis E virus | ? | Hepatitis E |
| Unknown | Astroviruses | 1 | Gastroenteritis, neonatal necrotizing enterocolitis |
| Papovaviridae | Papillomaviruses | 2 | Plantar warts |

1. The virus particle or virion consists of a genome, either RNA or DNA, that is surrounded by a protective protein shell called the capsid. This shell is itself often enclosed within an envelope that contains both protein and lipid.
2. Viruses replicate only inside specific host cells. They are totally dependent on the host cell's synthetic apparatus and energy sources, and are thus parasites at the genetic level.

## 4.1.2 Classification of animal viruses

The present universal system for virus taxonomy is set arbitrarily at the hierarchical levels of family, genus, and species by the International Committee on Taxonomy of Viruses (*1*). The fundamental criteria used for classification purposes are the type and strandedness of the nucleic acid of the viral genome and the presence or absence of a lipoprotein envelope.

Virus families, designated by terms ending in -viridae, represent clusters of genera of apparently common evolutionary origin. Virus genera are designated by terms ending in -virus and are based on common evolutionary origin and biophysicochemical or serological properties (see Table 4.1). Virus species have not been designated formally except for the family Adenoviridae, where the term is now defined on the basis of immunological distinctiveness.

## 4.1.3 Virus families occurring in water

Picornaviruses are 27–28 nm particles consisting of positive-sense single-stranded RNA enclosed in a protein coat of icosahedral symmetry, which are stable at pH 3; one member of this family, hepatitis A virus, is particularly stable, e.g. it can survive for some hours at pH 1. They resist inactivation by various environmental factors for a number of weeks, particularly when associated with sediments in natural waters. The genus *Enterovirus*, which is one of the three genera of the Picornaviridae family pathogenic to humans, contains six major groups: human polioviruses, human echoviruses, human coxsackievirus groups A and B, the new enterovirus serotypes 68–71, and, as mentioned above, hepatitis A virus.

The family Reoviridae contains six genera, two of which—human reoviruses (orthoreoviruses) and human rotaviruses—have been detected in polluted water. The virus particles are approximately 70 nm in diameter and have both an inner capsid 50–65 nm in size, of icosahedral symmetry, enclosing a double-stranded, segmented genome, and an outer one, in which striking differences are apparent in the different genera. The orthoreoviruses have a well-defined outer capsid, composed of hexagonal and pentagonal subunits. The rotavirus outer capsid lacks visible subunit structures. Both genera lose infectivity relatively slowly even at ambient temperatures and are stable over a wide range of pH values.

The family Adenoviridae contains two genera. The mammalian adenoviruses include 41 human species, subdivided on the basis of their biophysical, biochemical, biological, and immunological characteristics into six subgenera (A–F). The virion is a non-enveloped regular icosahedron (20 triangular surfaces and 12 vertices), which is 65–80 nm in diameter. A fibre-like structure projects from each of the vertices. The genome is a single linear molecule of double-stranded DNA.

Parvoviridae are among the smallest of the DNA animal viruses. The virion is 18–26 nm in diameter, is of icosahedral symmetry and has a single-stranded DNA genome. The family Parvoviridae contains three genera, for two of which, *Parvovirus* and *Dependovirus*, waterborne transmission is a possibility. The virion is extremely resistant to inactivation; it is stable between pH 3 and 9, and at 56 °C for 60 minutes. The genus *Dependovirus* (adeno-associated virus, AAV), has a relatively wide host range; infection is common in the general population. AAV only infects human cells cryptically; no overt disease has been observed.

The so-called "small round structured viruses", which include Norwalk virus, contain RNA and a single capsid polypeptide typical of caliciviruses; they are therefore currently included in the Caliciviridae family (see also p. 47).

Hepatitis E virus is an important cause of acute hepatitis in tropical and subtropical countries. Classification of this virus is difficult, but many have placed it among the Caliciviridae (2).

The Papovaviridae consist of several genera, among them the papilloma viruses. Papovaviridae are non-enveloped, icosahedral particles, 45–55 nm in diameter, which contain one molecule of double-stranded DNA. They are highly resistant to inactivating environmental factors. Natural transmission is presumed to be through contact, and the diseases that they cause have been associated with swimming-pools.

## 4.2 Routes of exposure

### 4.2.1 General considerations

Acute gastrointestinal and diarrhoeal illnesses continue to be the major waterborne diseases throughout the world. Rapid methodological advances have recently been made in the study of their etiology that have revolutionized the diagnosis of viral diarrhoeal diseases. Waterborne outbreaks due to viruses have now been recorded from developed and developing countries all over the world (2–5). Many different strains of viruses have been isolated from raw and treated drinking-water (6). Isolation from water does not prove beyond all possible doubt that water is a vehicle for the transmission of disease, although it does indicate that a hazard exists. Proper treatment and disinfection should result in drinking-water that is essentially virus-free. Epidemiological proof of the waterborne transmission of viral diseases is very difficult to obtain for a variety of reasons (7), including the following:
  - the symptoms may not resemble those of typical waterborne diseases;
  - asymptomatic carriage and excretion occur in a large proportion of those infected;

- some infections have long incubation periods, e.g. hepatitis caused by hepatitis A virus,
- waterborne transmission may be at a low level, and secondary spread may occur by other routes;
- suitably sensitive methods for detecting the infectious agent in water may be lacking.

Waterborne transmission has been unequivocally demonstrated for hepatitis A and hepatitis E viruses, rotaviruses and Norwalk virus, and the explosive epidemics that they cause have been well documented. For the other viruses included in Table 4.1, waterborne transmission is a probability but has not been definitely established.

Low-level transmission may occur in which small numbers of viruses present in drinking-water, either sporadically or continuously, produce asymptomatic infections that remain unrecognized. The person-to-person spread of such infections in the community could lead to disease outbreaks apparently unconnected with water. However, the existence of such a mechanism has not been confirmed.

In a prospective epidemiological study among city dwellers receiving bacteriologically satisfactory drinking-water, it was found that the group receiving water not treated by reverse osmosis at the point of use had 25% more gastrointestinal symptoms than those receiving water treated by this process (8). The symptoms observed were compatible with infection caused by the Norwalk virus or astroviruses, which were probably incompletely removed from the sewage-contaminated river water used as the source.

In some areas, water sources may be heavily polluted, and the water-treatment processes used may not be reliable. For this reason, and because of the large number of persons at risk, drinking-water must be regarded as having a very significant potential as a vehicle for the environmental transmission of enteric viruses. As with other microbial infections, enteric viruses may also be transmitted by contaminated food and aerosols, as well as by direct contact, the usual mode of transmission.

Schemes for the recycling of wastewater for domestic use are being considered in some cities, while in many others, water for potable supplies is obtained from contaminated surface sources containing a significant proportion of wastewater. The risk of viruses penetrating the water-treatment processes—including pretreatment storage and disinfection—must be carefully evaluated whenever wastewater is to be reused in this way.

## 4.2.2 Specific families of viruses

Enteroviruses have a worldwide distribution, their prevalence increasing during the warm months of the year in temperate climates. The epidemiology of these infections suggests that faecal-to-oral transmission is the major means of spread and that various types of enterovirus can give rise to large outbreaks when they are transmitted by the water route.

Rotaviruses and orthoreoviruses have been detected in sewage, rivers, and lakes and in treated drinking-water in some countries (9–12). Transmission occurs via the faecal-to-oral route. The infection is usually associated with sporadic cases, but several large waterborne outbreaks have been well documented (13, 14). The rotaviruses are of considerable public health importance as a common cause of acute diarrhoea, particularly in young children. They infect and multiply in mature or differentiated enterocytes located on the villi of the duodenum and small intestine, and are excreted in large numbers; as many as 1000 virus particles may be present per gram of faeces for approximately 8 days after the onset of symptoms.

Adenoviruses generally infect conjunctival, respiratory, and intestinal epithelium in addition to regional lymphoid tissue. Prolonged excretion of viruses both from the pharynx and from the intestinal tract has been described. Several species, particularly subgroups B, C, D and E, and serotypes 1, 2, 3, 4, 5, 6, 7 and 15, have been isolated from sewage, rivers, lakes, groundwater, and water used for drinking and swimming. Waterborne transmission occurs by the faecal-to-oral route, by inhalation of adenovirus aerosols into the lower respiratory tract, and by eye contact when the conjunctival surface is mildly irritated. Several large outbreaks of pharyngoconjunctival fever have been associated with swimming-pools (15, 16).

The use of electron microscopy for the examination of faecal specimens from persons with nonbacterial gastroenteritis resulted in many observations of small viruses ranging in size from 20 to 40 nm, the "small round structured viruses" already mentioned on p. 45. The first of these viruses to be described was the Norwalk agent which was detected in volunteers fed filtered faecal suspension obtained from patients in an outbreak of winter vomiting disease. Morphologically similar viruses known as the Hawaii, Wollan, Ditching, Parramatta, Snow Mountain and Montgomery County agents were subsequently found. Failure to culture any of these agents satisfactorily delayed definitive classification but, as previously noted, they are now assigned to the Caliciviridae family.

Norwalk virus infects the villi of the jejunum. Virus shedding in stools occurs during the first 72 hours after the onset of illness. The virus is transmitted by the faecal-to-oral route. Of all Norwalk-related outbreaks, water seems to be responsible for about 40%, the type of water involved including drinking-water supplies, recreational bathing water, and shellfish-harvesting water (17).

## 4.3 Health effects

Enteric viruses are capable of producing a wide variety of syndromes, including rashes, fever, gastroenteritis, myocarditis, meningitis, respiratory disease, and hepatitis (Table 4.1). In general, asymptomatic infections are common and the more serious manifestations rare. However, when drinking-water is contaminated with sewage, gastroenteritis and hepatitis may occur in epidemic proportions. Apart from these infections, there is little, if any, epidemiological evidence to show that adequately treated drinking-water is involved in the transmission of virus infections.

Gastroenteritis of viral origin may be associated with a variety of agents (Table 4.1). It is usually of 24–72 hours' duration with nausea, vomiting and diarrhoea; it occurs in susceptible individuals of all ages, but is most serious in the very young and very old, where dehydration and electrolyte imbalance can occur rapidly and threaten life if not corrected without delay.

Dependoviruses (adeno-associated virus), together with adenoviruses, have been recovered from surface water (18); it is therefore suspected that waterborne transmission of these viruses can occur.

Hepatitis A virus (human enterovirus 72) and enterically transmitted hepatitis E virus cause infections of the liver typically accompanied by lassitude, anorexia, weakness, nausea, vomiting, headache, abdominal discomfort, fever, dark urine, and jaundice. Hepatitis, if mild, may require only rest and restricted activities for a week or two, but when severe may cause death from liver failure, or may result in chronic disease of the liver. Severe hepatitis is tolerated less well with increasing age, and the fatality rate increases sharply beyond middle age. The mortality rate is higher among those with pre-existing malignancy and cirrhosis (19). A fulminant form leading to death within days occurs in 0.1–0.6% of cases. Hepatitis E infection in pregnant women has a high mortality rate. Local epidemics are usually traceable to contaminated food or water. The virus has been detected in polluted rivers (20) and in drinking-water (21). Several very large outbreaks of drinking-water-transmitted hepatitis have occurred in India (2), China (Mendong, personal communication), Algeria (22) and the former Soviet Union (23).

Adenoviruses are among the viral agents associated with acute nonbacterial infectious gastroenteritis. Of the various species, two (types 40 and 41) cannot routinely replicate in cell cultures and are called fastidious variants. Such fastidious adenoviruses have been found in many parts of the world and are probably second only to rotaviruses as a cause of gastroenteritis in young children. They tend to be endemic rather than epidemic although outbreaks have occurred. Cytopathogenic adenoviruses can easily be detected in all kinds of water, so that waterborne transmission of the fastidious variants has also been suspected (6).

Rotaviruses are responsible for a large proportion of severe episodes of diarrhoea in small children and infants, and may also cause gastroenteritis in the elderly (24). They are responsible for as much as 50% of the gastroenteritis in infants and children admitted to hospital during the cooler months of the year in temperate climates. Rotaviruses have occasionally been isolated from drinking-water in some countries, but more often from sewage (9, 25). Acute infection is characterized by the abrupt onset of severe watery diarrhoea with fever and vomiting. Dehydration and metabolic acidosis may develop, resulting in death if untreated. Those most severely infected and affected are between 6 and 24 months old.

The Norwalk virus usually causes self-limiting explosive epidemics of gastroenteritis that last for 24–48 hours, are community-wide, and involve school-age children, family contacts, and adults. Roughly one-third of such outbreaks of gastroenteritis can be attributed to the Norwalk virus. Infections result in delayed gastric emptying, nausea, vomiting, and abdominal cramps. About 50% of infected persons have associated diarrhoea; some have fever and chills. A transient lymphopenia has been observed. Norwalk and Norwalk-like viruses (small round structured viruses) primarily infect and cause disease in older children and adults, and have been responsible for a large number of outbreaks of acute infectious nonbacterial gastroenteritis. Infection may be spread by municipal water systems, semi-public water supplies, recreational swimming, and stored water (*4, 26, 27*) although other modes of transmission, including person-to-person spread, are usually more important.

## References

1.  Francki RIB et al. *Classification and nomenclature of viruses. Fifth report of the International Committee on Taxonomy of Viruses.* Vienna, Springer-Verlag, 1991 (Suppl. 2 to *Archives of virology*).

2.  Ticehurst J. Identification and characterization of hepatitis E virus. In: Hollinger FB, Lemon SM, Margolis HS, eds. *Viral hepatitis and liver disease.* Baltimore, Williams and Wilkins, 1991: 501-513

3.  Wong DC et al. Epidemic and endemic hepatitis in India: evidence for a non-A, non-B hepatitis virus aetiology. *Lancet*, 1980, ii:876-879.

4.  Hejkal TW et al. Viruses in a community water supply associated with an outbreak of gastroenteritis and infectious hepatitis. *Journal of the American Water Works Association*, 1982, 74:318-321.

5.  Murphy AM, Grohmann GS, Sexton MFH. Infectious gastroenteritis in Norfolk Island and recovery of viruses from drinking water. *Journal of hygiene (London)*, 1983, 91:139-146.

6.  Bitton G et al. *Survey of virus isolation data from environmental samples.* Cincinnati, OH, US Environmental Protection Agency, 1986 (Contract Report 68-03-3196).

7.  Rao VC, Melnick JL. *Environmental virology.* Wokingham, Van Nostrand Reinhold (UK), 1986:10-17 (Aspects of Microbiology No. 13).

8.  Payment P et al. A prospective epidemiological study of drinking water related gastrointestinal illnesses. *Water science and technology*, 1991, 24 (2):27-28.

9.  Bates J, Goddard MR, Butler W. The detection of rotaviruses in products of wastewater treatment. *Journal of hygiene (London)*, 1984, 93:639-643.

10. Dahling DR, Safferman RS, Wright BA. Isolation of enterovirus and reovirus from sewage and treated effluents in selected Puerto Rican communities. *Applied and environmental microbiology*, 1989, 55:503-506.

11. Gerba CP et al. *Virus removal during conventional drinking water treatment.* Cincinnati, OH, US Environmental Protection Agency, 1984 (Project Report, Grant No. CR 809331010).

12. Walter R et al. Interactions between biotic and abiotic factors and viruses in a water system. *Water science and technology*, 1985, 17:139-151.

13. Andersson Y, Stenstrom TA. Waterborne outbreaks in Sweden—causes and etiology. *Water science and technology*, 1987, 19:575-580.

14. Hopkins RS et al. A community waterborne gastroenteritis outbreak: evidence of rotavirus as the agent. *American journal of public health*, 1984, 74:263-265.

15. Foy HM, Cooney MK, Hatlen JB. Adenovirus type 3 epidemic associated with intermittent chlorination of a swimming pool. *Archives of environmental health*, 1968, 17:795-802.

16. D'Angelo LJ et al. Pharyngoconjunctival fever caused by adenovirus type 4: report of a swimming pool-related outbreak with recovery of virus from pool water. *Journal of infectious diseases*, 1979, 140:42-47.

17. Goodman RA et al. Norwalk gastroenteritis associated with a water system in a rural Georgia community. *Archives of environmental health*, 1982, 37:358-360.

18. Towianska A, Potajallo U. Human pathogenic viruses in waters of Lake Zarnowiekie (north Poland). *Bulletin of the Institute of Maritime and Tropical Medicine in Gdynia*, 1990, 41:149-155.

19. National Research Council. *Proceedings of a Symposium on Viral Hepatitis.* Washington, DC, National Academy Press, 1975.

20. Pana A et al. Isolation of Hepatitis A virus from polluted river water on FRP/3 cells. *Lancet*, 1987, ii(5):1328 (letter).

21. Gerba CP, Rose JB, Singh SN. Waterborne gastroenteritis and viral hepatitis. *Critical reviews in environmental control*, 1985, 15(3):213-235.

22. Belabbes EH et al. Epidemic non-A, non-B viral hepatitis in Algeria: strong evidence for its spreading by water. *Journal of medical virology*, 1985, 16:257-263.

23. Khukhlovich PA et al. The epidemiological problems of viral non-A, non-B hepatitis with a fecal-oral mechanism of infection transmission. *Zurnal mikrobiologii, epidemiologii i immunobiologii*, 1989, 5:42-47.

24. Flewett TH, Woode GN. The rotaviruses. *Archives of virology*, 1978, 57:1-23.

25. Bosch A et al. Non-seasonal distribution of rotavirus in Barcelona raw sewage. *Zentralblatt für Bakteriologie, Mikrobiologie und Hygiene, Reihe B*, 1988, 186:273-277.

26. Baron RC et al. Norwalk gastrointestinal illness. *American journal of epidemiology*, 1982, 115:163-172.

27. Sekine S et al. Prevalence of small structured virus infections in acute gastroenteritis outbreaks in Tokyo. *Microbiology and immunology*, 1989, 33:207-217.

# 5.
# Protozoa

Drinking-water plays a major role in the spread of three of the intestinal protozoa pathogenic for humans, namely *Giardia intestinalis* (syn. *G. lamblia*, the etiological agent of human giardiasis), *Cryptosporidium parvum* (human cryptosporidiosis), and *Entamoeba histolytica* (amoebic dysentery). *Balantidium coli* infection (balantidiasis) is uncommon, although the parasite has a worldwide distribution. These pathogenic intestinal protozoa can be transmitted to humans by any mechanism whereby material contaminated with faeces containing viable organisms from infected individuals can reach the mouth. However, infections with pathogenic *Naegleria fowleri* (naegleriasis or primary amoebic meningoencephalitis) and *Acanthamoeba* spp. (meningitis, keratitis) are associated primarily with recreation and the inhalation of warm soil-contaminated water, and are comparatively rare.

## 5.1 *Giardia*

### 5.1.1 General description

#### *Life cycle*

Organisms in the genus *Giardia* (also called *Lamblia*) are flagellated protozoa that parasitize the intestines of humans and animals. These flagellates have a simple two-stage life cycle consisting of the reproductive trophozoite stage and the environmentally resistant cyst stage. When ingested by a susceptible host, the cysts are induced to excyst by exposure to acid in the stomach and perhaps also by contact with enzymes or other as yet undefined digestants (*1*). After excysting, the trophozoite leaves the cyst wall behind and rapidly undergoes cytokinesis, splitting by binary fission into two daughter trophozoites (*2*) which are bilaterally symmetrical and vary in shape from ellipsoidal to pyriform (*3*). The anterior end is rounded and contains two nuclei, while the posterior end tends to be pointed. The dorsal side is convex, and the ventral side contains an adhesive or sucking disc by which the organism attaches itself to intestinal surfaces. Each trophozoite has two slender median rods or axostyles, four pairs of flagella, and a pair of median bodies. The trophozoites may be 9–21 μm long, 5–15 μm wide, and 2–4 μm thick.

Perhaps in response to population pressures, the trophozoites release their hold on the intestinal epithelium and enter the lumen. As they travel down the intestines, they are apparently induced to encyst by exposure to bile, alkaline pH, and possibly bacterial metabolites (4). The cysts are ovoid, 8–12 µm long by 7–10 µm wide, and contain the same structures (nuclei, axostyles, median bodies) as the trophozoites; however, up to four nuclei may be visible within each cyst. The cysts are discharged with the faeces and thereby returned to the environment.

The length of time that cysts can survive depends on the temperature. *G. intestinalis* cysts have survived for at least 77 days and *G. muris* cysts for at least 84 days when suspended in water at less than 10 °C. Above 20 °C, cyst inactivation is relatively rapid. Sharp decreases in cyst viability have been noted after 3 days' storage in water at 20 °C or after only 1 day at 37 °C. The thermal death point for *G. muris* cysts has been reported to be 54 °C, and *G. intestinalis* have been inactivated by exposure to 55 °C for 5 minutes. Cysts may be inactivated in water by bringing the temperature to boiling point (5–8).

### Host range

*Giardia* organisms are widely distributed in nature and have been reported as occurring in more than 40 species of animals including amphibians, birds, and mammals (9). However, whether or not giardiasis is, or can be, a zoonosis is debatable. Some investigators have reported infecting a variety of animals —including dog, beaver, muskrat, gerbil, and rat—with cysts from human sources (10–12), but others have been unable to infect mice, hamsters, rats, cats, and dogs with such cysts (13). However, all of them have been able to infect some species of animals with cysts derived from different ones. While there are anecdotal reports to suggest that humans may become infected with cysts from deer, beavers, and muskrats (14), no controlled studies on human volunteers inoculated with organisms from animal sources have yet been reported. It appears that some species of *Giardia* may be host-specific while others may not be. In addition, since at least some animals that inhabit watersheds can become infected with cysts from humans, they may act as intermediaries for human *Giardia* infection rather than as primary reservoirs. Methods are needed capable of differentiating between the cysts causing human infections and those found in environmental samples. Until such methods are developed, it would seem prudent, as has been suggested (15), to assume that humans may be susceptible to many of the *Giardia* infecting lower animals.

The North American literature strongly supports the concept that animal vectors have been the source of the contamination of watersheds and of waters all but inaccessible to humans.

## 5.1.2 Routes of exposure

As with other pathogenic intestinal protozoa, *Giardia* can be transmitted by any mechanism whereby material contaminated with faeces containing viable organisms from infected individuals can reach the mouth. Documented routes of exposure include drinking-water, recreational water, food, and person-to-person contact.

### *Water*

Epidemic giardiasis associated with contaminated drinking-water has been reported in the United States of America (*16*), Canada (*17*), England (*18*), Scotland (*19*), and Sweden (*20*). Drinking-water has also been implicated as the vehicle of transmission in outbreaks occurring among travellers in the former Soviet Union (*21*). The USA has experienced a great number of reported waterborne outbreaks, over 25 occurring between 1986 and 1988 (*22*). In some of the outbreaks, water supplies had been contaminated with human sewage; in others, faecal discharges from watershed animals were the suspected sources of the contamination. Surveys of such animals have shown very high *Giardia* prevalence in aquatic voles (*23*) and muskrats (*24*). Most of the outbreaks in the USA have been attributed to contaminated surface water treated only by disinfection (*16*). *Giardia* cysts can be inactivated by disinfection, but are among the most resistant waterborne pathogens; effective disinfection calls for consideration of the water pH, turbidity, and temperature, as well as controlling the disinfectant dose and contact time (*25*). The wide distribution of *Giardia* in humans and animals, the uncertainty concerning cross-species infectivity, the resistance of the cysts to inactivation by disinfection, and experience with the outbreaks led the USA to develop regulations on the disinfection of all surface water supplies in the country (*26*). Risk analysis, using a probabilistic model, suggests that an annual risk of infection of less than one per 10 000 population can be achieved for source waters with 0.7–70 cysts per 100 litres, when treatment to achieve a $10^3$–$10^5$-fold reduction is applied (*27*).

Endemic giardiasis has also been associated with the consumption of contaminated drinking-water in such diverse locations as the USA (*16*) and South Africa (*28*). In addition to endemic and epidemic giardiasis from drinking-water supplies, there have been reported outbreaks in the USA (*29*) and in Canada (*30*), affecting children and adults, caused by the ingestion of swimming-pool water. The source of contamination in these outbreaks was apparently related to defecation in the water by infected children.

### *Relative significance of routes of exposure*

Quantifying the degree of significance of the various routes of transmission of giardiasis is difficult because of a lack of information on the total prevalence or incidence of infection or disease. Bennett and co-workers (*31*), using published material and survey data from the National Center for Health Statistics, estimated that 60% of the cases of giardiasis occurring in the USA were waterborne. Kappus & Juranek (*32*) suggested that 45–50% of giardiasis cases in the USA were associated with drinking unfiltered municipal water. They also suggested that 40–45% of cases were associated directly or indirectly with person-to-person transmission at day-care centres, and that the remaining cases (about 10%) involved exposure while travelling, engaging in sexual practices that involve faecal exposure, or ingesting untreated surface water while hiking or camping. The contribution of waterborne as opposed to person-to-person transmission may be expected to vary from country to country depending on a number of factors including the extent of water treatment, the sanitation facilities, and local customs. However, apart from *Cryptosporidium* (see p. 56), *Giardia* probably has the greatest potential for transmission through drinking-water of all the waterborne parasitic protozoa since:

- cysts from humans are infective for a wide variety of domestic and wild animals and are widely distributed in the environment;
- some waterborne outbreaks have been attributed to the contamination of drinking-water by cysts of nonhuman origin;
- the cysts are highly resistant to disinfection.

## 5.1.3 Health effects

Although the pathogenicity of the organisms was for long controversial, it is now widely accepted that *Giardia* can cause disease, and Koch's postulates have been satisfied by experimental human infections (*33*). Much of the controversy apparently arose from the highly variable illness-to-infection ratio observed. Asymptomatic infections with *Giardia* have been reported to account for up to 76% of the total under epidemic conditions (*34*). The time between ingestion of the organism and the appearance of the parasite in the stool is about 9–14 days, while the incubation period may range from 1 to 75 days with a median value of 8–15 days (*35*). Symptomatic infections may be acute, subacute, or chronic, and the condition may last for months if not diagnosed and treated. Symptoms that have been commonly reported include diarrhoea, flatulence, foul-smelling stools, cramps, distension, fatigue, anorexia, nausea, weight loss, and vomiting. Intolerance to lactose may develop during the infection and persist even after the organism has been eradicated (*35*). Infection in children may interfere with growth and normal development (*36*), but mortality has rarely been reported in patients of any age.

The pathophysiological mechanisms in giardiasis remain to be clarified. As with the clinical effects, histopathological changes in the intestinal mucosa can cover a wide spectrum ranging from minimal to significant enteropathy with enterocyte damage, villus atrophy, and crypt hyperplasia (*37*).

No explanation can be given for the broad range of clinical and pathological effects observed but both parasite and host factors are probably involved. Strain variation in pathogenicity has been demonstrated in humans (*33*), while strain and host variations have been observed in animals (*38*). In addition to local effects that can be produced directly by the parasites, their metabolic activity (*39*), and secretion products, host factors that could contribute to the degree of tissue damage include nutritional status, systemic immune responses, and mucosal immunity (*37, 40*). *Giardia* isolated from humans and animals have been found to be associated with bacteria, virus-like particles and mycoplasma-like organisms (*41*). It has been suggested that these apparent symbionts may be transmitted via *Giardia* cysts. In addition, a double-standed RNA virus has been found in *Giardia* (*42*). Some isolates of *G. intestinalis* are susceptible to infection with this virus while others are not (*43*). What effect, if any, these associated organisms might have on the virulence of *Giardia* or on the pathogenesis of the disease is not known.

## 5.2 *Cryptosporidium* spp.

### 5.2.1 General description

*Cryptosporidium* spp. are intracellular coccidian parasites of the gastrointestinal and respiratory tracts of numerous animals, including mammals, birds, and fish, and have a worldwide distribution. At present, six species are known, namely *C. parvum* and *C. muris*, which infect mammals, *C. baileyi* and *C. meleagridis*, which infect birds, and *C. serpentis* and *C. nasorum*, which infect reptiles and fish, respectively. *C. parvum* is the major species responsible for clinical disease in humans and domestic animals (*44*). As with both *E. histolytica* and *G. intestinalis*, infection occurs by ingestion of the transmissive phase which, for *Cryptosporidium* spp., is the oocyst. Person-to-person transmission occurs (*45*), and oocysts from humans are infective for numerous mammals, including cattle and sheep (*46*), while both domestic and feral animals may be reservoirs of human infection (*47*). Infected humans can excrete $10^9$ oocysts a day, and calves and lambs can excrete up to $10^{10}$ oocysts daily for up to 14 days (*48*). The average density of oocysts in raw sewage has been estimated at 5000 per litre (*49*). The broad host range together with the high output of oocysts ensures a high level of contamination in the environment. *Cryptosporidium* is an obligate parasite that develops only within a living host cell; unlike the other protozoa transmitted by drinking-water, but in common with other coccidia, it has several characteristic developmental stages (*44*). Infection is initiated following ingestion of the oocyst, which contains four naked, motile sporozoites. These are released through the suture in the oocyst wall following exposure to trypsin and bile salts, and attach themselves intimately to the surface of adjacent epithelial cells. They develop within a parasitophagous vacuole which is intracellular but extracytoplasmic, initially as a fixed trophozoite, then through asexual and sexual stages to finally become oocysts.

*Cryptosporidium* completes its life cycle within a single host; however, unlike *E. histolytica* and *G. lamblia*, endogenous reinfection (autoinfection) occurs which, together with recycling of the asexual stage, allows parasite numbers to build up to a high level. In addition, external maturation of oocysts is not required, and the thin-walled oocysts, which account for up to 20% of the total, excyst during passage through the intestine, releasing sporozoites which further increase the infection. The majority of the oocysts become detached and sporulate during passage through the gut to become thick-walled oocysts which are infective when excreted. *C. parvum* oocysts are spherical; their modal size is 4.5 x 5.0 μm (range 4–6 μm).

In various surveys conducted throughout the world, *Cryptosporidium* infection in immunocompetent persons has been found in 26 countries, with a reported prevalence of 0.6-20% in developed countries and 4-20% in developing ones. The infection is more common in children than in adults (50). Among AIDS patients, cryptosporidiosis has a prevalence of 3-4% in the USA and over 50% in some African countries and Haiti. An asymptomatic carrier state exists, but the ratio of cases to carriers has not been determined. At present, no effective drug is available for the treatment of cryptosporidiosis.

## 5.2.2 Routes of exposure

As with other pathogenic intestinal protozoa, *Cryptosporidium* can be transmitted by any mechanism whereby material contaminated with faeces containing viable organisms from infected humans or animals can reach the mouth.

### *Drinking-water*

Humans and other mammals are reservoirs for infection, and the contamination of water supplies with either human or animal sewage can lead to the transmission of *Cryptosporidium* through drinking-water. Outbreaks have been traced to the contamination of drinking-water by both human and animal wastewaters (*51–54*). Oocysts can survive several months in water at 4 °C and are among the most chlorine-resistant pathogens known (*55*). Waterborne outbreaks of cryptosporidiosis have been reported from both the USA and the United Kingdom and, in most of the recently documented outbreaks, oocysts have been identified in drinking-water. Outbreaks have been associated with untreated drinking-water, water treated by chlorination only, and water subjected to conventional treatment (coagulation, sedimentation, sand filtration and chlorination). Because oocysts are only 4–6 μm in size, the extent to which those present in raw water are removed by various water-treatment processes is still unclear. As with other intestinal protozoa pathogenic to humans, the infective dose is thought to be small. When two primates were given a dose of 10 oocysts, disease was produced in both (*56*). Information both on oocyst survival in the environment and on resistance to disinfection is incomplete at present; however, oocysts lose their infectivity at temperatures below 0 °C or when kept at above 45 °C for 5–20 minutes (*55–57*).

Apart from *Giardia* (see p. 52), *Cryptosporidium* probably has the greatest potential for transmission through drinking-water of all the waterborne parasitic protozoa since:
- oocysts from humans are infective for a wide variety of domestic and wild animals, and are widely distributed in the environment;
- some waterborne outbreaks have been attributed to the contamination of drinking-water by oocysts of nonhuman origin;
- among the protozoa under consideration, *Cryptosporidium* spp. have the smallest and most chlorine-resistant oocysts.

### Other routes of exposure

Swimming-pools have been incriminated in the transmission of cryptosporidiosis (*54*), but the evidence for the outdoor recreational water route for the transmission of infection is circumstantial (*52, 53*). However, as oocysts can be detected in recreational waters, and such waters are being increasingly used for immersion sports, it is likely that the importance of this route of infection will increase in the future.

Since both animals and humans are reservoirs of infection and both *E. histolytica* and *G. intestinalis* can be transmitted by food, it seems likely that this may also be true for *Cryptosporidium* spp.

The transmission of *Cryptosporidium* infection between children and adults appears to be rare where good personal hygiene is practised. However, the transmission of infection among preschool children in day-care centres (*46, 58*) and similar institutions is probably common.

## 5.2.3 Health effects

### Immunocompetent patients

While infection may be asymptomatic, it is usually associated with diarrhoea (80–90% of cases). Gastrointestinal symptoms, which may be accompanied by an influenza-like illness (20–40% of cases), include vomiting, anorexia, and flatulence. Symptoms typically last 7–14 days, and prolonged excretion of oocysts is unusual.

### Immunocompromised patients

In patients with AIDS, other acquired abnormalities of T-lymphocytes, congenital hypogammaglobulinaemia, severe combined immunodeficiency syndrome, those receiving immunosuppressive drugs, and those with severe malnutrition, a severe cholera-like illness is produced, resulting in intractable nausea, weight loss, and severe dehydration (as much as 20 litres of liquid stool may be lost per day).

Except in those patients in whom the suppression of the immune system can be relieved by stopping immunosuppressant drugs, symptoms persist unabated until the patient dies (*59*).

## 5.3 *Entamoeba histolytica*

### 5.3.1 General description

*E. histolytica* is distributed worldwide and exists in trophozoite and cyst stages. Infection occurs by ingestion of cysts; these range in size from 10 to 20 μm (average 12 μm). Since *E. histolytica* is primarily a parasite of primates, humans are the reservoir of infection. Dysenteric individuals pass only trophozoites, which are adversely affected by environmental factors such as drying and changes in temperature and salt concentration, while most or all of the parasites in this active amoeboid stage are destroyed by gastric juice (*60*). Consequently, chronic cases and carriers who excrete cysts are more important sources of infection. Various surveys throughout the world have indicated a prevalence of 10–45% for *E. histolytica* infections and carriers can discharge up to $1.5 \times 10^7$ cysts daily (*61*).

### 5.3.2 Routes of exposure

Since humans are the primary reservoir for infection with *E. histolytica*, the contamination of water supplies with domestic sewage can lead to the transmission of this organism through drinking-water. Outbreaks have been traced to sewage contamination of drinking-water (*61*). The potential for waterborne transmission may be greater in the tropics, where the carrier rate sometimes exceeds 50%, as compared with more temperate regions where the prevalence in the general population is generally less than 10%. The cysts can survive for several months in water at 0 °C, 3 days at 30 °C, 30 minutes at 45 °C, and 5 minutes at 50 °C (*55*), and are extremely resistant to chlorination (*62*).

    *E. histolytica* may also be transmitted by food, including raw vegetables, and food handlers may be important in transmission (*61*). Although swimming-pools have not been definitely incriminated, they are a potential source.

    Of the intestinal protozoan pathogens, *E. histolytica* is the most prevalent worldwide. Person-to-person spread and contamination of food by infected food handlers appear to be the most significant means of transmission, although contaminated drinking-water also plays a role.

### 5.3.3 Health effects

Though most infections with *E. histolytica* are asymptomatic or cause only minor symptoms, deaths can occur. The usual clinical manifestations are gastroenteritis with symptoms ranging from mild diarrhoea to fulminating bloody dysentery. Liver abscess is the most common metastatic complication. Pathogenicity appears to depend both on strain virulence and on host factors, including the nutritional status of the individual and the associated bacterial flora (*61*).

## 5.4 *Balantidium coli*

### 5.4.1 General description

*Balantidium coli* is a ciliated organism of worldwide distribution; both the trophozoite and cyst stages can be infective for humans. The spherical to ovoid cysts are 40–60 μm in diameter, yellowish to greenish in colour, and have a two-membrane wall. Human infections usually occur as a result of the ingestion of food or water contaminated with faecal material from infected swine. Other hosts include lesser primates and, rarely, dogs and rats. *B. coli* is very common in swine but is considerably less prevalent in humans. Asymptomatic carrier infections can occur in humans and the world incidence is estimated at less than 0.7% (*60*).

### 5.4.2 Route of exposure

The only reported waterborne outbreak of balantidiasis occurred in the Truk District of Micronesia in 1971. It was concluded that the epidemic probably resulted from the contamination of water supplies by pig faeces when a devastating typhoon destroyed pig pens and precarious water-catchment facilities (*63*).

### 5.4.3 Health effects

The incidence of balantidiasis in humans is low, and direct contact with pigs appears to be the main route of transmission of the causative organism. The potential exists for the transmission of the organism in food and water contaminated with pig faeces.

Balantidiasis can present as an acute bloody dysentery, but an asymptomatic carrier state also occurs in humans (*60*).

## 5.5 *Naegleria* and *Acanthamoeba*

### 5.5.1 General description

Free-living amoebae cause severe human disease of waterborne origin. *Naegleria fowleri* is the etiological agent of primary amoebic meningoencephalitis (*64*). Although another species of *Naegleria, N. australiensis,* is known to produce fatal brain infection in experimental animals, no human cases due to this species have been reported (*65*). Various species of the genus *Acanthamoeba* cause keratitis, skin and pulmonary infections, and granulomatous amoebic meningitis (*66*). Infections by *Hartmannella* reported in the older literature were all due to *Acanthamoeba*. Infections with *N. fowleri* are almost always associated with recreational contact rather than with the drinking of water. *Acanthamoeba* eye infections are mostly related to inadequate cleaning or disinfection of contact lenses.

*Naegleria* spp. exist in three forms, namely as a trophozoite, a flagellate, and a cyst stage (*67*). The trophozoites (10–20 μm) move by eruptive pseudopod formation. They have a single nucleus with a central nucleolus, although binucleated and multinucleated forms do occur. A sexual stage is unknown, and reproduction is by simple binary fission. The trophozoite can transform into a flagellate stage with two anterior flagella. The flagellate does not divide but reverts to the trophozoite stage. Under adverse conditions, the trophozoite transforms into a circular cyst, 7–15 μm in diameter. Although the cyst is quite resistant to chlorination, prolonged contact does kill it.

*Acanthamoeba* spp. have two forms (*67*). The trophozoites (10–30 μm) are characterized by needle-like projections called filopodia or acanthopodia. Like *Naegleria*, they usually have a single nucleus with a central nucleolus, and reproduce by binary fission. In most species, the cyst stage (14–25 μm) is typically polygonal or starlike and has two easily distinguished cell walls. In some species, including the most virulent ones, the cyst is more or less rounded, and the two cell walls are difficult to discern. Cysts of *Acanthamoeba* are extremely resistant to chlorination.

Pathogenic species can be differentiated from nonpathogenic ones by pre-screening on cell lines and then by intranasal instillation of the cultured amoebae into mice. Different species of pathogenic *Naegleria* and *Acanthamoeba* can be identified by antigen, isoenzyme and/or DNA studies. *Naegleria fowleri* is typically thermophilic, growing in water at temperatures up to 45 °C. Pathogenic *Acanthamoeba* rarely thrive at such high temperatures.

## 5.5.2 Routes of exposure

Because of its thermophilic nature, *N. fowleri* is distributed worldwide in surface waters that are naturally heated by the sun or in industrial cooling waters and geothermal springs (*68*). Most infections are reported in industrialized countries. In Australia, many fatal cases occurred through the use of unfiltered, chlorinated water for washing and bathing (*69*). Cases in developing countries are most probably under-reported.

Some *Acanthamoeba* infections are related to water, but most, except for keratitis, occur in debilitated persons. Keratitis can occur following a minor trauma to the eye and subsequent washing, or as a result of wearing contact lenses. In particular, inadequate cleaning and disinfection of contact lenses favour the occurrence of *Acanthamoeba* keratitis. Contact lens cases appear to be breeding places for this organism.

*Acanthamoeba* can be found in all environments, and particularly frequently in chlorinated swimming-pools and drinking-water. Although airborne transmission of free-living amoebae does occur, the evidence for infection by this route is controversial.

## 5.5.3 Health effects

*Naegleria fowleri* causes fatal meningoencephalitis particularly in young and healthy individuals after swimming or activities causing infected water to be inhaled. The amoeba enters the brain by penetrating the olfactory mucosa and cribriform plate (*70*). The infection is very severe, and patients often die (5–10 days after penetration) before the infectious agent can be diagnosed. In addition, treatment is difficult, as only amphotericin B appears to be effective. Administration of other antibiotics together with amphotericin B might increase success rates. Although the infection remains rare (about 100 cases had been described up to 1980), new cases are encountered every year.

*Acanthamoeba* can cause diseases ranging from meningitis to pulmonary and wound infections, but few cases have been reported. However, the number of cases of keratitis increased considerably in the 1980s. While only 20 cases of keratitis were reported up to 1984, the number of cases in the USA had increased to over 200 by 1989 (*71*). Very few treatments are effective against *Acanthamoeba* infections, although keratitis cases can now be treated effectively; corneal transplants were usually necessary in the past.

*Legionella* bacteria can grow inside the cells of *Naegleria*, *Acanthamoeba* (*72*) and other free-living amoebae, and are protected against disinfection when inside the cysts of these amoebae. This is discussed further on p. 29.

# References

1. Bingham AK, Meyer EA. *Giardia* excystation can be induced *in vitro* in acidic solution. *Nature (London)*, 1979, 277:301-302.

2. Coggins JR, Schaefer FW. *Giardia muris*: scanning electron microscopy of *in vitro* excystation. *Experimental parasitology*, 1984, 57:62-67.

3. Levine ND. *Veterinary protozoology*. Ames, IA, Iowa State University Press, 1985.

4. Gillin FD et al. *Giardia lamblia*: the roles of bile, lactic acid, and pH in the completion of the life cycle *in vitro*. *Experimental parasitology*, 1989, 69:164-174.

5. Bingham AK, Jarroll EL, Meyer EA. *Giardia* sp: physical factors of excystation *in vitro*, and excystation vs eosin exclusion as determinants of viability. *Experimental parasitology*, 1979, 47:284-291.

6. Deregnier DP et al. Viability of *Giardia* cysts suspended in lake, river and tap water. *Applied and environmental microbiology*, 1989, 55:1223-1229.

7. Wickramanayake GB, Rubin AJ, Sproul OJ. Effects of ozone and storage temperature on *Giardia* cysts. *Journal of the American Water Works Association*, 1985, 77(8):74-77.

8.  Schaefer FW, Rice EW, Hoff JC. Factors promoting *in vitro* excystation of *Giardia muris* cysts. *Transactions of the Royal Society of Tropical Medicine and Hygiene*, 1984, 78:795-800.

9.  Cox FEG. Systematics of parasitic protozoa. In: Kreier JP, Baker JR, eds. *Parasitic protozoa*, Vol. 1. New York, Academic Press, 1991:55-80.

10. Davies RB, Hibler CP. Animal reservoirs and cross-species transmission of *Giardia*. In: Jakubowski W, Hoff JC, eds. *Waterborne transmission of giardiasis*. Cincinnati, OH, US Environmental Protection Agency, 1979: 104-126 (EPA-600/9-79-001).

11. Erlandsen SL et al. Cross-species transmission of *Giardia* spp.: inoculation of beavers and muskrats with cysts of human, beaver, mouse and muskrat origin. *Applied and environmental microbiology*, 1988, 54(11):2777-2785.

12. Belosevic M, Faubert GM. Animal models for infections with *G. duodenalis*-type organisms. In: Meyer EA, ed. *Human parasitic diseases*, Vol. 3. *Giardiasis*. Amsterdam, Elsevier, 1990:77-90.

13. Woo PTK, Paterson WB. *Giardia lamblia* in children in day-care centres in southern Ontario, Canada, and susceptibility of animals to *G. lamblia*. *Transactions of the Royal Society of Tropical Medicine and Hygiene*, 1986, 80:56-59.

14. Jakubowski W. The control of *Giardia* in water supplies. In: Meyer EA, ed. *Human parasitic diseases*. Vol. 3. *Giardiasis*. Amsterdam, Elsevier, 1990:335-353.

15. Meyer EA. The epidemiology of giardiasis. *Parasitology today*, 1985, 1(4):101-105.

16. Craun GF. Waterborne giardiasis. In: Meyer EA, ed. *Human parasitic diseases*, Vol. 3, *Giardiasis*. Amsterdam, Elsevier, 1990:257-293.

17. Wallis PM, Zammuto RM, Buchanan-Mappin JM. Cysts of *Giardia* spp. in mammals and surface waters in southwestern Alberta. *Journal of wildlife diseases*, 1986, 22:115-118.

18. Jephcott AE, Begg NT, Baker IA. Outbreak of giardiasis associated with mains water in the United Kingdom. *Lancet*, 1986, i:730-732.

19. Benton C et al. The incidence of waterborne and water-associated disease in Scotland from 1945 to 1987. *Water science and technology*, 1989, 21(3):125-129.

20. Neringer R, Andersson Y, Eitrem R. A water-borne outbreak of giardiasis in Sweden. *Scandinavian journal of infectious diseases*, 1987, 19:85-90.

21. Jokipii L, Jokipii AM. Giardiasis in travelers: a prospective study. *Journal of infectious diseases*, 1974, 130:295-299.

22. Levine WC, Stephenson WT, Craun GF. Waterborne disease outbreaks, 1986–1988. *Morbidity and mortality weekly report*, 1990, 39:1-13.

23. Pacha RE et al. Small rodents and other mammals associated with mountain meadows as reservoirs of *Giardia* spp. and *Campylobacter* spp. *Applied and environmental microbiology*, 1987, 53:1547-1579.

24. Erlandsen SL et al. Prevalence of *Giardia* in beaver and muskrat populations in northeastern states and Minnesota: detection of intestinal trophozoites at necropsy provides greater sensitivity than detection of cysts in faecal samples. *Applied and environmental microbiology*, 1990, 56:31-36.

25. Hoff JC. *Inactivation of microbial agents by chemical disinfectants.* Cincinnati, OH, US Environmental Protection Agency, 1986 (EPA-600/2-86-067).

26. US Environmental Protection Agency. National Primary Drinking Water Regulations; filtration, disinfection, turbidity, *Giardia lamblia*, viruses, *Legionella* and heterotrophic bacteria; final rule. *Federal register*, 1989, 54(124):27486-27541.

27. Rose JB, Haas CN, Regli S. Risk assessment and control of waterborne giardiasis. *American journal of public health*, 1991, 81:709-713.

28. Esrey SA et al. Drinking water source, diarrhoeal morbidity and child growth in villages with both traditional and improved water supplies in rural Lesotho, Southern Africa. *American journal of public health*, 1988, 78:1451-1455.

29. Porter JD et al. *Giardia* transmission in a swimming pool. *American journal of public health*, 1978:659-662.

30. Greensmith CT et al. Giardiasis associated with the use of a water slide. *Pediatric infectious disease journal*, 1988, 7:91-94.

31. Bennett JV et al. Infectious and parasitic diseases. *American journal of preventative medicine*, 1987, 3 (Suppl. 3):102-114.

32. Kappus K, Juranek DD. *Giardia* in the well. *Journal of the American Medical Association*, 1988, 259:1810 (letter).

33. Nash TE et al. Experimental human infection with *Giardia lamblia*. *Journal of infectious diseases*, 1987, 156:974-984.

34. Lopez CE et al. Waterborne giardiasis; a communitywide outbreak of disease and a high rate of asymptomatic infection. *American journal of epidemiology*, 1980, 112:495-507.

35. Smith JW, Wolfe MS. Giardiasis. *Annual review of medicine*, 1980, 31:373-383.

36. Farthing MJ et al. Natural history of *Giardia* infection of infants and children in rural Guatemala and its impact on physical growth. *American journal of clinical nutrition*, 1986, 43:395-405.

37. Ferguson A, Gillon J, Munro G. Pathology and pathogenesis of the intestinal mucosal damage in giardiasis. In: Meyer EA, ed. *Human parasitic diseases*, Vol. 3, *Giardiasis*. Amsterdam, Elsevier, 1990:155-173.

38. Visvesvara GS, Dickerson J, Healy GR. Variable infectivity of human-derived *Giardia lamblia* cysts for Mongolian gerbils (*Meriones unquiculatus*). *Journal of clinical microbiology*, 1988, 26:837-841.

39. Halliday CE, Clark C, Farthin MJ. *Giardia*–bile salt interactions *in vitro* and *in vivo*. *Transactions of the Royal Society of Tropical Medicine and Hygiene*, 1988, 82:428-432.

40. Farthing MJ. Immune responses in human giardiasis. *Saudi medical journal*, 1989, 10:1-8.

41. Feely DE et al. Ultra-structural evidence for the presence of bacteria, viral-like particles, and mycoplasma-like organisms associated with *Giardia* spp. *Journal of protozoology*, 1988, 35:151-158.

42. Wang AL, Wang CC. Discovery of a specific double-stranded RNA virus in *Giardia lamblia*. *Molecular and biochemical parasitology*, 1986, 21:269-276.

43. Miller RL, Wang AL, Wang CC. Identification of *Giardia lamblia* isolates susceptible and resistant to infection by the double-stranded RNA virus. *Experimental parasitology*, 1988, 66:118-123.

44. Current WL. The biology of *Cryptosporidium*. *American Society of Microbiology news*, 1988, 54:605-611.

45. Current WL et al. Human cryptosporidiosis in immunocompetent and immunodeficient persons. Studies of an outbreak and experimental transmission. *New England journal of medicine*, 1983, 308:1252-1257.

46. Fayer R. Ungar BL. *Cryptosporidium* spp. and cryptosporidiosis. *Microbiological reviews*, 1986, 50:458-483.

47. Centers for Disease Control. Human cryptosporidiosis—Alabama. *Morbidity and mortality weekly report*, 1982, 31:252-254.

48. Blewett DA. Quantitative techniques in *Cryptosporidium* research. In: Angus KW, Blewett DA, eds. *Cryptosporidiosis. Proceedings of the First International Workshop*, Edinburgh, The Animal Diseases Research Association, 1989:85-95.

49. Madore MS et al. Occurrence of *Cryptosporidium* oocysts in sewage effluent and selected surface waters. *Journal of parasitology*, 1987, 73:702-705.

50. Soave R, Johnson WD. *Cryptosporidium* and *Isospora belli* infections. *Journal of infectious diseases*, 1988, 157:225-229.

51. Hayes EB et al. Large community outbreak of cryptosporidiosis due to contamination of a filtered public water supply. *New England journal of medicine*, 1989, 320:1372-1376.

52. Casemore DP. Epidemiological aspects of human cryptosporidiosis. *Epidemiology and infection*, 1990, 104:1-28.

53. Gallaher MM et al. Cryptosporidiosis and surface water. *American journal of public health*, 1989, 79:39-42.

54. Department of the Environment, Department of Health. *Cryptosporidium in water supplies. Report of the Group of Experts.* London, Her Majesty's Stationery Office, 1990:37-45.

55. Smith HV et al. *The effect of free chlorine on the viability of Cryptosporidium spp. oocysts.* Medmenham, Water Research Centre, 1988 (Report PRU 2023-M).

56. Miller RA, Bronsdon MA, Morton WR. Experimental cryptosporidiosis in a primate model. *Journal of infectious diseases*, 1990, 161(2): 312-315.

57. Sherwood D et al. Experimental cryptosporidiosis in laboratory mice. *Infection and immunity*, 1982, 38:471-475.

58. Anderson BC. Moist heat inactivation of *Cryptosporidium* spp. *American journal of public health*, 1985, 75:1433-1434.

59. Soave R, Armstrong D. *Cryptosporidium* and cryptosporidiosis. *Reviews of infectious diseases*, 1986, 8:1012-1023.

60. Freeman BA. *Burrows textbook of microbiology*, 22nd ed. Philadelphia, Saunders Co., 1985.

61. *Prevention and control of intestinal parasitic infections: report of a WHO Expert Committee.* Geneva, World Health Organization, 1987 (WHO Technical Report Series, No. 749).

62. Hoff JC. Disinfection resistance of *Giardia* cysts: origins of current concepts and research in progress. In: Jakubowski W, Hoff JC, eds. *Waterborne transmission of giardiasis.* Cincinnati, OH, US Environmental Protection Agency, 1979:231-239 (EPA-600/9-79-001).

63. Walzer PD et al. Balantidiasis outbreak in Truk. *American journal of tropical medicine and hygiene*, 1973, 22:33-41.

64. Carter R. Description of a *Naegleria* sp. isolated from two cases of primary amoebic meningo-encephalitis, and of the experimental pathological changes induced by it. *Journal of pathology*, 1970, 100:217-244.

65. John DT, de Jonckheere JF. Isolation of *Naegleria australiensis* from an Oklahoma lake. *Journal of protozoology*, 1985, 32:571-575.

66. Hanssens M, de Jonckheere JF, de Meunynck C. *Acanthamoeba* keratitis. A clinico pathological case report. *International ophthalmology*, 1985, 7:203-213.

67. Page FC. *A new key to freshwater and soil Gymnamoeba*. Ambleside, Freshwater Biological Association, 1988.

68. de Jonckheere JF. Pathogenic and nonpathogenic *Acanthamoeba* spp. in thermally polluted discharges and surface waters. *Journal of protozoology*, 1981, 28:56-59.

69. Dorsch MM, Cameron AS, Robinson BS. The epidemiology and control of primary amoebic meningo-encephalitis with particular reference to South Australia. *Transactions of the Royal Society of Tropical Medicine and Hygiene*, 1983, 77:372-377.

70. John DT. Opportunistically pathogenic free-living amoebae. In: Kreir JP, Baker JR, eds. *Parasitic protozoa*. Vol. 3, New York, Academic Press, 1993:143-246.

71. Stehr-Green JK et al. The epidemiology of *Acanthamoeba* keratitis in the United States. *American journal of ophthalmology*, 1989, 107:331-336.

72. Rowbotham TJ. Preliminary report on the pathogenicity of *Legionella pneumophila* for freshwater and soil amoebae. *Journal of clinical pathology*, 1980, 33:1179-1183.

# 6.
# Helminths

The helminths or parasitic worms comprise two unrelated groups of organisms, namely flatworms belonging to the phylum Platyhelmintha, and roundworms belonging to the phylum Nematoda. Apart from the guinea worm, *Dracunculus medinensis*, which is transmitted solely by drinking-water, it is rare for any of those listed in Table 6.1 to be so transmitted. On the other hand, the continued use of poor-quality borehole or piped water is a major factor in the risk of acquiring the other helminth infections.

### Table 6.1 Helminths potentially transmitted by drinking-water

| Zoological classification | Species | Infective stage and usual mode of infection |
|---|---|---|
| Phylum Nematoda (roundworms) | *Dracunculus medinensis* | Larvae in cyclops ingested in water |
| | *Ascaris lumbricoides* | Eggs ingested from soil |
| | *Toxocara canis* | Eggs ingested from soil |
| | *Trichuris trichiura* | Eggs ingested from soil |
| | *Necator americanus* | Penetrative larvae in soil |
| | *Ancylostoma duodenale* | Penetrative larvae in soil |
| | *Strongyloides stercoralis* | Penetrative larvae in water |
| Phylum Platyhelmintha, class Trematoda (flukes) | *Schistosoma* spp. | Free-swimming cercarial larvae penetrate skin |
| | *Fasciola* spp. | Cercarial larvae encysted and ingested on vegetation |
| Class Cestoidea, subclass Cestoda (tapeworms) | *Taenia solium* | Cysticerci consumed in raw pork or wild boar |
| | *Echinococcus* spp. | Eggs ingested from soil |
| | *Spirometra* spp. | Larvae in cyclops ingested in water or from soil |

# 6.1 *Dracunculus medinensis*[1]

## 6.1.1 General description

The guinea worm is the longest nematode parasite of humans, the female worm measuring up to 700 mm in length. When the female is ready to discharge its embryos, its anterior end emerges from a blister, usually on the foot or lower limb, and releases many thousands of embryos when the affected part of the body is immersed in water. The male worms measure only 25 mm in length, remain in the tissues and so are never seen. Embryos can be released on several occasions on contact with water in ponds, or in large open step-wells, used as sources of drinking-water. After a few weeks the entire worm is expelled from the body. Embryos can live in water for about 3 days but, when ingested by certain species of freshwater cyclopoid Copepoda (Crustacea), penetrate into the haemocoelom, moult twice, and are infective to a new host in about 2 weeks. If the cyclops, which measure 0.5–2 mm in length, are swallowed in drinking-water, the larvae are released in the stomach, penetrate the intestinal and peritoneal walls, and inhabit the subcutaneous tissues. Mature gravid female worms emerge about 1 year after infection (*1*).

Infection with guinea worm is geographically limited to rural areas of India, Pakistan, and 16 countries in sub-Saharan Africa (Benin, Burkina Faso, Cameroon, Chad, Côte d'Ivoire, Ethiopia, Ghana, Kenya, Mali, Mauritania, Niger, Nigeria, Senegal, Sudan, Togo, and Uganda). The annual incidence of dracunculiasis is estimated to be less than 2 million cases; approximately 140 million people are at risk (*2*).

## 6.1.2 Routes of exposure

Drinking-water containing infected cyclops is the only source of infection with *Dracunculus*, which is therefore the only human parasite that can be eradicated solely by the provision of safe drinking-water. The eradication of guinea worm infection from the world by 1995 was a target of the International Drinking Water Supply and Sanitation Decade (1981–1990), and the World Health Assembly formally committed itself to this goal in 1991 (resolution WHA 44.5).

The disease occurs in rural areas where piped water supplies are not always available. Control is based principally on the provision of boreholes and safe wells, but also includes measures aimed at preventing contamination of water sources, filtering of water by consumers, and in some situations chemical treatment of ponds and open wells. There are no effective antihelminthic drugs for the clinical treatment of the infection.

Transmission is usually highly seasonal, depending on changes in water sources. For instance, transmission is highest in the early rainy season in a dry

---

[1] The valuable contribution made by Dr P.J.A. Ranque, Dracunculiasis Eradication, WHO, Geneva, in the preparation of this section is gratefully acknowledged.

savanna zone of Mali with under 800 mm annual rainfall, but in the dry season in the humid savanna area of southern Nigeria with over 1300 mm annual rainfall.

### 6.1.3 Health effects

As previously mentioned, when a female guinea worm emerges, it causes the formation of a blister, which bursts, and a portion of the worm is extruded. In about 50% of all cases, the whole worm is extruded in a few weeks, the lesion then heals rapidly, and disability is of limited duration. However, in the remaining cases, complications ensue, and the track of the worm becomes secondarily infected, leading to morbidity, which lasts for months. Mortality is extremely rare, but permanent disability can result from contractures of tendons and chronic arthritis; in 1988, it was estimated that, in Nigeria, there were 12 000 such cases annually out of more than 600 000 infections each year.

Usually only one worm emerges, but there may be two, three, or occasionally many. Worms do not survive for more than one transmission season, but there does not appear to be any acquired immunity, and the same individuals can be reinfected many times. Incidence rates in infected communities can be very high, 30% of the 14–45-year age group often becoming infected each year. The economic effect on agricultural productivity can be important: for instance, an 11% annual reduction in rice production has been reported from an area of eastern Nigeria, at a cost of US$ 20 million (3).

## 6.2 *Schistosoma*[1]

### 6.2.1 General description

*Schistosoma* spp. belong to the class of trematodes or flukes, whose infective larvae are able to penetrate the human skin or mucous membranes, causing schistosomiasis. They may be transmitted through drinking-water, but are more of a hazard when water is used for washing or bathing.

Schistosome eggs are excreted in the urine or faeces of an infected person, and break open on reaching fresh water, releasing a tiny parasite (a miracidium). This must penetrate a freshwater snail within 8–12 hours if it is to develop further. Once it has penetrated the snail, the parasite divides many times until, within 4–7 weeks or longer, depending on the type of parasite, thousands of new forms (cercariae) break out of the snail into the water. The cercariae can live for up to 48 hours, and can penetrate human skin within a few seconds.

After penetration, the young parasites migrate through the lymphatic system to the blood vessels of the portal system, affecting the intestine (intestinal schis-

---

[1] The valuable contribution made by Dr K.E. Mott, Schistosomiasis Control, WHO, Geneva, in the preparation of this section is gratefully acknowledged.

tosomiasis) or the blood vessels around the bladder (urinary schistosomiasis), and develop into male or female adult worms within about 4 weeks. The adult worms live less than 5 years on average, although they can live for up to 40 years. Of the eggs produced by the female worm—over 200 per day for some species—only about half leave the body in the faeces (intestinal schistosomiasis) or in the urine (urinary schistosomiasis), the rest remaining embedded in the body, where they damage important organs. Heavy infections with schistosomes, which occur mainly in children, cause the actual disease.

Intestinal schistosomiasis caused by *Schistosoma mansoni* occurs in 52 countries in Africa, the Eastern Mediterranean Region, the Caribbean, and South America. Oriental or Asiatic intestinal schistosomiasis, caused by the *S. japonicum* group of parasites (including *S. mekongi* in the Mekong river basin), is endemic in seven countries in the South-East Asia and Western Pacific Regions. (Another form of intestinal schistosomiasis caused by *S. intercalatum* has been reported from ten central African countries.) Urinary schistosomiasis, caused by *S. haematobium*, is endemic in 54 countries in the African and Eastern Mediterranean Regions.

## 6.2.2 Routes of exposure

Schistosome infections are acquired when infected water is used for domestic activities, bathing or washing, or while working in contact with water. Ingested cercariae can penetrate the buccal mucous membranes, but this is a relatively unimportant route of entry. If safe drinking-water is readily available it will be used for washing, thus reducing the need to use contaminated surface water.

While there is a real possibility of piped untreated surface water transmitting schistosomiasis, most transmission is from unpiped sources such as pools, wells, and cisterns. In regions where schistosomiasis is endemic, the construction of dams and large reservoirs often leads to an increase in the population of the aquatic snail host and thus favours the spread of the disease. There are also many examples of increased transmission of schistosomiasis as a result of irrigation, the most dramatic being found along the Nile valley in Egypt and Sudan (*4*).

Schistosome infections are a hazard of recreational and irrigational water use rather than of drinking-water. However, improvements in community water supplies will reduce the incidence of schistosomiasis, particularly in communities where incidence is high (*4, 5*).

## 6.2.3 Health effects

The human schistosomes are a cause of severe morbidity and sometimes death in the 200 million people infected worldwide. In terms of socioeconomic and public health importance in tropical and subtropical areas, the disease now ranks second to malaria (*4*).

In communities where it is endemic, the prevalence of infection is greatest in 10–14-year-old children; in many African communities over 70% of village children may be infected. Pathology is due mainly to the host's reaction to eggs that fail to escape. Primary lesions are mainly in the liver, intestine, and around the bladder, but the most severe pathological effects are the consequence of secondary damage to the upper urinary tract, bladder cancer, and liver fibrosis and its haemodynamic consequences.

Schistosomiasis has a significant effect on health (6). In infected people without clinical evidence of disease, it is estimated that 30 work days are lost per year as a result of *S. japonicum* infection and 4 work days per year as a result of *S. haematobium* infection. After a latency period of 5–15 years, approximately 10% of infected people will develop severe disease. An 18% reduction in the work output of persons with severe *S. mansoni* infection can be expected. A reduction of 12% or more in exercise capacity was found in children with *S. haematobium* infection in Zimbabwe, but this was recovered by 1 month after treatment. Similarly, a 7–10% improvement in exercise capacity was found in children with *S. haematobium* infection 1 month after treatment in Kenya (KE Mott, personal communication).

A specific type of bladder cancer occurs in countries where urinary schistosomiasis is endemic, and is the leading cause of death due to cancer in Egypt among men aged 20–44 years. Diseases of the central nervous system, affecting the spinal cord, are more frequent and cause more debility than is widely recognized, especially among migrants into endemic areas of *S. mansoni* transmission.

In persons with schistosomiasis and intercurrent hepatitis B or typhoid fever, the severity and duration of both increase markedly, with an increased risk of chronic liver disease.

Since a single cercaria is infective, there is no safe level and cercariae should be absent from drinking-water. In the absence of routine monitoring assays, reliance must be placed on preventive measures if a significant risk from drinking-water is suspected in an area. The cercariae have a free-living life of under 48 hours, and storage for this period renders water safe (7). It is likely that storage for 24 hours will greatly reduce infectivity. Slow sand filters, provided that they are properly operated, will remove the majority of cercariae, and disinfection at a residual level of 0.5 mg of free chlorine per litre for 1 hour will kill cercariae of the human schistosomes (8). A sounder approach is to use a source that does not contain the host snails and is not subject to excretal contamination.

## 6.3 Other helminths

A great variety of helminth eggs and larvae have been detected in drinking-water, and it is clear that none of those infective to humans should be present if the drinking-water is to be safe. However, the vast majority of such helminths are not primarily waterborne, and it is neither feasible nor necessary to monitor water for them on a routine basis (9).

Helminths that could conceivably be transmitted through drinking-water are listed in Table 6.1. *Fasciola* spp., which belong to the same class as the schistosomes (the Trematoda), are principally parasites of farm and domestic animals. The cercariae which emerge from freshwater snails encyst on water plants and infect humans if these are ingested. Some tapeworms (Cestoda) have very resistant eggs, and those of *Taenia solium* (the pork tapeworm) and *Echinococcus* spp. can develop in humans. Eggs are liberated from the gravid proglottids (segments), and are passed out in faeces. They can then be ingested from soil or on salad vegetables, although the normal route of infection with *T. solium* is the ingestion of raw pork containing the larval cysticercus stage. Eggs of *Echinococcus* have been recovered from wells in an area of East Africa and might be transmitted in drinking-water. Another tapeworm, *Spirometra,* has its tapeworm stage in carnivores, and two intermediate hosts, the first being a cyclopoid copepod and the second an amphibian, reptile, rodent or herbivore, depending on species. Humans occasionally act as intermediate hosts for the larvae (spargana) by ingesting first-stage larvae inside cyclops when drinking water from ponds.

The resistant eggs of various common, ubiquitous, intestinal nematode parasites of humans, such as *Ascaris* and *Trichuris* (and the common dog ascarid, *Toxocara,* the eggs of which can hatch in humans and the larvae cause visceral damage), are passed in faeces and normally ingested in soil or on salad vegetables. The eggs occasionally enter water but have a high relative density and settle quickly; drinking-water does not play an important part in their transmission.

Other intestinal nematode parasites which infect many millions of people in the tropics and subtropics are *Necator* and *Ancylostoma* (the hookworms) and *Strongyloides.* Eggs (or, in the case of *Strongyloides,* larvae) are passed in the faeces, and the larvae develop in the soil into an infective stage which can penetrate the skin of a new host. While the larvae of *Ancylostoma* are sometimes ingested on salad vegetables, there is little evidence that drinking-water is ever a source of infection for these soil-transmitted nematodes.

## References

1.  Muller R. *Dracunculus* and dracunculiasis. *Advances in parasitology,* 1971, 9:73-151.

2.  Drancunculiasis. Global surveillance summary, 1992. *Weekly epidemiological record,* 1993, 68(18):125-132.

3.  Edungbola LD et al. *Guinea worm control as a major contributor to self-sufficiency in rice production in Nigeria.* Lagos, Nigeria, UNICEF, 1987.

4.  *The control of schistosomiasis: second report of the WHO Expert Committee.* Geneva, World Health Organization, 1993 (WHO Technical Report Series, No. 830)

5.  Esrey SA et al. Effects of improved water supply and sanitation on ascariasis, diarrhoea, dracunculiasis, hookworm infection, schistosomiasis and trachoma. *Bulletin of the World Health Organization,* 1991, 69:609-621.

6. Hunter J et al. *Parasitic diseases in water resources development.* Geneva, World Health Organization, 1993.

7. Jones MF, Brady FJ. Survival of *Schistosoma japonicum* cercariae at various temperatures in several types of water. *National Institute of Health bulletin,* 1974, 189:131-136.

8. Coles GC, Mann H. Schistosomiasis and water works practice in Uganda. *East African medical journal,* 1971, 48:40-43.

9. Feachem RG et al. *Sanitation and disease. Health aspects of excreta and wastewater management.* Chichester, John Wiley & Sons, 1983 (World Bank Studies in Water Supply and Sanitation No. 3).

# 7.

# Toxins from cyanobacteria

Blooms of cyanobacteria (commonly called blue-green algae) are very common in lakes and reservoirs used for potable water supply. These bacteria are capable of producing various toxins which fall into the following three categories: (i) hepatotoxins produced in fresh water by *Microcystis*, *Oscillatoria* and *Anabaena*, and by *Nodularia* in brackish water; (ii) neurotoxins produced by species of *Anabaena*, *Oscillatoria*, *Nostoc*, *Cylindrospermum* and *Aphanizomenon*; (iii) lipopolysaccharides from a number of species (*1*).

The most commonly encountered are the hepatotoxins, which induce death by circulatory shock as a result of massive liver haemorrhage within 2–24 hours of oral intake of a sufficiently large quantity (*2–7*). At present, there are thought to be more than 13 variants of the toxin, which is a cyclic structure containing seven amino acids of relative molecular mass varying from about 800 to 1050. The best studied of these hepatotoxins is microcystin LR:R, which has a relative molecular mass of 994.

The $LD_{50}$ of microcystin LR:R has been shown to be about 30 µg/kg of body weight in mice by intraperitoneal injection (*8*). A lethal dose is about 1–2 µg of pure toxin per mouse; however, the toxicity by the oral route appears to be about an order of magnitude less. There appear to be no other toxicity data available on the pure toxin, although studies with diluted extracts of a toxic bloom, reported to contain 56.6 µg/ml of an unknown variant of microcystin, showed that liver damage could be induced in mice given a one-quarter dilution of the extract in their drinking-water for 1 year (*9*). Microcystin was not mutagenic in the Ames test (*10*), but purified microcystin LR inhibited protein phosphatase *in vitro* with the same potency and specificity as the tumour promoter okadaic acid (*11*).

The hepatotoxic cyclic peptide from *Nodularia*, termed nodularin, has a structure similar to that of microcystin, but contains only five amino acids. The oral $LC_{50}$ for mice has been determined as 67 µg/ml for females and 73 µg/ml for males receiving 4.5–7 ml of drinking-water per day containing crude extracts (*7*).

There are a number of unconfirmed reports of algal toxins in drinking-water supplies causing health problems, including an outbreak of hepatoenteritis in Palm Island, Australia (*12*). However, the most convincing evidence comes from an epidemiological study by Falconer et al. (*13*) of an Australian community in which raised serum enzymes indicative of mild, reversible liver damage were observed in hospital patients who drank water from a local reservoir with a very large toxic bloom of *Microcystis aeruginosa*. Recent surveys of large numbers of fresh waters worldwide, which produce heavy growths of cyanobacteria, have shown the presence of cyanobacterial toxins at over 60% of sites (*14*). Algal blooms may change from being nontoxic to toxic in a very short time, but there is at present no well established method for analysis of the toxin in drinking-water.

It has been reported that activated carbon removes microcystin to a significant extent (*15–17*) and that ozone at a dose of 1.0–1.5 mg/litre destroys toxicity (*17*) by converting microcystin into a less toxic substance (*18*). The use of algicides such as copper sulfate at the height of the bloom is not recommended, since this leads to a massive release of toxin into the water, and may have been responsible for the unusual problems seen on Palm Island (*12*).

At present, it is not clear how great a hazard algal toxins pose in drinking-water, and the data are insufficient to enable any guidelines to be drawn up. However, problems resulting from the progressive eutrophication of inland waters appear to be increasing and with them the likelihood of cyanobacterial blooms. This emphasizes the need for the protection of sources, and particularly of lakes and reservoirs, from discharges of nutrient-rich effluent.

## References

1. National Rivers Authority. *Toxic blue-green algae.* London, 1990 (Water Quality Series No. 2).

2. Eriksson E et al. Cell selective cytotoxicity of a peptide toxin from the cyanobacterium *Microcystis aeruginosa. Biochimica et biophysica acta*, 1987, 930:304-310.

3. Falconer IR, Buckley T, Runnegar MT. Biological half-life, organic distribution and excretion of [125]I-labelled toxic peptide from the blue-green algae *Microcystis aeruginosa. Australian journal of biological sciences*, 1986, 39:17-21.

4. Runnegar MT et al. Lethal potency and tissue distribution of [125]I-labelled toxic peptides from the blue-green alga *Microcystis aeruginosa. Toxicon*, 1986, 24:506-509.

5. Runnegar MT, Falconer IR. Effect of toxin from the cyanobacterium *Microcystis aeruginosa* on ultrastructural morphology and actin polymerization in isolated hepatocytes. *Toxicon*, 1986, 24:109-115.

6. Brooks WP, Codd GA. Distribution of *Microcystis aeruginosa* peptide toxin and interactions with hepatic microsomes in mice. *Pharmacology and toxicology*, 1987, 60:187-191.

7. Kiviranta J et al. Mouse oral toxicity of the cyanobacterium *Nodularia spumigena*, and inhibition of hepatotoxicity by hydrocortisone. *Acta pharmaceutica fennica*, 1990, 99:69-76.

8.  Lovell RA et al. Toxicity of intraperitoneal doses of microcystin-LR in two strains of male mice. *Journal of environmental pathology, toxicology and oncology*, 1989, 9:221-237.

9.  Falconer IR et al. Oral toxity of a bloom of the cyanobacterium *Microcystis aeruginosa* administered to mice over periods up to 1 year. *Journal of toxicology and environmental health*, 1988, 24:291-305.

10. Grabow WOK et al. *Microcystis aeruginosa* toxin: cell culture toxicity, haemolysis and mutagenicity assays. *Applied and environmental microbiology*, 1982, 43:1425-1433.

11. Mackintosh C et al. Cyanobacterial microcystin-LR is a potent and specific inhibitor of protein phosphatases 1 and 2A from both mammals and higher plants. *FEBS letters*, 1990, 264:187-192.

12. Hawkins PR et al. Severe hepatotoxicity caused by the tropical cyanobacterium (blue-green alga) *Cylindrospermopsis raciborskii* (Woloszynska) Seenaya and Subba Raju isolated from a domestic water supply reservoir. *Applied and environmental microbiology*, 1985, 50:1292-1295.

13. Falconer IR, Beresford AM, Runnegar MTC. Evidence of liver damage by toxin from a bloom of the blue-green alga, *Microcystis aeruginosa*. *Medical journal of Australia*, 1983, 1:511-514.

14. Codd GA, Bell SC, Brooks WP. Cyanobacterial toxins in water. *Water science and technology*, 1989, 21(3):1-13.

15. Falconer IR et al. Using activated carbon to remove toxicity from drinking water containing cyanobacterial blooms. *Journal of the American Water Works Association*, 1989, 81:102-105.

16. Himberg K et al. The effect of water treatment processes on the removal of hepatotoxins from *Microcystis* and *Oscillatoria* cyanobacteria: a laboratory study. *Water research*, 1989, 23:979-984.

17. Lahti K, Hiisvirta L. Removal of cyanobacterial toxins in water treatment processes: review of studies conducted in Finland. *Water supply*, 1989, 7:149-154.

18. Dahlem AM. *Structure/toxicity relationships and fate of low molecular weight peptide toxins of cyanobacteria*. Department of Veterinary Medical Science, Graduate College, University of Illinois at Urbana-Champaign, 1989 (PhD thesis).

# 8.
# Nuisance organisms

Nuisance organisms constitute a morphologically and physiologically diverse group, including planktonic and benthic cyanobacteria (blue-green algae), actinomycetes, iron, manganese, and sulfur bacteria, crustacea, and protozoa. These organisms cause problems when the conditions in reservoirs or distribution systems are such as to support their growth. Thus organic matter in drinking-water supports the growth of bacteria and fungi, which in turn will help to maintain populations of protozoa and crustacea. Many invertebrate animals can feed on bacteria, fungi, and protozoa. The content of organic compounds in treated water should therefore ideally be so low as to inhibit the growth of bacteria and to prevent that of other organisms during distribution.

## 8.1 Microbiological problems

Although the raw water itself does not usually contain large numbers of nuisance organisms, problems may develop during the water-treatment process. Nuisance organisms become concentrated on the surfaces and inside the beds of filters, where they autolyse and release cellular compounds that cause colour, turbidity, tastes, and odours. Activated carbon filters will, after a while, contain large amounts of organic matter, thus providing an excellent substrate for bacteria, which can create problems in the water supply, either by causing taste, odour, and turbidity, or microbiologically by increasing the colony counts of aerobic heterotrophic bacteria. Significant amounts of organic carbon can cause the growth of *Aeromonas* spp. in the distribution system during the warmer months of the year (see section 3.2.2). Large numbers of aerobic, heterotrophic bacteria in treated water can interfere with the interpretation of the tests for the coliform group by masking their presence or giving false positive reactions. A particular problem exists with some strains of *Aeromonas* spp., which produce acid and gas with coliform media, even at 44 °C.

Most of these nuisance organisms can be controlled relatively easily by care in operating water-treatment processes. Nutrient-rich raw water should be avoided if proper water treatment cannot be applied.

The compounds produced by nuisance organisms have low taste and odour thresholds, e.g. the earthy taints of geosmin (*trans*-1,10-dimethyl-*trans*-9-decadole) and MIB (2-methylisoborneol) produced by actinomycetes and cyanobacteria. These compounds cause problems in drinking-water at threshold values of 10 and 25 ng/litre respectively, and are therefore often the cause of complaints by consumers before they are detected by analytical methods. It is therefore advisable to use panels of trained judges of taste and odour so that the compounds can be detected and the necessary measures taken before they become a problem in the drinking-water supply. Another way to prevent nuisance organisms from causing taste and odour problems is by means of regular microscopic examination of the organisms present in the water. As soon as a group of organisms known to cause these problems becomes dominant, appropriate measures should be taken to deal with them.

Some of these organisms can also produce colour in drinking-water. Pigmented organisms, such as cyanobacteria and algae, can be crushed on filters, resulting in the release of pigments, while microalgae can pass through the filters and cause both coloration and turbidity.

If water contains ferrous or manganous salts, these can be oxidized by iron or manganese bacteria, resulting in rust-coloured or black deposits in storage tanks and on the walls of pipes in parts of the distribution system where the flow rate is low. If the flow rate is subsequently increased, however, these deposits can be loosened and transported to consumers. Rust-coloured deposits can stain laundry. The slurry will also contain organic deposits which can decompose to produce tastes and odours. Manganese-oxidizing microorganisms (bacteria, fungi, and, very rarely, protozoa) produce deposits in aquifers, wells, and water conduits, the problems caused by such deposits including reduced yield, clogging of slots in well pipes, increased turbulence in pipes resulting in reduced flow velocity, damage to equipment for measuring water flow, black-coloured water, stains on laundry, and problems with food-handling establishments. The deposits can contain heavy metals such as arsenic, lead, zinc, and copper. Bacteria can become attached to them, so that, if they are disturbed, the colony count of the water will be increased. Prevention is based on the removal of Mn(II) from raw water, if a value of about 0.1 mg/litre is exceeded.

Iron and sulfur bacteria may contribute to the corrosion of iron and steel well pipes and drinking-water mains. Such microbially mediated corrosion can occur as a consequence of:
- the adsorption of nutrients and the depletion of dissolved oxygen by the colonies of microorganisms that have accumulated at the metal surface;
- the liberation of corrosive metabolites, such as organic acids and other complex-forming compounds;
- the production of sulfuric acid from sulfides or elemental sulfur; and
- the inclusion of sulfate-reducing bacteria in the cathodic process under anaerobic conditions.

The presence of certain organisms in water may be an indication either of the corrosion of cast iron or of the biodeterioration of construction materials to form substances that support the growth of microorganisms. The latter include non-metallic materials, such as plastics, rubber-jointing compounds, and pipe-lining materials, which can provide organic nutrients and thus encourage the growth of microorganisms, sometimes including coliform organisms other than *Escherichia coli* and *Pseudomonas aeruginosa*. Deterioration can occur in pipelines carrying groundwater or surface water. Unchlorinated waters, or water in which the chlorine residual has disappeared, appear to support higher rates of attack than those in which a residual can be detected.

Nuisance organisms may also cause problems in groundwater sources by encrusting well screens, thus reducing yield and impairing the aesthetic quality of the supply. Their presence may also indicate organic pollution of the aquifer.

Routine monitoring of such nuisance organisms cannot be recommended because of their diverse nature and unpredictable occurrence, although bacteriologists should be aware that they can impair water quality. It is not practicable to specify any quantitative guideline values for nuisance microorganisms.

## 8.2 Problems caused by invertebrate animals

Invertebrate animals often infest shallow, open wells, from which supplies are drawn by bucket, but problems are not uncommon in large, public supplies. The animals derive their food from the bacteria, algae, and protozoa in the water or present on slimes on pipe and tank surfaces.

The types of animal concerned can be considered, for control purposes, as belonging to two groups. Firstly, there are free-swimming organisms in the water itself or on water surfaces, such as the crustacea *Gammarus pulex* (freshwater shrimp), *Crangonyx pseudogracilis*, *Cyclops* spp. and *Chydorus sphaericus*. Secondly, there are other animals that either move along surfaces or are anchored to them (such as *Asellus aquaticus* (water louse), snails, *Dreissena polymorpha* (the zebra mussel) and other bivalve molluscs, and the bryozoan *Plumatella* sp.), or inhabit slimes (such as *Nais* spp., nematodes and the larvae of chironomids) (*1*). In warm weather, slow sand filters can sometimes discharge the larvae of gnats (*Chironomus* and *Culex* spp.) into the water, if the top layer of the bed collapses, causing draw-down of unfiltered water.

The only health hazard positively identified arises in tropical countries where water fleas (*Cyclops*) are the intermediate host of the guinea worm (*Dracunculus medinensis*) (see section 6.1).

Penetration of waterworks and mains is more likely to be a problem when low-quality raw waters are abstracted and high-rate filtration processes used. Prechlorination assists in destroying animal life and in its removal by filtration but, if excessive, may produce chlorinated organic compounds and convert total organic carbon into a biodegradable form. Maintenance of chlorine residuals in the distribution system, the production of high-quality water, and the regular cleaning of water mains by flushing or swabbing will usually prevent infestation.

Bryozoan infestation can be treated with a shock dose of chlorine, maintained at 10 mg/litre for about 24 hours, followed by flushing. Permethrin treatment of water at an average dose of 0.01–0.02 mg/litre for 24–48 hours has been used to destroy *Asellus* and other crustacea, but treated water must not be discharged into watercourses, as it is rapidly toxic to fish and other aquatic life at this concentration (*2, 3*). The most effective procedure is to draw treated water into the main by opening hydrants downstream of the injection point. These are then closed, allowing sufficient contact time (ideally 24 hours) to paralyse the crustacea, after which the mains are cleared by flushing and swabbing. Persons using renal dialysis should not be supplied with permethrin-treated water, and those rearing fish should be warned not to replenish the culture tanks with mains water while it is being treated. The treated water can be safely discharged into sewers for treatment at sewage works (*2*).

## References

1. *Standard methods for the examination of water and wastewater*, 17th ed. Washington, DC, American Public Health Association, 1989.

2. Abram FSH et al. *Permethrin for the control of animals in water mains*. Medmenham, Water Research Centre, 1980 (TR 145).

3. Fawell JK. *An assessment of the safety in use of permethrin for disinfection of water mains*. Medmenham, Water Research Centre, 1987 (Report PRU 1412-M/1).

# 9.
# Microbial indicators of water quality

## 9.1 Rationale

The recognition that faecally polluted water is responsible for spreading enteric diseases led to the development of sensitive methods of verifying that drinking-water is free from faecal contamination. Even though many waterborne pathogens can now be detected, the methods are often difficult, relatively expensive, and time-consuming. Furthermore, pathogens are shed into water only from infected people and animals, and it is not possible to examine water for every possible pathogen that might be present. It is prudent to regard as unsafe all water that contains bacteria indicating faecal pollution, because of the risk that enteric pathogens may be present. The bacteria selected as indicators of faecal pollution should be universally present in the faeces of humans and warm-blooded animals in large numbers. Other desirable properties of faecal indicators are that they should be readily detected by simple methods and that they do not grow in natural waters. Furthermore, it is essential that their persistence in water and the extent to which they are removed by water treatment are similar to those of waterborne pathogens.

Examination for faecal indicator bacteria in drinking-water provides a very sensitive method of quality assessment. It is also important to determine the quality of the raw water, not only to assess the degree of pollution but also to enable the best local source to be selected and the best form of treatment chosen. Microbiological examination for faecal indicators is the most sensitive and specific method for detecting recent faecal pollution, i.e. pollution that is potentially dangerous, since simple chemical analysis is not adequate for this purpose. Water must be examined regularly and frequently because pollution is often intermittent and may not be detected if examination is limited to only one or a small number of samples. For this reason it is better to examine drinking-water frequently by means of a simple test rather than less often by several tests or a more complicated test. When personnel and facilities are limited, routine microbiological examination for evidence of faecal contamination must always be given first priority ( 1 ).

Microbiological examinations can also be carried out with other objectives than assessing the degree of faecal contamination. They may give information on the effectiveness with which specific groups of microorganisms have been removed by treatment processes; thus, if bacteriophages are present this may indicate that viruses have not been removed, and the presence of spores of sulfite-reducing clostridia also shows highly persistent microorganisms may have survived. Colony counts of aerobic, heterotrophic bacteria, or microscopic or indirect chemical methods (e.g. the assay of adenosine triphosphate by luminometry) may provide information on the availability of nutrients in the water that support bacterial growth, which may result in aesthetic problems or in the presence of opportunistic pathogens. For some of these latter organisms, specific culture methods are also being used, namely for *Pseudomonas aeruginosa*, *Legionella* and *Aeromonas* (see section 3.2); however, these should not be used routinely, but only when necessary to solve problems related to the occurrence of the organisms concerned.

## 9.2 Indicators of faecal contamination

The use of normal intestinal organisms as indicators of faecal pollution rather than the pathogens themselves is universally accepted for monitoring and assessing the microbial safety of water supplies. In practice, the criteria to be satisfied by an ideal indicator (see section 9.1) cannot all be met by any one organism. However, many of them are best fulfilled by *Escherichia coli*, and to a lesser extent by the thermotolerant coliform bacteria; *E. coli* is thus the indicator of choice when resources for supplementary microbiological examination are limited. Other microorganisms that satisfy some of these criteria, though not to the same extent as *E. coli* and the thermotolerant coliform organisms, can also be used as supplementary indicators of faecal pollution in certain circumstances.

Because enteroviruses and the cysts of some parasites are known to be more resistant than *E. coli* and coliform organisms to disinfection, the absence of these organisms in surface water that has only been disinfected will not necessarily indicate freedom from enteric viruses and the resting stages of *Cryptosporidium*, *Giardia*, amoebae, and other parasites.

The significance that can be attached to the presence or absence of particular faecal indicators varies with each organism and particularly with the degree to which that organism can be specifically associated with faeces. For example, some of the genera detected by the methods for enumeration of thermotolerant and total coliform bacteria have nonfaecal sources in the environment, e.g. in soil or decaying vegetation, or can even grow in the aquatic environment, thus limiting their usefulness as indicators of faecal contamination. Other bacterial indicators have useful properties which enable them to be used for particular purposes. For example, although the faecal streptococci and enterococci and the spores of sulfite-reducing clostridia, typified by *Clostridium perfringens*, are less numerous than coliforms in faecally polluted water, they have greater powers of survival and so may be used to confirm the presence of faecal contamination when *E. coli* is not found or to assess the efficiency of treatment processes. Anaerobic bacteria, such as bifidobacteria and the *Bacteroides fragilis* group, are more abundant than coliform organisms in faeces, but decay rapidly in water, and accepted standard methods for their detection and enumeration are not yet available. Full identification of these indicator organisms would require such an extensive series of tests as to be impracticable in routine monitoring.

## 9.2.1 *Escherichia coli*

*Escherichia coli* is abundant in human and animal faeces, where numbers may attain $10^9$ per gram of fresh faeces. It is found in sewage, treated effluents, and all natural waters and soils subject to recent faecal contamination, whether from humans, farm animals, or wild animals and birds. The presence of *E. coli* in water always indicates potentially dangerous contamination requiring immediate attention. Complete identification of *E. coli* is too complicated for routine use, hence certain tests have been evolved for identifying this organism rapidly with a high degree of certainty. Some of them are the subject of international and national standards and have been accepted for routine use, whereas others are still being developed or evaluated. Detection of *E. coli* on complex media entails incubation at the restrictive temperature of 44–45 °C in combination with demonstration of the production of acid and gas from lactose and of specific biochemical reactions such as indole production and β-glucuronidase activity, and the absence of urease activity. In other tests, chemically defined media with specific substrates for the growth and detection of enzymatic activities of *E. coli*, such as β-galactosidase and β-glucuronidase, are used. Confirmation of the presence of *E. coli*, as indicated by these methods, requires extensive biochemical identification or the use of alternative, commercially available test systems. Such confirmation is not recommended as a routine, but may be necessary to validate the use of routine tests under specific conditions.

## 9.2.2 Thermotolerant (faecal) coliform organisms

These are defined as the group of coliform organisms that are able to ferment lactose at 44–45 °C. They comprise the genus *Escherichia* and, to a lesser extent, species of *Klebsiella*, *Enterobacter*, and *Citrobacter*. Of these organisms, only *E. coli* is specifically of faecal origin, being always present in the faeces of humans, other mammals, and birds in large numbers, and rarely found in water or soil that has not been subject to faecal pollution. Thermotolerant coliforms other than *E. coli* may also originate from organically enriched water such as industrial effluents or from decaying plant materials and soils. In tropical and subtropical waters, thermotolerant coliform bacteria may occur without any obvious relation to human pollution and have been found on vegetation in a tropical rainforest (2). This means that the occurrence of the thermotolerant coliform group in subtropical or tropical waters or those enriched with organic wastes does not necessarily indicate faecal contamination by humans since they can originate from wild animals, including birds. However, their presence in waters in warm climates should not be ignored, as the basic assumption that pathogens may be present and that treatment has been inadequate still holds good.

Regrowth of thermotolerant coliform organisms in the distribution system is unlikely unless sufficient bacterial nutrients are present (biochemical oxygen demand (BOD) greater than 10 mg/litre) or unsuitable materials are in contact with the treated water, the water temperature is above 15 °C, and there is no free chlorine residual.

Thermotolerant coliforms are less reliable indicators of faecal contamination than *E. coli*, although under most circumstances their concentrations are directly related to *E. coli* concentrations in water. Their use for water-quality examination is therefore considered acceptable. Internationally standardized methods and media for their detection have been validated, and are relatively simple and widely available. When necessary, thermotolerant coliform isolates can be subjected to further confirmatory tests to detect those that are presumptive *E. coli*. Normally, a test for the ability to produce indole from tryptophan at 44 ± 0.5 °C is sufficient. The detection and identification of these organisms as faecal organisms or presumptive *E. coli* provide strong evidence of recent faecal contamination and of the need for immediate investigation.

Because thermotolerant coliform bacteria are readily detected by single-step methods, they have an important secondary role as indicators of the efficiency of individual water-treatment processes in removing faecal bacteria. They may therefore be used in assessing the degree of treatment necessary for waters of different quality and for defining performance targets for bacterial removal (see section 11.3).

## 9.2.3 Coliform organisms (total coliforms).

Coliform organisms have long been recognized as a suitable microbial indicator of drinking-water quality, largely because they are easy to detect and enumerate in water. The term "coliform organisms (total coliforms)" refers to Gram-negative, rod-shaped bacteria capable of growth in the presence of bile salts or other surface-active agents with similar growth-inhibiting properties, and able to ferment lactose at 35–37 °C with the production of acid, gas, and aldehyde within 24–48 hours. They are also oxidase-negative and non-spore-forming. These definitions have recently been extended by the development of rapid and direct enzymatic methods for enumerating and confirming members of the coliform group. By definition, coliform bacteria display β-galactosidase activity. Traditionally, coliform bacteria were regarded as belonging to the genera *Escherichia*, *Citrobacter*, *Enterobacter*, and *Klebsiella*. However, the group of coliform bacteria, as defined by modern taxonomical methods, is heterogeneous and includes lactose-fermenting bacteria which can be found in both faeces and the environment, namely in nutrient-rich waters, soil, decaying vegetation and drinking-water containing relatively high levels of nutrients. Examples of such species are *Enterobacter cloacae* and *Citrobacter freundii*.

The coliform group also contains species that are rarely, if ever, found in faeces and which can multiply in relatively good-quality drinking-water, e.g.

*Serratia fonticola*, *Rahnella aquatilis*, and *Buttiauxella agrestis*. Several lactose-fermenting species of *Serratia* and *Yersinia* can be isolated from uncontaminated water or soil. There are also many reports of the existence of non-lactose-fermenting but otherwise characteristic coliform bacteria. Lactose-negative strains which otherwise resemble the traditional coliform genera lack the lactose permease enzyme. They do, however, possess the β-galactosidase enzyme and will appear as coliform bacteria if a β-galactosidase test is applied. The existence of nonfaecal bacteria that fit the definition of coliform bacteria and of lactose-negative coliform bacteria limits the applicability of this group of bacteria as indicators of faecal pollution.

Coliform bacteria should not be detectable in treated water supplies and, if found, suggest inadequate treatment, post-treatment contamination, or excessive nutrients. In this sense, the coliform test can be used to assess treatment efficiency and the integrity of the distribution system. Although coliform organisms may not always be directly related to the presence of faecal contamination or pathogens in drinking-water, the coliform test is still useful for monitoring the microbial quality of public water supplies. If there is any doubt, especially when coliform organisms are found in the absence of faecal coliforms and *E. coli*, secondary indicator organisms may be used to determine whether faecal contamination is present; these include the faecal streptococci and sulfite-reducing clostridia, especially *Clostridium perfringens*.

## 9.2.4 Faecal streptococci

The term "faecal streptococci" refers to those streptococci generally present in the faeces of humans and animals. All possess the Lancefield group D antigen. Taxonomically, they belong to the genera *Enterococcus* and *Streptococcus*. The genus *Enterococcus* has recently been defined to include all streptococci sharing certain biochemical properties and having a wide tolerance of adverse growth conditions. It includes the species *E. avium*, *E. casseliflavus*, *E. cecorum*, *E. durans*, *E. faecalis*, *E. faecium*, *E. gallinarum*, *E. hirae*, *E. malodoratus*, *E. mundtii*, and *E. solitarius*. Most of these species are of faecal origin and can generally be regarded as specific indicators of human faecal pollution under many practical circumstances. They may, however, be isolated from the faeces of animals, whereas certain species and subspecies, such as *E. casseliflavus*, *E. faecalis* var. *liquefaciens*, *E. malodoratus*, and *E. solitarius* occur primarily on plant material. The taxonomy of enterococci has recently undergone important changes, and detailed knowledge of the ecology of many of the new species is lacking.

In the genus *Streptococcus*, only *S. bovis* and *S. equinus* possess the group D antigen and are members of the faecal streptococcus group. They occur mainly in animal faeces. Conventional media for the isolation and identification of faecal streptococci, such as m-enterococcus agar, KF-streptococcus agar, and azide-glucose broth, generally support the growth of all faecal streptococci. However, particularly in warm climates, other cocci may also develop on these media, so

86

that confirmatory tests are needed. More restrictive media that support the growth of the enterococci in particular have also been proposed and have been widely used in the USA (*3*). The applicability and specificity of these media need to be further tested under a wide range of conditions. Faecal streptococci rarely multiply in polluted water and are more persistent than *E. coli* and coliform bacteria. Their main value in assessing water quality is therefore as an additional indicator of treatment efficiency. Furthermore, streptococci are highly resistant to drying and may be valuable for purposes of routine control after new mains have been laid or distribution systems repaired, or for detecting pollution by surface run-off to groundwater or surface waters.

## 9.2.5 Sulfite-reducing clostridia

These are anaerobic, spore-forming organisms, of which the most characteristic, *Clostridium perfringens* (*C. welchii*), is normally present in faeces, though in much smaller numbers than *E. coli*. However, they are not exclusively of faecal origin and can be derived from other environmental sources. Clostridial spores can survive in water much longer than organisms of the coliform group and will resist disinfection. Their presence in disinfected waters may thus indicate deficiencies in treatment (*4*). In particular, the presence of *C. perfringens* in filtered supplies may be a sign of deficiencies in filtration practice, while *C. perfringens* spores may indicate the presence of protozoan cysts; because of their longevity, they are best regarded as indicating intermittent or remote contamination and thus are of special value. However, they are not recommended for the routine monitoring of distribution systems. Because they tend to survive and accumulate, they may be detected long after pollution has occurred and far from the source, and thus give rise to false alarms.

## 9.2.6 Bacteriophages

Bacteriophages are viruses that infect bacterial host cells. They usually consist of a nucleic acid molecule (genome) surrounded by a protein coat (capsid). Bacteriophages may contain either deoxyribonucleic acid (DNA) or ribonucleic acid (RNA) as the genome and may have a very simple, cubic structure or a more complex one with heads, tails, tail fibres, or other attachments. They are in the size range 25–100 nm. Bacteriophages have been proposed as indicators of water quality, particularly with respect to human enteric viruses, both because of their similar nature and because they are relatively easy to detect in water samples (*5*). Furthermore, data are accumulating showing the similarities between certain groups of bacteriophages and human enteric viruses in terms of survival in the aquatic environment and responses to water- and wastewater-treatment processes. Two groups of bacteriophages have been studied extensively in the context of viral indicators in water, namely the somatic coliphages, which infect standard *E. coli* host strains via cell wall (somatic) receptors, and the F-specific RNA bacteriophages which infect *E. coli* and related bacteria through the F- or sex-pili. Neither of these groups of organisms occurs in high concentration in faeces, but they are invariably found in sewage. They are used, therefore, primarily as an index of sewage contamination and, because of their high persistence as compared with bacterial indicators, as an additional indicator of treatment efficiency or groundwater protection.

### 9.2.7 Miscellaneous indicators

The bifidobacteria and the *Bacteroides fragilis* group are anaerobes which are specific to faeces, where they outnumber the coliform group. They do not survive or multiply in natural waters, and have been seen as an alternative to the coliform group in tropical and semitropical regions, where the latter can multiply in warm and organically enriched water (6). However, their numbers decline more rapidly then those of thermotolerant coliforms and *E. coli* in passing from faeces through sewage and into polluted waters, indicating that their rate of decay is greater than that of other bacterial indicators (6). This is a disadvantage, since bacteria in the coliform group are themselves more sensitive to decay than viral and protozoal pathogens. In addition, the methods of detecting them in water are not very reliable and have not been standardized.

## 9.3 Indicators of water quality and treatment efficacy

### 9.3.1 Heterotrophic plate counts (colony counts)

Heterotrophic plate counts may be used to assess the general bacterial content of water. They do not represent all the bacteria present in the water but only those able to grow and produce visible colonies on the media used and under the prescribed conditions of temperature and time of incubation. Colony counts are often determined following incubation at 22 °C and 37 °C to assess the relative proportions of naturally occurring water bacteria unrelated to faecal pollution and of bacteria derived from humans and warm-blooded animals, respectively. The count at 22 °C is of little sanitary value, but is useful in assessing the efficiency of water treatment, specifically the processes of coagulation, filtration, and disinfection, where the objective is to keep counts as low as possible. The 22 °C count may also be used to assess the cleanliness and integrity of the distribution system and the suitability of the water for use in the manufacture of food and drink, where high counts may lead to spoilage. Any increase in counts in the test at 37 °C as compared with those normally found may be an early sign of pollution.

### 9.3.2 *Aeromonas* spp. and *Pseudomonas aeruginosa*

Apart from heterotrophic plate counts, the use of other microorganisms, including *Aeromonas* and *Pseudomonas aeruginosa*, has been advocated as a means of assessing the hygienic quality of drinking-water (7, 8). However, neither examination for these organisms nor heterotrophic plate counts are essential for the routine monitoring of hygienic quality. They are of value in certain circumstances in giving an indication of the general cleanliness of the distribution system and in assessing the quality of bottled water. However, high heterotrophic plate counts and counts of these bacteria may interfere with the detection of *E. coli*, coliforms, and other bacterial indicators of faecal pollution.

## 9.4 Methods

### 9.4.1 Standard methods

Microbiological examination provides the most sensitive, although not the most rapid, indication of the pollution of drinking-water supplies. Because the growth medium and the conditions of incubation, as well as the nature and age of the water sample, can influence the species isolated and the count, the accuracy of microbiological examinations may vary. This means that the standardization of methods and of laboratory procedures is of great importance if uniform criteria for the microbiological quality of water are to be used in different laboratories and countries. International standard methods should be evaluated in local circumstances before being adopted in national surveillance programmes. Information is given here on established standard methods, particularly those of the International Organization for Standardization (ISO), Geneva (Table 9.1), to encourage their use. There are also other well established national standards, such as those of the American Public Health Association (APHA) (3) and of the United Kingdom (9). Established standard methods should be used for routine examinations.

Whatever method is chosen for the detection of *E. coli* and the coliform group, some means of "resuscitating" or recovering environmentally or disinfectant-damaged strains must be used, such as preincubation for a short time at a lower temperature (3, 9)

### 9.4.2 Methods for pathogenic bacteria, protozoa, and cytopathic enteroviruses

Although the direct search for specific pathogenic bacteria has no place in the routine microbiological examination of water, there are occasions when examination for intestinal pathogens may be necessary as, for example, during an epidemic, when pollution is suspected, or in the evaluation of a new source. The chances of detecting pathogens will be greater if large samples of water are examined, and if media selective for certain intestinal pathogens are used. Examination for bacterial pathogens will include some, if not all, of the following steps: concentration of the organisms in the sample, inoculation into enrichment broth, subculture onto selective agar media, and biochemical and serological

### Table 9.1 ISO standards for water quality

| Standard no. | Title |
|---|---|
| 5667-1:1980 | Sampling — Part 1: Guidance on the design of sampling programmes |
| 5667-2:1982 | Sampling — Part 2: Guidance on sampling techniques |
| 5667-3:1985 | Sampling — Part 3: Guidance on the preservation and handling of samples |
| 5667-4:1987 | Sampling — Part 4: Guidance on sampling from lakes, natural and man-made |
| 5667-5:1991 | Sampling — Part 5: Guidance on sampling of drinking-water and water used for food and beverage processing |
| 5667-6:1990 | Sampling — Part 6: Guidance on sampling of rivers and streams |
| 6222:1988 | Enumeration of viable micro-organisms—colony count by inoculation in or on a nutrient agar culture medium |
| 6461-1:1986 | Detection and enumeration of the spores of sulfite-reducing anaerobes (clostridia) — Part 1: Method by enrichment in a liquid medium |
| 6461-2:1986 | Detection and enumeration of the spores of sulfite-reducing anaerobes (clostridia) — Part 2: Method by membrane filtration |
| 7704:1985 | Evaluation of membrane filters used for microbiological analyses |
| 7899-1:1984 | Detection and enumeration of faecal streptococci — Part 1: Method by enrichment in a liquid medium |
| 7899-2:1984 | Detection and enumeration of faecal streptococci — Part 2: Method by membrane filtration |
| 8199:1988 | General guide to the enumeration of micro-organisms by culture |
| 8360-1:1988 | Detection and enumeration of *Pseudomonas aeruginosa* — Part 1: Method by enrichment in liquid medium |
| 8360-2:1988 | Detection and enumeration of *Pseudomonas aeruginosa* — Part 2: Membrane filtration method |
| 9308-1:1990 | Detection and enumeration of coliform organisms, thermotolerant coliform organisms and presumptive *Escherichia coli* — Part 1: Membrane filtration method |
| 9308-2:1990 | Detection and enumeration of coliform organisms, thermotolerant coliform organisms and presumptive *Escherichia coli* — Part 2: Multiple tube (most probable number) method |
| 6579:1990 | General guidance on methods for the detection of *Salmonella* |

examination of suspect colonies. Rather than rely on a single method, it is better to use as many methods as possible so that no opportunity to detect a pathogen is missed (*3, 9*). This is especially true for the detection of *Salmonella*, since no single method is suitable for all serotypes.

Isolation methods are available for *Salmonella* spp. (*3, 9*), *Shigella* spp. (*10*), *Vibrio cholerae* (*11*), *Yersinia enterocolitica* (*12*), *Campylobacter* spp. (*13–15*), *Legionella* spp. (*16, 17*), *P. aeruginosa* (*3, 9*), *Aeromonas* spp. (*18*), *Giardia* spp. (*19–22*), *Cryptosporidium* spp. (*21–23*), and *Naegleria* spp. (*24*).

Standard methods are now available for concentrating and recovering cytopatic enteroviruses from large volumes of water (i.e. in the range 10–1000 litres) (*3, 25–27*). A method for enumerating male-specific bacteriophages in water has been described (*28*), and some of the factors influencing their recovery have been reviewed (*5*).

# References

1. *Surveillance of drinking-water quality.* Geneva, World Health Organization, 1976 (WHO Monograph Series No. 63).

2. Rivera SC et al. Isolation of faecal coliforms from pristine sites in a tropical rain forest. *Applied and environmental microbiology,* 1988, 54:513-517.

3. *Standard methods for the examination of water and wastewater,* 17th ed. Washington, DC, American Public Health Association, 1989.

4. Kool HJ. Treatment processes applied in public water supply for the removal of microorganisms. In: James A, Evison L, eds. *Biological indicators of water quality.* Chichester, John Wiley & Sons, 1979:17.1-17.31.

5. Havelaar AH et al. Bacteriophages as model viruses in water quality control. IAWPRC Study Group on Health-related Water Microbiology. *Water research,* 1991, 25: 529-549.

6. Allsop K, Stickler DJ. An assessment of *Bacteroides fragilis* group organisms as indicators of human faecal pollution. *Journal of applied bacteriology,* 1985, 58: 95-99.

7. Feachem RG et al. *Sanitation and disease. Health aspects of excreta and wastewater management.* Baltimore, Johns Hopkins University Press, 1981 (World Bank Studies in Water Supply and Sanitation No. 3).

8. Geldreich EE. Current status of microbiological water quality criteria. *American Society for Microbiology news,* 1981, 47:23-27.

9. Department of Health and Social Security. *The bacteriological examination of drinking-water supplies 1982.* London, Her Majesty's Stationery Office, 1983 (Reports on Public Health and Medical Subjects No. 71)

10. Park CE et al. Improved procedure of selective enrichment of *Shigella* in the presence of *Escherichia coli* by use of 4-chloro-2-cyclopentylphenyl beta-D-galactopyranoside. *Canadian journal of microbiology,* 1977, 23:563-566.

11. *Guidelines for cholera control.* Geneva, World Health Organization, 1993.

12. Highsmith AK et al. Isolation of *Yersinia enterocolitica* from well water and growth in distilled water. *Applied and environmental microbiology,* 1977, 34:745-750.

13. Bolton FJ, Robertson L. A selective medium for isolating *Campylobacter jejuni/coli. Journal of clinical pathology,* 1982, 35:462-467.

14. Bolton FJ et al. A most probable number method for estimating small numbers of campylobacter in water. *Journal of hygiene (London),* 1982, 89:185-190.

15. Stelzer W. Untersuchungen zum Nachweis von *Campylobacter jejuni* und *C. coli* in Abwasser. [Detection of *Campylobacter jejuni* and *C. coli* in wastewater] *Zentralblatt für Mikrobiologie*, 1988, 143:47-54.

16. Colbourne JS, Trew RM. Presence of *Legionella* in London's water supplies. *Israel journal of medical sciences*, 1986, 22:633-639.

17. Dennis PJL. Isolation of legionellae from environmental specimens. In: Harrison TG, Taylor AG, eds. *A laboratory manual for Legionella*. Chichester, John Wiley & Sons, 1988:31-44.

18. Havelaar AG, During M, Versteeg JF. Ampicillin-dextrin agar medium for the enumeration of *Aeromonas* species in water by membrane filtration. *Journal of applied bacteriology*, 1987, 62:279-287.

19. Jakubowski W, Ericksen TH. Methods for detection of Giardia cysts in water supplies. In: Jakubowski W, Hoff JC, eds. *Waterborne transmission of giardiasis*. Cincinnati, OH, US Environmental Protection Agency, 1979:193-210 (EPA-600/9-79-001).

20. Sauch JF. Use of immunofluorescence and phase-contrast microscopy for detection and identification of *Giardia* cysts in water samples. *Applied and environmental microbiology*, 1985, 50:1434-1438.

21. Department of the Environment: Standing Committee of Analysts. *Isolation and identification of Giardia cysts, Cryptosporidium oocysts and free-living pathogenic amoebae in water*. London, Her Majesty's Stationery Office, 1990.

22. Lechevallier MW et al. Comparison of the zinc sulfate and immunofluorescence techniques for detecting *Giardia* and *Cryptosporidium*. *Journal of the American Water Works Association*, 1990, 82(9):75-82.

23. Ongerth JE, Stibbs HH. Identification of *Cryptosporidium* oocysts in river water. *Applied and environmental microbiology*, 1987, 53:672-676.

24. Wellings FM et al. Isolation and identification of pathogenic *Naegleria* from Florida lakes. *Applied and environmental microbiology*, 1977, 34:661-667.

25. Berg G et al. *USEPA manual of methods for virology*. Cincinnati, OH, US Environmental Protection Agency, 1984 (EPA-600/4-84-013).

26. Rao VC, Melnick JL. *Environmental virology*. Wokingham, Van Nostrand Reinhold (UK), 1986.

27. Hurst CJ et al. Detecting viruses in water. *Journal of the American Water Works Association*, 1989, 81(9):71-80.

28. Havelaar AH, Hogeboom WM. A method for the enumeration of male-specific bacteriophages in sewage. *Journal of applied bacteriology*, 1984, 56:439-447.

# 10.
# Microbiological criteria

## 10.1 Rationale

### 10.1.1 Overall strategy

A supply of drinking-water should be sufficient in quantity, wholesome, and not injurious to health. These requirements are all inter-related. The history of water-supply engineering has repeatedly shown that the provision of safe drinking-water is the most important step which can be taken to improve the health of a community by preventing the spread of waterborne disease.

Microbiological monitoring provides a sensitive indication of the extent to which source protection, treatment, and distribution are effective barriers to the transmission of infectious agents of waterborne disease at the time that the samples were taken. It is important to realize at the outset that microbiological integrity is provided by source protection and treatment, and that sudden loss of this integrity or steady deterioration may be missed if monitoring is not frequent enough. Proper design of sampling schemes is important.

The task of monitoring is properly that of the water-supply agency whereas surveillance—keeping public health and the safety and acceptability of water supplies under continuous review—is the duty of the local and national health authorities. Good communications between bodies responsible for monitoring and surveillance are essential. The user has an important role in preserving the quality of the water delivered to the premises through the proper design, construction, and maintenance of storage tanks, taps, and associated plumbing so as to prevent deterioration.

### 10.1.2 Treatment objectives and microbiological criteria

It is difficult with the epidemiological knowledge currently available to assess the risk to health presented by any particular level of pathogens in water, since this will depend equally on the infectivity and invasiveness of the pathogen and on the innate and acquired immunity of the individuals consuming the water. It is only prudent to assume, therefore, that no water in which pathogenic micro-organisms can be detected can be regarded as safe, however low the concentration.

Furthermore, only certain waterborne pathogens can be detected reliably and easily in water, and some cannot be detected at all. This has led over many years to the adoption of the concept of faecal indicator species (see section 9.2) and to universal agreement that the most specific and suitable bacteriological indicator of faecal pollution is *Escherichia coli*. Any water that contains *E. coli* must be regarded as faecally contaminated and unsafe, and requiring immediate remedial action.

Only strict attention to source protection and to the design and operation of efficient treatment and distribution will guarantee the exclusion of pathogens from drinking-water delivered to the consumer. For each water supply, the quality of the source water must guide the selection of the treatment processes, and due attention must be given to the ability of these processes to eliminate different pathogens (see Chapter 11). The microbiogical water criteria presented here provide the means for demonstrating that these measures have been satisfactory at the time of sampling. The selection and design of water-treatment processes capable of achieving the necessary reductions in faecal and pathogenic agents will ensure that, if properly operated, these systems will always be able to produce water of the desired quality. This strategy is the only one that can be adopted in the case of pathogens, such as *Giardia, Cryptosporidium,* and viruses, that are more resistant than *E. coli* to terminal disinfection.

## 10.1.3 Water supplies for small remote communities

The provision of water supplies to small remote communities encounters particular problems worldwide, in that location, available facilities, and financial constraints often mean that only untreated water can be supplied, treatment is limited in extent because only local resources are available, or monitoring is infrequent or impossible. In such circumstances, sanitary assessment of the supply is all-important, and it is recommended that such assessments should be carried out periodically and at least yearly. In addition, the guideline values recommended here should be regarded as a goal for the future, not an immediate requirement. The guideline values recommended for the elimination of hazards may be very difficult to achieve under some conditions, and must then be applied, together with adequate methods of excreta disposal, in an appropriate manner depending on those conditions and on the availability of resources. Unless other sources of risk are adequately controlled, the effect of providing pure water on the transmission of diarrhoeal diseases may not be achieved.

The particular problems of supplies for small remote communities and their management are the subject of Volume 3 of *Guidelines for drinking-water quality.*

## 10.2 Bacteriological quality

Guideline values for bacteriological quality are summarized in Table 10.1, but they should not be used uncritically without reference to the information given in the text. It is most important that the reasons for adopting them are properly understood.

## Table 10.1 Bacteriological quality of drinking-water [a]

| Organisms | Guideline value |
|---|---|
| **All water intended for drinking** | |
| *E. coli* or thermotolerant coliform bacteria [b, c] | Must not be detectable in any 100-ml sample |
| **Treated water entering the distribution system** | |
| *E.coli* or thermotolerant coliform bacteria [b] | Must not be detectable in any 100-ml sample |
| Total coliform bacteria | Must not be detectable in any 100-ml sample |
| **Treated water in the distribution system** | |
| *E. coli* or thermotolerant coliform bacteria [b] | Must not be detectable in any 100-ml sample |
| Total coliform bacteria | Must not be detectable in any 100-ml sample. In the case of large supplies, where sufficient samples are examined, must not be present in 95% of samples taken throughout any 12-month period. |

[a] Immediate investigative action must be taken if either *E. coli* or total coliform bacteria are detected. The minimum action in the case of total coliform bacteria is repeat sampling; if these bacteria are detected in the repeat sample, the cause must be determined by immediate further investigation.

[b] Although *E. coli* is the more precise indicator of faecal pollution, the count of thermotolerant coliform bacteria is an acceptable alternative. If necessary, proper confirmatory tests must be carried out. Total coliform bacteria are not acceptable indicators of the sanitary quality of rural water supplies, particularly in tropical areas where many bacteria of no sanitary significance occur in almost all untreated supplies.

[c] It is recognized that, in the great majority of rural water supplies in developing countries, faecal contamination is widespread. Under these conditions, the national surveillance agency should set medium-term targets for the progressive improvement of water supplies, as recommended in Volume 3 of *Guidelines for drinking-water quality*.

It is self-evident and unquestionable that water intended for drinking must not contain agents of waterborne disease. However, many pathogens, including bacteria, viruses, and parasites, are difficult or even impossible to detect. For this reason, as already explained in Chapter 9, microbial indicators of water quality, i.e. bacteria indicating either the potential for faecal pollution or that such pollution has occurred, are used, since their presence shows that pathogens could also be present. The most numerous of the faecal indicator bacteria is the coliform group, and the most suitable member of this group is *Escherichia coli*, since it alone is derived exclusively from the faeces of humans and warm-blooded animals. In practice, thermotolerant coliform organisms or *E. coli* should not be detectable in any 100-ml sample of any water intended for drinking.

A further reason for adopting this criterion is that it is readily achievable by water treatment. Efficient treatment, together with terminal disinfection, should yield water free from coliform organisms, no matter how polluted the original water may have been. Furthermore, in nearly all epidemics of waterborne disease, it can be shown that the bacteriological quality of the water was unsatisfactory and that there was evidence of contamination or a failure of terminal disinfection (*1*, *2*).

In practice, the fact that *E. coli* can be found in wild and domestic animals and birds is not important because they can also carry pathogens infectious for humans.

During the passage of water from the treatment works to the consumer, its bacteriological quality may deteriorate. Members of the coliform group may be present in inadequately treated supplies or those contaminated after leaving the treatment plant, as a result either of growth on unsuitable materials in contact with the water (those used for washers, packing materials, lubricants, plastics and plasticizers, for example) or of entry from soil or natural water through leaky valves and glands, repaired mains, or back-siphonage. This type of post-contamination will most probably be found when the water is untreated or undisinfected, or where there is limited or no residual disinfectant. The occasional occurrence of coliform organisms in water in the distribution system or untreated supplies in up to 5% of samples taken over any 12-month period, in the absence of *E. coli*, can be regarded as acceptable. It should be stressed that the regular occurrence of these organisms, as opposed to their occasional and sporadic detection, in such samples must be a cause of concern.

Bottled natural mineral waters constitute a special case; their quality is the subject of Codex Alimentarius standards. The water must be collected and bottled under conditions such that it will retain its original quality. When such water is marketed, the Codex standard specifies that it shall not contain *E. coli*, coliform bacteria, group D streptococci, or *Pseudomonas aeruginosa* in 250-ml samples, provision being made for re-examination if not more than two coliforms (but not *E. coli*) or group D streptococci are found in 250 ml (*3*).

## 10.3 Virological quality

### 10.3.1 Rationale

It is essential that drinking-water supplies should be essentially free of human enteric viruses so that the risk of transmission of waterborne viral disease is negligible. It must be assumed that any drinking-water supply subject to faecal contamination exposes consumers to the risk of viral disease. There are thus two approaches to preventing viral contamination of drinking-water, namely: (i) providing drinking-water from a source that is free of faecal contamination; and (ii) producing drinking-water from a faecally contaminated source by treating it in a manner capable of reducing enteric viruses to a negligible level.

Although methods of concentrating and detecting low levels of viruses in water are available, they are too complex, expensive, and time-consuming for routine monitoring. Furthermore, not all relevant viruses can be detected by the methods currently available. As a result, failure to detect viruses in even very large volumes of water does not prove that the water is virus-free and that consumers are not at risk of viral disease. In fact, a recent epidemiological–virological study indicated that drinking-water produced by conventional treatment from a faecally contaminated surface source might have been responsible for 25% of all gastrointestinal illness of probable viral etiology, even though the treated water was of acceptable microbiological quality (4).

Progress has recently been made in modelling, assessing, and predicting the risks of waterborne disease associated with drinking-water containing different concentrations of viruses and protozoan cysts (5). Although this has provided estimates of the health risks linked to the consumption of contaminated drinking-water, the modelling and risk analyses are based on limited dose–response data and require further refinement and verification; they are therefore not sufficiently developed to provide quantitative criteria for virus concentrations in drinking-water. Even if such health risk assessments for waterborne viruses were possible, the inability to monitor viruses in drinking-water reliably would preclude their practical application.

In the light of the foregoing, the guidelines for viruses in drinking-water presented in Table 10.2 are based on the probable virological quality of the source water and the required degree of treatment for source waters containing different levels of faecal contamination and hence different levels of viruses. The aim of these source-protection and water-treatment guidelines is to ensure that no viruses are present even in very large volumes of drinking-water.

## 10.3.2 Guidelines for groundwaters

If groundwater is obtained from a protected source and found to be free of faecal contamination, it can be assumed that the water is of acceptable virological quality for drinking if other essential criteria are met. The water source and its delivery system (casing, pump, pipes, and other appurtenances) must be free of faecal contamination from either surface (e.g. waste infiltration) or subsurface (e.g. septic tanks) sources. Specifically, the water must meet the guideline criteria for turbidity and pH (Table 10.2), bacteriological quality (Table 10.1), and parasitological quality (section 10.4)

Groundwater obtained from a protected source showing evidence of faecal contamination (1–20 E. coli per 100 ml) or exposed indirectly to obvious surface or subsurface sources of faecal contamination (e.g. wastewater infiltration of septic tanks) must be adequately disinfected to reduce enteric viruses to negligible levels. Adequate disinfection is defined (see Table 10.2) as the application of chlorine to achieve a free residual of at least 0.5 mg/litre after a minimum contact time of 30 minutes in water having a median turbidity not exceeding 1 NTU and a pH of <8.0, or an equivalent disinfection process in tems of virus inactivation. All such disinfection processes must produce at least 99.99% reduction of enteric viruses.

Groundwater sources and their delivery systems not adequately protected from either surface or subsurface faecal contamination, such as shallow dug wells

**Table 10.2 Recommended treatments for different water sources to produce water with negligible virus risk[a]**

| Type of source | Recommended treatment |
| --- | --- |
| **Ground water** | |
| Protected, deep wells; essentially free of faecal contamination | Disinfection[b] |
| Unprotected, shallow wells; faecally contaminated | Filtration and disinfection |
| **Surface water** | |
| Protected, impounded upland water; essentially free of faecal contamination | Disinfection |
| Unprotected impounded water or upland river; faecal contamination | Filtration and disinfection |
| Unprotected lowland rivers; faecal contamination | Pre-disinfection or storage, filtration, disinfection |
| Unprotected watershed; heavy faecal contamination | Pre-disinfection or storage, filtration, additional treatment and disinfection |
| Unprotected watershed; gross faecal contamination | Not recommended for drinking-water supply |

[a] For all sources, the median value of turbidity before terminal disinfection must not exceed 1 nephelometric turbidity unit (NTU) and must not exceed 5 NTU in single samples.

Terminal disinfection must produce a residual concentration of free chlorine of $\geq 0.5$ mg/litre after at least 30 minutes of contact in water at pH<8.0, or must be shown to be an equivalent disinfection process in terms of the degree of enterovirus inactivation (>99.99%).

Filtration must be either slow sand filtration or rapid filtration (sand, dual, or mixed media) preceded by adequate coagulation-flocculation (with sedimentation or flotation). Diatomaceous earth filtration or a filtration process demonstrated to be equivalent for virus reduction can also be used. The degree of virus reduction must be >90%.

Additional treatment may consist of slow sand filtration, ozonation with granular activated carbon absorption, or any other process demonstrated to achieve >99% enterovirus reduction.

[b] Disinfection should be used if monitoring has shown the presence of *E. coli* or thermotolerant coliform bacteria.

or other unsealed or uncased wells, may be used as drinking-water sources if their *E. coli* count does not exceed 2000 per 100 ml and the water is treated by filtration and disinfection. Unprotected groundwaters containing more than 2000 *E. coli* per 100 ml are considered grossly faecally contaminated and are not recommended as water-supply sources regardless of treatment, unless no higher-quality water sources are available. In this situation, the water must be treated by at least three unit processes each of which is individually capable of reducing viruses, as prescribed for contaminated surface water (see Table 10.2).

## 10.3.3 Guidelines for surface water sources

In general, surface waters are never completely pure and will always be subject to some degree of faecal contamination, so that treatment to reduce viruses to negligible levels will always be required. The quality of the source water in terms of the degree of faecal contamination (as defined by *E. coli* counts in the raw source water) will determine the degree of treatment required (see Table 10.2).

For source waters derived from protected watersheds essentially free of human faecal contamination, possibly subject only to low levels of faecal contamination from indigenous animals, and containing fewer than 20 *E. coli* per 100 ml, the required degree of treatment is adequate disinfection. However, it is essential that the source water should have a median turbidity not exceeding 1 NTU and a maximum turbidity not exceeding 5 NTU in single samples in order to ensure adequate virus inactivation by disinfection. Surface water sources that meet these virological criteria may nevertheless be contaminated with unacceptable levels of *Giardia* cysts and *Cryptosporidium* oocysts, neither of which can be adequately controlled by disinfection treatment to control viruses. If there is a risk of protozoal contamination, the source water may have to be treated by means of strictly controlled coagulation and filtration to ensure that these agents are removed. Where necessary, special investigations can be conducted to determine whether source water contamination by protozoan cysts or oocysts is probable or demonstrable.

Surface waters from inadequately protected watersheds contaminated by both human and animal faeces and containing 20–2000 *E. coli* per 100 ml must be treated by both filtration and disinfection in order to reduce enteric viruses to negligible levels. Because such waters are likely to contain protozoal cysts or oocysts as well as enteric viruses, filtration and disinfection must be adequate to control both of these classes of pathogens.

Surface waters from inadequately protected watersheds heavily contaminated by human and animal faeces and having *E. coli* counts of over 2000 per 100 ml but not more than 20 000 per 100 ml, will require extensive treatment consisting of filtration, disinfection, and at least one other process (e.g. long-term storage or an additional filtration or disinfection process) capable of producing additional reduction of viruses of >99%. Such surface waters are clearly inferior as sources of drinking-water and should be used only when no other source of higher quality is available. If such a source is used, the local authorities will have to bear the considerable burden of ensuring that the treatment is properly designed, operated, and maintained and that there is adequate monitoring and surveillance of the water system and its water quality to ensure a continuous supply of acceptable virological quality.

Surface waters from inadequately protected sources containing more than 20 000 *E. coli* per 100 ml are considered to be grossly faecally contaminated and hence unsuitable for drinking-water supply regardless of the extent and type of treatment. Production of drinking-water from such a source carries a great risk of inadequate virological quality and would be undertaken only under the most extraordinary circumstances.

## 10.4 Parasitological quality

It is not possible to set guideline values for pathogenic protozoa, helminths, and free-living organisms, other than that these agents should not be present in drinking-water, because only one or very few organisms are required for humans to become infected. The analytical methods for protozoan pathogens are expensive and time-consuming and cannot be recommended for routine use. Methods for concentrating the resting stages of *Giardia* and *Cryptosporidium* from large volumes of water are being standardized. When facilities are available for studying the incidence of these parasites in surface water, these methods could be used for measuring the efficiency of different water-treatment processes in removing them and the incidence of carriage of these parasites by animal vectors in the watershed. A better understanding of information on the epidemiology and zoonotic relationships of these parasites from the point of view of human health will then be possible.

The control of parasitic disease and of invertebrate animal life in water mains is best accomplished by means of appropriate treatment.

## 10.5 Monitoring

### 10.5.1 Approaches and strategies

The monitoring of drinking-water quality ideally consists of the following components:
- the control of quality on a routine basis to verify that treatment and distribution comply with the prescribed objectives and regulations;
- the surveillance, usually at specified intervals, of the entire water-supply system from source to consumer from the point of view of microbiological safety.

Continuous control is an integral part of the responsibilities of the water-supply agency, through which the waterworks management ensures the satisfactory performance of the treatment processes, the quality of the water produced and the absence of secondary contamination within the distribution network. In principle, an independent body should verify that the waterworks correctly performs its duties. This surveillance is usually the responsibility of the local, regional and national health authorities.

### 10.5.2 Sampling frequencies and procedures

The frequency of sampling will be determined by the resources available. The more frequently the water is examined, the more likely it is that chance contamination will be detected. Two main points should be noted. Firstly, the chance of detecting pollution which occurs periodically, rather than randomly, is increased if samples are taken at different times of the day and on different days of the week. Secondly, frequent examination by a simple method is more valuable than frequent examination by a complex test or series of tests. Sampling frequencies for raw water sources will depend on their overall quality, their size, the likelihood of contamination, and the season of the year. They should be established by local control agencies and are often specified in national regulations and guidelines. The results, together with information from the sanitary inspection of the gathering grounds, will often indicate whether increased vigilance is needed.

Sampling frequencies for treated water leaving the waterworks depend on the quality of the water source and the type of treatment. Minimum frequencies are one sample every 2 weeks for waterworks with a groundwater source, and one sample every week for waterworks with a surface water source.

The frequency of sampling should be greater where a large number of people are supplied because of the larger number of people at risk. Advice on the design of sampling programmes and on the frequency of sampling is given in ISO standards (see Table 9.1) and in many national regulations. The minimum number of samples to be taken each month for water in the distribution system is given for different population sizes in Table 10.3.

**Table 10.3 Minimum sampling frequencies for drinking-water in the distribution system**

| Population served | Samples to be taken monthly |
| --- | --- |
| Less than 5000 | 1 sample |
| 5000–100 000 | 1 sample per 5000 population |
| More than 100 000 | 1 sample per 10 000 population, plus 10 additional samples |

Samples should be taken at random intervals in each month from fixed points, such as pumping stations and tanks, from random locations throughout the distribution system and from taps connected directly to the mains in houses and large multioccupancy buildings, where there is a greater risk of contamination through cross-connections and back-siphonage. The frequency of sampling should be increased at times of epidemics, flooding, and emergency operations, or following interruptions of supply or repair work. With systems serving small communities, periodic sanitary surveys are likely to yield more information than infrequent sampling.

No general recommendation can be made for unpiped supplies and untreated water because the quality and likelihood of contamination will vary seasonally and with local conditions. The frequency should be established by the local control agency and reflect local conditions, including the results of sanitary surveys.

Detailed advice on the procedures to be used for sampling different sources of water or treatment plants and distribution systems and at the tap are given in Volume 3 of *Guidelines for drinking-water quality* and in standard methods (6, 7) (see Table 9.1). However, the following general points should be noted.

Care must be taken to ensure that samples are representative of the water to be examined and that no accidental contamination occurs during sampling. Sample collectors should therefore be trained and made aware of the responsible nature of their work. Samples should be clearly labelled with the site, date, time and other relevant information, and sent to the laboratory for analysis without delay.

If the water to be examined is likely to contain chlorine, chloramine, chlorine dioxide, or ozone, sodium thiosulfate should be added to neutralize any residual disinfectant. Properly controlled, the concentration of thiosulfate has no significant effect on the coliform organisms, including *E. coli*, either in chlorinated or in unchlorinated water samples during storage (6). If heavy metals, particularly copper, are present, chelating agents (e.g. edetic acid (EDTA) or nitrilotriacetic acid (NTA)) should also be added.

When samples of disinfected water are taken, the concentration of residual disinfectant at the sampling point and the pH should be determined at the time of collection.

When a number of samples are to be taken for various purposes from the same location, the sample for bacteriological examination should be collected first to avoid the risk of contamination of the sampling point.

Samples must be taken from different parts of the distribution system to ensure that all parts of it are tested. When streams, lakes, or cisterns are being sampled, the water must be taken from below the surface, away from banks, sides of tanks, and stagnant zones, and without stirring up sediments. Taps, sampling ports, and the orifices of pumps should, if possible, be disinfected and a quantity of water run to waste to flush out the stagnant water in the pipe before the sample is taken. Sampling ports in treatment processes and on water mains must be carefully sited to ensure that samples are representative. The length of pipework to the tap should be as short as possible.

The changes that may occur in the bacterial content of water on storage can be reduced to a minimum by ensuring that samples are not exposed to light and are kept cool, preferably between 4 and 10 °C, but not frozen. Examination should begin as soon as possible after sampling and certainly within 24 hours. If samples cannot be cooled, they must be examined within 2 hours of sampling. If neither condition can be met, the sample should not be analysed.

## 10.5.3 Surveillance programme requirements

Surveillance is the continuous and vigilant public health assessment and review of the safety and acceptability of drinking-water supplies. Each component of the drinking-water system—the source, treatment, storage, and distribution—must function without risk of failure. A failure in one part will jeopardize and nullify the effects of other parts that function perfectly, as well as the care that has been taken to ensure that they do so. Water is liable to contamination at all stages in the process of supply, hence the need for constant vigilance. At the same time, careful and intelligent assessment of likely sources of risk and breakdown is necessary before a supply system is planned and installed and, indeed, continuously thereafter, because of possible changes in conditions and potential sources of contamination. Contingency plans must be made to deal with any emergencies that may arise through natural or man-made disasters, such as accidents, wars, and civil commotions, or the cessation of supplies of essential chemicals used in treatment.

An essential part of surveillance is the establishment of a proper network for regulation and command. At government level, this means the establishment and enforcement of national standards, and the promulgation of national guidelines for achieving compliance with the laws and standards; for the water-supply agency, it means promotion of local codes of good waterworks practice together with formal instruction and training. A national inspectorate should be established to ensure that the legal requirements are met and standards complied with. This body should be separate from that representing the interests of the water provider.

Both the water provider and the inspectorate should have properly equipped laboratory facilities staffed by trained and properly qualified personnel, adequate facilities for sustaining at all times the level of monitoring required, and sufficient capacity to carry out additional examinations as required to meet special needs. Operational staff at the waterworks, should also be appropriately trained and qualified.

Lines of communication and command must be established at the outset and must be properly understood by all staff up to the highest levels. This will ensure the effective functioning of day-to-day operations and also that immediate remedial action is taken in emergencies and when contamination is discovered. Bacteriological failures must be acted on as soon as discovered, so that the microbiologist must have the authority to instruct the engineer and the operational staff to take the necessary action. The lines of communication needed in an emergency will be complex, involving not only different public bodies but also authorities responsible for different geographical regions. Appropriate instructions must be laid down and understood at each site.

The scope of surveillance, together with examples covering the points made in this section, has been considered in a separate WHO publication, which should be consulted (8). The importance of surveillance is highlighted repeatedly in official reports of serious outbreaks of waterborne disease, which usually reveal deficiencies in more than one area (1, 2, 9). Surveillance procedures are described further in Volume 3 of *Guidelines for drinking-water quality.*

The levels of surveillance of drinking-water quality differ widely in developing countries in line with the differences in economic development and the provision of community water supplies in those countries. Surveillance should be progressively developed and expanded by adapting the level to the local situation and economic resources, with gradual implementation, consolidation, and development to the level ultimately desired.

## 10.6 Action to be taken when contamination is detected

No surface water can be assumed to be free from enteric pathogens, including viruses and parasites, since they can be derived from wild or farm animals living in the catchment area as well as from human faecal contamination. The geographical and seasonal distribution of specific pathogens in natural waters can provide valuable information on the epidemiology of disease in animal populations and the routes of transmission to the human population. Such information also indicates the precautions needed to safeguard the sources of water and the degree of treatment needed.

The occurrence of any pathogenic agent, bacterial, viral, or animal, in a drinking-water supply is always a matter for the gravest concern, demanding immediate attention to treatment and to determining the cause. The examination of drinking-water for a particular pathogen will most probably be required when the water is suspected to be the cause of an outbreak of disease in the community supplied with the water. The finding of the causal agent of the disease in the water, together with the distribution of primary cases among those using it, prove that the supply is implicated, particularly if the disease is not found among those not using the water and not acquiring infection secondarily.

### 10.6.1 Bacterial indicators of faecal contamination

The finding of *Escherichia coli* in any sample of water intended for drinking is a matter for concern, since it indicates that the water has been recently contaminated by faecal material from humans or animals, and that there is a likelihood that pathogens will also be present. If the water is a treated piped supply, there is also the strongest reason for suspecting that there has been a breakdown in disinfection, treatment before disinfection has failed, or contaminated water has entered the system. Immediate action must be taken to discover the source of contamination and to increase the dosage of disinfectant so as to ensure that an adequate residual is present in the water delivered to the consumer, until the problem is overcome. Consideration should be given to telling consumers to boil water intended for drinking. If the quality of water leaving the works is satisfactory, ingress of contaminated water will most usually arise as a result either of damage to the distribution system or repairs to it, or through infiltration into underground service reservoirs or directly into the mains as a result of low pressure and back-siphonage or cross-connections. Where treatment is minimal, because source water is normally of high quality, sudden deterioration resulting from storms, flooding, or massive pollution incidents will mean that the disinfection applied is inadequate. Prior assessment of hazards by sanitary survey or by the establishment of "early-warning" monitoring systems in the catchment area will help avoid such events.

A finding of thermotolerant or total coliform bacteria in the presumptive test demands instant attention. The positively reacting tubes or colonies must be examined further using confirmatory tests, and for the presence of *E. coli*. The water must immediately be resampled from the same source. The waterworks engineer must be informed at once, so that investigations can be made to discover the source of the contamination. Such action must be regarded as the minimum. Where the failure concerns water leaving the treatment works, investigations and corrective action as outlined in the previous paragraph are necessary immediately and before the results of the confirmatory test are known.

The finding of total coliform organisms, in the absence of thermotolerant coliforms or *E. coli*, in a treated piped supply usually indicates post-treatment contamination, or growth on pipes or fittings, when the treated water entering the supply system is satisfactory. It suggests either that materials coming into contact with water, such as those used for pipes, washers, pipe sealants, and packings, or rubber and plastics used for other purposes, are supporting growth or that untreated water is entering the distribution network. Because total coliforms of nonfaecal origin can exist in natural waters, their presence can occasionally be tolerated in unpiped or untreated water, if thermotolerant coliform bacteria and *E. coli* are absent. If they are present repeatedly or in consecutive samples, as indicated in Table 10.1, action must be taken to improve the sanitary protection of the source.

In temperate or cold climates, the finding of total or thermotolerant coliform bacteria in the presumptive test leads in a high proportion of cases to confirmation of the presence of *E. coli* and therefore of evidence of faecal contamination. This may be less common in tropical and semitropical regions, particularly where the water is untreated. Nevertheless, the indication must not be ignored for the reasons given in section 9.2. If desired, the faecal origin of such coliform organisms can be confirmed using the faecal streptococcus and sulfite-reducing clostridia tests.

## 10.6.2 Miscellaneous indicators

Occasionally, and particularly where the source water is derived from lowland rivers and where the water temperatures in the distribution system are 20 °C or higher, *Aeromonas* spp. can occur and will interfere with the interpretation of the total coliform tests. At these temperatures and where the free chlorine residual is below 0.2 mg/litre, these bacteria are able to grow on assimilable organic carbon in the water. Similar significance attaches to the finding of *Pseudomonas aeruginosa* in supply systems. Both these organisms can occur in the absence of coliform bacteria and will interfere with the interpretation of the coliform tests. Their sanitary significance is unclear, although they can be opportunistically pathogenic and are undesirable where water is used in the manufacture of food and drink, or is supplied to hospitals. Measures to eradicate them must be taken, and may include eliminating unsatisfactory materials in contact with the water, cleaning distribution systems and plumbing in the buildings affected, and maintaining adequate residual disinfectant in the supply.

Bacteria recovered in colony counts at 22 °C are without sanitary significance. However, the occurrence of such bacteria in numbers exceeding 100 per

100 ml in piped water may indicate enrichment of the water with assimilable organic carbon. Large numbers are undesirable in water used for preparing food and drink or for bottling. Any increase in the numbers of colonies above normal levels when counts are made at 37 °C should be regarded with suspicion, since it may be caused by the onset of polluting conditions, particularly if not accompanied by an increase in the count at 22 °C. An increase in the count at 37 °C is often a valuable indication of undesirable changes and should prompt an investigation of the supply or of the gathering grounds, if the water is untreated.

The presence of macroscopic animal life in drinking-water is aesthetically objectionable if nothing else. With piped supplies, it is an indication that flushing and cleaning of the distribution system are needed (see section 8.2). Their occurrence may sometimes reflect unusually high water temperatures as, for example, when chironomid larvae are discharged from slow sand filters into the treated water.

# References

1. Galbraith NS et al. Water and disease after Croydon: a review of water-borne and water-associated diseases in the UK 1937-86. *Journal of the Institution of Water and Environmental Management*, 1987, 1:7-21.

2. Craun GF. Waterborne disease outbreaks in the United States of America: causes and prevention. *World health statistics quarterly*, 1992, 45: 192-199.

3. Codex Alimentarius Commission. *Codex standards for natural mineral waters.* Rome, Food and Agriculture Organization of the United Nations, 1994 (Codex Alimentarius Vol. XI, Part III).

4. Payment P et al. A randomized trial to evaluate the risk of gastrointestinal disease due to consumption of drinking-water meeting current microbiological standards. *American journal of public health*, 1991, 81:703-708.

5. Regli S et al. Modelling the risk from *Giardia* and viruses in drinking-water. *Journal of the American Water Works Association*, 1991, 83(11):76-84.

6. *Standard methods for the examination of water and wastewater*, 17th ed. Washington, DC, American Public Health Association, 1989.

7. *The bacteriological examination of drinking-water supplies 1982.* London, Her Majesty's Stationery Office, 1983 (Reports on Public Health and Medical Subjects No. 71).

8. *Surveillance of drinking-water quality.* Geneva, World Health Organization, 1976 (Monograph Series No. 63).

9. Short CS. The Bramham incident, 1980—an outbreak of water-borne infection. *Journal of the Institution of Water and Environmental Management*, 1988, 2:383-390.

# 11.

# Protection and improvement of water quality

The emphasis in this section is on protecting and improving the microbiological quality of drinking-water. It is a basic principle, long established as a result of the lessons learned from serious outbreaks of waterborne disease, that a single barrier to the spread of pathogenic organisms is not sufficient to ensure the purity of drinking-water (1, 2). Purity is not the only requirement, however; the drinking-water supply must also be capable of meeting the anticipated demand. Inadequate supply, together with geographical factors, often means that raw water of poor microbiological quality and possibly containing significant amounts of wastewater has to be used. A second principle is that to ensure that the drinking-water delivered to the consumer is free from pathogens, the level of treatment should be related to the degree of pollution expected in the source water. In the case of contaminated water sources, several treatment processes, designed primarily for such water will be necessary. Together, these processes will progressively remove pathogens and other contaminants from raw water and consistently produce a safe and wholesome supply of drinking-water. Ideally, safety should be achieved before the final treatment step, so that the failure of any one process will not result in waterborne disease, i.e. the system is fail-safe. The protection of the source from pollution and the provision of adequate and properly operated treatment processes constitute the essential barriers to the transmission of disease on which the supply of wholesome water depends (1, 2).

## 11.1 Water sources

### 11.1.1 Selection of sources

Before a new source of drinking-water supply is selected, it is important to ensure that: (1) the quality of the water is satisfactory or can be improved by treatment to make it suitable for drinking; (2) the source will yield enough water to meet the needs of the community not only under the normal conditions of the average annual cycle but also under conditions which are unusual but can be expected, say, once in 10 years; (3) under normal abstraction conditions, the change in local water flow patterns will not cause any unacceptable deterioration in the quality of the water abstracted; and (4) the water to be abstracted can be protected against pollution.

A full sanitary and microbiological survey of the catchment area should be carried out to locate all the sources of pollution. It may be that the treatment or diversion of a small polluting discharge could make a large potential source acceptable (*3*). If remote upland sources of surface waters are being considered, it is important to assess whether access by people or livestock can be prevented and whether wild animals are likely to be vectors of salmonellae, *Giardia*, and *Cryptosporidium*.

## 11.1.2 Source protection

In the past, isolation of the watershed from human activity was an important means of protecting a waterway or aquifer from contamination. The rising cost of land and increases in population have made this procedure more costly and difficult, especially when new sources must be found in an area that is already developed. It is still desirable for water suppliers to own or control the land to the extent that this is feasible (*1*).

Another line of defence is to prevent polluting activities in the area which may be a source of infection. This means, for instance, defining areas where sewage sludge may not be applied, and exercising strict control over discharges of sewage effluents and agricultural wastes, the location of sites for the dumping of garbage and toxic wastes, and drilling, mining, and quarrying. Control of such activities does not necessarily mean that they should be banned, but that, in the interests of public health, they should be licensed and open to inspection and monitoring whenever water quality could be affected. Where potentially harmful substances are handled or made, steps should be taken to ensure that any effluents are either adequately treated or conveyed safely over the catchment area (*3*).

Sources of groundwater such as springs and wells should be sited and constructed so as to be protected from surface drainage and flooding. Zones of groundwater abstraction should be fenced off to prevent public access, kept free from rubbish, and sloped to prevent the formation of pools in wet weather. Animal husbandry should be adequately controlled in such zones (*1, 3*).

Protection of open surface water is difficult. It may be possible to protect a reservoir from major human activity, but the protection of a river, if possible at all, may be feasible only over a limited stretch. Often it is necessary to accept existing and historical uses of a river or lake and to design the treatment accordingly. Adequate sewage treatment is important in preserving water quality at downstream intakes (*3*).

## 11.2 Treatment processes

The fundamental purpose of water treatment is to protect the consumer from pathogens and from impurities in the water that may be injurious to human health or offensive. Where appropriate, treatment should also remove impurities which, although not harmful to human health, may make the water unappealing to drink, damage pipes, plant, or other items with which the water may come into contact, or render operation more difficult or costly.

These purposes are achieved, as previously mentioned, by introducing successive barriers, such as coagulation, sedimentation (or flotation), and filtration, to remove pathogens and impurities. The final barrier is disinfection. The function of the entire system, and indeed of much of water treatment, may with some justification be regarded as that of conditioning the water for effective and reliable disinfection (3).

## 11.2.1 Storage

The storage of water in reservoirs creates favourable conditions for the self-purification of the stored water, but may also cause undesirable changes in water quality. The benefits of storage include the provision of a continuous supply of water, reduction in turbidity, reduction in pathogens through the action of sunlight and sedimentation, dilution of undesirable substances that may accidentally enter the intake, and oxidation of impurities. It also provides a buffer should pollution occur in the river. Undesirable conditions created by storage include those associated with the production of algae, pollution by birds and animals, evaporation, and the leaching of iron and manganese from soils and rocks (2, 3).

Reservoirs should either be constructed in series or designed to prevent short-circuiting, since this will enhance removal of pathogens and self-purification. The benefits of reservoir storage are greatest in the summer and when residence periods are about 3–4 weeks.

## 11.2.2 Presedimentation

Highly turbid surface water may require presedimentation before further treatment. Presedimentation basins are constructed in excavated ground or of steel or concrete. Such basins may be preceded by equipment for the addition of chemicals to provide partial coagulation during periods when the water is too turbid to clarify by sedimentation alone.

## 11.2.3 Prechlorination

Prechlorination to breakpoint has been widely used as an alternative to storage for water derived from lowland rivers and is also used when stored water contains much planktonic life. Its purpose is to reduce counts of faecal bacteria and pathogens, destroy animal life and algae, and oxidize ammoniacal nitrogen, iron, and manganese, thereby assisting in their removal. The combined and free chlorine which remains effectively discourages microbial activities, such as protozoal predation and nitrification, as well as microbial growth during subsequent filtration. When used to disinfect raw water, the oxidative effect of chlorine and even more of ozone will result in the partial conversion of total organic carbon into biodegradable organic carbon which, if not removed by biological activity during treatment (e.g. during slow sand or granular activated carbon filtration), can result in the growth of nuisance organisms during distribution. Prechlorination of organically enriched surface waters has been shown to produce a substantial increase in the content of trihalomethanes and is often a wasteful use of chlorine. It is important to balance the maintenance of the microbiological safety of drinking-water against possible hazards associated with the formation of such disinfection by-products.

## 11.2.4 Coagulation and flocculation

To remove particulate matter, a water-treatment plant will generally include equipment for coagulation and flocculation, followed by sedimentation and filtration.

Coagulation involves the addition of chemicals (e.g. aluminium sulfate, ferric sulfate) to neutralize the charges on particles and facilitate their agglomeration during the slow mixing provided in the flocculation step (1). Flocs thus formed co-precipitate, adsorb and entrap natural colour and mineral particles, and can bring about major reductions in counts of protozoa, faecal bacteria, pathogens, and viruses.

Coagulation and flocculation require a high level of operational skill. Chemical dosages and pH control must be correct, and the plant must be designed to ensure proper floc formation. Before it is decided to use coagulation as part of a treatment process, careful consideration must be given to the likelihood of process stability, the availability of regular supplies of chemicals, and the need for qualified personnel (3).

## 11.2.5 Sedimentation or flotation

The purpose of sedimentation is to permit settleable floc to be deposited and thus reduce the concentration of suspended solids that must be removed by filters (2). Flotation is an alternative to sedimentation, and has advantages when the amount of floc is small.

The factors that influence sedimentation include the size, shape, and weight of the floc, viscosity and hence the temperature of the water, the detention time, the number, depth, and areas of the basins, the surface overflow rate, the velocity of flow, and the inlet and outlet design (1, 2).

Arrangements must be made for the collection and safe disposal of sludge from sedimentation tanks.

## 11.2.6 Rapid filtration

Typically, rapid sand filters consist of 0.4–1.2 m of sand, usually of an effective size of 0.5–1.0 mm, supported by gravel and underdrains. In recent years, single-medium filters have often been replaced by dual-medium or multimedia ones. During filtration, residual particles of floc not removed by sedimentation are trapped in the interstices of the bed, and may induce further flocculation of particles. A limited amount of biological activity may also occur, if it is not suppressed by prechlorination or by high flow rates. Both sand and mixed-media filters are normally cleaned by reversal of the flow though the bed (backwashing). Backwash water is either discharged to the sewer or drying beds or recycled after removal of sludge.

The performance of rapid filters in removing microorganisms and turbidity varies over the duration of the run between backwashings. Immediately after backwashing, performance is poor, until the bed has compacted. In some plants, water is filtered and diverted for recycling for 15–30 min at the start of each filter run. In some waterworks, a 30-min slow start for each filter run is included to prevent the initial breakthrough. Performance will also deteriorate progressively when backwashing is needed, since floc may escape through the bed into the treated water, thereby increasing its turbidity. In view of the foregoing, proper supervision and control of filtration at the waterworks are essential.

## 11.2.7 Slow sand filtration

Typically, slow sand filters consist of 0.5–1.5 m of silica sand with an effective size of 0.3–0.6 mm. The upper layer of fine sand is supported on gravel and a system of underdrains.

Slow sand filtration is simpler to operate than rapid filtration, as frequent backwashing is not required (4, 5). It is therefore particularly suitable for developing countries and small rural systems, but is applicable only if sufficient land is available. On the other hand, the filters are readily clogged by algal blooms and do not remove heavy metals and many micropollutants efficiently. They effectively remove biodegradable organic carbon and oxidize ammonia.

When the filter is first brought into use, a microbial slime community (*schmutzdecke*) develops at the surface of the bed. This consists of bacteria, free-living ciliated protozoa and amoebae, crustacea, and invertebrate larvae acting in food chains, resulting in the oxidation of organic substances in the water and of ammoniacal nitrogen to nitrate. Pathogenic bacteria, viruses, and resting stages of parasites are removed, principally by adsorption on to the *schmutzdecke* and by subsequent predation. When correctly loaded and operated, slow sand filtration is capable of bringing about a great improvement in water quality (6). Slow sand filters, operated at a filtration rate of 1.1–4.2 m/day, were able to remove 97–99% of enteroviruses at water temperatures of 6–11 °C. This was somewhat greater than for *E. coli*, and removal was greatest when the water was warmest (7). A slow sand filter is more efficient than any other process in removing parasites (helminths and protozoa). Nevertheless, the effluent from such a filter might well contain a few *E. coli* and viruses, especially during the early phase of a filter run. It is usual to divert or recycle the filtered water produced immediately after commissioning or cleaning a filter bed until the *schmutzdecke* has been established and become effective.

## 11.2.8 Infiltration

Surface water can also be treated by infiltration of the raw or partly treated water into river banks or sand dunes, followed by underground passage; this is an effective means of removing undesirable microorganisms and viruses. Infiltration is applicable only in areas where suitable geological conditions exist. Pretreatment is required to prevent clogging of the infiltration area. In addition, water abstracted from the aquifer usually needs some additional treatment, such as aeration and filtration, to remove, e.g. iron and manganese present in anaerobic groundwater. The residence time underground should be as long as possible to obtain a water comparable in quality to groundwater.

## 11.2.9 Disinfection

The overall objective of disinfection is to ensure that the quality criteria specified in Table 10.1 (see p. 95) are always met.

Terminal disinfection of piped drinking-water supplies is of paramount importance and is almost universal, since it is the final barrier to the transmission of waterborne bacterial and viral diseases. Although chlorine and hypochlorite are most often used, water may also be disinfected with chloramines, chlorine dioxide, ozone, and ultraviolet irradiation (*3, 8*).

The efficacy of any disinfection process will depend on the degree of purity achieved by prior treatment, as disinfectants are highly active and will be neutralized to a greater or lesser extent by organic matter and readily oxidizable compounds in water. Microorganisms that are aggregated or adsorbed on to particulate matter will also be partly protected from disinfection. It is therefore recommended that the median turbidity of water before disinfection should not exceed 1 NTU; it should not exceed 5 NTU in any individual sample.

Practical experience has shown that the kinetics of the disinfection of drinking-water follow the first-order model of Chick's law, in which the fraction of the original population surviving, $x_t/x_o$, after treatment for a time $t$ is given by

$$x_t/x_o = e^{-kt},$$

where $k$ is the specific death rate. This law is based on the assumption that all the agents being removed are equally sensitive to the disinfectant and that they are randomly distributed and not clumped together.

The specific death rate with disinfection, $k$, or the contact time, $t$, required to kill a given percentage of the original population is usually proportional to the concentration, $C$, of disinfectant, as in Watson's empirical dilution law:

$$C^n t = k$$

where $k$ is a constant of proportionality and $n$ is the dilution exponent. For water disinfection, the value of $n$ is close to 1, and it is therefore convenient to express the product of the concentration and the time required to bring about 99% removal of a given agent as a $C \cdot t$ value. This must be done with caution, because it is assumed that Chick's law is followed and that the conditions of disinfection (temperature, pH, chemical composition of the water, its disinfectant demand, and the physiological state of the agents being disinfected) are constant (9). Table 11.1 lists $C \cdot t$ values for different agents and disinfectants, and shows that, of the microorganisms listed, *E. coli* is generally the most sensitive, that the three viruses differ in sensitivity not only among themselves but also to the different disinfectants, and that the parasites *Giardia* and *Cryptosporidium* are the most resistant (10–12). Table 11.1 also indicates that normal chlorination conditions (i.e. free chlorine residual of 0.5 mg/litre, a contact time of 30 min, pH less than 8.0, and water turbidity less than 1 NTU) can be expected to bring about reductions greatly in excess of 99% for *E. coli* and the viruses specified but not for the parasitic protozoa.

### Table 11.1 C.t values (mg.min/l) for 99% inactivation of various agents by disinfectants at 5 °C[a]

| Agent | Disinfectant | | | |
|---|---|---|---|---|
| | Free chlorine pH 6-7 | Preformed chloramine pH 8-9 | Chlorine dioxide pH 6-7 | Ozone pH 6-7 |
| *E.coli* | 0.034–0.05 | 95–180 | 0.4–0.75 | 0.02 |
| Poliovirus type 1 | 1.1–2.5 | 768–3740 | 0.2–6.7 | 0.1–0.2 |
| Hepatitis A virus | 1.8 | ca 590 | 1.7 | – |
| Rotavirus | 0.01–0.05 | 3810–6480 | 0.2–2.1 | 0.006–0.06 |
| *Giardia lamblia* cysts | 47–>150 | – | – | 0.5–0.6 |
| *Giardia muris* cysts | 30–630 | – | 7.2–18.5 | 1.8–2.0 |
| *Cryptosporidium parvum* oocysts | – | – | 6.5–8.9 | < 3.3–6.4 |
| *Cryptosporidium* oocysts from human faeces | $7.7 \times 10^6$–$8.7 \times 10^6$ | – | – | – |

[a] Calculated from data in references 10–12.

It is thus clear that great care is needed to ensure that the treatment processes preceding terminal disinfection are operated correctly to ensure the effective removal of pathogens. There are many instances of disinfection failure when turbidity was 5 NTU or more. It is therefore axiomatic that, for successful disinfection, turbidity should always be less than 5 NTU and preferably less than 1 NTU.

As with chemical disinfection, ultraviolet disinfection is more effective against vegetative bacteria than against viruses and bacterial spores, while protozoal cysts are the most resistant. Data show that the minimum dosage recommended, 16 mW.s/cm², is sufficient to inactivate more than 99.9% of vegetative

113

bacteria but not the other agents (*10*). Disinfection by ultraviolet radiation is applicable only to clear waters, since appreciable turbidity or dissolved organic carbon will attenuate the radiation. Although there is no residual effect of disinfection by ultraviolet radiation, this is not a drawback when the water has been treated to a high standard to remove biodegradable organic carbon and where the water distribution system is well maintained.

## 11.3 Choice of treatment

### 11.3.1 Microbiological conditions

In rural areas supplying small communities, protection of the source of water may be the only "treatment" possible. Such supplies are considered in detail in Volume 3 of *Guidelines for drinking-water quality*. In large communities, the demand for water is high and can often be met only by using sources of poor microbiological quality.

Two considerations are of paramount importance: firstly, the quality of drinking-water is totally dependent on protection of the source, treatment of the water, and maintenance of the integrity of the distribution system; and secondly, microbiological monitoring can influence water quality only if its findings, and those of the agency responsible for surveillance, are made known to the water engineer and any remedial measures necessary are implemented.

### 11.3.2 Treatment of groundwater

Groundwater extracted from well protected aquifers is usually free from pathogenic microorganisms, and the distribution of such groundwater without treatment is common practice in many countries. However, the catchment area must be protected by effective regulatory measures and the distribution system adequately protected against secondary contamination of the drinking-water. If the water, in its passage from source to consumer, cannot be protected at all times, disinfection and the maintenance of adequate chlorine residuals are imperative.

### 11.3.3 Treatment of surface water

The extent to which faecal bacteria, viruses, and parasites are removed by properly designed and operated equipment for flocculation, coagulation, sedimentation, and rapid filtration is equivalent to that achieved by slow sand filtration.

Additional treatment, such as ozonation, will have a considerable disinfecting action besides converting part of the total organic carbon into a biodegradable form. If it is followed by activated carbon treatment or other biological filtration stage, some of the biodegradable organic carbon will be removed by microbial activity, thus reducing the potential for aftergrowth of nuisance bacteria in distribution networks.

Disinfection should be regarded as obligatory for all piped supplies of surface water, even if derived from high-quality, unpolluted sources, since there should always be more than one barrier against the transmission of infection by a water supply. In large, properly run waterworks, the criteria for the absence of *E. coli* and coliform bacteria can then be met with a very high degree of probability.

Table 11.2 shows that conventional urban water treatment relies on pretreatment and terminal disinfection to remove much of the microbial contamination. Nevertheless, conventional treatment can be effectively operated as a three-stage multiple-barrier system involving: (1) coagulation and settling or flotation; (2) rapid filtration; and (3) terminal disinfection.

**Table 11.2 An example to illustrate the level of performance that can be achieved in removal of turbidity and thermotolerant coliform bacteria in conventional urban water treatment**

| Stage and process | Turbidity | | | Thermotolerant coliform bacteria | | |
|---|---|---|---|---|---|---|
| | Removal[a] (%) | Average loading (NTU)[b] | Maximum loading (NTU)[b] | Removal[a] (h) % | Average loading (per 100 ml) | Maximum loading (per 100 ml) |
| Micro-straining | NA[c] | NA | NA | NA | NA | NA |
| Pretreatment[d] | NA | NA | NA | >99.9 | 1000 | 10 000 |
| Coagulation/settling[e] | 90 | 50 | 300 | NA | NA | NA |
| Rapid filtration[e] | >80 | 5 | 30 | 80 | 1 | 10 |
| Terminal chlorination | NA | 1 | 5 | >99.9 | <1 | 2 |
| Mains distribution | NA | <1 | <5 | NA | <1 | <1 |

[a] Required performance.
[b] NTU, nephelometric turbidity units.
[c] NA, not applicable, Process not designed to remove turbidity and/or bacteria. Micro-straining removes micro-algae and zooplankton
[d] Pretreatments that can result in significant reductions in thermotolerant coliform bacteria are storage in reservoirs for 3–4 weeks, and pre-disinfection.
[e] Taken together, coagulation, settling, and rapid filtration should be expected to remove 99.9% of thermotolerant coliform bacteria.

Another approach to the application of the multiple-barrier principle has been applied in urban areas for supplies derived from rivers. It involves: (1) raw water storage (or plain sedimentation); (2) rapid sand filtration; (3) slow sand filtration; and (4) terminal disinfection. Steps 1–3 remove turbidity, while 1, 3 and 4 remove microbes. Infiltration, which is highly effective in removing bacteria, viruses, and organic carbon, has been used, notably in the Netherlands, as an additional process following storage and rapid filtration.

## 11.3.4 Small-scale treatment of surface water

The multiple-barrier concept, as applied in the treatment of surface water for urban supplies, can be adapted for use in rural and remote regions. A typical series of processes would include: (1) storage, sedimentation, or screening; (2)

triple-stage gravel prefiltration; (3) slow sand filtration; and (4) disinfection. Table 11.3 lists typical performance objectives for the removal of turbidity and thermotolerant coliform bacteria in such plants.

A detailed account of water treatment and supply for small remote communities is given in Volume 3 of *Guidelines for drinking-water quality*.

**Table 11.3 An example of performance objectives for removal of turbidity and thermotolerant coliform bacteria in small-scale water treatment**

| Stage and process | Turbidity | | | Thermotolerant coliform bacteria | | |
|---|---|---|---|---|---|---|
| | Removal[a] (%) | Average loading (NTU)[b] | Maximum loading (NTU)[b] | Removal[a] (h) % | Average loading (per 100 ml) | Maximum loading (per 100 ml) |
| Screening | NA[c] | NA | NA | NA | NA | NA |
| Plain sedimentation | 50 | 60 | 600 | 50 | 1000 | 10 000 |
| Gravel pre-filters (3-stage) | 80 | 30 | 300 | 90 | 500 | 5000 |
| Slow sand filter | >90 | 6 | 60 | 95 | 50 | 500 |
| Disinfection | NA | <1 | <5 | >99.9 | <3 | 25 |
| Distributed water | NA | <1 | <5 | NA | <1 | <1 |

[a] Required performance.
[b] NTU, nephelometric turbidity units.
[c] NA, not applicable. Process not designed to remove turbidity and/or bacteria.

## 11.4 Distribution networks

A distribution network transports water from the place of treatment to the consumer. Its design and size will be governed both by the topography and the location and size of the community. The aim is always to ensure that the consumer receives a sufficient and uninterrupted supply and that contamination is not introduced in transit. The shape of the network will be influenced by the location of consumers.

Distribution systems are especially vulnerable to contamination when the pressure falls, particularly in the intermittent supplies of many cities in developing countries. Suction is often created by direct pumping from the mains to private storage tanks, a practice which should be prohibited.

The bacteriological quality of water can deteriorate during distribution, and there are a number of places where contamination can be introduced. If the water contains significant assimilable organic carbon and adequate residual levels of disinfectant are not maintained, or if water mains are not flushed and cleaned frequently enough, growth of nuisance bacteria and other organisms can occur. Where the water contains appreciable assimilable organic carbon and where the water temperature exceeds 20 °C, a chlorine residual of 0.25 mg/litre may be required to prevent the growth of *Aeromonas* and other nuisance bacteria. Attached microorganisms may grow even in the presence of residual chlorine.

Underground storage tanks and service reservoirs must be inspected for deterioration and for infiltration of surface water and groundwater. It is desirable for the land enclosing underground storage tanks to be fenced off, both to prevent access by people and animals and to prevent damage to the structures.

Repair work on mains provides another opportunity for contamination to occur. Local loss of pressure may result in back-siphonage of contaminated water unless check valves are introduced into the consumers' water system at sensitive points, such as supplies to ornamental pools, garden irrigation, urinals, and water closets. When repairs to mains have been completed or when new mains are installed, it is essential that the pipes are cleaned, disinfected, and then emptied and refilled with mains water. The water should then be tested bacteriologically after 24 hours, and new mains should not be brought into service until the water quality is bacteriologically satisfactory. If the main has been damaged and water from a fractured sewer or drain may have entered, the situation is most serious and, in addition to chlorination of the water in the repaired main, the level of chlorination should be increased and the main not returned to service until the water quality is satisfactory. These and other actions to be taken should be specified both in national codes of practice and in local instructions to waterworks staff.

As already mentioned, microbial contamination can occur as a result of the use of unsuitable materials for items coming into contact with water; such materials include those used for washers, jointing and packing materials, pipe and tank lining compounds, and plastics used in pipes, tanks, and faucets, all of which can deteriorate to form substances that support the growth of microorganisms. Such materials should be subject to approval by the authority responsible for the water-supply system.

## References

1. Department of National Health and Welfare, Canada *Water treatment principles and applications: A manual for the production of drinking-water*. Ottawa, Canadian Government Publishing Centre, 1993.

2. Cox CR. *Operation and control of water treatment processes*. Geneva, World Health Organization, 1969.

3. Espinoza O, Benedek P, Warden J, eds. *Disinfection of rural and small-community water supplies: a manual for design and operation*. Copenhagen, WHO Regional Office for Europe, 1989.

4. Visscher JT et al. *Slow sand filtration for community water supply*. The Hague, International Reference Centre for Community Water Supply, 1987 (Technical Paper Series No. 24).

5.  Huisman L, Wood WE. *Slow sand filtration.* Geneva, World Health Organization, 1974.

6.  Pescod MB, Abouzaid H, Sundaresan BB. *Slow sand filtration, a low cost treatment for water supplies in developing countries.* Medmenham, Water Research Centre, 1986, (published on behalf of the WHO Regional Office for Europe).

7.  Slade JS. Enteroviruses in slow sand filtered water. *Journal of the Institution of Water Engineers and Scientists,* 1978, 32: 530-536.

8.  White GC. *Handbook of chlorination,* 2nd ed. New York, Van Nostrand Reinhold, 1985.

9.  Hoff JC. *Inactivation of microbial agents by chemical disinfectants.* Springfield, VA, National Technical Information Service, 1986 (PB 86-232586/AS).

10. Sobsey MD. Inactivation of health-related microorganisms in water by disinfection processes. *Water science and technology,* 1989, 21:179-195.

11. Peeters JE et al. Effect of disinfection of drinking-water with ozone or chlorine dioxide on survival of *Cryptosporidium parvum* oocysts. *Applied and environmental microbiology,* 1989, 55:1519-1522.

12. Smith HV et al. *The effect of free chlorine on the viability of Cryptosporidium spp. oocysts.* Medmenham, Water Research Centre, 1989 (PRU 2023-M).

# PART 2

## Chemical and physical aspects

# 12.
# Chemical and physical aspects: introduction

## 12.1 Background information used

The assessment of the toxicity of drinking-water contaminants has been made on the basis of published reports from the open literature, information submitted by governments and other interested parties, and unpublished proprietary data. In the development of the guideline values, existing international approaches to developing guidelines were carefully considered. Previous risk assessments developed by the International Programme on Chemical Safety (IPCS) in Environmental Health Criteria monographs, the International Agency for Research on Cancer (IARC), the Joint FAO/WHO Meetings on Pesticide Residues (JMPR), and the Joint FAO/WHO Expert Committee on Food Additives (JECFA) were reviewed. These assessments were relied upon except where new information justified a reassessment. The quality of new data was critically evaluated prior to their use in risk assessment.

## 12.2 Drinking-water consumption and body weight

Global data on the consumption of drinking-water are limited. In studies carried out in Canada, the Netherlands, the United Kingdom, and the United States of America, the average daily *per capita* consumption was usually found to be less than 2 litres, but there was considerable variation between individuals. As water intake is likely to vary with climate, physical activity, and culture, the above studies, which were conducted in temperate zones, can give only a limited view of consumption patterns throughout the world. At temperatures above 25 °C, for example, there is a sharp rise in fluid intake, largely to meet the demands of an increased sweat rate (*1*).

In developing the guideline values for potentially hazardous chemicals, a daily *per capita* consumption of 2 litres by a person weighing 60 kg was generally assumed. The guideline values set for drinking-water using this assumption do, on average, err on the side of caution. However, such an assumption may underestimate the consumption of water per unit weight, and thus exposure, for those living in hot climates as well as for infants and children, who consume more fluid per unit weight than adults.

The higher intakes, and hence exposure, for infants and children apply for only a limited time, but this period may coincide with greater sensitivity to some toxic agents and less for others. Irreversible effects that occur at a young age will have more social and public health significance than those that are delayed. Where it was judged that this segment of the population was at a particularly high risk from exposure to certain chemicals, the guideline value was derived on the basis of a 10-kg child consuming 1 litre per day or a 5-kg infant consuming 0.75 litre per day. The corresponding daily fluid intakes are higher than for adults on a body weight basis.

## 12.3 Inhalation and dermal absorption

The contribution of drinking-water to daily exposure includes direct ingestion as well as some indirect routes, such as inhalation of volatile substances and dermal contact during bathing or showering.

In most cases, the data were insufficient to permit reliable estimates of exposure by inhalation and dermal absorption of contaminants present in drinking-water. It was not possible, therefore, to address intake from these routes specifically in the derivation of the guideline values. However, that portion of the total tolerable daily intake (TDI) allocated to drinking-water is generally sufficient to allow for these additional routes of intake (see section 12.4.1). When there is concern that potential inhalation of volatile compounds and dermal exposure from various indoor water uses (such as showering) are not adequately addressed, authorities could adjust the guideline value.

## 12.4 Health risk assessment

There are two principal sources of information on health effects resulting from exposure to chemicals that can be used in deriving guideline values. The first is studies on human populations. The value of such investigations is often limited, owing to lack of quantitative information on the concentrations to which people are exposed or on simultaneous exposure to other agents. The second, and the one used most often, is toxicity studies using laboratory animals. Such studies are generally limited because of the relatively small number of animals used and the relatively high doses administered. Furthermore, there is a need to extrapolate the results to the low doses to which human populations are usually exposed.

In order to derive a guideline value to protect human health, it is necessary to select the most suitable experimental animal study on which to base the extrapolation. Data from well-conducted studies, where a clear dose–response relationship has been demonstrated, are preferred. Expert judgement was exercised in the selection of the most appropriate study from the range of information available.

## 12.4.1 Derivation of guideline values using a tolerable daily intake approach

For most kinds or toxicity, it is generally believed that there is a dose below which no adverse effects will occur. For chemicals that give rise to such toxic effects, a tolerable daily intake (TDI) can be derived as follows:

$$TDI = \frac{NOAEL \text{ or } LOAEL}{UF}$$

where  $NOAEL$  = no-observed-adverse-effect level,
     $LOAEL$  = lowest-observed-adverse-effect level,
     $UF$     = uncertainty factor.

The guideline value (GV) is then derived from the TDI as follows:

$$GV = \frac{TDI \times bw \times P}{C}$$

where  $bw$ = body weight (60 kg for adults, 10 kg for children, 5 kg for infants),
      $P$  = fraction of the TDI allocated to drinking-water,
      $C$  = daily drinking-water consumption (2 litres for adults, 1 litre for children, 0.75 litre for infants).

### Tolerable daily intake

The TDI is an estimate of the amount of a substance in food or drinking-water, expressed on a body weight basis (mg/kg or µg/kg of body weight), that can be ingested daily over a lifetime without appreciable health risk (2).

Over many years, JECFA and JMPR have developed certain principles in the derivation of acceptable daily intakes (ADIs). These principles have been adopted where appropriate in the derivation of TDIs used in developing guideline values for drinking-water quality (3, 4).

ADIs are established for food additives and pesticide residues that occur in food for necessary technological purposes or plant protection reasons. For chemical contaminants, which usually have no intended function in drinking-water, the term "tolerable daily intake" is seen as more appropriate than "acceptable daily intake", as it signifies permissibility rather than acceptability (3).

As TDIs are regarded as representing a tolerable intake for a lifetime, they are not so precise that they cannot be exceeded for short periods of time (4). Short-term exposure to levels exceeding the TDI is not a cause for concern, provided the individual's intake averaged over longer periods of time does not appreciably exceed the level set (5). The large uncertainty factors generally involved in establishing a TDI (see page 124) serve to provide assurance that exposure exceeding the TDI for short periods is unlikely to have any deleterious effects upon health. However, consideration should be given to any potential acute toxic effects that may occur if the TDI is substantially exceeded for short periods of time (4).

The calculated TDI was used to derive the guideline value, which was then rounded to one significant figure. In some instances, ADI values with only one significant figure set by JECFA or JMPR were used to calculate the guideline value (4). The guideline value was generally rounded to one significant figure to reflect the uncertainty in animal toxicity data and exposure assumptions made. More than one significant figure was used for guideline values only where extensive information on toxicity and exposure to humans provided greater certainty.

### No-observed-adverse-effect level and lowest-observed-adverse-effect level

The NOAEL is defined as the highest dose or concentration of a chemical in a single study, found by experiment or observation, that causes no detectable adverse health effect. Whenever possible, the NOAEL is based on long-term studies, preferably of ingestion in drinking-water. However, NOAELs obtained from short-term studies and studies using other sources of exposure (e.g., food, air) may also be used.

If a NOAEL is not available, a LOAEL may be used, which is the lowest observed dose or concentration of a substance at which there is a detectable adverse health effect. When a LOAEL is used instead of a NOAEL, an additional uncertainty factor is normally used (see below).

### Uncertainty factors

The application of uncertainty factors has been widely used in the derivation of ADIs for food additives, pesticides, and environmental contaminants. The derivation of these factors requires expert judgement and a careful sifting of the available scientific evidence.

In the derivation of the WHO drinking-water quality guideline values, uncertainty factors were applied to the lowest NOAEL or LOAEL for the response considered to be the most biologically significant and were determined by consensus among a group of experts using the approach outlined below:

| Source of uncertainty | Factor |
|---|---|
| Interspecies variation (animals to humans) | 1–10 |
| Intraspecies variation (individual variations) | 1–10 |
| Adequacy of studies or database | 1–10 |
| Nature and severity of effect | 1–10 |

Inadequate studies or databases include those that used a LOAEL instead of a NOAEL and studies considered to be shorter in duration than desirable. Situations in which the nature or severity of effect might warrant an additional uncertainty factor include studies in which the end-point was malformation of a fetus or in which the end-point determining the NOAEL was directly related to possible carcinogenicity. In the latter case, an additional uncertainty factor was applied for carcinogenic compounds for which a guideline value was derived using a TDI approach (see section 12.4.2). Factors lower than 10 were used, for example, for interspecies variation when humans are known to be less sensitive than the animal species studied.

The total uncertainty factor should not exceed 10 000. If the risk assessment would lead to a higher uncertainty factor, then the resulting TDI would be so imprecise as to lack meaning. For substances for which uncertainty factors were greater than 1000, guideline values are designated as provisional in order to emphasize the high level of uncertainty inherent in these values.

The selection and application of uncertainty factors are important in the derivation of guideline values for chemicals, as they can make a considerable difference to the values set. For contaminants for which there is relatively little uncertainty, the guideline value was derived using a small uncertainty factor. For most contaminants, however, there is great scientific uncertainty, and a large uncertainty factor was used. Hence, there may be a large margin of safety above the guideline value before adverse health effects result.

There is considerable merit in using a method that allows a high degree of flexibility. However, it is important that, where possible, the derivation of the uncertainty factor used in calculating a guideline value is clearly presented as part of the rationale. This helps authorities in using the guidelines, as the safety margin in allowing for local circumstances is clear. It also helps in determining the urgency and nature of the action required in the event that a guideline value is exceeded.

### Allocation of intake

Drinking-water is not usually the sole source of human exposure to the substances for which guideline values have been set. In many cases, the intake from drinking-water is small in comparison with that from other sources such as food and air. Guideline values derived using the TDI approach take into account exposure from all sources by apportioning a percentage of the TDI to drinking-water. This approach ensures that total daily intake from all sources (including drinking-water containing concentrations of the substance at or near the guideline value) does not exceed the TDI.

Wherever possible, data concerning the proportion of total intake normally ingested in drinking-water (based on mean levels in food, air, and drinking-water) or intakes estimated on the basis of consideration of physical and chemical properties were used in the derivation of the guideline values. Where such information was not available, an arbitrary (default) value of 10% for drinking-water was used. This default value is, in most cases, sufficient to account for additional routes of intake (i.e., inhalation and dermal absorption) of contaminants in water.

It is recognized that exposure from various media may vary with local circumstances. It should be emphasized, therefore, that the derived guideline values apply to a typical exposure scenario or are based on default values that may not be applicable for all areas. In those areas where relevant data on exposure are available, authorities are encouraged to develop context-specific guideline values that are tailored to local circumstances and conditions. For example, in areas where the intake of a particular contaminant in drinking-water is known to be much greater than that from other sources (i.e., air and food), it may be appropriate to allocate a greater proportion of the TDI to drinking-water to derive a guideline value more suited to the local conditions. In addition, in cases in which guideline values are exceeded, efforts should be made to assess the contribution of other sources to total intake; if practicable, exposure from these sources should be minimized.

## 12.4.2 Derivation of guideline values for potential carcinogens

The evaluation of the potential carcinogenicity of chemical substances is usually based on long-term animal studies. Sometimes data are available on carcinogenicity in humans, mostly from occupational exposure.

On the basis of the available evidence, IARC categorizes chemical substances with respect to their potential carcinogenic risk into the following groups (6) (for a detailed description of the classifications, see box on pp. 127–128):

Group 1   : the agent is carcinogenic to humans
Group 2A : the agent is probably carcinogenic to humans
Group 2B : the agent is possibly carcinogenic to humans
Group 3   : the agent is not classifiable as to its carcinogenicity to humans
Group 4   : the agent is probably not carcinogenic to humans.

In establishing the present guideline values for drinking-water quality, the IARC classification for carcinogenic compounds was taken into consideration. For a number of compounds, additional information was also available.

It is generally considered that the initiating event in the process of chemical carcinogenesis is the induction of a mutation in the genetic material (DNA) of somatic cells (i.e., cells other than ova or sperm). Because the genotoxic mechanism theoretically does not have a threshold, there is a probability of harm at any level of exposure. Therefore, the development of a TDI is considered inappropriate, and mathematical low-dose extrapolation is applied. On the other hand, there are carcinogens that are capable of producing tumours in animals or humans without exerting genotoxic activity, but acting through an indirect mechanism. It is generally believed that a threshold dose exists for these nongenotoxic carcinogens.

In order to make the distinction with respect to the underlying mechanism of carcinogenicity, each compound that has been shown to be a carcinogen was evaluated on a case-by-case basis, taking into account the evidence of genotox-

## Evaluation of carcinogenic risk to humans

IARC considers the body of evidence as a whole in order to reach an overall evaluation of the carcinogenicity for humans of an agent, mixture, or circumstance of exposure.

The agent, mixture, or exposure circumstance is described according to the wording of one of the following categories, and the designated group is given. The categorization of an agent, mixture, or exposure circumstance is a matter of scientific judgement, reflecting the strength of the evidence derived from studies in humans and in experimental animals and from other relevant data.

### Group 1. The agent (mixture) is carcinogenic to humans.
### The exposure circumstance entails exposures that are carcinogenic to humans.

This category is used when there is *sufficient evidence* of carcinogenicity in humans. Exceptionally, an agent (mixture) may be placed in this category when evidence in humans is less than sufficient but there is *sufficient evidence* of carcinogenicity in experimental animals and strong evidence in exposed humans that the agent (mixture) acts through a relevant mechanism of carcinogenicity.

### Group 2

This category includes agents, mixtures, and exposure circumstances for which, at one extreme, the degree of evidence of carcinogenicity in humans is almost sufficient, as well as those for which, at the other extreme, there are no human data but for which there is evidence of carcinogenicity in experimental animals. Agents, mixtures, and exposure circumstances are assigned to either group 2A (probably carcinogenic to humans) or group 2B (possibly carcinogenic to humans) on the basis of epidemiological and experimental evidence of carcinogenicity and other relevant data.

### Group 2A. The agent (mixture) is probably carcinogenic to humans.
### The exposure circumstance entails exposures that are probably carcinogenic to humans.

This category is used when there is *limited evidence* of carcinogenicity in humans and *sufficient evidence* of carcinogenicity in experimental animals. In some cases, an agent (mixture) may be classified in this category when there is *inadequate evidence* of carcinogenicity in humans and *sufficient evidence* of carcinogenicity in experimental animals and strong evidence that the carcinogenesis is mediated by a mechanism that also operates in humans. Exceptionally, an agent, mixture, or exposure circumstance may be classified in this category solely on the basis of *limited evidence* of carcinogenicity in humans.

> **Group 2B. The agent (mixture) is possibly carcinogenic to humans. The exposure circumstance entails exposures that are possibly carcinogenic to humans.**
>
> This category is used for agents, mixtures, and exposure circumstances for which there is *limited evidence* of carcinogenicity in humans and less than *sufficient evidence* of carcinogenicity in experimental animals. It may also be used when there is *inadequate evidence* of carcinogenicity in humans but there is *sufficient evidence* of carcinogenicity in experimental animals. In some instances, an agent, mixture, or exposure circumstance for which there is *inadequate evidence* of carcinogenicity in humans but *limited evidence* of carcinogenicity in experimental animals together with supporting evidence from other relevant data may be placed in this group.
>
> **Group 3. The agent (mixture or exposure circumstance) is not classifiable as to its carcinogenicity to humans.**
>
> This category is used most commonly for agents, mixtures, and exposure circumstances for which the evidence of carcinogenicity is inadequate in humans and inadequate or limited in experimental animals.
>
> Exceptionally, agents (mixtures) for which the evidence for carcinogenicity is inadequate in humans but sufficient in experimental animals may be placed in this category when there is strong evidence that the mechanism of carcinogenicity in experimental animals does not operate in humans.
>
> Agents, mixtures, and exposure circumstances that do not fall into any other group are also placed in this category.
>
> **Group 4. The agent (mixture) is probably not carcinogenic to humans.**
>
> This category is used for agents or mixtures for which there is *evidence suggesting lack of carcinogenicity* in humans and in experimental animals. In some instances, agents or mixtures for which there is *inadequate evidence* of carcinogenicity in humans but *evidence suggesting lack of carcinogenicity* in experimental animals, consistently and strongly supported by a broad range of other relevant data, may be classified in this group.

icity, the range of species affected, and the relevance to humans of the tumours observed in experimental animals.

For carcinogens for which there is convincing evidence to suggest a nongenotoxic mechanism, guideline values were calculated using a TDI approach, as described in section 12.4.1.

In the case of compounds considered to be genotoxic carcinogens, guideline values were determined using a mathematical model, and the guideline values presented in Volume 1 are the concentrations in drinking-water associated with an estimated upper bound excess lifetime cancer risk of $10^{-5}$ (one additional cancer case per 100 000 of the population ingesting drinking-water containing the substance at the guideline value for 70 years). Concentrations associated with estimated excess lifetime cancer risks of $10^{-4}$ and $10^{-6}$ can be calculated by multiplying and dividing, respectively, the guideline value by 10. These values are also presented in this volume to emphasize the fact that each country should select its own appropriate risk level. In cases in which the concentration associated with a $10^{-5}$ excess lifetime cancer risk is not practical because of inadequate analytical or treatment technology, a provisional guideline value was set at a practicable level and the estimated associated cancer risk presented.

Although several models exist, the linearized multistage model was generally adopted in the development of these guidelines. Other models were considered more appropriate in a few cases.

It should be emphasized, however, that guideline values for carcinogenic compounds computed using mathematical models must be considered at best as a rough estimate of the cancer risk. These models do not usually take into account a number of biologically important considerations, such as pharmacokinetics, DNA repair, or immunological protection mechanisms. However, the models used are conservative and probably err on the side of caution.

To account for differences in metabolic rates between experimental animals and humans—the former are more closely correlated with the ratio of body surface areas than with body weights—a surface area to body weight correction is sometimes applied to quantitative estimates of cancer risk derived on the basis of models for low-dose extrapolation. Incorporation of this factor increases the risk by approximately one order of magnitude (depending on the species upon which the estimate is based) and increases the risk estimated on the basis of studies in mice relative to that in rats. The incorporation of this factor is considered to be overly conservative, particularly in view of the fact that linear extrapolation most likely overestimates risk at low doses; indeed, Crump et al. (7) concluded that "all measures of dose except dose rate per unit of body weight tend to result in overestimation of human risk". Consequently, guideline values for carcinogenic contaminants were developed on the basis of quantitative estimates of risk that were not corrected for the ratio of surface area to body weight.

## 12.5 Mixtures

Chemical contaminants of drinking-water supplies are present together with numerous other inorganic and organic constituents. The guideline values were calculated separately for individual substances, without specific consideration of the potential for interaction of each substance with other compounds present. However, the large margin of safety incorporated in the majority of guideline values is considered to be sufficient to account for such potential interactions. In addition, the majority of contaminants will not be present at concentrations at or near their guideline value.

There may, however, be occasions when a number of contaminants with similar toxicological effects are present at levels near their respective guideline values. In such cases, decisions concerning appropriate action should be made, taking into consideration local circumstances. Unless there is evidence to the contrary, it is appropriate to assume that the toxic effects of these compounds are additive.

## 12.6 Format of monographs for chemical substances

The format adopted for the monographs in this publication is shown below. All of the headings may not, however, be required in every monograph.

**General description**
Identity
Physicochemical properties
Organoleptic properties
Major uses
Environmental fate

**Analytical methods**

**Environmental levels and human exposure**
Air
Water
Food
Estimated total exposure and relative contribution of drinking-water

**Kinetics and metabolism in laboratory animals and humans**

**Effects on laboratory animals and *in vitro* test systems**
Acute exposure
Short-term exposure
Long-term exposure
Reproductive toxicity, embryotoxicity, and teratogenicity
Mutagenicity and related end-points
Carcinogenicity

**Effects on humans**

**Guideline value**

## References

1.  International Commission on Radiological Protection. *Report of the Task Group on Reference Man.* New York, Pergamon Press, 1992 (ICRP No. 23).

2.  *Evaluation of certain veterinary drug residues in food: thirty-eighth report of the Joint FAO/WHO Expert Committee on Food Additives.* Geneva, World Health Organization, 1991 (WHO Technical Report Series, No. 815).

3.  *Principles for the safety assessment of food additives and contaminants in food.* Geneva, World Health Organization, 1987 (Environmental Health Criteria, No. 70).

4.   *Principles for the toxicological assessment of pesticide residues in food.* Geneva, World Health Organization, 1990 (Environmental Health Criteria, No. 104).

5.   *Evaluation of certain food additives and contaminants: thirty-third report of the Joint FAO/WHO Expert Committee on Food Additives.* Geneva, World Health Organization, 1989 (WHO Technical Report Series, No. 776).

6.   International Agency for Research on Cancer. *Occupational exposures to mists and vapours from strong inorganic acids; and other industrial chemicals.* Lyon, 1992 (IARC Monographs on the Evaluation of Carcinogenic Risks to Humans, Vol. 54).

7.   Crump K, Allen B, Shipp A. Choice of dose measures for extrapolating carcinogenic risk from animals to humans: an empirical investigation of 23 chemicals. *Health physics*, 1989, 57(Suppl.1):387-393.

# 13.
# Inorganic constituents and physical parameters

## 13.1 Aluminium

### 13.1.1 General description

#### *Identity*

Aluminium is a widespread and abundant element, accounting for some 8% of the earth's crust. It is found as a normal constituent of soils, plants, and animal tissues.

| Compound | CAS no. | Molecular formula |
|---|---|---|
| Aluminium | 7429-90-5 | Al |
| Aluminium oxide | 1344-28-1 | $Al_2O_3$ |
| Aluminium chloride (hexahydrate) | 7446-70-0 | $AlCl_3.6H_2O$ |
| Aluminium sulfate | 10043-01-3 | $Al_2(SO_4)_3$ |
| Aluminium hydroxide | 21645-51-2 | $Al(OH)_3$ |

#### *Physicochemical properties (1)*

| Property | Al | $Al_2O_3$ | $AlCl_3.6H_2O$ | $Al_2(SO_4)_3$ | $Al(OH)_3$ |
|---|---|---|---|---|---|
| Melting point (°C) | 660.37 | 2072 | 100 (decomposes) | 770 (decomposes) | 300 |
| Boiling point (°C) | 2467 | 2980 | - | - | - |
| Density at 20 °C ($g/cm^3$) | 2.702 | 3.965 | 2.398 | 2.71 | 2.42 |
| Water solubility (g/litre) | insoluble | insoluble | soluble | 31.3 at 0 °C | - |

#### *Organoleptic properties*

In the presence of aluminium, levels of iron normally too low to cause problems may produce obvious discoloration of water. The incidence of discoloration in distribution system water, and therefore the frequency of consumer complaints, increases if the aluminium level exceeds about 0.1–0.2 mg/litre in the final water.

### Major uses

Aluminium has many industrial and domestic applications. Its compounds are used as antacids, antiperspirants, food additives, and vaccine adjuvants. Aluminium salts are also widely used in water treatment as flocculants.

### Environmental fate

Aluminium is usually present in treated drinking-water in the form of reactive species of low relative molecular mass; in natural waters, it is usually associated with particulate matter or organic complexes of high relative molecular mass (2).

## 13.1.2 Analytical methods

Aluminium may be determined by colorimetry (lower detection limit 5 µg/litre) and by inductively coupled plasma emission spectrometry (lower detection limit 40 µg/litre).

## 13.1.3 Environmental levels and human exposure

### Air

Aluminium is present in air at nanogram per cubic metre levels as a result of the weathering of aluminosilicate rocks and emissions from industrial sources, automobiles, and cigarette smoke (3).

### Water

Aluminium may be present in natural waters as a consequence of leaching from soil and rock. In a survey of aluminium in raw waters in the USA, ranges of 14–290 µg/litre in groundwater and 16–1170 µg/litre in surface water were reported (4). In the United Kingdom, concentrations of 200–300 µg/litre were associated with low pH levels and 400–600 µg/litre with an afforested catchment (5).

Aluminium salts are used as coagulants in water treatment. Residual aluminium concentrations in finished waters are a function of the aluminium levels in the source water, the amount of aluminium coagulant used, and the efficiency of filtration of the aluminium floc. Where residual concentrations are high, aluminium may be deposited in the distribution system, and a gradual reduction with increasing distance from the treatment plant may then be observed. Disturbance of the deposits by changes in flow rate may increase aluminium levels at the tap and render the water aesthetically unacceptable (6).

### Food

The concentrations of aluminium in food vary widely depending on the nature of the foodstuffs. Studies suggest that aluminium leached from tea leaves can make a significant contribution to dietary intake (7). Use of food additives containing aluminium, such as preservatives, fillers, colouring agents, anticaking agents, emulsifiers, and baking powders, also increases dietary intake.

In addition to its presence in food *per se*, aluminium leaching from cooking utensils may represent a potential source of dietary exposure (8, 9). Use of aluminium by the food industry in containers and packaging constitutes another dietary source (10).

It should be noted that the ubiquitous nature of aluminium makes it difficult to ensure freedom from contamination throughout the various stages of analysis. The reported concentrations of aluminium in foodstuffs such as vegetables, which are readily contaminated with soil, appear to be decreasing as analytical techniques improve.

### Pharmaceuticals

The use of antacids, analgesics, and other aluminium-containing medications is a significant source of exposure for some individuals (11,12).

### Estimated total exposure and relative contribution of drinking-water

A value of 20 mg/day has been suggested as a "typical" daily aluminium intake (13,14). However, because of individual and geographical variations in eating and drinking habits, a range of 5–20 mg of aluminium per day is probably more realistic. Aluminium in drinking-water will usually contribute only a very small proportion of the total daily intake. If a contribution of 20 mg/day from food is assumed, an adult drinking 2 litres of water per day containing 200 µg of aluminium per litre would receive approximately 2% of his or her total intake from drinking-water.

## 13.1.4 Kinetics and metabolism in laboratory animals and humans

Studies suggest that less than 1% of dietary inorganic aluminium is absorbed (15, 16). Factors affecting absorption may include vitamin D and fluoride (17) and the presence of complexing agents (18). Aluminium, once absorbed, appears to bind to serum proteins (19); it is eliminated from the body by the kidneys (17). Individuals with renal insufficiency tend to accumulate aluminium as a consequence of their inability to excrete it via the kidneys (20).

## 13.1.5 Effects on laboratory animals and *in vitro* test systems

### Short-term exposure

Groups of 25 male Sprague-Dawley rats were fed diets containing basic sodium aluminium phosphates or aluminium hydroxide at mean aluminium doses ranging from 67 to 302 mg/kg of body weight per day for 28 days. No treatment-related effects on body weight, organ weights, haematology, and clinical chemistry were observed, and there was no evidence of increased aluminium concentrations in bone (21).

In a study in which rats received drinking-water containing aluminium nitrate for 1 month, elevated aluminium levels were found in the heart and spleen, and histological changes were apparent in the liver and spleen at doses of 54 and 108 mg of aluminium per kg of body weight per day. No adverse effects were observed at a dose level of 27 mg of aluminium per kg of body weight per day (22).

Rats fed diets containing aluminium hydroxide at 257 or 1075 mg of aluminium per kg of diet for 67 days, equivalent to 13 or 54 mg of aluminium per kg of body weight per day, exhibited elevated levels of aluminium in the tibia, liver, and kidneys. Reduced bone strengths were also noted at the highest dose level (23).

Groups of 10 female Sprague-Dawley rats received aluminium nitrate in their drinking-water at doses of 0, 360, 720, or 3600 mg/kg of body weight for 100 days (equivalent to 0, 26, 52, or 260 mg of aluminium per kg of body weight per day). The only effect observed was depression of body weight gain associated with reduced water and feed intake at the highest dose level. Organ weight, histopathology of the brain, heart, lungs, kidneys, liver, and spleen, haematology, and some clinical chemistry indices were also examined (24).

Rats given oral doses of 0.0025, 0.25, or 2.5 mg of aluminium per kg of body weight for 6 months exhibited some changes in behaviour and mild changes in the biochemistry of the testes at the highest dose level, but there were no significant effects at the lower doses (25).

In a study in which dogs (4 per sex per dose) were fed diets containing basic sodium aluminium phosphate at 0, 3000, 10 000, or 30 000 mg/kg (mean daily aluminium doses of 4, 10, 27, or 75 mg/kg of body weight for males and 3, 10, 22, or 80 mg/kg of body weight for females) for 26 weeks, mild histopathological changes were observed in the liver, kidney, and testes of males in the highest-dose group, whereas brain aluminium concentrations were slightly elevated in females given the highest dose. No effects were noted at the lower dose levels (26).

### Long-term exposure

Chronic oral intake of aluminium in the diet at doses of about 50 or 100 mg/kg of body weight per day decreased locomotor responses and slowed the acquisition of avoidance behaviour in rats (27). In other studies in rats, it was reported that

135

aluminium produced osteomalacia (28) and microcytic anaemia (29), initiated impairment of kidney function (30), and caused damage to the lysosomes in the liver, spleen, and kidneys (31).

### Reproductive toxicity, embryotoxicity, and teratogenicity

An increase in the aluminium content of the placenta and fetus was found when pregnant mice were given oral doses of aluminium chloride (equivalent to 0, 40, or 60 mg of aluminium per kg of body weight per day) on days 7–16 of gestation (32). No evidence of embryotoxicity or teratogenicity was found in a study of pregnant rats fed aluminium chloride in their diet on days 6–19 of gestation at doses of approximately 5 or 10 mg of aluminium per kg of body weight per day (33). A delay in weight gain and neuromotor development was reported in the offspring of rats given oral doses of aluminium chloride (equivalent to 155 or 192 mg of aluminium per kg of body weight per day) from day 8 of gestation to parturition (34).

Mouse dams fed a diet containing 500 or 1000 mg of aluminium per kg (equivalent to 75 or 150 mg/kg of body weight per day) exhibited neurotoxicity, and their offspring showed neurological changes consistent with maternal toxicity and subsequent delayed development (35). In a study in which groups of 10 pregnant rats were given oral doses of aluminium nitrate of 0, 180, 360, or 720 mg/kg of body weight per day from day 14 of gestation to day 21 of lactation, offspring of dams receiving the highest dose exhibited depressed body weight gain (36).

No evidence of impaired reproductive performance was observed in male rats receiving drinking-water containing aluminium chloride at doses of approximately 0.5, 5, or 50 mg of aluminium per kg of body weight per day for 90 days (37).

### 13.1.6 Effects on humans

In the early 1970s, a syndrome known as dialysis dementia was described in patients on dialysis, characterized by an insidious onset of altered behaviour, dementia, speech disturbance, muscular twitching, and convulsions, usually with a fatal outcome. Patients had markedly elevated serum aluminium levels with increased concentrations in many tissues, including the cerebral cortex (38). Investigations established a correlation between the aluminium concentration in the water used to prepare the dialysate fluid and the incidence of the syndrome (39, 40). Aluminium from other sources, such as phosphate-binding gels, albumin, and peritoneal dialysis fluid, may also result in elevated aluminium levels in patients on dialysis.

Aluminium has been implicated in the etiology of two severe neurodegenerative diseases, amyotrophic lateral sclerosis and parkinsonism dementia, observed at very high incidence among the Chamorro people of Guam. One hypothesis suggests that chronic nutritional deficiencies of calcium and magnesium might lead to increased absorption of aluminium, resulting in its deposition in neurons (*41*), with consequent interference with their structure and eventual formation of the neurofibrillary tangles in the brain that characterize these diseases (*42*).

In Alzheimer disease, the first recognizable symptoms are memory lapses, disorientation, confusion, and frequently depression. These symptoms mark the start of a progressive mental deterioration for which there is no treatment. Aluminium is one of numerous causal factors that have been proposed for this disease. The brains of Alzheimer patients appear to have elevated levels of aluminium in regions containing large numbers of neurofibrillary tangles (*43, 44*).

Several hypotheses have been put forward to explain the role of aluminium in Alzheimer disease. The normal blood–brain and cytoplasmic barriers to aluminium may be defective, allowing aluminium to enter the nuclei of brain neurons (*45*). The localization of aluminium in the amyloid plaque cores of Alzheimer brains has led to the proposition that aluminium might in some way be involved in initiating events leading to plaque formation (*46*). Aluminium present in the DNA-containing structures of nuclei from the affected regions of such brains may reduce transcription and account for disorders in many cellular processes (*47*). It has also been proposed that aluminium may interfere with calcium metabolism (*48*).

Few attempts have been made to study the relationship between Alzheimer disease and exposure to aluminium from an epidemiological point of view. Vogt (*49*) investigated the relationship between concentrations of aluminium in water and the frequency of Alzheimer disease in southern Norway. Rates of mortality associated with dementia listed as the cause of death on death certificates were found to correlate positively with concentrations of aluminium in the water of different geographical areas. However, this study had a number of weaknesses, including the use of data on raw water rather than on distributed supplies, dubious epidemiological statistics, and inadequate adjustment for other confounding factors.

In a further retrospective epidemiological study of Alzheimer disease and aluminium in drinking-water in Norway, it was concluded that a geographical association existed between aluminium in drinking-water and registered death rates from dementia (*50*). However, rates of dementia were also correlated with population density and other socioeconomic variables, so that the evidence provided by this study must be regarded as very weak.

An epidemiological study has been carried out in the United Kingdom in which exposure to aluminium from drinking-water was calculated from data provided by local water undertakings (*51*). Rates of Alzheimer disease were estimated from the records of computerized tomographic scanning units. Districts in which aluminium concentrations in drinking-water exceeded 0.01 mg/litre (four subsets: 0.02–0.04 mg/litre, 0.05–0.07 mg/litre, 0.08–0.11 mg/litre, and >0.11 mg/litre) were found to have an approximately 50% greater incidence of Alzheimer disease as compared with those in which aluminium concentrations were below 0.01 mg/litre (one set only). A slight but unconvincing increase in the rate of Alzheimer disease was found with increasing aluminium concentrations for patients aged 40–64 but not those aged 40–69. As all four sets of districts with aluminium concentrations above 0.01 mg/litre showed a higher, and similar, incidence of Alzheimer disease as compared with the set with concentrations below 0.01 mg/litre, the conclusions of this study seem to hinge on the ability of the data to represent adequately the incidence of Alzheimer disease in the latter group.

These three studies give some support to the hypothesis of a positive relationship between the concentration of aluminium in drinking-water and the incidence of Alzheimer disease. The results cannot be considered as conclusive, however, as there are particular difficulties in evaluating the relationship between aluminium and Alzheimer disease by epidemiological means, namely doubts as to the reliability of the data for aluminium exposure and the ability to identify accurately the frequency of Alzheimer disease in different areas, and the possibility of unknown confounding factors.

## 13.1.7 Conclusions

Aluminium is of low toxicity in laboratory animals, and JECFA established a provisional tolerable weekly intake (PTWI) of 7 mg/kg of body weight in 1988 (52). However, this was based on studies of aluminium phosphate (acidic), which is not the chemical form in which aluminium is present in drinking-water.

In some studies, aluminium appeared to be associated with the brain lesions characteristic of Alzheimer disease, and in a few ecological epidemiological studies the incidence of this disease has been associated with aluminium in drinking-water. These ecological analyses must be interpreted with caution and need to be confirmed by analytical epidemiological studies.

While further studies are needed, the balance of epidemiological and physiological evidence does not at present support a causal role for aluminium in Alzheimer disease. No health-based guideline value is therefore derived. However, a concentration of aluminium of 0.2 mg/litre in drinking-water provides a compromise between the practical use of aluminium salts in water treatment and discoloration of distributed water.

## References

1.  Lide DR, ed. *CRC handbook of chemistry and physics*, 73rd ed. Boca Raton, FL, CRC Press, 1992–93.

2.  Gardner MJ, Gunn AM. Bioavailability of aluminium from food and drinking-water. In: Lord Walton of Detchant, ed. *Alzheimer's disease and the environment.* London, Royal Society of Medicine Services, 1991 (Round Table Series 26).

3.  Jones KC, Bennet BG. *Exposure commitment assessments of environmental pollutants,* Vol. 4. *Aluminium.* London, University of London, Monitoring and Assessment Research Centre, 1985 (MARC Report No. 33).

4.  Miller RG et al. The occurence of aluminium in drinking-water. *Journal of the American Water Works Association,* 1984, 76(1):84-91.

5.  Bull KR, Hall JR. Aluminium in the rivers Esk and Duddon, Cumbria and their tributaries. *Environmental pollution (Series B),* 1986, 12:165-193.

6.  Ainsworth RG, Oliphant R, Ridgway JW. *The introduction of new water into old distribution systems.* Medmenham, Water Research Centre, 1980 (TR 146).

7.  Fairweather-Tait SJ, Moore GR, Fatemi SEJ. Low levels of aluminium in tea. *Nature,* 1987, 330:213.

8.  Vozam L. [Content of aluminium in the diet and its biological action.] *Voprosy pitanija,* 1962, 21:28 (in Russian).

9.  Trapp GA, Cannon JB. Aluminium pots as a source of dietary aluminium. *New England journal of medicine,* 1981, 304:172.

10. Greger JL. Aluminium content of the American diet. *Food technology,* 1985, 39:73-80.

11. Sorenson JRJ et al. Aluminium in the environment and human health. *Environmental health perspectives,* 1984, 8:3-95.

12. Spencer H et al. Effect of small doses of aluminum-containing antacids on calcium and phosphorus metabolism. *American journal of clinical nutrition,* 1982, 36:32-40.

13. Mertz W, ed. *Trace elements in human and animal nutrition,* 5th ed. New York, Academic Press, 1986–1987.

14. US Federation of American Societies for Experimental Biology. *Evaluation of the health aspects of aluminium compounds as food ingredients.* Washington, DC, 1975 (Report FDA BF-77 24; NTIS PB-262-655).

15. Gorsky JE et al. Metabolic balance of aluminum studied in six men. *Clinical chemistry,* 1979, 25:1739-1743.

16. Greger JL, Baier MJ. Excretion and retention of low or moderate levels of aluminium by human subjects. *Food chemistry and toxicology,* 1983, 21:473-477.

17. Alfrey AC. Aluminum metabolism. *Kidney international,* 1986, 29(18):8-11.

18. Slanina P et al. Dietary citric acid enhances adsorption of aluminum antacids. *Clinical chemistry,* 1986, 32:539-541.

19. Trapp GA. Plasma aluminum is bound to transferrin. *Life sciences*, 1983, 33:311-316.

20. Davenport A, Roberts NB. Serum aluminium levels in acute renal failure. *Lancet*, 1986, 2:1397-1398.

21. Hicks JS, Hackett DS, Sprague GL. Toxicity and aluminium concentration in bone following dietary administration of two sodium aluminium phosphate formulations in rats. *Food chemistry and toxicology*, 1987, 25:533-538.

22. Gomez M et al. Short-term oral toxicity study of aluminium in rats. *Archivos de farmacología y toxicología*, 1986, 12:144-151.

23. Greger JL, Gum ET, Bula EN. Mineral metabolism of rats fed various levels of aluminium hydroxide. *Biological trace element research*, 1986, 9:67-77.

24. Domingo JL et al. Nutritional and toxicological effects of short-term ingestion of aluminium by the rat. *Research communications in chemical pathology and pharmacology*, 1987, 56:409-419.

25. Krasovskii GN, Vasukovich LY, Chariev OG. Experimental study of biological effects of lead and aluminum following oral administration. *Environmental health perspectives*, 1979, 30:47-51.

26. Pettersen JC et al. Twenty-six week toxicity study with KASAL® (basic sodium aluminum phosphate) in beagle dogs. *Environmental and geochemical health*, 1990, 12:121-123.

27. Commissaris RL et al. Behavioral changes in rats after chronic aluminum and parathyroid hormone administration. *Neurobehaviorial toxicology and teratology*, 1982, 4:403-410.

28. Chan Y et al. Effects of aluminium on normal and uremic rats: tissue distribution, vitamin D metabolites, and quantitative bone histology. *Calcified tissue international*, 1983, 35:344-351.

29. Kaiser L et al. Microcytic anemia secondary to intraperitoneal aluminum in normal and uremic rats. *Kidney international*, 1984, 26:269-274.

30. Braunlich H et al. Renal effects of aluminium in uraemic rats and in rats with intact kidney function. *Journal of applied toxicology*, 1986, 6:55-59.

31. Stein G et al. Aluminium induced damage of the lysosomes in the liver, spleen and kidneys of rats. *Journal of applied toxicology*, 1987, 7:253-258.

32. Cranmer JM et al. Fetal-placental-maternal uptake of aluminium in mice following gestational exposure: effect of dose and route of administration. *Neurotoxicology*, 1986, 7:601-608.

33. McCormack KM et al. Effect of prenatal administration of aluminum and parathyroid hormone on fetal development in the rat. *Proceedings of the Society for Experimental Biology and Medicine*, 1979, 161:74-77.

34. Bernuzzi V, Desor D, Lehr PR. Effects of prenatal aluminum exposure on neuromotor maturation in the rat. *Neurobehavioral toxicology and teratology*, 1986, 8:115-119.

35. Golub MS et al. Maternal and developmental toxicity of chronic aluminum exposure in mice. *Fundamental and applied toxicology*, 1987, 8:346-357.

36. Domingo JL et al. Effects of oral aluminium administration on perinatal and postnatal development in rats. *Research communications in chemical pathology and pharmacology*, 1987, 57:129-132.

37. Dixon RL, Sherins RJ, Lee ID. Assessment of environmental factors affecting male fertility. *Environmental health perspectives*, 1979, 30:53-68.

38. Alfrey AC, Legendre GR, Kaehny WD. The dialysis encephalopathy syndrome. Possible aluminium intoxication. *New England journal of medicine*, 1976, 294:184-188.

39. Savory J, Wills MR. Dialysis fluids as a source of aluminium accumulation. *Contributions in nephrology*, 1984, 38:12-23.

40. Davison AM et al. Water supply aluminium concentration, dialysis dementia and effect of reverse-osmosis water treatment. *Lancet*, 1982, 2:785-787.

41. Garruto RM, Yase Y. Neurodegenerative disorders of the Western Pacific: the search for mechanisms of pathogenesis. *Trends in neurosciences*, 1986, 9:368-374.

42. Garruto RM, Yanagihara R, Carleton Gajdusek D. Models of environmentally induced neurological disease: epidemiology and etiology of amyotrophic lateral sclerosis and parkinsonism-dementia in the Western Pacific. *Environmental geochemistry and health*, 1990, 12(1/2):137-151.

43. Crapper DR, Krishnan SS, Quittkat S. Aluminium, neurofibrillary degeneration and Alzheimer's disease. *Brain*, 1976, 99:67-80.

44. Perl DP, Brody AR. Alzheimer's disease: X-ray spectrometric evidence of aluminum accumulation in neurofibrillary tangle-bearing neurons. *Science*, 1980, 208:297-299.

45. Crapper DR et al. Intranuclear aluminum content in Alzheimer's disease, dialysis encephalopathy and experimental aluminum encephalopathy. *Acta neuropathologica (Berlin)*, 1980, 50:19-24.

46. Candy J et al. Aluminosilicates and senile plaque formation in Alzheimer's disease. *Lancet*, 1986, i:354-357.

47. Crapper DR et al. Brain aluminum in Alzheimer's disease: influence of sample size and case selection. *Neurotoxicology*, 1980, 1(4):25-32.

48. Deary IJ, Hendrickson AE. Calcium and Alzheimer's disease. *Lancet*, 1986, 1:1219.

49. Vogt T. *Water quality and health—study of possible relation between aluminium in drinking-water and dementia.* Oslo, Central Bureau of Statistics of Norway, 1986 (Sosiale og Økonomiske Studier 61) (English abstract).

50. Flaten TP. *Geographical associations between aluminium in drinking-water and death rates with dementia (including Alzheimer's Disease), Parkinson's disease and amyotrophic lateral sclerosis in Norway.* Paper presented at the Workshop on Aluminium and Health, Oslo, Norway, 2-5 May 1988.

51. Martyn CN et al. Geographical relation between Alzheimer's disease and aluminium in drinking-water. *Lancet*, 1989, 1:59-62.

52. *Toxicological evaluation of certain food additives and contaminants.* Geneva, World Health Organization, 1989:113-154 (WHO Food Additives Series, No. 24).

# 13.2 Ammonia

## 13.2.1 General description

### Identity

CAS no.: 7664-41-7
Molecular formula: $NH_3$

In what follows, the term "ammonia" covers both the nonionized form ($NH_3$) and the ammonium cation ($NH_4^+$) unless stated otherwise.

### Physicochemical properties (1, 2)

| Property | Value |
| --- | --- |
| Melting point | -77.76 °C |
| Boiling point | -33.43 °C |
| Density of vapour | 0.6 g/litre at 20 °C |
| Water solubility | 421 g/litre at 20 °C; 706 g/litre at 0 °C |
| Vapour pressure | 882 kPa at 20 °C |

### Organoleptic properties

The threshold odour concentration of ammonia in water is approximately 1.5 mg/litre.[1] A taste threshold of 35 mg/litre has been proposed for the ammonium cation (1).

### Major uses

Ammonia is used in fertilizer and animal feed production and in the manufacture of fibres, plastics, explosives, paper, and rubber. It is used as a coolant, in metal processing, and as a starting product for many nitrogen-containing compounds (3). Ammonia and ammonium salts are used in cleansing agents and as food additives (1, 4), and ammonium chloride is used as a diuretic.[2]

### Environmental fate

On dissolution in water, ammonia forms the ammonium cation; hydroxyl ions are formed at the same time. The equilibrium constant of this reaction, $K_B$ is 1.78 x 10$^{-5}$ (3). The degree of ionization depends on the temperature, the pH, and the concentration of dissolved salts in the water.

The environmental cycling of nitrogen relies mainly on nitrate, followed by ammonia and the ammonium cation, which predominates. The ammonium cation is less mobile in soil and water than ammonia and is involved in the biological processes of nitrogen fixation, mineralization, and nitrification (2).

## 13.2.2 Analytical methods

Ammonia and ammonium cation at concentrations between 0.025 and 3 mg/litre can be determined by the indophenol reaction (1, 2, 5, 6). An ammonia-selective electrode can also be used, as can titrimetry, which is less sensitive (2, 5, 6).

## 13.2.3 Environmental levels and human exposure

### Air

Air in urban areas contains up to 20 µg of ammonia per m$^3$. Air in areas where farm animals are reared intensively may contain levels as high as 300 µg/m$^3$ (7).

---

[1] Source: *Hazardous Substances Data Bank: Ammonia.* Bethesda, MD, National Library of Medicine, 1990.

[2] Source: *Hazardous Substances Data Bank: Ammonium chloride.* Bethesda, MD, National Library of Medicine, 1990.

### Water

Natural levels in groundwaters are usually below 0.2 mg of ammonia per litre. Higher natural contents (up to 3 mg/litre) are found in strata rich in humic substances or iron or in forests (8). Surface waters may contain up to 12 mg/litre (1). Ammonia may be present in drinking-water as a result of disinfection with chloramines.

The presence of ammonia at higher than geogenic levels is an important indicator of faecal pollution (5). Taste and odour problems as well as decreased disinfection efficiency are to be expected if drinking-water containing more than 0.2 mg of ammonia per litre is chlorinated (9), as up to 68% of the chlorine may react with the ammonia and become unavailable for disinfection (10). Cement mortar used for coating the insides of water pipes may release considerable amounts of ammonia into drinking-water and compromise disinfection with chlorine (10).

The presence of elevated ammonia levels in raw water may interfere with the operation of manganese-removal filters because too much oxygen is consumed by nitrification, resulting in mouldy, earthy-tasting water (8). The presence of the ammonium cation in raw water may result in a drinking-water containing nitrite as the result of catalytic action (11) or the accidental colonization of filters by ammonium-oxidizing bacteria.

### Food

Ammonium is a natural component of many foods. Minor amounts of ammonium compounds (<0.001–3.2%) are also added to foods as acid regulators, stabilizers, flavouring substances, and fermentation aids (1).

### Estimated total exposure and relative contribution of drinking-water

The estimated daily ammonia intake through food and drinking-water is 18 mg, by inhalation less than 1 mg, and through cigarette smoking (20 cigarettes per day) also less than 1 mg. In contrast, 4000 mg of ammonia per day are produced endogenously in the human intestine (1).

## 13.2.4 Kinetics and metabolism in laboratory animals and humans

Ammonia is a key metabolite in mammals. It has an essential role in acid–base regulation and the biosynthesis of purines, pyrimidines, and non-essential amino acids (2). It is formed in the body by the deamination of amino acids in the liver, as a metabolite in nerve excitation and muscular activity, and in the gastrointestinal tract by the enzymatic breakdown of food components with the assistance of bacterial flora.[1] About 99% of metabolically produced ammonia is absorbed from the gastrointestinal tract and transported to the liver, where it is incorporated into urea as part of the urea cycle. Urea formed in the liver is absorbed by the blood, transferred to the kidney, and excreted in urine (2). Of the ammonia found in urine, two-thirds originates from the tubular epithelium of the kidney where, as a product of the glutaminase reaction, it maintains the acid–base equilibrium by the uptake of hydrogen ions (1).

## 13.2.5 Effects on laboratory animals and *in vitro* test systems

### *Acute exposure*

Oral $LD_{50}$ values for ammonium salts are in the range 350–750 mg/kg of body weight (4). Single doses of different ammonium salts at 200–500 mg/kg of body weight resulted in lung oedema, nervous system dysfunction, acidosis, and kidney damage (1).

### *Short-term exposure*

Animals subchronically exposed to different ammonium salts (75–360 mg/kg of body weight as the ammonium ion) in drinking-water exhibited physiological adaptation to induced acidosis, slight organ effects, or increased blood pressure (1, 2).

### *Long-term exposure*

In male Sprague-Dawley rats given drinking-water containing 1.5% ammonium chloride (about 478 mg of ammonium ion per kg of body weight per day) over a period of 330 days, significant decreases were found in bone mass, calcium content, and blood pH. The treated animals also had lower body weights and lower fat accumulation than controls (1).

### *Reproductive toxicity, embryotoxicity, and teratogenicity*

Oral administration of different ammonium compounds at doses of 100–200 mg/kg of body weight to impuberal female rabbits resulted in enlargement of the ovaries and uterus, hypertrophy of the breast with milk secretion, follicular ripening, and formation of the corpus luteum. A dose of 0.9% ammonium chloride (approximately 290 mg of ammonia per kg of body weight per day) in the drinking-water of pregnant rats inhibited fetal growth but had no teratogenic effects (1).

---

[1] Source: *Hazardous Substances Data Bank: Ammonia.* Bethesda, MD, National Library of Medicine, 1990.

### Mutagenicity and related end-points

At high concentrations, positive results in the Balb e/3T3-transformation test, the sex-linked dominant/lethal mutation test, and chromosomal aberrations in fibroblasts of Chinese hamsters were observed; other genotoxicity tests gave negative results (2).

### Carcinogenicity

There is no evidence that ammonia is carcinogenic (2).

## 13.2.6 Effects on humans

Ammonia has a toxic effect on healthy humans only if the intake becomes higher than the capacity to detoxify.

If ammonia is administered in the form of its ammonium salts, the effects of the anion must also be taken into account. With ammonium chloride, the acidotic effects of the chloride ion seem to be of greater importance than those of the ammonium ion (1). At a dose of more than 100 mg/kg of body weight per day (33.7 mg of ammonium ion per kg of body weight per day), ammonium chloride influences metabolism by shifting the acid–base equilibrium, disturbing the glucose tolerance, and reducing the tissue sensitivity to insulin (2).

## 13.2.7 Conclusions

Ammonia is not of direct importance for health in the concentrations to be expected in drinking-water. A health-based guideline has therefore not been derived.

Ammonia can, however, indicate faecal contamination, compromise disinfection efficiency, cause taste and odour problems, result in nitrite formation in distribution systems, and cause the failure of filters for the removal of manganese.

## References

1. *Ammonia*. Geneva, World Health Organization, 1986 (Environmental Health Criteria, No. 54).

2. *Summary review of health effects associated with ammonia.* Washington, DC, US Environmental Protection Agency, 1989 (EPA/600/8-89/052F).

3. Holleman AF, Wiberg E. *Lehrbuch der anorganischen Chemie.* [*Textbook of inorganic chemistry.*] Berlin, Walter de Gruyter, 1985.

4. Institut National de Recherche et de Sécurité de France (INRS). Ammoniac et solutions aqueuses, fiche toxicologique 16. *Cahiers de notes documentaires*, 1987, 128:461-465.

5.  International Organization for Standardization. *Water quality—determination of ammonium*. Geneva, 1984, 1986 (ISO5664:1984; ISO6778:1984; ISO7150-1:1984; ISO7150-2:1986).

6.  *Standard methods for the examination of water and wastewater*, 17th ed. Washington, DC, American Public Health Association/American Water Works Association/Water Pollution Control Federation, 1989.

7.  Ellenberg H, 1987. Cited in: Skeffington RA, Wilson EJ. Excess nitrogen deposition: issues for consideration. *Environmental pollution*, 1988, 54:159-184.

8.  Dieter HH, Möller R. Ammonium. In: Aurand K et al., eds. *Die Trinkwasser verordnung, Einführung und Erläuterungen.* [*The drinking-water regulations, introduction and explanations.*] Berlin, Erich-Schmidt Verlag, 1991:362-368.

9.  Weil D, Quentin KE. Bildung und Wirkungsweise der Chloramine bei der Trinkwasseraufbereitung. [Formation and mode of action of chloramines in drinking-water treatment.] 1. Teil (parts 1 and 2). *Zeitschrift für Wasser und Abwasser Forschung*, 1975, 8:5-16; 46-56.

10. Wendlandt E. Ammonium/Ammoniak als Ursache für Wiederverkeimungen in Trinkwasserleitungen. [Ammonium/ammonia as cause of bacterial regrowth in drinking-water pipes.] *Gas- und Wasserfach, Wasser-Abwasser*, 1988, 129:567-571.

11. Reichert J, Lochtmann S. Auftreten von Nitrit in Wasserversorgungssystemen. [Occurrence of nitrite in water distribution systems.] *Gas- und Wasserfach, Wasser-Abwasser*, 1984, 125:442-446.

# 13.3 Antimony

## 13.3.1 General description

### Identity

| Compound | CAS no. | Molecular formula |
|---|---|---|
| Antimony | 7440-36-0 | Sb |
| Potassium antimony tartrate | 28300-74-5 | $KSbOC_4H_4O_6$ |
| Sodium antimony tartrate | 34521-09-0 | $NaSbOC_4H_4O_6$ |
| Sodium antimony bis(pyrocatechol) 2,4-disulfate | 15489-16-4 | $C_{12}H_{18}Na_5O_{23}S_4Sb$ |

## *Physicochemical properties (1–3)*[1]

| Property | Sb | $KSbOC_4H_4O_6$ | $NaSbOC_4H_4O_6$ | $C_{12}H_{18}Na_5O_{23}S_4Sb$ |
|---|---|---|---|---|
| Melting point (°C) | 630.5 | 100 | – | – |
| Boiling point (°C) | 1635 | – | – | – |
| Density at 20 °C (g/cm³) | 6.691 | 2.6 | – | – |
| Vapour pressure at 886 °C (kPa) | 0.133 | – | – | – |
| Water solubility (g/litre) | insoluble | 83 | 666.7 | soluble |

## *Organoleptic properties*

Potassium antimony tartrate is odourless and has a sweet metallic taste (*2*).

## *Major uses*

Antimony is used in semiconductor alloys, batteries, antifriction compounds, ammunition, cable sheathing, flameproofing compounds, ceramics, glass, pottery, type castings for commercial printing, solder alloys, and fireworks. Some antimony compounds are used for the treatment of parasitic diseases and as pesticides (*1–3*).

## *Environmental fate*

Antimony may be present in the atmosphere in gaseous, vapour, and particulate forms. In water, it may undergo either oxidation or reduction, depending on the pH and the other ions present. Soluble forms tend to be quite mobile in water, whereas less soluble species are adsorbed onto clay or soil particles. Antimony may be leached from landfills and sewage sludge into groundwater, surface water, and sediment (*4*), from the last of which it can be released to the atmosphere through microbial activity under anaerobic conditions (*5*). More than half of the naturally occurring antimony in sediments is bound to extractable iron and aluminium (*6*). Antimony is only slightly bioaccumulated.

## 13.3.2 Analytical methods

Antimony can be determined by graphite furnace atomic absorption spectrometry (lower detection limit 0.8 µg/litre, EPA method 204.2) or inductively coupled plasma mass spectrometry (lower detection limit 0.02 µg/litre, EPA method 6020). Following separation of antimony(III) from antimony(V) using

---

[1] Source: *Hazardous Substances Data Bank*. Bethesda, MD, National Library of Medicine, 1990.

N-(p-methoxyphenyl)-2-furylacrylohydroxamic acid, the two species can be determined by electrothermal atomic absorption spectrometry at concentrations down to 0.01 µg/litre (7).

### 13.3.3 Environmental levels and human exposure

**Air**

Antimony was present in the air of four of 58 American cities at levels of 0.42–0.85 µg/m$^3$. Three of 29 nonurban areas had concentrations of 1–2 ng/m$^3$ (8). Smoking can result in antimony contamination of indoor air (9).

**Water**

Antimony has been identified in natural waters in both the antimony(III) and antimony(V) oxidation states and as methyl antimony compounds. It occurs in seawater at a concentration of about 0.2 µg/litre (10, 11). A survey in the USA found antimony in only three of 988 samples of finished drinking-water from groundwater sources, the concentrations ranging from 41 to 45 µg/litre (lower detection limit 9 µg/litre)(12). In a study of 3834 samples of drinking-water, antimony was found in 16.5% of samples, at concentrations ranging from 0.6 to 4 µg/litre (mean 1.87 µg/litre) (13).

**Food**

Trace quantities of antimony are present in the food supply, the concentration in the diet of a typical adult male being 9.3 µg/kg dry weight based on the analysis of food composites (14).

**Estimated total exposure and relative contribution of drinking-water**

The average intake of antimony by ingestion of food is about 18 µg/day (14); the corresponding figure for drinking-water will usually be less than 8 µg/day.

### 13.3.4 Kinetics and metabolism in laboratory animals and humans

Antimony is not readily absorbed from the gastrointestinal tract, regardless of valence state (15), absorption ranging from less than 5% in cows (16) to 15% in rats (17). Most of the antimony absorbed accumulates in the spleen, liver, and bone (18, 19). Transfer of antimony from maternal to fetal blood has been demonstrated (20). Trivalent antimony readily enters red blood cells, but pentavalent antimony does not (21, 22). Available data are insufficient to determine whether antimony(V) compounds are reduced to antimony(III) in vivo. Parenterally administered trivalent antimony was excreted via the faeces and urine in mice, white rats, hamsters, guinea-pigs, rabbits, dogs, and humans (23). Pentavalent antimony was excreted primarily in the urine. In cows, orally administered antimony trichloride was excreted primarily in the faeces (*16*). In adult males, 21.6–70% of the antimony administered daily was excreted in urine, only low levels (0.8–8.4%) being present in faeces. Pentavalent antimony was excreted in urine more rapidly than trivalent antimony (*22, 24*).

## 13.3.5 Effects on laboratory animals and *in vitro* test systems

### Acute exposure

The acute oral $LD_{50}$ values for potassium antimony tartrate in mice and rats range from 115 to 600 mg of antimony per kg of body weight, whereas an oral $LD_{50}$ of 15 mg of antimony per kg of body weight has been reported for rabbits (*4*).

### Short-term exposure

Four rabbits were given potassium antimony tartrate at 15 mg/kg of body weight per day (5.6 mg of antimony per kg of body weight per day) for 7–22 days (*25*). Small increases in nonprotein nitrogen in blood and urine and in mean urine ammonia nitrogen were observed, which the author interpreted as evidence of increased protein catabolism. Gross and microscopic examination showed haemorrhagic lesions in the stomach and small intestine, liver atrophy with fat accumulation and congestion, haemorrhage in the renal cortex, with some tubular necrosis. This study suggests a LOAEL of 5.6 mg/kg of body weight per day, based on minimal histological injury in tissues.

Male and female Wistar rats were given two antimony-containing pigments in the diet at concentrations up to 10 000 mg/kg (36 and 22 mg/kg of body weight per day, respectively) for 91 days. No effects on behaviour, food consumption, growth, mortality, haematology, clinical data, or organ weights were observed (*26*). No toxic effects were observed in rats given potassium antimony tartrate, potassium antimonate, antimony trioxide, or antimony pentoxide in food at doses ranging from 0.1 to 4 mg/day for 107 days (*1*).

### Long-term exposure

Potassium antimony tartrate (0 or 5 mg of antimony per litre) was administered in drinking-water to male and female Charles River CD mice from the time of weaning until death (*27*). Weight loss was observed in males after 18 months and decreased weight gain in females at 12 and 18 months, and life spans were decreased in females but not in males. No significant fatty degeneration of the liver was observed. This study suggests a LOAEL of 0.5 mg/kg of body weight per day.

In a companion study, potassium antimony tartrate (0 or 5 mg of antimony per litre) was administered in drinking-water to Long-Evans rats (50 per sex per dose) from the time of weaning until death (*28*). This corresponds to an average dose of 0.43 mg of antimony per kg of body weight per day, assuming a body weight of 0.35 kg and water consumption of 30 ml/day. No significant effects on glucosuria, proteinuria, fasting blood glucose levels, body weight, heart weight, or heart-to-body-weight ratio were observed. Mean longevity decreased in both sexes. Serum cholesterol levels were increased in male rats and decreased in female rats. Nonfasting blood glucose levels were lower in both sexes. Antimony accumulated in kidney, liver, heart, lung, and spleen, increasing with age and dose. This study identified a LOAEL of 0.43 mg of antimony per kg of body weight per day based on decreased longevity and altered blood glucose and serum cholesterol levels.

### Reproductive toxicity, embryotoxicity, and teratogenicity

Four ewes fed antimony potassium tartrate at a dose level of 2 mg/kg of body weight for 45 days or throughout gestation gave birth to normal, full-term lambs (*29*). Sterility and fewer offspring were observed in rats following inhalation exposures to antimony trioxide over 2 months (*1, 30*). In female rabbits and mice injected with sodium antimony tartrate or an unknown organic antimony compound over a period ranging from 16 to 77 days, some contraception, abortion, and fetal damage occurred, but sterility in male mice was not observed (*31*). No abnormalities were reported in Wistar rat fetuses whose mothers were given intramuscular injections of antimony dextran glycoside during gestation (*19*).

### Mutagenicity and related end-points

Antimony trichloride, antimony pentachloride, and antimony trioxide were mutagenic in the *Bacillus subtilis* (H17 and M45) *rec*-assay (*1, 32, 33*). Potassium and sodium antimony tartrate induced chromosomal aberrations in cultured human leukocytes (*34, 35*). Piperazine and potassium antimony tartrate induced chromosomal aberrations in rat bone marrow cells *in vivo* (*36*).

### Carcinogenicity

The effect of lifetime exposure to antimony on tumour frequency was investigated in Charles River CD mice given potassium antimony tartrate (0 or 5 mg of antimony per litre) in drinking-water from the time of weaning until death (*27*). Tumours (benign and malignant) were found in 34.8% of control animals (no explanation given) and 18.8% of the antimony-treated animals. The authors concluded that antimony exposure had no effect on the incidence or type of spontaneous tumours. In a companion study (*28*), no significant effects of antimony exposure on tumour frequency were observed in male or female rats.

Antimony trioxide and antimony ore concentrate were found to cause lung tumours in female rats exposed by inhalation (*1, 37, 38*).

## 13.3.6 Effects on humans

Acute antimony poisoning may result in vomiting, diarrhoea, and death (*39, 40*). Sodium stibogluconate given intravenously in a daily dose of 600 mg of antimony(V) for 10 days to 16 patients with skin lesions caused by parasitic protozoa did not adversely affect either glomerular or renal function (*41*). Trivalent and pentavalent antimony compounds affected the ECGs of patients being treated for schistosomiasis (*42, 43*).

Six adult males who had worked in an antimony smelter for 2–13 years exhibited no signs of adverse cardiac, bladder, kidney, or haematological effects, nor were there any reported effects on general health (*1, 44*). Workmen in a plant where antimony trisulfide was used exhibited increased blood pressure (14 of 113), significant changes in their ECGs (37 of 75), and ulcers (7 of 111 as compared with 15 out of 1000 in the total plant population) (*1, 45*). Female workers employed in an antimony plant showed an increased incidence of spontaneous late abortions (12.5%) as compared with female workers not exposed to antimony dust (4.1%) (*30*).

Workers exposed for 9–31 years to dust containing a mixture of antimony trioxide and antimony pentoxide in an antimony smelting plant (*1, 46*) exhibited symptoms such as chronic coughing, bronchitis, and emphysema, conjunctivitis, staining of frontal tooth surface, inactive tuberculosis, and pleural adhesions. "Antimony dermatitis" characterized by vesicular or pustular lesions was seen in more than half the exposed workers.

## 13.3.7 Provisional guideline value

In its overall evaluation based on inhalation exposure, IARC concluded that antimony trioxide is possibly carcinogenic to humans (Group 2B) and antimony trisulfide is not classifiable as to its carcinogenicity to humans (Group 3) (*1*).

In a limited lifetime study in which rats were exposed to antimony in drinking-water at a single dose level of 0.43 mg of antimony per kg of body weight per day, decreased longevity and altered blood levels of glucose and cholesterol were observed (*28*). The incidence of benign or malignant tumours was not affected. Using an uncertainty factor of 500 (100 for inter- and intraspecies variation and 5 for the use of a LOAEL instead of a NOAEL), a TDI of 0.86 µg/kg of body weight can be calculated. An allocation of 10% of the TDI to drinking-water gives a concentration of 0.003 mg/litre (rounded figure), which is below the practical limit of quantitative analysis.

A provisional guideline value for antimony has therefore been set at a practical quantification level of 0.005 mg/litre. This results in a margin of safety of approximately 250-fold for potential health effects, based on the LOAEL of 0.43 mg/kg of body weight per day observed in the limited lifetime study in rats.

## References

1.  International Agency for Research on Cancer. *Some organic solvents, resin monomers and related compounds, pigments and occupational exposures in paint manufacture and painting.* Lyon, 1989:291-305 (IARC Monographs on the Evaluation of Carcinogenic Risks to Humans, Vol. 47).

2.  Hawley GG. *The condensed chemical dictionary,* 10th ed. New York, Van Nostrand Reinhold, 1981.

3.  Weast RC, Astle MJ, Beyer WH, eds. *CRC handbook of chemistry and physics,* 70th ed. Boca Raton, FL, CRC Press, 1989.

4.  Callahan MA, Slimak MW, Gable NW. *Water-related environmental fate of 129 priority pollutants,* Vol. 1. *Final report.* Cincinnati, OH, US Environmental Protection Agency, 1979 (EPA-440/14-79-029A and B).

5.  Brannon JM, Patrick WH Jr. Fixation and mobilization of antimony in sediments. *Environmental pollution, Series B,* 1985, 9:107-126.

6.  Crecelius EA, Bothner MH, Carpenter R. Geochemistries of arsenic, antimony, mercury, and related elements in sediments of Puget Sound. *Environmental science and technology,* 1975, 9:325-333.

7.  Abbassi SA. Sub-micro determination of antimony(III) and antimony(V) in natural and polluted waters and total antimony in biological materials by flameless AAS following extractive separation with *N-p*-methoxy-phenyl-2-furylacrylohydroxamic acid. *Analytical letters,* 1989, 22(1):237-255.

8.  US Environmental Protection Agency. *Computer printout of air monitoring data for selected inorganics from the Aerometric Information Retrieval System (AIRS).* Research Triangle Park, NC, Office of Air Quality Planning and Standards, 1988.

9.  Gerhardsson L et al. Antimony in lung, liver, and kidney tissue from deceased smelter workers. *Scandinavian journal of work, environment and health,* 1983, 8:201-208.

10. Andreae MO, Asmode J, Van't Dack L. Determination of antimony(III), antimony(V) and methylantimony species in natural waters by atomic absorption spectrometry with hydride generation. *Analytical chemistry,* 1981, 53:1766-1771.

11. Byrd JT, Andreae MO. Distribution of arsenic and antimony in species in the Baltic Sea. *Transactions of the American Geophysical Union,* 1982, 63:71 (abstract).

12. Longtin JP. *Status report—national inorganics and radionuclides survey.* Cincinnati, OH, US Environmental Protection Agency, Office of Drinking Water, 1985.

13. *Antimony: an environmental and health effects assessment.* Washington, DC, US Environmental Protection Agency, Office of Drinking Water, 1984.

14. *Draft toxicological profile for antimony and compounds.* Atlanta, GA, US Department of Health and Human Services, Agency for Toxic Substances and Disease Registry, 1990.

15. Felicetti SA, Thomas RG, McClellan RC. Metabolism of two valence states of inhaled antimony in hamsters. *American Industrial Hygiene Association journal,* 1974, 35:292-300.

16. Van Bruwaene RE et al. Metabolism of antimony-124 in lactating cows. *Health physics,* 1982, 43:733-738.

17. Moskalev YI. Materials on the distribution of radioactive antimony. *Medical radiology,* 1959, 4(3):6-13.

18. Westrick ML. Physiologic responses attending administration of antimony, alone or with simultaneous injections of thyroxin. *Proceedings of the Society for Experimental Biology and Medicine,* 1953, 82:6-60.

19. Casals JB. Pharmacokinetic and toxicological studies of antimony dextran glycoside (RL-712). *British journal of pharmacology,* 1972, 46:281-288.

20. Leffler P, Nordström S. *Metals in maternal and fetal blood. Investigation of possible variations of the placental barrier function.* Vällingby, Statens Vattenfallsverk, 1984 (Project KOL-HÄLSA-MILJÖ, KHM-TR-71, DE83751427).

21. Molokhia MM, Smith H. The behaviour of antimony in blood. *Journal of tropical medicine and hygiene,* 1969, 72:222-225.

22. Otto GF, Maren TH, Brown HW. Blood levels and excretion rates of antimony in persons receiving trivalent and pentavalent antimonials. *American journal of hygiene,* 1947, 46:193-211.

23. Otto GF, Maren TH. VI. Studies on the excretion and concentration of antimony in blood and other tissues following the injection of trivalent and pentavalent antimonials into experimental animals. *American journal of hygiene,* 1950, 51:370-385.

24. Lippincott SW et al. A study of the distribution and fate of antimony when used as tartar emetic and fuadin in the treatment of American soldiers with schistosomiasis japonica. *Journal of clinical investigation,* 1947, 26:370-378.

25. Pribyl E. On the nitrogen metabolism in experimental subacute arsenic and antimony poisoning. *Journal of biological chemistry,* 1927, 74:775-781.

26. Bomhard E et al. Subchronic oral toxicity and analytical studies on nickel rutile yellow and chrome rutile yellow with rats. *Toxicology letters,* 1982, 14:189-194.

27. Schroeder HA et al. Zirconium, niobium, antimony and fluorine in mice: effects on growth, survival and tissue levels. *Journal of nutrition,* 1968, 95:95-101.

28. Schroeder HA, Mitchener M, Nason AP. Zirconium, niobium, antimony, vanadium and lead in rats: life term studies. *Journal of nutrition*, 1970, 100:59-68.

29. James LF, Lazar VA, Binns W. Effects of sublethal doses of certain minerals on pregnant ewes and fetal development. *American journal of veterinary research*, 1966, 27:132-135.

30. Beljaeva AP. [The effect of antimony on reproductive function.] *Gigiena truda i professional'nye zabolevanija*, 1967, 11(1):32-37 (in Russian).

31. Hodgson EC, Vardon AC, Singh Z. Studies of the effects of antimony salts on conception and pregnancy in animals. *Indian journal of medical research*, 1927, 15:491-495.

32. Kanematsu N, Kada T. Mutagenicity of metal compounds. *Mutation research*, 1978, 53:207-208.

33. Kanematsu N, Hara M, Kada T. *Rec* assay and mutagenicity studies on metal compounds. *Mutation research*, 1980, 77:109-116.

34. Paton GR, Allison AC. Chromosome damage in human cell cultures induced by metal salts. *Mutation research*, 1972, 16:332-336.

35. Hashem N, Shawki R. Cultured peripheral lymphocytes: one biologic indicator of potential drug hazard. *African journal of medical science*, 1976, 5(2):155-163.

36. El Nahas S, Temtamy SA, deHondt HA. Cytogenetic effect of two antimonial antibilharzial drugs: tartar emetic and bilharcid. *Environmental mutagenesis*, 1982, 4:83-91.

37. Watt WD. Chronic inhalation toxicity of antimony trioxide: validation of the threshold limit value. *Dissertation abstracts international, B*, 1983, 44:739.

38. Groth DH et al. Carcinogenic effects of antimony trioxide and antimony ore concentrate in rats. *Journal of toxicology and environmental health*, 1986, 18:607-626.

39. Kaplan E, Korff FA. Antimony in food poisoning. *Food research*, 1937, 1:529-536.

40. Miller JM. Poisoning by antimony: a case report. *Southern medical journal*, 1982, 75:592.

41. Jolliffe DS. Nephrotoxicity of pentavalent antimonials. *Lancet*, 1985, i:584.

42. Schroeder EF, Rose FA, Mast H. Effect of antimony on the electrocardiogram. *American journal of medical science*, 1946, 212:697-706.

43. Chulay JD, Spencer HC, Mugambi M. Electrocardiographic changes during treatment of leishmaniasis with pentavalent antimony (sodium stibogluconate). *American journal of tropical medicine and hygiene*, 1985, 34:702-709.

44. Oliver T. The health of antimony oxide workers. *British medical journal*, 1933, i:1094-1095.

45. Brieger H et al. Industrial antimony poisoning. *Industrial medicine and surgery*, 1954, 23:521-523.

46. Potkonjak V, Pavlovich M. Antimoniosis: a particular form of pneumoconiosis. I. Etiology, clinical and X-ray findings. *International archives of occupational and environmental health*, 1983, 51:199-207.

## 13.4 Arsenic

### 13.4.1 General description

#### *Identity*

Arsenic exists in oxidation states of -3, 0, 3, and 5. It is widely distributed throughout the earth's crust, most often as arsenic sulfide or as metal arsenates and arsenides.

| Compound | CAS no. | Molecular formula |
|---|---|---|
| Arsenic | 7440-38-2 | As |
| Arsenic trioxide | 1327-53-3 | $As_2O_3$ |
| Arsenic pentoxide | 1303-28-2 | $As_2O_5$ |
| Arsenic sulfide | 1303-33-9 | $As_2S_3$ |
| Dimethylarsinic acid | 75-60-5 | $(CH_3)_2AsO(OH)$ |
| Lead arsenate | 10102-48-4 | $PbHAsO_4$ |
| Potassium arsenate | 7784-41-0 | $KH_2AsO_4$ |
| Potassium arsenite | 10124-50-2 | $KAsO_2 \cdot HAsO_2$ |

## Physicochemical properties (1, 2)

| Compound | Melting point (°C) | Boiling point (°C) | Density (g/cm³) | Water solubility (g/l) |
|---|---|---|---|---|
| As | 613 | – | 5.727 at 14 °C | insoluble |
| $As_2O_3$ | 312.3 | 465 | 3.738 | 37 at 20 °C |
| $As_2O_5$ | 315 (decomposes) | – | 4.32 | 1500 at 16 °C |
| $As_2S_3$ | 300 | 707 | 3.43 | $5 \times 10^{-4}$ (at 18 °C) |
| $(CH_3)_2AsO(OH)$ | 200 | – | – | 829 at 22 °C |
| $PbHAsO_4$ | 720 (decomposes) | – | 5.79 | very slightly soluble |
| $KH_2AsO_4$ | 288 | – | 2.867 | 190 at 6 °C |
| $KAsO_2 HAsO_2$ | – | – | – | soluble |

## Major uses

Arsenicals are used commercially and industrially as alloying agents in the manu-facture of transistors, lasers, and semiconductors, as well as in the processing of glass, pigments, textiles, paper, metal adhesives, wood preservatives, and ammu-nition. They are also used in the hide tanning process and, to a limited extent, as pesticides, feed additives, and pharmaceuticals.

## Environmental fate

Arsenic is introduced into water through the dissolution of minerals and ores, from industrial effluents, and via atmospheric deposition (3–5). In well oxygen-ated surface waters, arsenic(V) is generally the most common species present (6, 7); under reducing conditions, such as those often found in deep lake sedi-ments or groundwaters, the predominant form is arsenic(III) (8, 9). An increase in pH may increase the concentration of dissolved arsenic in water (10).

## 13.4.2 Analytical methods

A silver diethyldithiocarbamate spectrophotometric method is available for the determination of arsenic: the detection limit is about 1 µg/litre (11). Graphite furnace atomic absorption spectroscopy in combination with high-pressure liquid chromatography can also be used to determine various arsenic species (6).

### 13.4.3 Environmental levels and human exposure

*Air*

Arsenic concentrations in air range from 0.4 to 30 ng/m$^3$ (*12–14*); higher concentrations are present in the vicinity of industrial sources (*12, 15*).

*Water*

The level of arsenic in natural waters generally varies between 1 and 2 µg/litre (*3*). Concentrations may be elevated, however, in areas containing natural sources; values as high as 12 mg/litre have been reported (*16*).

*Food*

Fish and meat are the main sources of dietary intake of arsenic (*17*); levels ranging from 0.4 to 118 mg/kg have been reported in marine fish sold for human consumption, and concentrations in meat and poultry can be as high as 0.44 mg/kg (*18*).

The mean daily intake of arsenic in food for adults has been estimated to range from 16.7 to 129 µg (*17, 19–21*); the corresponding figures for infants and children are 1.26–15.5 µg (*22, 23*).

On the basis of data on the arsenic content of various foodstuffs (*20, 24*), it can be estimated that approximately 25% of the intake of arsenic from food is inorganic and 75% is organic.

*Estimated total exposure and relative contribution of drinking-water*

The estimated mean daily intake of arsenic from food is approximately 40 µg, about 10 µg of which is inorganic arsenic. The mean daily intake of arsenic from drinking-water will generally be less than 10 µg, based on a concentration of arsenic in drinking-water in areas without natural sources of less than 5 µg/litre and an average daily consumption of 2 litres of drinking-water. The estimated intake from air is generally less than 1 µg.

### 13.4.4 Kinetics and metabolism in laboratory animals and humans

Ingested elemental arsenic is poorly absorbed and largely eliminated unchanged. Soluble arsenic compounds are rapidly absorbed from the gastrointestinal tract (*3*); arsenic(V) and organic arsenic are rapidly and almost completely eliminated via the kidneys (*25–27*). Inorganic arsenic may accumulate in skin, bone, and muscle (*28*); its half-life in humans is between 2 and 40 days (*29*).

Arsenic(III) is eliminated from the body by the rapid urinary excretion of nonmethylated arsenic in both the trivalent and pentavalent forms and by detoxification by sequential methylation of arsenic(III) in the liver to monomethylarsonic acid (MMAA) and dimethylarsinic acid (DMAA) (*30, 31*). Limited short-term studies on humans indicate that the capacity to methylate inorganic arsenic is progressively, but not completely, saturated when daily intake exceeds 0.5 mg (*32*).

In humans, inorganic arsenic does not appear to cross the blood–brain barrier; however, transplacental transfer of arsenic in humans has been reported (*33*).

## 13.4.5 Effects on laboratory animals and *in vitro* test systems
### *Long-term exposure*

There were significant reductions in cardiac output and stroke volume in male Wistar rats and female New Zealand rabbits ingesting drinking-water containing 50 μg of arsenic(III) per ml for 18 and 10 months, respectively. In contrast, there was no effect on cardiac function in rats following ingestion of the same concentration of arsenic(V) for 18 months (*34*).

### *Reproductive toxicity, embryotoxicity, and teratogenicity*

Teratogenic effects of arsenic in chicks, golden hamsters, and mice have been reported (*35, 36*). Arsenate was teratogenic in the offspring of pregnant hamsters following exposure on days 4–7 of gestation by minipump implantation (*37*); the threshold blood level for teratogenesis was 4.3 μmol/kg (*38*). The specific form of arsenic responsible for teratogenesis is not known, but it may be arsenite (*39*).

### *Mutagenicity and related end-points*

Arsenic does not appear to be mutagenic in bacterial and mammalian assays, although it can induce chromosome breakage, chromosomal aberrations, and sister chromatid exchange in a linear, dose-dependent fashion in a variety of cultured cell types, including human cells (*24, 40*). Arsenic(III) is about an order of magnitude more potent than arsenic(V) in this respect (*24*).

### *Carcinogenicity*

Arsenic has not been found to be carcinogenic in animal bioassays, with one exception. In a study of the potential of arsenic compounds to act as promoters, a significant increase in the incidence of kidney tumours was observed in male Wistar rats injected intraperitoneally with a single dose of diethylnitrosamine (30 mg/kg) and, from day 7, given the maximum tolerated dose (160 mg/litre) of arsenic(III) in drinking-water for 25 weeks (*41*).

## 13.4.6 Effects on humans

Although the results of available studies indicate that arsenic may be an essential element for several animal species (e.g. goats, rats, and chicks), there is no evidence that it is essential for humans (*24*).

The acute toxicity of arsenic compounds in humans is predominantly a function of their rate of removal from the body. Arsine is considered to be the most toxic form, followed by the arsenites [arsenic(III)], the arsenates [arsenic(V)] and organic arsenic compounds. Lethal doses in humans range from 1.5 mg/kg of body weight (diarsenic trioxide) to 500 mg/kg of body weight (DMAA) (*42*). Acute arsenic intoxication associated with the ingestion of well-water containing 1.2 and 21.0 mg of arsenic per litre has been reported (*43, 44*).

Early clinical symptoms of acute intoxication include abdominal pain, vomiting, diarrhoea, muscular pain, and weakness, with flushing of the skin. These symptoms are often followed by numbness and tingling of the extremities, muscular cramping, and the appearance of a papular erythematous rash (*45*). Within a month, symptoms may include burning paraesthesias of the extremities, palmoplantar hyperkeratosis, Mee's lines on fingernails, and progressive deterioration in motor and sensory responses (*45–47*).

Signs of chronic arsenicalism, including dermal lesions, peripheral neuropathy, skin cancer, and peripheral vascular disease, have been observed in populations ingesting arsenic-contaminated drinking-water (*48–55*). Dermal lesions were the most commonly observed symptoms, occurring after minimum exposure periods of approximately 5 years. Effects on the cardiovascular system were observed in children consuming arsenic-contaminated water (mean concentration 0.6 mg/litre) for an average of 7 years (*51, 52*).

In a large study conducted in China (Province of Taiwan), a population of 40 421 was divided into three groups based on the arsenic content of their well-water (high, >0.60 mg/litre; medium, 0.30–0.59 mg/litre; and low, <0.29 mg/litre) (*48*). There was a clear dose–response relationship between exposure to arsenic and the frequency of dermal lesions, "blackfoot disease" (a peripheral vascular disorder), and skin cancer. However, several methodological weaknesses (e.g. investigators were not "blinded") complicate the interpretation of the results. In addition, the possibility that other compounds present in the water supply might have been responsible for blackfoot disease was not considered. It has been suggested, for example, that humic acid in artesian well-water is the cause of the disease, not arsenic (*56*).

In a study in which cancer mortality was examined in relation to the arsenic content of contaminated drinking-water in the same villages of China (Province of Taiwan) and at the same three levels, there were significant dose–response relationships for age-adjusted rates for cancers of the bladder, kidney, skin, and lung in both sexes and cancers of the prostate and liver in males (*57*). A study in which the ecological correlations between the arsenic level of well-water and mortality from various malignant neoplasms in China (Province of Taiwan) were examined demonstrated a significant association with the arsenic level in well-water for cancers of the liver, nasal cavity, lung, skin, bladder, and kidney in both males and females and for prostate cancer in males (58).

In an investigation of the association between cancer incidence and the ingestion of arsenic-contaminated water in a limited area of China (Province of Taiwan), standardized mortality ratios (SMRs) for cancers of the bladder, kidney, skin, lung, liver, and colon were significantly elevated in the area of arsenic contamination. The SMRs for all but colon cancer also correlated well with the prevalence rate for blackfoot disease (59). In a case–control study of 204 subjects who died of cancer (69 of bladder, 76 of lung, and 59 of liver cancer) and 368 community controls matched for age and sex, the odds ratios of developing these cancers for those who had used artesian well-water for 40 or more years were 3.90, 3.39, and 2.67, respectively. Dose–response relationships were observed for all three cancer types by duration of exposure, and the odds ratios were not changed significantly when several other risk factors were taken into consideration in logistic regression analysis (60). A Technical Panel on Arsenic established by the US Environmental Protection Agency concluded that, although these studies demonstrated a qualitative relationship between the ingestion of arsenic-contaminated water and internal cancers, the data were not sufficient to enable the dose–response relationship to be assessed (24).

In a study conducted in Mexico, the health status of the populations of two rural towns was examined, the towns differing in the average arsenic concentration of their water supplies, which was 0.41 ± 0.114 mg/litre ("exposed") in the first and 0.005 ± 0.007 mg/litre ("control") in the second (54). The prevalence of nonspecific symptoms, such as nausea, abdominal pain, and diarrhoea, was significantly higher in the "exposed" population; the relative risks for these symptoms ranged from 1.9 to 4.8, while that of developing cutaneous lesions ranged from 3.6 to 36. The prevalence of skin cancer in the "exposed" population in Mexico was 6.4%, as compared with 1.06% in the population with similar exposure in China (Province of Taiwan) (0.30–0.59 mg/litre group) (48). This study suffered from methodological weaknesses; for example, the investigators were not blinded and drinking-water was assumed to be the only source of arsenic.

In a case–control study of 270 children with congenital heart disease and 665 healthy children, maternal consumption during pregnancy of drinking-water containing detectable arsenic concentrations was associated with a three-fold increase in the occurrence of coarctation of the aorta (the prevalence odds ratio adjusted for all measured contaminants and source of drinking-water was 3.4 with 95% confidence limits of 1.3–8.9) (35). However, no adjustment was made for maternal age, socioeconomic status, or previous reproductive history, and exposure was not determined directly.

In a case–control study in Massachusetts of 286 women with spontaneous abortions and 1391 women with live births, elevated odds ratios for miscarriages were associated with exposure to arsenic in drinking-water (61). The odds ratio for spontaneous abortion, adjusted for maternal age, educational level, and history of prior spontaneous abortion, for women exposed to undetectable concentrations, 0.8–1.3 µg/litre, and 1.4–1.9 µg/litre of arsenic in their drinking-water were 1.0, 1.1, and 1.5, respectively. Again, however, exposure was determined indirectly, and it would be desirable to follow up these preliminary results in studies designed to assess exposure more accurately.

## 13.4.7 Provisional guideline value

Inorganic arsenic compounds are classified by IARC in Group 1 (carcinogenic to humans) on the basis of sufficient evidence for carcinogenicity in humans and limited evidence for carcinogenicity in animals (62). No adequate data on the carcinogenicity of organic arsenicals were available. The guideline value has been derived on the basis of estimated lifetime cancer risk.

Data on the association between internal cancers and ingestion of arsenic in drinking-water are limited and insufficient for quantitative assessment of an exposure–response relationship (24). However, based on the increased incidence of skin cancer observed in the population in China (Province of Taiwan), the US Environmental Protection Agency has used a multistage model that is both linear and quadratic in dose to estimate the lifetime skin cancer risk associated with the ingestion of arsenic in drinking-water. With this model and data on males (24), the concentrations of arsenic in drinking-water associated with estimated excess lifetime skin cancer risks of $10^{-4}$, $10^{-5}$, and $10^{-6}$ are 1.7, 0.17, and 0.017 µg/litre, respectively.

It should be noted, however, that these values may overestimate the actual risk of skin cancer because of possible simultaneous exposure to other compounds in the water and possible dose-dependent variations in metabolism that could not be taken into consideration. In addition, the concentration of arsenic in drinking-water at an estimated skin cancer risk of $10^{-5}$ is below the practical quantification limit of 10 µg/litre.

A value of 13 µg/litre may be derived (assuming a 20% allocation to drinking-water) on the basis of the provisional maximum tolerable daily intake (PMTDI) of inorganic arsenic of 2 µg/kg of body weight set by the Joint FAO/WHO Expert Committee on Food Additives (JECFA) in 1983 and confirmed as a provisional tolerable weekly intake (PTWI) of 15 µg/kg of body weight in 1988 (63). JECFA noted, however, that the margin between the PTWI and intakes reported to have toxic effects in epidemiological studies was narrow.

With a view to reducing the concentration of arsenic in drinking-water, a provisional guideline value of 0.01 mg/litre is recommended. The estimated excess lifetime risk of skin cancer associated with exposure to this concentration is 6 x $10^{-4}$.

# References

1. Lide DR, ed. *CRC handbook of chemistry and physics*, 73rd ed. Boca Raton, FL, CRC Press, 1992–93.

2. International Agency for Research on Cancer. *Some metals and metallic compounds.* Lyon, 1980 (IARC Monographs on the Evaluation of Carcinogenic Risk to Humans, Vol. 23).

3. Hindmarsh JT, McCurdy RF. Clinical and environmental aspects of arsenic toxicity. *CRC critical reviews in clinical laboratory sciences*, 1986, 23:315-347.

4. *Arsenic.* Geneva, World Health Organization, 1981 (Environmental Health Criteria, No. 18).

5. Nadakavukaren JJ et al. Seasonal variation of arsenic concentration in well water in Lane County, Oregon. *Bulletin of environmental contamination and toxicology*, 1984, 33:264-269.

6. Irgolic KJ. *Speciation of arsenic compounds in water supplies.* Research Triangle Park, NC, US Environmental Protection Agency, 1982 (EPA-600/S1-82-010).

7. Cui CG, Liu ZH. Chemical speciation and distribution of arsenic in water, suspended solids and sediment of Xiangjiang River, China. *Science of the total environment*, 1988, 77:69-82.

8. Welch AH, Lico MS, Hughes JL. Arsenic in ground water of the western United States. *Ground water*, 1988, 26:333-347.

9. Lemmo NV et al. Assessment of the chemical and biological significance of arsenical compounds in a heavily contaminated watershed. Part 1. The fate and speciation of arsenical compounds in aquatic environments–a literature review. *Journal of environmental science and health*, 1983, A18:335.

10. Slooff W et al., eds. *Integrated criteria document arsenic.* Bilthoven, Netherlands, National Institute of Public Health and Environmental Protection, 1990 (report no. 710401004).

11. International Organization for Standardization. *Water quality—determination of total arsenic.* Geneva, 1982 (ISO 6595-1982).

12. Ball AL, Rom WN, Glenne B. Arsenic distribution in soils surrounding the Utah copper smelter. *American Industrial Hygiene Association journal*, 1983, 44:341.

13. Environmental Applications Group Ltd. *Identification of sources of inhalable particulates in Canadian urban areas. Final report.* Ottawa, Environment Canada, 1984.

14. Environment Canada. *Tables of inhalable particulate and inorganic compound concentrations in 2 monitoring stations (Windsor and Walpole Island) in the Windsor/Walpole Air Monitoring Network in Ontario.* Ottawa, 1988.

15. *Air quality guidelines for Europe.* Copenhagen, WHO Regional Office for Europe, 1987 (European Series No. 23).

16. Grinspan D, Biagini R. [Chronic endemic regional hydroarsenicism. The manifestations of arsenic poisoning caused by drinking water.] *Medicina cutanea Ibero-Latino-Americana*, 1985, 13:85-109 (in Spanish).

17. Gartrell MJ et al. Pesticides, selected elements, and other chemicals in adult total diet samples, October 1980–March 1982. *Journal of the Association of Official Analytical Chemists*, 1986, 69:146-159.

18. Bureau of Chemical Safety (Canada). *Food/field monitoring project FM-35.* Ottawa, Department of National Health and Welfare, 1983.

19. Dabeka RW, McKenzie AD, Lacroix GMA. Dietary intakes of lead, cadmium, arsenic and fluoride by Canadian adults: a 24-hour duplicate diet study. *Food additives and contaminants*, 1987, 4:89-101.

20. Hazell T. Minerals in foods: dietary sources, chemical forms, interactions, bioavailability. *World review of nutrition and dietetics*, 1985, 46:1-123.

21. Zimmerli B, Bosshard E, Knutti R. [Occurrence and health risk evaluation of toxic trace elements in the diet.] *Mitteilungen aus dem Gebiete der Lebensmitteluntersuchung und Hygiene*, 1989, 80:490 (in German).

22. Nabrzyski M, Gajewska R, Lebiedzinska A. [Arsenic content of daily diets of children and adults.] *Rocznik Panstwowego Zakladu Higieny*, 1985, 36:113-118 (in Polish).

23. Gartrell MJ et al. Pesticides, selected elements, and other chemicals in infant and toddler total diet samples, October 1980–March 1982. *Journal of the Association of Official Analytical Chemists*, 1986, 69:123-145.

24. Risk Assessment Forum. *Special report on ingested inorganic arsenic. Skin cancer; nutritional essentiality.* Washington, DC, US Environmental Protection Agency, 1988 (EPA-625/3-87/013).

25. Buchet JP, Lauwerys R, Roels H. Comparison of the urinary excretion of arsenic metabolites after a single oral dose of sodium arsenite, monomethylarsonate, or dimethylarsinate in man. *International archives of occupational and environmental health*, 1981, 48:71-79.

26. Luten JB, Riekwel-Booy G, Rauchbaar A. Occurrence of arsenic in plaice (*Pleuronectes platessa*), nature of organo-arsenic compound present and its excretion by man. *Environmental health perspectives*, 1982, 45:165-170.

27. Tam GK et al. Excretion of a single oral dose of fish-arsenic in man. *Bulletin of environmental contamination and toxicology*, 1982, 28:669-673.

28. Ishinishi N et al. Arsenic. In: Friberg L et al., eds. *Handbook on the toxicology of metals*, 2nd ed. Vol. II. Elsevier, Amsterdam, 1986:43-73.

29. Pomroy C et al. Human retention studies with $^{74}$As. *Toxicology and applied pharmacology*, 1980, 53:550-556.

30. Lovell MA, Farmer JG. Arsenic speciation in urine from humans intoxicated by inorganic arsenic compounds. *Human toxicology*, 1985, 4:203-214.

31. Buchet JP, Lauwerys R. Study of inorganic arsenic methylation by rat liver *in vitro*: relevance for the interpretation of observations in man. *Archives of toxicology*, 1985, 57:125-129.

32. Buchet JP, Lauwerys R, Roels H. Urinary excretion of inorganic arsenic and its metabolites after repeated ingestion of sodium metaarsenite by volunteers. *International archives of occupational and environmental health*, 1981, 48:111-118.

33. Gibson RS, Gage LA. Changes in hair arsenic levels in breast and bottle fed infants during the first year of infancy. *Science of the total environment*, 1982, 26:33-40.

34. Carmignani M, Boscolo P, Castellino N. Metabolic fate and cardiovascular effects of arsenic in rats and rabbits chronically exposed to trivalent and pentavalent arsenic. *Archives of toxicology*, 1985, 8 (Suppl.):452-455.

35. Zierler S et al. Chemical quality of maternal drinking water and congenital heart disease. *International journal of epidemiology*, 1988, 17:589-594.

36. Hood RD, Bishop SL. Teratogenic effects of sodium arsenate in mice. *Archives of environmental health*, 1972, 24:62-65.

37. Ferm VH, Hanlon DP. Constant rate exposure of pregnant hamsters to arsenate during early gestation. *Environmental research*, 1985, 37:425-432.

38. Hanlon DP, Ferm VH. Concentration and chemical status of arsenic in the blood of pregnant hamsters during critical embryogenesis. 1. Subchronic exposure to arsenate utilizing constant rate administration. *Environmental research*, 1986, 40:372-379.

39. Hanlon DP, Ferm VH. Concentration and chemical status of arsenic in the blood of pregnant hamsters during critical embryogenesis. 2. Acute exposure. *Environmental research*, 1986, 40:380-390.

40. Jacobson-Kram D, Montalbano D. The reproductive effects assessment group's report on the mutagenicity of inorganic arsenic. *Environmental mutagenesis*, 1985, 7:787-804.

41. Shirachi DY, Tu SH, McGowan JP. *Carcinogenic potential of arsenic compounds in drinking water.* Research Triangle Park, NC, US Environmental Protection Agency, 1986 (EPA-600/S1-86/003).

42. Buchet JP, Lauwerys RR. Evaluation of exposure to inorganic arsenic. *Cahiers de médecine du travail,* 1982, 19:15.

43. Wagner SL et al. Skin cancer and arsenical intoxication from well water. *Archives of dermatology,* 1979, 115:1205-1207.

44. Feinglass EJ. Arsenic intoxication from well water in the United States. *New England journal of medicine,* 1973, 288:828-830.

45. Murphy MJ, Lyon LW, Taylor JW. Subacute arsenic neuropathy: clinical and electrophysiological observations. *Journal of neurology, neurosurgery and psychiatry,* 1981, 44:896-900.

46. Wesbey G, Kunis A. Arsenical neuropathy. *Illinois medical journal,* 1981, 150:396-398.

47. Fennell JS, Stacy WK. Electrocardiographic changes in acute arsenic poisoning. *Irish journal of medical science,* 1981, 150:338-339.

48. Tseng WP. Effects of dose-response relationship of skin cancer and blackfoot disease with arsenic. *Environmental health perspectives,* 1977, 19:109-119.

49. Tseng WP et al. Prevalence of skin cancer in an endemic area of chronic arsenicism in Taiwan. *Journal of the National Cancer Institute,* 1968, 40:453-463.

50. Borgoño JM, Greiber R. Epidemiological study of arsenicism in the city of Antofagasta. In: Hemphill DD, ed. *Trace substances in environmental health, V. A symposium,* Columbia, University of Missouri Press, 1972:13-24.

51. Zaldivar R. A morbid condition involving cardio-vascular, broncho-pulmonary, digestive and neural lesions in children and young adults after dietary arsenic exposure. *Zentralblatt für Bakteriologie und Hygiene, Abteilung I: Originale,* 1980, B170:44-56.

52. Zaldivar R, Ghai GL. Clinical epidemiological studies on endemic chronic arsenic poisoning in children and adults, including observations on children with high- and low-intake of dietary arsenic. *Zentralblatt für Bakteriologie und Hygiene, Abteilung I: Originale,* 1980, B170:409-421.

53. Valentine JL et al. Arsenic effects on human nerve conduction. In: Gawthorne JM, Howell JM, White CL, eds. *Proceedings of the 4th International Symposium on Trace Element Metabolism in Man and Animals, Perth, Western Australia, 11-15 May 1981.* Berlin, Springer-Verlag, 1982:409.

54. Cebrian ME et al. Chronic arsenic poisoning in the north of Mexico. *Human toxicology*, 1983, 2:121-133.

55. Hindmarsh JT et al. Electromyographic abnormalities in chronic environmental arsenicalism. *Journal of analytical toxicology*, 1977, 1:270-276.

56. Lu FJ. Blackfoot disease: arsenic or humic acid? *Lancet*, 1990, 336(8707):115-116.

57. Wu MM et al. Dose-response relation between arsenic concentration in well water and mortality from cancers and cardiovascular diseases. *American journal of epidemiology*, 1989, 130:1123-1132.

58. Chen CJ, Wang CJ. Ecological correlation between arsenic level in well water and age-adjusted mortality from malignant neoplasms. *Cancer research*, 1990, 50:5470-5474.

59. Chen CJ et al. Malignant neoplasms among residents of a blackfoot disease-endemic area in Taiwan: high-arsenic artesian well water and cancers. *Cancer research*, 1985, 45:5895-5899.

60. Chen CJ et al. A retrospective study on malignant neoplasms of bladder, lung and liver in blackfoot disease endemic area of Taiwan. *British journal of cancer*, 1986, 53:399-405.

61. Aschengrau A, Zierler S, Cohen A. Quality of community drinking water and the occurrence of spontaneous abortion. *Archives of environmental health*, 1989, 44:283-290.

62. International Agency for Research on Cancer. *Overall evaluations of carcinogenicity: an updating of IARC Monographs volumes 1–42*. Lyon, 1987:100-106. (IARC Monographs on the Evaluation of Carcinogenic Risks to Humans, Suppl. 7).

63. Joint FAO/WHO Expert Committee on Food Additives. *Toxicological evaluation of certain food additives and contaminants*. Cambridge, Cambridge University Press, 1989:155-162 (WHO Food Additives Series, No. 24).

## 13.5 Asbestos

### 13.5.1 General description

***Identity***

Asbestos is a general term for fibrous silicate minerals containing iron, magnesium, calcium, or sodium. These can be divided into two main groups, namely serpentine (e.g. chrysotile) and amphibole (e.g. amosite, crocidolite, and tremolite).

## *Physicochemical properties*

Chrysotile is easily degraded by strong acids, whereas amphiboles are more resistant. The various forms of asbestos are generally resistant to alkali. The chemical nature and crystalline structure of asbestos impart to it a number of characteristics, including high tensile strength, durability, flexibility, and resistance to heat and chemicals (*1*).

## *Major uses*

Asbestos, particularly chrysotile, is used in a large number of applications, particularly in construction materials, such as asbestos-cement (A/C) sheet and pipe, electrical and thermal insulation, and friction products, such as brake linings and clutch pads (*1*).

## 13.5.2 Analytical methods

The method of choice for the quantitative determination of asbestos in ambient air and water is transmission electron microscopy (TEM) with identification by energy-dispersive X-ray analysis and selected-area electron diffraction (TEM/SAED). However, TEM/SAED is costly, and preliminary screening with TEM alone (*2*), which has a detection limit of below 0.1 million fibres per litre (MFL) in water (*3*), is therefore often used.

## 13.5.3 Environmental levels and human exposure
### *Air*

Mean chrysotile concentrations at 24 locations in southern Ontario (Canada) ranged from <2 to 11 fibres longer than 5 μm per litre. Concentrations at 10 remote rural locations were all below the detection limit in this study (<2 fibres/litre) (*1, 4*). Levels in samples from downtown and suburban locations in Stockholm (Sweden) were in the range 1–3 fibres longer than 5 μm per litre (*1, 4*).

Airborne asbestos may be released from tapwater in the home. Mean airborne asbestos concentrations were significantly higher (1.7 ng/m$^3$) in three homes with water containing elevated concentrations of asbestos than in three control homes (0.31 ng/m$^3$); however, the difference in concentration was due primarily to increased numbers of short fibres (<1 μm), which are considered to pose little health risk. Moreover, all the fibre concentrations found in this limited study were within the range of those measured in indoor and outdoor air in other investigations (*5*). Negligible amounts of asbestos fibres were released to air from water containing 40 ± 10 MFL via a conventional drum-type humidifier (*6*).

## Water

Asbestos is introduced into water by the dissolution of asbestos-containing minerals and ores as well as from industrial effluents, atmospheric pollution, and A/C pipes in water-distribution systems. Exfoliation of asbestos fibres from A/C pipes is related to the aggressiveness of the water supply (*3*). Although A/C piping is used in about 19% of water-distribution systems in Canada, erosion of such piping appeared to contribute measurably to the asbestos content of water supplies at only two of 71 locations surveyed (*7*). In contrast, high levels of asbestos have been recorded in association with the severe deterioration of A/C pipe containing chrysotile and crocidolite in Woodstock, New York (USA) (*8*).

Chrysotile was the predominant type of asbestos detected in a national survey of the water supplies of 71 communities in Canada; concentrations varied from not detectable (<0.1 MFL) to 2000 MFL, while median fibre lengths were in the range 0.5–0.8 µm. It was estimated that concentrations were >1 MFL in the water supplies of 25% of the population, >10 MFL for 5% of the population, and >100 MFL for 0.6% of the population. Concentrations were higher in raw than in treated water (*7*).

The results of a number of surveys indicate that most of the population of the USA consumes drinking-water containing asbestos in concentrations below 1 MFL (*9*). In 1974, concentrations of optically visible fibres up to 33 MFL were detected in drinking-water supplies in the Netherlands (*10*). The results of a survey of asbestos concentrations in raw and treated waters in the United Kingdom suggest that most drinking-waters contain asbestos fibres in concentrations varying from not detectable up to 1 MFL (*11*).

## Food

The asbestos content of solid foodstuffs has not been well studied because of the lack of a simple, reliable analytical method. Foods that contain soil particles, dust, or dirt probably contain asbestos fibres; crude estimates suggest that the intake of asbestos in food may be significant in comparison with that in drinking-water (*12*). Concentrations of 0.151 MFL and 4.3–6.6 MFL in beer and 1.7–12.2 MFL in soft drinks have been reported (*13*).

## 13.5.4 Kinetics and metabolism in laboratory animals and humans

Information on the transmigration of ingested asbestos through the gastrointestinal tract to other tissues is contradictory (*1, 3*). Available data indicate that penetration, if it occurs at all, is extremely limited.

## 13.5.5 Effects on laboratory animals and *in vitro* test systems

### Reproductive toxicity, embryotoxicity, and teratogenicity

Administration of 4–400 mg of chrysotile per kg of body weight to CD-1 mice on days 1–15 of pregnancy did not affect the survival of the progeny. *In vitro* administration did not interfere with implantation on transfer of exposed blastocysts to recipient females but did result in a decrease in post-implantation survival. The authors concluded that asbestos was not teratogenic in these studies (*14*).

### Mutagenicity and related end-points

Although not mutagenic, all types of asbestos have induced chromosomal aberrations in *in vitro* studies (*15*). In *in vivo* studies, a single oral administration of chrysotile did not increase the frequency of micronuclei in mice, and there was no increase in chromosomal aberrations in monkeys following oral administration of chrysotile by gavage (*10*).

### Carcinogenicity

Although the carcinogenicity of inhaled asbestos is well established, there is no conclusive evidence that ingested asbestos is carcinogenic (*1, 3, 16*). In a series of extensive investigations involving treatment groups of 250 animals of each sex (*17–19*), no treatment-related increases in tumour incidence were observed in Syrian golden hamsters fed 1% amosite or short-range (98% shorter than 10 µm) or intermediate-range (65% longer than 10 µm) chrysotile, or in Fischer 344 rats fed 1% tremolite or amosite or short-range chrysotile in the diet over their lifetime. Although the incidence of benign epithelial neoplasms in the gastrointestinal tract in male Fischer 344 rats fed 1% intermediate-range chrysotile was significantly increased as compared with that in pooled controls from contemporary lifetime asbestos feeding studies in the same laboratory, the increase was not statistically significant in comparison with the data for concurrent controls and was limited to one sex.

## 13.5.6 Effects on humans

The health hazards associated with the inhalation of asbestos in the occupational environment have long been recognized and include asbestosis, bronchial carcinoma, malignant mesothelioma of the pleura and peritoneum, and possibly cancers of the gastrointestinal tract and larynx. In contrast, little convincing evidence has been found of the carcinogenicity of ingested asbestos in epidemiological studies of populations supplied with drinking-water containing high concentrations of asbestos (*1, 15, 19–26*). Moreover, the ability of asbestos fibres ingested in drinking-water to migrate through the walls of the gastrointestinal tract in sufficient numbers to cause adverse local or systemic effects is the subject of considerable disagreement (*1, 27, 28*).

In ecological population studies (*1, 20, 22–25*) (i.e. studies in which individual exposures were not estimated and population mobility was not adequately addressed), no consistent evidence was found of an association between cancer mortality or incidence and the ingestion of asbestos in drinking-water. In an analytical epidemiological (case–control) study that was inherently more sensitive than the ecological studies, there was no consistent evidence of a cancer risk associated with the ingestion of asbestos in drinking-water in Puget Sound, where levels up to 200 MFL were observed (*26*).

## 13.5.7 Conclusions

Although asbestos is a known human carcinogen by the inhalation route, available epidemiological studies do not support the hypothesis that an increased cancer risk is associated with the ingestion of asbestos in drinking-water. Moreover, in extensive feeding studies in animals, asbestos has not consistently increased the incidence of tumours of the gastrointestinal tract. There is therefore no consistent, convincing evidence that ingested asbestos is hazardous to health, and it is concluded that there is no need to establish a guideline value for asbestos in drinking-water.

## References

1.  *Asbestos and other natural mineral fibres.* Geneva, World Health Organization, 1986 (Environmental Health Criteria, No. 53).

2.  Pitt R. Asbestos as an urban area pollutant. *Journal of the Water Pollution Control Federation*, 1988, 60:1993-2001.

3.  Toft P et al. *Asbestos in drinking-water.* Ottawa, Ontario, Canada, Department of National Health and Welfare, Health Protection Branch, 1984 (CRC critical reviews in environmental control).

4.  Chatfield E. *Measurement of asbestos fibre concentrations in ambient atmospheres.* Report prepared for the Royal Commission on Matters of Health and Safety Arising from the Use of Asbestos in Ontario. Toronto, Ontario, Canada, 1983.

5.  Webber JS, Syrotynski S, King MV. Asbestos-contaminated drinking water: its impact on household air. *Environmental research*, 1988, 46:153-167.

6.  Meranger JC, Reid WW, Davey ABC. The transfer of asbestos from water to air via a portable drum-type home humidifier. *Canadian journal of public health*, 1979, 70:276-278.

171

7. Chatfield EJ, Dillon MJ. *A national survey for asbestos fibres in Canadian drinking water supplies.* Ottawa, Canada, Department of National Health and Welfare, 1979 (Environmental Health Directorate Report 79-EHD-34).

8. Webber JS, Covey JR, King MV. Asbestos in drinking water supplied through grossly deteriorated A-C pipe. *Journal of the American Water Works Association*, 1989, 81:80.

9. Millette JR et al. Asbestos in water supplies of the United States. *Environmental health perspectives*, 1983, 53:45-48.

10. Montizaan GK, Knaap AG, van der Heijden CA. Asbestos: toxicology and risk assessment for the general population in The Netherlands. *Food chemistry and toxicology*, 1989, 27:53-63.

11. Conway DM, Lacey RF. *Asbestos in drinking water. Results of a survey.* Medmenham, Water Research Centre, 1984 (Technical Report TR202).

12. Rowe JN. Relative source contributions of diet and air to ingested asbestos exposure. *Environmental health research*, 1983, 53:115-120.

13. Cunningham HM, Pontefract RD. Asbestos fibres in beverages and drinking water. *Nature (London)*, 1971, 232:332-333.

14. Schneider U, Maurer RR. Asbestos and embryonic development. *Teratology*, 1977, 15:273-279.

15. International Agency for Research on Cancer. *Overall evaluations of carcinogenicity: an updating of IARC Monographs volumes 1–42.* Lyon, 1987:106-116 (IARC Monographs on the Evaluation of Carcinogenic Risks to Humans, Suppl. 7).

16. DHHS Working Group. Report on cancer risks associated with the ingestion of asbestos. *Environmental health perspectives*, 1987, 72:253-265.

17. McConnell EE et al. Chronic effects of dietary exposure to amosite and chrysotile asbestos in Syrian golden hamsters. *Environmental health perspectives*, 1983, 53:11-25.

18. McConnell EE et al. Chronic effects of dietary exposure to amosite asbestos and tremolite in F344 rats. *Environmental health perspectives*, 1983, 53:27-44.

19. National Toxicology Program. *Toxicology and carcinogenesis studies of chrysotile asbestos in F344 rats.* Research Triangle Park, NC, US Department of Health and Human Services, 1985 (NIH Publication No. 86-2551; Technical Report No. 295).

20. Toft P et al. Asbestos and drinking water in Canada. *Science of the total environment*, 1981, 18:77-89.

21. Conforti PM et al. Asbestos in drinking water and cancer in the San Francisco Bay area: 1969-1974 incidence. *Journal of chronic diseases*, 1981, 34:211-224.

22. Sigurdson EE et al. Cancer morbidity investigations: lessons from the Duluth study of possible effects of asbestos in drinking water. *Environmental research*, 1981, 25:50-61.

23. Meigs JW et al. Asbestos cement pipe and cancer in Connecticut 1955-1974. *Journal of environmental health*, 1980, 42:187.

24. Millette JR et al. Epidemiology study of the use of asbestos-cement pipe for the distribution of drinking water in Escambia County, Florida. *Environmental health perspectives*, 1983, 53:91-98.

25. Sadler TD et al. The use of asbestos-cement pipe for public water supply and the incidence of cancer in selected communities in Utah. *Journal of community health*, 1984, 9:285-293.

26. Polissar L, Severson RK, Boatman ES. A case control study of asbestos in drinking water and cancer risk. *American journal of epidemiology*, 1984, 119:456-471.

27. Boatman ES et al. Use of quantitative analysis of urine to assess exposure to asbestos fibres in drinking water in the Puget Sound region. *Environmental health perspectives*, 1983, 53:131-139.

28. Carter RE, Taylor WF. Identification of a particular amphibole asbestos fibre in tissues of persons exposed to a high oral intake of the mineral. *Environmental research*, 1980, 21:85-93.

# 13.6 Barium

## 13.6.1 General description

### *Identity*

Barium is present as a trace element in both igneous and sedimentary rocks. Although it is not found free in nature (*1*), it occurs in a number of compounds, most commonly barium sulfate (barite) and, to a lesser extent, barium carbonate (witherite).

| Compound | CAS no. | Molecular formula |
|---|---|---|
| Barium sulfide | 21109-95-5 | BaS |
| Barium chloride | 10361-37-2 | $BaCl_2$ |
| Barium oxide | 1304-28-5 | BaO |
| Barium hydroxide | 17194-00-2 | $Ba(OH)_2$ |
| Barium bromide | 10553-31-8 | $BaBr_2$ |
| Barium nitrate | 10022-31-8 | $Ba(NO_3)_2$ |
| Barium nitrite | 13465-94-6 | $Ba(NO_2)_2$ |
| Barium sulfate | 7727-43-7 | $BaSO_4$ |
| Barium acetate | 543-80-6 | $Ba(C_2H_3O_2)_2$ |

## Physicochemical properties (2, 3)

| Compound | Melting point (°C) | Boiling point (°C) | Density (g/cm³) | Water solubility (g/l) |
|---|---|---|---|---|
| BaS | 1200 | – | 4.25 | readily soluble |
| $BaCl_2$ | 960 | 1560 | 3.856 at 24 °C | 310 at 0 °C |
| BaO | 1923 | 2000 | 5.32–5.72 | 15 at 0 °C |
| $Ba(OH)_2$ | 77.9 | 800 | 2.18 at 16 °C | 38.9 at 20 °C |
| $BaBr_2$ | 847 | decomposes | 4.781 at 24 °C | 980 at 0 °C |
| $Ba(NO_3)_2$ | 592 | decomposes | 3.24 at 23 °C | 92 at 20 °C |
| $Ba(NO_2)_2$ | 217 | decomposes | 3.23 | 675 at 20 °C |
| $BaSO_4$ | 1580 | – | 4.50 at 15 °C | 0.00285 at 30 °C |
| $Ba(C_2H_3O_2)_2$ | – | – | 2.47 | 770 at 26 °C |

## Major uses

Barium compounds, including barium sulfate and barium carbonate, are used in the plastics, rubber, electronics, and textiles industries, in ceramic glazes and ena-mels, in glass-making, brick-making, and paper-making, as a lubricant additive, in pharmaceuticals and cosmetics, in case-hardening of steel, and in the oil and gas industry as a wetting agent for drilling mud (4, 5).

## Environmental fate

Barium in water comes primarily from natural sources. The acetate, nitrate, and halides are soluble in water, but the carbonate, chromate, fluoride, oxalate, phos-phate, and sulfate are quite insoluble. The solubility of barium compounds in-creases as the pH level decreases (1).

Organic barium compounds are ionic and are hydrolysed in water (6). The concentration of barium ions in natural aquatic systems is limited by the pres-ence of naturally occurring anions and possibly also by the adsorption of these ions onto metal oxides and hydroxides (7).

## 13.6.2 Analytical methods

Barium concentrations in water may be determined by atomic absorption spectroscopy, using either direct aspiration into an air–acetylene flame (detection limit 2 µg/litre) or atomization in a furnace (detection limit 100 µg/litre) (1). Barium in water may also be determined by inductively coupled plasma atomic emission spectrometry, the detection limits being equivalent or superior to those of flame atomic absorption spectroscopy (8).

## 13.6.3 Environmental levels and human exposure

### Air

Barium is generally present in air in particulate form as a result of industrial emissions, particularly in combustion of coal and diesel oil and waste incineration. Concentrations ranging from 0.0015 to 0.95 µg/m$^3$ have been reported. The estimated respiratory intake for an adult male is in the range 0.03–22 µg/day (US Environmental Protection Agency, unpublished data, 1984).

### Water

The concentration of barium in groundwater in the Netherlands was measured at 60 locations; the mean and maximum concentrations were 0.23 and 2.5 mg/litre, respectively (9).

Barium concentrations in distributed drinking-water in Canada were found to range from not detectable (detection limit 5 µg/litre) to 600 µg/litre, with a median value of 18 µg/litre; in 86% of the 122 locations surveyed, the concentrations were below 100 µg/litre (10). In 83% of 262 locations surveyed in the Netherlands in 1983, barium concentrations in drinking-water were below 50 µg/litre; the maximum concentration found was below 200 µg/litre (11). In a study of the water supplies of cities in the USA, a median value of 43 µg/litre was reported; in 94% of all determinations the concentrations found were <100 µg/litre (12). Levels of barium in municipal water supplies in Sweden varied from 1 to 20 µg/litre (12).

If an average daily water consumption of 2 litres and a concentration of about 30 µg/litre are assumed, the daily intake of barium from drinking-water is approximately 60 µg.

### Food

Most foods contain less than 0.002 mg of barium per gram (13). Some cereal products and nuts may contain high levels: e.g. bran flakes, 0.0039 mg/g; pecans, 0.0067 mg/g; and Brazil nuts, up to 4 mg/g (14).

The long-term mean dietary barium intake for adults has been found to be 0.75 mg/day (range 0.44–1.8 mg/day), including food and fluids (*15*); 0.6 mg/day from total diet (*12*); and 1.24 mg/day (range 0.65–1.8 mg/day) for food only (*16*).

### Estimated total exposure and relative contribution of drinking-water

On the basis of the above considerations, the mean daily intake of barium from food, water, and air is estimated to be slightly more than 1 mg/day, food being the primary source for the non-occupationally exposed population. However, where barium levels in water are high, drinking-water may contribute significantly to barium intake.

## 13.6.4 Kinetics and metabolism in laboratory animals and humans

Soluble barium salts are most readily absorbed, although insoluble compounds may also be absorbed to a significant extent (*17, 18*). The degree of absorption of barium from the gastrointestinal tract also depends on the animal species, the contents of the gastrointestinal tract, diet, and age (*17–19*).

Barium is rapidly transported in blood plasma, principally to bone (*20*). Elevated barium/calcium ratios were found in the teeth of children exposed to drinking-water containing 10 mg of barium per litre (*21*). It has been reported that barium crosses the placental barrier in humans (*16*).

The faecal route of excretion of barium is the most important in humans and animals (*22*); in humans, 20% of an ingested dose is excreted in the faeces and 7% in the urine within 24 hours (*12, 20*).

## 13.6.5 Effects on laboratory animals and *in vitro* test systems

### Acute exposure

The oral $LD_{50}$ of barium chloride in rats is reported to be 118 mg/kg of body weight (*23*).

### Short-term exposure

No effects on blood pressure were seen in Sprague-Dawley rats exposed to 100 mg of barium per litre as barium chloride in drinking-water (equivalent to 1.5 mg/kg of body weight per day) for up to 20 weeks (*24*). In the same series of studies, no changes were seen in blood pressure in hypertension-susceptible Dahl and uninephrectomized rats exposed for 16 weeks to up to 1000 mg of barium per litre in distilled water or 0.9% saline. At 1000 mg/litre, however, ultrastructural changes in the glomeruli of the kidney were discernible by electron microscopy. In addition, no significant electrocardiographic changes during (-)-nor-epinephrine challenge were observed in Sprague-Dawley rats ingesting drinking-water containing 250 mg of barium per litre for 5 months (24).

### Long-term exposure

In a study on the lifetime exposure of Long-Evans rats to 5 mg of barium per litre as barium acetate in drinking-water, the only significant effect reported was an increase in proteinuria in males (25). In a similar study in which 5 mg of barium per litre as barium acetate was administered in drinking-water to Charles River CD mice over their entire life span, there was a slight reduction in the survival of males, but no effects on body weight gain, oedema, or blanching of incisor teeth (26). No histopathological effects were found in 34 tissues of male and female Sprague-Dawley rats exposed to 1, 10, 100, or 250 mg of barium per litre as barium chloride in drinking-water for up to 68 weeks (24).

Groups of female Long-Evans rats were exposed to 1, 10, or 100 mg of barium per litre as barium chloride in drinking-water for 1, 4, or 16 months (27), equivalent to average doses of 0.051, 0.51, and 5.1 mg of barium per kg of body weight per day (2). Mean systolic pressure remained unchanged in animals exposed to the lowest dose for 16 months. At the intermediate dose, there were mean increases in blood pressure of 0.533–0.933 kPa (4–7 mmHg) by 8 months, which persisted thereafter. In rats receiving the highest dose, significant and persistent increases in mean systolic pressure of 1.60 kPa (12 mmHg) were seen after only 1 month, gradually increasing to a mean of 2.13 kPa (16 mmHg) after 16 months of exposure. Rates of cardiac contraction, electrical excitability, and high-energy phosphate and phosphorylation potential were decreased. As increases in systolic pressure of 0.533-0.933 kPa (4–7 mmHg) are deemed small enough not to constitute an adverse effect, the NOAEL can be considered to be 0.51 mg of barium per kg of body weight per day, and the LOAEL is 5.1 mg of barium per kg of body weight per day.

It has been estimated that a 0.1–1% increase in the clinical incidence of coronary heart disease in the USA over a 6-year period could result from a 2kPa (15 mmHg) increase in mean systolic blood pressure. Although a 0.67 kPa (5 mmHg) increase in systolic blood pressure would have virtually no short-term clinical implications for those aged 35 years and younger, such an increase may become a difference of nearly 1.33 kPa (10 mmHg) by age 65, which would increase the average risk of a heart attack by 14% in the USA (28).

### Reproductive toxicity, embryotoxicity, and teratogenicity

No studies on the reproductive, embryotoxic, or teratogenic effects of the ingestion of barium in food or drinking-water were found. In contrast, the inhalation of barium carbonate dust adversely affected spermatogenesis in male rats exposed to 22.6 mg/m$^3$, and shortened the estrous cycle and disturbed the morphological structure of the ovaries in female rats exposed to 13.4 and 3.1 mg/m$^3$ for 4 months (*29*).

### Mutagenicity and related end-points

Barium chloride did not increase the frequency of mutation in repair-deficient strains of *Bacillus subtilis* (*30*) or induce errors in viral DNA transcription *in vitro* (*31*).

### Carcinogenicity

In extremely limited lifetime bioassays of rats and mice exposed to 5 mg/litre in drinking-water, no evidence was found on gross examination at autopsy to show that barium is carcinogenic (*25, 26*).

## 13.6.6 Effects on humans

Barium is not considered to be an essential element for human nutrition (*16*).

At high concentrations, barium causes vasoconstriction by its direct stimulation of arterial muscle, peristalsis as a result of the violent stimulation of smooth muscle, and convulsions and paralysis following stimulation of the central nervous system (*32*). Depending on the dose and solubility of the barium salt, death may occur in a few hours or a few days. The acute toxic oral dose of barium chloride for humans is 0.2–0.5 g; the estimated acute lethal oral dose is between 3 and 4 g (*33*). Repeated exposures to barium chloride in table salt are believed to have caused recurrent outbreaks of "pa-ping" disease (a transient paralysis resembling familial periodic paralysis) in China (*34*), but recovery was usually rapid (*12*).

The prevalence of dental caries was reported to be significantly lower in 39 children from a community ingesting drinking-water containing 8–10 mg of barium per litre as compared with that in 36 children from another community ingesting drinking-water containing <0.03 mg/litre (*35*). However, the study population was small, and dental examinations were not conducted in a blind manner.

Associations between the barium content of drinking-water and mortality from cardiovascular disease have been observed in several ecological epidemiological studies. Significant negative correlations between barium concentrations in drinking-water and mortality from atherosclerotic heart disease (*36*) and total cardiovascular disease (*37*) have been reported. Conversely, significantly higher sex- and age-adjusted death rates for "all cardiovascular diseases" and "heart disease" have been reported in an unspecified number of Illinois communities with high concentrations of barium in drinking-water (2–10 mg/litre) as compared with those with low concentrations (<0.2 mg/litre) in 1971–75 (*38*). There were, however, several confounding factors; although the communities were matched for demographic characteristics and socioeconomic status, population mobility differed between the communities with high and low barium levels. Moreover, it was not possible to control for the use of water softeners in the home (*39*).

The results of the ecological study in Illinois were not confirmed in a cross-sectional study of the prevalence of cardiovascular disease in 1175 adult residents of West Dundee, Illinois (mean barium concentration in drinking-water 7.3 mg/litre, range 2–10 mg/litre), as compared with 1203 adult residents of McHenry (mean concentrations of barium in drinking-water 0.1 mg/litre) (*40*). The socioeconomic status and demographic characteristics of the populations in the two towns were similar. Blood pressures of all participants were measured, and data on the occurrence of cardiovascular, cerebrovascular, and renal disease and possible confounding factors were obtained by means of questionnaires administered by trained survey workers. There were no significant differences between the two populations in the prevalence of hypertension, stroke, and heart and kidney disease, even when the use of water softeners, medication, duration of exposure, smoking, and obesity were taken into account. The authors concluded that blood pressure in adults does not appear to be adversely affected even following prolonged ingestion of drinking-water containing more than 7 mg of barium per litre.

In a recent clinical study, 11 "healthy" men were exposed to barium (as barium chloride) in drinking-water (0 mg/litre for 2 weeks, 5 mg/litre for the next 4 weeks, and 10 mg/litre for the last 4 weeks) (*41*). Attempts were made to control several of the risk factors for cardiovascular disease, including diet, exercise, smoking, and alcohol consumption, throughout the study period (although subjects were not continuously monitored in this regard). No consistent indication of any adverse effects was found. There was, however, a trend towards an increase in serum calcium between 0 and 5 mg/litre, which persisted at 10 mg/litre; for total calcium, normalized for differences in albumin level, this increase was statistically significant. The authors suggested that the increase would not be expected to be clinically important. The lack of adverse effects observed in this study may be attributable to the small number of subjects included or the short period of exposure.

## 13.6.7 Guideline value

As there is no evidence that barium is carcinogenic (*12*), the guideline value for barium in drinking-water is derived using the TDI approach.

In the most sensitive epidemiological study conducted to date, there were no significant differences in blood pressure or in the prevalence of cardiovascular disease between a population drinking water containing a mean barium concentration of 7.3 mg/litre and one whose water contained a concentration of 0.1 mg/litre (*40*). Using the NOAEL of 7.3 mg/litre obtained from this study and an uncertainty factor of 10 to account for intraspecies variation, a guideline value of 0.7 mg/litre (rounded figure) can be derived for barium in drinking-water.

This value is close to that derived from the results of toxicological studies in animal species. A TDI of 51 µg/kg of body weight can be calculated, based on a NOAEL of 0.51 mg/kg of body weight per day in a chronic study in rats (*27*) and incorporating uncertainty factors of 10 for intraspecies variation and 1 for interspecies variation, as the results of a well-conducted epidemiological study (*40*) indicate that humans are not more sensitive than rats to barium in drinking-water. The value derived from this TDI, based on a 20% allocation to drinking-water, is 0.3 mg/litre (rounded figure).

## References

1.  Office of Drinking Water. *Health advisory–barium*. Washington, DC, US Environmental Protection Agency, 1985.

2.  Office of Drinking Water. *Drinking water criteria document for barium*. Washington, DC, US Environmental Protection Agency, 1985.

3.  Lide DR, ed. *CRC handbook of chemistry and physics*, 73rd ed. Boca Raton, FL, CRC Press, 1992–93.

4.  Brooks SM. Pulmonary reactions to miscellaneous mineral dusts, man-made mineral fibers, and miscellaneous pneumoconioses. In: Merchant JA, ed. *Occupational respiratory diseases*. Cincinnati, OH, US Department of Health and Human Services, Appalachian Laboratory for Occupational Safety and Health, 1986:401-458 (DHHS (NIOSH) Publication No. 86-102).

5.  Miner S. *Preliminary air pollution survey of barium and its compounds. A literature review*. Raleigh, NC, US Department of Health, Education, and Welfare, National Air Pollution Control Administration, 1969.

6.  Cotton FA, Wilkinson G. *Advanced inorganic chemistry: comprehensive text*, 4th ed. New York, NY, John Wiley, 1980:286.

7.  Hem JD. *Study and interpretation of the chemical characteristics of natural water. US Geologic Survey sampling data*, Washington, DC, US Government Printing Office, 1959 (Water Supply Paper 1473).

8.  Laboratory Services Branch. *The determination of trace metals in surface waters by ICP-AAS*. Toronto, Canada, Ontario Ministry of the Environment, 1988.

9.  Van Duijvenbooden W. *The quality of ground water in the Netherlands*. Bilthoven, Netherlands, National Institute of Public Health and Environmental Protection, 1989 (RIVM Report No. 728820001).

10. Subramanian KS, Méranger JC. A survey for sodium, potassium, barium, arsenic, and selenium in Canadian drinking water supplies. *Atomic spectroscopy*, 1984, 5:34-37.

11. Fonds AW, Van Den Eshof AJ, Smit E. *Integrated criteria document barium*. Bilthoven, Netherlands, National Institute of Public Health and Environmental Protection, 1987 (RIVM Report No. 218108004).

12. *Barium*. Geneva, World Health Organization, 1990 (Environmental Health Criteria No. 107).

13. Gormican A. Inorganic elements in foods used in hospital menus. *Journal of the American Dietetic Association*, 1970, 56:397-403.

14. Mertz W, ed. *Trace elements in human and animal nutrition*, 5th ed. New York, NY, Academic Press, 1986:418-420.

15. International Commission on Radiological Protection. *Report of the task group on reference man*. New York, NY, Pergamon Press, 1975 (Publication 23).

16. Schroeder HA, Tipton IH, Nason P. Trace metals in man: strontium and barium. *Journal of chronic diseases*, 1972, 25:491-517.

17. McCauley PT, Washington IS. Barium bioavailability as the chloride, sulfate, or carbonate salt in the rat. *Drug and chemical toxicology*, 1983, 6:209-217.

18. Clavel JP et al. Intestinal absorption of barium during radiological studies. *Therapie*, 1987, 42(2):239-243.

19. Taylor DM, Bligh PH, Duggan MH. The absorption of calcium, strontium, barium and radium from the gastrointestinal tract of the rat. *Biochemical journal*, 1962, 83:25-29.

20. National Research Council. *Drinking water and health*, Vol. 1. Washington, DC, National Academy of Sciences, 1977.

21. Miller RG et al. Barium in teeth as indicator of body burden. In: Calabrese EJ, Tuthill RW, Condie L, eds. *Inorganics in drinking water and cardiovascular disease*. Princeton, NJ, Princeton Scientific Publishing Co., 1985: 211–219 (Advances in modern environmental toxicology, Vol. 9).

22. Ohanian EV, Lappenbusch WL. *Problems associated with toxicological evaluations of barium and chromium in drinking water*. Washington, DC, US Environmental Protection Agency, Office of Drinking Water, 1983.

23. National Institute of Occupational Safety and Health. *Registry of Toxic Effects of Chemical Substances (RTECS)* (database). Washington, DC, US Department of Health and Human Services, 1989.

24. McCauley PT et al. Investigations into the effect of drinking water barium on rats. In: Calabrese EJ, Tuthill RW, Condie L, eds. *Inorganics in drinking water and cardiovascular disease*. Princeton, NJ, Princeton Scientific Publishing Co., 1985: 197–210 (Advances in modern environmental toxicology, Vol. 9).

25. Schroeder HA, Mitchener M. Life-term studies in rats: effects of aluminum, barium, beryllium and tungsten. *Journal of nutrition*, 1975, 105:421-427.

26. Schroeder HA, Mitchener M. Life-term effects of mercury, methyl mercury and nine other trace elements on mice. *Journal of nutrition*, 1975, 105:452-458.

27. Perry HM et al. Cardiovascular effects of chronic barium ingestion. *Trace substances and environmental health*, 1983, 16:155-164.

28. Wilkins JR, Calabrese EJ. Health implications of a 5 mmHg increase in blood pressure. *Toxicology and industrial health*, 1985, 1:13-28.

29. Tarasenko NY, Pronin OA, Silayev AA. Barium compounds as industrial poisons (an experimental study). *Journal of hygiene, epidemiology, microbiology, and immunology*, 1977, 21:361-373.

30. Nishioka H. Mutagenic activities of metal compounds in bacteria. *Mutation research*, 1975, 31:186-189.

31. Loeb L, Sirover M, Agarwal S. Infidelity of DNA synthesis as related to mutagenesis and carcinogenesis. In: *Advances in experimental medicine and biology*, 1978, 91:103. Cited in US Environmental Protection Agency. *Health effects assessment for barium*. Washington, DC, 1984.

32. Stockinger HE. The metals. In: Clayton GD, Clayton FE, eds. *Patty's industrial hygiene and toxicology*, 3rd ed. Vol. 2A. New York, NY, John Wiley, 1981:1493-2060.

33. Reeves AL. Barium. In: Friberg L, Nordberg GF, Vouk VB, eds. *Handbook on the toxicology of metals*. 2nd ed. Amsterdam, Elsevier/North Holland Biomedical Press, 1986:84-94.

34. Shankle R, Keane JR. Acute paralysis from barium carbonate. *Archives of neurology*, 1988, 45(5):579-580.

35. Zdanowicz JA et al. Inhibitory effect of barium on human caries prevalence. *Community dentistry and oral epidemiology*, 1987, 15:6-9.

36. Schroeder HA, Kramer LA. Cardiovascular mortality, municipal water, and corrosion. *Archives of environmental health*, 1974, 28:303-311.

37. Elwood PC, Abernethy M, Morton M. Mortality in adults and trace elements in water. *Lancet*, 1974, 2:1470-1472.

38. Brenniman GR et al. Cardiovascular disease death rates in communities with elevated levels of barium in drinking water. *Environmental research*, 1979, 20:318-324.

39. National Research Council. *Drinking water and health*, Vol. 4. Washington, DC, National Academy Press, 1982:167-170.

40. Brenniman GR, Levy PS. Epidemiological study of barium in Illinois drinking water supplies. In: Calabrese EJ, Tuthill RW, Condie L, eds. *Inorganics in water and cardiovascular disease*. Princeton, NJ, Princeton Scientific Publishing Co., 1985:231-240.

41. Wones RG, Stadler BL, Frohman LA. Lack of effect of drinking water barium on cardiovascular risk factors. *Environmental health perspectives*, 1990, 85:355-359.

# 13.7 Beryllium

## 13.7.1 General description

### *Identity*

Beryllium is an alkaline earth metal and a constituent of many common minerals, such as beryl and beryllonite (*1*).

### *Physicochemical properties (2)*

| Property | Value |
| --- | --- |
| Physical state | Grey solid |
| Melting point | 1278 °C |
| Boiling point | 2970 °C |
| Density | 1.848 g/cm$^3$ at 20 °C |

### *Organoleptic properties*

A taste detection threshold of 0.24 g/litre has been reported for beryllium chloride (*3*).

### *Major uses*

Beryllium and its alloys have a number of important uses, mostly based on their heat resistance; these include use in space vehicles, X-ray equipment, and electrical components (*1*).

## 13.7.2 Analytical methods

Beryllium is determined directly in acidified aqueous samples by electrothermal atomization atomic absorption spectrophotometry. Other metals, such as iron, magnesium, aluminium, and manganese, can interfere with the method. The detection range for beryllium is 0.22–4 µg/litre (*4*). Other methods include

183

graphite furnace and flame atomic absorption spectroscopy (5) and gas chromatography with electron capture detection (6).

## 13.7.3 Environmental levels and human exposure

### Air

Beryllium is released to air principally as a result of the combustion of fossil fuels (7). However, it is infrequently detected in the atmosphere, and concentrations are usually less than 5 ng/m$^3$ (8).

### Water

Beryllium enters natural waters through the weathering of rocks, atmospheric fallout, and industrial and municipal discharges (1). Concentrations in natural waters are generally less than 1 µg/litre (1, 7). Beryllium is rarely detected in drinking-water and then only at very low concentrations. In a large-scale survey in the United States, mean and maximum concentrations of 0.2 and 1.2 µg/litre, respectively, were reported (9).

### Food

The beryllium content of various foodstuffs has been reported to be in the range 0.06–0.17 mg/kg (10). A typical dietary intake has been reported as 100 µg/day, although in a study in the United Kingdom it was estimated that the dietary intake could be less than 15 µg/day (1).

### Estimated total exposure and relative contribution of drinking-water

The major route of exposure of the general population to beryllium is through food, the contribution from air being negligible in comparison. If a daily intake in the diet of 100 µg of beryllium in adults and a beryllium concentration in drinking-water of 1 µg/litre are assumed, the total contribution from water would be 2% (1). At lower dietary levels, the relative contribution from drinking-water would be increased.

## 13.7.4 Kinetics and metabolism in laboratory animals and humans

Beryllium and its compounds are not readily absorbed via the oral route, as they tend to form insoluble compounds at physiological pH (11). Following exposure to the chloride and sulfate, less than 1% and 20% respectively of ingested beryllium was absorbed in experimental animals (1, 12). Negligible amounts of beryllium are absorbed through the intact skin (1). Absorbed oral doses are distributed to the gastrointestinal tract, liver, blood, and kidney, and are ultimately stored in bone (12,13). Inhaled or ingested beryllium is excreted mainly in the faeces (14).

## 13.7.5 Effects on laboratory animals and *in vitro* test systems

### Acute exposure

In general, beryllium compounds are less acutely toxic in animals via the oral route than via other routes of administration ($1$). Oral $LD_{50}$s of 18–200 mg/kg of body weight have been reported in rodents for a number of beryllium compounds ($1$).

### Long-term exposure

In a lifetime study, Long-Evans male and female rats were exposed to 5 mg of beryllium sulfate per litre in drinking-water. Other than a slight depression in the growth of males from 2 to 6 months of age, there were no changes in gross or microscopic pathology, clinical chemistry, or urine analysis ($15$). Similarly, in a lifetime study in Charles River mice given beryllium sulfate at 5 mg/litre in their drinking-water, slight effects on female body weight were seen. No other treatment-related effects were observed ($16$).

### Reproductive toxicity, embryotoxicity, and teratogenicity

No studies are available on the repoductive toxicity of beryllium following ingestion, However, the chloride and oxide have been found to be fetotoxic after intratracheal administration and embryotoxic after intravenous administration ($17$).

### Mutagenicity and related end-points

Beryllium does not appear to be mutagenic in various *Salmonella typhimurium* strains ($18$). It has been shown to interact with DNA ($19$) and to cause gene mutations ($20$), chromosomal aberrations, and sister chromatid exchange in cultured mammalian somatic cells ($21$). Sister chromatid exchange has also been reported in mouse macrophages ($22$). Dose-dependent positive transformation was induced in mammalian cell lines ($23$), although beryllium did not induce DNA repair in rat hepatocytes ($24$). It did not increase the incidence of micronucleated polychromic erythrocytes in the bone marrow of mice *in vivo* ($18$).

### Carcinogenicity

Beryllium compounds administered by injection or inhalation can induce malignant tumours in laboratory animals ($1$). However, animal studies are inadequate to evaluate whether beryllium compounds are carcinogenic by oral administration. In two lifetime studies, rats and mice ingesting beryllium in drinking-water at a concentration of 5 mg/litre did not show a significant increase in tumours as compared with controls ($15,16$). In another study in which Wistar rats were fed beryllium at 5, 50, or 500 mg/kg of diet, no treatment-related increase in tumours as compared with controls was observed ($1$).

## 13.7.6 Effects on humans

No studies are available on the health effects of ingested beryllium. However, as gastrointestinal absorption is poor, toxicity is expected to be low via this route. Inhalation of beryllium compounds during occupational exposure has been shown to cause acute pneumonitis and chronic pulmonary granulomatosis, also known as chronic beryllium disease (25). There is evidence that the chronic disease is immunologically mediated (25). When insoluble beryllium compounds have become embedded in the skin, allergic-type dermatitis and granulomatous skin ulcerations have been reported, as also has conjunctivitis (1).

IARC has classified beryllium and beryllium compounds as being probably carcinogenic to humans (Group 2A), on the basis of occupational exposure and inhalation studies in laboratory animals (25). However, the epidemiological studies that led to this conclusion have been criticized (26).

## 13.7.7 Conclusions

There are no suitable oral data on which a toxicologically supportable guideline value could be based. However, the very low concentrations of beryllium normally found in drinking-water seem unlikely to pose a hazard to consumers.

## References

1. *Beryllium.* Geneva, World Health Organization, 1990 (Environmental Health Criteria, No. 106).

2. International Agency for Research on Cancer. *Some metals and metallic compounds.* Lyon, 1980: 143-204 (IARC Monographs on the Evaluation of Carcinogenic Risks to Humans, Vol. 23).

3. Stahl WH. *Compilation of odour and taste threshold values data.* Philadelphia, PA, American Society for Testing and Materials, 1973.

4. Antimony, arsenic, beryllium, chromium, cobalt, copper, gallium, germanium, indium, nickel, selenium, silver, thallium, vanadium and zinc by electrothermal AAS. In: *Methods for the examination of water and associated material.* London, Her Majesty's Stationery Office, 1988.

5. Makhnev YA et al. [Atomic absorption spectrometric determination of beryllium in natural and waste waters after chemical preconcentration.] *Journal of analytical chemistry of the USSR,* 1986, 41(7), Part 1:905-910 (in Russian).

6. Measures CI, Edmond JM. Determination of beryllium in natural waters in real time using electron capture detection gas chromatography. *Analytical chemistry,* 1986, 58(9):2065-2069.

7.  Skilleter DN. Beryllium. In: Fishbein L, Furst A, Mehlman MA, eds. *Genotoxic and carcinogenic metals: environmental and occupational occurrence and exposure.* Princeton, NJ, Princeton Scientific Publishing Co., 1987: 61-86 (Advances in Modern Environmental Toxicology, Vol. 11).

8.  Fishbein L. Overview of analysis of carcinogenic and/or mutagenic metals in biological and environmental samples. 1. Arsenic, beryllium, cadmium, chromium and selenium. *International journal of environmental and analytical chemistry,* 1984, 17(2):113-170.

9.  National Academy of Sciences. *Drinking water and health.* Washington, DC, National Research Council, 1977.

10. Meehan WR, Smythe LE. Occurrence of beryllium as a trace element in environmental materials. *Environmental science and technology,* 1967, 1:839-844.

11. Lefevre ME, Joel DD. Distribution of label after intragastric administration of beryllium-7 labelled carbon to weanling and aged mice. *Proceedings of the Society for Experimental Biology and Medicine,* 1986, 182(1):112-119.

12. Berry JP, Escaig F, Galle P. Study of the intracellular localisation of beryllium by analytical ion microscopy. *Comptes rendus hebdomadaires des séances de l'Académie des Sciences,* Série 3, 1987, 304(10):239-243.

13. Watanabe K et al. [Biotoxicity and beryllium distribution in organs by oral administration of beryllium compounds for long periods. II. Experimental study on oral administration of beryllium compounds.] *Rodo kagaku,* 1985, 61(5):235-246 (in Japanese). (*Chemical abstracts,* CA103(13)99963w).

14. Rhoads K, Sanders CL. Lung clearance, translocation, and acute toxicity of arsenic, beryllium, cadmium, cobalt, lead, selenium, vanadium, and ytterbium oxides following deposition in the rat lung. *Environmental research,* 1985, 36:359-378.

15. Schroeder HA, Mitchener M. Life-term studies in rats: effects of aluminum, barium, beryllium and tungsten. *Journal of nutrition,* 1975, 105(4):421-427.

16. Schroeder HA, Mitchener M. Life-term effects of mercury, methyl mercury and nine other trace metals on mice. *Journal of nutrition,* 1975, 105:452-458.

17. Selivanova LN, Savinova TB. [Effects of beryllium chloride and oxide on the sexual function of female rats and the development of their progeny.] *Gigiena i sanitarija,* 1986, 8:44-46 (in Russian).

18. Ashby J et al. Studies on the genotoxicity of beryllium sulphate *in vitro* and *in vivo.* *Mutation research,* 1990, 240(3):217-225.

19. Kubinski H, Gutzke GE, Kubinski ZO. DNA-cell-binding (DCB) assay for suspected carcinogens and mutagens. *Mutation research,* 1981, 89:95-136.

20. Miyaki M et al. Mutagenicity of metal cations in cultured cells from Chinese hamster. *Mutation research*, 1979, 68:259-263.

21. Larramendy ML, Popescu NC, Di Paolo JA. Induction by inorganic metal salts of sister chromatid exhanges and chromosome aberrations in humans and Syrian hamster strains. *Environmental mutagenesis*, 1981, 3:597-606.

22. Anderson O. Effect of coal combustion products and metal compounds on sister chromatid exchange (SCE) in a macrophage like cell line. *Environmental health perspectives*, 1983, 47:239-253.

23. Dunkel VC et al. Comparative neoplastic transformation responses of BALB/3T3 cells, Syrian hamster embryo cells, and Rauscher murine leukemia virus-infected Fischer 344 rat embryo cells to chemical compounds. *Journal of the National Cancer Institute*, 1981, 67:1303-1312.

24. Williams GM, Laspia MF, Dunkel VC. Reliability of the hepatocyte primary culture DNA repair test in testing of coded carcinogens and non-carcinogens. *Mutation research*, 1982, 97:359-370.

25. International Agency for Research on Cancer. *Overall evaluations of carcinogenicity: an updating of IARC Monographs volumes 1-42.* Lyon, 1987:127-128 (IARC Monographs on the Evaluation of Carcinogenic Risks to Humans, Suppl. 7).

26. Reeves AL. Beryllium: toxicological research of the last decade. *Journal of the American College of Toxicology*, 1989, 8(7):1307-1313.

# 13.8 Boron

## 13.8.1 General description

### Identity

Boron is widely distributed in the environment, borax, kernite, and tourmaline being three of the more commonly mined boron minerals. The chemical forms of boron in nature include boric acid and more condensed species such as tetraborate (*1*).

### Physicochemical properties (2)

| Property | Boron | Boric acid ($H_3BO_3$) | Borax ($Na_2B_4O_7\,10H_2O$) |
|---|---|---|---|
| Physical state | solid | solid | solid |
| Melting point (°C) | 2300 | 169 | 75 |
| Density (g/cm³) | 2.35 | 1.43 | 1.73 |
| Water solubility (g/litre) | insoluble | 63.5 | 20.1 (cold) |

## Major uses

Elemental boron and its carbides are used in composite structural materials, high-temperature abrasives, special-purpose alloys, and steel-making. Boron halides are used as catalysts in the manufacture of magnesium alloy products, metal refining, and rocket fuels. Boron hydrides are used as reductants, to control heavy metal discharges in wastewater, as catalysts, and in jet and rocket fuels (*1*, *2*).

Boric acid and borates are used in glass manufacture and as wood and leather preservatives, flame retardants, cosmetic products, and neutron absorbers for nuclear installations. Boric acid, borates, and perborates have been used as mild antiseptics or bacteriostats in eyewashes, mouthwashes, burn dressings, and nappy rash powders, although boric acid is not now regarded as effective for this purpose. Borax is used extensively as a cleaning compound, and borates are applied as agricultural fertilizers. Boron compounds are also used as algicides, herbicides, and insecticides (*1*, *2*).

## Environmental fate

The environmental chemistry of boron is not well understood. In water, the predominant species is probably boric acid, which does not dissociate readily at physiological pH (*3*).

## 13.8.2 Analytical methods

Boron can be determined by atomic absorption using either direct aspiration into a flame or a furnace technique, the latter having greater sensitivity. Inductively coupled plasma atomic emission spectroscopy can also be used. Detection limits range from 1.25 to 5 µg/litre (*2*, *4*). At concentrations between 0.01 and 1 mg/litre, boron can be determined by spectrometric techniques (*5*).

## 13.8.3 Environmental levels and human exposure

### Air

The presence of boron in the atmosphere has been attributed to sea spray, volcanic activity, accumulation in dust, and industrial pollution. Boron concentrations of 0.17 µg/m$^3$ have been reported in ocean air (*3*).

### Water

The concentration of boron in seawater ranges from 4 to 5 mg/litre as boric acid. In Canadian coastal waters, boron levels are in the range 3.7–4.3 mg/litre. Estuarine waters are rich in boron, as it can be transported from the sea (*3*). Boron concentrations in surface waters in the USA range from 0 to 6.5 mg/litre, although most are below 1 mg/litre (3). In northern Italy, boron concentrations in lake waters are below 0.09 mg/litre and, in about 65% of river water samples, close to natural background levels (0.1 mg/litre) (6).

In selected drinking-water supplies in the USA, boron levels were found to be between 0 and 0.74 mg/litre (median 0.12 mg/litre). High levels were attributed to seawater intrusion and fertilizers (3). Average boron concentrations in 3842 samples of treated and distributed water in Canada surveyed in 1987–89 ranged from 0.042 to 235 µg/litre, the maximum being 570 µg/litre (7). In the Netherlands, levels of boron in all drinking-water plants in 1984 varied from <0.005 to 0.61 mg/litre (median 0.02 mg/litre) (4). In selected drinking-water supplies in the former USSR, boron levels were 0–6.0 mg/litre (8). In Sierra Leone, boron levels in nine different drinking-water sources were in the range 4.6–18.1 mg/litre. The highest levels were found in pipe-borne untreated and stream water (9). Levels of boron in 37 brands of mineral water ranged from <0.005 to 4.2 mg/litre; in seven samples, the level was above 1 mg/litre (10).

## Food

As a constituent of foodstuffs, boron occurs mainly in plant tissues, legumes containing the highest concentrations (25–50 µg/g dry weight), followed by fruits and vegetables (5–20 µg/g) and cereals and grains (1–5 µg/g). In animal muscle and soft tissues, concentrations are well below 1 µg/g. Cow's milk normally contains 0.5–1.0 mg/litre, the level depending on the boron intake of the cow. Beverages contain variable amounts of boron: coffee, 0.16 mg/litre; apple juice, 1.2 mg/litre; orange juice, 0.53 mg/litre; and lemon juice, 0.59 mg/litre (3, 11).

## Estimated total exposure and relative contribution of drinking-water

The total daily boron intake in normal human diets was reported to vary from 2.1 to 4.3 mg/day in 1965 and from 1.3 to 4.4 mg/day in 1972 (2). In Canada, this intake was estimated to be 1–3 mg for an adult, depending on the number of boron-containing vegetables in the diet. The contribution from drinking-water was estimated at 0.24 mg/day, based on the median value measured in the USA (3). The contribution to boron intake from air is negligible. The total daily intake can therefore be estimated to be between 1 and 5 mg.

## 13.8.4 Kinetics and metabolism in laboratory animals and humans

Boron in food or administered as soluble borate (borax) or boric acid is rapidly and almost completely absorbed. Over 93% of a single oral dose of 750 mg of boric acid administered to human volunteers was recovered in the urine within 96 h (2). Between 50% and 66% of boric acid administered orally to rabbits

(17.1–119.9 mg of boron per kg of body weight per day) was excreted in the urine (2). Absorption through intact skin is poor but is much greater through damaged skin (12). Transplacental distribution has been reported (2).

## 13.8.5 Effects on laboratory animals and *in vitro* test systems

### Acute exposure

Boric acid and borax have a low acute oral toxicity; $LD_{50}$ values for mice, rats, and dogs range from 2000 to over 6000 mg/kg of body weight (7,13). Signs of acute toxicity for both borax and boric acid include depression, ataxia, convulsions, and death; kidney degeneration and testicular atrophy are also observed (1).

### Short-term exposure

After repeated oral administration of borax or boric acid to rats and dogs, growth inhibition, organ weight changes, and testicular atrophy were the most striking effects. In 90-day studies with rats and dogs at doses ranging from 17.5 to 5250 mg of boron per kg of food (as borax or boric acid), no clear NOAEL could be established (13).

In a 13-week study, mice were fed diets containing boric acid at 1200–20 000 mg/kg of food. At high doses (≥5000 mg/kg of food), increased mortality and degeneration or atrophy of the seminiferous tubules were observed. In all dose groups, extramedullary haemapoiesis of the spleen of minimal to mild severity was seen (14).

### Long-term exposure

No effects were observed on body weight and longevity in a limited lifetime study in which Swiss mice received 5 mg of boron per litre (as sodium metaborate) in their drinking-water (2).

In a study in which B6C3F$_1$ mice received 0, 2500, or 5000 mg of boric acid per kg in the diet for 103 weeks, mortality was significantly increased in both treatment groups. At the highest dose, testicular atrophy and interstitial cell hyperplasia were observed in male mice (14).

Male and female Sprague-Dawley rats were fed diets containing 0, 117, 350, or 1170 mg of boron per kg of food (as borax or boric acid) for 2 years. At the highest dose, increased brain and thyroid weights, decreased body and testes weights, and histopathological alterations of the testes were observed. The NOAEL in this study was 350 mg of boron per kg of food (equivalent to 17.5 mg of boron per kg of body weight per day) (13).

When dogs were fed 0, 58, 117, or 350 mg of boron per kg in the diet (as borax or boric acid) for 2 years, no effects were observed on body weight, food consumption, organ weights, clinical parameters, and histopathology. Dogs fed a diet containing 1170 mg of boron per kg of food (as borax) for 38 weeks exhibited severe testicular atrophy and spermatogenic arrest by week 26. The NOAEL in this study was 350 mg of boron per kg of food (equivalent to 8.8 mg of boron per kg of body weight per day) (*13*).

### Reproductive toxicity, embryotoxicity, and teratogenicity

In a 90-day drinking-water study with male rats, the highest dose of 6.0 mg of boron per litre (as borax) (0.426 mg of boron per kg of body weight per day) had no effects on fertility and reproduction or on the weight of the testes, prostate, or seminal vesicles. Fructose, zinc, and acid phosphatase levels in the prostate were unaltered (*15*).

In a 90-day feeding study in rats with borax (dose levels 0, 25, 50, and 100 mg of boron per kg of body weight per day), a LOAEL of 25 mg of boron per kg of body weight per day was established based on dose-dependent tubular germinal aplasia (*16*).

In a multigeneration study, 0, 117, 350, or 1170 mg of boron per kg of food (as borax or boric acid) was administered to male and female rats (*13*). At the highest dose, rats were found to be sterile, males showed atrophied testes in which spermatozoa were absent, and females showed decreased ovulation (NOAEL 350 mg of boron per kg of food, equivalent to 17.5 mg of boron per kg of body weight per day).

### Mutagenicity and related end-points

The mutagenic activity of boric acid was examined in the *Salmonella typhimurium* and mouse lymphoma assays with negative results. No induction of sister chromatid exchange or chromosomal aberrations was observed in Chinese hamster ovary cells (*14*). Sodium borate did not cause gene mutations in the *S. typhimurium* preincubation assay (*2*). Borax was not mutagenic in cell transformation assays with Chinese hamster cells, mouse embryo cells, and human fibroblasts (*17*).

### Carcinogenicity

Tumour incidence was not enhanced in studies in which B6C3F$_1$ mice received 0, 2500, or 5000 mg of boric acid per kg of food for 103 weeks (*14*) or Sprague-Dawley rats were fed diets containing 0, 117, 350, or 1170 mg of boron per kg of food (as borax or boric acid) for 2 years (*13*).

## 13.8.6 Effects on humans

Acute boron poisoning has been reported after the application of dressings, powders, or ointments containing borax and boric acid to large areas of burned or abraded skin; the lowest reported dermal lethal dose of boric acid is 8600 mg/kg of body weight (1505 mg of boron per kg of body weight). Ingestion has also been the cause of acute boron poisoning; the lowest reported oral dose of boric acid causing such poisoning is 640 mg/kg of body weight (112 mg of boron per kg of body weight) (1, 16). Symptoms of boron poisoning include gastrointestinal disturbances, erythematous skin eruptions, and signs of central nervous system stimulation followed by depression (1, 3).

Chronic exposure to boric acid and tetraborates such as borax leads to gastrointestinal irritation, with loss of appetite, nausea, and vomiting, and the appearance of an erythematous rash (12, 16). In a human nutrition study in postmenopausal women in which basal diets supplying 0.25 mg of boron per day were supplemented with 3 mg of boron per day for 119 days, reduced urinary calcium and magnesium excretion and elevated steroid levels were reported (2).

## 13.8.7 Guideline value

As mutagenicity studies gave negative results and carcinogenicity has not been observed, a TDI of 88 µg/kg of body weight was derived by applying an uncertainty factor of 100 (for intra- and interspecies variation) to a NOAEL for testicular atrophy of 8.8 mg of boron per kg of body weight per day in a 2-year diet study in dogs (13). This gives a guideline value for boron of 0.3 mg/litre (rounded figure) if 10% of the TDI is allocated to drinking-water. It should be noted, however, that the intake of boron from food is poorly characterized and that drinking-water treatment does not appear to be very effective in removing it.

## References

1.   Larsen LA. Boron. In: Seiler HG, Sigel H, eds. *Handbook on toxicity of inorganic compounds*, New York, NY, Marcel Dekker, 1988.

2.   Office of Drinking Water. *Draft drinking water health advisory document on boron*. Washington, DC, US Environmental Protection Agency, 1989.

3.   Department of National Health and Welfare (Canada). *Guidelines for Canadian drinking water quality 1978, supporting documentation*. Ottawa, 1978.

4.   Fonds AW, van den Eshof AJ, Smit E. *Integrated criteria document boron*, Bilthoven, The Netherlands, National Institute of Public Health and Environmental Protection, 1987 (Report no. 218108004).

5. International Organization for Standardization. *Water quality—determination of borate—spectrometric method using azomethine-H.* Geneva, 1990 (ISO 9390:1990).

6. Tartari G, Camusso M. Boron content in freshwaters of Northern Italy. *Water, air, and soil pollution,* 1988, 38:409-417.

7. Health and Welfare (Canada). *Guidelines for Canadian drinking water quality. Supporting documentation.* Ottawa, 1990.

8. Centre of International Projects of SCST (State Committee for Science and Technology). [*Boron and its inorganic compounds.*] Moscow, 1989 (in Russian).

9. Nonie SE, Randle K. Boron content of the Freetown drinking water. *Journal of radioanalytical nuclear chemistry, letters,* 1987, 118(4):269-275.

10. Allen HE, Halley-Henderson MA, Hass CN. Chemical composition of bottled mineral water. *Archives of environmental health,* 1989, 44(2):102-116.

11. Mazza B et al. The boron content of industrially produced orange and lemon juices. *Essenze derivati agrumari,* 1982, 51(3):217-227.

12. Browning E. *Toxicity of industrial metals,* 2nd ed. London, Butterworth, 1969:90.

13. Weir RJ, Fisher RS. Toxicologic studies on borax and boric acid. *Toxicology and applied pharmacology,* 1972, 23:351-364.

14. National Toxicology Program. *Toxicology and carcinogenesis studies of boric acid (CAS No. 10043-35-3) in B6C3F$_1$ mice (feed studies).* Research Triangle Park, NC, US National Institutes of Health, 1987 (Technical Report Series 324; NIH Publ. No. 88-2580).

15. Dixon RL, Sherins RJ, Lee IP. Assessment of environmental factors affecting male fertility. *Environmental health perspectives,* 1979, 30:53-68.

16. Stokinger HE. Boron. In: Clayton GD, Clayton FE, eds. *Patty's industrial hygiene and toxicology,* Vol. IIB, *Toxicology,* 3rd ed. New York, Wiley, 1981:2978-3005.

17. Dixon RL, Lee IP, Sherins RJ. Methods to assess reproductive effects of environmental chemicals: studies of cadmium and boron administered orally. *Environmental health perspectives,* 1976, 13:59-67.

# 13.9 Cadmium

## 13.9.1 General description

### Identity

Cadmium is a metal with an oxidation state of +2. It is chemically similar to zinc and occurs naturally with zinc and lead in sulfide ores.

### Physicochemical properties (1–3)

| Property | Value |
|---|---|
| Physical state | Soft white solid |
| Density | 8.64 g/cm$^3$ |
| Melting point | 320.9 °C |
| Boiling point | 765 °C at 100 kPa |
| Solubility | Soluble in dilute nitric and concentrated sulfuric acids |

### Major uses

Cadmium metal is used mainly as an anticorrosive, electroplated on to steel. Cadmium sulfide and selenide are commonly used as pigments in plastics. Cadmium compounds are used in electric batteries, electronic components, and nuclear reactors (2, 4).

### Environmental fate

Fertilizers produced from phosphate ores constitute a major source of diffuse cadmium pollution. The solubility of cadmium in water is influenced to a large degree by its acidity; suspended or sediment-bound cadmium may dissolve when there is an increase in acidity (2). In natural water, cadmium is found mainly in bottom sediments and suspended particles (4).

## 13.9.2 Analytical methods

Cadmium can be determined by atomic absorption spectroscopy using either direct aspiration into a flame or a furnace spectrometric technique. The detection limit is 5 µg/litre with the flame method and 0.1 µg/litre with the furnace procedure (1, 5).

## 13.9.3 Environmental levels and human exposure

### Air

Cadmium is present in ambient air in the form of particles in which cadmium oxide is probably an important constituent (4). Annual average concentrations in four cities in Germany in 1981–82 were 1–3 ng/m$^3$. In the Netherlands, annual average concentrations in 1980–83 were 0.7–2 ng/m$^3$. Levels are generally higher in the vicinity of metallurgical plants. In industrial areas in Belgium, annual average levels in 1985–86 were 10–60 ng/m$^3$ (2). For the general population not living in such areas, cadmium intakes from air are unlikely to exceed 0.8 μg/day (6).

Cigarette smoking increases cadmium concentrations inside houses. The average daily exposure from cigarette smoking (20 cigarettes a day) is 2–4 μg of cadmium (2).

### Water

Cadmium concentrations in unpolluted natural waters are usually below 1 μg/litre (4). Median concentrations of dissolved cadmium measured at 110 stations around the world were <1 μg/litre, the maximum value recorded being 100 μg/litre in the Rio Rimao in Peru (7). Average levels in the Rhine and Danube in 1988 were 0.1 μg/litre (range 0.02–0.3 μg/litre) (8) and 0.025 μg/litre (9), respectively. In the sediments near Rotterdam harbour, levels in mud varied from 1 to 10 mg/kg dry weight in 1985–86, down from 5–19 mg/kg dry weight in 1981 (2).

Contamination of drinking-water may occur as a result of the presence of cadmium as an impurity in the zinc of galvanized pipes or cadmium-containing solders in fittings, water heaters, water coolers, and taps. Drinking-water from shallow wells in areas of Sweden where the soil has been acidified contained concentrations of cadmium approaching 5 μg/litre (4). In Saudi Arabia, mean concentrations of 1–26 μg/litre were found in samples of potable water, some of which were taken from private wells or cold corroded pipes (10). Levels of cadmium could be higher in areas supplied with soft water of low pH, as this would tend to be more corrosive in plumbing systems containing cadmium. In the Netherlands, in a survey of 256 drinking-water plants in 1982, cadmium (0.1–0.2 μg/litre) was detected in only 1% of the drinking-water samples (2).

### Food

Food is the main source of cadmium intake from nonoccupationally exposed people. Crops grown in polluted soil or irrigated with polluted water may contain increased concentrations, as may meat from animals grazing on contaminated pastures (3). Animal kidneys and livers concentrate cadmium. Levels in fruit, meat, and vegetables are usually below 10 μg/kg, in liver 10–100 μg/kg, and in kidney 100–1000 μg/kg. In cereals, levels are about 25 μg/kg wet weight. In 1980–88, average cadmium levels in fish were 20 μg/kg wet weight. High levels were found in shellfish (200–1000 μg/kg) (11).

Based on cadmium levels measured in 1977–84, the estimated daily intake in food by the Netherlands population is 20 μg/person (3). The dietary daily intake of cadmium has also been estimated to be in the range 10–35 μg (11). In contaminated areas in Japan, daily intakes in 1980 were in the range 150–250 μg, based on measurements of cadmium in faeces (4).

### Estimated total exposure and relative contribution of drinking-water

Food is the main source of nonoccupational exposure to cadmium, with dietary daily intakes, as stated above, in the range 10–35 μg. The intake from drinking-water is usually less than 2 μg/day (6). Smoking will increase the daily intake of cadmium. In western Europe, the USA, and Australia, the average daily oral intake of cadmium by nonsmokers living in unpolluted areas is 10–25 μg (12).

## 13.9.4 Kinetics and metabolism in laboratory animals and humans

Absorption via the gastrointestinal tract is influenced by the solubility of the cadmium compound concerned. In healthy persons 3–7% of the cadmium ingested is absorbed; in iron-deficient people, this figure can reach 15–20% (13). Absorbed cadmium enters the bloodstream and is transported to other parts of the body. After binding to metallothionein, it is filtered in the kidney through the glomerulus into the primary urine, then reabsorbed in the proximal tubular cells, where the cadmium–metallothionein bond is broken. The unbound cadmium stimulates the production of new metallothionein, which binds cadmium in the renal tubular cells, thereby preventing the toxic effects of free cadmium. If the metallothionein-producing capacity is exceeded, damage to the proximal tubular cells occurs, the first sign of this effect being low-molecular-weight proteinuria (4).

Tissue cadmium concentrations increase with age. Both kidney and liver act as cadmium stores; 50–85% of the body burden is stored in kidney and liver, 30–60% being stored in the kidney alone. The biological half-life in humans is in the range 10–35 years. Because of the considerable age-related accumulation of cadmium in the body, only a small part of the cadmium absorbed will be excreted in the urine. About 0.007% of the body burden is excreted daily by adults, but individual variation is large (6, 12, 13).

## 13.9.5 Effects on laboratory animals and *in vitro* test systems

### Acute exposure

Cadmium compounds have a moderate acute oral toxicity; oral $LD_{50}$ values for mice and rats range from 60 to over 5000 mg/kg of body weight. Major effects are desquamation of epithelium, necrosis of the gastric and intestinal mucosa, and dystrophic changes of liver, heart, and kidneys (13).

## Short-term exposure

After repeated oral administration, the critical effect in animals is a characteristic lesion of the proximal tubules of the kidneys resulting in impaired tubular resorption and consequent urinary excretion of low-molecular-weight proteins. In rhesus monkeys, a NOAEL of 3 mg of cadmium per kg of diet (given as cadmium chloride) was found for these effects, which were also produced by repeated oral administration to rats of doses of 10 mg of cadmium per litre in drinking-water or 10 mg/kg of diet (given as cadmium chloride) and above. Effects on bone (osteoporosis) were also frequently seen at doses of 10–30 mg of cadmium per kg of diet or 10 mg/litre and above in drinking-water. Effects on the liver, haematopoietic system, and immune system have also been reported (13).

## Reproductive toxicity, embryotoxicity, and teratogenicity

Studies on oral exposure have not provided evidence of teratogenic effects at dose levels below those that were toxic to maternal animals. Fetotoxic and embryotoxic effects were also observed only at toxic dose levels. In a multigeneration study in rats, dose levels up to 100 mg/kg of diet did not cause effects on reproduction. In four-generation studies, 1 mg of cadmium per litre in drinking-water and 0.125 mg of cadmium per kg in the diet caused effects on fertility in mice and rats, respectively. Mild testicular changes in rats were seen after oral administration of 50 mg of cadmium per kg of body weight for 15 months. No effects were seen at 5 mg/kg of body weight or when rats were exposed to 70 mg/litre in their drinking-water for 70 days (13).

## Mutagenicity and related end-points

Both negative and positive results have been reported with regard to DNA degradation, decreased fidelity of DNA synthesis, microbial DNA repair, gene mutations, and chromosomal abnormalities in mammalian cell cultures, higher plants, and intact animals. It should be noted that the positive results were often weak and seen at high concentrations that also caused cytotoxicity (13).

## Carcinogenicity

An oral carcinogenicity study in rats with cadmium chloride (1–50 mg of cadmium per kg of diet) did not reveal significantly increased tumour incidence. In long-term oral toxicity studies in rats, no increase in tumour incidence was seen (13). Lung tumours were induced in rats following the inhalation of inorganic cadmium compounds (13,14).

## 13.9.6 Effects on humans

The estimated lethal oral dose for humans is 350–3500 mg of cadmium; a dose of 3 mg of cadmium has no effects on adults (13).

With chronic oral exposure, the kidney appears to be the most sensitive organ. Cadmium affects the resorption function of the proximal tubules, the first symptom being an increase in the urinary excretion of low-molecular-weight proteins, known as tubular proteinuria (13) (see also section 13.9.4). Intakes of 140–255 µg of cadmium per day have been associated with low-molecular-weight proteinuria in the elderly; the minimum (critical) level of cadmium in the human renal cortex, related to the first sign of tubular dysfunction, varied from 100 to 450 mg/kg wet weight (6). The estimated critical concentration in the renal cortex at which the prevalence of low-molecular-weight proteinuria would reach 10% in the general population is about 200 mg/kg; this would be reached after a daily dietary intake of about 175 µg per person for 50 years, as calculated by regression analysis of cadmium intake and mean kidney cadmium concentration in various countries (6). It was estimated that a daily intake of 100 µg of cadmium per person would lead to the critical cadmium concentration in the renal cortex being exceeded in 2% of the population (6). More severe cadmium damage may also involve the glomeruli, giving rise to increased inulin clearance. Other possible effects include aminoaciduria, glucosuria, and phosphaturia. Disturbances in the renal handling of phosphorus and calcium may cause resorption of minerals from bone, which can result in the development of kidney stones and osteomalacia.

Many cases of itai-itai disease (osteomalacia with various grades of osteoporosis accompanied by severe renal tubular disease) and low-molecular-weight proteinuria have been reported among people living in contaminated areas in Japan and exposed to cadmium via food and drinking-water. The daily intake of cadmium in the most heavily contaminated areas amounted to 600–2000 µg/day; in other less heavily contaminated areas, daily intakes of 100–390 µg/day have been found (12). A relationship between chronic occupational exposure to cadmium or chronic oral exposure to cadmium via the diet in contaminated areas and hypertension could not be demonstrated (13).

Epidemiological studies of people chronically exposed to cadmium via the diet as a result of environmental contamination have not shown an increased cancer risk. The results of studies of chromosomal aberrations in the peripheral lymphocytes of patients with itai-itai disease exposed chronically to cadmium via the diet were contradictory. No reliable studies on reproductive, teratogenic, or embryotoxic effects in humans are available. Epidemiological studies of humans exposed by inhalation to relatively high cadmium concentrations in the workplace showed some evidence of an increased lung cancer risk, but a definite conclusion could not be reached (13).

## 13.9.7 Guideline value

There is some evidence that cadmium is carcinogenic by the inhalation route, and IARC has classified cadmium and cadmium compounds in Group 2A (*15*). However, there is no evidence of carcinogenicity by the oral route, and no clear evidence that cadmium is genotoxic.

On the assumption of an absorption rate for dietary cadmium of 5% and a daily excretion rate of 0.005% of body burden, JECFA concluded that, if levels of cadmium in the renal cortex are not to exceed 50 mg/kg, the total intake of cadmium should not exceed 1 µg/kg of body weight per day. The provisional tolerable weekly intake (PTWI) was therefore set at 7 µg/kg of body weight in 1989 (*6*), and reconfirmed in 1993 (*16*). It is recognized that the margin between the PTWI and the actual weekly intake of cadmium by the general population is small, namely less than 10-fold, and that this margin may be even smaller in smokers. A guideline value for cadmium of 0.003 mg/litre is established based on an allocation of 10% of the PTWI to drinking-water.

## References

1.  Ware GW, ed. Cadmium. USEPA Office of Drinking Water health advisories. *Reviews of environmental contamination and toxicology*, 1989, 107:25-37.

2.  Ros JPM, Slooff W, eds. *Integrated criteria document cadmium*. Bilthoven, Netherlands, National Institute of Public Health and Environmental Protection, 1987 (Report no. 758476004).

3.  International Agency for Research on Cancer. *Cadmium, nickel, some epoxides, miscellaneous industrial chemicals and general considerations on volatile anaesthetics*. Lyon, 1976: 39-74 (IARC Monographs on the Evaluation of the Carcinogenic Risk of Chemicals to Man, Vol. 11).

4.  Friberg L, Nordberg GF, Vouk VB, eds. *Handbook of the toxicology of metals*, Vol. II. Amsterdam, Elsevier, 1986:130-184.

5.  International Organization for Standardization. *Water quality—determination of cadmium*. Geneva, 1985, 1986 (ISO 5961:1985; ISO 8288:1986).

6.  World Health Organization. *Toxicological evaluation of certain food additives and contaminants*. Cambridge, Cambridge University Press, 1989:163-219 (WHO Food Additives Series, No. 24).

7.  World Health Organization/United Nations Environment Programme. *GEMS—Global fresh water quality*. Oxford, Blackwell Reference, 1989.

8.  Arbeitsgemeinschaft Rhein-Wasserwerke e.V. *45. Jahresbericht 1988.* [*45th annual report, 1988.*] Düsseldorf, 1988.

9.  Arbeitsgemeinschaft Wasserwerke Bodensee-Rhein. *20. Jahresbericht 1988.* [*20th annual report, 1988.*] Karlsruhe, 1988.

10. Mustafa HT et al. Cadmium and zinc concentrations in the potable water of the eastern provinces of Saudi Arabia. *Bulletin of environmental contamination and toxicology,* 1988, 40:462-467.

11. Galal-Gorchev H. Dietary intake of pesticide residues, cadmium, mercury and lead. *Food additives and contaminants,* 1991, 8:793-806.

12. *Cadmium.* Geneva, World Health Organization, 1992 (Environmental Health Criteria, No. 134).

13. Krajnc EI et al. *Integrated criteria document. Cadmium—Effects. Appendix.* Bilthoven, Netherlands, National Institute of Public Health and Environmental Protection, 1987 (Report no. 758476004).

14. Oldiges H, Hochrainer P, Glaser U. Long-term inhalation study with Wistar rats and four cadmium compounds. *Toxicological and environmental chemistry,* 1989, 19:217-222.

15. International Agency for Research on Cancer. *Overall evaluations of carcinogenicity: an updating of IARC Monographs volumes 1–42.* Lyon, 1987:139-142 (IARC Monographs on the Evaluation of Carcinogenic Risk to Humans, Suppl. 7).

16. *Evaluation of certain food additives and contaminants: forty-first report of the Joint FAO/WHO Expert Committee on Food Additives.* Geneva, World Health Organization, 1993 (WHO Technical Report Series, No. 837).

# 13.10 Chloride

## 13.10.1 General description

### Identity

Chlorides are widely distributed in nature as salts of sodium ($NaCl$), potassium ($KCl$), and calcium ($CaCl_2$).

### Physicochemical properties (1)

| Salt | Solubility in cold water (g/litre) | Solubility in hot water (g/litre) |
|---|---|---|
| Sodium chloride | 357 | 391 |
| Potassium chloride | 344 | 567 |
| Calcium chloride | 745 | 1590 |

### Organoleptic properties

The taste threshold of the chloride anion in water is dependent on the associated cation. Taste thresholds for sodium chloride and calcium chloride in water are in the range 200–300 mg/litre (*2*). The taste of coffee is affected if it is made with water containing a chloride concentration of 400 mg/litre as sodium chloride or 530 mg/litre as calcium chloride (*3*).

### Major uses

Sodium chloride is widely used in the production of industrial chemicals such as caustic soda, chlorine, sodium chlorite, and sodium hypochlorite. Sodium chloride, calcium chloride, and magnesium chloride are extensively used in snow and ice control. Potassium chloride is used in the production of fertilizers (*4*).

### Environmental fate

Chlorides are leached from various rocks into soil and water by weathering. The chloride ion is highly mobile and is transported to closed basins or oceans.

## 13.10.2 Analytical methods

A number of suitable analytical techniques are available for chloride in water, including silver nitrate titration with chromate indicator (*5*), mercury(II) nitrate titration with diphenylcarbazone indicator, potentiometric titration with silver nitrate, automated iron(III) mercury(II) thiocyanate colorimetry, chloride ion-selective electrode, silver colorimetry, and ion chromatography. Limits of detection range from 50 µg/litre for colorimetry to 5 mg/litre for titration (*6*).

## 13.10.3 Environmental levels and human exposure

### Air

Exposure to chloride in air has been reported to be negligible (*4*).

### Water

Chloride in surface and groundwater originates from both natural and anthropogenic sources, such as run-off containing road de-icing salts, the use of inorganic fertilizers, landfill leachates, septic tank effluents, animal feeds, industrial effluents, irrigation drainage, and seawater intrusion in coastal areas (*4*).

The mean chloride concentration in several rivers in the United Kingdom was in the range 11–42 mg/litre during 1974–81 (*7*). Evidence of a general increase in chloride concentrations in groundwater and drinking-water has been found (*8*), but exceptions have also been reported (*9*). In the USA, aquifers prone to seawater intrusion have been found to contain chloride at concentrations ranging from 5 to 460 mg/litre (*10*), whereas contaminated wells in the Philippines have been reported to have an average chloride concentration of 141 mg/litre (*11*). Chloride levels in unpolluted waters are often below 10 mg/litre and sometimes below 1 mg/litre (*4*).

Chloride in water may be considerably increased by treatment processes in which chlorine or chloride is used. For example, treatment with 40 g of chlorine per $m^3$ and 0.6 mol of iron chloride per litre, required for the purification of groundwater containing large amounts of iron(II), or surface water polluted with colloids, has been reported to result in chloride concentrations of 40 and 63 mg/litre, respectively, in the finished water (*8*).

## Food

Chloride occurs naturally in foodstuffs at levels normally less than 0.36 mg/g. An average intake of 100 mg/day has been reported when a salt-free diet is consumed. However, the addition of salt during processing, cooking, or eating can markedly increase the chloride level in food, resulting in an average dietary intake of 6 g/day, which may rise to 12 g/day in some cases (*4*).

## Estimated total exposure and relative contribution of drinking-water

If a daily water consumption of 2 litres and an average chloride level in drinking-water of 10 mg/litre are assumed, the average daily intake of chloride from drinking-water would be approximately 20 mg per person (*4*), but a figure of approximately 100 mg/day has also been suggested (*8*). Based on these estimates and the average dietary (not salt-free) intake of 6 g/day, drinking-water intake accounts for about 0.33–1.6% of the total intake.

## 13.10.4 Kinetics and metabolism in laboratory animals and humans

In humans, 88% of chloride is extracellular and contributes to the osmotic activity of body fluids. The electrolyte balance in the body is maintained by adjusting total dietary intake and by excretion via the kidneys and gastrointestinal tract. Chloride is almost completely absorbed in normal individuals, mostly from the proximal half of the small intestine. Normal fluid loss amounts to about 1.5–2 litres/day, together with about 4 g of chloride per day. Most (90–95%) is excreted in the urine, with minor amounts in faeces (4–8%) and sweat (2%) (*4*).

## 13.10.5 Effects on laboratory animals and *in vitro* test systems

### *Acute exposure*

The oral $LD_{50}$ values for calcium chloride, sodium chloride, and potassium chloride in the rat have been reported as 1000, 3000, and 2430 mg/kg of body weight, respectively (8).

### *Short-term exposure*

The toxicity of chlorides depends on the cation present; that of chloride itself is unknown. Although excessive intake of drinking-water containing sodium chloride at concentrations above 2.5 g/litre has been reported to produce hypertension (12), this effect is believed to be related to the sodium ion concentration.

## 13.10.6 Effects on humans

A normal adult human body contains approximately 81.7 g of chloride. On the basis of a total obligatory loss of chloride of approximately 530 mg/day, a dietary intake for adults of 9 mg of chloride per kg of body weight has been recommended (equivalent to slightly more than 1 g of table salt per person per day). For children up to 18 years of age, a daily dietary intake of 45 mg of chloride per kg of body weight should be sufficient (4). A dose of 1 g of sodium chloride per kg of body weight was reported to have been lethal in a 9-week-old child (8).

Chloride toxicity has not been observed in humans except in the special case of impaired sodium chloride metabolism, e.g. in congestive heart failure (13). Healthy individuals can tolerate the intake of large quantities of chloride provided that there is a concomitant intake of fresh water. Little is known about the effect of prolonged intake of large amounts of chloride in the diet. As in experimental animals, hypertension associated with sodium chloride intake appears to be related to the sodium rather than the chloride ion (4).

## 13.10.7 Other considerations

Chloride increases the electrical conductivity of water and thus its corrosivity. In metal pipes, chloride reacts with metal ions to form soluble salts (8), thus increasing levels of metals in drinking-water. In lead pipes, a protective oxide layer is built up, but chloride enhances galvanic corrosion (14). It can also increase the rate of pitting corrosion of metal pipes (8).

## 13.10.8 Conclusions

Chloride concentrations in excess of about 250 mg/litre can give rise to detectable taste in water, but the threshold depends on the associated cations. Consumers can, however, become accustomed to concentrations in excess of 250 mg/litre. No health-based guideline value is proposed for chloride in drinking-water.

## References

1. Weast RC, ed. *CRC handbook of chemistry and physics*, 67th ed. Boca Raton, FL, CRC Press, 1986.

2. Zoeteman BCJ. *Sensory assessment of water quality.* New York, NY, Pergamon Press, 1980.

3. Lockhart EE, Tucker CL, Merritt MC. The effect of water impurities on the flavour of brewed coffee. *Food research,* 1955, 20:598.

4. Department of National Health and Welfare (Canada). *Guidelines for Canadian drinking water quality. Supporting documentation.* Ottawa, 1978.

5. International Organization for Standardization. *Water quality—determination of chloride.* Geneva, 1989 (ISO 9297:1989).

6. Department of the Environment. *Methods for the examination of waters and associated materials: chloride in waters, sewage and effluents 1981.* London, Her Majesty's Stationery Office, 1981.

7. Brooker MP, Johnson PC. Behaviour of phosphate, nitrate, chloride and hardness in 12 Welsh rivers. *Water research,* 1984, 18(9):1155-1164.

8. *Sodium, chlorides, and conductivity in drinking water: a report on a WHO working group.* Copenhagen, WHO Regional Office for Europe, 1978 (EURO Reports and Studies 2).

9. Gelb SB, Anderson MP. Sources of chloride and sulfate in ground water beneath an urbanized area in Southeastern Wisconsin (Report WIS-WRC-81-01 NTIS). *Chemical abstracts,* 1981, 96(2):11366g.

10. Phelan DJ. *Water levels, chloride concentrations, and pumpage in the coastal aquifers of Delaware and Maryland.* Washington, DC, US Geological Survey, 1987 (USGS Water Resources Investigations Report 87-4229; Dialog Abstract No. 602039).

11. Morales EC. Chemical quality of deep well waters in Cavite, Philippines. *Water quality bulletin,* 1987, 12(1):43-45.

12. Fadeeva VK. [Effect of drinking-water with different chloride contents on experimental animals.] *Gigiena i sanitarija*, 1971, 36(6):11-15 (in Russian). (Dialog
Abstract No. 051634).

13. Wesson LG. *Physiology of the human kidney.* New York, NY, Grune and Stratton,
1969:591 (cited in ref. 4).

14. Gregory R. Galvanic corrosion of lead solder in copper pipework. *Journal of the Institute of Water and Environmental Management*, 1990, 4(2):112-118.

# 13.11 Chromium

## 13.11.1 General description

### Identity

Chromium is widely distributed in the earth's crust. It can exist in oxidation
states of +2 to +6. Soils and rocks may contain small amounts of chromium,
almost always in the trivalent state.

### Physicochemical properties (1–4)

| Property | Cr | $CrCl_3$ | $K_2CrO_4$ | $Cr_2O_3$ | $CrO_3$ |
|---|---|---|---|---|---|
| Melting point (°C) | 1857 | 1152 | 968.3 | 2266 | 196 |
| Boiling point (°C) | 2672 | – | – | 4000 | – |
| Solubility (g/litre) | insoluble | slightly soluble | 790 | insoluble | 624 |
| Density (g/cm³) | 7.14 | 2.76 | 2.73 | 5.21 | 2.70 |

### Major uses

Chromium and its salts are used in the leather tanning industry, the manufacture
of catalysts, pigments and paints, fungicides, the ceramic and glass industry, and
in photography, and for chrome alloy and chromium metal production, chrome
plating, and corrosion control (*1, 3, 4*).

### Environmental fate

The distribution of compounds containing chromium(III) and chromium(VI)
depends on the redox potential, the pH, the presence of oxidizing or reducing
compounds, the kinetics of the redox reactions, the formation of chromium(III)
complexes or insoluble chromium(III) salts, and the total chromium concentration. In the environment, chromium(VI) occurs mostly as $CrO_4^{2-}$ or $HCrO_4^-$,
and chromium(III) as $Cr(OH)_n^{(3-n)+}$. In soil, chromium(III) predominates.
Chromium(VI) can easily be reduced to chromium(III) by organic matter, for example, and its occurrence in soil is often the result of human activities. In water,

chromium(III) is a positive ion that forms hydroxides and complexes, and is adsorbed at relatively high pH values. In surface waters, the ratio of chromium(III) to chromium(VI) varies widely, and relatively high concentrations of the latter can be found locally. In general, chromium(VI) salts are more soluble than those of chromium(III), making chromium(VI) relatively mobile.

In air, chromium is present in the form of aerosols. It can be removed from the atmosphere by wet and dry deposition. Both trivalent and hexavalent chromium are released into the air. Because of analytical difficulties, data on chromium speciation in ambient air are rarely available, but the proportion present as chromium(VI) has been estimated as 0.01–30%, based on one study (4).

## 13.11.2 Analytical methods

Methods for the determination of chromium in biological and environmental samples are developing rapidly, and all early results (especially for the lower chromium levels) should be interpreted with caution.

Many techniques can be used for the determination of total chromium, including atomic absorption spectroscopy, emission spectroscopy, X-ray fluorescence, and neutron activation analysis. Detection limits for atomic absorption spectroscopy are in the range 0.05–0.2 µg/litre (5).

For determining chelated chromium or the hexavalent or trivalent form only, such methods as gas chromatography (with various detection techniques), polarography, and spectrophotometry can be used (3–5). The determination of chromium species is currently a very sophisticated procedure, and few analytical data are available (4).

## 13.11.3 Environmental levels and human exposure

### Air

In arctic air, chromium concentrations of 5–70 pg/m$^3$ have been measured. Ambient air at most stations in the USA contained very little chromium; mean levels were generally below 300 ng/m$^3$, and median levels less than 20 ng/m$^3$ (6). In non-industrialized areas, concentrations above 10 ng/m$^3$ are uncommon (7). Concentrations in urban areas are 2–4 times higher than regional background concentrations (8). The mean concentration of total chromium in air in the Netherlands varied from 2 to 5 ng/m$^3$ (4).

As a result of smoking, indoor air concentrations can be 10–400 times greater than outdoor concentrations (approximately 1000 ng/m$^3$).

## Water

The average concentration of chromium in rainwater is in the range 0.2–1 µg/litre (*4, 9–11*). Natural chromium concentrations in seawater of 0.04–0.5 µg/litre have been measured (*3*). In the North Sea, a concentration of 0.7 µg/litre was found (*4*).

The natural total chromium content of surface waters is approximately 0.5–2 µg/litre and the dissolved chromium content 0.02–0.3 µg/litre (*4, 10, 12*). Chromium concentrations in antarctic lakes increase with depth from <0.6 to 30 µg/litre (*13*). Most surface waters contain between 1 and 10 µg of chromium per litre. In general, the chromium content of surface waters reflects the extent of industrial activity. In surface waters in the USA, levels up to 84 µg/litre have been found (*1*); in central Canada, surface water concentrations ranged from 0.2 to 44 µg/litre.[1] In the Rhine, chromium levels are below 10 µg/litre (*14*), and in 50% of the natural stream waters in India the concentration is below 2 µg/litre (*9*).

In general, the chromium concentration in groundwater is low (<1 µg/litre). In the Netherlands, a mean concentration of 0.7 µg/litre has been measured, with a maximum of 5 µg/litre (*4*). In India, 50% of 1473 water samples from dug wells contained less than 2 µg/litre (*9*). In groundwater in the USA, levels up to 50 µg/litre have been reported; in shallow groundwater, median levels of 2–10 µg/litre have been found (*1,15*). Most supplies in the USA contain less than 5 µg/litre. In 1986, levels in 17 groundwater supplies and one surface water supply exceeded 50 µg/litre (*1*).

Approximately 18% of the population of the USA are exposed to drinking-water levels between 2 and 60 µg/litre and <0.1% to levels between 60 and 120 µg/litre (*1*). In the Netherlands, the chromium concentration of 76% of the supplies was below 1 µg/litre and of 98% below 2 µg/litre (*16*). A survey of Canadian drinking-water supplies gave an overall median level of 2 µg of chromium per litre, with maxima of 14 µg/litre (raw water) and 9 µg/litre (treated water) (*17*).

## Food

Food contains chromium at concentrations ranging from <10 to 1300 µg/kg (*4, 18, 19*). Highest concentrations have been found in meat, fish, fruit, and vegetables (*18*). Utensils used in the preparation of food may contribute to chromium levels.

## Estimated total exposure and relative contribution of drinking-water

Mean chromium intakes from food and water range from 52 to 943 µg/day (*3*). The estimated total intake of chromium from air, water, and food by the general

---

[1] Data from the National Water Quality Data Bank (NAQUADAT), Inland Waters Directorate, Environment Canada, 1985.

population in the United Kingdom is in the range 78–106 µg/day. Food contributed 93–98% of the total intake and water 1.9–7%. The contribution from air was negligible (*18*). In the Netherlands, the estimated mean daily chromium intake is 100 µg, with a range of 50–200 µg (*4*).

In general, food appears to be the major source of intake. Drinking-water intake can, however, contribute substantially when total chromium levels are above 25 µg/litre.

## 13.11.4 Kinetics and metabolism in laboratory animals and humans

Oral exposure studies in animals found that <0.5–6% of chromium compounds was absorbed; in human studies, the corresponding figure could be as much as 10%. Absorption depends on chromium speciation; chromium(VI) appears to be absorbed from the gastrointestinal tract to a greater extent than chromium(III). Tissue chromium levels of rats exposed to chromium(VI) (as potassium chromate) in drinking-water were 4–15 times higher than those of rats exposed to chromium(III) (as the trichloride). The absorption of chromium(VI) is lowered by partial intragastric reduction to chromium(III) (*20*). Mean fractional absorption values of 5% and 25% have been estimated for the gastrointestinal absorption of chromium(III) and chromium(VI) species and of organic chromium in food ("biologically incorporated"), respectively (*21*). A fractional absorption value of 5% is considered to be a good estimate for the gastrointestinal absorption of soluble inorganic chromium compounds, but 0.5% is more appropriate for that of insoluble inorganic chromium compounds such as chromium trioxide pigment (*20*).

Once absorbed, the fate of chromium will depend on the oxidation state. Chromium(VI) readily penetrates cell membranes, but chromium(III) does not. Chromium is therefore found in both erythrocytes and plasma after gastrointestinal absorption of chromium(VI) but exclusively in the plasma after that of chromium(III). Once transported through the cell membrane, chromium(VI) is rapidly reduced to chromium(III), which subsequently binds to macromolecules. In animal studies, chromium was found to accumulate mainly in liver, kidneys, spleen, and bone marrow after both oral and parenteral administration of different compounds, the distribution depending on the speciation. In humans, the highest concentrations are found in hilar lymph nodes and lungs, followed by spleen, liver, and kidneys (*20*), and tissue chromium levels decline with age. In both laboratory animals and humans, water-soluble compounds can be converted into insoluble compounds with long residence times.

After oral exposure to chromium compounds, especially those of chromium(III), chromium is recovered almost entirely in the faeces because of the poor absorption rate. Animal studies show that urine is the major route of elimination of absorbed chromium. In a 1-year balance study in which two humans had mean daily dietary intakes of 200 and 290 µg of chromium, 60% and 40% of the total amount excreted were recovered in the urine and faeces, respectively (*20*).

## 13.11.5 Effects on laboratory animals and *in vitro* test systems

### *Acute exposure*

Oral $LD_{50}$ values in rats were in the range 20–250 mg of chromium(VI) per kg of body weight and 185–615 mg of chromium(III) per kg of body weight, based on tests with dichromates and chromic compounds, respectively (*20*).

### *Short-term exposure*

Three-month-old inbred BD rats (5–14 per sex per dose) were exposed for 90 days, 5 days per week, to 0, 2%, or 5% of insoluble, nonhydrated chromium(III) oxide ($Cr_2O_3$) pigment in feed (*22*). The dose levels are equivalent to 0, 480, and 1210 mg of chromium(III) per kg of body weight per day (*20*). Survival, feed intake, body and organ weights, blood analysis, and the macroscopic and microscopic appearance of major organs were not affected. The only effect observed was a dose-related decrease in liver and spleen weights, ranging from 15% to 35% (*22*).

### *Long-term exposure*

Chromium(III)
In a 1-year study, 5-week-old Sprague-Dawley albino rats (9 males and 12 females) were exposed to 25 mg of chromium(III) per litre (as chromium trichloride, $CrCl_3$) in drinking-water, equivalent to 2.5 mg of chromium(III) per kg of body weight per day. Feed consumption, body weight gain, and the gross and microscopic appearance of tissues were not affected. The only effect observed was some accumulation of chromium in various tissues (*23*).

Chromium(VI)
In a 1-year study, 5-week-old albino Sprague-Dawley rats (8–12 per sex per dose) were exposed to dose levels up to 25 mg of chromium(VI) per litre (as potassium chromate) in drinking-water. The highest dose is equivalent to 2.5 mg of chromium(VI) per kg of body weight per day. Feed consumption, body weight gain, blood parameters, and the gross and microscopic appearance of organs were not affected. The only effects observed were decreased water consumption (20%) and accumulation of chromium in various tissues (*23*).

In a limited lifetime toxicity study in which Swiss mice of the Charles River CD strain (54 per sex) were exposed from weaning until death to 5 mg of chromium(VI) per litre (as potassium chromate) in drinking-water, survival parameters and body weight were not affected (*24*). Exposure of NMRI mice in a

29-month three-generation study to 135 mg of chromium(VI) per litre (as potassium chromate) in drinking-water did not affect survival or growth (25).

### Reproductive toxicity, embryotoxicity, and teratogenicity

In a 90-day study with limited numbers of 3-month-old inbred BD rats, exposure of male and female animals for 60 days prior to mating and through gestation to dose levels of 0, 2%, or 5% insoluble, nonhydrated chromium(II) oxide pigment in feed did not result in embryotoxicity or fetotoxicity or teratogenicity (22). In studies with hamsters and mice, parenteral administration of chromium(III) or chromium(VI) during gestation did result in embryotoxicity or fetotoxicity and teratogenicity. These effects appear to be associated with maternal toxicity, but definitive conclusions cannot be reached (20).

### Mutagenicity and related end-points

Chromium(VI) compounds cause mutations and allied effects such as chromosomal aberrations in a wide range of prokaryotic and eukaryotic test systems, both *in vitro* and *in vivo*. Chromium(III) compounds are not active in similar systems, or only at high, cytotoxic concentrations. It has therefore been concluded that chromium(VI) is mutagenic, whereas chromium(III) is not.

The mutagenic activity of chromium(VI) is decreased or abolished by reducing agents such as human gastric juice and rat liver microsomal fraction. Inactive chromium(III) compounds are not converted into mutagens by biological systems, but only by treatment with strong oxidizing agents. The difference between the mutagenic action of chromium(VI) and chromium(III) can be explained by differences in physicochemical properties. Although chromium(VI), which readily penetrates cell membranes, is the causative agent, there are strong indications that chromium(III) or intermediates such as chromium(V) formed during the intracellular reduction of chromium(VI) are the genetically active agents that form ligands with macromolecules such as DNA (20).

### Carcinogenicity

In a lifetime carcinogenicity study in which 3-month-old inbred male and female BD rats (60 per dose) were exposed, 5 days per week for 600 days, to 0, 2%, or 5% of insoluble, nonhydrated chromium(III) oxide pigment in feed, tumour incidence was not affected (22). The highest dose is equivalent to 1210 mg of chromium(III) per kg of body weight per day(20).

In a limited lifetime carcinogenicity study, Swiss mice of the Charles River CD strain (54 per sex) were exposed from weaning until death to 5 mg of chromium(VI) per litre (as potassium chromate) in drinking-water. According to the authors (24), the study suggested that chromium(VI) is carcinogenic, but the very limited data reported do not allow evaluation (20).

Exposure of NMRI mice in a 29-month three-generation study to 135 mg of chromium(VI) per litre (as potassium chromate) in drinking-water did not result in carcinogenic activity in the stomach (25).

The carcinogenicity of chromium, especially with regard to lung tumours, has also been investigated in a number of inhalation studies; in other studies, the chromium was administered by implantation or injection. Based on all the available studies, it has been concluded that there is sufficient evidence in experimental animals for the carcinogenicity of calcium, lead, strontium, and zinc chromates (chromium(VI)); limited evidence for the carcinogenicity of chromium trioxide (chromic acid) and sodium dichromate; and inadequate evidence for the carcinogenicity of other chromium(VI) and chromium(III) compounds and of metallic chromium (2, 26).

## 13.11.6 Effects on humans

### Requirements

The daily chromium requirement for adults is estimated to be 0.5–2 μg of absorbable chromium(III). If a fractional absorption value of 25% for "biologically incorporated" chromium(III) in food is assumed, this is provided by a daily dietary intake of 2–8 μg of chromium(III), equivalent to 0.03–0.13 μg of chromium(III) per kg of body weight per day for a 60-kg adult (20).

### Acute exposure

Ingestion of 1–5 g of "chromate" (not further specified) resulted in severe acute effects such as gastrointestinal disorders, haemorrhagic diathesis, and convulsions. Death may occur following cardiovascular shock (20).

### Mutagenicity

In some occupational studies, increased incidences of genotoxic effects such as chromosomal aberrations and sister chromatid exchanges have been found in workers exposed to chromium(VI) compounds (20).

### Carcinogenicity

In epidemiological studies, an association has been found between occupational exposure to chromium(VI) compounds and mortality due to lung cancer. On the basis of these studies, it has been concluded that there is sufficient evidence of respiratory carcinogenicity in humans exposed to chromium(VI) in these occupational settings. Data on lung cancer risk in other chromium-associated occupational settings and for cancer at sites other than the lungs are considered to be insufficient. The epidemiological data do not allow an evaluation of the relative contributions to carcinogenic risk of metallic chromium, chromium(III), and chromium(VI) or of soluble versus insoluble chromium compounds, but it appears that exposure to a mixture of chromium(VI) compounds of different solubilities results in the highest risk to humans (2, 26).

IARC has classified chromium(VI) in Group 1 (carcinogenic to humans) and metallic chromium and chromium(III) in Group 3 (not classifiable as to their carcinogenicity to humans) (2, 26).

## 13.11.7 Provisional guideline value

In principle, because the health effects are determined largely by the oxidation state, different guideline values for chromium(III) and chromium(VI) should be derived. However, current analytical methods and the variable speciation of chromium in water favour a guideline value for total chromium.

Because of the carcinogenicity of chromium(VI) by the inhalation route and its genotoxicity, the current guideline value of 0.05 mg/litre has been questioned, but the available toxicologial data do not support the derivation of a new value. As a practical measure, 0.05 mg/litre, which is considered to be unlikely to give rise to significant risks to health, has been retained as the provisional guideline value until additional information becomes available and chromium can be re-evaluated.

## References

1. Office of Drinking Water. *Health advisory—chromium*. Washington, DC, US Environmental Protection Agency, 1987.

2. International Agency for Research on Cancer. *Some metals and metallic compounds.* Lyon, 1980:205-323 (IARC Monographs on the Evaluation of the Carcinogenic Risk of Chemicals to Humans, Vol. 23).

3. *Chromium*. Geneva, World Health Organization, 1988 (Environmental Health Criteria No. 61).

4. Slooff W et al. *Integrated criteria document chromium*. Bilthoven, Netherlands, National Institute of Public Health and Environmental Protection, 1989 (Report no. 758701002).

5. International Organization for Standardization. *Water quality—determination of total chromium*. Geneva, 1990 (ISO 9174:1990).

6. Environmental Monitoring Systems Laboratory. *Frequency distributions by site/year for chromium, the results of samples collected at National Air Surveillance Network sites.* Research Triangle Park, NC, US Environmental Protection Agency, 1984.

7. National Academy of Sciences. *Drinking water and health*, Vol. 3. Washington, DC, National Academy Press, 1980.

8. Nriagu JO, Nieboer E, eds. *Chromium in the natural and human environments*. New York, NY, John Wiley, 1988.

9. Handa BK. Occurrence and distribution of chromium in natural waters of India. *Advances in environmental science and technology*, 1988, 20:189-214.

10. Xingzhen Q, Xiuxia L. [Investigation on the natural background values and states of elements in natural water from the upper reaches of the Nenjiang river.] *Kexue tongbao*, 1987, 32(14):983-987 (in Chinese).

11. Barrie LA et al. On the concentration of trace metals in precipitation. *Atmospheric environment*, 1987, 21(5):1133-1135.

12. Shiller AM, Boyle EA. Variability of dissolved trace metals in the Mississippi River. *Geochimica et cosmochimica acta*, 1987, 51(12):3273-3277.

13. Masuda N et al. Trace element distributions in some saline lakes of the Vestfold Hills, Antarctica. *Hydrobiologia*, 1988, 165:103-114.

14. RIWA. *De samenstelling van het Rijnwater in 1986 en 1987*. [*Composition of the water of the Rhine in 1986 and 1987*.] Amsterdam, 1989.

15. Deverel SJ, Millard SP. Distribution and mobility of selenium and other trace elements in shallow ground water of the Western San Joaquin Valley, California. *Environmental science and technology*, 1988, 22:697-702.

16. Fonds AW, van den Eshof AJ, Smit E. *Water quality in the Netherlands*. Bilthoven, Netherlands, National Institute of Public Health and Environmental Protection, 1987 (Report no. 218108004).

17. Méranger JC, Subramanian KS, Chalifoux C. A national survey of cadmium, chromium, copper, lead, zinc, calcium, and magnesium in Canadian drinking water supplies. *Environmental science and technology*, 1979, 13:707-711.

18. Ministry of Agriculture, Fisheries and Food. *Survey of aluminium, antimony, chromium, cobalt, indium, nickel, thallium and tin in food. 15. Report of the Steering Group on Food Surveillance; The Working Party on the Monitoring of Foodstuffs for Heavy Metals*. London, Her Majesty's Stationery Office, 1985.

19. Agency for Toxic Substances and Disease Registry. *Toxicological profile for chromium*. Washington, DC, US Public Health Service, 1989 (ATSFDR/TP-88/10).

20. Janus JA, Krajnc EI. *Integrated criteria document chromium: effects. Appendix*. Bilthoven, Netherlands, National Institute of Public Health and Environmental Protection, 1990.

21. Thorne MC et al. *Pharmacodynamic models of selected toxic chemicals in man*, Vol. 1. *Review of metabolic data*. Lancaster, MTP Press, 1986.

22. Ivankovic S, Preussmann R. Absence of toxic and carcinogenic effects after adminis-tration of high doses of chromic oxide pigment in subacute and long-term feeding experiments in rats. *Food and cosmetics toxicology*, 1975, 13:347-351.

23. MacKenzie RD et al. Chronic toxicity studies. II. Hexavalent and trivalent chromi-um administered in drinking water to rats. *Archives of industrial health*, 1958, 18:232-234.

24. Schroeder HA, Mitchener M. Scandium, chromium(VI), gallium, yttrium, rhodium, palladium, indium in mice: effects on growth and life span. *Journal of nutrition*, 1971, 101:1431-1438.

25. Borneff I et al. [Carcinogenic substances in water and soil. XXII. Mouse drinking study with 3,4-benzpyrene and potassium chromate.] *Archiv für Hygiene*, 1968, 152(68):45-53 (in German).

26. International Agency for Research on Cancer. *Chromium, nickel and welding*. Lyon, 1990 (IARC Monographs on the Evaluation of Carcinogenic Risks to Humans, Vol. 49).

# 13.12 Colour

## 13.12.1 General description

### *Identity*

The appearance of colour in water is caused by the absoption of certain wave-lengths of normal light by coloured substances ("true" colour) and by the scatter-ing of light by suspended particles; combined, these constitute "apparent" colour (*1–3*). Treatment removes much of the suspended matter from drinking-water, and most of the remaining discoloration arises from true colour, which is general-ly substantially less than apparent colour (*4*).

### *Organoleptic properties*

It has been suggested that the organic matter (primarily humic and fulvic acids) usually responsible for the colour of drinking-water give it an earthy smell and taste, but there is no conclusive evidence for this. Highly coloured polluted water will frequently have an objectionable taste, but the precise causal relationship is unknown. It is known that the organic colouring material in water stimulates the growth of many aquatic microorganisms, some of which are directly responsible for the production of odour in water (*5*).

## 13.12.2 Analytical methods

There are essentially two methods for the measurement of colour intensity in potable water: visual comparison with standards, and absorbance analysis (6).

In the visual comparison method, colour is measured in true colour units (TCU, or Hazen units), 1 TCU being defined as the colour produced by 1 mg of platinum per litre (as chloroplatinic acid) in the presence of 2 mg of cobalt(II) chloride per litre (4, 6). The colour of a filtered water sample is measured by visual comparison with a series of standards of known TCU. This method was designed for use in the determination of the colour of naturally (yellow-brown) coloured water and is difficult to apply to other colours. As the colour of natural surface waters generally increases with increasing pH (1), it is recommended that the pH of a colour sample be recorded together with the colour measurement (4, 6).

Absorbance analysis involves filtration through a cellulose-acetate membrane and subsequent spectrophotometric measurement of the absorbance of the filtrate (6).

## 13.12.3 Environmental levels and human exposure

### Water

As already mentioned, colour in natural waters is due mainly to organic matter, particularly dissolved humic and fulvic acids, which originate from soil, peat, and decaying vegetation. In addition, inorganic iron and manganese are present in some groundwaters and surface waters and may impart a red and black hue, respectively. Highly coloured wastewaters, in particular from the pulp, paper, dye, and textile industries, can also produce coloured waters.

Discoloration of potable water may arise from the dissolution of iron (red) or copper (blue) in distribution pipes, which can be enhanced by bacteriological processes. Microbiological action can also produce "red water", resulting from the oxidation of iron(II) to iron(III) by "iron bacteria". Similarly, black discoloration may result from the action of bacteria capable of oxidizing dissolved manganese to give insoluble forms.

## 13.12.4 Effects on laboratory animals and *in vitro* test systems

### Short-term exposure

A low-ash preparation of soil fulvic acid was supplied in drinking-water at concentrations of 10, 100, or 1000 mg/litre to male rats for periods of up to 90 days (Becking & Yagminas, 1978, unpublished data). No significant changes in body weight, food and water intake, organ/body weight ratios, or tissue histology were observed. The same fulvic acid preparation given daily for 14 days to rats by gavage at a dosage of 1000 mg/kg of body weight was not lethal but did reduce the rate of weight gain and cause slight changes in kidney enzyme concentrations.

Drinking-water containing nonchlorinated (total organic carbon (TOC) concentration 1.0 g/litre) and chlorinated humic substances (TOC 0.1, 0.5, 1.0 g/litre) was administered to groups of male Sprague-Dawley rats for a period of 90 days (7). The average body weight gain and terminal body weight were decreased significantly by 1.0 g/litre chlorinated humic substances and slightly by 0.5 g/litre chlorinated humic and 1.0 g/litre nonchlorinated humic substances. No significant differences were observed in food consumption. However, fluid consumption was significantly decreased by 1.0 g/litre nonchlorinated and 1.0 or 0.5 g/litre chlorinated humic substances, namely by 14%, 16%, and 17%, respectively. The most significant finding of this study was the increased incidence and severity of haematuria in the group receiving 1.0 g/litre chlorinated humic substances. These studies suggest that there is minimal risk from exposure to chlorination by-products of humic acids as far as target organ effects are concerned.

### Mutagenicity and related end-points

Chlorinated and nonchlorinated humic acids (TOC 1 g/litre in distilled water) were tested for mutagenic activity by both *in vitro* and *in vivo* assays. In the Ames test, the results showed positive mutagenic activity only after chlorination, whereas induction of sister chromatid exchange was observed with both chlorinated and nonchlorinated humic acids. In contrast, in the *in vivo* studies, no evidence was found of mutagenic activity for both chlorinated and nonchlorinated samples (8).

## 13.12.5 Effects on humans

Colour-producing organic substances are not themselves thought to be harmful to health. However, they can react with chlorine to produce undesirable levels of chlorination by-products, including trihalomethanes.

Most metals readily form complexes with humic substances in water, which can greatly increase their solubility (9,10). For example, naturally occurring humic substances in water may increase the solubility of iron by a factor of up to 109 (10).

The bioavailability and human toxicity of complexes between humic material and such toxic metals as aluminium, copper, cadmium, and mercury have been investigated in only a small number of studies (11).

## 13.12.6 Conclusions

The colour of drinking-water is usually due to the presence of coloured organic acids (humic and fulvic) associated with the humus fraction of soil. Colour is strongly influenced by the presence of iron and other metals, either as natural impurities or as corrosion products. It may also result from the contamination of the water source with industrial effluents and may be the first indication of a hazardous situation. The source of colour in a water supply should be investigated, particularly if a substantial change takes place. Colours below 15 TCU are usually acceptable to consumers, but acceptability may vary according to local circumstances. No health-based guideline value is proposed for colour in drinking-water.

## References

1.  Black AP, Christman RF. Characteristics of colored surface water. *Journal of the American Water Works Association*, 1963, 55:753.

2.  Black AP, Hannah SA. Measurement of low turbidities. *Journal of the American Water Works Association*, 1965, 57:901.

3.  Conner KJ, Stiff MJ. *The characteristics and chemical treatment of soluble humic colour in water. III. Simulation of chemical treatment.* Medmenham, Water Research Centre, 1987 (WRC Report 543-S).

4.  American Public Health Association. *Standard methods for the examination of water and wastewater*, 17th ed. Washington, DC, 1989.

5.  Prakash A. Humic substances and aquatic productivity. In: Povoledo D, Golterman HL, eds. *Humic substances 1972*. Wageningen, Netherlands, Pudoc, 1975:259-268.

6.  International Organization for Standardization. *Water quality examination and determination of colour.* Geneva, 1985 (ISO 7887:1985).

7.  Condie LW, Laurie RD, Bercz JP. Subchronic toxicology of humic acid following chlorination in the rat. *Journal of toxicology and environmental health*, 1985, 15:305-314.

8.  Meier JR, Bull RJ. Mutagenic properties of drinking water disinfectants and by-products. In: Jolley RL et al., eds, *Water chlorination, chemistry, environmental impact and health effects*, Vol. 5. Chelsea, MI, Lewis Publishers, 1985:207-249.

9.  Chiou CT et al. Water solubility enhancement of some organic pollutants and pesticides by dissolved humic and fulvic acids. *Environmental science and technology*, 1986, 20:502-508.

10. Shapiro J. Effect of yellow organic acids on iron and other metals in water. *Journal of the American Water Works Association*, 1964, 56:1062.

11. Petersen RC et al. Health aspects of humic compounds in acid environments. *Water quality bulletin*, 1986, 11(1):44-49.

## 13.13 Copper

### 13.13.1 General description

#### *Identity*

Widely used copper compounds include $CuCl_2·2H_2O$ (CAS no. 7447-39-4), $Cu(NO_3)_2·3H_2O$ (CAS no. 10031-43-3), and $CuSO_4·5H_2O$ (CAS no. 7758-99-8).

#### *Physicochemical properties (1, 2)*

| Compound | Water solubility (g/litre) |
|---|---|
| $CuCl_2·2H_2O$ | 710 at 0 °C; 1080 at 100 °C |
| $Cu(NO_3)_2·3H_2O$ | 1380 at 0 °C; 12 700 at 100 °C |
| $CuSO_4·5H_2O$ | 320 at 0 °C; 2030 at 100 °C |

#### *Organoleptic properties*

Dissolved copper imparts a colour and an unpleasant astringent taste to drinking-water (3). Staining of laundry and plumbing fixtures occurs when copper concentrations in water exceed 1 mg/litre. The taste threshold is above 5 mg/litre, although taste is detectable in distilled water at 2.6 mg/litre (4). The organoleptic threshold of dissolved $Cu^{2+}$ is 0.8–1.0 mg/litre in mineral water and 2.4–3.2 mg/litre in 5 mmol/litre saccharose (5).

#### *Major uses*

Copper is an important heat and electrical conductor. It is also used for water pipes, roof coverings, household goods, and chemical equipment, in the arts, and in many alloys (e.g. brass and bronze). Copper oxides, chlorides, sulfates, ethano-ates, bromides, and carbonates are widely used in pest control, as inorganic dyes, as feed additives, in photography, in seed disinfectants, as fungicides and algi-cides, and in electroforming (1, 2, 6).

#### *Environmental fate*

Monovalent copper is unstable in aqueous solution. Only those copper(I) com-pounds that are insoluble in water ($Cu_2O$, $Cu_2S$) and certain copper(I) com-plexes are stable in aqueous environments. Cu(II) forms complexes with both inorganic and organic ligands such as ammonium and chloride ions and humic acids (2).

## 13.13.2 Analytical methods

The most important methods for the determination of copper and their detection limits are atomic absorption spectrometry with flame detection (1.5 µg/litre) or in the graphite furnace (60 ng/litre); pulse inverse voltammetry (1 ng/litre); spectral photometry (100 µg/litre); neutron activation (0.2 ng of copper per 500 mg solid sample); and emission spectroscopy (0.5 µg/litre) (6, 7).

## 13.13.3 Environmental levels and human exposure

### Air

Copper concentrations in air in rural areas in the USA and Europe are normally below 10 ng/m$^3$. In urban areas, concentrations may be as high as 1500 ng/m$^3$ (6, 8), although levels around 25 ng/m$^3$ have also been found (6).

### Water

Natural copper concentrations in drinking-water are around a few micrograms per litre (6). Depending on such properties as hardness, pH, anion concentrations, oxygen concentration, temperature, and the technical conditions of the pipe system (1, 6), water from copper pipes may contain several milligrams of copper per litre (1, 9). In a sample of water for human consumption which had remained stagnant for 12 h, an extreme level of 22 mg of copper per litre was found (10).

### Food

Foods especially rich in copper (10–100 mg/kg) are veal and pig, sheep, and calf liver. Chocolate and chocolate products, tea, and coffee (dry) can also contain more than 10 mg of copper per kg. Other foods may contain up to 10 mg/kg (nuts), median values being around 2 mg/kg (1, 11).

### Estimated total exposure and relative contribution of drinking-water

Copper is ingested by humans mainly via food and drinking-water. In two 24-h intake studies in the Netherlands, the average daily copper intake per person was 1.2–1.4 mg (1). Intakes of 1.82–2.38 mg/day (11) and less than 0.95 mg/day (duplicate study) (12) have been reported in the western and eastern parts of Germany, respectively; intakes in the USA were 2-4 mg/day (6). Drinking-water can contribute a significant proportion of the daily copper intake if it has flowed through copper installations (1, 6).

### 13.13.4 Kinetics and metabolism in laboratory animals and humans

Up to 100% copper absorption was observed in newborn rats. After weaning, absorption rates fell in various animal species to below 10% (*13*). Estimated values for intestinal copper absorption in humans vary between 25% and 65% (*13*). In adults, the absorption and retention rates of copper depend on the daily intake and, as a consequence, copper overload is unlikely. In a balance study with bottle-fed infants, absorption and retention rates were 23.9% and 21.9% of intake, respectively (*14*).

Copper is an essential element. Balance studies on adults suggest that a copper intake of 1–5 mg/day, corresponding to 20–80 µg/kg of body weight per day (*15, 16*) is required. The normal copper content in the adult is 1–2 mg/kg of body weight. In neonates, the liver contains over 90% of the total body copper (4–5 mg/kg of body weight); the copper concentration in the newborn liver is 6–10-fold higher than in the adult liver (*17*) but decreases during the first 3 months of life (*18*).

Normal copper concentrations in plasma are 0.9–1.3 mg/litre (*17*). Of this, 5–10% is bound to albumin and 90–95% specifically to the copper transport protein ceruloplasmin (*8, 13*). In the liver, copper is bound mainly to metallothionein but also to functionally specific enzymes (*19*); glutathione serves as a buffer to trap free copper ions that would otherwise be toxic (*20*). Partial saturation of metallothionein with copper and zinc in the liver of the newborn depends on the cytosolic zinc:copper ratio (*18*).

About 1 mg of copper per day is transported to the tissues bound to ceruloplasmin (*15, 16*). Excretion takes place primarily via the faeces; urine contains only 0.5–3% of the daily intake (*6, 21, 22*).

### 13.13.5 Effects on laboratory animals and *in vitro* test systems

**Acute exposure**

Depending on the animal species and the anion of the copper salt administered, oral $LD_{50}$s vary between 15 (guinea-pig: $CuCl_2$) and 416 (rats: $Cu(OH)Cl$; $Cu_2O$) mg/kg of body weight (*13, 21, 22*).

**Short-term exposure**

In most studies with rodents, copper given orally in doses of up to 50 mg/kg of body weight for less than 1 year caused either no effects or adaptation to copper exposure with transient signs of toxicity. No such adaptation was observed in rabbits, pigs, and sheep (*13, 21, 22*), the last-named being especially sensitive to some of the acute effects of excess copper intake.

## Long-term exposure

In two oral studies, NOAELs of 5 mg/kg of body weight per day (1 year; dog) and 160 mg/kg of body weight per day (2 years; rat) were found for the end-points liver functional changes (dog) and various macroscopic and microscopic pathological parameters (rat). In a 16-month rabbit study, a LOAEL of 12 mg/kg of body weight per day was estimated for cirrhosis-like hepatic changes (*21, 22*).

## Reproductive toxicity, embryotoxicity, and teratogenicity

Copper gluconate given orally to mice and rats at 30 mg/kg of body weight per day on days 6–14 and 5–15 of gestation, respectively, was neither embryotoxic nor teratogenic. In another assay with comparable exposure, the fertility of rats was not affected. A much higher NOAEL was reported with copper sulfate for skeletal deformations of fetuses from exposed mothers, but reduced maternal food intake could not be ruled out as the cause (*6, 21, 22*).

## Mutagenicity and related end-points

The results of mutagenicity tests are inconclusive (*6*). Positive results from *in vitro* tests using free copper ions are not applicable to the *in vivo* situation, where copper is always tightly bound to low- and high-molecular-weight ligands (*18, 19*).

## Carcinogenicity

Based on the results of a number of animal studies involving oral and intraperitoneal exposure to various copper compounds, it is generally agreed that copper and its salts are not animal carcinogens (*6, 21, 22*).

## 13.13.6 Effects on humans

### Acute exposure

The lethal oral dose for adults lies between 50 and 500 mg of copper(II) salt per kg of body weight. Vomiting, diarrhoea, nausea, and some acute symptoms presumably due to local irritation by ingested copper(II) ions have been described in several case reports (*6, 21, 22*). The estimated concentration of copper(II) in drinking-water or beverages that can lead to symptoms of this type is 30 mg/litre but may vary with the binding and chemical form of copper present.

### Short-term exposure

Copper pipes in haemodialysis devices have caused systemic copper poisoning in patients (*21, 22*). Drinking-water from a new copper kettle used over a period of 3 months for the preparation of food and beverages may have been responsible for a strongly enhanced serum copper level, behavioural changes, diarrhoea, and progressive loss of strength in a 15-month-old child (*23*).

A 14-month-old infant died of micronodular liver cirrhosis, probably due to pre- and postnatal exposure to up to 6.8 mg of copper per litre in the very acid water that had flowed through a copper installation and had been used to prepare the infant's feed (*24*). A total of 22 similar cases of early childhood liver cirrhosis have been described in two limited areas in Germany (*25*). The estimated daily copper intake that might have triggered the cirrhosis in the infants' early months of life (*26*) is at least 900 µg/kg of body weight, about 10 times their daily requirement (*21, 22*).

### Long-term exposure

In hepatolenticular degeneration (Wilson disease) which is caused by reduced copper excretion in the bile, the normal daily copper intake of a few milligrams is enough to trigger liver cirrhosis and excessive copper accumulation in many organs, but only after several years of exposure (*6, 27*). The copper status of the healthy liver of neonates during the first few months of life is comparable to that of a person suffering from Wilson disease (*28*), which may explain why infants are more sensitive to factors that threaten copper homoeostasis than are older children and adults (*25*).

In a recent Finnish report, it was claimed that a positive correlation existed between coronary heart disease incidence and the plasma copper level under conditions of selenium malnutrition (*29*). The duration and source of the excessive copper exposure in this study were not specified.

### 13.13.7 Provisional guideline value

Based on a NOAEL of 5 mg/kg of body weight per day for the end-point liver toxicity in a rather old 1-year study in dogs and in the light of the essentiality of copper, a provisional maximum tolerable daily intake (PMTDI) of 0.5 mg/kg of body weight was established by JECFA in 1982 (*21, 22*). An allocation of 10% of the PMTDI to drinking-water gives a guideline value of 2 mg of copper per litre (rounded figure). Although this study did not take into account the differences in copper metabolism in the neonate, a concentration of 2 mg/litre should provide a sufficient margin of safety for bottle-fed infants because their copper intake from other sources is usually low. In view of the remaining uncertainties regarding copper toxicity in humans, however, this guideline value is considered provisional. Copper can give rise to taste problems, but the taste should be acceptable at the health-based provisional guideline value.

# References

1.  Slooff W et al., eds. *Integrated criteria document copper.* Bilthoven, Netherlands, National Institute of Public Health and Environmental Protection, 1989 (Report no. 758474009).

2.  Holleman AF, Wiberg E. *Lehrbuch der anorganischen Chemie.* [*Textbook of inorganic chemistry.*] Berlin, Walter de Gruyter, 1985.

3.  Page GG. Contamination of drinking water by corrosion of copper tubes. *New Zealand journal of sciences,* 1973, 16:349.

4.  Cohen JM et al. Taste threshold concentrations of metals in drinking water. *Journal of the American Water Works Association,* 1960, 52:660-670.

5.  Béguin-Bruhin Y et al. Threshold concentration of copper in drinking water. *Lebensmittel-Wissenschaft und Technologie,* 1983, 16:22-26.

6.  *Summary review of the health effects associated with copper: health issue assessment.* Cincinnati, OH, US Environmental Protection Agency, 1987 (EPA 600/8-87/001).

7.  International Organization for Standardization. *Water quality—determination of cobalt, nickel, copper, zinc, cadmium and lead.* Geneva, 1986 (ISO 8288:1986).

8.  Friberg L, Nordberg GF, Vouk VB, eds. Copper. In: *Handbook on the toxicology of metals.* Amsterdam, Elsevier, 1986:233-254.

9.  Alam I, Sadiq M. Metal contamination of drinking water from corrosion of distribution pipes. *Environmental pollution,* 1989, 57:167-178.

10. *Bericht des Bayrischen Staatsministeriums des Innern an den Bayrischen Landtag über Gesundheitsgefährdungen durch kupferhaltiges Trinkwasser.* [*Report of the Bavarian Ministry of the Interior to the Bavarian Parliament on health risks from copper in drinking water.*] Munich, 1989 (Az. IE3-5305-10/17/89).

11. Deutsche Gesellschaft für Ernährung e.V. *Material zum Ernährungsbericht.* [*Materials for the German nutrition report.*] Frankfurt, 1980.

12. Anke M. Trace element intake (zinc, manganese, copper, molybdenum, iodine and nickel) of humans in Thuringia and Brandenburg of the Federal Republic of Germany. *Journal of trace elements and electrolytes in health and disease,* 1991, 5(2): 69-74.

13. Janus JA et al. *Integrated criteria document copper: effects.* Bilthoven, Netherlands, National Institute of Public Health and Environmental Protection, 1989 (Appendix to report no. 758474009).

14. Ziegler EE et al. Zink-, Kupfer- und Bleibilanzen bei normalen Säuglingen. [Zinc, copper and lead balances in normal infants.] In: Gladtke E, ed. *Spurenelemente—Analytik, Umsatz, Bedarf, Mangel und Toxikologie.* [*Trace elements—analysis, turnover, requirements, deficiency and toxicology.*] Stuttgart, Georg Thieme Verlag, 1979:56-67.

15. Epstein O. Liver copper in health and disease. *Postgraduate medical journal,* 1983, 59:88-94.

16. Davis GK, Mertz W. Copper. In: Mertz W, ed. *Trace elements in human and animal nutrition,* 5th ed. New York, NY, Academic Press, 1986:301-364.

17. Lentner C, ed. *Geigy scientific tables.* Vol. 1. *Units of measurement, body fluids, composition of the body, nutrition,* 8th ed. Basel, Ciba-Geigy, 1981.

18. Klein D et al. Metallothionein, copper and zinc in fetal and neonatal human liver: changes during development. *Toxicology letters,* 1991, 56:61-67.

19. Cousins RJ. Absorption, transport and hepatic metabolism of copper and zinc: special reference to metallothionein and ceruloplasmin. *Physiological reviews,* 1985, 65:238-309.

20. Freedman JH, Ciriole MR, Peisach J. The role of glutathione in copper metabolism and toxicity. *Journal of biological chemistry,* 1989, 264:5598-5605.

21. *Evaluation of certain food additives and contaminants:* twenty-sixth report of the Joint FAO/WHO Expert Committee on Food Additives. Geneva, World Health Organization, 1982:31-32 (WHO Technical Report Series, No. 683).

22. Joint FAO/WHO Expert Committee on Food Additives. *Toxicological evaluation of certain food additives.* Cambridge, Cambridge University Press, 1982:265-296. (WHO Food Additives Series, No. 17).

23. Salmon MA, Wright T. Chronic copper poisoning presenting as pink disease. *Archives of disease in childhood,* 1971, 46:108-110.

24. Walker-Smith J, Blomfield J. Wilson's disease or chronic copper poisoning? *Archives of disease in childhood,* 1973, 48:476-479.

25. Eife R et al. Die frühkindliche Leberzirrhose als Folge der chronischen Kupferintoxikation. [Early childhood cirrhosis as the consequence of chronic copper intoxication.] *Bundesgesundheitsblatt,* 1991, 34:327-329.

26. O'Neill NC, Tanner MS. Uptake of copper from brass vessels by bovine milk and its relevance to Indian childhood cirrhosis. *Journal of pediatric gastroenterology and nutrition,* 1989, 9:167-172.

27. Scheinberg IH. Human health effects of copper. In: Nriagu JO, ed. *Copper in the environment,* Vol. 2. New York, NY, John Wiley, 1979:17-31.

28. Linder MC, Munro HN. Iron and copper metabolism during development. *Enzyme*, 1973, 15:111-138.

29. Salonen JT et al. Interactions of serum copper, selenium, and low density lipoprotein cholesterol in atherogenesis. *British medical journal*, 1991, 302:756-760.

## 13.14 Cyanide

### 13.14.1 General description

Almost all of the recent literature on cyanide has resulted from interest in the root crop cassava, which provides a major part of the diet for between 300 and 500 million people living in developing countries in the tropics and subtropics. If not properly prepared, cassava can contain very high levels of cyanide, and outbreaks of disease have been associated with its consumption.

### 13.14.2 Analytical methods

Cyanide can be determined in water by both titrimetric and photometric techniques, with a detection limit of 2 µg/litre (*1*).

### 13.14.3 Environmental levels and human exposure

**Water**

Cyanides are occasionally found in drinking-water, primarily as a consequence of industrial contamination.

**Food**

A recent study suggests that dietary exposure to cyanide is considerably greater in developing countries than in developed ones. For a group of 73 subjects in Liberia consuming cassava, the mean daily intake of cyanide ion was calculated to be 0.61 mg/kg of body weight (*2*). Although insufficient data are available from which to calculate the average daily intake in developed countries, it is very unlikely to be of this magnitude.

### 13.14.4 Kinetics and metabolism in laboratory animals and humans

Cyanide ion is readily absorbed by the gastrointestinal tract and is rapidly converted into thiocyanate by the enzyme rhodanese. Oral and subcutaneous doses of cyanide in rats are excreted as thiocyanate, primarily in the urine (*3, 4*). Golden hamsters exposed to cyanide by subcutaneous infusion appeared to excrete only a relatively small percentage (10–15%) of the dose as thiocyanate in the urine (5), perhaps because rhodanese activity in hamsters is lower than in rats, and hence they are less able to convert cyanide into thiocyanate (6).

## 13.14.5 Effects on laboratory animals and in vitro test systems

### Short-term exposure

A reduction in feed consumption and body weight gain was noted in a group of six male and two female African rats fed diets containing potassium cyanide at 2500 mg/kg for 84 days. No effects on the pathology of the thyroid, liver, kidney, and spleen or on serum total proteins, albumin, aspartate aminotranferase, and alanine aminotransferase were observed, but serum urea concentration was elevated (7).

Addition of potassium cyanide at a concentration of 200 mg/litre to the drinking-water of a group of seven male Sprague-Dawley rats produced a slight elevation in liver weight but had no effect on body weight gain after 21 days. Addition of potassium cyanide to the diet at 200 mg/kg had no effect on either parameter. However, there was evidence that cyanide added to the diet was quickly lost or bound, and hence actual exposure was likely to have been less than anticipated. This study also showed that cyanide offers some protection against selenium toxicity in rats, possibly through the formation of the SeCN ion (8).

Six weanling pigs were fed a diet containing potassium cyanide (500 mg of cyanide per kg) for 56 days. A reduction in feed intake was noted, but there was no effect on body weight gain. There were no effects on the weights of several organs examined except for some evidence of an increase in thyroid weight. Pathological examination of a range of tissues revealed no treatment-related effects (9).

Pigs were fed diets of cassava containing 0, 96, or 400 mg of cyanide per kg for 72 days. A lowering of serum thyroxine was noted at both dose levels. There were no effects on serum total protein, albumin, alanine aminotransferase, and aspartate aminotransferase, but serum urea was elevated (10).

Erythrocyte glucose-6-phosphate dehydrogenase activity was significantly depressed in miniature swine receiving oral doses of 1.2 mg of cyanide ion per kg of body weight per day from week 0 to week 12, but activity returned to control levels after week 16. At lower doses of 0.4 and 0.7 mg of cyanide ion per kg of body weight per day, enzyme inhibition was initially delayed; by week 20, activity was significantly lower than in controls and the highest dose group (11).

The effects of cyanide on behaviour were studied in pigs given oral doses of 0, 0.4, 0.7, or 1.2 mg of cyanide ion per kg of body weight per day for 6 months. Exposure to cyanide was reported to produce increasing ambivalence and slower response times to stimuli with increasing dose. Behaviours demanding high energy tended to be affected more readily than those demanding low energy. An effect on glucose metabolism was suggested as a possible explanation for this finding. A reduction in serum thyroxine and, more notably, in triiodothyronine levels was found at all three doses (12). However, clear effects were observed only at the highest dose.

A group of 10 male rats was fed a 10% casein diet containing added methionine, vitamin $B_{12}$, iodine, and potassium cyanide (1500 mg/kg) for nearly 1 year. Compared with a control group not receiving cyanide, depression of body weight gain was observed throughout the study, but there were no deaths or clinical signs of toxicity. Depression of both plasma thyroxine and the thyroxine secretion rate, suggestive of depressed thyroid function, was evident at 4 months but less so after 1 year. At autopsy, the animals were found to have enlarged thyroids, which may have been the mechanism of adaptation. Some differences in the histopathology of the spinal cord, notably the white matter, were also found between controls and cyanide-treated animals (13).

Chicks were fed diets containing up to 30% cassava root meal for 28 days. The cassava root meal itself contained 300 mg of total cyanide per kg. No effects on survival, feeding performance, body weight gain, or haematology were noted. The additional inclusion of 3% cassava foliage meal (containing 156 mg of total cyanide per kg and 20 µg of aflatoxin per kg) resulted in depression of body weight gain (14).

## Reproductive toxicity, embryotoxicity, and teratogenicity

A group of 20 pregnant female rats was fed cassava diets with added potassium cyanide (500 mg/kg) for about 20 days. After parturition, dams and offspring were continued on the diet for the 21-day lactation period. Some pups were also continued on the diet for a further 28 days post-weaning. No effects on gestation, lactation performance, or growth of offspring were seen. However, if offspring from dams not treated with cyanide were exposed during the post-weaning period only, depression of both body weight gain and feed intake as compared with untreated controls was observed (15).

Groups of six pregnant pigs were fed diets of cassava to which cyanide at levels of 0, 250, or 500 mg/kg (as potassium cyanide) was added until parturition, after which sows and offspring returned to a standard diet for a 56-day lactation period. Dietary cyanide had no effect on the numbers or weights of fetuses. A slight elevation of maternal thyroid weight was noted. Pathological changes were also observed in this organ in animals receiving the highest dose level (16). This study suggests that effects may occur in the pig at doses an order of magnitude lower than that found in short-term studies on the rat.

Pregnant golden hamsters were exposed to sodium cyanide (0.126–0.1295 mmol/kg per hour) on days 6–9 of gestation by infusion via subcutaneously implanted osmotic minipumps. High incidences of resorptions and malformations were seen in the offspring, the most common abnormalities being neural tube defects (5).

## 13.14.6 Effects on humans

Cyanide may lower vitamin $B_{12}$ levels and hence exacerbate vitamin $B_{12}$ deficiency. It has also been linked to an increased incidence of goitre (cretinism) in Zaire through effects on iodine uptake by the thyroid. Those with nutritional inadequacy or inborn metabolic errors are particularly vulnerable (17). Chronic effects on the thyroid and particularly on the nervous system were observed in some populations as a consequence of the consumption of inadequately processed cassava containing high levels of cyanide. This problem seems to have decreased significantly in the West African populations in which it was widely reported following a change in processing methods and a general improvement in nutritional status.

## 13.14.7 Guideline value

There are a very limited number of toxicological studies suitable for use in deriving a guideline value. There is, however, some indication in the literature that pigs may be more sensitive than rats. Only one study is available in which a clear effect level was observed, at 1.2 mg/kg of body weight per day, in pigs exposed for 6 months (12). The effects observed were on behavioural patterns and serum biochemistry.

Using the LOAEL from this study and applying an uncertainty factor of 100 to reflect inter- and intraspecies variation (no additional factor for a LOAEL was considered necessary because of doubts over the biological significance of the observed changes), a TDI of 12 µg/kg of body weight was calculated.

An allocation of 20% of the TDI to drinking-water is made because exposure to cyanide from other sources is normally small and because exposure from water is only intermittent. This results in a guideline value of 0.07 mg/litre (rounded figure), which is considered to be protective for both acute and long-term exposure.

## References

1.  International Organization for Standardization. *Water quality—determination of cyanide.* Geneva, 1984 (ISO 6703-1:1984).

2.  Jackson LC. Possible adaptation to serum thiocyanate overload associated with chronic sublethal dietary cyanide ingestion. *Human biology,* 1988, 60:615-622.

3.  Okoh PN. Excretion of [14]C-labelled cyanide in rats exposed to chronic intake of potassium cyanide. *Toxicology and applied pharmacology,* 1983, 70:335-339.

4.  Okoh PN, Pitt GAJ. The metabolism of cyanide and the gastrointestinal circulation of the resulting thiocyanate under conditions of chronic cyanide intake in the rat. *Canadian journal of physiology and pharmacology,* 1982, 60:381-386.

5. Doherty PA, Ferm VH, Smith RP. Congenital malformations induced by infusion of sodium cyanide in the golden hamster. *Toxicology and applied pharmacology*, 1982, 64:456-464.

6. Himwich WA, Saunders JP. Enzymatic conversion of cyanide to thiocyanate. *American journal of physiology*, 1948, 158:348-354.

7. Tewe OO. Effect of dietary cyanide on the performance, metabolism and pathology of the African rat (*Cricetomys gambianus* Waterhouse). *Nutrition reports international*, 1982, 26:529-536.

8. Palmer IS, Olson OE. Partial prevention by cyanide of selenium poisoning in rats. *Biochemical and biophysical research communications*, 1979, 90:1379-1386.

9. Tewe OO, Maner JH. Cyanide, protein and iodine interactions in the performance, metabolism and pathology of pigs. *Research in veterinary science*, 1980, 29:271-276.

10. Tewe OO et al. Effect of varying dietary cyanide levels on serum thyroxine and protein metabolites in pigs. *Nutrition reports international*, 1984, 30:1249-1253.

11. Jackson LC, Chandler JP, Jackson RT. Inhibition and adaptation of red cell glucose-6-phosphate dehydrogenase (G6PD) *in vivo* to chronic sublethal dietary cyanide in an animal model. *Human biology*, 1986, 58:67-77.

12. Jackson LC. Behavioral effects of chronic sublethal dietary cyanide in an animal model: implications for humans consuming cassava (*Manihot esculenta*). *Human biology*, 1988, 60:597-614.

13. Philbrick DJ et al. Effect of prolonged cyanide and thiocyanate feeding in rats. *Journal of toxicology and environmental health*, 1979, 5:579-592.

14. Gomez G, Aparicio MA, Wilhite CC. Relationship between dietary cassava cyanide levels and broiler performance. *Nutrition reports international*, 1988, 37:63-75.

15. Tewe OO, Maner JH. Long-term and carry-over effect of dietary inorganic cyanide (KCN) in the life cycle performance and metabolism of rats. *Toxicology and applied pharmacology*, 1981, 58:1-7.

16. Tewe OO, Maner JH. Performance and pathophysiological changes in pregnant pigs fed cassava diets containing different levels of cyanide. *Research in veterinary science*, 1981, 30:147-151.

17. Wilson J. Cyanide in human disease: a review of clinical and laboratory evidence. *Fundamental and applied toxicology*, 1983, 3:397-399.

# 13.15 Fluoride

## 13.15.1 General description

### Identity

Fluorine is a fairly common element that does not occur in the elemental state in nature because of its high reactivity. It accounts for about 0.3 g/kg of the earth's crust and exists in the form of fluorides in a number of minerals, of which fluorspar, cryolite, and fluorapatite are the most common. The oxidation state of the fluoride ion is -1.

### Physicochemical properties (1, 2)

| Property | Sodium fluoride (NaF) | Hydrogen fluoride (HF) |
|---|---|---|
| Physical state | White, crystalline powder | Colourless liquid or gas with biting smell |
| Melting point (°C) | 993 | -83 |
| Boiling point (°C) | 1695 at 100 kPa | 19.5 |
| Density (g/cm$^3$) | 2.56 | – |
| Water solubility | 42 g/litre at 10 °C | Readily soluble below 20 °C |
| Acidity | – | Strong acid in liquid form; weak acid dissolved in water |

### Major uses

Inorganic fluorine compounds are used in aluminium production, as a flux in the steel and glass fibre industries, and in the production of phosphate fertilizers (which contain an average of 3.8% fluorine), bricks, tiles, and ceramics. Fluosilicic acid is used in municipal water fluoridation schemes (1).

### Environmental fate

Although sodium fluoride is soluble in water (1), aluminium, calcium, and magnesium fluorides are only sparingly so (3).

## 13.15.2 Analytical methods

Fluoride is usually determined by means of an ion-selective electrode, which makes it possible to measure the total amount of free and complex-bound fluoride dissolved in water. The method can be used for water containing at least 20 µg/litre (2). For rainwater in which fluoride was present at a concentration of 10 µg/litre, a detection limit of 1 µg/litre was reported (4).

A method using a fluoride-selective electrode and an ion analyser to determine fluoride at levels of 0.05–0.4 mg/litre has been described (5). With a slight modification, the method can be used to measure fluoride at 0.4–2.0 mg/litre.

## 13.15.3 Environmental levels and human exposure

### Air

Natural background concentrations are of the order of 0.5 ng/m³. If anthropo-genic emissions are included, worldwide background concentrations are of the order of 3 ng/m³. In the Netherlands, concentrations in areas without sources are 30–40 ng/m³, rising to 70 ng/m³ in areas with many sources (2). In a survey of fluoride in the air of some communities in the USA and Canada, concentrations were in the range 0.02–2.0 µg/m³ (6). In some provinces of China, fluoride con-centrations in indoor air ranged from 16 to 46 µg/m³ owing to the indoor com-bustion of high-fluoride coal for cooking and for drying and curing food (7).

### Water

Traces of fluoride are present in many waters; higher concentrations are often as-sociated with underground sources. In seawater, a total fluoride concentration of 1.3 mg/litre has been reported (2). In areas rich in fluoride-containing minerals, well-waters may contain up to about 10 mg of fluoride per litre. The highest nat-ural level reported is 2800 mg/litre. Fluorides may also enter a river as a result of industrial discharges (2). In groundwater, fluoride concentrations vary with the type of rock that the water flows through but do not usually exceed 10 mg/litre (3). In the Rhine in the Netherlands, levels are below 0.2 mg/litre. In the Meuse, concentrations fluctuate (0.2–1.3 mg/litre) as a result of variations in industrial processes (2).

Fluoride concentrations in the groundwater of some villages in China were greater than 8 mg/litre (8, 9). In Canada, fluoride levels in drinking-water of <0.05–0.2 mg/litre (nonfluoridated) and 0.6–1.1 mg/litre (fluoridated) have been reported in municipal waters; in drinking-water prepared from well-water, levels up to 3.3 mg/litre have been reported. In the USA, 0.2% of the population is exposed to more than 2.0 mg/litre (3). In the Netherlands, year-round aver-ages for all drinking-water plants are below 0.2 mg/litre (2). In some African countries where the soil is rich in fluoride-containing minerals, levels in drinking-water are relatively high (e.g. 8 mg/litre in the United Republic of Tanzania) (3).

### Food

Virtually all foodstuffs contain at least traces of fluoride. All vegetation contains some fluoride, which is absorbed from soil and water. The highest levels in field-grown vegetables are found in curly kale (up to 40 mg/kg fresh weight) and endive (0.3–2.8 mg/kg fresh weight) (2). Other foods containing high levels in-clude fish (0.1–30 mg/kg) and tea (2, 3). High concentrations in tea can be caused by high natural concentrations in tea plants or by the use of additives during growth or fermentation. Levels in dry tea can be 3–300 mg/kg (average

100 mg/kg), so that 2–3 cups of tea contain approximately 0.4–0.8 mg (*2, 6*). In areas where water with a high fluoride content is used to prepare tea, the intake via tea can be several times greater.

### Dental uses

For dental purposes, fluoride preparations may contain low (0.25–1 mg per tablet; 1000–1500 mg of fluorine per kg of toothpaste) or high concentrations (liquids containing 10 000 mg/litre and gels containing 4000–6000 mg/kg are used for local applications) (*2*).

### Estimated total exposure and relative contribution of drinking-water

Levels of daily exposure to fluoride depend mainly on the geographical area. In the Netherlands, the total daily intake is calculated to be 1.4–6.0 mg of fluoride. Food seems to be the source of 80–85% of fluoride intake; intake from drinking-water is 0.03–0.68 mg/day and from toothpaste 0.2–0.3 mg. For children, the total intake via food and water is decreased because of lower consumption. Intake of food and water relative to body weight is higher, however, and is further increased by the swallowing of toothpaste or fluoride tablets (up to 3.5 mg of fluoride per day) (*2*).

Daily intakes ranging from 0.46 to 3.6–5.4 mg/day have been reported in several studies (*6*). Daily exposure in volcanic areas (e.g. the United Republic of Tanzania) may be as high as 30 mg for adults, mainly from drinking-water intake (J.E.M. Smet, personal communication, 1990). In areas with relatively high concentrations in groundwater, drinking-water becomes increasingly important as a source of fluoride. In some counties in China where coal has a high fluoride content, the average daily intake of fluoride ranged from 0.3 to 2.3 mg via air and from 1.8 to 8.9 mg via food (*10*).

### 13.15.4 Kinetics and metabolism in laboratory animals and humans

After oral uptake, water-soluble fluorides are rapidly and almost completely absorbed in the gastrointestinal tract. Fluorides less soluble in water are absorbed to a lesser degree. Absorbed fluoride is transported via the blood; with prolonged intake of fluoride from drinking-water, concentrations in the blood are the same as those in drinking-water, a relationship that remains valid up to a concentration in drinking-water of 10 mg/litre. Distribution of fluoride is a rapid process. It is incorporated into teeth and bones; there is virtually no storage in soft tissues. Incorporation into teeth and skeletal tissues is reversible; after cessation of exposure, mobilization from these tissues takes place. Fluoride is excreted via urine, faeces, and sweat (*3, 6, 11*).

## 13.15.5 Effects on laboratory animals and *in vitro* test systems
### *Long-term exposure*

Most long-term studies are limited. In drinking-water studies with sodium fluoride, effects on skeletal tissues were observed. In a 2-year study in rats and mice (25 or 175 mg of sodium fluoride per litre of drinking-water), dentine discoloration and dysplasia developed at both dose levels; osteosclerosis in the long bones was seen in the high-dose females only (*12*). In another recent 2-year oral study in rats, there were effects on the teeth (ameloblastic dysplasia, fractured and malformed incisors, enamel hypoplasia) and bones (subperiosteal hyperkeratosis) at all dose levels, including the lowest of 4 mg of sodium fluoride per kg of body weight per day (*13*).

### *Mutagenicity and related end-points*

Many mutagenicity studies have been carried out with fluorides (usually sodium fluoride). Tests on bacteria and insects were negative, as were *in vivo* studies (*11*, *12*, *14*). In mammalian cells *in vitro*, fluoride causes genetic damage (including chromosomal aberrations) at cytotoxic concentrations only ($\geqslant$10 mg/litre), the mechanism for which is not known. This genetic effect is probably of limited revelance for practical human exposures (*11*).

### *Carcinogenicity*

IARC evaluated the available studies in 1987 and concluded that the limited data provided inadequate evidence of carcinogenicity in experimental animals (*14*). In a recent study in which rats and mice were given sodium fluoride in drinking-water at 11, 45, or 79 mg/litre (as fluoride ion), only the incidence of osteosarcomas in the bones of male rats increased (incidences 0/80, 0/51, 1/50, and 3/80 in the controls, low-, mid-, and high-dose groups, respectively). This increase was considered to provide equivocal evidence for a carcinogenic action in male rats; the study yielded no evidence for such an action in female rats or in male or female mice (*12*). In another recent study, no carcinogenic effect was observed in rats given sodium fluoride in the diet at dose levels of 4, 10, or 25 mg/kg of body weight per day for 2 years (*13*).

## 13.15.6 Effects on humans

Fluorine is probably an essential element for both animals and humans. For humans, however, the essentiality has not been demonstrated unequivocally, and no data indicating the minimum nutritional requirement are available. To produce signs of acute fluoride intoxication, minimum oral doses of at least 1 mg of fluoride per kg of body weight were required (*11*).

Many epidemiological studies of possible adverse effects of the long-term ingestion of fluoride via drinking-water have been carried out. These studies clearly establish that fluoride primarily produces effects on skeletal tissues (bones and teeth). Low concentrations provide protection against dental caries, especially in children. This protective effect increases with concentration up to about 2 mg of fluoride per litre of drinking-water; the minimum concentration of fluoride in drinking-water required to produce it is approximately 0.5 mg/litre.

Fluoride may give rise to mild dental fluorosis (prevalence: 12–33%) at drinking-water concentrations between 0.9 and 1.2 mg/litre (15). This has been confirmed in numerous studies, including a recent large-scale survey carried out in China (16), which showed that, with drinking-water containing 1 mg of fluoride per litre, dental fluorosis was detectable in 46% of the population examined. As a rough approximation, for areas with a temperate climate, manifest dental fluorosis occurs at concentrations above 1.5–2 mg of fluoride per litre of drinking-water. In warmer areas, dental fluorosis occurs at lower concentrations in the drinking-water because of the greater amounts of water consumed (3, 6, 10). It is also possible that, in areas where fluoride intake via routes other than drinking-water (e.g. air, food) is elevated, dental fluorosis develops at concentrations in drinking-water below 1.5 mg/litre (10).

Fluoride can also have more serious effects on skeletal tissues. Skeletal fluorosis (with adverse changes in bone structure) is observed when drinking-water contains 3–6 mg of fluoride per litre. Crippling skeletal fluorosis develops where drinking-water contains over 10 mg of fluoride per litre (6). The US Environmental Protection Agency considers a concentration of 4 mg/litre to be protective against crippling skeletal fluorosis (17).

Several epidemiological studies are available on the possible association between fluoride in drinking-water and cancer rates among the population. IARC evaluated these studies in 1982 and 1987 and considered that they provided inadequate evidence of carcinogenicity in humans (1,14). The results of several epidemiological studies on the possible adverse effects of fluoride in drinking-water on pregnancy outcome are inconclusive (3, 6, 11).

It is known that persons suffering from certain forms of renal impairment have a lower margin of safety for the effects of fluoride than the average person. The data available on this subject are, however, too limited to allow a quantitative evaluation of the increased sensitivity to fluoride toxicity of such persons (3, 11).

## 13.15.7 Guideline value

In 1987, IARC classified inorganic fluorides in Group 3 (14). Although there was equivocal evidence of carcinogenicity in one study in male rats, extensive epidemiological studies have shown no evidence of it in humans (12).

There is no evidence to suggest that the guideline value of 1.5 mg/litre set in 1984 needs to be revised. Concentrations above this value carry an increasing risk of dental fluorosis, and much higher concentrations lead to skeletal fluorosis. The value is higher than that recommended for artificial fluoridation of water supplies (*18*). In setting national standards for fluoride, it is particularly important to consider climatic conditions, water intake, and intake of fluoride from other sources (e.g. from food and air). In areas with high natural fluoride levels, it is recognized that the guideline value may be difficult to achieve in some circumstances with the treatment technology available.

## References

1.  International Agency for Research on Cancer. *Some aromatic amines, anthraquinones and nitroso compounds, and inorganic fluorides used in drinking-water and dental preparations.* Lyon, 1982:237-303 (IARC Monographs on the Evaluation of the Carcinogenic Risk of Chemicals to Humans, Vol. 27).

2.  Slooff W et al., eds. *Basisdocument fluoriden.* Bilthoven, Netherlands, National Institute of Public Health and Environmental Protection, 1988 (Report no. 758474005).

3.  Office of Drinking Water. *Drinking water criteria document on fluoride.* Washington, DC, US Environmental Protection Agency, 1985 (TR-823-5).

4.  Barnard WR, Nordstrom DK. Fluoride in precipitation. i. Methodology with fluoride-selective electrode. *Atmospheric environment*, 1982, 16:99.

5.  Liu JW et al. Measurement of low level fluoride in water and water-based products using a fluoride electrode and an ion analyzer with automatic calibration program. *Journal of micronutrient analysis*, 1987, 3:295-305.

6.  *Fluorine and fluorides.* Geneva, World Health Organization, 1984 (Environmental Health Criteria, No. 36).

7.  Cao SR, Li YF. The evaluation of indoor air quality in areas of endemic fluorosis caused by coal combustion. In: *Proceedings of the XIX Conference of the International Society for Fluoride Research, Kyoto, Japan, 1992.* Kyoto, Department of Hygiene and Public Health, Osaka Medical College, 1992:38.

8.  Fuhong R, Shuqin J. Distribution and formation of high-fluorine groundwater in China. *Environmental geology and water science*, 1988, 12(1):3-10.

9.  *Drinking water atlas of China.* Beijing, China Cartographic Publishing House, 1990:91-92.

10. Cao SR et al. Study on preventive and control measures on coal-combustion type endemic fluorosis in three Gorges areas in China. (Proceedings of the Fourth National Academic Conference on Endemic Fluorosis.) *Chinese journal of endemic disease*, 1992, II(Suppl.):6-21 (in Chinese).

11. Janssen PJCM, Janus JA, Knaap AGAC. *Integrated criteria document fluorides—effects.* Bilthoven, Netherlands, National Institute of Public Health and Environmental Protection, 1988 (Appendix to Report no. 75847005).

12. National Institutes of Health. *Toxicology and carcinogenesis studies of sodium fluoride (CAS no. 7681-49-4) in F344/N rats and B6C3F₁ mice.* Research Triangle Park, NC, 1990 (NIH Publication No. 90-2848; National Toxicology Program Technical Report 393).

13. Maurer JK et al. Two-year carcinogenicity study of sodium fluoride in rats. *Journal of the National Cancer Institute*, 1990, 82:1118-1126.

14. International Agency for Research on Cancer. *Overall evaluations of carcinogenicity: an updating of IARC monographs volumes 1-42.* Lyon, 1987:208-210 (IARC Monographs on the Evaluation of Carcinogenic Risks to Humans, Suppl. 7).

15. Dean HT. Epidemiological studies in the United States. In: Moulton FR, ed. *Fluorine and dental health.* Washington, DC, American Association for the Advancement of Science, 1942 (AAAS Publication No. 19).

16. Chen CJ et al. *A nationwide survey on drinking water quality and waterborne diseases in China.* Beijing, Institute of Environmental Health and Monitoring, Chinese Academy of Preventive Medicine, 1988:95-99 (in Chinese).

17. US Environmental Protection Agency. National primary drinking water regulations; fluoride; final rule and proposed rule. *Federal register*, 1985, 50(220):47142-47171.

18. Murray JJ, ed. *Appropriate use of fluorides for human health.* Geneva, World Health Organization, 1986.

# 13.16 Hardness

## 13.16.1 General description

### *Identity*

Water hardness is the traditional measure of the capacity of water to react with soap, hard water requiring considerably more soap to produce a lather. It is not caused by a single substance but by a variety of dissolved polyvalent metallic ions, predominantly calcium and magnesium cations, although other cations, e.g. barium, iron, manganese, strontium and zinc, also contribute. Hardness is most commonly expressed as milligrams of calcium carbonate equivalent per litre, water containing less than 60 mg of calcium carbonate per litre generally being considered as soft. Although hardness is caused by cations, it may also be discussed in terms of carbonate (temporary) and noncarbonate (permanent) hardness.

## Sources

The principal natural sources of hardness in water are dissolved polyvalent metallic ions from sedimentary rocks, seepage, and run-off from soils. Calcium and magnesium, the two principal ions, are present in many sedimentary rocks, the most common being limestone and chalk. They are also present in a wide variety of industrial products and are common constituents of food. As mentioned above, a minor contribution to the total hardness of water is also made by other polyvalent ions, e.g. aluminium, barium, iron, manganese, strontium, and zinc.

## Organoleptic properties

The taste threshold for the calcium ion is in the range 100–300 mg/litre, depending on the associated anion, but higher concentrations are acceptable to consumers. Hardness levels above 500 mg/litre are generally considered to be aesthetically unacceptable, although this level is tolerated in some communities (1).

## 13.16.2 Environmental levels and human exposure

### Water

Concentrations of up to 100 mg of calcium per litre are fairly common in natural sources of water; sources containing over 200 mg of calcium per litre are rare. Magnesium salts are soluble, natural water sources typically containing concentrations of up to 10 mg/litre. Such sources rarely contain more than 100 mg of magnesium per litre, and it is usually calcium hardness that predominates (2).

In drinking-water, hardness is in the range 10–500 mg of calcium carbonate per litre (3). Estimated daily intakes of 2.3 and 52.1 mg of magnesium in soft- and hard-water areas, respectively, have been reported, based on adults drinking 2 litres of water per day (4).

### Food

Virtually all foods contain calcium and magnesium, and dietary intake is the principal route of exposure. Typical diets provide about 1000 mg of calcium per day and 200–400 mg of magnesium per day. Dairy products are a particularly rich source of calcium, whereas magnesium tends to be associated more with meat and foodstuffs of plant origin (4–6).

### Estimated total exposure and relative contribution of drinking-water

The typical dietary contribution of calcium and magnesium is over 80% of the total daily intake. Of this, approximately 30% of calcium and 35% of magnesium will be absorbed. For calcium and magnesium, the typical contribution from water is 5–20% (2, 5, 6).

## 13.16.3 Effects on humans

There does not appear to be any convincing evidence that water hardness causes adverse health effects in humans. In contrast, the results of a number of epidemiological studies have suggested that water hardness may protect against disease. However, the available data are inadequate to prove any causal association.

### Cardiovascular disease

In most large-scale studies, an inverse relationship between the hardness of drinking-water and cardiovascular disease has been reported (7–13). However, no such association has been found in some studies (14, 15), and in those involving small geographical areas a clear association is often not found (16).

The extent to which confounding variables, such as climatic, socioeconomic, or major risk factors, may account for the inverse relationship is unclear. Nevertheless, in a number of studies, a weak inverse relationship was reported after allowance was made for climatic and socioeconomic factors (17) and after major risk factors such as hypertension, smoking habits, and elevated serum lipids were taken into account (18, 19). An inverse relationship between hardness and cardiovascular disease had been reported in men after allowing for climatic and certain social factors, but only up to about 170 mg of calcium carbonate per litre (20).

A variety of hypotheses have been proposed to explain the possible inverse association (21–27). However, none has been fully substantiated, nor has a particular element been found to be conclusively associated with cardiovascular disease.

### Other health effects

The results of several studies have suggested that a variety of other diseases are also inversely correlated with the hardness of water, including anencephaly (28, 29) and various types of cancer (30, 31). However, the significance of these results is unclear, and it has been suggested that the associations may reflect disease patterns that can be explained by social, climatological, and environmental factors, rather than by the hardness of the water. Some data suggest that very soft waters with a hardness of less than 75 mg/litre may have an adverse effect on mineral balance, but detailed studies are not available.

## 13.16.4 Other considerations

Depending on the interaction of other factors, such as pH and alkalinity, water with a hardness above approximately 200 mg/litre may cause scale deposition in the distribution system, as well as increased soap consumption. In contrast, soft water, with a hardness less than about 100 mg/litre, has a greater tendency to cause corrosion of pipes, resulting in the presence of certain heavy metals, such as cadmium, copper, lead and zinc, in drinking-water (2). The degree to which such corrosion and solubilization of metals occurs also depends on the pH, alkalinity, and dissolved oxygen concentration.

## 13.16.5 Conclusions

Although a number of epidemiological studies have shown a statistically significant inverse relationship between the hardness of drinking-water and cardiovascular disease, the available data are inadequate to permit the conclusion that the association is causal. No health-based guideline value for water hardness is proposed.

## References

1.  Zoeteman BCJ. *Sensory assessment of water quality.* Oxford, Pergamon Press, 1980.

2.  National Research Council. *Drinking water and health.* Washington, DC, National Academy of Sciences, 1977.

3.  Marier JR, Neri LC, Anderson TW. *Water hardness, human health, and the importance of magnesium.* Ottawa, National Research Council of Canada, 1979.

4.  Neri LC et al. Magnesium and certain other elements and cardiovascular disease. *Science of the total environment*, 1985, 42:49-75.

5.  *Trace elements in human nutrition*: report of a WHO Expert Committee. Geneva, World Health Organization, 1973 (WHO Technical Report Series, No. 532).

6.  Neri LC, Johansen HL. Water hardness and cardiovascular mortality. *Annals of the New York Academy of Sciences*, 1978, 304:203-221.

7.  Anderson TW et al. Ischemic heart disease, water hardness and myocardial magnesium. *Canadian Medical Association journal*, 1975, 113:119-203.

8.  Masironi R, Pisa Z, Clayton D. Myocardial infarction and water hardness in the WHO myocardial infarction registry network. *Bulletin of the World Health Organization*, 1979, 57:291-299.

9.  Leoni V, Fabiani L, Ticchiarelli L. Water hardness and cardiovascular mortality rate in Abruzzo, Italy. *Archives of environmental health*, 1985, 40(5):274-278.

10. Zeighami EA et al. Drinking water inorganics and cardiovascular disease: a case–control study among Wisconsin farmers. In: Calabrese EJ, Tuthill RW, Condie L, eds. *Advances in modern toxicology—inorganics in drinking water and cadiovascular disease.* Princeton, NJ, Princeton Scientific Publishing, 1985.

11. Smith WC, Crombie IK. Coronary heart disease and water hardness in Scotland—is there a relationship? *Journal of epidemiology and community health*, 1987, 41:227-228.

12. Kubis M. The relationship between water hardness and the occurrence of acute myocardial infarction. *Acta Universitatis Palackianae Olomucensis Facultatis Medicae*, 1985, 111:321-324.

13. Dzik AJ. Cerebrovascular disease mortality rates and water hardness in North Dakota. *South Dakota journal of medicine*, 1989, 42(4):5-7.

14. MacKinnon AU, Taylor SH. Relationship between sudden coronary deaths and drinking water hardness in five Yorkshire cities and towns. *International journal of epidemiology*, 1980, 9(3):247-249.

15. Sonneborn M et al. Health effects of inorganic drinking water constituents, including hardness, iodide and fluoride. *CRC critical reviews on environmental control*, 1983, 13(1):1-22.

16. Meyer DH, Williams G. Mortality from all causes and from ischemic heart disease in Australian capital cities. *Medical journal of Australia*, 1977, 2:504-506.

17. Pocock SJ et al. British Regional Heart Study: geographic variations in cardiovascular mortality and the role of water quality. *British medical journal*, 1980, 280:1243-1249.

18. Nerbrand C et al. Cardiovascular mortality and morbidity in seven counties in Sweden in relation to water hardness and geological settings. The project: myocardial infarction in mid-Sweden. *European heart journal*, 1992, 13(6):721-727.

19. Shaper AG et al. British Regional Heart Study: cardiovascular risk factors, in middle-aged men in 24 towns. *British medical journal*, 1981, 283:179-186.

20. Lacey RF, Shaper AG. Changes in water hardness and cardiovascular death-rates. *International journal of epidemiology*, 1984, 134:18-24.

21. Pomrehn PR. Softened water usage and blood pressure. In: Calabrese EJ, Tuthill RW, Condie L, eds. *Advances in modern toxicology—Inorganics in drinking water and cardiovascular disease*. Princeton, NJ, Princeton Scientific Publishing, 1985.

22. Alexa L et al. [An assessment of minerals in drinking water from the Iasi County and the incidence of cardiovascular disease.] *Revista de igiena bacteriologie, virusologie, parazitologie, epidemiologie, pneumoftiziologie, Seria bacteriologie, virusologie, parazitologie, epidemiologie*, 1988, 37(1):35-43 (in Romanian).

23. Hopps HC, Feder GL. Chemical qualities of water that contribute to human health in a positive way. *Science of the total environment*, 1986, 54:207-216.

24. Luoma H et al. Risk of myocardial infarction in Finnish men in relation to fluoride, magnesium, and calcium concentration in drinking water. *Acta medica Scandinavica*, 1983, 213: 171-176.

25. Marier JR, Neri LC. Quantifying the role of magnesium in the interrelationship between human mortality/morbidity and water hardness. *Magnesium*, 1985, 4(2-3):53-59.

26. Singh RB. Effect of dietary magnesium supplementation in the prevention of coronary heart disease and sudden cardiac death. *Magnesium trace elements*, 1990, 9:143-151.

27. Derry CW, Bourne DE, Sayed AR. The relationship between the hardness of treated water and cardiovascular disease mortality in South African urban areas. *South African medical journal*, 1990, 77:522-524.

28. Crawford MD, Gardner MJ, Sedgwick PA. Infant mortality and hardness of local water supplies. *Lancet*, 1972, 1(758):988-992.

29. Bound JP et al. The incidence of anencephalus in the Fylde Peninsula 1956–1976 and changes in water hardness. *Journal of epidemiology and community health*, 1981, 35(2):102-105.

30. Zemla B.[Geographical incidence of gastric carcinoma in relation to hardness of water for drinking and household needs.] *Wiadomości lekarskie*, 1980, 33(13): 1027-1031 (in Polish).

31. Wigle DT et al. Contaminants in drinking water and cancer risks in Canadian cities. *Canadian journal of public health*, 1986, 77(5):335-342.

## 13.17 Hydrogen sulfide

### 13.17.1 General description

#### Identity

CAS no.: 7783-06-4
Molecular formula: $H_2S$

#### Physicochemical properties (1, 2)[1]

| Property | Value |
| --- | --- |
| Physical appearance | Colourless gas |
| Melting point | -85.5 °C |
| Boiling point | -60.7 °C |
| Density | 1.54 g/litre at 0 °C |
| Water solubility | 4370 ml/litre at 0 °C; 1860 ml/litre at 40 °C |
| Vapour pressure | 1875 kPa at 20 °C |

---

[1] Conversion factor in air: 1 mg/m$^3$ = 0.670 ppm.

## Organoleptic properties

Hydrogen sulfide has an offensive "rotten eggs" odour that is detectable at very low concentrations in air, below 8 $\mu g/m^3$ (*3*). At concentrations of 50–150 $mg/m^3$ in air, it has a deceptively sweet smell; above this range, it deadens the sense of smell (*4*). In water, the taste and odour thresholds for hydrogen sulfide are estimated to be between 0.05 and 0.1 mg/litre. The taste and odour threshold for sulfides is about 0.2 mg/litre (*5*).

## Major uses

The major uses of hydrogen sulfide include its conversion into sulfur and sulfuric acid and the manufacture of inorganic sulfides, thiophenes, thiols, thioaldehydes, and thioketones. It is used in dye manufacture, tanning, the production of wood-pulp, chemical processing, and the manufacture of cosmetics. Spring waters that contain elevated concentrations of hydrogen sulfide are used for therapeutic medicinal baths (*1*).

## Environmental fate

Hydrogen sulfide is formed when soluble sulfides are hydrolysed in water. In water, hydrogen sulfide dissociates, forming monohydrogensulfide(1-) (HS⁻) and sulfide ($S^{2-}$) ions. The relative concentrations of these species are a function of the pH of the water, hydrogen sulfide concentrations increasing with decreasing pH. At pH 7.4, about one-third exists as undissociated hydrogen sulfide and the remainder largely as the monohydrogensulfide(1-) anion (*6*). The sulfide is present in appreciable concentrations above pH 10 (*1*). In well aerated water, hydrogen sulfide is readily oxidized to sulfates and biologically oxidized to elemental sulfur. In anaerobic water, microbial reduction of sulfate to sulfide can occur (*7*).

## 13.17.2 Analytical methods

Hydrogen sulfide is traditionally determined using an acid displacement procedure (*8, 9*); the hydrogen sulfide is displaced by acidification, followed by analysis by gas chromatography using a flame photometric detector. The procedure has been used for water, sewage, and effluents containing 0–2.0 mg of sulfide per litre with a detection limit of about 0.25 mg of sulfur per litre (*9*). An estimated lower detection limit of 0.06 mg/litre has been reported for a similar method (*10*). The methylene blue colorimetric method is another standard analytical procedure for hydrogen sulfide determination, at concentrations ranging between 0.1 and 20 mg/litre (*11*). A number of methods have been developed for the determination of sulfide (*11, 12*).

### 13.17.3 Environmental levels and human exposure

*Air*

Hydrogen sulfide is present in air primarily as a result of natural emissions. Concentrations generally vary from 0.1 to 1 $\mu g/m^3$ in ambient air, although concentrations above 100 $\mu g/m^3$ have been reported near industrial plants (*3*). An estimated daily intake of 2–20 $\mu g$ can be calculated on the assumption that 20 $m^3$ of air containing hydrogen sulfide at natural concentrations is inhaled.

*Water*

Most of the hydrogen sulfide present in raw waters is derived from natural sources and industrial processes. It is particularly noticeable in some groundwaters, depending on source rock mineralogy and the microorganisms present (*13*). In the USA, a maximum concentration of 500 $\mu g$ of undissociated hydrogen sulfide per litre has been reported in fresh water (*14*).

*Food*

A number of foodstuffs and drinks may contain sulfides. However, estimation of exposure from food is complicated by the formation of sulfides in cooked foods. Levels in heated dairy products range from 0.8 mg/litre in skimmed milk (0.1% fat) to 1.84 mg/litre in cream (30.5% fat). The hydrogen sulfide content of cooked meat ranges from 0.276 mg/kg for beef to 0.394 mg/kg for lamb. Hydrogen sulfide is formed principally from the sulfur-containing amino acids in meat protein, levels being higher in anaerobically packaged meat. Dimethyl sulfide is used in the manufacture of jellies, candy, soft drinks, and cream in the United Kingdom, where the maximum probable intake has been estimated at 1.7 mg/day (*15*).

### 13.17.4 Kinetics and metabolism in laboratory animals and humans

Hydrogen sulfide and soluble alkali sulfides are rapidly absorbed following ingestion (*7*). Inhaled hydrogen sulfide has been shown to be distributed to the brain, liver, kidneys, pancreas, and small intestine (*16*). It is metabolized mainly by the liver, the two routes being oxidation to sulfate and methylation to methanethiol and dimethyl sulfide (*17*). Sulfides and sulfates are rapidly excreted via the kidneys in experimental animals, but a small proportion of the sulfides may also be excreted via the lungs. Some metallic sulfides are excreted in the faeces (*1*).

## 13.17.5 Effects on laboratory animals and *in vitro* test systems

### *Acute exposure*

Oral $LD_{50}$ values of 205 and 208 mg/kg of body weight were reported in the mouse and rat, respectively, for sodium sulfide (Registry of Toxic Effects of Chemical Substances, 1989, unpublished data).

### *Short-term exposure*

Dimethyl sulfide given daily at an oral dose of 250 mg/kg of body weight for 14 weeks was found to produce no ill effects in rats. This dose is equivalent to a daily intake of 15 g by a 60-kg adult. However, hydrogen sulfide has been reported to be more toxic than dimethyl sulfide by a factor of 50 (*18*).

### *Reproductive toxicity, embryotoxicity, and teratogenicity*

The ingestion of "thermal" mineral water containing 4–12 mg of hydrogen sulfide per litre was embryotoxic in rats, whereas water containing 2–3 mg/litre had no effect. However, the significance of these findings is doubtful, as few experimental details were published and the mineral water contained numerous other substances (*19*). No effects on pregnancy were seen other than a dose-dependent increase in delivery time in female rats exposed to 112 mg/m³ hydrogen sulfide from day 6 of gestation until day 21 postpartum. In addition, no significant effects on the growth and development of pups were seen (*20*).

### *Mutagenicity and related end-points*

Hydrogen sulfide was not mutagenic in *Salmonella typhimurium* strains TA97, TA98, or TA100, with or without metabolic activation (*21*). Chromosomal aberrations have been reported in the bone marrow of adult rats exposed to 10 mg/m³ for 3–4 months (*22*). Hydrogen sulfide has been shown to increase the mutagenicity of hydrogen peroxide in *S. typhimurium* strain TA102 (*23*). This may be significant where hydrogen peroxide is employed as an oxidizing agent in water-treatment processes.

### *Carcinogenicity*

In a study in which Charles River CD male and female rats were given 9 or 18 mg of sodium sulfide per kg of body weight in water by gavage in either the presence or absence of a 1% thyroid extract at least twice a week for 78 weeks, no evidence of carcinogenicity was found. Because of the high mortality in all treated and control groups, the validity of the results is questionable (*24*).

## 13.17.6 Effects on humans

No data are available on the oral toxicity of hydrogen sulfide. However, alkali sulfides irritate mucous membranes and can cause nausea, vomiting, and epigastric pain following ingestion. The oral dose of sodium sulfide fatal to humans has been estimated at 10–15 g (*1*).

When inhaled, hydrogen sulfide is highly acutely toxic to humans (*25*). Its rapid mode of action involves the formation of a complex with the iron(III) ion of the mitochondrial metalloenzyme cytochrome oxidase, thereby blocking oxidative metabolism (*4, 25*). Other enzymes reported to be inhibited by sulfides are succinate dehydrogenase, adenosinetriphosphatase, DOPA oxidase, carbonic anhydrase, dipeptidase, benzamidase, and some enzymes containing iron such as catalase and peroxidases (*1*). Reduction of disulfide bridges in proteins has been suggested as a mechanism whereby enzyme function could be altered (*3*). Irritation of the eyes and respiratory tract can be observed at concentrations of 15–30 mg/m$^3$, and concentrations of 700–1400 mg/m$^3$ can cause unconsciousness and respiratory paralysis resulting in death (*3*).

Few studies on prolonged exposure to low concentrations of hydrogen sulfide have been undertaken. In one study, the reticulocytes of 17 workers engaged in wood-pulp production who were exposed to low levels of hydrogen sulfide and methylthiols were analysed (*26*). The activities of a number of enzymes involved in the haem biosynthetic pathway were inhibited, although the mechanism is unclear.

## 13.17.7 Conclusions

The taste and odour threshold for hydrogen sulfide in water has been estimated to be as low as 0.05 mg/litre. Although oral toxicity data are lacking, it is unlikely that anyone could consume a harmful dose of hydrogen sulfide in drinking-water. Consequently, no health-based guideline value is proposed. However, hydrogen sulfide should not be detectable in drinking-water by taste or odour.

## References

1.  *Hydrogen sulfide.* Geneva, World Health Organization, 1981 (Environmental Health Criteria, No. 19).

2.  Macaluso P. Hydrogen sulfide. In: *Encyclopedia of chemical technology.* Vol. 19, 2nd ed. New York, NY, John Wiley, 1969:375.

3.  *Air quality guidelines for Europe.* Copenhagen, WHO Regional Office for Europe, 1987.

4.  Patwardhan SA, Abhyankar SM. Toxic and hazardous gases. IV. *Colourage*, 1988, 35(12):15-18.

5. National Health and Welfare Canada. *Guidelines for Canadian drinking-water quality—supporting documentation*. Ottawa, 1978.

6. US National Research Council. *Subcommittee on hydrogen sulfide*. Baltimore, MD, University Park Press, 1979.

7. Mance G, O'Donnell AR, Campbell JA. *Proposed environmental quality standards for List 11 substances in water: sulphide*. Medmenham, Water Research Centre, 1988 (ESSL, TR 257).

8. Standing Committee on Analysis. *Sulphide in waters and effluents*. London, Her Majesty's Stationery Office, 1983.

9. Hawke DJ et al. Determination of sulphides in water and effluents using gas chromatography. *Analyst*, 1985, 110:269-272.

10. Ballinger D, Lloyd A. A method for the determination of sulfides in water, sewage and effluents. *Water pollution control*, 1981:648-654.

11. American Public Health Association. *Standard methods for the examination of water and wastewater*, 17th ed. Washington, DC, 1989.

12. Caron F, Kramer JR. Gas chromatographic determination of volatile sulfides at trace levels in natural freshwaters. *Analytical chemistry*, 1989, 61:114-118.

13. Carpenter AB et al. *Influence of mineralogy and microorganisms on iron and sulfide concentrations in groundwater*. Springfield, VA, US National Technical Information Service, 1971:38 (NTIS PB 205773).

14. Torrans EL, Clemens HP. Physiological and biochemical effects of acute exposure of fish to hydrogen sulfide. *Comparative biochemistry and physiology*, 1982, 71:183-190.

15. Kraft AA, Brant AW, Ayres JC. Detection of hydrogen sulfide in packaged meats and broken-out shell eggs. *Food technology*, 1956, 10:443-444.

16. Voigt GE, Muller P. The histochemical effect of hydrogen sulphide poisoning. *Acta histochemica*, 1955, 1:223.

17. Weisinger RA, Jakoby WB. S-methylation: thiol S-methyltransferase. In: Jakoby WB, ed. *Enzymatic basis of detoxification*, Vol. 2. New York, NY, Academic Press, 1980:131.

18. Susman JL et al. Pulmonary excretion of hydrogen sulfide, methanethiol, dimethyl sulfide and dimethyl disulfide in mice. *Drug and chemical toxicology*, 1978, 1(4):327-338.

19. Beruashvili TA. [Hygienic evaluation of hydrogen sulfide-containing thermal waters used in hot water supply systems.] *Gigiena i sanitarija*, 1980, 6:11-13 (in Russian).

20. Hayden LJ, Goeden H, Roth SH. Growth and development in the rat during sub-chronic exposure to low levels of hydrogen sulfide. *Toxicology and industrial health*, 1990, 6:389-401.

21. Hughes TJ, Sparacine C, Frazier S. *Validation of chemical and biological techniques for evaluation of vapours in ambient air/mutagenicity testing of (12) vapour-phase compounds*. Washington, DC, US Environmental Protection Agency, 1984 (Report EPA-600/1-84-005; Order no. PB84-164219).

22. Bariliak IR, Vasil'eva IA. [Antimitotic and cytogenetic activity of small concentrations of carbon disulfide and hydrogen sulfide.] *Citologija genetika*, 1974, 8(2):126-129 (in Russian).

23. Berglin EH, Carlsson J. Effect of hydrogen sulfide on the mutagenicity of hydrogen peroxide in *Salmonella typhimurium* strain TA102. *Mutation research*, 1986, 175(1):5-9.

24. Weisburger EK et al. Carcinogenicity tests of certain environmental and industrial chemicals, *Journal of the National Cancer Institute*, 1981, 67(1):75-89.

25. Gosselin RE, Smith RP, Hodge HC. Hydrogen sulfide. In: *Clinical toxicology of commercial products*, 5th ed. Baltimore, MD, Williams and Wilkins, 1984:III-198-III-202.

26. Tenhunen R, Savolainen H, Jappinen P. Changes in haem synthesis associated with occupational exposure to organic sulphides. *Clinical science*, 1983, 64:187-191.

# 13.18 Iron

## 13.18.1 General description

### *Identity*

Iron is the second most abundant metal in the earth's crust, of which it accounts for about 5%. Elemental iron is rarely found in nature, as the iron ions $Fe^{2+}$ and $Fe^{3+}$ readily combine with oxygen- and sulfur-containing compounds to form oxides, hydroxides, carbonates, and sulfides. Iron is most commonly found in nature in the form of its oxides (*1, 2*).

### *Physicochemical properties (3)*

| Property | Value |
|---|---|
| Melting point | 1535 °C |
| Specific gravity | 7.86 at 25 °C |

## Organoleptic properties

Iron (as $Fe^{2+}$) concentrations of 40 µg/litre can be detected by taste in distilled water. In a mineralized spring water with a total dissolved solids content of 500 mg/litre, the taste threshold value was 0.12 mg/litre. In well-water, iron concentrations below 0.3 mg/litre were characterized as unnoticeable, whereas levels of 0.3–3 mg/litre were found acceptable (E. Dahi, personal communication, 1991).

In drinking-water supplies, iron(II) salts are unstable and are precipitated as insoluble iron(III) hydroxide, which settles out as a rust-coloured silt. Anaerobic groundwaters may contain iron(II) at concentrations of up to several milligrams per litre without discoloration or turbidity in the water when pumped directly from a well, although turbidity and colour may develop in piped systems at iron levels above 0.05–0.1 mg/litre. Staining of laundry and plumbing may occur at concentrations above 0.3 mg/litre (4).

Iron also promotes undesirable bacterial growth ("iron bacteria") in water-works and distribution systems, resulting in the deposition of a slimy coating on the piping (4).

## Major uses

Iron is used as constructional material, *inter alia* for drinking-water pipes. Iron oxides are used as pigments in paints and plastics. Other compounds are used as food colours and for the treatment of iron deficiency in humans. Various iron salts are used as coagulants in water treatment.

## Environmental fate

Aeration of iron-containing layers in the soil can affect the quality of both groundwater and surface water if the groundwater table is lowered or nitrate leaching takes place. Dissolution of iron can occur as a result of oxidation and decrease in pH.

## 13.18.2 Analytical methods

Iron in water can be determined by atomic absorption spectrometry (detection limit 1 µg/litre) or by colorimetric methods (detection limit 5 µg/litre) (5).

## 13.18.3 Environmental levels and human exposure

### Air

In remote areas, iron levels in air are about 50–90 ng/m³; at urban sites, levels are about 1.3 µg/m³. Concentrations up to 12 µg/m³ have been reported in the vicinity of iron- and steel-producing plants (6).

## Water

The median iron concentration in rivers has been reported to be 0.7 mg/litre. In anaerobic groundwater where iron is present in the form of iron(II), concentrations will usually be 0.5–10 mg/litre, but concentrations up to 50 mg/litre can sometimes be found (6). Concentrations of iron in drinking-water are normally less than 0.3 mg/litre but may be higher in countries where various iron salts are used as coagulating agents in water-treatment plants and where cast iron, steel, and galvanized iron pipes are used for water distribution.

## Food

Iron occurs as a natural constituent in plants and animals. Liver, kidney, fish, and green vegetables contain 20–150 mg/kg, whereas red meats and egg yolks contain 10–20 mg/kg. Rice and many fruits and vegetables have low iron contents (1–10 mg/kg).

## Estimated total exposure and relative contribution of drinking-water

Reported daily intakes of iron in food — the major source of exposure — range from 10 to 14 mg (7, 8). Drinking-water containing 0.3 mg/litre would contribute about 0.6 mg to the daily intake. Intake of iron from air is about 25 µg/day in urban areas.

## 13.18.4 Kinetics and metabolism in humans

Iron is an essential trace element in living organisms. The data in this section are derived from studies in humans only; laboratory animals are not acceptable models because they have much higher intakes than humans and do not absorb iron compounds in the same way (6).

Most iron is absorbed in the duodenum and upper jejunum (9). Absorption depends on the individual's iron status and is regulated so that excessive amounts of iron are not stored in the body (10). Total body iron in adult males and females is usually about 50 and 34–42 mg/kg of body weight, respectively (10). The largest fraction is present as haemoglobin, myoglobin, and haem-containing enzymes. The other major fraction is stored in the body as ferritin and haemosiderin, mainly in the spleen, liver, bone marrow, and striated muscle (6).

Daily losses of iron in adults are small (1 mg/day) and due mainly to cell exfoliation. About two-thirds of this loss occurs from the gastrointestinal tract and most of the remainder from the skin. Iron losses in urine and sweat are negligible (11). In adult females, there is an additional iron loss of about 15–70 mg each month in menstrual blood (12).

## 13.18.5 Effects on laboratory animals and *in vitro* test systems

### *Acute exposure*

Wide variations in toxicity have been reported for different iron salts and animal species. Oral $LD_{50}$s for iron salts are about 300–600 mg/kg of body weight in the mouse and about 800–2000 mg/kg of body weight in the rat (*13*). The effects of toxic doses of iron include depression, rapid and shallow respiration, coma, convulsions, respiratory failure, and cardiac arrest.

### *Reproductive toxicity, embryotoxicity, and teratogenicity*

Iron compounds were not teratogenic in the chicken embryo test (*14*). In a study of iron(II) sulfate and iron(III) sodium diphosphate in mice and rats, neither maternal toxicity nor teratogenic effects were found (*14,15*). In an eight-generation reproduction study in rats, iron oxide was not toxic at an estimated intake of 25 mg of iron per day, and reproductive performance was better than expected (*14,15*). In a five-generation study, iron dextran administered by intramuscular injection had no effect on litter size or growth (*16*).

### *Mutagenicity and related end-points*

A number of iron(II) and iron(III) salts have been tested for mutagenicity in *Saccharomyces cerevisiae* strain D-4 and *Salmonella typhimurium* strains TA1535, TA1537, and TA1538, with and without metabolic activation. Iron(II) lactate, iron(III) diphosphate, iron(III) orthophosphate, and iron(III) sodium diphosphate were inactive in all systems used. Iron(II) sulfate was active in the suspension tests with activation. Iron(II) gluconate was mutagenic for indicator strain TA1538 in activation tests with primate liver preparations (*14*). Iron dextran did not induce chromosomal aberrations in human leukocyte cultures (*17*).

### *Carcinogenicity*

Iron dextran complex repeatedly injected subcutaneously or intramuscularly was considered by IARC to be carcinogenic to animals (*18*).

## 13.18.6 Effects on humans

Iron is an essential element in human nutrition. Estimates of the minimum daily requirement for iron depend on age, sex, physiological status, and iron bioavailability and range from about 10 to 50 mg/day (*12*).

The average lethal dose of iron is 200–250 mg/kg of body weight, but death has occurred following the ingestion of doses as low as 40 mg/kg of body weight (*6*). Autopsies have shown haemorrhagic necrosis and sloughing of areas of mucosa in the stomach with extension into the submucosa. Chronic iron overload results primarily from a genetic disorder (haemochromatosis) characterized by increased iron absorption and from diseases that require frequent transfusions (*10*). Adults have often taken iron supplements for extended periods without deleterious effects (*10*), and an intake of 0.4–1 mg/kg of body weight per day is unlikely to cause adverse effects in healthy persons (*19*).

## 13.18.7 Conclusions

Anaerobic groundwaters may contain iron(II) at concentrations up to several milligrams per litre without discoloration or turbidity in the water when directly pumped from a well. Taste is not usually noticeable at iron concentrations below 0.3 mg/litre, although turbidity and colour may develop in piped systems at levels above 0.05–0.1 mg/litre. Laundry and sanitary ware will stain at iron concentrations above 0.3 mg/litre.

Iron is an essential element in human nutrition. Estimates of the minimum daily requirement for iron depend on age, sex, physiological status, and iron bioavailability and range from about 10 to 50 mg/day.

As a precaution against storage of excessive iron in the body, JECFA established a provisional maximum tolerable daily intake (PMTDI) in 1983 of 0.8 mg/kg of body weight (*14*), which applies to iron from all sources except for iron oxides used as colouring agents, and iron supplements taken during pregnancy and lactation or for specific clinical requirements. Allocation of 10% of this PMTDI to drinking-water gives a value of about 2 mg/litre, which does not present a hazard to health. The taste and appearance of drinking-water will usually be affected below this level, although iron concentrations of 1–3 mg/litre can be acceptable for people drinking anaerobic well-water.

No health-based guideline value for iron is proposed.

## References

1.  Elinder C-G. Iron. In: Friberg L, Nordberg GF, Vouk VB, eds. *Handbook on the toxicology of metals*, Vol. II. Amsterdam, Elsevier, 1986:276-297.

2.  Knepper WA. Iron. In: *Kirk-Othmer encyclopedia of chemical technology*, Vol. 13. New York, NY, Wiley Interscience, 1981:735-753.

3.  Budavari S, O'Neill M, Smith A, eds. *The Merck index*, 11th ed. Rahway, NJ, Merck, 1989.

4.  Department of National Health and Welfare (Canada). *Nutrition recommendations. The report of the Scientific Review Committee.* Ottawa, 1990.

5.  International Organization for Standardization. *Water quality—determination of iron.* Geneva, 1988 (ISO 6332:1988).

6. National Research Council. *Iron*. Baltimore, MD, University Park Press, 1979.

7. National Food Agency of Denmark. *Food monitoring in Denmark*. Copenhagen, 1990 (Publication No. 195).

8. National Research Council. *Recommended dietary allowances*, 10th ed. Washington, DC, National Academy Press, 1989.

9. Dalman PR. Iron. In: Brown ML, ed. *Present knowledge in nutrition*, 6th ed. Washington, DC, International Life Sciences Institute, Nutrition Foundation, 1990.

10. Bothwell TH et al. *Iron metabolism in man*. Oxford, Blackwell, 1979.

11. Green RW et al. Body iron excretion in man. A collaborative study. *American journal of medicine*, 1968, 45:336-353.

12. *Requirements of vitamin A, iron, folate and Vitamin B$_{12}$. Report of a Joint FAO/WHO Expert Consultation*. Rome, Food and Agriculture Organization of the United Nations, 1988 (FAO Food and Nutrition Series, No. 23).

13. Weaver LC et al. Comparative toxicology of iron compounds. *American journal of medical science*, 1961, 241:296-302.

14. Joint FAO/WHO Expert Committee on Food Additives. *Toxicological evaluation of certain food additives and food contaminants*. Cambridge, Cambridge University Press, 1983 (WHO Food Additives Series, No. 18).

15. Life Sciences Research Office. *Evaluation of the health aspects of iron and iron salts as food ingredients*. Washington, DC, Food and Drug Administration, 1980 (PB80-178676).

16. Fisch RO et al. Potential toxicity of iron overload in successive generations of rats. *American journal of clinical nutrition*, 1975, 28:136-139.

17. Paton GR, Allison AC. Chromosome damage in human cell culture induced by metal salts. *Mutation research*, 1972, 16:332-336.

18. International Agency for Research on Cancer. *Overall evaluations of carcinogenicity: an updating of IARC monographs volumes 1-42*. Lyon, 1987:226 (IARC Monographs on the Evaluation of Carcinogenic Risks to Humans, Suppl. 7).

19. Finch CA, Monsen ER. Iron nutrition and the fortification of food with iron. *Journal of the American Medical Association*, 1972, 219:1462-1465.

## 13.19 Lead

### 13.19.1 General description

#### *Identity*

Lead is the commonest of the heavy elements, accounting for 13 mg/kg of the earth's crust. Several stable isotopes of lead exist in nature, including, in order of abundance, [208]Pb, [206]Pb, [207]Pb, and [204]Pb.

#### *Physicochemical properties*

| Property | Value |
| --- | --- |
| Physical state | Soft metal |
| Melting point | 327 °C |

#### *Major uses*

Lead is used in the production of lead acid batteries, solder, alloys, cable sheathing, pigments, rust inhibitors, ammunition, glazes, and plastic stabilizers (*1*). Tetraethyl and tetramethyl lead are important because of their extensive use as antiknock compounds in petrol, but their use for this purpose has been almost completely phased out in North America and western Europe, though not in eastern Europe or many developing countries. From a drinking-water perspective, the almost universal use of lead compounds in plumbing fittings and as solder in water-distribution systems is important. Lead pipes may be used in older distribution systems and plumbing (*2*).

### 13.19.2 Analytical methods

Atomic absorption spectrometry and anodic stripping voltammetry are the methods most frequently used for determining the levels of lead in environmental and biological materials. Detection limits of less than 1 µg/litre can be achieved by means of atomic absorption spectrometry (*3*). Because corrosion of plumbing systems is an important source of excessive lead in drinking-water, lead levels in water should be measured at the tap, rather than at the drinking-water source, when estimating human exposure.

### 13.19.3 Environmental levels and human exposure

#### *Air*

Concentrations of lead in air depend on a number of factors, including proximity to roads and point sources. Annual geometric mean concentrations measured at more than 100 stations across Canada declined steadily from 0.74 µg/m$^3$ in 1973 to 0.10 µg/m$^3$ in 1989 (*4, 5*), reflecting the decrease in the use of lead additives in petrol. Typical quarterly averages for urban areas without significant point sources in the USA in 1987 were in the range 0.1–0.3 µg/m$^3$; in the vicinity of major point sources, such as lead smelters and battery plants, air levels typically ranged from 0.3 to 4.0 µg/m$^3$ (6). Levels at three locations in Barcelona (Spain) during the winter of 1985 ranged from 0.9 to 2.5 µg/m$^3$ (7), presumably reflecting heavy use of leaded petrol. The overall means in London and in a rural area of Suffolk in 1984–85 were 0.50 µg/m$^3$ (range 0.23–0.82) and 0.10 µg/m$^3$ (range 0.05–0.17), respectively (8). Levels of lead in 1983 in the Norwegian Arctic, an area remote from urban influences, varied between 0.1–0.3 and 0.3–9.0 ng/m$^3$ (9).

If an average concentration in air of 0.2 µg/m$^3$ is assumed, the intake of lead from air can be calculated to range from 0.5 µg/day for an infant to 4 µg/day for an adult.

## *Water*

With the decline in atmospheric emissions of lead since the introduction of legislation restricting its use in fuels, water has assumed new importance as the largest controllable source of lead exposure in the USA (10).

Lead is present in tapwater to some extent as a result of its dissolution from natural sources but primarily from household plumbing systems in which the pipes, solder, fittings, or service connections to homes contain lead. PVC pipes also contain lead compounds that can be leached from them and result in high lead concentrations in drinking-water. The amount of lead dissolved from the plumbing system depends on several factors, including the presence of chloride and dissolved oxygen, pH, temperature, water hardness, and standing time of the water, soft, acidic water being the most highly plumbosolvent (11, 12). Although lead can be leached from lead piping indefinitely, it appears that the leaching of lead from soldered joints and brass taps decreases with time (10). Soldered connections in recently built homes fitted with copper piping can release enough lead (210–390 µg/litre) to cause intoxication in children (13). The level of lead in drinking-water may be reduced by corrosion-control measures such as the addition of lime and the adjustment of the pH in the distribution system from < 7 to 8–9 (14,15).

In 1988, it was estimated that a lead level of 5 µg/litre was exceeded in only 1.1% of public water-distribution systems in the USA (16). A more recent review of lead levels in drinking-water in the USA found the geometric mean to be 2.8 µg/litre (10). The median level of lead in drinking-water samples collected in five Canadian cities was 2.0 µg/litre (17). A recent study in Ontario (Canada) found that the average concentration of lead in water actually consumed over a one-week sampling period was in the range 1.1–30.7 µg/litre, with a median level of 4.8 µg/litre (18). In the United Kingdom in 1975–76, there was virtually no lead in the drinking-water in two-thirds of households, but in 10% of homes in England and 33% in Scotland levels were above 50 µg/litre (2). In Glasgow

(Scotland), where the water was known to be plumbosolvent, the lead concentration in about 40% of the samples exceeded 100 µg/litre (*19*).

If a concentration of 5 µg/litre in drinking-water is assumed, the total intake of lead from this source can be calculated to range from 3.8 µg/day for an infant to 10 µg/day for an adult.

## Food

Prepared food contains small but significant amounts of lead. The lead content is increased when the water used for cooking or the cooking utensils contain lead, or the food, especially if acidic, has been stored in lead-ceramic pottery ware or lead-soldered cans. The intake of lead from lead-soldered cans is declining as the use of lead-free solders becomes more widespread in the food processing industry (*2, 20*).

A number of estimates based on figures for per capita consumption have been made of the daily dietary lead intake, e.g. 27 µg/day in Sweden (*21* ); 66 µg/day in Finland (*22*); and 23 µg/day for a 2-year-old in the USA (*23*). Estimates obtained from duplicate diet studies are in the same range and include a mean dietary intake for all food and drink of about 40 µg/day for mothers and 30 µg/day for children aged 5–7 years in England (*8*) and 53.8 µg/day (0.8 µg/kg of body weight per day) for the intake of lead from food for adolescents and adults in Canada (*17*). Lead intakes for adults were 90 µg/day in Belgium, 24 µg/day in Sweden, and 177 µg/day in Mexico, based on faecal monitoring of lead (*24*). In some countries, dietary intakes as high as 500 µg/day have been reported (*20*). The regular consumption of wine can also result in a significant increase in lead intake; an average level of 73 µg/litre has been reported (*25*).

## Other routes of exposure

Soil and household dust are significant sources of lead exposure for small children (*6, 26, 27*), but the levels are highly variable, ranging from <5 µg/g to tens of milligrams per gram in contaminated areas. As lead is immobile, levels in contaminated soils will remain essentially unchanged unless action is taken to decontaminate them (*28*). The highest lead concentrations usually occur in surface soil at depths of 1–5 cm.

In a 2-year study in England during 1984 and 1985, the geometric mean concentrations of lead in road dust collected in the vicinity of two London schools and in a rural area were 1552–1881 and 83–144 µg/g, respectively. For household dusts in London and in a rural area of Suffolk for 3 consecutive years (1983–85) the geometric mean concentrations were 857 and 333 µg/g, respectively (*8*). Household dust concentrations were 332 µg/g in an Edinburgh study (*29*) and 424 µg/g in one in Birmingham (*30*).

The amount of soil ingested by children aged 1–3 years is about 40–55 mg/day (*27, 31, 32*). A comprehensive study of a group of 2-year-old urban children indicated an intake of lead from dust of 42 µg/day, almost twice the dietary lead intake (*30*). Studies in inner-city areas in the USA have shown that peeling paint or dust originating from leaded paint during removal may contribute significantly to children's exposure to lead (*33*).

### Estimated total exposure and relative contribution of drinking-water

More than 80% of the daily intake of lead is derived from the ingestion of food, dirt, and dust. At 5 µg/litre, the average daily intake of lead from water forms a relatively small proportion of the total daily intake for children and adults but a significant one for bottle-fed infants. Such estimates have a wide margin of error, as it is not known to what extent the general public flushes the system before using tapwater; in addition, the stagnation time (and hence the lead level) is highly variable (*10*). The contribution of ingested dust and dirt to the total intake is known to vary with age, peaking around 2 years (*32*).

## 13.19.4 Kinetics and metabolism in laboratory animals and humans

Adults absorb approximately 10% of the lead contained in food (*6*), but young children absorb 4–5 times as much (*34, 35*); the gastrointestinal absorption of lead from ingested soil and dust by children has been estimated to be close to 30% (*26*). Absorption is increased when the dietary intakes of iron or calcium and phosphorus are low (*36–38*). Iron status is particularly important, as children from disadvantaged homes are more likely to suffer from anaemia, further increasing their absorption of lead (*39*).

The principal vehicle for the transport of lead from the intestine to the various body tissues is the red blood cell (*40*), in which lead is bound primarily to haemoglobin and has a special affinity for the beta, delta and, in particular, fetal gamma chains (*41*). Following its absorption, lead appears both in a soft tissue pool consisting of the blood, liver, lungs, spleen, kidneys, and bone marrow, which is rapidly turned over, and in a more slowly turned over skeletal pool. The half-life of lead in blood and soft tissues is about 36–40 days for adults (*42*), so that blood lead concentrations reflect only the intake of the previous 3–5 weeks. In the skeletal pool, the half-life of lead is approximately 17–27 years (*42, 43*). In adults, some 80–95% of the total body burden of lead is found in the skeleton, as compared with about 73% in children (*44, 45*). The biological half-life of lead may be considerably longer in children than in adults (*46*). Under conditions of extended chronic exposure, a steady-state distribution of lead between various organs and systems usually exists (*6*), and the blood lead concentration can therefore be used as a reasonably good indicator of exposure from all sources (*47*); the relationship between them is generally thought to be curvilinear in character (*2, 19*).

Placental transfer of lead occurs in humans as early as week 12 of gestation, and uptake of lead by the fetus continues throughout development (*48*). The concentration of lead in umbilical cord blood is 80–100% of the maternal blood lead level; the same applies to blood lead in the fetus (*49–52*).

Inorganic lead is not metabolized in the body. Unabsorbed dietary lead is eliminated in the faeces, and lead that is absorbed but not retained is excreted unchanged via the kidneys or through the biliary tract (*53*). Metabolic balance studies in infants and young children indicated that, at intakes greater than 5 µg/kg of body weight per day, net retention of lead averaged 32% of intake, whereas retention was negative (i.e. excretion exceeded intake) at intakes less than 4 µg/kg of body weight per day (*35*). No increases in blood lead were observed in infants with low exposure to other sources of lead and mean dietary intakes of 3–4 µg/kg of body weight per day (*54*), thus confirming the metabolic data.

## 13.19.5 Effects on laboratory animals and *in vitro* test systems

### Neurological effects

Research on young primates has demonstrated that exposure to lead results in significant behavioural and cognitive deficits, e.g. impairment of activity, attention, adaptability, learning ability, and memory, as well as increased distractibility. Such effects have been observed following postnatal exposure of monkeys to lead for 29 weeks in amounts resulting in blood lead levels ranging from 10.9 to 33 µg/dl (*55*). These effects persisted into early adulthood, even after levels in the blood had returned to 11–13 µg/dl, and were maintained for the following 8–9 years (*56*). Studies on small groups of monkeys dosed continuously from birth onwards with 50 or 100 µg/kg of body weight per day showed that at 7–8 years of age there were still significant deficits in both short-term memory and spatial learning (*57*).

### Reproductive toxicity, embryotoxicity, and teratogenicity

Effects on sperm counts and on the testicles (testicular atrophy) in male rats and on estrous cycles in female rats have been observed at blood lead levels above 30 µg/100 ml (*58, 59*).

### Mutagenicity and related end-points

Results of studies on the genotoxicity of lead are conflicting (*54, 60–62*), but most suggest that some lead salts are genotoxic. Lead chloride, ethanoate, oxide, and tetroxide were inactive in mutagenicity tests on a number of prokaryotes and fungi, including *Salmonella typhimurium* and *Saccharomyces cerevisiae*. *In vitro* tests on human cells were positive for chromosomal damage in one case and negative in two others. *In vivo* short-term tests on mice, rats, cattle, and monkeys were positive in three cases (dominant lethal test and chromosome damage to bone marrow cells) but negative in five others (*60, 61*).

## Carcinogenicity

Renal tumours have been induced in rats, mice, and hamsters exposed orally to high levels of lead ethanoate, subacetate, or phosphate in the diet. In one study, 5, 18, 62, 141, 500, 1000, or 2000 mg of lead per kg of diet (about 0.3, 0.9, 3, 7, 27, 56, and 105 mg/kg of body weight per day) were fed to rats for 2 years. Renal tumours (mostly tubular epithelial adenomas) developed in male rats at 500, 1000, and 2000 mg/kg, but only at 2000 mg/kg in female rats (*53, 62, 63*).

## 13.19.6 Effects on humans

Lead is a cumulative general poison, infants, children up to 6 years of age, the fetus, and pregnant women being the most susceptible to adverse health effects. Its effects on the central nervous system can be particularly serious.

## Acute and long-term exposure

Overt signs of acute intoxication include dullness, restlessness, irritability, poor attention span, headaches, muscle tremor, abdominal cramps, kidney damage, hallucinations, and loss of memory, encephalopathy occurring at blood lead levels of 100–120 µg/dl in adults and 80–100 µg/dl in children. Signs of chronic lead toxicity, including tiredness, sleeplessness, irritability, headaches, joint pains, and gastrointestinal symptoms, may appear in adults at blood lead levels of 50–80 µg/dl. After 1–2 years of exposure, muscle weakness, gastrointestinal symptoms, lower scores on psychometric tests, disturbances in mood, and symptoms of peripheral neuropathy were observed in occupationally exposed populations at blood lead levels of 40–60 µg/dl (*6*).

Renal disease has long been associated with lead poisoning; however, chronic nephropathy in adults and children has not been detected below blood lead levels of 40 µg/dl (*64, 65*). Damage to the kidneys includes acute proximal tubular dysfunction and is characterized by the appearance of prominent inclusion bodies of a lead–protein complex in the proximal tubular epithelial cells at blood lead concentrations of 40–80 µg/dl (*66*).

There are indications of increased hypertension at blood lead levels greater than 37 µg/dl (*67*). A significant association has been established, without evidence of a threshold, between blood lead levels in the range 7–34 µg/dl and high diastolic blood pressure in people aged 21–55, based on data from the second US National Health and Nutrition Examination Survey (NHANES II) (*68, 69*). The significance of these results has been questioned (*70*).

Lead interferes with the activity of several of the major enzymes involved in the biosynthesis of haem (*6*). The only clinically well-defined symptom associated with the inhibition of haem biosynthesis is anaemia (*40*), which occurs only at blood lead levels in excess of 40 µg/dl in children and 50 µg/dl in adults (*71*). Lead-induced anaemia is the result of two separate processes: the inhibition of haem synthesis and an acceleration of erythrocyte destruction (*40*). Enzymes involved in the synthesis of haem include δ-aminolaevulinate synthetase (whose activity is indirectly induced by feedback inhibition, resulting in accumulation of δ-aminolaevulinate, a neurotoxin) and δ-aminolaevulinic acid dehydratase (δ-ALAD), coproporphyrinogen oxidase, and ferrochelatase, all of whose acitivities are inhibited (*6, 40*). The activity of δ-ALAD is a good predictor of exposure at both environmental and industrial levels, and inhibition of its activity in children has been noted at a blood lead level as low as 5 µg/dl (*72*); however, no adverse health effects are associated with its inhibition at this level.

Inhibition of ferrochelatase by lead results in an accumulation of erythrocyte protoporphyrin (EP), which indicates mitochondrial injury (*47*). NOAELs for increases in EP levels in infants and children exist at about 15–17 µg/dl (*73–75*). In adults, the NOAEL for increases in EP levels ranged from 25 to 30 µg/dl (*76*); for females alone, the NOAEL ranged from 20 to 25 µg/dl, which is closer to that observed for children (*74, 77, 78*). Changes in growth patterns in infants younger than 42 months of age have been associated with increased levels of EP; persistent increases in levels led initially to a rapid gain in weight but subsequently to a retardation of growth (*79*). An analysis of the NHANES II data showed a highly significant negative correlation between the stature of children aged 7 years and younger and blood lead levels in the range 5–35 µg/dl (*80*).

Lead has also been shown to interfere with calcium metabolism, both directly and by interfering with the haem-mediated generation of the vitamin D precursor 1,25-dihydroxycholecalciferol. A significant decrease in the level of circulating 1,25-dihydroxycholecalciferol has been demonstrated in children whose blood lead levels were in the range 12–120 µg/dl, with no evidence of a threshold (*81,82*). Tissue lead content is increased in calcium-deficient persons, a fact that assumes great importance in the light of the increased sensitivity to lead exposure that could result from the calcium-deficient status of pregnant women. It has also been demonstrated that interactions between calcium and lead were responsible for a significant portion of the variance in the scores on general intelligence ratings, and that calcium influenced the deleterious effect of lead (*83*). The regulatory enzyme brain protein, kinase C, is stimulated *in vitro* by picomolar lead concentrations (an effect similar to that produced by micromolar calcium concentrations), levels that could be expected from environmental exposure (*84*).

Several lines of evidence demonstrate that both the central and peripheral nervous systems are the principal targets for lead toxicity. The effects include sub-encephalopathic neurological and behavioural effects in adults, and there is also electrophysiological evidence of effects on the nervous system of children at blood lead levels well below 30 µg/dl. Aberrant electroencephalograph readings were significantly correlated with blood levels down to 15 µg/dl (*85, 86*). Significant reductions in maximal motor nerve conduction velocity (MNCV) have been observed in children aged 5–9 years living near a smelter, with a threshold occurring at a blood lead level around 20 µg/dl; a 2% decrease in the MNCV was seen for every 10 µg/dl increase in the blood lead level (87). The auditory nerve may be a target for lead toxicity, in view of reports of reduced hearing acuity in children (88). In the NHANES II survey in the USA, the association with blood lead was highly significant at all levels from 5 to 45 µg/dl for children 4–19 years old, with a 10-20% increased likelihood of an elevated hearing threshold for persons with a blood lead level of 20 µg/dl as compared with 4 µg/dl (89). The NHANES II data also showed that blood lead levels were significantly associated with the age at which infants first sat up, walked, and started to speak. Although no threshold existed for the age at which the child first walked, thresholds existed at the 29th and 28th percentile of lead rank for the age at which the child sat up and spoke, respectively (89).

### Reproductive effects

Gonadal dysfunction in men, including depressed sperm counts, has been associated with blood lead levels of 40–50 µg/dl (90–93). Reproductive dysfunction may also occur in females occupationally exposed to lead (6, 61).

Epidemiological studies have shown that exposure of pregnant women to lead increases the risk of preterm delivery. In a study of 774 pregnant women in Port Pirie who were followed to the completion of their pregnancy, the relative risk of preterm delivery was more than four times higher among women with blood lead levels above 14 µg/dl than in those with 8 µg or less per dl (94).

Elevated cord blood lead levels were associated with minor malformations, such as angiomas, syndactylism, and hydrocele, in about 10% of all babies. The relative risk of malformation doubled at blood lead levels of about 7–10 µg/dl, and the incidence of any defect increased with increasing cord lead levels over the range 0.7–35.1 µg/dl (95).

### Mutagenicity

Cytogenetic studies in humans exposed to lead (blood lead levels > 40 µg/dl) have given conflicting results; chromatid and chromosomal aberrations, breaks, and gaps were reported in 9 of 16 studies but not in the remainder (60, 61).

### Carcinogenicity

The carcinogenicity of lead in humans has been examined in several epidemiological studies, which either have been negative or have shown only very small excess mortalities from cancers. In most of these studies, there were either concurrent exposures to other carcinogenic agents or other confounding factors such as smoking that were not considered (60, 61). A study on 700 smelter workers (mean blood level 79.7 µg/litre) and battery factory workers (mean blood level 62.7 µg/litre) indicated an excess of deaths from cancer of the digestive and respiratory systems (96), the significance of which has been debated (97, 98). There was also a nonsignificant increase in urinary tract tumours in production workers. In a study on lead smelter workers in Australia, no significant increase in cancers was seen, but there was a substantial excess of deaths from chronic renal disease (99). IARC considers that the overall evidence for carcinogenicity in humans is inadequate (60).

### Neurological effects in infants and children

A number of cross-sectional and longitudinal epidemiological studies have been designed to investigate the possible detrimental effects that exposure of young children to lead might have on their intellectual abilities and behaviour. These studies have been concerned with documenting effects arising from exposure to "low" levels of lead (i.e. blood lead < 40 µg/dl), at which overt clinical symptoms are absent. Several factors affect the validity of the conclusions drawn from them (100), including the statistical power of the study, the effect of bias in the selection of study and control populations, the choice of parameter used to evaluate lead exposure, the temporal relationship between exposure measurement and psychological evaluations, the extent to which the neurological and behavioural tests used can be quantified accurately and reproducibly, which confounding covariates are included in any multiple regression analysis, and the effect of various nutritional and dietary factors, such as iron and calcium intake (39).

### Cross-sectional studies

A number of cross-sectional studies have been carried out in which many of the above factors were taken into account. In one such study in the USA, a group of 58 children aged 6–7 years with "high" dentine lead levels (corresponding to a blood lead level of approximately 30–50 µg/dl) performed significantly less well than 100 children from a "low" lead group (mean blood lead level 24 µg/dl). The children's performance was measured using the Wechsler intelligence test in addition to other visual and auditory tests and teachers' behavioural ratings (101). There was a significant difference of 4 points and a uniform downward shift in IQ scores. Although this study found that a child in the group with "high" dentine lead was three times more likely to have an IQ of 80 or lower than one in the "low" lead group, it was claimed in a 1986 review that the effect was statistically significant only for children with the highest lead levels in dentine (blood lead > 40 µg/dl) (6).

A similar study in which lead in dentine was used as the indicator of exposure was carried out on a cohort of 400 children in the United Kingdom (102). There were several consistent but nonsignificant differences between the high- and low-lead groups similar to those observed in the American study, including

IQ decrements of about 2 points and poorer scores in behaviour indices. In the British study, mean blood lead levels in the "high" exposure group (15.1 µg/dl) were lower than the mean of the "low" group (24 µg/dl) in the American study, which may explain why the results lacked statistical significance. The results of studies on children in Germany (*103–105*) were similar to those of the British study, in that the effect of lead on behaviour was only of borderline significance.

In another study (*106*) involving 500 Edinburgh schoolchildren aged 6–9 years, a small (up to 5 points in the British Ability Scales) but significant negative relationship was found between blood lead levels and intelligence scores, reading skills, and number skills. There was a dose–response relationship in the range 5.6–22.1 µg/dl. The effect of lead was small compared with that of several of the other 33 variables considered. A series of studies (*107–109*) on about 800 children in the United Kingdom with blood lead levels between 4 and 32 µg/dl failed to find any significant associations between lead and indices of intelligence and behaviour after socioeconomic and family characteristics were taken into account. It was suggested that lead might have a noticeable effect only when other factors predisposing to social disadvantage (particularly low socioeconomic status or poor home environment) are present (*108–110*).

In a cross-sectional study in Lavrion (Greece) involving 509 primary school-children living near a lead smelter, blood lead levels between 7.4 and 63.9 µg/dl (mean 23.7 µg/dl) were recorded (*111*). When the IQ was measured by means of the revised Wechsler Intelligence Scale for Children and due account taken of 17 potential confounders, a significant association was found between blood lead levels and IQ, with a threshold at about 25 µg/dl. Attentional performance was also associated with blood lead levels in two different tests, but no threshold level was found. This study was part of a multicentre collaborative international study on schoolchildren sponsored by WHO and the Commission of the European Communities (*112*). A more or less uniform protocol was used, and quality assurance procedures were applied to the exposure analyses. The most consistent associations were for visual–motor integration as measured by the Bender Gestalt test and for reaction performance as measured by the Vienna Reaction Device. The results of many of the remaining tests were inconsistent. The degree of association between lead exposure and outcome was very weak (<0.8%), even in the statistically significant cases.

The cross-sectional studies are, on balance, consistent in demonstrating statistically significant associations between blood lead levels of 30 µg/dl or more and IQ deficits of about 4 points. Although there were associations between lower blood lead levels and IQ deficits of about 2 points, these were only marginally statistically significant, except in the Edinburgh study. It is particularly difficult to determine minimum levels above which significant effects occur.

## Longitudinal studies

Longitudinal studies have the advantage as compared with cross-sectional studies that more precise estimates of exposure can be made; in addition, the reversibility of the effects and the temporal sequence of causality can be investigated. However, such studies also have certain disadvantages: for example, repeated psychometric testing may lead to artefactual results, and there may also be problems of bias associated with attrition within the study population.

The possible relationship between low-level lead exposure during the fetal period and in early childhood and later effects on infant and child development has been investigated in at least six prospective studies, in the USA (Boston, Cincinnati, and Cleveland), Australia (Port Pirie, Sydney), and Scotland (Glasgow). Broadly similar methodologies were used in all the studies to facilitate comparisons. The Bayley Scales of Infant Development or subsets of this test were used to evaluate early cognitive development in verbal and performance skills in infants and young children, whereas the McCarthy Scales of Children's Abilities (MSCA) were used in most studies on older children. In all the studies, except that in Glasgow, the average maternal and cord blood lead concentrations were less than 10 μg/dl (range 6.0–9.5 μg/dl).

In the Boston Lead Study, three groups of infants and young children were classified according to umbilical cord blood lead concentrations, the levels in the low-, middle-, and high-lead groups being < 3, 6–7, and 10–25 μg/dl (mean 14.6 μg/dl), respectively. Children were tested twice a year from age 6 months to almost 5 years (*113, 114*). After controlling for 12 potential confounders, a significant inverse relationship was demonstrated between fetal exposure, measured as lead levels in cord blood, and mental development at age 2, as measured by the Bayley Mental Development Index (MDI). There was no significant correlation with the children's current blood lead levels, all of which were less than 8.8 μg/dl. However, the results of testing at almost 5 years, using the McCarthy Scales, showed an attenuation of this association. At 57 months, only the association between intelligence scores and blood lead 3 years previously, at age 2, remained significant after controlling for confounding variables (*114*).

In a longitudinal study involving 305 pregnant women in Cincinnati (*115*), an inverse relationship was found between either prenatal or neonatal blood lead levels and performance in terms both of the Bayley Psychomotor Development Index (PDI) and the Bayley MDI at the ages of 3 and 6 months for both male infants and infants from the poorest families. The mean blood lead levels for neonates and their mothers were 4.6 and 8.2 μg/dl, respectively, and all blood lead levels were below 30 μg/dl. Multiple regression analysis for boys only showed that, for every increment of 1 μg/dl in the prenatal blood lead level, the covariate-adjusted Bayley MDI at 6 months of age decreased by 0.84 points. The inverse relationship between MDI and prenatal blood lead disappeared at age 1, because it was accounted for, and mediated through, the effect of lead on birth weight; however, the Bayley PDI was still significantly related to maternal blood lead (*116*).

In a prospective study of design similar to that of the Boston study, undertaken at Port Pirie, a lead smelter town in Australia, 537 children were studied from birth to 4 years (*117*). The cohort was divided into four groups on the basis of maternal and umbilical blood lead, which ranged from a geometric mean of 0.21 to 0.72 µmol/litre (4.3–14.9 µg/dl). The mean blood lead level varied from 9.1 µg/dl at mid-pregnancy to 21.3 and 19 µg/dl at 2 and 4 years, respectively. The integrated postnatal average blood lead level was 19.1 µg/dl. At 6, 15, 24, and 36 months, the developmental status of the child was assessed by means of the Bayley MDI; the MSCA were used at 4 years. At each age, a consistent but weak inverse relationship was found between concurrent postnatal blood lead levels and MSCA scores; no allowance was made for possible confounding factors. No such relationship was found for perinatal blood lead. After 18 covariates considered to be potential confounders were incorporated in the multivariate analysis, the integrated blood lead level showed the strongest inverse relation with the General Cognitive Index (GCI) score (a subset of the McCarthy Scales) at age 4 years, which suggests that the detrimental effect of lead on child development is cumulative during early childhood. Repeated analysis restricted to children whose blood lead levels were below 25 µg/dl showed that the inverse relationship with the GCI score was as strong for this group as for the cohort as a whole, thus demonstrating the absence of a clear threshold below which a detrimental effect of lead on child development does not occur.

A number of prospective studies have failed to show any consistent association between mental development and blood lead, either during the perinatal period or in early childhood. In a study carried out on extremely socially disadvantaged mothers and infants in Cleveland, Ohio (USA), no relationship was found between blood lead at any time and language development, MDI, or the results of the Stanford-Binet IQ test at age 3 years, after confounding factors, the most important of which was the care-giving environment, were taken into account. In this cohort, half the mothers had alcohol-related problems, and the average maternal IQ was 79 (*118*). In a second Australian study carried out in Sydney on a relatively prosperous population of 318 mothers and children, no association was found between blood lead in the mother or the child at any age and mental or motor deficits at age 4 years, after account was taken of six covariates, including the HOME score (a measure of the care-giving environment) (*119*). A third negative study was that carried out in Glasgow (Scotland), where the primary exposure was to high lead levels in water which were dramatically reduced by corrosion-control measures shortly after the children were born. The cohort was divided into high, medium, and low groups, on the basis of maternal blood lead, with means of 33.1, 17.7, and 7.0 µg/dl, respectively. Although the expected decrements in scores in the Bayley MDI and PDI were observed at ages 1 and 2 years as lead exposure increased, they could be better accounted for by birth weight, home environment, and socioeconomic status, as shown by stepwise multiple regression analysis (*120*).

The results of the prospective studies have been somewhat disappointing because of the inconsistency between studies. It appears that prenatal exposure may have early effects on mental development, but that these do not persist up to age 4, at least not as shown by the tests so far used. There are indications that these early effects may be mediated through birth weight or other factors. Several studies have indicated that the generally higher exposures of children in the 18–36-month age range may be negatively associated with mental development, but this, too, has not been confirmed by other studies.

## 13.19.7 Guideline value

The evidence for the carcinogenicity of lead in humans is inconclusive because of the limited number of studies, the small cohort sizes, and the failure to take adequate account of potential confounding variables. However, an association has been demonstrated experimentally between the ingestion of lead salts and renal tumours. Lead and inorganic lead compounds have therefore been placed in Group 2B of the IARC classification, namely possible human carcinogen (evidence inadequate in humans, sufficient in animals) (60).

As there is evidence from human studies that adverse effects other than cancer may occur at very low lead levels, and that a guideline thus derived would also be protective for carcinogenic effects, it is considered appropriate to derive the guideline using the TDI approach.

In 1986, JECFA established a provisional tolerable weekly intake (PTWI) of 25 µg of lead per kg of body weight (equivalent to 3.5 µg/kg of body weight per day) for infants and children which took account of the fact that lead is a cumulative poison so that any increase in the body burden of lead should be avoided (71). The PTWI was based on metabolic studies in infants (35, 54) showing that a mean daily intake of 3–4 µg/kg of body weight was not associated with an increase in blood lead levels or in the body burden of lead, whereas an intake of 5 µg/kg of body weight or more resulted in lead retention. This PTWI was reconfirmed by JECFA in 1993 and extended to all age groups (121).

On the assumption of a 50% allocation to drinking-water for a 5-kg bottle-fed infant consuming 0.75 litres of drinking-water per day, the guideline value is 0.01 mg/litre. As infants are considered to be the most sensitive subgroup of the population, this guideline value will also be protective for other age groups.

Lead is exceptional in that most lead in drinking-water arises from plumbing in buildings and the remedy consists principally of removing plumbing and fittings containing it. This requires time and money, and it is recognized that not all water will meet the guideline immediately. Meanwhile, all other practical measures to reduce total exposure to lead, including corrosion control, should be implemented.

## References

1.  *Lead—environmental aspects.* Geneva, World Health Organization, 1989 (Environmental Health Criteria, No. 85).

2.  Quinn MJ, Sherlock JC. The correspondence between U.K. 'action levels' for lead in blood and in water. *Food additives and contaminants,* 1990, 7:387-424.

3.  International Organization for Standardization. *Water quality—determination of cobalt, nickel, copper, zinc, cadmium and lead.* Geneva, 1986 (ISO 8288:1986).

4.  Environment Canada. *National air pollution surveillance annual summary 1988.* Ottawa, 1989 (Report EPS 7/AP/19).

5.  Environmental Protection Service. *Urban air quality trends in Canada, 1970-79.* Ottawa, Environment Canada, 1981 (Report EPS 5-AP-81-14).

6.  US Environmental Protection Agency. *Air quality criteria for lead.* Research Triangle Park, NC, 1986 (Report EPA-600/8-83/028F).

7.  Tomas X et al. Application of pattern recognition to speciation data of heavy metals in suspended particulates of urban air. *Journal of chemometrics,* 1988, 3:139.

8.  Strehlow CD, Barltrop D. Temporal trends in urban and rural blood lead concentrations. *Environmental geochemistry and health,* 1987, 9:74.

9.  Pacyna JM, Ottar B. Transport and chemical composition of the summer aerosol in the Norwegian Arctic. *Atmospheric environment,* 1985, 19:2109.

10. Levin R, Schock MR, Marcus AH. Exposure to lead in U.S. drinking water. In: *Proceedings of the 23rd Annual Conference on Trace Substances in Environmental Health,* Cincinnati, OH, US Environmental Protection Agency, 1989.

11. Schock MR. Understanding lead corrosion control stategies. *Journal of the American Water Works Association,* 1989, 81:88.

12. Schock MR. Causes of temporal variability of lead in domestic plumbing systems. *Environmental monitoring and assessment,* 1990, 15:59.

13. Cosgrove E et al. Childhood lead poisoning: case study traces source to drinking water. *Journal of environmental health,* 1989, 52:346.

14. Moore MR et al. Maternal lead levels after alterations to water supply. *Lancet,* 1981, 2:203-204.

15. Sherlock JC et al. Reduction in exposure to lead from drinking water and its effect on blood lead concentration. *Human toxicology,* 1984, 3:383-392.

16. US Environmental Protection Agency. National primary drinking water regulations for lead and copper. *Federal register*, 1988, 53:31515-31578.

17. Dabeka RW, McKenzie AD, Lacroix GMA. Dietary intakes of lead, cadmium, arsenic and fluoride by Canadian adults: a 24-hour duplicate diet study. *Food additives and contaminants*, 1987, 4:89-101.

18. Department of National Health and Welfare (Canada). *Guidelines for Canadian drinking water quality: supporting documentation. Lead.* Ottawa, 1992.

19. Sherlock JC, Quinn MJ. Relationship between blood lead concentrations and dietary lead intake in infants: the Glasgow Duplicate Diet Study 1979-1980. *Food additives and contaminants*, 1986, 3:167-176.

20. Galal-Gorchev H. Dietary intake of pesticide residues, cadmium, mercury and lead. *Food additives and contaminants*, 1991, 8(6):793-806.

21. Slorach SA et al. Intake of lead, cadmium and certain other metals via a typical Swedish weekly diet. *Vår Föda*, 1983, 35 (Suppl. 1).

22. Varo P, Kovistoinen P. Mineral element composition of Finnish foods. XII. General discussion and nutritional evaluation. *Acta agriculturae scandinavica*, 1980, Suppl. 22:165.

23. Gunderson EL. FDA Total Diet Study, April 1982-April 1984, dietary intakes of pesticides, selected elements, and other chemicals. *Journal of the Association of Official Analytical Chemists*, 1988, 71:1200-1209.

24. Karolinska Institute. *Global Environmental Monitoring System (GEMS) assessment of human exposure to lead: comparison between Belgium, Malta, Mexico and Sweden.* Stockholm, 1985.

25. Elinder C-G et al. Wine—an important source of lead exposure. *Food additives and contaminants*, 1988, 5:641-644.

26. Drill S et al. *The environmental lead problem: an assessment of lead in drinking water from a multi-media perspective.* Washington, DC, US Environmental Protection Agency, 1979 (Report EPA-570/9-79-003).

27. Clausing P, Brunekreef B, van Wijnen JH. A method for estimating soil ingestion by children. *International archives of occupational and environmental health*, 1987, 59:73-82.

28. Centers for Disease Control. *Preventing lead poisoning in young children.* Atlanta, GA, Department of Health and Human Services, 1985:7-19 (Publ. No. 99-2230).

29. Raab GM, Laxen DPH, Fulton M. Lead from dust and water as exposure sources for children. *Environmental geochemistry and health*, 1987, 9:80.

30. Davies DJA et al. Lead intake and blood lead in two-year-old U.K. urban children. *Science of the total environment*, 1990, 90:13-29.

31. Calabrese EJ et al. How much soil do young children ingest: an epidemiologic study. *Regulatory toxicology and pharmacology*, 1989, 10:123-137.

32. Van Wijnen JH, Clausing P, Brunekreef B. Estimated soil ingestion by children. *Environmental research*, 1990, 51:147-162.

33. Mushak P, Crocetti AF. Determination of numbers of lead-exposed American children as a function of lead source: integrated summary of a report to the U.S. Congress on childhood lead poisoning. *Environmental research*, 1989, 50:210-229.

34. Alexander FW. The uptake of lead by children in differing environments. *Environmental health perspectives*, 1974, 7:155-159.

35. Ziegler EE et al. Absorption and retention of lead by infants. *Pediatric research*, 1978, 12:29-34.

36. Van Barneveld AA, Van den Hamer CJA. Drinking water hardness, trace elements and cardiovascular diseases: main effects of Ca and Mg on metabolism of Mn, Pb and Cd in mice. *Nutrition research*, 1985, Suppl. 1:345.

37. Blake KC, Barbezat GO, Mann M. Effect of dietary constituents on the gastro-intestinal absorption of [203]Pb in man. *Environmental research*, 1983, 30:182.

38. Blake KC, Mann M. Effects of calcium and phosphorus on the gastrointestinal absorption of [203]Pb in man. *Environmental research*, 1983, 30:188-194.

39. Mahaffey KR. Nutritional factors in lead poisoning. *Nutrition reviews*, 1981, 39–353.

40. Moore MR. Haematological effects of lead. *Science of the total environment*, 1988, 71:419-431.

41. Ong CN, Lee WR. High affinity of lead for foetal haemoglobin. *British journal of industrial medicine*, 1980, 37:292-298.

42. Rabinowitz MB, Wetherill CW, Kopple JD. Kinetic analysis of lead metabolism in healthy humans. *Journal of clinical investigations*, 1976, 58:260-270.

43. Holtzman RB. Application of radiolead to metabolic studies. In: Nriagu JO, ed. *The biogeochemistry of lead in the environment. Part B*. Amsterdam, Elsevier/North Holland Biomedical Press, 1978:37.

44. Alessio L, Foa V. In: Alessio L et al., eds. *Human biological monitoring of industrial chemicals series.* Luxembourg, Commission of the European Communities, 1983:107.

45. Barry PSI. Distribution and storage of lead in human tissues. In: Nriagu JO, ed. *The biogeochemistry of lead in the environment. Part B.* Amsterdam, Elsevier/North Holland Biomedical Press, 1978:97.

46. Succop PA, O'Flaherty EJ, Bornschein RL. A kinetic model for estimating changes in the concentration of lead in the blood of young children. In: Lindberg SE, Hutchinson TC, eds. *Heavy metals in the environment.* Vol. 2. Edinburgh, CEP Consultants, 1987:289.

47. Mushak P et al. Prenatal and postnatal effects of low-level lead exposure: integrated summary of a report to the U.S. Congress on childhood lead poisoning. *Environmental research*, 1989, 50:11-36.

48. Barltrop D. Transfer of lead to the human foetus. In: Barltrop D, Burland WL, eds. *Mineral metabolism in paediatrics.* Oxford, Blackwell Scientific Publications, 1969:135-151.

49. Angell NF, Lavery JP. The relationship of blood lead levels to obstetric outcome. *American journal of obstetrics and gynecology*, 1982, 142:40-46.

50. Moore MR et al. Some studies of maternal and infant lead exposure in Glasgow. *Scottish medical journal*, 1982, 27:113-122.

51. Gershanik JJ, Brooks GG, Little JA. Blood lead values in pregnant women and their offspring. *American journal of obstetrics and gynecology*, 1974, 119:508-511.

52. Lacey RF. Lead in water, infant diet and blood: the Glasgow Duplicate Diet Study. *Science of the total environment*, 1985, 41:235-257.

53. Syracuse Research Corporation. *Toxicological profile for lead.* Atlanta, GA, Agency for Toxic Substances and Disease Registry (ATSDR), US Public Health Service and US Environmental Protection Agency, 1990.

54. Rye JE et al. Dietary intake of lead and blood lead concentration in early infancy. *American journal of diseases of children*, 1983, 137:886-891.

55. Rice DC. Primate research: relevance to human learning and development. *Developmental pharmacology and therapeutics*, 1987, 10:314-327.

56. Gilbert SG, Rice DC. Low-level lifetime lead exposure produces behavioral toxicity (spatial discrimination reversal) in adult monkeys. *Toxicology and applied pharmacology*, 1987, 91:484-490.

57. Rice DC, Karpinski KF. Lifetime low-level lead exposure produces deficits in delayed alternation in adult monkeys. *Neurotoxicology and teratology*, 1988, 10:207-214.

58. Hilderbrand DC et al. Effect of lead acetate on reproduction. *American journal of obstetrics and gynecology*, 1973, 115:1058-1065.

59. Chowdhury AR, Dewan A, Gandhi DN. *Toxic effect of lead on the testes of rat. Biomedica biochimica acta*, 1984, 43:95-100.

60. International Agency for Research on Cancer. *Overall evaluations of carcinogenicity: an updating of IARC monographs volumes 1–42.* Lyon, 1987:230-232 (IARC Monographs on the Evaluation of Carcinogenic Risks to Humans, Suppl. 7).

61. International Agency for Research on Cancer. *Some metals and metallic compounds.* Lyon, 1980:23 (IARC Monographs on the Evaluation of Carcinogenic Risks to Humans, Vol. 23).

62. Marcus WL. Lead health effects in drinking water. *Toxicology and industrial health*, 1986, 2:363-407.

63. Azar A, Trochimowicz HJ, Maxfield ME. Review of lead studies in animals carried out at Haskell Laboratory: two-year feeding study and response to hemorrhage study. In: Barth D et al., eds. *Environmental health aspects of lead. Proceedings of an International Symposium. October 1972, Amsterdam, The Netherlands.* Luxembourg, Commission of the European Communities, 1973:199-210.

64. Campbell BC et al. Renal insufficiency associated with excessive lead exposure. *British medical journal*, 1977, 1:482-485.

65. Lilis R et al. Lead effects among secondary lead smelter workers with blood lead below 80 microgram/100 mL. *Archives of environmental health*, 1977, 32:256-266.

66. Ritz E, Mann J, Wiecek A. Does lead play a role in the development of renal insufficiency? *Contributions to nephrology*, 1988, 64:43-48.

67. Pocock SJ et al. Blood lead concentration, blood pressure, and renal function. *British medical journal*, 1984, 289:872-874.

68. Harlan WR et al. Blood lead and blood pressure. Relationship in the adolescent and adult US population. *Journal of the American Medical Association*, 1985, 253:530-534.

69. Pirkle JL et al. The relationship between blood levels and blood pressure and its cardiovascular risk implications. *American journal of epidemiology*, 1985, 121:246-258.

70. Gartside PS. The relationship between blood lead levels and blood pressure and its cardiovascular risk implications. *American journal of epidemiology*, 1986, 124:864-867 (letter).

71. Joint FAO/WHO Expert Committee on Food Additives. *Toxicological evaluation of certain food additives and contaminants*. Cambridge, Cambridge University Press, 1987:223-255 (WHO Food Additives Series, No. 21).

72. Granick JL et al. Studies in lead poisoning. II. Correlation between the ratio of activated to inactivated delta-aminolevulinic acid dehydratase of whole blood and the blood lead level. *Biochemical medicine*, 1973, 8:149-159.

73. Piomelli S et al. Threshold for lead damage to heme synthesis in urban children. *Proceedings of the National Academy of Sciences of the United States of America*, 1982, 79:3335-3339.

74. Roels H et al. Impact of air pollution by lead on the heme biosynthetic pathway in school-age children. *Archives of environmental health*, 1976, 31:310-316.

75. Rabinowitz MB, Leviton A, Needleman HL. Occurrence of elevated protoporphyrin levels in relation to lead burden in infants. *Environmental research*, 1986, 39:253-257.

76. Grandjean P, Lintrup J. Erythrocyte-Zn-protoporphyrin as an indicator of lead exposure. *Scandinavian journal of clinical and laboratory investigation*, 1978, 38:669-675.

77. Toriumi H, Kawai M. Free erythrocyte protoporphyrin (FEP) in a general population, workers exposed to low-level lead, and organic-solvent workers. *Environmental research*, 1981, 25:310-316.

78. Zielhuis RL. Dose–response relationships for inorganic lead. *International archives of occupational and environmental health*, 1975, 35 (1):1-18.

79. Angle CR, Kuntzelman DR. Increased erythrocyte protoporphyrins and blood lead—a pilot study of childhood growth patterns. *Journal of toxicology and environmental health*, 1989, 26:149-156.

80. Schwartz J, Angle C, Pitcher H. Relationship between childhood blood lead levels and stature. *Pediatrics*, 1986, 77:281-288.

81. Rosen JF et al. Reduction in 1,25-dihydroxyvitamin D in children with increased lead absorption. *New England journal of medicine*, 1980, 302:1128-1131.

82. Mahaffey KR et al. Association between age, blood lead concentration, and serum 1,25-hydroxycholecalciferol levels in children. *American journal of clinical nutrition*, 1982, 35:1327-1331.

83. Lester ML, Horst RL, Thatcher RW. Protective effects of zinc and calcium against heavy metal impairment of children's cognitive function. *Nutrition and behaviour*, 1986, 3:145.

84. Markovac J, Goldstein GW. Picomolar concentrations of lead stimulate brain protein kinase C. *Nature*, 1988, 334:71-73.

85. Otto DA et al. Effects of age and body lead burden on CNS function in young children. I. Slow cortical potentials. *Electroencephalography and clinical neurophysiology*, 1981, 52:229-239.

86. Otta DA et al. Effects of low to moderate lead exposure on slow cortical potentials in young children: two-year follow-up study. *Neurobehavioural toxicology and teratology*, 1982, 4:733-737.

87. Schwartz J et al. Threshold effect in lead-induced peripheral neuropathy. *Journal of pediatrics*, 1988, 112:12-17.

88. Robinson G et al. Effects of low to moderate lead exposure on brainstem auditory evoked potentials in children. In: *Neurobehavioural methods in occupational and environmental health*. Copenhagen, WHO Regional Office for Europe, 1985:177-182 (Environmental Health Series No. 3).

89. Schwartz J, Otto D. Blood lead, hearing thresholds, and neurobehavioral development in children and youth. *Archives of environmental health*, 1987, 42:153-160.

90. Lancranjan I. Reproductive ability of workmen occupationally exposed to lead. *Archives of environmental health*, 1975, 30:396-401.

91. Wildt K, Eliasson R, Berlin M. Effects of occupational exposure to lead on sperm and semen. In: Clarkson TW, Nordberg GF, Sager PR, eds. *Reproductive and developmental toxicity of metals. Proceedings of a joint meeting, May 1982, Rochester, N.Y.* New York, Plenum Press, 1983:279-300.

92. Cullen MR, Kayne RD, Robins JM. Endocrine and reproductive dysfunction in men associated with occupational inorganic lead intoxication. *Archives of environmental health*, 1984, 39:431-440.

93. Assennato G et al. Sperm count suppression without endocrine dysfunction in lead-exposed men. *Archives of environmental health*, 1986, 41:387-390.

94. McMichael AJ et al. The Port Pirie cohort study: maternal blood lead and pregnancy outcome. *Journal of epidemiology and community health*, 1986, 40:18-25.

95. Needleman HL et al. The relationship between prenatal exposure to lead and congenital anomalies. *Journal of the American Medical Association*, 1984, 251:2956-2959.

96. Cooper WC, Gaffey WR. Mortality of lead workers. *Journal of occupational medicine,* 1975, 17:100-107.

97. Kang HK, Infante PR, Carra JS. Occupational lead exposure and cancer. *Science,* 1980, 20(1):935-936 (letter).

98. Cooper WC, Wong O, Kheifets L. Mortality among employees of lead battery plants and lead producing plants, 1947-1980. *Scandinavian journal of work, environment and health,* 1985, 11:331-345.

99. McMichael AJ, Johnson HM. Long-term mortality profile of heavily-exposed lead smelter workers. *Journal of occupational medicine,* 1982, 24:375-378.

100. Smith M. The effects of low-level lead exposure on children. In: Smith MA, Grant LD, Sors AI, eds. *Lead exposure and child development: an international assessment.* Boston, MA, Kluwer Academic Publishers, 1989:3.

101. Needleman HL et al. Deficits in psychologic and classroom performance of children with elevated dentine lead levels. *New England journal of medicine,* 1979, 300:689-695.

102. Smith M et al. The effects of lead exposure on urban children: the Institute of Child Health/Southampton study. *Developmental medicine and child neurology,* 1983, 25 (Suppl.47):1-54.

103. Winneke G, Hrdina KG, Brockhaus A. Neuropsychological studies in children with elevated tooth-lead concentrations. I. Pilot study. *International archives of occupational and environmental health,* 1982, 51:169-183.

104. Winneke G, Kraemer U. Neuropsychological effects of lead in children: interactions with social background variables. *Neuropsychobiology,* 1984, 11:195-202.

105. Winneke G et al. Neuropsychological studies in children with elevated tooth-lead concentrations. II. Extended study. *International archives of occupational and environmental health,* 1983, 51:231-252.

106. Fulton M et al. Influence of blood lead on the ability and attainment of children in Edinburgh. *Lancet,* 1987, 1:1221-1226.

107. Lansdown RG et al. Blood-lead levels, behaviour, and intelligence: a population study. *Lancet,* 1974, i:538-541.

108. Lansdown R et al. The relationship between blood-lead concentrations, intelligence, attainment and behaviour in a school population: the second London study. *International archives of occupational and environmental health,* 1986, 57:225-235.

109. Harvey PG et al. Blood lead, behaviour, and intelligence test performance in preschool children. *Science of the total environment,* 1984, 40:45-60.

110. Yule W, Rutter M. Effect of lead on children's behaviour and cognitive performance: a critical review. In: Mahaffey KR, ed. *Dietary and environmental lead: human health effects*. Amsterdam, Elsevier Science Publishers, 1985.

111. Hatzakis A et al. Psychometric intelligence and attentional performance deficits in lead-exposed children. In: Linberg SE, Hutchinson TC, eds. *Heavy metals in the environment*, Vol. 1. Edinburgh, CEP Consultants, 1987:204-209.

112. Winneke G et al. Results from the European multicenter study on lead neurotoxicity in children: implications for risk assessment. *Neurotoxicology and teratology*, 1990, 12:553-559.

113. Bellinger D et al. Longitudinal analyses of prenatal and postnatal lead exposure and early cognitive development. *New England journal of medicine*, 1987, 316:1037-1043.

114. Bellinger D et al. Low-level lead exposure and child development; assessment at age five of a cohort followed from birth. In: Lindberg SE, Hutchinson TC, eds. *Heavy metals in the environment*, Vol. 1. Edinburgh, CEP Consultants, 1987:49-53.

115. Dietrich KN et al. Low-level fetal lead exposure effect on neurobehavioral development in early infancy. *Pediatrics*, 1987, 80:721-730.

116. Dietrich KN et al. Neurobehavioural effects of foetal lead exposure; the first year of life. In: Smith MA, Grant LD, Sors AI, eds. *Lead exposure and child development, an international assessment*. Dordrecht, Kluwer Academic Publishers, 1989:320.

117. McMichael AJ et al. Port Pirie cohort study: environmental exposure to lead and children's abilities at the age of four years. *New England journal of medicine*, 1988, 319:468-475.

118. Ernhart CB, Greene T. Low-level lead exposure in the prenatal and early preschool periods: language development. *Archives of environmental health*, 1990, 45:342-354.

119. Cooney GH et al. Low-level exposures to lead: the Sydney lead study. *Developmental medicine and child neurology*, 1989, 31:640-649.

120. Moore MR, Bushnell IWR, Goldberg A. A prospective study of the results of changes in environmental lead exposure in children in Glasgow. In: Smith MA, Grant LD, Sors AI, eds. *Lead exposure and child development, an international assessment*. Dordrecht, Kluwer Academic Publishers, 1989:371.

121. *Evaluation of certain food additives and contaminants: forty-first report of the Joint FAO/WHO Expert Committee on Food Additives*. Geneva, World Health Organization, 1993 (WHO Technical Report Series, No. 837).

# 13.20 Manganese

## 13.20.1 General description

### Identity

| Compound | CAS no. | Molecular formula |
|---|---|---|
| Manganese | 7439-96-5 | Mn |
| Manganese(II) chloride | 7773-01-5 | $MnCl_2$ |
| Trimanganese tetroxide | 1317-35-7 | $Mn_3O_4$ |
| Manganese dioxide | 1313-13-9 | $MnO_2$ |
| Potassium permanganate | 7722-64-7 | $KMnO_4$ |

Manganese, one of the more abundant metals in the earth's crust, usually occurs together with iron. The most environmentally important manganese compounds are those that contain $Mn^{2+}$, $Mn^{4+}$, and $Mn^{7+}$ (1).

### Physicochemical properties (1)

| Property | Mn | $MnCl_2$ | $Mn_3O_4$ | $MnO_2$ | $KMnO_4$ |
|---|---|---|---|---|---|
| Melting point (°C) | 1244 | 650 | 1564 | – | – |
| Boiling point (°C) | 1962 | 1190 | – | – | – |
| Density (g/cm³) | 7.20 | 2.97 | 4.86 | 5.03 | 2.70 |
| Water solubility (g/litre) | Insoluble | 723 | Insoluble | Insoluble | 63.8 |

### Organoleptic properties

At concentrations exceeding 0.1 mg/litre, the manganese ion imparts an undesirable taste to beverages and stains plumbing fixtures and laundry (2). When manganese(II) compounds in solution undergo oxidation, manganese is precipitated, resulting in encrustation problems. Even at about 0.02 mg/litre, manganese will form coatings on piping that may later slough off as a black precipitate (3). In addition, certain nuisance organisms concentrate manganese and give rise to taste, odour, and turbidity problems in distributed water (2, 4).

### Major uses

Manganese is used principally in the manufacture of iron, steel, and other alloys. Manganese dioxide and other manganese compounds are used in products such as batteries, glass, and fireworks. Potassium permanganate is used as an oxidant for cleaning, bleaching, and disinfection purposes (5).

### Environmental fate

Elemental and inorganic forms of manganese may be present in the atmosphere as suspended particulates (6). In surface waters, manganese occurs in both dissolved and suspended forms. Anaerobic groundwater often contains elevated levels of dissolved manganese. The divalent form predominates in most water at pH 4–7, but more highly oxidized forms may occur at higher pH values or result from microbial oxidation (5). Manganese can be adsorbed onto soil to an extent depending on the organic content and cation exchange capacity of the latter. It can bioaccumulate in lower but not higher organisms, so that biomagnification in food-chains is not significant (1).

## 13.20.2 Analytical methods

Atomic absorption spectrophotometry is used for determining manganese concentrations in microlitre samples (7). Inductively coupled argon-plasma optical emission spectrometry has a detection limit of around 2 µg/litre for manganese (8). Colorimetric methods are also used in water analysis and have detection limits of about 10 µg/litre (9).

## 13.20.3 Environmental levels and human exposure

### Air

Concentrations of manganese average 5 ng/m$^3$ in the ambient air of nonindustrialized areas and up to 33 ng/m$^3$ in industrialized areas. Source-dominated air levels may reach 0.13 µg/m$^3$ or above (5).

### Water

Manganese concentrations in lakes and rivers around the world range from 0.001 to about 0.6 mg/litre (6).[1] Higher levels in aerobic waters are usually associated with industrial pollution. Reducing conditions in groundwater and some lakes and reservoirs are conducive to high levels: up to 1.3 mg/litre in neutral water and 9.6 mg/litre in acidic water (5). In the USA, in a number of public drinking-water surveys, mean manganese levels ranging from 0.004 to 0.03 mg/litre were reported (1, 5). In Germany, the drinking-water supplied to 90% of all households contained less than 0.02 mg of manganese per litre (10).

### Food

Manganese was found in dairy products at levels of 0.02–0.5 mg/kg; levels in meats, fish, and eggs were in the range 0.1–4 mg/kg. Higher levels were found in

---

[1] Also based on data from the National Water Quality Data Bank (NAQUADAT), Ottawa, Environment Canada, Inland Waters Directorate, 1976.

vegetables (0.41–6.61 mg/kg), grains and cereals (0.41–41 mg/kg), and nuts (18–47 mg/kg). A cup of tea can contain 0.4–1.3 mg of manganese (*1*).

### *Estimated total exposure and relative contribution of drinking-water*

The greatest exposure to manganese is usually from food. Adults consume between 2 and 20 mg/day in the diet, the upper end of the range being associated with a vegetarian diet (*11,12*). The average daily manganese nutrient requirement for normal physiological function is estimated to be 2–5 mg for adults (*13*). Infants consume 2.5–25 µg/kg of body weight per day during the first 6 months of life (*6*).

Manganese intake from drinking-water is normally substantially lower than that from food. At typical drinking-water levels of 4–30 µg/litre, the intake of manganese would range from 8 to 60 µg/day for an adult. Other sources indicate that manganese intake from water can be an order of magnitude higher (*5*). Drinking mineral water regularly can add significantly to manganese intake (*14*). Exposure to manganese from air is generally several orders of magnitude lower than that from the diet, about 0.1–3 µg, depending on the distance from the source.

## 13.20.4 Kinetics and metabolism in laboratory animals and humans

Absorption of manganese across the gastrointestinal tract is regulated by normal physiological processes that maintain manganese homoeostasis. Typically, about 3–8% of an ingested dose is absorbed (*15*), but absorption may be greater for young animals and infants (*16*). The absorption of manganese is intimately linked to that of iron, iron-deficient diets leading to an increased absorption of both iron and manganese (*15*). Absorption is inversely related to the level of calcium in the diet (*11*) and directly related to that of potassium (*17*).

Manganese is present in all tissues of the body, the highest levels usually being found in the liver, kidney, pancreas, and adrenals (*18,19*). It accumulates preferentially in certain regions of the brain in young animals and infants (*20, 21*). Manganese can also be detected in human hair (*22*).

Manganese does not appear to be covalently linked to any organometallic compounds in the body. It may undergo changes in oxidation state (*23*). Manganese is a constituent of the enzymes pyruvate carboxylase and superoxide dismutase, is required as a cofactor in a number of enzyme systems, and plays a role in flavoprotein function and the synthesis of sulfated mucopolysaccharides, cholesterol, and haemoglobin (*24, 25*).

Manganese is almost entirely excreted in the faeces, only a small proportion (0.1–2%) being eliminated in the urine. In humans, elimination is biphasic, with half-lives of 13 and 34 days (*15, 26*).

## 13.20.5 Effects on laboratory animals and *in vitro* test systems

### Acute exposure

Oral LD$_{50}$s ranging from 400 to 830 mg/kg of body weight have been reported for different forms of manganese (*1*, *5*).

### Short-term exposure

The central nervous system is the chief target for manganese. Doses ranging from 1 to 150 mg/kg of body weight per day produced a number of neurological effects in rats and mice, mainly involving alterations in neurotransmitter and enzyme levels in the brain. These changes were sometimes accompanied by clinical signs, such as incoordination and changes in activity level (*1*). Increased turnover of striatal catecholamines may be responsible for hyperactivity in early manganese intoxication (*27*).

### Long-term exposure

Chronic ingestion of 1–2 mg of manganese per kg of body weight per day produced changes in appetite and reduction in haemoglobin synthesis in rabbits, pigs, and cattle (*25*). Transient effects on biogenic amine levels and activities of dopamine β-hydroxylase and monoamine oxidase in rat brain have been noted with long-term exposures to manganese (*28–30*). An increase in physical activity level and a transient increase in dopaminergic function were observed in rats given 40 mg/kg of body weight per day for 65 weeks (*31*). Weakness and rigidity were observed in monkeys given oral doses of 25 mg/kg of body weight per day for 18 months (*32*).

### Reproductive toxicity, embryotoxicity, and teratogenicity

Several studies in rats and mice indicate that the ingestion of manganese can delay reproductive maturation in male animals. Testosterone levels were reduced in male rats given an oral dose of 13 mg of manganese per kg of body weight per day for 100–224 days (*33*), while delayed growth of the testes was observed in young rats ingesting 140 mg of manganese per kg of body weight per day for 90 days (*34*). These effects do not appear to be severe enough to affect sperm morphology or male reproductive function (*33, 35, 36*). In rats chronic parenteral administration of manganese produced marked degenerative changes in the seminiferous tubules, resulting in infertility (*37*).

### Mutagenicity and related end-points

Manganese produced an increased frequency of mutations in *Salmonella typhimurium* strain TA1537, *Photobacterium fischeri*, and *Escherichia coli*, as well as in *Saccharomyces cerevisiae*, mouse lymphoma cells, and hamster embryo cells, in both cases without metabolic activation. In *in vivo* assays, manganese increased both the frequency of mutations in *Drosophila melanogaster* and the number of chromosomal aberrations in rat bone marrow and spermatogonial cells (*1*).

### Carcinogenicity

A 2-year oral study in rats and mice produced equivocal evidence of increased tumour incidence (*35, 36*). In male rats given oral manganese doses of 86, 290, or 930 mg/kg of body weight per day, the incidence of pancreatic cancer was slightly increased (4/50 for each dose, as compared with no tumours of this type in the control group) (*35*). Female mice given 810 mg/kg of body weight per day showed a small increase in pituitary adenomas, although the incidence of tumours of this type was within the range of historical control values (*36*).

Several studies in animals suggest that manganese may have an anticarcinogenic effect. It has been reported to inhibit the metabolic activation of aminoazodyes (*38*).

## 13.20.6 Effects on humans

Manganese is an essential element for many living organisms, including humans. Accordingly, adverse health effects can be caused by inadequate intake. Manganese-deficient animals exhibit impaired growth, skeletal abnormalities, reproductive deficits, ataxia of the newborn, and defects in lipid and carbohydrate metabolism (*5, 6, 25*). Although no specific manganese-deficiency syndrome has been described in humans, an association between manganese deficiency and disorders such as anaemia, bone changes in children, and lupus erythematosus has been suggested (*39*).

The neurological effects of inhaled manganese have been well documented in humans chronically exposed to elevated levels in the workplace. The syndrome known as "manganism" is characterized by weakness, anorexia, muscle pain, apathy, slow speech, monotonous tone of voice, emotionless "mask-like" facial expression, and slow clumsy movement of the limbs. In general, these effects are irreversible. The minimal exposure level producing neurological effects is not certain but is probably in the range 0.1–1 mg/m$^3$ (*1*).

By the oral route, manganese is often regarded as one of the least toxic elements, although there is some controversy as to whether the neurological effects observed with inhalation exposures also occur with oral ones.

In 1941, in an epidemiological study in Japan, adverse effects were seen in humans consuming manganese dissolved in drinking-water, probably at a concentration close to 28 mg/litre (*38*). The manganese was derived from 400 dry-cell batteries buried near a drinking-water well. A total of 16 cases of poisoning were reported, the symptoms including lethargy, increased muscle tone, tremor, and mental disturbances. The most severe effects were seen in elderly people, but only minor ones in children. The concentrations of other metals, especially zinc, were also excessive, and it was never unequivocally established whether manganese alone was responsible for the disease.

An epidemiological study was conducted in Greece to investigate the possible correlation between manganese exposure from water and neurological effects in elderly people (40). The levels of manganese were 3.6–14.6 µg/litre in the control area and 81–282 µg/litre and 1800–2300 µg/litre in the test areas. The authors concluded that progressive increases in the manganese concentration in drinking-water are associated with progressively higher prevalences of neurological signs of chronic manganese poisoning and higher manganese concentrations in the hair of older persons. However, no data were given on exposure from other sources such as food and dust, and little information was provided on nutritional status and other possible confounding variables.

In one area of Japan, a manganese concentration of 0.75 mg/litre in the drinking-water supply had no apparent adverse effects on the health of consumers (41). No signs of toxicity were observed in patients given 30 mg of manganese citrate (9 mg of manganese) per day for many months (11).

## 13.20.7 Provisional guideline value

The intake of manganese can be as high as 20 mg/day without apparent ill effects. With an intake of 12 mg/day, a 60-kg adult would receive 0.2 mg/kg of body weight per day. An uncertainty factor of 3 is applied to allow for the possible increased bioavailability of manganese from water, and 20% of the intake is allocated to water. This gives a value of 0.4 mg/litre.

Although no single study is suitable for use in calculating a guideline value, the weight of evidence from actual daily intake and from studies in laboratory animals given drinking-water in which neurotoxic and other effects were observed supports the view that a provisional health-based guideline value of 0.5 mg/litre should be adequate to protect public health.

It should be noted that manganese may be objectionable to consumers if it is deposited in water mains and causes water discoloration. Although concentrations below 0.1 mg/litre are usually acceptable to consumers, this may vary with local circumstances.

## References

1. Agency for Toxic Substances and Disease Registry. *Toxicological profile for manganese*. Atlanta, GA, US Department of Health and Human Services, 1992.

2. Griffin AE. Significance and removal of manganese in water supplies. *Journal of the American Water Works Association*, 1960, 52:1326.

3. Bean EL. Potable water—quality goals. *Journal of the American Water Works Association*, 1974, 66:221.

4. Wolfe RS. Microbial concentration of iron and manganese in water with low concentrations of these elements. *Journal of the American Water Works Association*, 1960, 52:1335.

5. Environmental Criteria and Assessment Office. *Health assessment document for manganese.* Cincinnati, OH, US Environmental Protection Agency, 1984 (EPA-600/8-83-013F).

6. *Manganese.* Geneva, World Health Organization, 1981 (Environmental Health Criteria, No. 17).

7. Slavin S, Barnett WB, Kahn HL. The determination of atomic absorption detection limits by direct measurement. *Atomic absorption news letter*, 1972, 11:37-41.

8. Inductively coupled plasma-atomic emission spectrometric method for trace element analysis of water and wastes. Method 200.7. *Code of federal regulations* (Appendix C to Part 136), 1987:512-523.

9. International Organization for Standardization. *Water quality—determination of manganese.* Geneva, 1986 (ISO 6333:1986).

10. *Umwelt-Survey,* Vol. IIIb. [*Environment survey.*] Berlin, Bundesgesundheitsamt, 1991 (WaBoLu-Heft No. 3/1991).

11. Schroeder HA, Balassa JJ, Tipton IH. Essential trace metals in man: manganese. A study in homeostasis. *Journal of chronic diseases*, 1966, 19:545-571.

12. Pennington JAT et al. Mineral content of foods and total diets: the selected minerals in foods survey, 1982 to 1984. *Journal of the American Dietetic Association*, 1986, 86:876-891.

13. National Academy of Sciences. *Recommended dietary allowances*, 10th ed. Washington, DC, National Academy Press, 1989.

14. Dieter HH et al. Manganese in natural mineral waters from Germany. *Die Nahrung-Food*, 1992, 36:476-483.

15. Sandstrom B et al. Manganese absorption and metabolism in man. *Acta pharmacologia toxicologia*, 1986, 59(Suppl.):60-62.

16. Keen CL, Bell JG, Lonnerdal B. The effect of age on manganese uptake and retention from milk and infant formulas in rats. *Journal of nutrition*, 1986, 116:395-402.

17. Office of Research and Development. *Scientific and technical assessment report on manganese.* Washington, DC, US Environmental Protection Agency, 1975 (EPA-600/6-75-002).

18. Tipton IH, Cook MJ. Trace elements in human tissue. Part II. Adult subjects from the United States. *Health physics*, 1963, 9:103-145.

19. Sumino K et al. Heavy metals in normal Japanese tissues: amounts of 15 heavy metals in 30 subjects. *Archives of environmental health*, 1975, 30:487-494.

20. Kontur PJ, Fechtur LD. Brain regional manganese levels and monoamine metabolism in manganese-treated neonatal rats. *Neurotoxicology and teratology*, 1988, 10:295-303.

21. Zlotkin SH, Buchanan BE. Manganese intakes in intravenously fed infants. *Biological trace element research*, 1986, 9:271-279.

22. Fergusson JE, Holzbecher J, Ryan DE. The sorption of copper(II), manganese(II), zinc(II) and arsenic(III) onto human hair and their desorption. *Science of the total environment*, 1983, 26:121-135.

23. Gibbons RA et al. Manganese metabolism in cows and goats. *Biochimica biophysica acta*, 1976, 444:1-10.

24. National Research Council. *Manganese*. Washington, DC, National Academy of Sciences, Committee on Medical and Biological Effects of Environmental Pollutants, 1973.

25. Hurley LS, Keen CL. Manganese. In: Mertz N, ed. *Trace elements in human and animal nutrition*, Vol. 1. 5th ed. New York, NY, Academic Press, 1987:185-223.

26. *Recommended health-based limits on occupational exposure to heavy metals: report of a WHO Study Group*. Geneva, World Health Organization, 1980 (WHO Technical Report Series, No. 647).

27. Chandra SV. Psychiatric illness due to manganese poisoning. *Acta psychiatrica Scandinavica*, 1983, 303 (Suppl.):49-54.

28. Eriksson H, Lenngren S, Heilbronn E. Effect of long-term administration of manganese on biogenic amine levels in discrete striatal regions of rat brain. *Archives of toxicology*, 1987, 59:426-431.

29. Lai JC, Leung TK, Lim L. Differences in the neurotoxic effects of manganese during development and aging: some observations on brain regional neurotransmitter and non-neurotransmitter metabolism in a developmental rat model of chronic manganese encephalopathy. *Neurotoxicology*, 1984, 5:37-47.

30. Subhash MN, Padmashree TS. Regional distribution of dopamine $\beta$-hydroxylase and monoamine oxidase in the brains of rats exposed to manganese. *Food chemistry and toxicology*, 1990, 28:567-570.

31. Nachtman JP, Tubben RE, Conmissaris RL. Behavioral effects of chronic manganese administration in rats: locomotor activity studies. *Neurobehavioral toxicology and teratology*, 1986, 8:711-715.

32. Gupta SK, Murthy RC, Chandra SV. Neuromelanin in manganese-exposed primates. *Toxicology letters*, 1980, 6:17-20.

33. Laskey JW et al. Effects of chronic manganese ($Mn_3O_4$) exposure on selected reproductive parameters in rats. *Journal of toxicology and environmental health*, 1982, 9:677-687.

34. Gray LE, Laskey JW. Multivariate analysis of the effects of manganese on the reproductive physiology and behavior of the male house mouse. *Toxicology and environmental health*, 1980, 6:861-867.

35. Hejtmancik M et al. *The chronic study of manganese sulfate monohydrate (CAS no. 10034-96-5) in F344 rats.* Research Triangle Park, NC, National Toxicology Program, 1987.

36. Hejtmancik M et al. *The chronic study of manganese sulfate monohydrate (CAS no. 10034-96-5) in B6C3F$_1$ mice.* Research Triangle Park, NC, National Toxicology Program, 1987.

37. Chandra SV, Tandon SK. Enhanced manganese toxicity in iron-deficient rats. *Environmental physiology and biochemistry*, 1973, 3:230-235.

38. Kawamura R et al. Intoxication by manganese in well water. *Kitasato archives of experimental medicine*, 1941, 18:145-171.

39. Pier SM. The role of heavy metals in human health. *Texas reports on biology and medicine*, 1975, 33:85-106.

40. Kondakis XG et al. Possible health effects of high manganese concentration in drinking water. *Environmental health perspectives*, 1989, 44(3):175-178.

41. Suzuki Y. Environmental contamination by manganese. *Japanese journal of industrial health*, 1970, 12:529-533.

## 13.21 Mercury

### 13.21.1 General description

#### Physicochemical properties

| Property | Value |
|---|---|
| Physical state | Dense, silvery-white metal; liquid at normal temperatures and pressures |
| Vapour pressure | 0.16 Pa at 20 °C |
| Stability | Carbon–mercury bond in organic mercury compounds is chemically stable |

#### Major uses

Mercury is used for the cathode in the electrolytic production of chlorine and caustic soda, in electrical appliances (lamps, arc rectifiers, mercury cells), in industrial and control instruments (switches, thermometers, barometers), in laboratory apparatus, in dental amalgams, and as a raw material for various mercury compounds. The latter are used as fungicides, antiseptics, preservatives, pharmaceuticals, electrodes, and reagents.

#### Environmental fate

The solubility of mercury compounds in water varies: elemental mercury vapour is insoluble, mercury(II) chloride is readily soluble, mercury(I) chloride much less soluble, and mercury sulfide has a very low solubility.

Methylation of inorganic mercury has been shown to occur in columns of fresh water and in seawater (1), and bacteria (*Pseudomonas* spp.) isolated from mucous material on the surface of fish and soil were able to methylate mercury under aerobic conditions. Some anaerobic bacteria that possess methane synthetase are also capable of mercury methylation (2). Once methylmercury[1] is released from microbes, it enters the food chain as a consequence of rapid diffusion and tight binding to proteins in aquatic biota. The enzymology of $CH_3Hg^+$ hydrolysis and mercury(II) ion reduction is now understood in some detail. Environmental levels of methylmercury depend on the balance between bacterial methylation and demethylation (3).

---

[1] The generic term "methylmercury" is used throughout this text to refer to monomethylmercury compounds.

## 13.21.2 Analytical methods

Inorganic mercury is determined by flameless atomic absorption spectrometry (4). Cold vapour atomic absorption spectrometry and atomic fluorescence spectrometry have detection limits of 50 and 1 ng/litre, respectively.

Gas chromatography is commonly used for the determination of alkyl-mercury compounds. The neutron activation procedure is regarded as the most accurate and is generally used as the reference method (3).

## 13.21.3 Environmental levels and human exposure

### Air

Mercury levels in air are in the range 2–10 ng/m$^3$.

### Water

Inorganic mercury

Levels of mercury in rainwater are in the range 5–100 ng/litre, but mean levels as low as 1 ng/litre have been reported (3). Naturally occurring levels of mercury in groundwater and surface water are less than 0.5 µg/litre, although local mineral deposits may produce higher levels in groundwater. In 16 groundwaters and 16 shallow wells surveyed in the USA, mercury levels exceeded the maximum contaminant level of 2 µg/litre set by the US Environmental Protection Agency for drinking-water (5). An increase in the mercury concentration up to 5.5 µg/litre was reported for wells in Izu Oshima Island (Japan), where volcanic activity is frequent (6). The concentration range for mercury in drinking-water is the same as in rain, with an average of about 25 ng/litre (3).

Organic mercury

In a contaminated lake system in Canada, methylmercury was found to constitute a varying proportion of total mercury, depending on the lake (3). There have been no reports of methylmercury in drinking-water.

### Food

Food is the main source of mercury in non-occupationally exposed populations. Fish and fish products account for most of the organic mercury in food. The average daily intake of mercury from food is in the range 2–20 µg/day, but may be much higher in regions where ambient waters have become contaminated with mercury and where fish constitute a high proportion of the diet (7).

### Estimated total exposure and relative contribution of drinking-water

On the assumption of an ambient air level of 10 ng/m$^3$, the average daily intake of inorganic mercury by inhalation would amount to about 0.2 µg. If a level in drinking-water of 0.5 µg/litre is assumed, the average daily intake of inorganic mercury from this source would amount to about 1 µg. The average daily intake of mercury from food is in the range 2–20 µg/day.

## 13.21.4 Kinetics and metabolism in laboratory animals and humans

### Inorganic mercury

About 7–8% of ingested inorganic mercury in food is absorbed; absorption from water may be 15% or less, depending on the compound. About 80% of inhaled metallic mercury vapour is retained by the body, whereas liquid metallic mercury is poorly absorbed via the gastrointestinal tract. Inhaled aerosols of inorganic mercury are deposited in the respiratory tract and absorbed to an extent depending on particle size (8).

Inorganic mercury compounds are rapidly accumulated in the kidney, the main target organ for these compounds. The biological half-time is very long, probably years, in both animals and humans. Mercury salts are excreted via the kidney, liver, intestinal mucosa, sweat glands, and salivary glands, and milk; the most important routes are via the urine and faeces (8).

### Organic mercury

Dimethylmercury is almost completely absorbed through the gastrointestinal tract; after absorption it rapidly appears in the blood where, in humans, 80–90% is bound to red cells. Demethylation of methylmercury to inorganic mercury occurs at a slow but significant rate. The greater intrinsic toxicity of methylmercury as compared with inorganic mercury is due to its lipid solubility, which enables it to cross biological membranes more easily, and especially to enter the brain, spinal cord, and peripheral nerves, and to cross the placenta (3).

Most methylmercury is excreted in the inorganic form. The site and mechanism of demethylation are still not well understood (3).

## 13.21.5 Effects on laboratory animals and in vitro test systems

### Inorganic mercury

Short-term exposure

The toxic effects of inorganic mercury compounds are seen mainly in the kidney. Lesions in the proximal tubular cells were detected after a single intraperitoneal injection of 1 µmol of mercury(II) chloride per kg of body weight (0.2 mg/kg of body weight as mercury) in male rats. Accumulation of mercury in the kidneys, however, indicated that the absorption efficiency was much greater than that expected from the gastrointestinal tract (9).

When rats were given mercury(II) chloride (3 mg/kg of body weight) by gavage twice a week for 60 days, examination by immunofluorescence showed that deposits for IgC were present in the renal glomeruli. Morphological lesions of the ileum and colon were also observed, with abnormal deposits of IgA in the basement membranes of the intestinal glands and of IgG in the basement membranes of the lamina propria (10).

When rats were exposed to mercury(II) chloride (1 mg/kg of body weight per day) by intubation or subcutaneous injection for up to 11 weeks, the rate of body weight gain decreased after 20 days, and actual weight loss occurred after 65–70 days. There were also neuropathological effects, first detected after 2 weeks, namely peripheral vacuolization of cells in the dorsal root ganglia, followed by the development of multiple small lesions in the ganglia (11).

A single dose of 1 mg/kg of body weight of mercury(II) chloride or methylmercury(II) chloride, either orally or by subcutaneous injection, resulted in leakage of dye into the nervous parenchyma within 12 h, indicating that these compounds can increase the permeability of the blood–brain barrier (11).

## Long-term exposure

Rats injected subcutaneously 3 times weekly for up to 8 months with doses of inorganic mercury ranging from 0.05 to 2.5 mg/kg of body weight per injection (0.02–1.07 mg/kg of body weight per day) developed renal damage. This was characterized by an initial production of antiglomerular basement membrane antibodies, followed by the appearance of immune complex deposits in the glomerular tufts and small renal arteries accompanied by proteinuria and hypoalbuminaemia (12).

## Reproductive toxicity, embryotoxicity, and teratogenicity

Controlled mating tests in which male mice were injected with single doses of mercury(II) chloride (1 mg of mercury per kg of body weight) showed a significant decrease in fertility as compared with controls (13). Normal fertility was restored after about 2 months.

Gradual changes in testicular tissues were noted in rats treated with mercury(II) chloride at doses of 0.05 or 0.1 mg/kg of body weight intraperitoneally over 90 days (14). There was a decrease in seminiferous tubule diameter, spermatogenic cell counts, and Leydig's cell nuclear diameter as compared with controls.

Of female hamsters given a total of 3–4 mg of mercuric chloride during the first estrous cycle, 60% did not ovulate by day 1 of the third cycle (15). Ovulation was inhibited in female hamsters injected with mercury(II) chloride at high doses (6.4 or 12.8 mg of mercury per kg of body weight) during day 1 of the estrous cycle (16). Female hamsters injected with 1 mg of mercury(II) chloride per day during one estrous cycle exhibited significantly higher levels of follicle-stimulating hormone in their pituitaries as compared with controls (17).

Pregnant Wistar rats were exposed intravenously to mercury(II) chloride on different days of gestation. At mid-gestation, the minimum effective teratogenic dose of mercury (0.79 mg/kg of body weight) was high in relation to the maternal $LD_{50}$, and the incidence of fetal malformations, mainly brain defects, was 23% in all live fetuses. In rats of different gestational ages, uptake of $Hg^{2+}$ by the fetuses at this dose level decreased sharply between days 12 and 13 (18).

## Organic mercury

### Short-term exposure

In rats fed methylmercury dicyandiamide 5 days per week for 59 days, extensive damage to the renal cortex occurred with extensive inflammatory reaction surrounding the tubules and some early fibrosis even at the lowest dose of 0.6 mg/kg of body weight per day (19). Tubular degeneration of the kidney was also evident after subcutaneous injection of 10 mg/kg of body weight per day into rats for 7 consecutive days (20). In contrast to the effects of high doses of methylmercury on rats, kidney damage was not reported in cats exposed to 0.45 mg/kg of body weight (21) or in monkeys exposed to either 0.05 mg/kg of body weight per day (22) or to doses resulting in blood levels of up to 4 µg of mercury per ml of blood (23).

In cats, convulsions occurred after 60–83 days of exposure to 0.45 mg of methylmercury per kg of body weight per day; they were preceded 4–11 days earlier by progressive behavioural changes. Kittens were fed commercially available tuna contaminated with 0.3–0.5 mg of methylmercury(II) chloride per kg for 11 months. The total mercury intake over the period averaged 6.3 mg per cat or about 19 µg/day. Neurological disturbances were observed in three kittens after 7–11 months (24).

Squirrel monkeys were exposed for periods of up to 35 days to repeated oral doses of methylmercury(II) nitrate mixed with food or by stomach tube. The threshold for both behavioural and central nervous system pathology occurred at blood mercury concentrations in the range 0.75–1.2 mg/litre (25).

### Long-term exposure

In a study in which cats were fed methylmercury(II) chloride in a fish diet at doses of 0.003, 0.008, 0.020, 0.046, 0.074, or 0.176 mg/kg of body weight per day, 7 days a week for 2 years, detectable neurological impairment occurred in the group given 0.046 mg/kg of body weight per day after 60 weeks; this concentration was the lowest at which such impairment occurred. Pathological changes in the nervous system were restricted to the brain and dorsal root ganglia and were not seen at doses below 0.074 mg/kg of body weight per day (26).

Stumptail, pigtail, and squirrel monkeys were given methylmercury(II) chloride in food for periods in excess of 1000 days. This dosage regime was designed to maintain the blood mercury level at 1–4 mg/litre of blood. The critical effects seen were reduced sensitivity to visual stimuli at low luminescence and tremor on reaching for a small object. All monkeys with a blood concentration above 2 mg/litre developed symptoms with latent periods ranging from less then 20 to 200 days (23).

Cynomolgus monkeys were fed methylmercury from birth at doses of 0.05 mg/kg of body weight per day for 3–4 years. Blood concentrations of mercury peaked at 1.2–1.4 mg/litre, then declined after weaning to a steady level of 0.6–0.9 mg/litre. No overt signs of toxicity were noted but, when tested after 3–4 years, the monkeys exhibited impaired spatial vision under conditions of both high and low luminescence (22).

## Reproductive toxicity, embryotoxicity, and teratogenicity

Mice were given single doses of 3.6, 5.3, 8, 12, 18, or 27 mg of methyl-mercury(II) chloride per kg of body weight at 9.5, 12.5, or 15.5 days post-fertilization (27). The trend among $F_1$ females towards an adverse effect of dose on litter size, although not statistically significant, was in the direction to be expected if methylmercury(II) chloride can affect oogenesis in females exposed during fetal life.

A single dose of 2, 3, or 4 mg of mercury(II) ethanoate (about 1.3–2.5 mg of mercury) was injected intravenously in three groups of female hamsters on day 8 of gestation (28). The exposed groups showed resorption frequencies of 12, 34, and 52%, respectively, as compared with 4% in the controls.

High doses of methylmercury given to pregnant rodents produced cleft palate (29, 30). Prenatal exposure of rats can produce renal functional abnormalities detectable in offspring at 42 days of age (31).

Female rats were injected with 0, 6, or 10 mg of methylmercury(II) chloride per kg of body weight on gestational days 6–9 (32). Dams given 10 mg/kg of body weight either failed to give birth or the young were stillborn. External morphology was normal in rats given either of the two lower doses. Methylmercury produced hydrocephalus, decreased thickness of the cerebral cortex in the parietal section, and increased thickness of the hippocampus in the occipital section; with these exceptions, the brains of mercury-treated rats showed normal development.

Hamsters were given either 10 mg of methylmercury per kg of body weight on gestational day 10 or 2 mg/kg on gestational days 10–15 (33, 34). In the neonatal cerebellar cortex, degenerative changes such as accumulation of lysosomes and areas of floccular cytoplasmic degradation were frequently observed in the neuroblast granular layer as well as in more differentiated neural elements in the molecular and internal granular layers. Pyknotic nuclei were seen singly and in groups throughout the external granular layer of treated animals. In the adult cerebellum, focal areas of astrogliosis were observed in the molecular layer of treated animals.

## Mutagenicity and related end-points

Animal and cell culture studies confirm that methylmercury damages chromosomes if given orally at a dose of 5 mg/kg of body weight to pregnant mice

(*16, 35*), intraperitoneally at 2 mg/kg of body weight daily for 3 weeks to adult hamsters (*36*), and intraperitoneally at 10 mg/kg of body weight to ovulating Syrian hamsters (*37*). Methylmercury at low concentrations (0.05–0.1 μmol/litre) has been reported to interfere with gene expression in *in vitro* cultures of glioma cells (*38*). Non-disjunction and sex-linked recessive lethal mutations were induced in *Drosophila melanogaster* by treatment with methylmercury (*39*).

Carcinogenicity
Groups of mice were fed 15 or 30 mg of methylmercury per kg of diet for up to 78 weeks. The majority of the 30 mg/kg group died from neurotoxicity by week 26. Histopathological examination of kidney tissue from all animals surviving after 53 weeks revealed renal tumours in 13 of 16 males in the 15 mg/kg group. Of these, 11 were classified as adenocarcinomas and two as adenomas (*40*).

## 13.21.6 Effects on humans

### *Inorganic mercury*

Acute exposure
Mercury will cause severe disruption of any tissue with which it comes into contact in sufficient concentration, but the two main effects of mercury poisoning are neurological and renal disturbances. The former is characteristic of poisoning by methyl- and ethylmercury(II) salts, in which liver and renal damage are of relatively little significance, the latter of poisoning by inorganic mercury.

In general, however, the ingestion of acute lethal toxic doses of any form of mercury will result in the same terminal signs and symptoms, namely shock, cardiovascular collapse, acute renal failure, and severe gastrointestinal damage. Acute oral poisoning results primarily in haemorrhagic gastritis and colitis; the ultimate damage is to the kidney. Clinical symptoms of acute intoxication include pharyngitis, dysphagia, abdominal pain, nausea and vomiting, bloody diarrhoea, and shock. Later, swelling of the salivary glands, stomatitis, loosening of the teeth, nephritis, anuria, and hepatitis occur (*41*).

Ingestion of 500 mg of mercury(II) chloride causes severe poisoning and sometimes death in humans (*42*). Acute effects result from the inhalation of air containing mercury vapour at concentrations in the range 0.05–0.35 mg/m$^3$ (*43, 44*). Exposure for a few hours to 1–3 mg/m$^3$ may give rise to pulmonary irritation and destruction of lung tissue and occasionally to central nervous systems disorders (*45*).

Dermal exposure to alkyl mercurials may give rise to acute toxic dermatitis and eczematous changes.

Long-term exposure
Many studies involving the observation of more than 1000 individuals indicate that the classical signs and symptoms of elemental mercury vapour poisoning (objective tremors, mental disturbances, and gingivitis) may be expected to

appear after chronic exposure to air mercury concentrations above 0.1 mg/m$^3$ (8). Nonspecific neurological and physiological symptoms were also associated with lower exposure levels.

Considerable mercury exposure of children of workers at a thermometer plant has been reported (46). The median urine mercury level of 23 such children was 25 µg/litre as compared with 5 µg/litre in 39 controls. No signs of mercury intoxication were seen on clinical examination or reported by parents (3).

## Organic mercury

The adverse health effects of occupational exposure to alkylmercury compounds constitute what is known as the Hunter-Russel syndrome (concentric constriction of the visual field, ataxia, dysarthria, etc.); this was seen in four workers exposed to methylmercury fungicide (47).

Methyl- and ethylmercury compounds have been the cause of the largest number of cases of mercury poisoning and of fatalities in the general population as a result of the consumption of contaminated fish or of bread prepared from cereals treated with alkylmercury fungicides. The earliest effects are nonspecific, e.g. paraesthesia, malaise, and blurred vision. These are followed by concentric constriction of the visual field, deafness, dysarthria, and ataxia. In the worst cases, the patient may go into coma and ultimately die. At high doses, methylmercury affects the peripheral nervous system in human subjects (48).

The two major epidemics of methylmercury poisoning in Japan, in Minamata Bay and in Niigata, both known as Minamata disease, were caused by the industrial release of methylmercury and other mercury compounds into Minamata Bay and into the Agano River, followed by accumulation of the mercury in edible fish. The maximum blood level of methylmercury without adverse health effects was estimated to be 0.33 µg/ml based on the epidemiological study of the Minamata disease endemic area (49). By 1971, a total of 269 cases of Minamata disease had been reported in Minamata and Niigata, of which 55 proved fatal. By March 1989, 2217 cases of Minamata disease had been officially recognized in Minamata and 911 cases in Niigata (50).

The largest recorded epidemic caused by the ingestion of contaminated bread prepared from wheat and other cereals treated with alkyl (methyl- or ethyl-) mercury fungicides took place in the winter of 1971–72 in Iraq, and resulted in the admission of over 6000 patients to hospital and over 500 deaths (51). Previous epidemics have occurred in Guatemala, Iraq, and Pakistan, and on a limited scale in other countries (3, 8, 52).

The Cree Indians of northern Quebec were also known to be exposed to methylmercury through the consumption of contaminated local fish. The relationship between measures of exposure and neurological abnormalities was studied in two communities. A positive association was found between neurological abnormalities and methylmercury exposure in both communities, but the relationship was statistically significant only in one of them (53, 54).

The first indication of possible congenital Minamata disease was the unusual occurrence of cerebral palsy-like conditions in nine infants in the endemic areas (population about 1700) during 21 months. These infants had severe cerebral involvement (palsy and mental retardation); mild or no symptoms of poisoning were seen in their mothers, although there is a possibility that slight symptoms might have been overlooked (*3*).

According to an epidemiological study of an outbreak in Iraq, the clinical picture was dose-dependent. In those who were exposed to high maternal blood levels of methylmercury, the picture was one of cerebral palsy indistinguishable from that resulting from other causes (microcephaly, hyper-reflexia, and gross motor and mental impairment, associated with blindness or deafness). Milder forms were not easy to diagnose during the first few months of life, but became clearer with time. The cases showed mainly psychomotor impairment and persistence of pathological reflexes (*53*, *55–57*). The relationship between prenatal exposure to methylmercury and neurological and developmental abnormalities was also studied. Abnormality of the tendon reflex was positively associated with methylmercury exposure only in boys, without a dose–response relationship (*58*). Findings in the milder cases were quite similar to those associated with the minimal brain syndrome (*3*).

Marsh et al. (*59*) demonstrated a dose–response relationship between the deteriorated neurological score in children and the maximum mercury concentration during gestation in a single strand of maternal head hair.

## 13.21.7 Guideline value

Almost all mercury in uncontaminated drinking-water is thought to be in the form of $Hg^{2+}$. Thus, it is unlikely that there is any direct risk of the intake of organic mercury compounds, and especially of alkylmercurials, as a result of the ingestion of drinking-water. However, there is a real possibility that methylmercury will be converted into inorganic mercury.

In 1972, JECFA established a provisional tolerable weekly intake (PTWI) of 5 µg/kg of body weight of total mercury, of which no more than 3.3 µg/kg of body weight should be present as methylmercury (*60*). This PTWI was reaffirmed in 1978 (*61*). In 1988, JECFA reassessed methylmercury, as new data had become available; it confirmed the previously recommended PTWI for the general population, but noted that pregnant women and nursing mothers were likely to be at greater risk from the adverse effects of methylmercury. The available data were considered insufficient, however, to allow a specific methylmercury intake to be recommended for this population group (*62*, *63*).

To be on the conservative side, the PTWI for methylmercury was used to derive a guideline value for inorganic mercury in drinking-water. As the main exposure is from food, 10% of the PTWI was allocated to drinking-water. The guideline value for total mercury is 0.001 mg/litre (rounded figure).

# References

1. *Mercury—environmental aspects.* Geneva, World Health Organization, 1989 (Environmental Health Criteria, No. 86).

2. Wood JM, Wang HK. Microbial resistance to heavy metals. *Environmental science and technology*, 1983, 17:82a-90a.

3. *Methylmercury.* Geneva, World Health Organization, 1990 (Environmental Health Criteria, No. 101).

4. International Organization for Standardization. *Water quality—determination of total mercury by flameless atomic absorption spectrometry.* Geneva, 1983, 1984 (ISO 5666-1,2:1983; -3:1984).

5. Ware GW, ed. Mercury. USEPA Office of Drinking Water health advisories. *Reviews of environmental contamination and toxicology*, 1989, 107:93-102.

6. Magara Y et al. Effects of volcanic activity on heavy metal concentration in deep well water. In: *Technical Papers Water Nagoya '89; 7th Regional Conference and Exhibition of Asia-Pacific.* International Water Supply Association, 1989:411-419.

7. Galal-Gorchev H. Dietary intake of pesticide residues, cadmium, mercury, and lead. *Food additives and contaminants*, 1991, 8:793-806.

8. *Inorganic mercury.* Geneva, World Health Organization, 1991 (Environmental Health Criteria, No. 118).

9. Miura K, Mori R, Imura N. Effects of selenium on mercury-induced renal lesions and on subcellular mercury distribution. *Ecotoxicology and environmental safety*, 1981, 5:351-367.

10. Andres P. IgA-IgG disease in the intestine of brown Norway rats ingesting mercuric chloride. *Clinical immunology and immunopathology*, 1984, 30:488-494.

11. Chang L, Hartmann HA. Blood–brain barrier dysfunction in experimental mercury intoxication. *Acta neuropathologica*, 1972, 21:179-184.

12. Makker SP, Aikawa M. Mesangial glomerulonephropathy with deposition of IgG, IgM and C3 induced by mercuric chloride. A new model. *Laboratory investigation*, 1979, 41:45-50.

13. Lee IP, Dixon RL. Effects of mercury on spermatogenesis studied by velocity sedimentation cell separation and serial mating. *Journal of pharmacology and experimental therapeutics*, 1975, 194:171-181.

14. Chowdhury AR et al. Histomorphometric and biochemical changes in the testicular tissues of rats treated with mercuric chloride. *Biomedica biochimica acta*, 1986, 45:949-956.

15. Lamperti AA, Printz RH. Localization, accumulation, and toxic effects of mercuric chloride on the reproductive axis of the female hamster. *Biology of reproduction*, 1974, 11:180-186.

16. Watanabe T, Shimada T, Endo A. Effects of mercury compounds on ovulation and meiotic and mitotic chromosomes in female golden hamster. *Teratology*, 1982, 25:381-384.

17. Lamperti A, Niewenhuis R. The effects of mercury on the structure and function of the hypothalamo-pituitary axis in the hamster. *Cell and tissue research*, 1976, 170: 315-324.

18. Holt D, Webb M. The toxicity and teratogenicity of mercuric mercury in the pregnant rat. *Archives of toxicology*, 1986, 58:243-248.

19. Magos L et al. Tissue levels of mercury in autopsy specimens of liver and kidney. *Bulletin of the World Health Organization*, 1976, 53(Suppl.):93-96.

20. Klein R et al. A model of acute methyl mercury intoxication in rats. *Archives of pathology*, 1972, 93:408-418.

21. Chang LW et al. Neurological changes in cats following long-term diet of mercury contaminated tuna. *Acta neuropathologica (Berlin)*, 1974, 27:171-176.

22. Rice DC, Gilbert SG. Early chronic low-level methyl mercury poisoning in monkeys impairs spatial vision. *Science*, 1982, 216:759-761.

23. Evans HL, Garman RH, Weiss B. Methylmercury: exposure duration and regional distribution as determinants of neurotoxicity in non-human primates. *Toxicology and applied pharmacology*, 1977, 41:15-33.

24. Albaus L et al. Toxicity for cats of methyl mercury in contaminated fish from Swedish lakes and of methyl mercury hydroxide added to fish. *Environmental research*, 1972, 5:425-442.

25. Berlin MH, Nordberg G, Hellberg J. The uptake and distribution of methyl mercury in the brain of *Saimari sciuresus* in relation to behavioral and morphological changes. In: Miller MW, Clarkson TW, eds. *Mercury, mercurials and mercaptans*. Springfield, IL, Charles C. Thomas, 1973:187-205.

26. Charbonneau SM et al. Chronic toxicity of methyl mercury in the adult cat. Interim report. *Toxicology*, 1976, 5:337-349.

27. Gates AH, Doherty RA, Cox C. Reproduction and growth following prenatal methylmercuric chloride exposure in mice. *Fundamental and applied toxicology*, 1986, 7:486-493.

28. Gale TF, Ferm VH. Embryopathic effects of mercuric salts. *Life sciences*, 1971, 10:1341-1347.

29. Lee M et al. Effect of sodium selenite on methylmercury-induced cleft palate in the mouse. *Environmental research*, 1979, 19:39-48.

30. Harper K, Burns R, Erickson RP. Genetic aspects of the effects of methylmercury in mice: the incidence of cleft palate and concentrations of adenosine 3':5' cyclic monophosphate in tongue and palatal shelf. *Teratology*, 1981, 23:397-401.

31. Smith MA. The effect of heavy metals on the cytoplasmic fine structure of *Skeletonema costatum* (Bacillariophyta). *Protoplasma*, 1983, 116:14-23.

32. Kutscher CL et al. Effects of the high methylmercury dose used in the collaborative behavioral teratology study on brain anatomy. *Neurobehavioral toxicology and teratology*, 1985, 7:775-777.

33. Reuhl KR, Chang LW, Townsend JW. Pathological effects of *in utero* methylmercury exposure on the cerebellum of the golden hamster. I. Early effects upon the neonatal cerebellar cortex. *Environmental research*, 1981, 26:281-306.

34. Reuhl KR, Chang LW, Townsend JW. Pathological effects of *in utero* methylmercury exposure on the cerebellum of the golden hamster. II. Residual effects on the adult cerebellum. *Environmental research*, 1981, 26:307-327.

35. Curle DC et al. Methylmercury toxicity: *in vivo* evaluation of teratogenesis and cytogenic changes. *Anatomischer Anzeiger (Jena)*, 1983, 153:69-82.

36. Gilbert MM et al. Protective effect of vitamin E on genotoxicity of methylmercury. *Journal of toxicology and environmental health*, 1983, 12:767-773.

37. Mailhes JB. Methylmercury effects on Syrian hamster metaphase II oocyte chromosomes. *Environmental mutagenesis*, 1983, 5:679-686.

38. Ramanujam M, Prasad KM. Alterations in gene expression after chronic treatment of glioma cells in culture with methylmercuric chloride. *Biochemical pharmacology*, 1979, 28:2979-2984.

39. Magnusson J, Ramel G. Genetic variation in the susceptibility to mercury and other metal compounds in *Drosophila melanogaster*. *Teratogenesis, carcinogenesis, and mutagenesis*, 1986, 6:4.

40. Mitsumori K et al. Carcinogenicity of methylmercury chloride in ICR mice: preliminary note on renal carcinogens. *Cancer letters*, 1981, 12:305-310.

41. Stockinger HE. The metals. In: Clayton GD, Clayton FE, eds. *Patty's industrial hygiene and toxicology,* Vol. 2A, 3rd ed. New York, NY, John Wiley & Sons, 1981: 1769-1792.

42. Bidstrup FL. *Toxicity of mercury and its compounds.* Amsterdam, Elsevier, 1964.

43. Nielsen-Kudsk F. Absorption of mercury vapour from the respiratory tract in man. *Acta pharmacologica,* 1972, 23:250.

44. Teisinger J, Fiserova-Bergerova V. Pulmonary retention and excretion of mercury vapours in man. *Industrial medicine and surgery,* 1965, 34:580.

45. Skerfving S, Vostal J. Symptoms and signs of intoxication. In: Friberg L, Vostal J, eds. *Mercury in the environment.* Cleveland, OH, CRC Press, 1972:93.

46. Hudson PJ et al. Elemental mercury exposure among children of thermometer plant workers. *Pediatrics,* 1987, 79:935-938.

47. Hunter D, Russel DS. Focal cerebral and cerebellar atrophy in a human subject to dose of organic mercury compounds. *Journal of neurology, neurosurgery and psychiatry,* 1954, 17:235-241.

48. Rustam H et al. Evidence for a neuromuscular disorder in methylmercury poisoning. *Archives of environmental health,* 1975, 30:190-195.

49. Kitamura M. [Methylmercury accumulation in human tissues.] *Advances in neurological sciences,* 1974, 18:825-834 (in Japanese).

50. Japan Environmental Agency. *Quality of the environment in Japan–1989.* Tokyo, 1989:242-243.

51. Bakir F et al. Methylmercury poisoning in Iraq. *Science,* 1973, 181:230-241.

52. Greenwood MR. Methylmercury poisoning in Iraq. An epidemiological study of the 1971-1972 outbreak. *Journal of applied toxicology,* 1985, 5:148-159.

53. McKeown-Eyssen GE, Ruedy J, Neims A. Methylmercury exposure in northern Quebec. I. Neurologic findings in adults. *American journal of epidemiology,* 1983, 118:461-469.

54. McKeown-Eyssen GE, Ruedy J. Prevalence of neurological abnormality in Cree Indians exposed to methylmercury in northern Quebec. *Clinical and investigative medicine,* 1983, 6:161-169.

55. Marsh DO et al. Fetal methylmercury poisoning: New data on clinical and toxicological aspects. *Transactions of the American Neurology Association,* 1977, 102:69-71.

56. Marsh DO et al. Fetal methylmercury poisoning: clinical and toxicological data on 29 cases. *Annals of neurology*, 1980, 7:348-353.

57. Marsh DO et al. Dose-response relationship for human fetal exposure to methylmercury. *Clinical toxicology*, 1981, 18:1311-1318.

58. McKeown-Eyssen CE, Ruedy J, Neims A. Methyl mercury exposure in northern Quebec. II. Neurologic findings in children. *American journal of epidemiology*, 1983, 118:470-479.

59. Marsh DO et al. Fetal methylmercury poisoning, relationship between concentration in single strands of maternal hair and child effects. *Archives of neurology*, 1987, 44:1017-1022.

60. *Evaluation of certain food additives and the contaminants mercury, lead, and cadmium*: sixteenth report of the Joint FAO/WHO Expert Committee on Food Additives. Geneva, World Health Organization, 1972 (WHO Technical Report Series, No. 505).

61. *Evaluation of certain food additives and contaminants*: twenty-second report of the Joint FAO/WHO Expert Committee on Food Additives. Geneva, World Health Organization, 1978 (WHO Technical Report Series, No. 631).

62. Joint FAO/WHO Expert Committee on Food Additives. *Toxicological evaluation of certain food additives and contaminants*. Cambridge, Cambridge University Press, 1989:295-328 (WHO Food Additives Series, No. 24).

63. *Evaluation of certain food additives and contaminants*: thirty-third report of the Joint FAO/WHO Expert Committee on Food Additives. Geneva, World Health Organization, 1989 (WHO Technical Report Series, No. 776).

## 13.22 Molybdenum

### 13.22.1 General description

**Physicochemical properties** (1, 2)

| Property | Value |
| --- | --- |
| Melting point | 2610 °C |
| Boiling point | 5560 °C |
| Density | 10.2 g/cm$^3$ |
| Vapour pressure | 0.133 kPa at 3102 °C |
| Water solubility | insoluble |

**Organoleptic properties**

Ammonium molybdate imparts a slightly astringent taste to water at concentrations above about 10 mg of molybdenum per litre (2).

## Major uses

Molybdenum is used in the manufacture of special steels, in electrical contacts, spark plugs, X-ray tubes, filaments, screens, and grids for radio valves, and in the production of tungsten, glass-to-metal seals, nonferrous alloys, and pigments. Molybdenum disulfide has unique properties as a lubricant additive. Molybdenum compounds are used in agriculture either for the direct treatment of seeds or in the formulation of fertilizers to prevent molybdenum deficiency (*1, 3, 4*).

## Environmental fate

Molybdenum disulfide is sparingly soluble in water but is readily oxidized to give more soluble molybdates, which are stable in water in the absence of a reducing agent (*2*).

## 13.22.2 Analytical methods

Molybdenum can be determined by graphite furnace atomic absorption spectroscopy with a detection limit of 0.25 μg/litre. Inductively coupled plasma atomic emission spectroscopy has a detection limit of 2 μg/litre (*5*).

## 13.22.3 Environmental levels and human exposure

### Air

Human intake of airborne molybdenum is not likely to be a major exposure pathway (*6*).

### Water

Molybdenum was present in 32.7% of surface water samples from 15 major river basins in the USA at concentrations ranging from 2 to 1500 μg/litre (mean 60 μg/litre) (*7, 8*). Levels in groundwater ranged from undetectable to 270 μg/litre in another survey in the USA (*9*).

In a survey of finished water supplies in the USA, concentrations ranged from undetectable to 68 μg/litre (median 1.4 μg/litre) (*10*). In another survey of 380 finished water samples from across the USA, 29.9% contained measurable concentrations of molybdenum, with a mean of 85.9 μg/litre and a range of 3–1024 μg/litre (*8*).

Levels of molybdenum in drinking-water do not usually exceed 10 μg/litre (*11*). However, in areas near molybdenum mining operations, the molybdenum concentration in finished water can be as high as 200 μg/litre. Tapwater concentrations as high as 580 μg/litre have been reported in Colorado (*6*).

### Food

Legumes, grains, and organ meats are good food sources of molybdenum; fruits, root and stem vegetables, and muscle meat are relatively poor ones (*12,13*).

### Estimated total exposure and relative contribution of drinking-water

Molybdenum intakes in the USA range from 240 µg/day for adult men to 100 µg/day for women. Average intake is higher in those on low incomes (*13, 14*). In most areas, molybdenum intake via drinking-water will not exceed 20 µg/day (*11*).

## 13.22.4 Kinetics and metabolism in laboratory animals and humans

The rate of gastrointestinal absorption of molybdenum is influenced by its chemical form and the animal species. Hexavalent molybdenum is readily absorbed following oral administration, the amount absorbed being higher in non-ruminants than in ruminants (*15–17*). Tetravalent molybdenum is not readily absorbed (*15*). In humans, 30–70% of dietary molybdenum is absorbed from the gastrointestinal tract (*18,19*).

Following gastrointestinal absorption, molybdenum rapidly appears in the blood and most organs. Highest concentrations are found in the liver, kidneys, and bones (*15, 16, 20*). Molybdenum crosses the placental barrier (*21*). There is no apparent bioaccumulation of molybdenum in human tissues (*20*).

In rodents, molybdenum compounds are excreted largely in the urine, and only to a small extent in faeces (*15,16*). In ponies, cattle, and sheep, molybdenum excretion is generally divided between faeces and urine, owing to less complete gastrointestinal absorption (*17, 22, 23*). Molybdenum intake and excretion are balanced in most nonruminant species, including humans (*20*).

## 13.22.5 Effects on laboratory animals and *in vitro* test systems

### Short-term exposure

Oral subchronic $LD_{50}$s for molybdenum(VI) oxide, calcium molybdate, and ammonium molybdate in rats were 125, 101, and 330 mg of molybdenum per kg of body weight per day, respectively (*15*). Death occurred over a period of 8–232 days.

In animals, molybdenum interacts in a complex manner with copper and sulfate by a mechanism which is as yet unknown. Animals on copper-deficient diets are generally more susceptible to molybdenum toxicity than those on copper-adequate diets. Dietary sulfate protects nonruminants against the symptoms of poisoning; if the animals are copper-deficient, however, it can intensify them (*24, 26*).

In a study in which Holtzman rats (4 per dose) were fed diets containing hydrogen molybdate at 75 or 300 mg/kg (7.5 or 30 mg of molybdenum per kg of body weight per day), molybdenum significantly inhibited growth and increased copper and molybdenum concentrations in liver. These effects were reduced or reversed by the addition of sulfate (25). An enlargement of the femorotibial joint and a thickening of the epiphysis of the femur and tibia were observed at both doses. This study suggests a LOAEL of 7.5 mg of molybdenum per kg of body weight per day, based on body weight loss and bone deformities.

Three weanling guinea-pigs were fed a low-copper basal diet with dietary additions of 0, 200, 500, 1000, or 2000 mg of molybdenum (8, 20, 40, or 80 mg/kg of body weight per day) for 8 weeks (27). An increase in molybdenum in the blood, liver, and kidneys was observed with increasing dietary molybdenum levels. An increase in copper was also observed in the blood and kidneys with increasing molybdenum intake; at the two highest doses, there was a decrease in liver copper concentrations.

Weanling Long-Evans rats receiving dietary sodium molybdate (50 or 80 mg of molybdenum per kg of body weight per day) over 5–8 weeks developed diarrhoea, while weight gain decreased and copper levels in the liver increased (28).

In ruminants, sulfate tends to increase the toxicity of molybdenum even in the absence of copper deficiency (26, 29, 30). Molybdenum concentrations of 10 mg/kg of body weight in the ruminant diet resulted in tissue copper depletion, potentiated by dietary sulfate (31).

A total of 12 male Holstein calves (3 per group) received ammonium molybdate at 0, 1, 10, or 50 mg of molybdenum per litre (average daily doses of < 0.01, 0.07, 0.7, or 3.7 mg of molybdenum per kg of body weight per day) in drinking-water for 21 days (32). No effects on growth were observed, but nonceruloplasmin copper was significantly elevated and copper uptake from plasma into liver was less than the endogenous loss in calves receiving the highest dose. The author suggested that the minimum toxic concentration of molybdenum is between 10 and 50 mg/litre, so that the NOAEL would be 0.07 mg/kg of body weight per day.

The effects of dietary molybdenum (1.7 g/day) were tested in four Holstein cows that were on low copper intake (30). None of the animals showed overt signs of toxicity after 6 months. After the molybdenum intake was increased to 3.4 g/day (7 mg/kg of body weight per day), one cow developed severe diarrhoea and exhibited signs of lethargy, cessation of milk synthesis, and general emaciation. When the molybdenum dose was increased to 5.1 g/day (10 mg/kg of body weight per day), two of three cows exhibited diarrhoea and emaciation. The addition of 0.26% sulfate greatly increased the severity of molybdenum toxicity. Dietary molybdenum increased the content of copper in the kidney and brain but decreased it in the liver. The kidney and spleen concentrated molybdenum to a greater degree than the liver or other organs.

### Reproductive toxicity, embryotoxicity, and teratogenicity

Five pairs of Charles River CD mice received 10 mg of molybdenum per litre (as molybdate) (about 1.5 mg of molybdenum per kg of body weight per day) in deionized drinking-water for up to 6 months (*33*). Excess fetal mortality was observed; there were 15 (of 238) dead pups in the $F_1$ generation and 7 (of 242) dead pups, five dead litters, and one maternal death in the $F_2$ generation. The experiment was discontinued after the $F_3$ generation because of the elevated incidence of deaths of offspring and parents and infertility.

Four pregnant Cheviot ewes given diets supplemented with 50 mg of molybdenum per day (as ammonium molybdate) gave birth to four lambs, three of which exhibited ataxia (*34*). Histological examination revealed degenerative changes in the cytoarchitecture of the cerebral cortex and demyelination of the cortex and spinal cord, lesions similar to those described by other investigators as "swayback".

The effects of dietary molybdenum on reproductive ability and pup growth during lactation were studied in Long-Evans rats fed diets containing 0.1, 2, 8, or 14 mg of molybdenum per kg of body weight per day and either 5 or 20 mg of copper per kg for 13 weeks (*35*). The reduced number of litters at the two highest molybdenum concentrations was attributed to the apparent infertility of males in the groups concerned as a result of varying degrees of degeneration of the seminiferous tubules. Lactating mothers at the two highest doses lost less weight during lactation than females in the lower-dose groups, and there were indications that pups from mothers exposed to the highest dose of molybdenum gained less weight at weaning than other pups; these effects were probably due to reductions in milk production associated with high maternal dietary intake of molybdenum. The NOAEL was 2 mg/kg of body weight per day.

Molybdenum administered orally by capsule for 129 days to two male Holstein calves at doses between 4.1 and 7.8 mg/kg of body weight per day caused a gradual disappearance of the spermatogenic and interstitial tissue. The LOAEL was 4.1 mg/kg of body weight per day (*36*). Female sheep fed a diet low in copper (1 mg/kg) and high in both molybdenum (25 mg/kg) and sulfate (0.53%) exhibited signs of reproductive failure (*37*).

### Mutagenicity and related end-points

Ammonium molybdate was mutagenic in two of three *Escherichia coli* strains. Molybdenum(V) chloride was negative and ammonium molybdate strongly positive in the *Bacillus subtilis rec*-assay using DNA repair-competent H17 and repair-deficient M45 strains (*38*). Ammonium and sodium molybdates were neither mutagenic nor recombinogenic in the *Saccharomyces cerevisiae* reverse mutation and gene conversion assays (*39*).

## Carcinogenicity

Although a significantly increased incidence of lung adenomas was observed in strain A mice injected intraperitoneally with molybdenum(VI) oxide (*40*), this study has no direct relevance to molybdenum intake via drinking-water. Recent studies suggest that molybdenum may act to prevent certain forms of cancer induced by *N*-nitroso compounds, e.g. oesophageal, forestomach, and mammary gland cancer, in laboratory animals (*41, 42*).

## 13.22.6 Effects on humans

Molybdenum is considered to be an essential trace element in both animals and humans. Safe and adequate intake levels have been suggested for various segments of the population, namely 0.015–0.04 mg/day for infants, 0.025–0.15 mg/day for children aged 1–10, and 0.075–0.25 mg/day for all individuals above the age of 10 (*43*).

An infant with inborn deficiency of the molybdoenzymes sulfite oxidase and xanthine dehydrogenase exhibited abnormal distribution of urinary metabolites, neurological disorders, dislocated ocular lenses, and failure to thrive (*44*). A Crohn disease patient receiving total parenteral nutrition developed tachycardia, tachypnoea, severe headaches, night blindness, nausea, vomiting, central scotomas, generalized oedema, lethargy, disorientation, and coma; these symptoms were attributed to dietary molybdenum deficiency resulting in impaired function of the two molybdoenzymes (*45*).

Urinary levels of molybdenum and copper and serum levels of uric acid and ceruloplasmin appeared to be affected by molybdenum levels in drinking-water over a 2-year period (*12*). The low-molybdenum group consisted of 42 individuals from Denver, Colorado (USA), where the molybdenum concentration in drinking-water ranged from 1 to 50 µg/litre. The high-molybdenum group consisted of 13 college students from Golden, Colorado, where the drinking-water molybdenum concentrations were equal to or greater than 200 µg/litre. Plasma molybdenum levels were within the normal range among subjects in the low-molybdenum group, and no adverse health effects were observed in these subjects. Higher daily urinary molybdenum was associated with higher molybdenum intake: the mean urinary molybdenum for the Denver subjects was 87 µg/day compared with 187 µg/day for those from Golden. Higher mean serum ceruloplasmin (401 v. 30 mg per 100 ml) and lower mean serum uric acid (4.4 v. 5.3 mg per 100 ml) were also associated with the higher molybdenum intake. Because no adverse effects were seen in either group, this study suggested a NOAEL for molybdenum in drinking-water of 200 µg/litre.

Evidence to support the suggestion that the molybdenum intake may have influenced serum ceruloplasmin was provided by a follow-up study of 13 students in Golden, Colorado, 2 years after the initial study. During this time, the average concentration of molybdenum in the Golden water supply decreased to

40 µg/litre (12). At this lower level of molybdenum in the drinking-water, serum molybdenum was nearly identical to the mean for the Denver residents. Serum ceruloplasmin was within the normal range of 20–35 µg/dl. Although serum uric acid levels increased, this was believed to be the result of alcohol consumption. There were no significant differences in urinary copper levels.

An epidemiological study involving 557 subjects in India indicated that a form of lower-limb osteoporosis may be associated with the high molybdenum content of the cereals consumed by the population (46).

The results of a cross-sectional study of 400 persons in two settlements of a molybdenum-rich province of the former Soviet Union suggested that the high incidence (18–31%) of a gout-like disease was associated with high intake of molybdenum (10–15 mg/day). The disease was characterized by joint pains in the legs and hands, enlargement of the liver, disorders of the gastrointestinal tract, liver, and kidney, increased blood levels of molybdenum and uric acid, increased xanthine oxidase activity, decreased blood levels of copper, and increased urinary copper. An increased synthesis of the molybdoenzyme xanthine oxidase resulting from high dietary molybdenum levels was proposed as the mechanism for this disorder (47).

A cross-sectional study was conducted with 25 workers at a molybdenum smelter in Denver, Colorado, exposed to molybdenum in dust (predominantly molybdenum(VI) oxide and other soluble oxides). The calculated minimum daily body burden was 0.15 mg/kg of body weight per day. High levels of molybdenum were present in the blood of 15 workers (up to 300 µg/litre) and in the urine of 12 of 14 workers (up to 11 mg/litre) (48). Mean serum ceruloplasmin and uric acid were higher for workers than controls. According to answers to medical questionnaires, six workers had upper respiratory infections in the 2 weeks prior to the questionnaire, and 15 reported joint pains, back pains, headaches, or skin or hair changes.

## 13.22.7 Guideline value

No data are available on the carcinogenicity of molybdenum by the oral route. In a 2-year study of humans exposed via drinking-water, the NOAEL was found to be 0.2 mg/litre (12), but there are some concerns about the quality of this study. Although an uncertainty factor of 10 would normally be applied to reflect intraspecies variation, it is recognized that molybdenum is an essential element, and a factor of 3 is therefore considered to be adequate. This gives a guideline value of 0.07 mg/litre (rounded figure), which is in the same range as that derived on the basis of the results of toxicological studies in animals and is consistent with the essential daily requirement for molybdenum.

# References

1.  Weast RC, ed. *Handbook of chemistry and physics*, 67th ed. Cleveland, OH, CRC Press, 1986.

2.  Asmanguljan TA. [Determination of the maximum permissible concentration of molybdenum in open bodies of water.] *Gigiena i sanitarija*, 1965, 30:1-5 (in Russian).

3.  Climax Molybdenum Co. *Molybdenum chemicals*, Greenwich, CT, 1973:1-7 (Bulletin Cdb-16).

4.  Stokinger HE. *Encyclopedia of occupational health and safety*, 3rd rev. ed. Geneva, International Labour Organisation, 1983, 2:1403-1404.

5.  American Public Health Association. *Standard methods for the examination of water and wastewater*. 17th ed. Washington, DC, 1989.

6.  Chappell WR. *Transport and biological effects of molybdenum in the environment. Progress report.* Boulder, CO, University of Colorado and Colorado State University, 1973.

7.  National Academy of Sciences. *Drinking water and health*. Washington, DC, 1977:279-285.

8.  Kopp JF, Kroner RC. *Trace metals in waters of the United States. A five-year summary of trace metals in rivers and lakes of the United States (Oct. 1, 1962-Sept. 30, 1967)*. Cincinnati, OH, US Department of the Interior, Federal Water Pollution Control Administration, 1967.

9.  Kehoe RA, Chalak J, Largent EJ. The concentration of certain trace metals in drinking waters. *Journal of the American Water Works Association*, 1944, 36:637-644.

10. Durfor CN, Becker E. *Public water supplies of the 100 largest cities in the United States*. Washington, DC, US Geological Survey, 1964 (Water Supply Paper No. 1812).

11. Greathouse DG, Osborne RH. Preliminary report on nationwide study of drinking water and cardiovascular diseases. *Journal of environmental pathology and toxicology*, 1980, 4(2-3):65-76.

12. Chappel WR et al. *Human health effects of molybdenum in drinking water.* Cincinnati, OH, US Environmental Protection Agency, 1979 (EPA-600A-79-006).

13. Tsongas TA et al. Molybdenum in the diet: an estimate of average daily intake in the United States. *American journal of clinical nutrition*, 1980, 33:1103-1107.

14. Pennington JAT, Young BE, Wilson D. Nutritional elements in U.S. diets: results from the total diet study, 1982 to 1986. *Journal of the American Dietetic Association*, 1989, 89:659-664.

15. Fairhall LT et al. *The toxicity of molybdenum*. Washington, DC, US Government Printing Office, 1945:1-35 (Public Health Service Bulletin No. 293).

16. Kosarek LJ. *The kinetics of molybdenum99 gastrointestinal absorption and tissue elimination in the rat*. Boulder, CO, University of Colorado, 1976 (Master's thesis).

17. Miller JK et al. Comparison of 99Mo metabolism in young cattle and swine. *Journal of animal science*, 1972, 34:846-850.

18. Engel RW, Price NO, Miller RF. Copper, manganese, cobalt and molybdenum balance in pre-adolescent girls. *Journal of nutrition*, 1967, 92:197-204.

19. Robinson MF et al. Metabolic balance of zinc, copper, cadmium, iron, molybdenum and selenium in young New Zealand women. *British journal of nutrition*, 1973, 30:195-205.

20. Schroeder HA, Balassa JJ, Tipton IH. Essential trace metals in man: molybdenum. *Journal of chronic diseases*, 1970, 23:481-499.

21. Meinel B et al. Contents of trace elements in the human liver before birth. *Biologia neonatorum*, 1979, 36:225-232.

22. Cymbaluk NF et al. Influence of dietary molybdenum on copper metabolism in ponies. *Journal of nutrition*, 1981, 111:96-106.

23. Kelleher CA et al. The absorption of labelled molybdenum compounds in sheep fitted with re-entrant cannulae in the ascending duodenum. *Journal of comparative pathology*, 1983, 93:83-92.

24. Gray LF, Daniel LJ. Effect of the copper status of the rat on the copper–molybdenum–sulfate interaction. *Journal of nutrition*, 1964, 84:31-37.

25. Miller RF, Price NO, Engel RW. Added dietary inorganic sulfate and its effects upon rats fed molybdenum. *Journal of nutrition*, 1956, 60:539-547.

26. Suttle NF. The nutritional significance of the Cu:Mo interrelationship to ruminants and non-ruminants. In: Hemphill DD, ed. *Trace substances in environmental health*, Vol. VII. Columbia, MO, University of Missouri, 1974:245-249.

27. Arthur D. Interrelationships of molybdenum and copper in the diet of the guinea pig. *Journal of nutrition*, 1965, 87:69-76.

28. Cox D et al. Influence of excess dietary molybdenum on rat and calf liver and heart enzymes. *Journal of nutrition*, 1960, 70:63-68.

29. Campbell CM et al. Effects of molybdenum and copper relationship on early weaned calves. In: Chappell WR, Petersen KK, eds. *Molybdenum in the environment*, Vol. I. New York, NY, Marcel Dekker, 1976:75-84.

30. Huber JT, Price NO, Engel RW. Response of lactating dairy cows to high levels of dietary molybdenum. *Journal of animal science*, 1971, 32:364-367.

31. Suttle NF. The role of thiomolybdates in the nutritional interactions of copper, molybdenum and sulfur: fact or fantasy? *Annals of the New York Academy of Science*, 1980, 355:195-207.

32. Kincaid RL. Toxicity of ammonium molybdate added to drinking water of calves. *Journal of dairy science*, 1980, 63:608-610.

33. Schroeder HA, Mitchener M. Toxic effects of trace elements on the reproduction of mice and rats. *Archives of environmental health*, 1971, 23:102-106.

34. Mills CF, Fell BF. Demyelination in lambs born of ewes maintained on high intakes of sulphate and molybdate. *Nature*, 1960, 185:20-22.

35. Jeter MA, Davis GK. The effect of dietary molybdenum upon growth, hemoglobin, reproduction and lactation of rats. *Journal of nutrition*, 1954, 54:215-220.

36. Thomas JW, Moss S. The effect of orally administered molybdenum on growth, spermatogenesis, and testes histology of young dairy bulls. *Journal of dairy science*, 1951, 34:929-934.

37. Suttle NF, Field AC. Effect of intake of copper, molybdenum and sulphate on copper metabolism in sheep. IV. Production of congenital and delayed swayback. *Journal of comparative pathology*, 1969, 79:453-464.

38. Nishioka H. Mutagenic actitvities of metal compounds in bacteria. *Mutation research*, 1975, 31:185-189.

39. Singh I. Induction of reverse mutation and mitotic gene conversion by some metal compounds in *Saccharomyces cerevisiae*. *Mutation research*, 1983, 117:149-152.

40. Stoner GD et al. Tests for carcinogenicity of metallic compounds by the pulmonary tumor response in strain A mice. *Cancer research*, 1976, 36:1744-1747.

41. Luo XM, Wei HJ, Yang SP. Inhibitory effects of molybdenum on esophageal and forestomach carcinogenesis in rats. *Journal of the National Cancer Institute*, 1983, 71:75-80.

42. Wei HJ, Luo XM, Yang SP. Effects of molybdenum and tungsten on mammary carcinogenesis in SD rats. *Journal of the National Cancer Institute*, 1985, 74(2):469-473.

43. National Academy of Sciences. *Recommended dietary allowances*, 10th ed. Washington, DC, National Academy Press, 1989:243-246, 284.

44. Johnson JL et al. Inborn errors of molybdenum metabolism: combined deficiencies of sulfite oxidase and xanthine dehydrogenase in a patient lacking the molybdenum cofactor. *Proceedings of the National Academy of Sciences*, 1980, 77:3715-3719.

45. Abumrad NN et al. Amino acid intolerance during prolonged total parenteral nutrition reversed by molybdate therapy. *American journal of clinical nutrition*, 1981, 34:2551-2559.

46. Krishnamachari KA, Krishnaswamy K. An epidemiological study of the syndrome of genu valgum among residents of endemic areas for fluorosis in Andhra Pradesh. *Indian journal of medical research*, 1974, 62:1415-1423.

47. Koval'skij VV, Jarovaja GA, Šmavonjan DM. [Changes of purine metabolism in man and animals under conditions of molybdenum biogeochemical provinces.] *Žurnal obščej biologij*, 1961, 22:179-191 (in Russian).

48. Walravens PA et al. Biochemical abnormalities in workers exposed to molybdenum dust. *Archives of environmental health*, 1979, 34:302-308.

## 13.23 Nickel

### 13.23.1 General description

#### Identity

Nickel occurs as a mixture of five natural stable isotopes, with relative atomic masses of 58, 60, 61, 62, and 64.

#### Physicochemical properties

| Property | Value |
|---|---|
| Melting point | 1453 °C |
| Boiling point | 2732 °C |
| Density (g/cm$^3$) | 8.90 at 25 °C |

#### Major uses

Nickel is used in a large number of alloys, including stainless steel, in batteries, chemicals, and catalysts, and in the electrolytic coating of items such as chromium-plated taps and fittings used for tapwater.

### Environmental fate

The nickel ion combines with oxygen-, nitrogen-, and sulfur-containing compounds and forms an extensive series of complexes in solution, including hydroxides, carbonates, carboxylic acids, phosphates, amines, and thiols (*1*). In aqueous solution, nickel occurs mostly as the green hexa-aquanickel(II) ion, $Ni(H_2O)_6^{2+}$ (*2*). The nickel ion content of groundwater may increase as a result of the oxidation of natural nickel-containing ferrosulfide deposits. Oxidation can occur if the groundwater table is lowered or if nitrate is leached from the soil.

## 13.23.2 Analytical methods

Nickel can be determined by atomic absorption spectrophotometry; the detection limit is 50 ng/litre (*3*).

## 13.23.3 Environmental levels and human exposure

### Air

Inhalation of airborne nickel may result in a total pulmonary exposure of 0.5 µg/day. The pulmonary exposure of a person smoking 20 cigarettes may be 4 µg/day (*4*).

### Water

Nickel concentrations in drinking-water around the world are normally below 20 µg/litre, although levels up to several hundred micrograms per litre in groundwater and drinking-water have been reported (*5, 6*). Nickel concentrations in drinking-water may be increased if raw waters are polluted by natural or industrial nickel deposits or if leaching from nickel–chromium plated taps and fitting occurs. Levels up to 1000 µg/litre have been reported in first-run water that had remained in the tap overnight (*4*).

### Food

The natural nickel content of various food items varies from 0 to 10 mg/kg. Nickel concentrations of more than 1 mg/kg have been found in cocoa, chocolate, soya beans, soy products, other dried legumes, nuts, oatmeal, and buckwheat. Nickel may be leached from kitchen utensils by acidic boiling water (*4*).

### Estimated total exposure and relative contribution of drinking-water

The average daily intake of nickel from food is between 100 and 300 µg and probably lower than 150 µg. A diet containing large amounts of food items in which nickel is present at concentrations above 1 mg/kg may result in a daily intake of 900 µg (*4*). Intake from food exceeds that from drinking-water (about 40 µg/day) and air (<5 µg/day).

### 13.23.4 Kinetics and metabolism in laboratory animals and humans

In humans, absorption of soluble nickel from drinking-water may be 40 times higher than that of nickel from food (*7*). Intestinal absorption may be increased several-fold by chelating agents such as disulfiram (*6*). Nickel penetrates the skin very slowly (*7*). It appears to be distributed to all organs, primary accumulation taking place in the kidneys, lungs, and liver. The formation of lipophilic nickel complexes can alter the distribution, and lead to much higher deposition in the brain than under normal conditions (*6*). Nickel is able to pass through the human placenta (*4*). It is excreted mainly through the urine. The estimated mean elimination half-time for serum is about 60 h (*8*).

### 13.23.5 Effects on laboratory animals and *in vitro* test systems

#### Acute exposure

Oral $LD_{50}$s of nickel in mice or rats are in the range 67–139 mg/kg of body weight (*1*).

#### Long-term exposure

In a 2-year study, dogs were fed nickel chloride in the diet at doses of approximately 3, 29, or 70 mg of nickel per kg of body weight per day. Depressed body weight gain, altered organ-to-body-weight ratios, and histopathological effects in the lungs were observed at the highest dose. The NOAEL was 29 mg of nickel per kg of body weight per day (*9*).

In a 2-year study with Wistar rats fed nickel chloride in the diet at doses of approximately 5, 50, or 125 mg of nickel per kg of body weight per day, depressed body weight gain and altered organ-to-body-weight ratios were observed at the two highest doses, but there were no effects on haematology or histopathology. The NOAEL was 5 mg of nickel per kg of body weight per day (*9*).

#### Reproductive toxicity, embryotoxicity, and teratogenicity

In a three-generation study in rats given 12.5, 25, or 50 mg of nickel per kg of body weight per day in drinking-water, a higher incidence of stillbirths was observed in all groups in the first generation; decreased body weights of weanlings were seen in all generations at the highest dose (*9*).

## Mutagenicity and related end-points

The nickel ion has been observed to enter cells and bind to DNA and RNA. Nickel has given positive results in tests with *Salmonella typhimurium*, *Corynebacterium*, and *Escherichia coli*. DNA damage has been observed in mammalian cells after *in vivo* exposure of Sprague-Dawley rats and *in vitro* exposure of Chinese hamster ovary (CHO) cells. Inhibition of DNA synthesis and induction of DNA repair have been shown in CHO cells. At nickel levels similar to those experienced by heavily exposed workers, sister chromatid exchange in peripheral blood lymphocytes, cell transformation *in vitro* in hamster cells and in human bronchial epithelial cells, and chromosomal aberrations in hamster cells were observed (*10*).

## Carcinogenicity

IARC has evaluated the data on pulmonary exposure to soluble nickel compounds and has concluded that the evidence for a carcinogenic effect in animals is limited. Several experimental investigations have demonstrated that a number of nickel compounds are carcinogenic after administration via various parenteral routes (e.g. inhalation, intramuscular injection, intrarenal injection). Together, these studies suggest that some nickel compounds, especially nickel sulfide, possess carcinogenic potential (*11*).

## 13.23.6 Effects on humans

Acute nickel intoxications are rare, and most reported cases are the result of industrial exposure to nickel carbonyl. Of 32 electroplating workers who inadvertently drank water heavily contaminated with nickel sulfate and chloride (1.63 g of nickel per litre), 20 developed symptoms (e.g. nausea, vomiting, abdominal discomfort, diarrhoea, giddiness, lassitude, headache, cough, shortness of breath) that typically lasted for a few hours but persisted for 1–2 days in seven cases. The nickel doses that caused symptoms were estimated to be in the range 7.1–35.7 mg/kg of body weight. Laboratory tests showed elevated levels of blood reticulocytes, urine albumin, and serum bilirubin. All the workers recovered rapidly without evident sequelae (*8*). Similar symptoms were observed in 23 patients at plasma nickel concentrations of approximately 3 mg/litre following exposure to nickel-containing water during haemodialysis. The nickel was leached from a nickel-plated, stainless-steel water-heating tank. In another accident, a 2-year-old girl died after swallowing 2.2–3.3 g of nickel as sulfate crystals (*10*).

Several epidemiological studies have suggested a risk of nasal, sinus, and lung cancer in workers in the nickel-producing industry by inhalation of soluble nickel at concentrations in excess of 1 mg/m$^3$ and of less soluble forms at concentrations greater than 10 mg/m$^3$ (*12*). IARC has recently re-evaluated the epidemiological data on respiratory exposure and found that sufficient human data are available to conclude that inhaled nickel sulfate is carcinogenic to humans (*11*).

Nickel is also a common skin allergen. The prevalence of nickel sensitivity is about 8–14.5% for adult women and about 1% for men. About 50% of nickel-sensitive women develop hand eczema, which in severe cases may cause incapacitation. Although only continued dermal exposures to nickel can lead to sensitization, subsequent dermal application or oral intake of extremely low doses of nickel may provoke eczema in sensitized individuals. Single oral doses of 36–80 µg of nickel per kg of body weight in lactose capsules have been shown to exacerbate hand eczema. In a study in which natural dietary nickel was ingested daily at a dose level of 8.3 µg/kg of body weight for 5 days, a worsening of vesicular hand eczema was observed in 10 out of 12 patients (*13*).

## 13.23.7 Guideline value

The guideline value is based on a dietary study in rats that showed a NOAEL of 5 mg/kg of body weight per day for altered organ-to-body-weight ratios (*9*). A TDI of 5 µg/kg of body weight was derived using an uncertainty factor of 1000, made up of 100 for inter- and intraspecies variation and an additional factor of 10 to compensate for the lack of adequate studies on long-term toxicity and reproductive effects, the lack of data on carcinogenicity by the oral route (although both the soluble and the sparingly soluble compounds of nickel are now considered to be human carcinogens in relation to pulmonary exposure), and a much higher intestinal absorption when taken on an empty stomach in drinking-water than when taken together with food.

With an allocation of 10% of the TDI to drinking-water, the health-based guideline value is 0.02 mg/litre (rounded figure), which should provide sufficient protection for nickel-sensitive individuals.

## References

1. Coogan TP et al. Toxicity and carcinogenicity of nickel compounds. *CRC critical reviews in toxicology*, 1989, 19(4):341-384.

2. Grandjean P, Andersen O, Nielsen GD. Nickel. In: Alessio L et al., eds. *Biological indicators for the assessment of human exposure to industrial chemicals*, Vol. 5. Ispra, Commission of the European Communities, 1988:59-80 (EUR 11478 EN).

3. International Organization for Standardization. *Water quality–determination of cobalt, nickel, copper, zinc, cadmium and lead*. Geneva, 1986 (ISO 8288:1986).

4. Grandjean P, Nielsen GD, Andersen O. Human nickel exposure and chemobiokinetics. In: Menne T, Maibach HI, eds. *Nickel and the skin: immunology and toxicology*. Boca Raton, FL, CRC Press, 1989:9-34.

5. Grandjean P. Human exposure to nickel. In: Sunderman FW Jr, ed. *Nickel in the human environment.* Lyon, International Agency for Research on Cancer, 1984:469-485 (IARC Scientific Publications No. 53).

6. McNeely MD, Nechay MW, Sunderman FW Jr. Measurements of nickel in serum and urine as indices of environmental exposure to nickel. *Clinical chemistry*, 1972, 18:992-995.

7. Sunderman FW et al. Nickel absorption and kinetics in human volunteers. *Proceedings of the Society for Experimental Biology and Medicine*, 1989, 191:5-11.

8. Sunderman FW et al. Acute nickel toxicity in electroplating workers who accidentally ingested a solution of nickel sulfate and nickel chloride. *American journal of industrial medicine*, 1988, 14:257-266.

9. Ambrose AM et al. Long term toxicologic assessment of nickel in rats and dogs. *Journal of food science and technology*, 1976, 13:181-187.

10. *Nickel.* Geneva, World Health Organization, 1991 (Environmental Health Criteria, No. 108).

11. International Agency for Research on Cancer. *Chromium, nickel, and welding.* Lyon, 1990:257-445 (IARC Monographs on the Evaluation of Carcinogenic Risks to Humans, Volume 49).

12. Doll R et al. Report of the international committee on nickel carcinogenesis in man. *Scandinavian journal of work, environment and health*, 1990, 16:1-84.

13. Nielsen GD et al. Nickel-sensitive patients with vesicular hand eczema: oral challenge with a diet naturally high in nickel. *British journal of dermatology*, 1990, 122:299-308.

## 13.24 Nitrate and nitrite

### 13.24.1 General description

#### *Identity*

Nitrate and nitrite are naturally occurring ions that are part of the nitrogen cycle. The nitrate ion ($NO_3^-$) is the stable form of combined nitrogen for oxygenated systems; although chemically unreactive, it can be reduced by microbial action. The nitrite ion ($NO_2^-$) contains nitrogen in a relatively unstable oxidation state; chemical and biological processes can further reduce nitrite to various compounds or oxidize it to nitrate (*1*).

## Physicochemical properties (1)

| Property | Nitrate | Nitrite |
|---|---|---|
| Acid | Conjugate base of strong acid $HNO_3$; $pK_a = -1.3$ | Conjugate base of weak acid $HNO_2$; $pK_a = 3.4$ |
| Salts | Very soluble in water | Very soluble in water |
| Reactivity | Unreactive | Reactive; oxidizes antioxidants, $Fe^{2+}$ of haemoglobin to $Fe^{3+}$, and primary amines; nitrosates several amines and amides |
| Conversion to nitrogen | 1 mg $NO_3^-$/litre = 0.226 mg $NO_3^-$-N/litre | 1 mg $NO_2^-$/litre = 0.304 mg $NO_2^-$-N/litre |

## Major uses

Nitrate is used mainly in inorganic fertilizers. It is also used as an oxidizing agent and in the production of explosives and purified potassium nitrate for glass making. Sodium nitrite is used as a food preservative, especially in cured meats. Nitrate is sometimes added to serve as a reservoir for nitrite.

## Environmental fate

In soil, fertilizers containing inorganic nitrogen and wastes containing organic nitrogen are first decomposed to give ammonia, which is then oxidized to nitrite and nitrate. The nitrate is taken up by plants during their growth and used in the synthesis of organic nitrogenous compounds. Surplus nitrate readily moves with groundwater (2, 3). Under aerobic conditions, it percolates in large quantities into the aquifer because of the small extent to which degradation or denitrification occurs. Under anaerobic conditions, nitrate may be denitrified or degraded almost completely to nitrogen.

The presence of high or low water tables, the amount of rainwater, the presence of other organic material, and other physicochemical properties are also important in determining the fate of nitrate in soil (4). In surface water, nitrification and denitrification may also occur, depending on the temperature and pH. The uptake of nitrate by plants, however, is responsible for most of the nitrate reduction in surface water.

Nitrogen compounds are formed in the air by lightning or discharged into it from industrial processes, motor vehicles, and intensive agriculture. Nitrate is present in air primarily as nitric acid and inorganic aerosols, as well as nitrate radicals and organic gases or aerosols. These are removed by wet and dry deposition.

## 13.24.2 Analytical methods

The methods used for the measurement of nitrate in water are usually based on photometric analysis after reduction to nitrite. Detection limits range from 3 to 220 µg of nitrate per litre (*5, 6*).

## 13.24.3 Environmental levels and human exposure

### Air

Atmospheric nitrate concentrations ranging from 0.1 to 0.4 µg/m$^3$ have been reported, the lowest concentrations being found in the South Pacific (*7*). Higher concentrations ranging from 1 to 40 µg/m$^3$ have also been reported, with annual means of 1–8 µg/m$^3$. Mean monthly nitrate concentrations in air in the Netherlands vary from 1 to 14 µg/m$^3$ (*8*). Indoor nitrate aerosol concentrations of 1.1–5.6 µg/m$^3$ were found to be related to outdoor concentrations (*9*).

### Water

Concentrations of nitrate in rainwater of up to 5 mg/litre[1] have been observed in industrial areas (*2*). In rural areas, concentrations are somewhat lower.

The nitrate concentration in surface water is normally low (0–18 mg/litre), but can reach high levels as a result of agricultural run-off, refuse dump run-off, or contamination with human or animal wastes. The concentration often fluctuates with the season and may increase when the river is fed by nitrate-rich aquifers. Nitrate concentrations have gradually increased in many European countries in the last few decades and have sometimes doubled over the past 20 years. In the United Kingdom, for example, an average annual increase of 0.7 mg/litre has been observed in some rivers (*10*).

The natural nitrate concentration in groundwater under aerobic conditions is a few milligrams per litre and depends strongly on soil type and on the geological situation. In the USA, naturally occurring levels do not exceed 4–9 mg/litre for nitrate and 0.3 mg/litre for nitrite (*3*). As a result of agricultural activities, the nitrate concentration can easily reach several hundred milligrams per litre (*5*). For example, concentrations of up to 1500 mg/litre were found in the groundwater in an agricultural area of India (*11*).

In the USA, nitrates are present in most surface water and groundwater supplies at levels below 4 mg/litre; levels exceed 20 mg/litre in about 3% of the surface waters and 6% of the groundwaters. In 1986, a nitrate concentration of 44 mg/litre (10 mg nitrate-nitrogen per litre) was exceeded in 40 surface water and 568 groundwater supplies. Nitrite levels were not surveyed but are expected to be much lower than 3.3 mg/litre (*3*).

---

[1] Unless otherwise stated, concentrations in water are expressed as mg of nitrate ($NO_3^-$) per litre and mg of nitrite ($NO_2^-$) per litre.

The increasing use of artificial fertilizers, the disposal of wastes (particularly from animal farming), and changes in land use are the main factors responsible for the progressive increase in nitrate levels in groundwater supplies over the last 20 years. In Denmark and the Netherlands, for example, nitrate concentrations are increasing by 0.2–1.3 mg/litre per year in some areas (5). Because of the delay in the response of groundwater to changes in soil, some endangered aquifers have not yet shown the increase expected from the increased use of nitrogen fertilizer or manure; once the nitrate reaches them, these aquifers will remain contaminated for decades, even if there is a substantial reduction in the nitrate loading of the surface.

In most countries, nitrate levels in drinking-water derived from surface water do not exceed 10 mg/litre. In some areas, however, concentrations are higher as a result of run-off and the discharge of sewage effluent and certain industrial wastes. In 15 European countries, the percentage of the population exposed to nitrate levels in drinking-water above 50 mg/litre ranges from 0.5 to 10% (5,12); this corresponds to nearly 10 million people. Individual wells in agricultural areas throughout the world are especially vulnerable, and nitrate levels in the water often exceed 50 mg/litre.

### Food

Vegetables and cured meat are in general the main sources of nitrate and nitrite in the diet, but small amounts may be present in fish and dairy products. Meat products may contain <2.7–945 mg of nitrate per kg and <0.2–64 mg of nitrite per kg, and dairy products <3–27 mg of nitrate per kg and <0.2–1.7 mg of nitrite per kg (12). Most vegetables and fruits contain 200–2500 mg of nitrate per kg (2). The nitrate content of vegetables can be affected by the processing of the food, the use of fertilizers, and growing conditions. Vegetables such as beetroot, lettuce, radish, and spinach often contain concentrations above 2500 mg/kg, especially when they are cultivated in greenhouses.

### Estimated total exposure and relative contribution of drinking-water

Air pollution appears to be a minor source. In general, vegetables will be the main source of nitrate intake when levels in drinking-water are below 10 mg/litre (3,12,13). When levels in drinking-water exceed 50 mg/litre, drinking-water will be the major source of total nitrate intake, especially for bottle-fed infants. In the Netherlands, the average population exposure is approximately 140 mg of nitrate per day (including the nitrate in drinking-water). The contribution of drinking-water to the nitrate intake is up to 14% from 80% of the supplies and up to 45% from 5% of them. For the bottle-fed infant, daily intake from formula made with water containing 50 mg of nitrate per litre would average about 8.3–8.5 mg of nitrate per kg of body weight per day.

The mean dietary intakes determined by the duplicate portion technique (*14*) range from 43 to 131 mg of nitrate per day and from 1.2 to 3 mg of nitrite per day. Estimates of the total nitrate intake based on the proportion of nitrate excreted in the urine (*15*) range from 39 to 268 mg/day, the higher values applying to vegetarian and nitrate-rich diets (*12*). According to the US Environmental Protection Agency, the average nitrate intake from food of males is approximately 40–100 mg/day. The daily nitrite intake ranges from 0.3 to 2.6 mg/day, primarily from cured meat (*16*).

## 13.24.4 Kinetics and metabolism in laboratory animals and humans

Ingested nitrate is readily and completely absorbed from the upper small intestine. Nitrite may be absorbed directly both from the stomach and the upper small intestine. Part of the ingested nitrite is reduced in the mouth or reacts with gastric contents prior to absorption.

Nitrate is rapidly distributed throughout the tissues. Approximately 25% of ingested nitrate is actively secreted into saliva, where it is partly (20%) reduced to nitrite by the oral microflora; nitrate and nitrite are then swallowed and re-enter the stomach. Bacterial reduction of nitrate may also take place in other parts of the human gastrointestinal tract but not normally in the stomach; exceptions are reported in humans with low gastric acidity, such as artificially fed infants and certain patients in whom hydrochloric acid secretion is lower than normal. In rats, active secretion and reduction of nitrate in saliva are virtually absent. Total nitrate reduction in rats is probably less than in humans.

Absorbed nitrite is rapidly oxidized to nitrate in the blood. Nitrite in the bloodstream is involved in the oxidation of haemoglobin to methaemoglobin: the $Fe^{2+}$ present in the haem group is oxidized to its $Fe^{3+}$ form, and nitrite binds firmly to this oxidized haem. Nitrite has been shown to cross the placenta and cause the formation of fetal methaemoglobin in rats. It may react in the stomach with nitrosatable compounds (e.g secondary and tertiary amines or amides in food) to form *N*-nitroso compounds. Such endogenous nitrosation has been shown to occur in human as well as animal gastric juice both *in vivo* and *in vitro*, mostly at higher pH values.

The major part of the ingested nitrate is eventually excreted in urine as nitrate, ammonia, or urea, faecal excretion being negligible. Little nitrite is excreted (*1, 5, 17*). The excess nitrate excretion that has often been observed after low nitrate and nitrite intake originates from endogenous synthesis, which amounts, in normal healthy humans, to 1 mmol/day on average, corresponding to 62 mg of nitrate per day or 14 mg of nitrate-nitrogen per day. Gastrointestinal infections increase nitrate excretion enormously, as a result, at least in part, of increased endogenous (nonbacterial) nitrate synthesis, probably induced by activation of the mammalian reticuloendothelial system (*5,17*).

## 13.24.5 Effects on laboratory animals and *in vitro* test systems
### *Acute exposure*

The acute oral toxicity of nitrate to laboratory animals is low to moderate: $LD_{50}$ values of 1600–9000 mg of sodium nitrate per kg of body weight have been reported. Ruminants are more sensitive to the effects of nitrate owing to high nitrate reduction in the rumen; the $LD_{50}$ for cows was 450 mg of sodium nitrate per kg of body weight. Nitrite is more toxic: $LD_{50}$ values of 85–220 mg of sodium nitrite per kg of body weight have been reported for mice and rats (*17*).

### *Short-term exposure*

In a 13-week study in which nitrite was given to rats in drinking-water, a dose-related hypertrophy of the adrenal zona glomerulosa was observed at all dose levels (100, 300, 1000, or 3000 mg of potassium nitrite per litre of drinking-water, corresponding to 54–1620 mg of nitrite per litre). Increased methaemoglobin levels were seen only in the highest dose group (*18*). Studies designed to clarify the etiology of this hypertrophy and its significance and to establish a no-effect level are currently in progress.

### *Long-term exposure*

The only observed effect of nitrate in rats after 2 years of oral dosage was growth inhibition; this was seen at dietary concentrations of 5% sodium nitrate and upwards. The NOAEL in this study was 1%, which corresponds to 500 mg of sodium nitrate per kg of body weight.

One of the long-term effects of nitrite reported in a variety of animal species is vitamin A deficiency; this is probably caused by the direct reaction of nitrite with the vitamin. The most important effect reported in long-term animal studies was an increase in methaemoglobin level, accompanied by histopathological changes in the lungs and heart, in rats receiving nitrite in drinking-water for 2 years. The LOAEL, which gave a methaemoglobin level of 5%, was 1000 mg of sodium nitrite per litre; the NOAEL was 100 mg/litre, corresponding to 10 mg of sodium nitrite per kg of body weight (*17*).

### *Reproductive toxicity, embryotoxicity, and teratogenicity*

The reproductive behaviour of guinea-pigs was impaired only at very high nitrate concentrations (30 000 mg/litre); the NOAEL was 10 000 mg/litre.

Nitrite appeared to cause fetotoxicity in rats at drinking-water concentrations (corresponding to 200–300 mg of sodium nitrite per kg of body weight) causing increased maternal methaemoglobin levels. However, after similar doses in feed in other studies, no embryotoxic effects were observed in rats. Teratogenic effects were not reported (*17*).

## Mutagenicity and related end-points

Nitrate is not mutagenic in bacteria and mammalian cells *in vitro*. Chromosomal aberrations were observed in the bone marrow of rats after oral nitrate uptake, but this could have been due to exogenous *N*-nitroso compound formation. Nitrite is mutagenic. It causes morphological transformations in *in vitro* systems; mutagenic activity was also found in a combined *in vivo–in vitro* experiment with Syrian hamsters. The results of *in vivo* experiments were controversial (*17*).

## Carcinogenicity

Nitrate is not carcinogenic in laboratory animals. Some studies in which nitrite was given to mice or rats in the diet showed slightly increased tumour incidences; however, the possibility of exogenous *N*-nitroso compound formation in these studies could not be excluded. In studies in which nitrite was given simultaneously with a nitrosatable compound, tumours were produced characteristic of the presumed corresponding *N*-nitroso compound. However, this was seen only at extremely high nitrite levels, of the order of 1000 mg/litre of drinking-water. At lower nitrite levels, tumour incidences resembled those of control groups treated with the nitrosatable compound only. On the basis of adequately performed and reported studies, it may be concluded that nitrite itself is not carcinogenic in laboratory animals (*17*).

## 13.24.6 Effects on humans

### Methaemoglobinaemia

The toxicity of nitrate to humans is thought to be solely the consequence of its reduction to nitrite. The major biological effect of nitrite in humans is its involvement in the oxidation of normal heamoglobin to methaemoglobin, which is unable to transport oxygen to the tissues. The reduced oxygen transport becomes clinically manifest when methaemoglobin concentrations reach 10% of that of haemoglobin and above; the condition, called methaemoglobinaemia, causes cyanosis and, at higher concentrations, asphyxia. The normal methaemoglobin level in humans is less than 2%, and in infants under 3 months of age less than 3%. The haemoglobin of young infants is more susceptible to methaemoglobin formation than that of older children and adults. Other groups especially susceptible to methaemoglobin formation include pregnant women and people deficient in glucose-6-phosphate dehydrogenase or methaemoglobin reductase.

Some cases of methaemoglobinaemia have been reported in adults consuming high doses of nitrate by accident or as a medical treatment. Fatalities were reported after single intakes of 4–50 g of nitrate, many of which occurred among special risk groups in whom gastric acidity was reduced. In a controlled study, an oral dose of 7–10.5 g of ammonium nitrate and an intravenous dose of 9.5 g of sodium nitrate did not cause increased methaemoglobin levels in adults (*17*).

Few cases of methaemoglobinaemia have been reported in older children. A correlation study among children aged 1–8 years in the USA showed that there was no difference in methaemoglobin levels between 64 children consuming high-nitrate well-water (22–111 mg of nitrate-nitrogen per litre) and 38 children consuming low-nitrate water (<10 mg of nitrate-nitrogen per litre). These concentrations correspond to 100–500 and 44 mg of nitrate per litre, respectively. All the methaemoglobin levels were within the normal range, suggesting that older children are relatively insensitive to the effects of nitrate (19).

Cases of methaemoglobinaemia related to low nitrate intake appear to be restricted to infants. In studies in which a possible association between clinical cases of infant methaemoglobinaemia or subclinically increased methaemoglobin levels and nitrate concentrations in drinking-water was investigated, a significant relationship was usually found, most clinical cases occurring at nitrate levels of 50 mg/litre and above, and almost exclusively in infants under 3 months of age (20). In most of these studies, no account was taken of the additional intake of nitrate or nitrite from other sources or of infections, which may increase endogenous nitrate synthesis; infections in which nitrate-reducing bacteria are involved result in massive endogenous nitrite production. Some cases of infant methaemoglobinaemia have indeed been described in which increased endogenous nitrite synthesis as a result of gastrointestinal infection appeared to be the only causative factor. As most cases of infant methaemoglobinaemia reported in the literature have been associated with the consumption of private and often bacterially contaminated well-water, the involvement of infections is highly probable. Most of these studies may therefore be less suitable from the point of view of the quantitative assessment of the risk of nitrate intake for healthy infants. On the other hand, bottle-fed infants have a high probability of developing gastrointestinal infections because of their low gastric acidity; this is an additional reason to treat them as a special risk group.

A few controlled studies on healthy infants have been reported. Methaemoglobin levels above 3% were found in infants receiving formula mixed with water containing more than 60 mg of nitrate per litre. Cyanosis appeared to occur only at doses above 50 mg of nitrate per kg of body weight (or approximately 300 mg/litre of drinking-water). However, the relevance of these studies to quantitative risk assessment is also questionable, as they were all short-term studies on small groups of infants of ages only partially falling within those of the special risk group, i.e. less than 3 months (1,5,12,17).

## Carcinogenicity

Nitrite was shown to react with nitrosatable compounds in the human stomach to form *N*-nitroso compounds, most of which have been found to be carcinogenic in all the animal species tested, so that they are probably also carcinogenic to humans, although data from a number of epidemiological studies are only suggestive. Nevertheless, a link between cancer risk and endogenous nitrosation as a result of high nitrate and/or nitrite intake is possible.

Several reviews of epidemiological studies have been published, most of which are geographical correlation studies relating estimated nitrate intake to gastric cancer risk. The US National Research Council found some suggestion of an association between high nitrate intake and gastric and/or oesophageal cancer (16). However, individual exposure data were lacking and several other plausible causes of gastric cancer were present. In a later WHO review (5), some of the earlier associations appeared to be weakened following the introduction of individual exposure data or after adjustment for socioeconomic factors. No convincing evidence was found of an association between gastric cancer and the consumption of drinking-water in which nitrate concentrations of up to 45 mg/litre were present. No firm evidence was found at higher levels either, but an association could not be excluded because of the inadequacy of the data available. More recent geographical correlation and occupational exposure studies also failed to demonstrate a clear relationship between nitrate intake and gastric cancer risk; however, a case–control study in Canada, in which dietary exposure to nitrate and nitrite was estimated in detail, showed that exogenous nitrite intake, largely from preserved meat, was significantly associated with the risk of developing gastric cancer (12).

It has been clearly established that the intake of certain dietary components present in vegetables, such as vitamins C and E, decreases the risk of gastric cancer. This is generally assumed to be at least partly due to the resulting decrease in the formation of N-nitroso compounds. It is possible that any effect of a high nitrate intake per se is masked in correlation studies by the antagonizing effects of simultaneously consumed dietary components. However, the absence of any link with cancer in occupational exposure is not in agreement with this theory.

The known increased risk of gastric cancer under conditions of low gastric acidity could be associated with the endogenous formation of N-nitroso compounds. High mean levels of N-nitroso compounds, as well as high nitrite levels, were found in the gastric juice of achlorhydric patients, who must therefore be considered as a special risk group for gastric cancer from the point of view of nitrate and nitrite intake (5,12,16,17).

### Other effects

Congenital malformations have been related to a high nitrate level in drinking-water in Australia; however, these observations were not confirmed. Other studies also failed to demonstrate a relationship between congenital malformations and nitrate intake (5,12).

Studies relating cardiovascular effects to nitrate levels in drinking-water gave inconsistent results (5).

Possible relationships between nitrate intake and effects on the thyroid have also been studied, as it is known that nitrate competitively inhibits iodine uptake.

However, there is no clear evidence that nitrate is an etiological factor in human goitre (5).

## 13.24.7 Guideline values

Experiments suggest that neither nitrate nor nitrite acts directly as a carcinogen in animals, but there is some concern about a possible increased risk of cancer in humans from the endogenous and exogenous formation of $N$-nitroso compounds, many of which are carcinogenic in animals. Suggestive evidence relating dietary nitrate exposure to cancer, especially gastric cancer, has been provided by geographical correlation or ecological epidemiological studies, but the results have not been confirmed by more definitive analytical studies. It must be recognized that many factors in addition to environmental nitrate exposure may be involved.

In summary, the epidemiological evidence for an association between dietary nitrate and cancer is insufficient, and the guideline value for nitrate in drinking-water is established solely to prevent methaemoglobinaemia, which depends on the conversion of nitrate to nitrite. Although bottle-fed infants of less than 3 months of age are most susceptible, occasional cases have been reported in some adult populations.

Extensive epidemiological data support the current guideline value for nitrate-nitrogen of 10 mg/litre. However, this value should not be expressed in terms of nitrate-nitrogen but as nitrate itself which is the chemical entity of health concern, and the guideline value for nitrate is therefore 50 mg/litre.

As a result of recent evidence of the presence of nitrite in some water supplies, it was concluded that a guideline value for nitrite should be proposed. However, the available animal studies are not appropriate for the establishment of a firm NOAEL for methaemoglobinaemia in rats. A pragmatic approach was therefore adopted in which a relative potency for nitrite and nitrate with respect to methaemoglobin formation of 10:1 (on a molar basis) was assumed. On this basis, a provisional guideline value for nitrite of 3 mg/litre is proposed. Because of the possibility of the simultaneous occurrence of nitrite and nitrate in drinking-water, the sum of the ratios of the concentrations of each to its guideline value should not exceed 1, i.e.:

$$\frac{C_{nitrite}}{GV_{nitrite}} + \frac{C_{nitrate}}{GV_{nitrate}} \leqslant 1$$

where $C$ = concentration
$GV$ = guideline value.

## References

1.  ICAIR Life Systems, Inc. *Drinking water criteria document on nitrate/nitrite, final draft.* Washington, DC, US Environmental Protection Agency, Office of Drinking Water, 1987.

2.  Van Duijvenbooden W, Matthijsen AJCM. *Integrated criteria document nitrate.* Bilthoven, Netherlands, National Institute of Public Health and Environmental Protection, 1989 (Report no. 758473012).

3.  Office of Drinking Water. *Estimated national occurrence and exposure to nitrate and nitrite in public drinking water supplies.* Washington, DC, US Environmental Protection Agency, 1987.

4.  Van Duijvenbooden W, Loch JPG. Nitrate in the Netherlands: a serious threat to groundwater. *Aqua*, 1983, 2:59-60.

5.  *Health hazards from nitrate in drinking water. Report on a WHO meeting, Copenhagen, 5-9 March 1984.* Copenhagen, WHO Regional Office for Europe, 1985 (Environmental Health Series, No. 1).

6.  International Organization for Standardization. *Water quality–determination of nitrate.* Geneva, 1986, 1988 (ISO 7890-1,2:1986; 3:1988).

7.  Prospero JM, Savoie DL. Effect of continental sources on nitrate concentrations over the Pacific Ocean. *Nature*, 1989, 339(6227):687-689.

8.  Janssen LHJM, Visser H, Roemer FG. Analysis of large scale sulphate, nitrate, chloride and ammonium concentrations in the Netherlands using an aerosol measuring network. *Atmospheric environment*, 1989, 23(12):2783-2796.

9.  Yocom JE. Indoor/outdoor air quality relationships: a critical review. *Journal of the Air Pollution Control Association*, 1982, 32:500-606.

10. Young CP, Morgan-Jones M. A hydrogeochemical survey of the chalk groundwater of the Banstead area, Surrey, with particular reference to nitrate. *Journal of the Institute of Water Engineers and Scientists*, 1980, 34:213-236.

11. Jacks G, Sharma VP. Nitrogen circulation and nitrate in ground water in an agricultural catchment in southern India. *Environmental geology*, 1983, 5(2):61-64.

12. European Chemical Industry Ecology and Toxicology Centre. *Nitrate and drinking water.* Brussels, 1988 (Technical Report No. 27).

13. Chilvers C, Inskip H, Caygill C. A survey of dietary nitrate in well-water users. *International journal of epidemiology*, 1984, 13:324-331.

14. *Guidelines for the study of dietary intake of chemical contaminants.* Geneva, World Health Organization, 1985 (WHO Offset Publication, No. 87).

15. Bartholomew B et al. Possible use of urinary nitrate as a measure of total nitrate intake. *Proceedings of the Nutrition Society*, 1979, 38:124a.

16. National Academy of Sciences. *The health effects of nitrate, nitrite and N-nitroso compounds. Part 1 of a two-part study by the Committee on Nitrite and Alternative Curing Agents in Food. Report by the US National Research Council.* Washington, DC, National Academy Press, 1981.

17. Speijers GJA et al. *Integrated criteria document nitrate–effects.* Bilthoven, The Netherlands, National Institute of Public Health and Environmental Protection, 1989 (Report no. 758473012).

18. Til HP et al. Evaluation of the oral toxicity of potassium nitrite in a 13-week drinking-water study in rats. *Food chemistry and toxicology*, 1988, 26(10):851-859.

19. Craun GF, Greathouse DG, Gunderson DH. Methemoglobin levels in young children consuming high nitrate well water in the United States. *International journal of epidemiology*, 1981, 10:309-317.

20. Walton G. Survey of literature relating to infant methemoglobinemia due to nitrate-contaminated water. *American journal of public health*, 1951, 41:986-996.

## 13.25 Dissolved oxygen

### 13.25.1 Organoleptic properties

Depletion of dissolved oxygen in water supplies can encourage the microbial reduction of nitrate to nitrite and sulfate to sulfide, giving rise to odour problems. It can also cause an increase in the concentration of iron(II) in solution. Water containing dissolved oxygen at below 80–85% saturation has been reported to lead to an increase in the incidence of consumer complaints relating particularly to colour (resulting from the corrosion of metal pipes) (*1*).

### 13.25.2 Analytical methods

The two commonly used methods of measuring oxygen concentrations in water are the iodometric method and the electrochemical probe or dissolved oxygen meter (*2, 3*).

### 13.25.3 Environmental levels

#### Water

The amount of dissolved oxygen present in water depends on the latter's physical and chemical characteristics (particularly temperature and salinity). The saturation concentration of dissolved oxygen decreases as the temperature and salinity increase. In fresh water at 5, 10, and 20 °C, the saturation concentrations are 12.8, 11.3, and 9.1 mg/litre, respectively (2).

## 13.25.6 Effects on humans

There are no reported health effects arising directly from a deficiency of dissolved oxygen in potable water or from its complete absence. Indirect effects may result from organoleptic problems, from exposure to high concentrations of corrosion products (e.g. iron, cadmium, lead, zinc), and from anaerobic conditions (see the section on hydrogen sulfide).

## 13.25.5 Conclusions

The dissolved oxygen content of water is influenced by the raw water temperature, composition, treatment, and any chemical or biological processes taking place in the distribution system. A dissolved oxygen content substantially lower than its saturation concentration may indicate that undesirable processes are occurring, which may adversely affect water quality. It is therefore desirable that dissolved oxygen levels be maintained as near saturation as possible. No health-based guideline value is recommended.

## References

1. Ridgway J. *WHO drinking water guidelines revision: organoleptic aspects of drinking water quality.* Medmenham, Water Research Centre, 1981 (WRC Report ER 403-M).

2. International Organization for Standardization. *Water quality–determination of dissolved oxygen–iodometric method.* Geneva, 1983 (ISO 5813:1983).

3. International Organization for Standardization. *Water quality–determination of dissolved oxygen–electrochemical probe method.* Geneva, 1990 (ISO 5814:1990).

## 13.26 pH

### 13.26.1 General description

The pH of a solution is the negative common logarithm of the hydrogen ion activity:

$$pH = -\log (H^+)$$

In dilute solutions, the hydrogen ion activity is approximately equal to the hydrogen ion concentration.

The pH of water is a measure of the acid–base equilibrium and, in most natural waters, is controlled by the carbon dioxide–bicarbonate–carbonate equilibrium system. An increased carbon dioxide concentration will therefore lower pH, whereas a decrease will cause it to rise. Temperature will also affect the equilibria and the pH. In pure water, a decrease in pH of about 0.45 occurs as the temperature is raised by 25 °C. In water with a buffering capacity imparted by bicarbonate, carbonate, and hydroxyl ions, this temperature effect is modified. The pH of most raw water lies within the range 6.5–8.5 (*1*).

## 13.26.2 Analytical methods

The pH of an aqueous sample is usually measured electrometrically with a glass electrode. Temperature has a significant effect on pH measurement (*1, 2*).

## 13.26.3 Relationship with water-quality parameters

The pH is of major importance in determining the corrosivity of water. In general, the lower the pH, the higher the level of corrosion. However, pH is only one of a variety of factors affecting corrosion (*3–8*).

## 13.26.4 Effects on laboratory animals

When solutions differing in pH were injected into the abdominal skin of mice, skin irritation was manifested at pH 10 after 6 h (*9*). In the rabbit, intracutaneous skin irritation was observed above pH 9.0 (*9*). In addition, a pH above 10 has been reported to be an irritant to the eyes of rabbits (*9*). No significant eye effects were reported in rabbits exposed to water of pH 4.5 (*10*).

## 13.26.5 Effects on humans

Exposure to extreme pH values results in irritation to the eyes, skin, and mucous membranes. Eye irritation and exacerbation of skin disorders have been associated with pH values greater than 11. In addition, solutions of pH 10–12.5 have been reported to cause hair fibres to swell (*10*). In sensitive individuals, gastrointestinal irritation may also occur. Exposure to low pH values can also result in similar effects. Below pH 4, redness and irritation of the eyes have been reported, the severity of which increases with decreasing pH. Below pH 2.5, damage to the epithelium is irreversible and extensive (*10*). In addition, because pH can affect the degree of corrosion of metals as well as disinfection efficiency, it may have an indirect effect on health.

## 13.26.6 Conclusions

Although pH usually has no direct impact on water consumers, it is one of the most important operational water-quality parameters. Careful attention to pH control is necessary at all stages of water treatment to ensure satisfactory water clarification and disinfection. For effective disinfection with chlorine, the pH should preferably be less than 8. The pH of the water entering the distribution system must be controlled to minimize the corrosion of water mains and pipes in household water systems. Failure to do so can result in the contamination of drinking-water and in adverse effects on its taste, odour, and appearance.

The optimum pH will vary in different supplies according to the composition of the water and the nature of the construction materials used in the distribution system, but is often in the range 6.5–9.5. Extreme pH values can result from accidental spills, treatment breakdowns, and insufficiently cured cement mortar pipe linings.

No health-based guideline value is proposed for pH.

## References

1.  American Public Health Association. *Standard methods for the examination of water and wastewater*, 17th ed. Washington, DC, 1989.

2.  *The measurement of electrical conductivity and laboratory determination of the pH value of natural, treated and wastewaters.* London, Her Majesty's Stationery Office, 1978.

3.  Nordberg GF, Goyer RA, Clarkson TW. Impact of effects of acid precipitation on toxicity of metals. *Environmental health perspectives*, 1985, 68:169-180.

4.  McClanahan MA, Mancy KH. Effect of pH on the quality of calcium carbonate film deposited from moderately hard and hard water. *Journal of the American Water Works Association*, 1974, 66(1):49-53.

5.  Langelier WF. Chemical equilibria in water treatment. *Journal of the American Water Works Association*, 1946, 38(2):169-178.

6.  Webber JS, Covey JR, King MV. Asbestos in drinking water supplied through grossly deteriorated A-C pipe. *Journal of the American Water Works Association*, 1989, 81(2):80-85.

7.  Murrel NE. Impact of metal solders on water quality. In: *Proceedings of the Annual Conference of the American Water Works Association*, Part 1, Denver, CO, AWWA, 1987:39-43.

8.  Stone A et al. The effects of short-term changes in water quality on copper and zinc corrosion rates. *Journal of the American Water Works Association*, 1987, 79(2):75-82.

9. Rose P. *Alkaline pH and health: a review prepared for the Water Research Centre.* Medmenham, Water Research Centre, 1986 (Water Research Centre Report No. LR 1178-M).

10. World Health Organization Working Group. Health impact of acidic deposition. *Science of the total environment,* 1986, 52:157-187.

## 13.27 Selenium

### 13.27.1 General description

#### Identity

Selenium is present in the earth's crust, often in association with sulfur-containing minerals. It can assume four oxidation states (-2, 0, +4, +6) and occurs in many forms, including elemental selenium, selenites and selenates (*1*).

#### Physicochemical properties (1)

| Property | Value |
|---|---|
| Physical state | Grey metallic/red amorphous powder or vitreous form |
| Boiling point | 685 °C |
| Water solubility | Insoluble |

#### Organoleptic properties

Many selenium compounds are odoriferous, some having an odour of garlic (*1*).

#### Environmental fate

Acid and reducing conditions reduce inorganic selenites to elemental selenium, whereas alkaline and oxidizing conditions favour the formation of selenates. Selenites and selenates are usually soluble in water. Elemental selenium is insoluble in water and not rapidly reduced or oxidized in nature. In alkaline soils, selenium is present as water-soluble selenate and is available to plants; in acid soils, it is usually found as selenite bound to iron and aluminium oxides in compounds of very low solubility (*2*).

### 13.27.2 Analytical methods

Atomic absorption spectrometry with hydride generation is the most convenient method of determining selenium in drinking-water. If 10-ml samples are used for routine analysis, the detection limit is about 0.5 µg/litre. Lower levels can be determined if larger sample volumes are used (*3*).

## 13.27.3 Environmental levels and human exposure

### *Air*

The level of selenium (mostly bound to particles) in most urban air ranges from 0.1 to 10 ng/m$^3$, but higher levels may be found in certain areas, e.g. in the vicinity of copper smelters (*4*).

### *Water*

The levels of selenium in groundwater and surface water range from 0.06 to about 400 µg/litre (*5–7*); in some areas, levels in groundwater may approach 6000 µg/litre (*8*). Concentrations increase at high and low pH as a result of conversion into compounds of greater solubility in water. Levels of selenium in tapwater samples from public water supplies around the world are usually much less than 10 µg/litre (*9,10*). Drinking-water from a high-selenium area in China was reported to contain 50–160 µg/litre (*1*).

### *Food*

Vegetables and fruits are mostly low in selenium content (<0.01 mg/kg). Levels of selenium in meat and seafood are about 0.3–0.5 mg/kg. Grain and cereal products usually contain <0.01–0.67 mg/kg. Great variations in selenium content have been reported in China, where those of corn, rice, and soya beans in high- and low-selenium areas were 4–12 and 0.005–0.01 mg/kg, respectively (*1, 2*).

### *Estimated total exposure and relative contribution of drinking-water*

Foodstuffs constitute the main source of selenium for the general population. Daily dietary intake varies considerably according to geographical area, food supply, and dietary habits. Recommended daily intakes have been set at 1.7 µg/kg of body weight in infants and 0.9 µg/kg of body weight in adults (*11*).

Most drinking-water contains much less than 10 µg/litre, except in certain seleniferous areas. A level of 1 µg/litre corresponds to an intake of 2 µg of selenium per day. Thus, given an intake from food of about 60 µg/day, the relative contribution from drinking-water is small. Even in high-selenium areas, the relative contribution of selenium from drinking-water may be small in comparison with that from locally produced food (*1*).

The intake of selenium by the general population from air and smoking appears to be insignificant and has been estimated to be less than 1–2 µg/day (*12*).

## 13.27.4 Kinetics and metabolism in laboratory animals and humans

Most water-soluble selenium compounds and selenium from food are effectively absorbed in the gastrointestinal tract (*13*). Elemental selenium (*14*) and selenium sulfide (*15*) are poorly absorbed. After absorption, water-soluble selenium compounds appear to be rapidly distributed to most organs, the highest concentrations being in kidney, liver, spleen, and testes (*16,17*).

Selenium compounds are biotransformed into excretable metabolites, including unknown as well as methylated selenides and trimethylselenonium ion at higher doses (*1, 12, 13, 18*). Selenites may react with metals in the body to form metal selenides (*12*). Most (49–70%) selenium is excreted in urine (*19*). In humans, selenite is eliminated in three phases, with half-lives of 1, 8–20, and 100 days, respectively (*13*).

Selenium is an essential trace element for many species, including humans (*2, 11, 20*). It is incorporated into proteins via a specific selenocysteine tRNA with co-translational synthesis of selenocysteine from phosphoserine tRNA and inorganic selenium (*20, 21*). Selenium is found as selenocysteine in glutathione peroxidase (*2, 20*) and is incorporated into other proteins, such as tetraiodothyronine deiodinase and selenoprotein P (*20, 22, 23*). (-)-Selenomethionine from food is apparently nonspecifically incorporated into proteins in competition with (-)-methionine.

## 13.27.5 Effects on laboratory animals and *in vitro* test systems

### Acute exposure

Selenite, selenate, selenocysteine, and selenomethionine are highly toxic and kill laboratory animals in single doses of 1.5–6 mg/kg of body weight (*1,12*).

### Long-term exposure

Signs of selenium deficiency in many farm and laboratory animals include degenerative changes in several organs, growth retardation, and failure to reproduce (*2,24*).

In rats, 5 mg of selenium per kg of diet may result in growth reduction (*25, 26*). At a dietary level of 6.4 mg of selenium per kg (given as selenite), liver changes and splenomegaly occurred. At 8 mg of selenium per kg, anaemia, pancreatic enlargement, and increased mortality were observed (*25*). Based on growth retardation, apparently caused by reduced secretion of growth hormone from the anterior pituitary gland as a result of local selenium accumulation (*27*), a NOAEL of about 0.4 mg of selenium per kg of body weight per day was suggested. Hepatotoxic effects have also been described following dietary administration of selenium (*28, 29*). Based on both growth retardation and organ toxicity, a LOAEL of 0.03 mg/kg of body weight per day has been suggested.

The syndromes "blind staggers" and "alkali disease" have been described in livestock and are associated with the consumption of selenium in accumulator plants (*30*).

### Reproductive toxicity, embryotoxicity, and teratogenicity

Selenate, selenite, and the amino acids selenocysteine and selenomethionine are teratogenic in avian species (*31*) and fish (*32*). Teratogenicity has also been observed in sheep (*33*) and pigs (*34*). In recent studies on monkeys (*Macaca fascicularis*) fed selenomethionine (25, 150 or 300 µg/kg of body weight per day) during organogenesis, no signs of teratogenicity were observed (*35*).

Adverse effects of selenate (3 mg/litre in drinking-water) on reproduction in mice and rats have been reported (*36*), but there are also two negative reports on the effects of selenite in hamsters and mice (*37*). Only at doses associated with overt maternal poisoning and nutritional deprivation was evidence of seleno-methionine-induced embryonic or fetal toxicity observed in rabbits and hamsters (*38, 39*).

### Mutagenicity and related end-points

A weak base-pair substitution mutagenic activity has been demonstrated for both selenite and selenate in *Salmonella typhimurium* strain TA100 (*40,41*). Selenite, selenate, and selenide induced unscheduled DNA synthesis, sister chromatid exchange, and chromosomal aberrations in cell cultures *in vitro*, often in the presence of glutathione (*42–44*). In one *in vivo* study, chromosomal aberrations and increased sister chromatid exchange were seen in hamster bone marrow cells after selenite treatment, but only at toxic doses (*45*).

### Carcinogenicity

Early studies in which tumours were seen in test animals (*46,47*) have been seriously questioned because of study limitations (*48*), and several evaluators have found the data to be inconclusive. In two studies on mice, there was either no increase or a decrease in the incidence of tumours after the administration of selenite or selenate (3 mg of selenium per litre of drinking-water) (*49*) or selenium oxide (2 mg of selenium per litre of drinking-water) (*50*). Further data indicate an anticarcinogenic effect of selected selenium compounds. Viewed collectively, these data seem to show that the compounds studied will not act as carcinogens at low or moderate doses (*12*).

Selenium sulfide given by gavage resulted in hepatocellular carcinomas in rats and mice (*51*) but caused no increased incidence in tumours when applied to the skin of mice (*52*).

## 13.27.6 Effects on humans

In humans, few reports of clinical signs of selenium deficiency are available. It has been suggested that it may be a factor in endemic cardiomyopathia (Keshan disease) and possibly also in the joint and muscle disease (Kaschin-Beck disease) in the Keshan region of China (1,12).

Acute oral doses of selenite and other selenium compounds cause symptoms such as nausea, diarrhoea, abdominal pain, chills, tremor, numbness in limbs, irregular menstrual bleeding, and marked hair loss (12,53).

High dietary intakes of selenium have been investigated in selenium-rich areas of South Dakota, USA. Symptoms in people with high urinary selenium levels included gastrointestinal disturbances, discoloration of the skin, and decayed teeth (54).

Children living in a seleniferous area in Venezuela exhibited more pathological nail changes, loss of hair, and dermatitis than those living in Caracas (55). Based on Chinese data on blood level–intake relationships (56), their estimated daily intake was about 0.66 mg of selenium. However, the groups concerned differed nutritionally in several ways.

In China, endemic selenium intoxication has been studied by Yang and colleagues (57). Morbidity was 49% among 248 inhabitants of five villages where the daily intake was about 5 mg of selenium. The main symptoms were brittle hair with intact follicles, lack of pigment in new hair, thickened and brittle nails, and skin lesions. Symptoms of neurological disturbances were observed in 18 of the 22 inhabitants of one heavily affected village only. Those affected recovered once diets were changed following evacuation from the areas concerned.

In a follow-up study, Yang et al. studied a population of about 400 individuals with average daily intakes ranging from 62 to 1438 µg (56, 58). Clinical signs of selenosis (hair or nail loss, nail abnormalities, mottled teeth, skin lesions, and changes in peripheral nerves) were observed in 5 of 439 adults having a mean blood selenium of 1346 µg/litre, corresponding to a daily intake of 1260 µg of selenium. A decrease in prothrombin time and in the concentration of glutathione in blood were seen at dietary intakes exceeding 750–850 µg.

In a recent study, 142 subjects from geographical areas where the average selenium intake was 239 µg/day (68–724 µg/day) were examined over 2 years (59) An association between selenium intake and alanine aminotransferase (ALAT) levels in serum was observed but considered to be clinically insignificant. None of the effects, including nail abnormalities, were related to selenium intake.

One case of selenium toxicity directly attributable to a water source has been reported. A family was exposed for about 3 months to well-water containing 9 mg of selenium per litre. They suffered from loss of hair, weakened nails, and mental symptoms, but recovered when they stopped using the water from the well concerned (33).

Two individuals received about 350 and 600 µg of selenium per day via diet and selenium-containing yeast for 18 months. Marginal haematological changes and a borderline increase in ALAT levels were seen (*60*). In a small group of patients with rheumatoid arthritis receiving daily supplements of 256 µg of selenium in selenium-enriched yeast in addition to selenium from food for 6 months, levels of selenium in serum and erythrocytes were increased considerably in comparison with those in a group receiving placebo (*61*).

## 13.27.7 Guideline value

Except for selenium sulfide, which does not occur in drinking-water, selenium does not appear to be carcinogenic. IARC has placed selenium and selenium compounds in Group 3 (*62*). Selenium compounds have been shown to be genotoxic in *in vitro* systems with metabolic activation. There was no evidence of teratogenic effects in monkeys. Long-term exposure in rats may result in growth retardation and liver pathology.

In humans, the toxic effects of long-term selenium exposure are manifested in nails, hair, and liver. Data from China indicate that clinical and biochemical (decreased liver prothrombin synthesis) signs occur at a daily intake above 0.8 mg. Daily intakes by Venezuelan children with clinical signs were estimated at about 0.66 mg on the basis of their blood levels and the Chinese data on the relationships between blood level and intake. Effects on the synthesis of a liver protein were also seen in a small group of patients with rheumatoid arthritis given selenium at a rate of 0.25 mg/day (total daily intake from all sources about 0.35 mg). No clinical or biochemical signs of selenium toxicity were reported in a group of 142 persons with a mean daily intake of 0.24 mg (maximum 0.72 mg) from food. However, the liver enzyme ALAT was positively correlated within reference values with selenium intake.

On the basis of these data, the NOAEL in humans was estimated to be about 4 µg/kg of body weight per day, on the assumption that soluble selenium salts in drinking-water may be more toxic than organic-bound selenium in food. The recommended daily intake of selenium is 0.9 µg/kg of body weight for adults. An allocation of 10% of the NOAEL in humans to drinking-water gives a health-based guideline value of 0.01 mg/litre (rounded figure).

## References

1. *Selenium.* Geneva, World Health Organization, 1987 (Environmental Health Criteria, No. 58).

2. National Research Council. *Selenium in nutrition.* Washington, DC, National Academy Press, 1983.

3. Verlinden M, Deelstra H, Adriaenssens E. The determination of selenium by atomic absorption spectrometry: a review. *Talanta*, 1981, 28:637.

4. Zoller WH, Reamer DC. Selenium in the atmosphere. In: *Proceedings of the Symposium on Selenium and Tellurium in the Environment.* Pittsburgh, PA, Industrial Health Foundation, 1976:54-66.

5. Lindberg P. Selenium determination in plant and animal material, and in water. *Acta veterinaria Scandinavica*, 1968, Suppl. 23.

6. Smith MJ, Westfall BB. Further field studies on the selenium problem in relation to public health. *US public health report*, 1937, 52:1375-1384.

7. Scott RC, Voegeli PT Jr. *Radiochemical analysis of ground and surface water in Colorado.* Boulder, Colorado Water Conservation Board, 1961 (Basic Data Report 7).

8. Cannon HG. *Geochemistry of rocks and related soils and vegetation in the Yellow Cat area, Grand County, Utah.* Washington, DC, US Geological Survey, 1964 (Bulletin No. 1176).

9. National Academy of Sciences. *Selenium.* Washington, DC, 1976.

10. National Academy of Sciences. *Drinking water and health.* Washington, DC, 1977.

11. National Research Council. *Recommended dietary allowances*, 10th ed. Washington, DC, National Academy Press, 1989.

12. Högberg J, Alexander J. Selenium. In: Friberg L, Nordberg GF, Vouk VB, eds. *Handbook on the toxicology of metals*, Vol. 2, 2nd ed. Amsterdam, Elsevier, 1986:482-520.

13. Bopp BA, Sonders RC, Kesterson JW. Metabolic fate of selected selenium compounds in laboratory animals and man. *Drug metabolism reviews*, 1982, 13:271-318.

14. Medinsky MA. A simulation model describing the metabolism of inhaled and ingested selenium compounds. *Toxicology and applied pharmacology*, 1981, 59:54-63.

15. Cummins LM, Kimura ET. Safety evaluation of selenium sulfide antidandruff shampoos. *Toxicology and applied pharmacology*, 1971, 20:89-96.

16. Brown DG, Burk RF. Selenium retention in tissues and sperm of rats fed a torula yeast diet. *Journal of nutrition*, 1973, 103:102-108.

17. Thomassen Y, Aaseth J. Selenium in human tissues. In: Ihnat M, ed. *Occurrence and distribution of selenium.* Boca Raton, FL, CRC Press, 1986.

18. Palmer IS, Olson OE. Relative toxicities of selenite and selenate in the drinking-water of rats. *Journal of nutrition*, 1974, 104:306-314.

19. Levander OA. Selenium in foods. In: *Proceedings of the Symposium on Selenium and Tellurium in the Environment.* Pittsburgh, PA, Industrial Health Foundation, 1976:26-53.

20. Böck A et al. Selenoprotein synthesis: an expansion of the genetic code. *Trends in biochemical science*, 1991, 16:463-467.

21. Mullenbach GT et al. Selenocysteine's mechanism of incorporation and evolution revealed in cDNAs of three glutathione peroxidases. *Protein engineering*, 1988, 2:239-246.

22. Yang JG, Hill KE, Burk RF. Dietary selenium intake controls rat plasma selenoprotein P concentration. *Journal of nutrition*, 1989, 119:1010-1012.

23. Deagen JT, Beilstein MA, Whanger PD. Chemical forms of selenium in selenium containing proteins from human plasma. *Journal of inorganic biochemistry*, 1991, 41:261-268.

24. Diplock AT. Metabolic aspects of selenium action and toxicity. *CRC critical reviews in toxicology*, 1976, 4(3):271-329.

25. Halverson AW, Palmer IS, Guss PL. Toxicity of selenium to post-weanling rats. *Toxicology and applied pharmacology*, 1966, 9:477-484.

26. Ip C. Prophylaxis of mammary neoplasia by selenium supplementation in the initiation and promotion phases of chemical carcinogenesis. *Cancer research*, 1981, 41:4386-4390.

27. Thorlacius-Ussing O. Selenium-induced growth retardation. *Danish medical bulletin*, 1990, 37:347-358.

28. Harr JR, Muth OH. Selenium poisoning in domestic animals and its relationship to man. *Clinical toxicology*, 1972, 5:175-186.

29. Harr JR et al., Selenium toxicity in rats. II. Histopathology. In: Muth OH et al, ed. *Selenium in biomedicine*. Westport, CT, AVI Publishing, 1967:153-178.

30. Shamberger RJ. *Biochemistry of selenium*. New York, NY, Plenum Press, 1983.

31. Hoffman DJ, Ohlendorf HM, Aldrich TW. Selenium teratogenesis in natural populations of aquatic birds in central California. *Archives of environmental contamination and toxicology*, 1988, 17:519-525.

32. Birge WJ et al. Fish and amphibian embryos–a model system for evaluating teratogenicity. *Fundamental and applied toxicology*, 1983, 3:237-242.

33. Rosenfeld I, Beath OA. *Selenium, geobotany, biochemistry, toxicity and nutrition*. New York, NY, Academic Press, 1964.

34. Wahlström RC, Olson OG. The effect of selenium on reproduction in swine. *Journal of animal science*, 1959, 18:141-145.

35. Tarantal AF et al. Developmental toxicity of L-selenomethionine in *Macaca fascicularis. Fundamental and applied toxicology*, 1991, 16:147-160.

36. Schroeder HA, Mitchener M. Selenium and tellurium in rats: effect on growth, survival and tumors. *Journal of nutrition*, 1971, 101:1531-1540.

37. Nobunaga T, Satoh H, Suzuki T. Effects of sodium selenite on methyl mercury embryotoxicity and teratogenicity in mice. *Toxicology and applied pharmacology*, 1979, 47:79-88.

38. Berschneider F et al. [Fetal and maternal damage to rabbits following application of sodium selenite, injectable Ursoselevit, and Ursoselevit premix.] *Monatshefte für Veterinärmedizin*, 1977, 8:299-304 (in German).

39. Ferm VH et al. Embryotoxicity and dose-response relationships of selenium in hamsters. *Reproductive toxicology*, 1990, 4:183-190.

40. Löfroth G, Ames BN. Mutagenicity of inorganic compounds in *Salmonella typhimurium*: arsenic, chromium, and selenium. *Mutation research*, 1978, 53:65-66.

41. Noda M, Takano T, Sakurai H. Mutagenic activity of selenium compounds. *Mutation research*, 1979, 66:175-179.

42. Khalil AM. The induction of chromosome aberrations in human purified peripheral blood lymphocytes following *in vitro* exposure to selenium. *Mutation research*, 1989, 224:503-506.

43. Ray JH, Altenburg LC. Sister-chromatid exchange induction by sodium selenite: dependence on the presence of red blood cells or red blood cell lysate. *Mutation research*, 1978, 54:343-354.

44. Whiting RF, Wei L, Stich HF. Unscheduled DNA synthesis and chromosome aberrations induced by inorganic and organic selenium compounds in the presence of glutathione. *Mutation research*, 1980, 78:159-169.

45. Norppa H, Westermark T, Knuutila S. Chromosomal effects of sodium selenite *in vivo. Hereditas*, 1980, 93:101-105.

46. Inne JR et al. Bioassay of pesticides and industrial chemicals for tumorigenicity in mice: a preliminary note. *Journal of the National Cancer Institute*, 1969, 42:1101-1114.

47. Volgarev MN, Tscherkes LA. Further studies in tissue changes associated with sodium selenate. In: Muth OH et al., ed. *Selenium in biomedicine*. Westport, CT, AVI Publishing, 1967:179-184.

48. International Agency for Research on Cancer. *Some aziridines, N-, S- and O-mustards and selenium.* Lyon, 1975:245-259 (IARC Monographs on the Evaluation of the Carcinogenic Risk of Chemicals to Man, Volume 9).

49. Schroeder HA, Mitchener M. Selenium and tellurium in mice. Effects on growth, survival, and tumours. *Archives of environmental health,* 1972, 24:66-71.

50. Schrauzer GN, Ishmael D. Effects of selenium and of arsenic on the genesis of spontaneous mammary tumors in inbred C$_3$H mice. *Annals of clinical laboratory science,* 1974, 4:441-447.

51. *Bioassay of selenium sulfide for possible carcinogenicity (gavage study).* Bethesda, MD, US Department of Health and Human Services, National Cancer Institute, 1980 (Technical Report Series 194).

52. *Bioassay of selenium sulfide for possible carcinogenicity (dermal study).* Bethesda, MD, US Department of Health and Human Services, National Cancer Institute, 1980 (Technical Report Series 197).

53. Sioris LJ, Cuthrie K, Pentel PR. Acute selenium poisoning. *Veterinary and human toxicology,* 1980, 22:364.

54. Smith MJ, Westfall BB. Further field studies on the selenium problem in relation to public health. *US public health report,* 1937, 52:1375-1384.

55. Jaffe WG. Effect of selenium intake in humans and in rats. In: *Proceedings of the Symposium on Selenium and Tellurium in the Environment.* Pittsburgh, PA, Industrial Health Foundation, 1976:188-193.

56. Yang G et al. Studies of safe maximal daily dietary selenium intake in a seleniferous area in China. Part I. *Journal of trace elements and electrolytes in health and disease,* 1989, 3:77-87.

57. Yang GQ et al. Endemic selenium intoxication of humans in China. *American journal of clinical nutrition,* 1983, 37:872-881.

58. Yang G et al. Studies of safe maximal daily dietary selenium intake in a seleniferous area in China. Part II. *Journal of trace elements and electrolytes in health and disease,* 1989, 3:123-130.

59. Longnecker MP et al. Selenium in diet, blood and toenails in relation to human health in a seleniferous area. *American journal of clinical nutrition,* 1991, 53:1288-1294.

60. Schrauzer GN, White DA. Selenium in human nutrition: dietary intakes and effects of supplementation. *Bioinorganic chemistry,* 1978, 8:303-318.

61. Tarp U et al. Selenium treatment in rheumatoid arthritis. *Scandinavian journal of rheumatology*, 1985, 14(4):364-368.

62. International Agency for Research on Cancer. *Overall evaluations of carcinogenicity: an updating of IARC monographs volumes 1-42.* Lyon, 1987:71 (IARC Monographs on the Evaluation of Carcinogenic Risks to Humans, Suppl. 7).

## 13.28 Silver

### 13.28.1 General description

#### *Identity*

Silver (CAS no. 7440-22-4) is present in silver compounds primarily in the oxidation state +1 and less frequently in the oxidation state +2. A higher degree of oxidation is very rare. The most important silver compounds from the point of view of drinking-water are silver nitrate ($AgNO_3$, CAS no. 7761-88-8) and silver chloride (AgCl, CAS no. 7783-90-6).

#### *Physicochemical properties (1)*

| Property | $AgNO_3$ | AgCl |
|---|---|---|
| Colour | White | White, darkens when exposed to light |
| Melting point (°C) | 212 | 455 |
| Water solubility at 25°C (g/litre) | 2150 | 0.00186 |

#### *Major uses*

The electrical and thermal conductivity of silver are higher than those of other metals. Important alloys are formed with copper, mercury, and other metals. Silver is used in the form of its salts, oxides, and halides in photographic materials and alkaline batteries, or as the element in electrical equipment, hard alloys, mirrors, chemical catalysts, coins, table silver, and jewellery. Soluble silver compounds may be used as external antiseptic agents (15–50 µg/litre), as bacteriostatic agents (up to 100 µg/litre), and as disinfectants (>150 µg/litre) (2).

#### *Environmental fate*

Silver occurs in soil mainly in the form of its insoluble and therefore immobile chloride or sulfide. As long as the sulfide is not oxidized to the sulfate, its mobility and ability to contaminate the aquatic environment are negligible. Silver in river water is "dissolved" by complexation with chloride and humic matter (3).

## 13.28.2 Analytical methods

The detection limit of the spectrographic and colorimetric method with dithizone is 10 µg of silver per litre for a 20-ml sample. The detection limit of atomic absorption spectroscopy (graphite furnace) is 2 µg of silver per litre, and of neutron activation analysis, 2 ng of silver per litre (*4*).

## 13.28.3 Environmental levels and human exposure

### Air

Ambient air concentrations of silver are in the low nanogram per cubic metre range (*5*).

### Water

Average silver concentrations in natural waters are 0.2–0.3 µg/litre. Silver levels in drinking-water in the USA that had not been treated with silver for disinfection purposes varied between "non-detectable" and 5 µg/litre. In a survey of Canadian tapwater, only 0.1% of the samples contained more than 1–5 ng of silver per litre (*5*). Water treated with silver may have levels of 50 µg/litre or higher (*4*); most of the silver will be present as nondissociated silver chloride.

### Food

Most foods contain traces of silver in the 10–100 µg/kg range (*6*).

### Estimated total exposure and relative contribution of drinking-water

The median daily intake of silver from 84 self-selected diets, including drinking-water, was 7.1 µg (*6*). Higher figures have been reported in the past, ranging from 20 to 80 µg of silver per day (*7*). The relative contribution of drinking-water is usually very low. Where silver salts are used as bacteriostatic agents, however, the daily intake of silver from drinking-water can constitute the major route of oral exposure.

## 13.28.4 Kinetics and metabolism in laboratory animals and humans

Silver may be absorbed via the gastrointestinal tract, lungs, mucous membranes, and skin lesions (*5*). The absorption rate of colloidal silver after oral application can be as high as 5% (*8*). Most of the silver transported in blood is bound to globulins (*5*). In tissues, it is present in the cytosolic fraction, bound to metallothionein (*9*). Silver is stored mainly in liver and skin and in smaller amounts in other organs (*5, 10*). The biological half-life in humans (liver) ranges from several to 50 days (*9*).

The liver plays a decisive role in silver excretion, most of what is absorbed being excreted with the bile in the faeces. In mice, rats, monkeys, and dogs, cumulative excretion was in the range 90–99%. Silver retention was about 10% in the dog, <5% in the monkey, and <1% in rodents (*10*). In humans, under normal conditions of daily silver exposure, retention rates between 0 and 10% have been observed (*5*).

## 13.28.5 Effects on laboratory animals and *in vitro* test systems

### Acute exposure

Oral $LD_{50}$ values between 50 and 100 mg/kg of body weight have been observed for different silver salts in mice (*11*).

### Short-term exposure

Hypoactive behaviour was observed in mice that had received 4.5 mg of silver per kg of body weight per day for 125 days (*12*).

### Long-term exposure

After 218 days of exposure, albino rats receiving approximately 60 mg of silver per kg of body weight per day via their drinking-water exhibited a slight greyish pigmentation of the eyes, which later intensified (*13*). Increased pigmentation of different organs, including the eye, was also observed in Osborne-Mendel rats after lifetime exposure to the same dose (*14*). Antagonistic effects between silver and selenium, involving the selenium-containing enzyme glutathione peroxidase, were observed in Holtzman rats (*15*).

### Mutagenicity and related end-points

In the *rec*-assay with *Bacillus subtilis*, there were no indications that silver chloride was mutagenic (*16*). Reverse mutations in *Escherichia coli* were not induced by silver nitrate (*17*). In the DNA repair test with cultivated rat hepatocytes, silver nitrate solution was positive only at a moderately toxic concentration (*18*). Silver nitrate increased the transformation rate of SA7-infected embryonic cells of Syrian hamsters (*19*).

### Carcinogenicity

Silver dust suspended in trioctanoin injected intramuscularly into Fischer 344 rats of both sexes was not carcinogenic (*20*).

## 13.28.6 Effects on humans

The estimated acute lethal dose of silver nitrate is at least 10 g (*21*).

The only known clinical picture of chronic silver intoxication is that of argyria, a condition in which silver is deposited on skin and hair, and in various organs following occupational or iatrogenic exposure to metallic silver and its compounds, or the misuse of silver preparations. Pigmentation of the eye is considered the first sign of generalized argyria (*21*). Striking discoloration, which occurs particularly in areas of the skin exposed to light, is attributed to the photochemical reduction of silver in the accumulated silver compounds, mainly silver sulfide. Melanin production has also been stimulated in some cases (*22, 23*).

It is difficult to determine the lowest dose that may lead to the development of argyria. A patient who developed a grey pigmentation in the face and on the neck after taking an unknown number of anti-smoking pills containing silver ethanoate was found to have a total body silver content of 6.4 ± 2 g (*22*). It has been reported that intravenous administration of only 4.1 g of silver arsphenamine (about 0.6 g of silver) can lead to argyria (*24*). Other investigators concluded that the lowest intravenous dose of silver arsphenamine causing argyria in syphilis patients was 6.3 g (about 0.9 g of silver) (*21*). It should be noted that syphilis patients suffering from argyria were often already in a bad state of health and had been treated with bismuth, mercury, or arsphenamine in addition to silver.

## 13.28.7 Conclusions

Argyria has been described in syphilitic patients in poor health who were therapeutically dosed with a total of about 1 g of silver in the form of silver arsphenamine together with other toxic metals. There have been no reports of argyria or other toxic effects resulting from the exposure of healthy persons to silver.

On the basis of present epidemiological and pharmacokinetic knowledge, a total lifetime oral intake of about 10 g of silver can be considered as the human NOAEL. As the contribution of drinking-water to this NOAEL will normally be negligible, the establishment of a health-based guideline value is not deemed necessary. On the other hand, special situations may exist where silver salts are used to maintain the bacteriological quality of drinking-water. Higher levels of silver, up to 0.1 mg/litre (a concentration that gives a total dose over 70 years of half the human NOAEL of 10 g), could then be tolerated without risk to health.

## References

1. Holleman AF, Wiberg E. *Lehrbuch der anorganischen Chemie.* [*Textbook of inorganic chemistry.*] Berlin, Walter de Gruyter, 1985.

2. National Academy of Sciences. *Drinking water and health.* Washington, DC, 1977:289-292.

3. Whitlow SI, Rice DL. Silver complexation in river waters of central New York. *Water research*, 1985, 19:619-626.

4. Fowler BA, Nordberg GF. Silver. In: Friberg L, Nordberg GF, Vouk VB, eds. *Handbook on the toxicology of metals.* Amsterdam, Elsevier, 1986:521-531.

5. US Environmental Protection Agency. *Ambient water quality criteria for silver.* Washington, DC, 1980 (EPA 440/5-80-071).

6. Gibson RS, Scythes CA. Chromium, selenium and other trace element intake of a selected sample of Canadian premenopausal women. *Biological trace element research*, 1984, 6:105.

7. National Academy of Sciences. *Drinking water and health*, Vol. 4. Washington, DC, 1982.

8. Dequidt J, Vasseur P, Gromez-Potentier J. Étude toxicologique expérimentale de quelques dérivés argentiques. 1. Localisation et élimination. *Bulletin de la Société de Pharmacie de Lille*, 1974, 1:23-35 (cited in reference 5).

9. Nordberg GF, Gerhardsson L. Silver. In: Seiler HG, Sigel H, Sigel A, eds. *Handbook on the toxicity of inorganic compounds.* New York, NY, Marcel Dekker, 1988:619-624.

10. Furchner JE, Richmond GR, Drake GA. Comparative metabolism of radionuclides in mammals. IV. Retention of silver-110m in the mouse, rat, monkey, and dog. *Health physics*, 1968, 15:505-514.

11. Goldberg AA, Shapiro M, Wilder E. Antibacterial colloidal electrolytes: the potentiation of the activities of mercuric-, phenylmercuric- and silver ions by a colloidal sulphonic anion. *Journal of pharmacy and pharmacology*, 1950, 2:20-26.

12. Rungby J, Danscher G. Hypoactivity in silver exposed mice. *Acta pharmacologica et toxicologica*, 1984, 55:398-401.

13. Olcott CT. Experimental argyrosis. V. Hypertrophy of the left ventricle of the heart. *Archives of pathology*, 1950, 49:138-149.

14. Olcott CT. Experimental argyrosis. III. Pigmentation of the eyes of rats following ingestion of silver during long periods of time. *American journal of pathology*, 1947, 23:783-789.

15. Wagner PA, Hoekstra WG, Ganther HE. Alleviation of silver toxicity by selenite in the rat in relation to tissue glutathione peroxidase. *Proceedings of the Society of Experimental Biology and Medicine*, 1975, 148:1106-1110.

16. Nishioka H. Mutagenic activities of metal compounds in bacteria. *Mutation research*, 1975, 31:185-189.

17. Demerec M, Bertani G, Flint J. A survey of chemicals for mutagenic action on *E. coli*. *The American naturalist*, 1951, 85:119-136.

18. Denizeau F, Marion M. Genotoxic effects of heavy metals in rat hepatocytes. *Cell biology and toxicology*, 1989, 5:15-25.

19. Casto BC, Meyers J, DiPaolo JA. Enhancement of viral transformation for evaluation of the carcinogenic or mutagenic potential of inorganic salts. *Cancer research*, 1979, 39:193-198.

20. Furst A, Schlauder MC. Inactivity of two noble metals as carcinogens. *Journal of environmental pathology and toxicology*, 1977, 1:51-57.

21. Hill WR, Pillsbury DM. *Argyria, the pharmacology of silver*. Baltimore, MD, Williams and Wilkins, 1939 (cited in reference 5).

22. East BW et al. Silver retention, total body silver and tissue silver concentrations in argyria associated with exposure to an anti-smoking remedy containing silver acetate. *Clinical and experimental dermatology*, 1980, 5:305-311.

23. Westhofen M, Schäfer H. Generalized argyrosis in man: neurological, ultrastructural and X-ray microanalytic findings. *Archives of otorhinolaryngology*, 1986, 243:260-264.

24. Gaul LE, Staud AH. Clinical spectroscopy. Seventy cases of generalized argyrosis following organic and colloidal silver medication. *Journal of the American Medical Association*, 1935, 104:1387-1390.

# 13.29 Sodium

## 13.29.1 General description

### *Identity*

| Compound | CAS no. | Molecular formula |
|---|---|---|
| Sodium | 7440-23-5 | Na |
| Sodium chloride | 7647-14-7 | NaCl |
| Sodium carbonate | 492-19-8 | $Na_2CO_3$ |
| Sodium hypochlorite | 7681-52-9 | NaOCl |
| Sodium metasilicate | 1344-09-8 | $Na_2SiO_3$ |

### Physicochemical properties *(1–5)*

| Property | Na | NaCl | $Na_2CO_3$ | NaOCl | $Na_2SiO_3$ |
|---|---|---|---|---|---|
| Melting point (°C) | 97.83 | 801 | 851 | – | – |
| Boiling point (°C) | 886 | 1413 | decomposes | – | – |
| Density at 20 °C (g/cm³) | 0.71 | 2.17 | 2.53 | – | – |
| Vapour pressure (kPa) | 0.133 | – | – | – | – |
| Water solubility at 0°C (g/l) | reacts violently | 357 | 71 | infinitely soluble | soluble |

### Organoleptic properties

The taste threshold for sodium in water depends on the associated anion and the temperature of the solution. At room temperature, the threshold values are about 20 mg/litre for sodium carbonate, 150 mg/litre for sodium chloride, 190 mg/litre for sodium nitrate, 220 mg/litre for sodium sulfate, and 420 mg/litre for sodium bicarbonate *(6)*.

### Major uses

Metallic sodium is used in the manufacture of tetraethyl lead and sodium hydride, in titanium production, as a catalyst for synthetic rubber, as a laboratory reagent, as a coolant in nuclear reactors, in electric power cables, in non-glare lighting for roads, and as a heat-transfer medium in solar-powered electric generators *(3)*. Sodium salts are used in water treatment, including softening, disinfection, corrosion control, pH adjustment, and coagulation *(7)*, in road de-icing and in the paper, glass, soap, pharmaceutical, chemical, and food industries.

### Environmental fate

Sodium salts are generally highly soluble in water and are leached from the terrestrial environment to groundwater and surface water. They are nonvolatile and will thus be found in the atmosphere only in association with particulate matter.

## 13.29.2 Analytical methods

Sodium concentrations can be determined by direct aspiration atomic absorption spectroscopy *(8)*. Detection limits of 2 and 40 µg/litre can be achieved with flame atomic absorption spectrometry and inductively coupled plasma atomic emission spectrometry, respectively.

## 13.29.3 Environmental levels and human exposure

### Air

The sodium levels in ambient air are low in comparison with those in food or water.

### Water

The sodium ion is ubiquitous in water. Most water supplies contain less than 20 mg of sodium per litre, but in some countries levels can exceed 250 mg/litre. Saline intrusion, mineral deposits, seawater spray, sewage effluents, and salt used in road de-icing can all contribute significant quantities of sodium to water. In addition, water-treatment chemicals, such as sodium fluoride, sodium bicarbonate, and sodium hypochlorite, can together result in sodium levels as high as 30 mg/litre. Domestic water softeners can give levels of over 300 mg/litre, but much lower ones are usually found (6).

In a survey of 2100 water samples in the USA in 1963–1966, the sodium ion concentrations found were in the range 0.4–1900 mg/litre; in 42% of the samples, the concentrations were in excess of 20 mg/litre, but in 5% they were greater than 250 mg/litre. In a later survey of 630 water-supply systems in the same country, the sodium ion concentrations found ranged from less than 1 to 402 mg/litre, with similar distribution of values (9).

### Food

Sodium is naturally present in all foods and may be added during food processing. Fresh fruit and vegetables contain sodium at concentrations in the range <10–1000 mg/kg; cereals and cheese may contain as much as 10–20 g/kg; and human and cows' milk contains 180 and 770 mg/litre, respectively (6, 10).

### Estimated total exposure and relative contribution of drinking-water

Food is the main source of daily exposure to sodium, primarily as sodium chloride. The estimation of daily intake from food is difficult because of the wide variation in concentrations and the fact that many people add salt to their food. In western Europe and North America, the estimated overall consumption of dietary sodium chloride is 5–20 g/day (2–8 g of sodium per day), the average being 10 g/day (4 g of sodium) (6). People on a low-sodium diet need to restrict their sodium intake to less than 2 g/day (9). The consumption of drinking-water containing 20 mg of sodium per litre would lead to a daily intake of about 40 mg of sodium.

## 13.29.4 Kinetics and metabolism in laboratory animals and humans

Virtually all of the sodium present in water and foods is rapidly absorbed from the gastrointestinal tract. Sodium is the principal cation found in the extracellular body fluids; only small amounts are found within cells (*11*). Some is found in bone, where it acts as a sodium reservoir in maintaining the blood pH.

The level of sodium in extracellular fluids is carefully maintained by the kidney and determines the volume of these fluids (*9*). Sodium balance is controlled through a complex interrelated mechanism involving both the nervous and hormonal systems (*12*). Sodium is excreted principally in the urine in amounts reflecting the dietary intake (*11*).

## 13.29.5 Effects on laboratory animals and *in vitro* test systems

### Acute exposure

The $LD_{50}$ values for rats and mice for sodium ion as the chloride salt are 1180 mg/kg of body weight and 1572 mg/kg of body weight, respectively. An $LD_{50}$ of 3147 mg/kg of body weight was reported for rabbits (*13*).

### Long-term exposure

Hypertension has been clearly demonstrated in different species of animals given high levels of sodium chloride in their diet (*6*). Despite the usual reservations about extrapolating animal results to humans, the consistency of the animal data suggests that they should not be ignored.

Ingestion of a high-salt diet resulted in hypertension in female Sprague-Dawley rats (*14*). Approximately 75% of 159 rats fed diets containing 8% sodium chloride (equal to 3597 mg of sodium ion per kg of body weight per day) for 12–15 months exhibited hypertension (systolic blood pressure >18.7 kPa (140 mmHg)) within 6–9 months of the initiation of the diet regimen; the mean blood pressure of these animals increased with age. Rats maintained on a low-salt diet (0.35% sodium chloride, equal to 157 mg of sodium ion per kg of body weight per day) did not exhibit a corresponding increase in blood pressure with age.

### Reproductive toxicity, embryotoxicity, and teratogenicity

The reproductive effects of the sodium ion were studied in three strains of pregnant rats (SHR, WKY, and Sprague-Dawley) fed diets containing either 0.4 or 8.0% sodium chloride (equal to 208 and 4196 mg of sodium ion per kg of body weight per day) throughout gestation and lactation (*15*). Their offspring were also placed on low- or high-sodium diets. Pregnancy rates were decreased in the high-salt diet group, by 38% in SHR rats and 66% in WKY rats. Although slight nonsignificant increases in systolic blood pressure were noted in high-salt WKY dams, significant decreases were observed in their SHR counterparts. SHR pups fed the high sodium level from high-salt dams had significantly higher blood pressure than offspring from all other groups after 11.5 weeks of exposure and exhibited high morbidity and mortality from peripheral capillary haemorrhage and stroke. Maternal high-salt diets caused depression of postnatal growth in all strains of rats studied.

No developmental effects were observed in the offspring of pregnant mice, rats, or rabbits given oral doses of sodium chloride equivalent to 189, 147, and 147 mg of sodium ion per kg of body weight, respectively, on days 6–15 (mice and rats) or 6–18 (rabbits) of gestation (*15,16*).

### Mutagenicity and related end-points

Sodium (as sodium chloride) produced gene mutations in mouse lymphocyte assays, induced unscheduled DNA synthesis in rats, and caused cytogenetic aberrations in hamster ovaries and lung cells as well as DNA damage in hamster ovaries and mouse lymphocytes (*13*). The overall importance of these findings is reduced because very high dose levels of sodium ion were used.

### Carcinogenicity

It is unlikely that sodium alone is carcinogenic. However, a high-salt diet may enhance the carcinogenic potency of chemicals such as $N$-methyl-$N'$-nitro-$N$-nitrosoguanidine in drinking-water by causing irritation of the gastroduodenal tract, thus increasing the exposure of epithelial cells to the carcinogen and resulting in an increased incidence of gastric tumours (*17*).

## 13.29.6 Effects on humans

Although it is generally agreed that sodium is essential to human life, there is no agreement on the minimum daily requirement. However, it has been estimated that a total daily intake of 120–400 mg will meet the daily needs of growing infants and young children, and 500 mg those of adults (*18*).

In general, sodium salts are not acutely toxic because of the efficiency with which mature kidneys excrete sodium. However, acute effects and death have been reported following accidental overdoses of sodium chloride (*6*). Acute effects may include nausea, vomiting, convulsions, muscular twitching and rigidity, and cerebral and pulmonary oedema (*12,19*). Excessive salt intake seriously aggravates chronic congestive heart failure, and ill effects due to high levels of sodium in drinking-water have been documented (*6*).

The effects on infants are different from those in adults because of the immaturity of infant kidneys. Infants with severe gastrointestinal infections can suffer from fluid loss, leading to dehydration and raised sodium levels in the plasma (hypernatraemia); permanent neurological damage is common under such conditions. Addition of cows' milk or tapwater containing high levels of sodium to solid food may exacerbate the effects (2, 6).

The relationship between elevated sodium intake and hypertension has been the subject of considerable scientific controversy. Although short-term studies have suggested that such a relationship does exist (20), most people in western Europe and North America ingest a high-salt diet from infancy yet do not exhibit persistent hypertension until the fourth decade (6). Whereas reducing the sodium intake can reduce the blood pressure of some individuals with hypertension, this is not effective in all cases (21). In addition, some data for both humans and animals suggest that the action of sodium may be at least partly modified by the level of the accompanying anion as well as that of other cations (22, 23). Although several studies suggest that high levels of sodium in drinking-water are associated with increased blood pressure in children (24, 25), in other studies no such association has been found (26, 27, 28).

A particularly striking observation is that, in "nonwesternized" populations, diets are low in sodium, the prevalence of hypertension is very low, and blood pressure does not increase with age. Although it is tempting to conclude that a causal relationship exists, a number of differences between "westernized" and "nonwesternized" populations might account for the difference. However, the good agreement between these results and those of other studies gives further support to a direct link between raised sodium intake and hypertension (6).

Although there is an association between hypertension and certain diseases, such as coronary heart disease, genetic differences in susceptibility, possibly protective minerals (potassium and calcium), and methodological weaknesses in experiments make it difficult to quantify the relationship, and sodium in drinking-water generally makes only a small contribution to total dietary sodium. No firm conclusions can therefore be drawn at present as to the importance of sodium in drinking-water and its possible association with disease.

## 13.29.7 Conclusions

Sodium salts are found in virtually all food (the main source of daily exposure) and drinking-water. Sodium levels in the latter are typically less than 20 mg/litre but can markedly exceed this in some countries. On the basis of existing data, no firm conclusions can be drawn concerning the possible association between sodium in drinking-water and the occurrence of hypertension. No health-based guideline value is therefore proposed. However, sodium may affect the taste of drinking-water at levels above about 200 mg/litre.

# References

1.  Stockinger HE. The metals. In: Clayton GD, Clayton FE, *Patty's industrial hygiene and toxicology. Vol. 2A. Toxicology.* New York, NY, John Wiley, 1981:2056-2057.

2.  Sax NI. *Dangerous properties of industrial materials*, 4th ed. New York, NY, Van Nostrand Reinhold, 1975:1101.

3.  Sax NI, Lewis RJ, eds. *Hawley's condensed chemical dictionary*, 11th ed. New York, NY, Van Nostrand Reinhold, 1987:1050-1051.

4.  Sittig M. *Handbook of toxic and hazardous chemicals and carcinogens*, 2nd ed. Park Ridge, NJ, Noyes Publications, 1981:792-793.

5.  Budavari S, O'Neil M, Smith A, eds. *The Merck index*, 11th ed. Rahway, NJ, Merck, 1989:1355.

6.  *Sodium, chlorides and conductivity in drinking water.* Copenhagen, WHO Regional Office for Europe, 1979 (EURO Reports and Studies, No. 2).

7.  National Academy of Sciences. *Drinking water and health*, Vol. 3. Washington, DC, National Academy Press, 1980:283-293.

8.  Andreae MO, Asmode J, Van't Dack L. Determination of sodium in natural waters by atomic absorption spectrometry with hydride generation. *Analytical chemistry*, 1981, 53:1766-1771.

9.  National Academy of Sciences. *Drinking water and health.* Washington, DC, National Academy Press, 1977:400-411.

10. Diem K, Lentner C, eds. *Documenta Geigy. Scientific tables*, 7th ed. Basel, Ciba-Geigy 1970:688.

11. Guthrie HA. *Introductory nutrition*, 7th ed. St Louis, MO, Times Mirror/Mosby College Publishing, 1989.

12. Department of National Health and Welfare (Canada). *Guidelines for Canadian drinking water quality. Supporting documentation.* Ottawa, 1992.

13. National Institute of Occupational Safety and Health. *Registry of Toxic Effects of Chemical Substances (RTECS).* Washington, DC, US Department of Health and Human Services, 1991 (NIOSH Publication 91-101-2).

14. Dahl LK. Possible role of salt intake in the development of essential hypertension. In: Cottier P, Bock KD, eds. *Essential hypertension: an international symposium.* Heidelberg, Springer-Verlag, 1960:53-65.

15. Karr-Dullien V, Bloomquist E. The influence of prenatal salt on the development of hypertension by spontaneously hypertensive rats (SHR) (40462). *Proceedings of the Society for Experimental Biology and Medicine*, 1979, 160:421-425.

16. Fregly MJ. Sodium and potassium. *Annual review of nutrition*, 1981, 1:69-93.

17. Takahashi M et al. Effect of high salt diet on rat gastric carcinogenesis induced by *N*-methyl-*N'*-nitro-*N*-nitrosoguanidine. *Gann*, 1983, 74:28-34.

18. National Research Council. *Recommended dietary allowances*, 10th ed. Washington, DC, National Academy Press, 1989.

19. Elton NW, Elton WJ, Narzareno JP. Pathology of acute salt poisoning in infants. *American journal of clinical pathology*, 1963, 39:252-264.

20. Luft FC et al. Cardiovascular and humoral responses to extremes of sodium intake in normal black and white men. *Circulation*, 1979, 60:697-706.

21. Laragh JH, Pecker MS. Dietary sodium and essential hypertension: some myths, hopes and truths. *Annals of internal medicine*, 1983, 98:735-743.

22. Kurtz TW, Morris RC Jr. Dietary chloride as a determinant of "sodium-dependent" hypertension. *Science*, 1983, 222:1139-1141.

23. Morgan TO. The effect of potassium and bicarbonate ions on the rise in blood pressure caused by sodium chloride. *Clinical science*, 1982, 63:407s.

24. Tuthill RW, Calabrese EJ. Drinking water sodium and blood pressure in children: a second look. *American journal of public health*, 1981, 71:722-729.

25. Fatula MI. The frequency of arterial hypertension among persons using water with an elevated sodium chloride content. *Soviet medicine*, 1967, 30:134-136.

26. Tuthill RW, Calabrese EJ. The Massachusetts blood pressure study. Part 4. Modest sodium supplementation and blood pressure change in boarding school students. In: *Advances in modern environmental toxicology. Vol. IX. Inorganics in drinking water and cardiovascular disease.* Princeton, NJ, Princeton Scientific Publishing Co., 1985:69.

27. Pomrehn PR et al. Community differences in blood pressure levels and drinking water sodium. *American journal of epidemiology*, 1983, 118:60-71.

28. Armstrong BK et al. Water sodium and blood pressure in rural school children. *Archives of environmental health*, 1982, 37:236-245.

# 13.30 Sulfate

## 13.30.1 General description

### Identity

Sulfates occur naturally in numerous minerals, including barite ($BaSO_4$), epsomite ($MgSO_4 \cdot 7H_2O$), and gypsum ($CaSO_4 \cdot 2H_2O$) (*1*).

### Organoleptic properties

Reported taste threshold concentrations in drinking-water are 250–500 mg/litre (median 350 mg/litre) for sodium sulfate, 250–1000 mg/litre (median 525 mg/litre) for calcium sulfate, and 400–600 mg/litre (median 525 mg/litre) for magnesium sulfate (*2*). In a survey of 10–20 people, the median concentrations that could be detected by taste were 237, 370, and 419 mg/litre for the sodium, calcium, and magnesium salts, respectively (*3*). Concentrations of sulfates at which 50% of panel members considered the water to have an "offensive taste" were approximately 1000 and 850 mg/litre for calcium and magnesium sulfate, respectively (*4*).

Addition of calcium and magnesium sulfate (but not sodium sulfate) to distilled water was found to improve the taste; an optimal taste was found at 270 and 90 mg/litre for calcium and magnesium sulfate, respectively (*4*).

### Major uses

Sulfates and sulfuric acid products are used in the production of fertilizers, chemicals, dyes, glass, paper, soaps, textiles, fungicides, insecticides, astringents, and emetics. They are also used in the mining, wood-pulp, metal, and plating industries, in sewage treatment, and in leather processing (*1*). Aluminium sulfate (alum) is used as a sedimentation agent in the treatment of drinking-water. Copper sulfate has been used for the control of algae in raw and public water supplies (*5*).

### Environmental fate

Sulfates are discharged into water from mines and smelters, and from kraft pulp and paper mills, textile mills, and tanneries. Sodium, potassium, and magnesium sulfates are all soluble in water, whereas calcium and barium sulfates and many heavy metal sulfates are less soluble. Atmospheric sulfur dioxide, formed by the combustion of fossil fuels and in metallurgical roasting processes, may contribute to the sulfate content of surface waters. Sulfur trioxide, produced by the photolytic or catalytic oxidation of sulfur dioxide, combines with water vapour to form dilute sulfuric acid, which falls as "acid rain" (*6*).

## 13.30.2 Analytical methods

Sulfate in aqueous solutions may be determined by a gravimetric method in which sulfate is precipitated as barium sulfate; the method is suitable for sulfate concentrations above 10 mg/litre (7).

## 13.30.3 Environmental levels and human exposure

### Air

Levels of sulfate in air in Ontario (Canada) have been found to range from 3.0 to 12.6 µg/m³, with a mean of 7.0 µg/litre (8). In a nationwide survey in the USA, sulfate concentrations in air ranged from 0.5 to 228 µg/m³, the means ranging from 0.8 to 31.5 µg/m³ (US Environmental Protection Agency, unpublished data, 1984). The average daily intake of sulfate from air, based on these means and on the assumption that 20 m³ of air is inhaled daily, would be in the range 0.02–0.63 mg.

### Water

Sulfate concentrations in rain in Canada varied between 1.0 and 3.8 mg/litre in 1980 (9). An annual mean value of about 6 mg/litre in precipitation over central Europe has been reported (10). Levels of sulfate in rain and surface water correlate with emission levels of sulfur dioxide from anthropogenic sources (11).

Seawater contains about 2700 mg of sulfate per litre (12). According to GEMS/WATER, a global network of water monitoring stations, typical sulfate levels in fresh water are in the vicinity of 20 mg/litre and range from 0 to 630 mg/litre in rivers, the highest values being found in Belgium and Mexico, from 2 to 250 mg/litre in lakes (the highest value is found in Mexico), and from 0 to 230 mg/litre in groundwater (the highest values are found in Chile and Morocco) (13). Levels of sulfate in rivers in western Canada ranged from 1 to 3040 mg/litre, most concentrations being below 580 mg/litre (Environment Canada, unpublished data, 1984). Levels of sulfate in groundwater in the Netherlands were below 150 mg/litre (14).

The mean sulfate level in municipal drinking-water supplies may be increased by treatment. Thus it was 12.5 mg/litre in untreated water in municipal water supplies in Ontario but 22.5 mg/litre in treated water (Ontario Ministry of the Environment, unpublished data, 1987). Levels in central Canada are particularly high; in Saskatchewan, median levels of 368 and 97 mg/litre were found in treated drinking-water from groundwater and surface water supplies, respectively, with a range of 3–2170 mg/litre (Saskatchewan Environment and Public Safety, unpublished data, 1989). In the Netherlands, the sulfate concentration of drinking-water from 65% of water-treatment plants was below 25 mg/litre in 1985 (14).

Based on the mean sulfate concentration of 22.5 mg/litre in Ontario and an average daily consumption of 2 litres of drinking-water, the average daily intake from this source would be 45 mg. However, in areas with much higher sulfate levels in drinking-water, such as Saskatchewan, daily intake from this source could be over 4000 mg.

### Food

No data on the sulfate content of foodstuffs were found; however, sulfates are used as additives in the food industry (*15*). The estimated average daily intake of sulfate in food in the USA is 453 mg, based on data on food consumption and reported usage of sulfates as additives (*16,17*). Sulfites and sulfides are also present in food.

### Estimated total exposure and relative contribution of drinking-water

The average daily intake of sulfate from drinking-water, air, and food is approximately 500 mg, food being the major source. However, in areas with drinking-water supplies containing high levels of sulfate, drinking-water may constitute the principal source of intake.

## 13.30.4 Kinetics and metabolism in laboratory animals and humans

About 30% of an oral dose of 13.9 g of magnesium sulfate heptahydrate administered in four equal hourly doses (*18*) and 43.5% of a similarly administered dose of 18.1 g of sodium sulfate decahydrate (*19*) were recovered in the urine of humans within 24 h. It was estimated that approximately 73% of calcium and magnesium sulfate administered to adult male Wistar rats in the diet was absorbed (*20*). The amount ingested, the nature of the accompanying anion, and the presence of certain dietary components influence the amount of sulfate absorbed. Low doses are generally absorbed well; at high doses (such as those used to induce catharsis), the absorptive capacity is probably exceeded, so that much of the dose is excreted in the faeces.

## 13.30.5 Effects on laboratory animals and *in vitro* test systems

### Acute exposure

The minimum lethal dose of magnesium sulfate in mammals is reported to be 200 mg/kg of body weight (*21*).

### Short-term exposure

In short-term (28-day) studies, there were no adverse effects other than diarrhoea in weanling pigs drinking water containing 3000 mg of sulfate per litre (*22*). Cattle can tolerate concentrations of sodium sulfate in their drinking-water up to

353

2610 mg/litre (corresponding to 527 mg/kg of body weight per day) for periods up to 90 days with no signs of toxicity except for changes in methaemoglobin and sulfhaemoglobin levels (23). However, 69 of 200 yearling calves, 22 of which subsequently died, developed polioencephalomalacia following the ingestion of a protein supplement containing 1.5% organic sulfate and drinking-water containing 1814 mg of sulfate per litre (24).

Groups of 20 male and 20 female Sprague-Dawley rats were given either tapwater or bottled mineral water containing sulfate at concentrations of 9–10, 280, or 1595 mg/litre for 90 days. No gastrointestinal disturbances or other effects were noted in any group, based on the evaluation of biochemical and haematological parameters as well as a histopathological examination (25).

## 13.30.6 Effects on humans

Sulfate is one of the least toxic anions. The lethal dose for humans as potassium or zinc sulfate is 45 g (21).

Ingestion of 8 g of sodium sulfate and 7 g of magnesium sulfate caused catharsis in adult males (18,19). Cathartic effects are commonly experienced by people consuming drinking-water containing sulfate in concentrations exceeding 600 mg/litre (26,27), although it is reported that with time humans can adapt to higher concentrations (28). Dehydration has also been reported as a common side-effect following the ingestion of large amounts of magnesium or sodium sulfate (29).

## 13.30.7 Conclusions

The major physiological effects resulting from the ingestion of large quantities of sulfate are catharsis, dehydration, and gastrointestinal irritation. Water containing magnesium sulfate at levels above 600 mg/litre acts as a purgative in humans. The presence of sulfate in drinking-water can also result in a noticeable taste; the lowest taste threshold concentration for sulfate is approximately 250 mg/litre, as the sodium salt. Sulfate may also contribute to the corrosion of distribution systems.

In the light of the above considerations, no health-based guideline value for sulfate in drinking-water is proposed. However, because of the gastrointestinal effects resulting from the ingestion of drinking-water containing high sulfate levels, it is recommended that health authorities be notified of sources of drinking-water that contain sulfate concentrations in excess of 500 mg/litre.

## References

1. Greenwood NN, Earnshaw A. *Chemistry of the elements.* Oxford, Pergamon Press, 1984.

2.  National Academy of Sciences. *Drinking water and health*. Washington, DC, National Research Council, 1977.

3.  Whipple GC. *The value of pure water*. New York, NY, John Wiley, 1907. Cited in: Committee on Water Quality Criteria. *Water quality criteria 1972*. Washington, DC, National Academy of Sciences, National Academy of Engineering, 1972.

4.  Zoeteman BCJ. *Sensory assessment of water quality*. New York, NY, Pergamon Press, 1980.

5.  McGuire MJ et al. Controlling attached blue-green algae with copper sulphate. *Journal of the American Water Works Association*, 1984, 76:60.

6.  Delisle CE, Schmidt JW. The effects of sulphur on water and aquatic life in Canada. In: *Sulphur and its inorganic derivatives in the Canadian environment*. Ottawa, National Research Council of Canada, 1977 (NRCC No. 15015).

7.  International Organization for Standardization. *Water quality–determination of sulfate*. Geneva, 1990 (ISO 9280:1990).

8.  Air Quality Assessment Unit. *Appendix to annual report on air quality in Ontario*. Etobicoke, Ontario Ministry of the Environment, 1987.

9.  Franklin CA et al. Health risks from acid rain: a Canadian perspective. *Environmental health perspectives*, 1985, 63:155-168.

10. World Health Organization/United Nations Environment Programme, GEMS (Global Environment Monitoring System). *Global freshwater quality*. Oxford, Alden Press, 1989.

11. Keller W, Pitblade JR. Water quality changes in Sudbury area lakes: a comparison of synoptic surveys in 1974–1976 and 1981–1983. *Water, air and soil pollution*, 1986, 29:285.

12. Hitchcock DR. Biogenic contributions to atmospheric sulphate levels. In: *Proceedings of the 2nd National Conference on Complete Water Re-use*. Chicago, IL, American Institute of Chemical Engineers, 1975.

13. UNEP/WHO/UNESCO/WMO. *GEMS/WATER data summary 1985–1987*. Burlington, Canada Centre for Inland Waters, 1990.

14. Van Dijk-Looijaard AM, Fonds AW. *Integrated criteria document sulfate*. Bilthoven, Netherlands, National Institute of Public Health and Environmental Protection, 1985 (RIVM Report No. 718612001).

15. Codex Alimentarius Commission. *Food additives*. Rome, Food and Agriculture Organization of the United Nations, 1992 (Codex Alimentarius Vol.I).

16. Informatics, Inc. *GRAS (generally recognized as safe) food ingredients: ammonium ion.* Washington, DC, National Technical Information Service, 1973 (US Department of Commerce PB-221-235).

17. Subcommittee on Research of GRAS (Generally Recognized as Safe) List (Phase II). *Food ingredients.* Washington, DC, National Academy of Sciences, 1972 (DHEW No. FDA 70-22).

18. Morris ME, Levy G. Absorption of sulfate from orally administered magnesium sulfate in man. *Journal of toxicology–clinical toxicology,* 1983, 20:107-114.

19. Cocchetto DM, Levy G. Absorption of orally administered sodium sulfate in humans. *Journal of pharmaceutical sciences,* 1981, 70:331-333.

20. Whiting SJ, Cole DE. Effect of dietary anion composition on acid-induced hypercalciuria in the adult rat. *Journal of nutrition,* 1986, 116:388-394.

21. Arthur D. Little, Inc. *Inorganic chemical pollution of freshwater.* Washington, DC, US Environmental Protection Agency, 1971 (Water Pollution Control Research Series No. DPV 18010).

22. Paterson DW et al. Effects on sulfate in water on swine reproduction and young pig performance. *Journal of animal science,* 1979, 49:664-667.

23. Digesti RD, Weeth HJ. A defensible maximum for inorganic sulfate in drinking water of cattle. *Journal of animal science,* 1976, 42:1498-1502.

24. Hibbs CM, Thilsted JP. Toxicosis in cattle from contaminated well water. *Veterinary and human toxicology,* 1983, 25:253-254.

25. Würzner HP. Exposure of rats during 90 days to mineral water containing various amounts of sulphate. *Zeitschrift für Ernährungswissenschaft,* 1979, 18:119-127.

26. Chien L et al. Infantile gastroenteritis due to water with high sulfate content. *Canadian Medical Association journal,* 1968, 99:102-104.

27. US Department of Health, Education, and Welfare. *Drinking water standards–1962.* Washington, DC, US Government Printing Office, 1962 (Public Health Service Publication No. 956).

28. US Environmental Protection Agency. National primary drinking water regulations; synthetic organic chemicals, inorganic chemicals and microorganisms; proposed rule. *Federal register,* 1985, 50(219):46936.

29. Fingl E. Laxatives and cathartics. In: Gilman AG et al., eds. *Pharmacological basis of therapeutics.* New York, NY, MacMillan Publishing, 1980.

## 13.31 Taste and odour

### 13.31.1 Sources in drinking-water

Taste and odour in drinking-water can be caused by microorganisms, or be of human origin, as in the contamination of water supplies with chemicals. Problems can also be caused by some water-treatment processes or by substances leached from water pipe or storage facility linings.

### *Inorganic constituents*

Compounds in water that are perceived as giving it a taste are generally inorganic substances present in concentrations much higher than those of organic pollutants. The salt concentration in water should be approximately the same as in saliva for the water to taste neutral (*1*). The concentrations of sodium, magnesium, and calcium chloride at which 50% of a tasting panel found an offensive taste were 465, 47, and 350 mg/litre, respectively (*2*).

Of the ions that may be present in water, iron can be tasted in distilled water at a concentration of about 0.05 mg/litre, copper at about 2.5 mg/litre, manganese at about 3.5 mg/litre, and zinc at about 5 mg/litre (*3*). Iron, in particular, is suspected of affecting the taste of water in practice (*4*).

### *Organic constituents*

Organic compounds can cause organoleptic effects in water (*5*) at taste and odour threshold concentrations that can vary from milligrams to nanograms per litre. The compounds concerned include humic substances, hydrophilic acids, carboxylic acids, peptides and amino acids, carbohydrates, and hydrocarbons (*6*).

### *Biological constituents*

The organisms most often linked to taste and odour problems are actinomycetes and various types of algae, but other aquatic organisms, such as protozoa and fungi, have been implicated from time to time.

Earthy-musty tastes and odours are produced by certain cyanobacteria (blue-green algae), actinomycetes, and a few fungi. The substances produced by actinomycetes and cyanobacteria that cause tastes and odours in drinking-water have been extensively discussed in the literature (*7–10*) and include geosmin, methyl-isoborneol (MIB) and cardin-4-ene-1-ol. Growing algae produce numerous volatile and nonvolatile organic substances, including aliphatic alcohols, aldehydes, ketones, esters, thioesters, and sulfides.

Occasionally, taste and odour problems in water are caused by other bacteria, fungi, zooplankton, and nemathelminthes. *Ferrobacteria* in water-distribution systems may produce tastes and odours (*11*), and somes species of *Pseudomonas* can cause a swampy odour (*12*), whereas others can convert sulfur-containing amino acids into hydrogen sulfide, methylthiol, and dimethylpolysulfide (*13*).

## Man-made pollution

Halogenated hydrocarbon solvents are the synthetic contaminants of drinking-water most frequently found because of the huge amounts produced, and their very diffuse use, chemical and biological stability, volatility, and negligible adsorption by soil and sediments.

## Production during water treatment

Water treatment often includes storage, slow sand filtration, or activated carbon filtration. Mircoorganisms can grow in the equipment used for these purposes and can then cause tastes and odours. The biological degradation of organic compounds in raw water can also lead to the production of substances such as phenols, aldehydes, and alkylbenzenes that cause taste and odour problems (*14*). In addition, the chemicals used in water treatment as coagulants, oxidants, or disinfectants can interact with organic compounds in water and occasionally produce tastes and odours.

Ozone is one of the most efficient agents in removing tastes and odours, but its use can lead to the formation of intermediate reaction products (*15*). In particular the formation of aliphatic aldehydes, which has been frequently reported in the literature (*16*), leads to the development of fruity, fragrant, and orange-like odours (*17*).

The free halogens used as water disinfectants can produce undesirable tastes and odours in the water. For chlorine residuals, threshold values vary significantly with pH: 75 µg/litre at pH 5 as compared with 450 µg/litre at pH 9 (*18*). Hypochlorous acid, hypochlorite ion, monochloramine, and dichloramine have odour thresholds ranging from 0.15 to 0.65 mg/litre (*19*).

Taste and odour problems that develop in water-treatment plants are frequently an indirect consequence of chlorination (*20*). The odour threshold values of chlorinated by-products are generally significantly lower than those of the original products; for example, odour thresholds for phenol, 4-chlorophenol, and 2,4-dichlorophenol are 1000–5000, 0.5–1200, and 2–210 µg/litre, respectively.

## 13.31.2 Analytical methods

Water evaluation panels are used to obtain early warnings and descriptions of taste and odour problems. Such panels may consist of a few members who meet regularly and have been specially trained, or of many untrained consumers (sometimes hundreds). It was concluded in one study that the results of evaluations by large consumer panels could be used to optimize the treatment process at a water-treatment plant, and it was suggested that panel evaluation should become a routine control method where contaminated surface water was used as the raw water source (*21*).

## 13.31.3 Health aspects

Odour in potable water may be indicative of some form of pollution of the water or of malfunction during water treatment or distribution and should not be accepted without knowledge of the exact cause. The senses of taste and smell may be more sensitive than the best available analytical instrumentation, and a description of the taste and odour of a water sample can be obtained only by the sensory analysis of that sample. Such an analysis is an important contribution to the subsequent chemical identification of the pollutant.

## 13.31.4 Conclusions

Since tastes and odours in drinking-water may be indicative of some form of pollution or malfunction during water treatment or distribution, investigations to determine their cause are necessary and the appropriate health authorities should be consulted, particularly if there is a sudden or substantial change. An unusual taste or odour might be an indication of the presence of potentially harmful substances.

The taste and odour of drinking-water should not be offensive to the consumer. However, there is enormous variation in the level and quality of taste and odour that are regarded as acceptable.

No health-based guideline value is proposed for taste and odour.

## References

1.  Bartoshuk LM. NaCl thresholds in man: thresholds for water taste or NaCl taste? *Journal of comparative physiology*, 1974, 87(2):310-325.

2.  Zoeteman BCJ. *Sensory assessment and chemical composition of drinking water*. The Hague, Van der Gang, 1978.

3.  Water Research Centre. *A guide to solving water quality problems in distribution systems*. Medmenham, 1981.

4.  Cohen JM et al. Taste threshold concentration of metals in drinking water. *Journal of the American Water Works Association*, 1960, 52(5):660-670.

5.  National Academy of Sciences. *Drinking water and health*. Washington, DC, 1977.

6.  Thurmann EJ. *Organic geochemistry of natural waters*. Amsterdam, Netherlands, Martinus Nijhoff, 1985.

7. Woods S et al. Microbes as a source of earthy flavours in potable water–a review. *International biodeterioration bulletin*, 1983, 19:3-16.

8. Gerber NN. Volatile substances from actinomycetes: their role in the odor pollution of water. *CRC critical reviews in microbiology*, 1979, 7:191-214.

9. Cross T. Aquatic actinomycetes: a critical survey of the occurrence, growth, and role of actinomycetes in aquatic habitats. *Journal of applied bacteriology*, 1981, 50:397-423.

10. Slater GP , Block VC. Volatile compounds of the cyanophyceae–a review. *Water science and technology*, 1983, 15(6/7):181-190.

11. MacKenthun KM, Keup LE. Biological problems encountered in water supplies. *Journal of the American Water Works Association*, 1970, 62(8):520-526.

12. Wajon JE et al. *The occurrence and control of swampy odour in the water supply of Perth, Western Australia.* Bentley, Western Australia, School of Applied Chemistry, Western Australia Institute of Technology, 1985.

13. Whitfield FB, Freeman D. Off-flavours in crustaceans caught in Australian coastal water. *Water science and technology*, 1983, 15(6/7):85-95.

14. Linden AC, Thijsse GJE. The mechanism of microbial oxidation of petroleum hydrocarbons. *Advances in enzymology*, 1965, 27:469-546.

15. Glaze WH. Reaction products of ozone: a review. *Environmental health perspectives*, 1986, 69:151.

16. Anselme C et al. *Removal of tastes and odors by the ozone-granular activated carbon water treatment processes.* Paper presented at the 7th Ozone World Congress, International Ozone Association, Tokyo, 1985.

17. Suffet IH et al. Removal of tastes and odors by ozonation. In: *Proceedings of the American Water Works Association Annual Conference, Seminar on Ozonation.* Denver, CO, AWWA, 1986.

18. Brayan PE et al. Taste threshold of halogens in the Delaware river. *Journal of the American Water Works Association*, 1973, 65(5):363-368.

19. Krasner SW, Barret SE. Aroma and flavor characteristics of free chlorine and chloramines. In: *Proceedings of the American Water Works Association Water Quality Treatment Conference*, Denver, CO, AWWA, 1984.

20. Burttschell RH et al. Chlorine derivatives of phenol causing taste and odor. *Journal of the American Water Works Association*, 1959, 51(2):205-214.

21. De Greef E et al. Drinking water contamination and taste assessment by large consumer panels. *Water science and technology*, 1983, 15(6/7):13-24.

## 13.32 Tin and inorganic tin compounds

### 13.32.1 General description

#### Identity

Tin in its most common form is a silvery white metal. Of the various tin-bearing minerals cassiterite is an oxide, while the remainder are complex sulfides. Tin forms two series of compounds, namely those of bivalent (tin(II)) and quadrivalent tin (tin(IV)). The most important inorganic compounds of tin are the oxides, chlorides, fluorides, and halogenated sodium stannates and stannites. Tin can form one to four covalent bonds with carbon (1, 2).

#### Physicochemical properties

| Property | Value |
|---|---|
| Melting point | 232 °C |
| Boiling point | 2260–2270 °C at 100 kPa |
| Density | 7.3 g/cm$^3$ |
| Water solubility | insoluble |

#### Major uses

Approximately 50% of the world production of tin is used for plating. Tin coatings are used for food containers and food-processing equipment. Tin is also used in alloys, such as solders, bronzes, and pewters. Inorganic tin compounds are used as pigments in the ceramic and textile industry (3).

### 13.32.2 Analytical methods

Total tin is determined by atomic absorption spectrometry (AAS) either with direct aspiration into a flame or a furnace technique. The graphite furnace AAS procedure is highly sensitive. Picric acid, a simple and very efficient matrix modifier, greatly improves the determination of tin in toluene solution by furnace AAS. When combined with toluene–tropolone extraction from acidified aqueous solutions, this procedure lowers the detection limit for inorganic tin from 1 µg/litre to 0.01 µg/litre (4).

### 13.32.3 Environmental levels and human exposure

#### Air

The background level of tin in air is about 0.01 µg/m$^3$, increasing to 0.3 µg/m$^3$ in urban areas and to 5 µg/m$^3$ near industrial emissions (1, 5).

361

## Water

The concentration of tin in rivers, estuaries, and oceans is generally less than 5 ng/litre, but the use of organotin biocides can produce significantly higher concentrations (e.g. 26–91 ng/litre near the California coast, 200–3300 ng/litre in Lake Michigan) (1). In seawater, levels of 0.3–980 ng/litre have been found. In rivers, levels were 6–10 ng/litre, but 300 ng/litre was found in the Rhine (6).

Levels of <42–295 µg/litre were found in 37 different bottled mineral waters (7). A mean range of 1.1–2.2 µg/litre (maximum 30 µg/litre) was found in a survey of water supplies in the USA. Values greater than 1–2 µg/litre are exceptional (5).

## Food

Most natural foods contain tin in trace amounts, but concentrations are increased by the use of organotin pesticides and the storage of liquids in cans (1). In most unprocessed foods, tin levels are generally less than 1 µg/g. Higher concentrations are found in canned foods as a result of the dissolution of the tin coating or tin plate, the levels depending largely on the type and acidity of the food, the presence of oxidants, the duration and temperature of storage, and the presence of air in the can headspace. Tin concentrations in foodstuffs in unlacquered cans frequently exceed 100 µg/g but are below 25 µg/g in lacquered cans (3, 5).

Low tin levels have been found in flour (10 ng/g), dried milk (50 ng/g), spinach (20 ng/g), and fish (4–8 µg/g); higher levels were reported in canned fruit (30–100 µg/g) and canned grapefruit juice (245–260 µg/g) (6). Vegetables grown on soils of high tin content contained less than 1 µg/g. Diets consisting of fresh vegetables, meat, and cereals contributed less than 1 mg to the daily intake (1).

## Estimated total exposure and relative contribution of drinking-water

Food, particularly canned food, represents the major route of human exposure to tin. Intake from this source varies widely and for some segments of the population can reach several milligrams per kilogram of body weight (3). Estimates of the mean daily intake of tin are numerous (e.g. 0.1–100 mg; 0.2–17 mg; 3.6 mg; 1.5–8.8 mg) (3, 5, 8). In a study on duplicate portions of the 24-hour diet in the Netherlands, the median daily intake of tin was 0.21 mg in 1976–78 (range <0.08–17.4 mg) and 1984–85 (range <0.09–9.81 mg) (9).

The contribution of air to the daily intake of humans is less than 1 µg per person. For the general population, drinking-water is not a significant source of tin. Based on a maximum value of 2 µg/litre, its contribution will be 4 µg (1, 3, 5).

## 13.32.4 Kinetics and metabolism in laboratory animals and humans

Both tin and inorganic tin compounds are poorly absorbed from the gastrointestinal tract; in most studies, absorption was less than 5%, although values as high as 20% have been reported (5). Gastrointestinal absorption is influenced by the oxidation state; studies with radiolabelled tin in the rat indicated that absorption of tin(II) was four times greater than that of tin(IV) (2.8 and 0.6%, respectively). The anion may also influence the rate of absorption (10). Highest tissue concentrations of tin after both oral and parenteral administration were found in bone (principal site of distribution), kidney, and liver (5).

Absorbed tin is excreted primarily via the kidneys, and only to a smaller extent via the bile (8). Rats given oral doses of different tin salts excreted 50% of the absorbed tin in the first 48 h. Following intravenous administration of tin(II) or tin(IV) salts to rats, 12% of the tin(II) and only 4% of the tin(IV) appeared in the faeces, indicating that the biliary toute is probably more important in the elimination of tin(II) (94% within 24 h) than of tin(IV) compounds (10).

Half-times ranging from 3 to 4 months and from 34 to 40 days were reported in the bones of rats after intramuscular and oral administration, respectively. Elimination of tin(II) chloride after intraperitoneal and intravenous administration to the mouse, rat, monkey, and dog was a four-component process that was similar in all the species studied, the half-time for the longest component being over 3 months (5).

## 13.32.5 Effects on laboratory animals and *in vitro* test systems

### Acute exposure

The acute toxicity of metallic tin and inorganic tin compounds (except tin hydrides) to animal species is low; the oral $LD_{50}$ values for tin(II) chloride for mice and rats are 250 and 700 mg/kg of body weight, respectively. The rabbit is less sensitive, the oral $LD_{50}$ being 10 000 mg/kg of body weight (5). Tin hydrides, like many other metallic hydrides, are highly toxic to animals; they exert their effects mainly on the central nervous system (11). High doses of inorganic tin compounds (of the order of the $LD_{50}$) affect the central nervous system, producing effects such as ataxia, muscular weakness, and central nervous system depression (5). The species-related differences illustrated by the $LD_{50}$ values are apparent even at low levels of exposure. The cat was found to be more sensitive to the oral administration of tin than either the dog or the rat; vomiting and diarrhoea were observed only in cats after oral administration of tin-containing fruit beverages (>5.4 mg of tin per kg of body weight) or a complex of tin(IV) chloride and sodium citrate (9 mg of tin per kg of body weight) (12).

## Short-term exposure

In 4- or 13-week feeding studies with rats given various tin salts (including tin(II) chloride) or tin oxides at dose levels of 50–10 000 mg/kg of food, doses above 3000 mg/kg caused anaemia, changes in a number of enzyme activities, and extensive damage to liver and kidney, particularly with the more soluble tin salts (e.g. the chloride, orthophosphate and sulfate) (*12,13*). When male weanling rats were given doses of up to 3 mg of tin per kg of body weight (as tin(II) chloride) at 12-h intervals for 90 days, an increase in acid phosphatase activity and a decrease in the calcium content and compressive strength of the femur were observed (*14*).

## Long-term exposure

Two drinking-water studies with mice were carried out (*12*): in the first the mice received 1000 or 5000 mg of tin per litre as sodium chlorostannate or 5000 mg of tin per litre as tin(II) oleate for 1 year; in the second study, mice were given 5 mg of tin per litre as tin(II) chloride over their lifetime. In neither study were any effects on growth rates or survival observed.

In a 115-week study, rats were exposed to 0, 200, 400, or 800 mg of tin per kg of food as tin(II) chloride. Anaemia was observed in weeks 4 and 13 at each treatment level, but not during the second year of the study. At autopsy, the only effect noted was a slight increase in the relative spleen weight at 400 and 800 mg/kg, but no histopathological changes were seen. A slightly increased tin content in the bones was seen at the highest dose level only. The NOAEL in this study was 400 mg/kg of food, equivalent to 20 mg/kg of body weight per day (*12*).

## Reproductive toxicity, embryotoxicity, and teratogenicity

Testicular degeneration was observed in rats receiving 10 mg of tin(II) chloride per kg in the feed for 13 weeks (*13*). Tin(II) chloride with casein in an aqueous medium at dose levels of 0, 200, 400, or 800 mg/kg of feed did not affect the reproductive performance of rats, although a transient anaemia was observed in the offspring before weaning (*12*).

Low transplacental transfer of tin was observed after the feeding of different tin salts (in amounts corresponding to tin levels of up to 500 mg/kg in the diet) to pregnant rats; no effects were seen in the fetuses (*5*).

Tin(II) chloride (at doses of up to 50 mg/kg of body weight) was not teratogenic or fetotoxic in mice, rats, and golden hamsters (*5*).

## Mutagenicity and related end-points

Tin(II) chloride was found not to be mutagenic in a *rec*-assay in *Bacillus subtilis* (*15*).

*Carcinogenicity*

In an oral carcinogenicity study with B6C3F$_1$ mice (dose levels 0, 1000, or 2000 mg of tin(II) chloride per kg of food), a dose-related significant increase in the incidence of hepatocellular adenomas and/or carcinomas was found in females. However, the highest incidence was within the historical range for female B6C3F$_1$ mice (*15*).

In a long-term feeding study in rats given sodium chlorostannate, three malignant tumours were observed at sacrifice, but the treatment groups were rather small (*13*). In a study with F-344 rats receiving 0, 1000, or 2000 mg of tin(II) chloride per kg of diet for 105 weeks, no increased tumour incidences were observed (*15*). No effects on tumour incidence were observed in long-term studies with rats given tin in drinking-water or in food (*12*).

## 13.32.6 Effects on humans

Vomiting, diarrhoea, fatigue, and headache were often observed following the consumption of canned products (tin concentrations as low as 150 mg/kg in canned beverages and 250 mg/kg in other canned foods) (*12*). In contrast, no toxic effects were noted in nine male volunteers consuming packaged military rations (tin contents ranging from 13 to 204 mg/kg) for successive 24-day periods and in two other studies on human volunteers who ate canned food with tin content ranging from 250 to 700 mg/kg for periods of 6–30 days (*5*). There is no evidence of adverse effects in humans associated with chronic exposure to tin (*12,14*).

## 13.32.7 Conclusions

The low toxicity of tin and inorganic tin compounds is the result largely of its low absorption, low tissue accumulation, and rapid excretion, primarily in the faeces. It was concluded that, because of the low toxicity of inorganic tin, a tentative guideline value could be derived three orders of magnitude greater than the normal tin concentration in drinking-water. The presence of tin in drinking-water does not, therefore, represent a hazard to human health. For this reason, the establishment of a numerical guideline value for inorganic tin is not deemed necessary.

## References

1. Magos L. Tin. In: Friberg L, Nordberg GF, Vouk V, eds. *Handbook on the toxicology of metals*, 2nd ed. Amsterdam, Elsevier Science Publishers, 1986:568-593.

2. Stokinger HE. Tin. In: Clayton GD, Clayton FE, eds. *Patty's industrial hygiene and toxicology*, Vol. IIa, *Toxicology*. 3rd ed. New York, NY, John Wiley, 1978:1940-1968.

3. Joint FAO/WHO Expert Committee on Food Additives. *Toxicological evaluation of certain food additives and contaminants*. Cambridge, Cambridge University Press, 1989:329-336 (WHO Food Additives Series, No. 24).

4. Pinel et al. Determination of trace amounts of total tin in water using extraction followed by graphite furnace atomic absorption spectrometry with an oxidising matrix modifier. *Journal of analytical atomic spectroscopy*, 1988, 3(3):475-477.

5. *Tin and organotin compounds–a preliminary review*. Geneva, World Health Organization, 1980 (Environmental Health Criteria, No. 15).

6. Weber G. The importance of tin in the environment. *Zeitschrift für analytische Chemie*, 1985, 321:217-224.

7. Allen HE, Halley-Henderson MA, Hass CN. Chemical composition of bottled mineral water. *Archives of environmental health*, 1989, 44(2):102-116.

8. Mance G et al. *Proposed environmental quality standards for list II substances–inorganic tin*. Medmenham, Water Research Centre, 1988 (TR254).

9. Vaessen HA, Van Ooik A. I*ntegrated criteria document tin*. Bilthoven, Netherlands, National Institute of Public Health and Environmental Protection, 1988 (Report No. 338474006).

10. Hiles RA. Absorption, distribution and excretion of inorganic tin in rats. *Toxicology and applied pharmacology*, 1974, 27:366-379.

11. Browning E. *Toxicity of industrial metals*, 2nd ed. London, Butterworth, 1969.

12. Joint FAO/WHO Expert Committee on Food Additives. *Toxicological evaluation of certain food additives and contaminants*. Cambridge, Cambridge University Press, 1982:297-319 (WHO Food Additives Series, No. 17).

13. De Groot AP, Feron VJ, Til HP. Short-term toxicity studies on some salts and oxides of tin in rats. *Food and cosmetics toxicology*, 1973, 11:19-30.

14. Yamaguchi M, Saito R, Okada S. Dose-effect of inorganic tin on biochemical indices in rats. *Toxicology*, 1980, 16:267-273.

15. National Toxicology Program. *Carcinogenesis bioassay of stannous chloride*. Bethesda, MD, National Institutes of Health, 1982 (DHHS Publication No. (NIH) 82-1787).

## 13.33 Total dissolved solids

### 13.33.1 General description

#### *Identity*

Total dissolved solids (TDS) is the term used to describe the inorganic salts and small amounts of organic matter present in solution in water. The principal constituents are usually calcium, magnesium, sodium, and potassium cations and carbonate, hydrogencarbonate, chloride, sulfate, and nitrate anions.

#### *Organoleptic properties*

The presence of dissolved solids in water may affect its taste (*1*). The palatability of drinking-water has been rated by panels of tasters in relation to its TDS level as follows: excellent, less than 300 mg/litre; good, between 300 and 600 mg/litre; fair, between 600 and 900 mg/litre; poor, between 900 and 1200 mg/litre; and unacceptable, greater than 1200 mg/litre (*1*). Water containing extremely low concentrations of TDS may be unacceptable because of its flat, insipid taste.

### 13.33.2 Analytical methods

The method of determining TDS in water supplies most commonly used is the measurement of specific conductivity with a conductivity probe that detects the presence of ions in water. Conductivity measurements are converted into TDS values by means of a factor that varies with the type of water (*2,3*). The practical quantification limit for TDS in water by this method is 10 mg/litre (M. Forbes, personal communication, 1988). High TDS concentrations can also be measured gravimetrically, although volatile organic compounds are lost by this method (*4*). The constituents of TDS can also be measured individually.

### 13.33.3 Environmental levels and human exposure

#### *Water*

TDS in water supplies originate from natural sources, sewage, urban and agricultural run-off, and industrial wastewater. Salts used for road de-icing can also contribute to the TDS loading of water supplies.

Concentrations of TDS from natural sources have been found to vary from less than 30 mg/litre to as much as 6000 mg/litre (*5*), depending on the solubilities of minerals in different geological regions. Thus values, expressed as the sum of the constituents, were below 500 mg/litre in 36 of 41 rivers monitored in Canada (*6*) while, in a survey of the Great Lakes, levels ranged from 65 to 227 mg/litre (*7*). The levels of TDS in all of the Great Lakes except Lake Superior have increased in the past 70 years, by 50–60 mg/litre in Lakes Erie and Ontario (*7–10*). Between 1960 and 1980, a threefold increase in TDS was observed in

367

the Kent River, Australia (5). Between 1955 and 1970, a tenfold increase in the salinity of the groundwater at Burlington, MA, was noted, resulting from road de-icing. The use of de-icing chemicals was prohibited thereafter (5).

## 13.33.4 Effects on humans

No recent data on health effects associated with the ingestion of TDS in drinking-water appear to exist; however, associations between various health effects and hardness, rather than TDS content, have been investigated in many studies (see page 237).

In early studies, inverse relationships were reported between TDS concentrations in drinking-water and the incidence of cancer (11), coronary heart disease (12), arteriosclerotic heart disease (13), and cardiovascular disease (14,15). Total mortality rates were also reported to be inversely correlated with TDS levels in drinking-water (15,16).

It was reported in a summary of a study in Australia that mortality from all categories of ischaemic heart disease and acute myocardial infarction was increased in a community with high levels of soluble solids, calcium, magnesium, sulfate, chloride, fluoride, alkalinity, total hardness, and pH when compared with one in which levels were lower (17). No attempts were made to relate mortality from cardiovascular disease to other potential confounding factors.

The results of a limited epidemiological study in the former Soviet Union indicated that the average number of "cases" of inflammation of the gallbladder and gallstones over a 5-year period increased with the mean level of dry residue in the groundwater (18). It should be noted, however, that the number of "cases" varied greatly from year to year in one district, as did the concentration of dry residue in each district, and no attempt was made to take possible confounding factors into account.

## 13.33.5 Other considerations

Certain components of TDS, such as chlorides, sulfates, magnesium, calcium, and carbonates, affect corrosion or encrustation in water-distribution systems (4). High TDS levels (>500 mg/litre) result in excessive scaling in water pipes, water heaters, boilers, and household appliances such as kettles and steam irons (19). Such scaling can shorten the service life of these appliances (20).

## 13.33.6 Conclusions

Reliable data on possible health effects associated with the ingestion of TDS in drinking-water are not available. The result of early epidemiological studies suggest that even low concentrations of TDS in drinking-water may have beneficial effects, although adverse effects have been reported in two limited investigations.

Water containing TDS concentrations below 1000 mg/litre is usually acceptable to consumers, although acceptability may vary according to circumstances. However, the presence of high levels of TDS in water may be objectionable to consumers owing to the resulting taste and to excessive scaling in water pipes, heaters, boilers, and household appliances (see also the section on hardness, page 237). Water with extremely low concentrations of TDS may also be unacceptable to consumers bacause of its flat, insipid taste; it is also often corrosive to water-supply systems.

In areas where the TDS content of the water supply is very high, the individual constituents should be identified and the local public health authorities consulted. No health-based guideline value is proposed for TDS. However, drinking-water guidelines are available for some of its constituents, including boron, fluoride, and nitrate.

## References

1. Bruvold WH, Ongerth HJ. Taste quality of mineralized water. *Journal of the American Water Works Association*, 1969, 61:170.

2. International Organization for Standardization. *Water quality–determination of electrical conductivity*. Geneva, 1985 (ISO 7888:1985).

3. Singh T, Kalra YP. Specific conductance method for *in situ* estimation of total dissolved solids. *Journal of the American Water Works Association*, 1975, 67(2):99.

4. Sawyer CN, McCarty PL. *Chemistry for sanitary engineers*, 2nd ed. New York, McGraw-Hill, 1967 (McGraw-Hill Series in Sanitary Science and Water Resources Engineering).

5. WHO/UNEP, GEMS. *Global freshwater quality*. Oxford, Alden Press, 1989.

6. Department of Fisheries and Environment (Canada), Water Quality Branch. *Surface water quality in Canada. An overview*. Ottawa, 1977.

7. Upper Lakes Reference Group. *The waters of Lake Huron and Lake Superior. Report to the International Joint Commission*, Vols. I-III, Parts A and B. Windsor, Canada, International Joint Commission, 1977.

8. Beeton AM. *Indices of Great Lakes eutrophication*. Ann Arbor, MI, University of Michigan, Great Lakes Research Division, 1966:1-8 (Publication No. 15).

9. Kormondy EJ. *Concepts of ecology*. Englewood Cliffs, NJ, Prentice-Hall, 1969:182-183.

10. Vaughn JC, Reed PA. Qualtity status of southern Lake Michigan. *Journal of the American Water Works Association*, 1972, 62:103.

11. Burton AC, Cornhill JF. Correlation of cancer death rates with altitude and with the quality of water supply of the 100 largest cities in the United States. *Journal of toxicology and environmental health*, 1977, 3(3):465-478.

12. Schroeder HA. Relation between mortality from cardiovascular disease and treated water supplies. Variation in states and 163 largest municipalities. *Journal of the American Medical Association*, 1960, 172:1902.

13. Schroeder HA. Municipal drinking water and cardiovascular death rates. *Journal of the American Medical Association*, 1966, 195:81-85.

14. Sauer HI. Relationship between trace element content of drinking water and chronic disease. In: Trace metals in water supplies: occurrence, significance and control. *University of Illinois Bulletin*, 1974, 71(108):39.

15. Craun GF, McGabe LJ. Problems associated with metals in drinking water. *Journal of the American Water Works Association*, 1975, 67:593.

16. Crawford MD, Gardner MJ, Morris JN. Mortality and hardness of water. *Lancet*, 1968, 1:1092.

17. Meyers D. Mortality and water hardness. *Lancet*, 1975, 1:398-399.

18. Popov VV. [On the question of a possible relationship between morbidity of the population with cholelithiasis and cholecystitis and the salt content and hardness of drinking-water.] *Gigiena i sanitarija*, 1968, 33(6):104-105 (in Russian).

19. Tihansky DP. Economic damages from residential use of mineralized water supply. *Water resources research*, 1974, 10(2):145.

20. McQuillan RG, Spenst PG. The addition of chemicals to apartment water supplies. *Journal of the American Water Works Association*, 1976, 68:415.

## 13.34 Turbidity

### 13.34.1 General description

#### *Identity*

Turbidity is caused by the presence in water of particulate matter, such as clay, silt, colloidal particles, and plankton and other microscopic organisms, and is a measure of the water's ability to scatter and absorb light. This depends on a number of factors, such as the number, size, shape, and refractive index of the particles and the wavelength of the incident light (*1*).

## Sources

The particles that cause turbidity in water vary in size between 1 nm and 1 mm (*2*). They can be divided into three classes: clay particles, which have an upper particle size limit of about 0.002 mm diameter; organic particles produced by the decomposition of plant and animal debris; and fibrous particles, e.g. those of minerals such as asbestos.

Soil particles, produced by the erosion of the land surface, have been found to constitute the major part of the suspended material in most natural waters. The coarser sand and silt fractions are wholly or partially coated with organic material. Phyllosilicate clay particles, as well as non-clay material, such as iron and aluminium oxides and hydroxides, quartz, amorphous silica, carbonates, and feldspar, constitute the clay fraction. Clay and organic material are often associated as a "clay–organic" complex. Humic substances have a much higher ion exchange capacity than inorganic clays, and their effects often predominate (*3*).

The accumulation of large numbers of microorganisms has been reported to produce turbid water. Examples include summer blooms of algae in surface water, algal debris, and the detritus from iron bacteria in distribution systems (*3*).

## 13.34.2 Analytical methods

A number of methods may be used to measure water turbidity, but nephelometry and turbidimetry form the basis of present standard methods (*4–6*).

## 13.34.3 Environmental levels and human exposure

All natural waters are turbid, surface waters generally more than groundwater. Raw water turbidity has been reported to range from less than 1 to more than 1000 NTU (nephelometric turbidity units) (*3*). As processes such as simple filtration or coagulation, sedimentation, and filtration are effective in removing turbidity, drinking-water concentrations are usually less than 1 NTU. If turbidity is present in higher concentrations, it may be as a consequence of inadequate treatment or the resuspension of sediment in the distribution system (*7*). It may also be due to the presence of inorganic particulate matter in some groundwaters.

## 13.34.4 Relationship with water quality parameters

The turbidity of water is related to or affects many other indicators of drinking-water quality. For example, there is a relationship between high turbidity and the appearance, colour, taste, and odour of both raw and filtered waters. It is reported that 50% of colour in water is due to a "colloidal fraction" of humic substances. This, however, is not true colour, which is the colour remaining after removal of turbidity (*6*).

Turbidity can have a significant effect on the microbiological quality of drinking-water. Its presence can interfere with the detection of bacteria and viruses in drinking-water (8); more importantly, turbid water has been shown to stimulate bacterial growth (2) since nutrients are adsorbed on to particulate surfaces, thereby enabling the attached bacteria to grow more rapidly than those in free suspension.

The main problem associated with turbidity is its effect on disinfection, because high levels have been shown to protect microorganisms from the action of disinfectants (8–10) and to increase the chlorine and oxygen demand (11). Coliform bacteria have been found in waters of turbidity between 4 and 84 NTU, free chlorine residuals between 0.1 and 0.5 mg/litre, and a minimum contact time of 30 min (3). In turbid water, *Escherichia coli* has been shown to be protected in the presence of chlorine levels of 0.35 mg/litre or greater (3).

The adsorptive capacity of some suspended particulates can lead to the presence of undesirable inorganic and organic compounds in drinking-water. Most important in this respect is the organic or humic component of turbidity. For example, herbicides such as 2,4-D, paraquat, and diquat can be adsorbed on to clay–humic particulates, the adsorption being greatly influenced by metal cations present in the humic material. In addition, the strength of the bonds in some metal–humate complexes in the turbidity fraction may complicate the measurement of trace metals in natural waters, resulting in an underestimation of the metal concentrations.

## 13.34.5 Effects on humans

The consumption of highly turbid water may constitute a health risk, because, as mentioned above, excessive turbidity can protect pathogenic microorganisms from the effects of disinfectants, stimulate the growth of bacteria in distribution systems, and increase the chlorine demand. In addition, the adsorptive capacity of some particulates may lead to the presence of harmful inorganic and organic compounds in drinking-water.

## 13.34.6 Conclusions

The appearance of water with a turbidity of less than 5 NTU is usually acceptable to consumers, although this may vary with local circumstances. However, because of its microbiological effects, it is recommended that turbidity be kept as low as possible. No health-based guideline value for turbidity is proposed.

The impact of turbidity on disinfection efficiency is discussed in section 11.2.9.

# References

1.  Katz EL. The stability of turbidity in raw water and its relationship to chlorine demand. *Journal of the American Water Works Association*, 1986, 78(2):72-75.

2.  McCoy WF, Olson BH. Relationship among turbidity, particle counts and bacteriological quality within water distribution lines. *Water research*, 1986, 20(8):1023-1029.

3.  Department of National Health and Welfare (Canada). *Guidelines for Canadian drinking water quality*. Ottawa, 1991.

4.  *Methods for the examination of water and associated materials: colour and turbidity of waters*. London, Her Majesty's Stationery Office, 1981.

5.  International Organization for Standardization. *Water quality—determination of turbidity*. Geneva, 1990 (ISO 7027:1990).

6.  American Public Health Association. *Standard methods for the examination of water and wastewater*, 17th ed. Washington, DC, 1989.

7.  Elliot T. Turbidity: the final element in assessing water quality. *Power*, 1986, 130(10):65-66.

8.  LeChevallier MW, Evans TM, Seidler RJ. Effect of turbidity on chlorination efficiency and bacterial persistence in drinking water. *Applied and environmental microbiology*, 1981, 42(1):159-167.

9.  Hoff JC. *The relationship of turbidity to disinfection of potable water. Evaluation of the microbiology standards for drinking water*. Washington, DC, US Environmental Protection Agency, 1978:103 (EPA-570/9-78-OOL).

10. Tracy HW, Camarena VM, Wing F. Coliform persistence in highly chlorinated waters. *Journal of the American Water Works Association*, 1966, 158:1151.

11. Reilly K. Relationship of bacterial counts with turbidity and free chlorine in two distribution systems. *Journal of the American Water Works Association*, 1983, 75(6):309-312.

## 13.35 Uranium[1]

### 13.35.1 General description

#### *Identity*

Uranium occurs naturally in the +2, +3, +4, +5 and +6 oxidation states, the last of these being the most common. In nature, uranium(VI) is commonly associated with oxygen as the uranyl ion, $UO_2^{2+}$. Naturally occurring uranium ([nat]U) is a mixture of three radionuclides ([234]U, [235]U, and [238]U), all of which decay by both alpha and gamma emissions (*1, 2*). Uranium is widespread in nature, occurring in granites and various other mineral deposits (*1, 3*).

| Compound | CAS no. | Molecular formula |
|----------|---------|-------------------|
| Uranium | 7440-61-1 | U |
| Uranyl ethanoate | 541-09-3 | $C_4H_6O_6U$ |
| Uranyl chloride | 7791-26-6 | $Cl_2O_2U$ |
| Uranyl nitrate | 36478-76-9 | $N_2O_8U$ |
| Uranium dioxide | 1344-57-6 | $UO_2$ |

#### *Physicochemical properties (1)*

| Compound | Melting point (°C) | Boiling point (°C) | Density at 20 °C (g/cm³) | Water solubility (g/l) |
|----------|--------------------|--------------------|--------------------------|------------------------|
| U | 1132 | 3818 | 19.0 | insoluble |
| $C_4H_6O_6U$ | 110 | 275 (decomposes) | 2.9 | 76.94 |
| $Cl_2O_2U$ | 578 | (decomposes) | – | 3200 |
| $N_2O_8U$ | 60.2 | 118 | 2.8 | soluble |
| $UO_2$ | 2878 | – | 10.96 | insoluble |

#### *Major uses*

Uranium is used mainly as fuel in nuclear power stations.

#### *Environmental fate*

Uranium is present in the environment as a result of leaching from natural deposits, release in mill tailings, emissions from the nuclear industry, the combustion of coal and other fuels, and the use of phosphate fertilizers that contain uranium.

---

[1] This review addresses only the chemical aspects of uranium toxicity. Information on the derivation of a guideline value based on radiological effects is presented in Chapter 17, page 908.

## 13.35.2 Analytical methods

Uranium in water is most commonly measured by solid fluorometry with either laser excitation or ultraviolet light following fusion of the sample with a pellet of carbonate and sodium fluoride (detection limit 0.1 µg/litre) (4). It can also be determined by inductively coupled plasma mass spectrometry (detection limit 0.1 µg/litre) (5).

## 13.35.3 Environmental levels and human exposure

### Air

Reported mean levels of uranium in ambient air are 0.02 ng/m$^3$ in Tokyo (6) and 0.08 ng/m$^3$ in New York City (7). On the assumption of a daily respiratory volume of 20 m$^3$ and a concentration in air of 0.05 ng/m$^3$, the daily intake of uranium from air would be about 1 ng. Tobacco smoke (from two packets of cigarettes per day) contributes up to 50 ng of uranium (8).

### Water

Uranium concentrations in drinking-water in Canadian cities are generally less than 1 µg/litre but have exceeded 8 µg/litre; concentrations were below the detection limit of 0.05 µg/litre in about 50% of samples taken (9). Uranium concentrations of up to 700 µg/litre have been found in private supplies in Canada (10, 11). The mean concentration of uranium in drinking-water in New York City ranged from 0.03 to 0.08 µg/litre (12); in five Japanese cities, the mean level in potable water supplies was 0.009 µg/litre (13).

The daily uranium intake from water in Finland is estimated to be 2.1 µg (14), and from drinking-water in Salt Lake City (USA) 1.5 µg (15). On the basis of the results of the survey of Canadian cities (9), the daily intake of uranium in drinking-water is likely to be approximately 0.1 µg.

### Food

Uranium has been detected in a variety of foodstuffs, the highest concentrations being found in shellfish and lower levels in fresh vegetables, cereals, and fish. The average per capita intake of uranium in food has been reported to be 1.3 µg/day (7) and 2–3 µg/day (15) in the USA and 1.5 µg/day in Japan (13).

In a review of naturally occurring sources of radioactive contamination in food, dietary intakes of $^{238}$U were found to range from 12 to 45 mBq/day in several European countries, from 11 to 60 mBq/day in Japan (the higher values were found in uranium mining areas), and from 15 to 17 mBq/day in the United States. The average daily dietary intake was of the order of 20 mBq, or about 4 µg. It was often difficult to determine whether these dietary intakes included that from drinking-water, and it was emphasized that the latter has sometimes been found to be equal to that from diet (*16*).

### Estimated total exposure and relative contribution of drinking-water

The daily intake of uranium from each source for adults is estimated to be: air, 0.001 µg; food, 1.4 µg; water, 0.1 µg. The total daily intake is therefore approximately 1.5 µg, most of which comes from food.

## 13.35.4 Kinetics and metabolism in laboratory animals and humans

The average human gastrointestinal absorption of uranium is 1–2% (*17*). Only 0.06% of ingested uranium was absorbed in Sprague-Dawley rats and New Zealand white rabbits fed *ad libitum* and having free access to drinking-water containing up to 600 mg of uranyl nitrate hexahydrate per litre for up to 91 days (*18*). Absorption increased with dose in starved rats given uranium by gavage; absorption ranged from 0.06 to 2.8% for doses of 0.03 and 45 mg of uranium per kg of body weight, respectively (*19*).

Following ingestion, uranium rapidly appears in the bloodstream (*19*), where it is associated primarily with the red cells (*20*) and forms a nondiffusible uranyl–albumin complex in equilibrium with a diffusible ionic uranyl hydrogen-carbonate complex ($UO_2HCO_3^+$) in the plasma (*21*). Clearance from the bloodstream is rapid, and the uranium subsequently accumulates in the kidneys and skeleton (*19*). The skeleton is the major site of uranium accumulation (*17*); the uranyl ion replaces calcium in the hydroxyapatite complex of bone crystals (*11*).

Once equilibrium is attained in the skeleton, uranium is excreted in the urine and faeces. Urinary excretion in humans has been found to account for approximately 1% of total excretion, averaging 4.4 µg/day (*15*), the rate depending in part on the pH of tubular urine (*21*). Under alkaline conditions, most of the uranyl hydrogencarbonate complex is stable and is excreted in the urine. If the pH is low, the complex dissociates to a variable degree, and the uranyl ion may then bind to cellular proteins in the tubular wall.

The estimated overall elimination half-life of uranium under conditions of normal daily intake is between 180 and 360 days (*11*).

## 13.35.5 Effects on laboratory animals and *in vitro* test systems

### Acute exposure

Reported oral $LD_{50}$s of uranyl ethanoate for rats and mice are 204 and 242 mg/kg of body weight, respectively (*22*). Among the most common signs of acute toxicity are piloerection, significant weight loss, and haemorrhages in the eyes, legs, and nose.

The most common renal injury caused by uranium in experimental animals is damage to the proximal convoluted tubules, predominantly in the distal two-thirds (*21*). At doses not high enough to destroy a critical mass of kidney cells, the effect is reversible, as some of the lost cells are replaced. However, the new epithelial lining differs morphologically, and possibly functionally, from normal tubular epithelium (*17,21*). Regeneration of the injured tubular epithelium begins 2–3 days after exposure (*21*). There is some evidence that tolerance may develop following repeated exposure to uranium (*23–25*).

## Short-term exposure

A total of 40 male Sprague-Dawley rats given 0, 2, 4, 8, or 16 mg of uranyl ethanoate dihydrate per kg of body weight per day (equivalent to doses of 0, 1.1, 2.2, 4.5, or 9.0 mg of uranium per kg of body weight per day) in drinking-water for 4 weeks exhibited a variety of biochemical effects, including increases in blood glucose levels at or above 4 mg/kg of body weight per day, decreases in aspartate aminotransferase and alanine aminotransferase values at or above 8 mg/kg of body weight per day, increases in several other haematological parameters at 16 mg/kg of body weight per day, and increases in total protein levels in all treated groups (*26*). The authors considered the NOAEL to be 2 mg/kg of body weight per day (1.1 mg of uranium per kg of body weight per day).

Preliminary results are available for a series of studies in which rats and rabbits were exposed to uranyl ion in drinking-water (A. Gilman, unpublished data, 1991). Groups of 15 male and 15 female weanling Sprague-Dawley rats consumed water containing 0.001 (control), 0.9, 4.8, 24, 120, or 600 mg of uranyl nitrate hexahydrate per litre (equivalent to doses of 0.00005, 0.06, 0.3, 1.5, 7.5, and 37 mg of uranium per kg of body weight per day in males, and 0.00005, 0.08, 0.4, 2, 10, and 54 mg of uranium per kg of body weight per day in females) for 90 days. A dose-related increase in the incidence and severity of kidney lesions, namely necrosis of the epithelial cells lining the proximal convoluted tubules, and the appearance of small vesicles in the cell lumen, were observed in all groups of treated male rats. The only renal lesions in females appeared in the highest dose group. The LOAEL for adverse effects on the kidney in male rats, based on the frequency and degree of degenerative lesions in the epithelium of the proximal convoluted tubule, was considered to be 4.8 mg/litre (or 0.3 mg of uranium per kg of body weight per day). Minor effects in the lowest dose group (0.9 mg/litre, or 0.06 mg of uranium per kg of body weight per day) were not considered to be adverse, as minor damage to the tubular epithelium appears to be partially reversible (*17, 21*). The reason for the difference in sensitivity between males and females is not clear, but it did not appear to be due to differences in pharmacokinetics, since accumulation of uranium in renal tissue did not differ significantly between the two sexes at all doses.

In a similar study, groups of 10 male New Zealand white rabbits were given uranyl nitrate hexahydrate in drinking-water at concentrations of 0.001 (control), 0.9, 4.8, 24, 120, or 600 mg/litre (determined to be equivalent to doses of 0, 0.05, 0.2, 0.9, 4.8, and 28.7 mg of uranium per kg of body weight per day) for 91 days (A. Gilman, unpublished data, 1991). Degenerative renal changes, namely pyknosis of nuclei in proximal convoluted tubules accompanied by vacuolation of tubules resulting in epithelial destruction in severely affected animals, and mild inflammatory changes were observed in the animals drinking water containing 24, 120, or 600 mg of uranyl nitrate hexahydrate per litre. There were histopathological changes in the thyroid gland at 24 and 600 mg/litre and mild hepatic changes in all dose groups. The LOAEL was considered to be 24 mg/litre (0.9 mg of uranium per kg of body weight per day). It should be noted, however, that these rabbits were not *Pasteurella*-free, and four of them contracted a *Pasteurella* infection during the course of the study. There were no dose-related changes in groups of 10 female *Pasteurella*-free rabbits drinking water containing <0.001 (control), 4.8, 24, or 600 mg of uranyl nitrate hexahydrate per litre (equivalent to doses of 0, 0.5, 1.3, and 43 mg of uranium per kg of body weight per day) for 91 days.

In an additional study in *Pasteurella*-free male New Zealand white rabbits, groups of 5–8 animals were given <0.001, 24, or 600 mg of uranyl nitrate hexahydrate per litre in drinking-water for 91 days, with a recovery period of up to 91 days (A. Gilman, unpublished data, 1991). Although minor histopathological lesions were seen in the thyroid, aorta, liver, and kidney, male rabbits did not respond as dramatically as those in the earlier study. It is possible that the *Pasteurella*-free rabbits are less sensitive to the effects of uranyl ion in drinking-water than the non-*Pasteurella*–free strain. The LOAEL for the *Pasteurella*-free rabbits was considered to be 600 mg/litre (43 mg of uranium per kg of body weight per day). The generally mild lesions observed following 91 days of exposure were less frequently reported in animals kept for 91 days after exposure ceased. Repair responses were observed in the tissues of some animals, suggesting that the mild lesions reported may be largely reversible.

### Long-term exposure

In an early series of experiments, very high doses (up to 20% in the diet) of a variety of uranium compounds were fed to rats, dogs, and rabbits in the diet for periods ranging from 30 days to 2 years (*27*). On the basis of very limited histopathological investigations, renal damage was reported in each species.

### Reproductive toxicity, embryotoxicity, and teratogenicity

Adverse reproductive effects, in terms of total number of litters and average number of young per litter, were reported in rats given 2% uranyl nitrate for 7 months (*27*).

### *Carcinogenicity*

Although bone cancer has been induced in experimental animals by injection or inhalation of soluble compounds of high-specific-activity uranium isotopes or mixtures of uranium isotopes, no carcinogenic effects have been reported in animals ingesting soluble or insoluble uranium compounds (*17*).

## 13.35.6 Effects on humans

Nephritis is the primary chemically induced effect of uranium in humans (*28*).

Little information is available on the chronic health effects of exposure to environmental uranium in humans. In Nova Scotia (Canada), clinical studies were performed on 324 persons exposed to variable amounts of naturally occurring uranium in drinking-water (up to 0.7 mg/litre) supplied from private wells. No relationship was found between overt renal disease or any other symptomatic complaint and exposure to uranium. However, a trend towards increasing excretion of urinary $\beta_2$-microglobulin and increasing concentration of uranium in well-water was observed; this raises the possibility that an early tubular defect was present and suggests that this parameter might be useful as an index of subclinical toxicity. The group with the highest uranium concentrations in well-water failed to follow this trend, but this was attributed to the fact that most of the individuals in this group had significantly reduced their consumption of well-water by the time that the measurements were made, leading to the conclusion that the suspected tubular defect might well be rapidly reversible (*10,11*).

## 13.35.7 Conclusions

Adequate short- and long-term studies on the chemical toxicity of uranium are not available, and a guideline value for uranium in drinking-water was therefore not derived. Until such information becomes available, it is recommended that the limits for the radiological characteristics of uranium be used (see Chapter 17). Based on these limits, the equivalent for natural uranium is approximately 0.14 mg/litre.

## References

1.  Lide DR, ed. *CRC handbook of chemistry and physics*. Boca Raton, FL, CRC Press, 1992-93.

2.  Cothern CR, Lappenbusch WL. Occurrence of uranium in drinking water in the US. *Health physics*, 1983, 45:89-99.

3.  Roessler CE et al. Uranium and radium-226 in Florida phosphate materials. *Health physics*, 1979, 37:269-267.

4.  Kreiger HL, Whittaker EL. *Prescribed procedures for measurement of radioactivity in drinking water*. Washington, DC, US Environmental Protection Agency, 1980 (EPA-600/4-80-032) (cited in: Blanchard RL et al. Radiological sampling and analytical methods for national primary drinking water regulations. *Health physics*, 1985, 48(5):587-600).

5.  Boomer DW, Powell MJ. Determination of uranium in environmental samples using inductively coupled plasma mass spectrometry. *Analytical chemistry*, 1987, 59:2810-2813.

6.  Hirose K, Sugimura Y. Concentration of uranium and the activity ratio of $^{234}$U/$^{238}$U in surface air: effect of atmospheric burn-up of Cosmos-954. *Meteorology and geophysics*, 1981, 32:317 (cited in reference 12).

7.  Fisenne IM et al. The daily intake of $^{234,235,238}$U, $^{228,230,232}$Th and $^{226,228}$Ra by New York City residents. *Health physics*, 1987, 53:357-363.

8.  Lucas HF, Markun F. Thorium and uranium in blood, urine and cigarettes. In: *Argonne National Laboratory Radiation Physics Division Annual Report*, Part 2. Argonne, IL, Argonne National Laboratory, 1970:47-52 (ANL-7760).

9.  Radiation Protection Bureau (Canada). *Environmental radioactivity in Canada*. Ottawa, Environmental Health Directorate, Department of National Health and Welfare, 1979-1985.

10. Moss MA et al. Uranium in drinking water–report on clinical studies in Nova Scotia. In: Brown SS, Savory J, eds. *Chemical toxicology and clinical chemistry of metals*. London, Academic Press, 1983:149-152.

11. Moss MA. *Chronic low level uranium exposure via drinking water–clinical investigations in Nova Scotia*. Halifax, Nova Scotia, Dalhousie University, 1985 (MSc thesis).

12. Fisenne IM, Welford GA. Natural U concentrations in soft tissues and bone of New York City residents. *Health physics*, 1986, 50(6):739-746.

13. Nozaki T et al. Neutron activation analysis of uranium in human bone, drinking water and daily diet. *Journal of radioanalytical chemistry*, 1970, 6:33-40.

14. Kahlos H, Asikainen M. Internal radiation doses from radioactivity of drinking water in Finland. *Health physics*, 1980, 39:108-111.

15. Singh NP et al. Daily U intake in Utah residents from food and drinking water. *Health physics*, 1990, 59(3):333-337.

16. Harley JH. Naturally occurring sources of radioactive contamination. In: Harley JH, Schmidt GD, Silini G, eds. *Radionuclides in the food chain*. Berlin, Springer-Verlag, 1988.

17. Wrenn ME et al. Metabolism of ingested U and Ra. *Health physics*, 1985, 48:601-633.

18. Tracy BL et al. Absorption and retention of uranium from drinking water by rats and rabbits. *Health physics*, 1992, 62(1):65-73.

19. La Touche YD, Willis DL, Dawydiak OI. Absorption and biokinetics of U in rats following an oral administration of uranyl nitrate solution. *Health physics*, 1987, 53:147-162.

20. Fisenne IM, Perry PM. Isotopic U concentration in human blood from New York City donors. *Health physics*, 1985, 49:1272-1275.

21. Berlin M, Rudell B. Uranium. In: Friberg L, Nordberg GF, Vouk VB, eds. *Handbook on the toxicology of metals*. Amsterdam, Elsevier/North Holland Biomedical Press, 1979:623-637.

22. Domingo JL et al. Acute toxicity of uranium in rats and mice. *Bulletin of environmental contamination and toxicology*, 1987, 39:168-174.

23. Durbin PW, Wrenn ME. Metabolism and effects of uranium in animals. In: *Conference on occupational health experience with uranium*, Washington, DC, US Energy Research and Development Administration, 1976:68-129 (available from National Technical Information Service).

24. Campbell DCC. *The development of an animal model with which to study the nephrotoxic effects of uranium-contaminated drinking water*. Halifax, Nova Scotia, Dalhousie University, 1985 (MSc thesis).

25. Yuile CL. Animal experiments. In: Hodge HC et al., eds. *Handbook of experimental pharmacology*, Vol. 36. *Uranium, plutonium, transplutonic elements*. Berlin, Springer-Verlag, 1973:165-195.

26. Ortega A et al. Evaluation of the oral toxicity of uranium in a 4-week drinking-water study in rats. *Bulletin of environmental contamination and toxicology*, 1989, 42:935-941.

27. Maynard EA, Hodge HC. Studies of the toxicity of various uranium compounds when fed to experimental animals. In: Voegtlin C, ed. *Pharmacology and toxicology of uranium compounds*. New York, McGraw-Hill, 1949:309-376.

28. Hursh JB, Spoor NL. Data on man. In: Hodge HC et al., eds., *Handbook of experimental pharmacology*, Vol. 36, *Uranium, plutonium, transplutonic elements*. Berlin, Springer-Verlag, 1973:197-240.

## 13.36 Zinc

### 13.36.1 General description

#### Identity

Zinc occurs in small amounts in almost all igneous rocks. The principal zinc ores are sulfides, such as sphalerite and wurzite (1). The natural zinc content of soils is estimated to be 1–300 mg/kg (2).

#### Physicochemical properties

| Property | Value |
|---|---|
| Physical state | Bluish-white metal |
| Melting point | 419.58 °C |
| Boiling point | 907 °C |
| Density (g/cm$^3$) | 7.14 at 20 °C |

#### Organoleptic properties

Zinc imparts an undesirable astringent taste to water. Tests indicate that 5% of a population could distinguish between zinc-free water and water containing zinc at a level of 4 mg/litre (as zinc sulfate). The detection levels for other zinc salts were somewhat higher. Water containing zinc at concentrations in the range 3–5 mg/litre also tends to appear opalescent and develops a greasy film when boiled (3).

#### Major uses

Zinc is used in the production of corrosion-resistant alloys and brass, and for galvanizing steel and iron products. Zinc oxide, used in rubber as a white pigment, for example, is the most widely used zinc compound. Peroral zinc is occasionally used to treat zinc deficiency in humans. Zinc carbamates are used as pesticides (1).

### 13.36.2 Analytical methods

Atomic absorption spectrophotometry is the most widely used method for the determination of zinc. The detection limit of the direct air–acetylene flame method is 50 µg/litre (4). Low concentrations can be measured by chelating zinc with ammonium pyrrolidine dithiocarbamate and extracting it with methyl isobutyl ketone (detection limit 0.5–1 µg/litre) (5).

### 13.36.3 Environmental levels and human exposure

#### Air

In rural areas, atmospheric zinc concentrations are typically between 10 and 100 ng/m$^3$, whereas levels in urban areas commonly fall within the range 100–500 ng/m$^3$ (2). Mean concentrations of zinc associated with particulate matter in ambient air in Canada were 85 ng/m$^3$ (6) and in Finland, 170 ng/m$^3$ (7).

## Water

In natural surface waters, the concentration of zinc is usually below 10 µg/litre, and in groundwaters, 10–40 µg/litre (1). In tapwater, the zinc concentration can be much higher as a result of the leaching of zinc from piping and fittings (2). The most corrosive waters are those of low pH, high carbon dioxide content, and low mineral salts content. In a Finnish survey of 67% of public water supplies, the median zinc content in water samples taken upstream and downstream of the waterworks was below 20 µg/litre; much higher concentrations were found in tapwater, the highest being 1.1 mg/litre (8). Even higher zinc concentrations (up to 24 mg/litre) were reported in a Finnish survey of water from almost 6000 wells (9).

## Food

Protein-rich foods, such as meat and marine organisms, contain high concentrations of zinc (10–50 mg/kg wet weight), whereas grains, vegetables, and fruit are low in zinc (usually <5 mg/kg) (1).

## Estimated total exposure and relative contribution of drinking-water

Values of 5–22 mg have been reported in studies on the average daily intake of zinc in different areas (1). The zinc content of typical mixed diets of North American adults varies between 10 and 15 mg/day (10). In Finland, the average daily intake of zinc from foodstuffs is calculated to be 16 mg (11). The recommended dietary allowance for adult men is set at 15 mg/day, for adult women 12 mg/day, for formula-fed infants 5 mg/day, and for preadolescent children 10 mg/day (12,13).

Drinking-water usually makes a negligible contribution to zinc intake unless high concentrations of zinc occur as a result of the corrosion of piping and fittings. Under certain circumstances, tapwater can provide up to 10% of the daily intake (9,14).

## 13.36.4 Kinetics and metabolism in laboratory animals and humans

Absorption of ingested zinc is highly variable (10–90%) and is affected by a number of factors. Homoeostatic mechanisms exist for the gastrointestinal absorption and excretion of zinc. High zinc concentrations are found in prostate, bone, muscle, and liver. Excretion takes place mainly (75%) via the gastrointestinal tract, and only to a smaller extent via urine and sweat. The biological half-time of retained zinc in humans is of the order of 1 year (1).

Zinc is an essential element in all living organisms. Nearly 200 zinc-containing enzymes have been identified, including many dehydrogenases, aldolases, peptidases, polymerases, and phosphatases (*15*).

## 13.36.5 Effects on laboratory animals and *in vitro* test systems

### Acute exposure

Acute oral $LD_{50}$ values in rats are reported to be as follows: zinc chloride 350, zinc sulfate 2950, and zinc ethanoate 2510 mg/kg of body weight (*16*).

### Long-term exposure

Zinc toxicosis has been documented in various mammalian species, including ferrets, sheep, cattle, pigs, horses, and dogs, mostly taking the form of copper deficiency caused by excessive zinc intake (*1,17*). Signs of toxicosis among a herd of 95 calves began to appear when calves were fed 1.2–2 g of zinc per day and exposed to a cumulative zinc intake of 42–70 g per calf (*18*). A high-zinc diet has been shown to induce hypocalcaemia and bone resorption in rats (*19*).

The antagonistic effects of zinc on the toxic effect of other metals, including cadmium, lead, and nickel, has been described in several reports (*20–22*).

### Carcinogenicity

One study with rats given zinc ethanoate (1.5 g of zinc per litre) in drinking-water indicated that there was an increase in the number of metastases following the intravenous injection of cells from a benzpyrene-induced sarcoma (*23*).

## 13.36.6 Effects on humans

Nutritional zinc deficiency in humans has been reported in a number of countries (*24–27*).

Acute toxicity results from the ingestion of excessive amounts of zinc salts, either accidentally or deliberately as an emetic or dietary supplement. Vomiting usually occurs after the consumption of more than 500 mg of zinc sulfate. Mass poisoning has been reported following the drinking of acidic beverages kept in galvanized containers; fever, nausea, vomiting, stomach cramps, and diarrhoea occurred 3–12 h after ingestion. Food poisoning attributable to the use of galvanized zinc containers in food preparation has also been reported; symptoms occurred within 24 h and included nausea, vomiting, and diarrhoea, sometimes accompanied by bleeding and abdominal cramps (*1*).

Manifest copper deficiency, which is the major consequence of the chronic ingestion of zinc (*13*), has been caused by zinc therapy (150–405 mg/day) for coeliac disease, sickle cell anaemia, and acrodermatitis enteropathica (*28–30*). Impairment of the copper status of volunteers by the dietary intake of 18.5 mg of zinc per day has been reported (*31*). Zinc supplementation of healthy adults with 20 times the recommended dietary allowance for 6 weeks resulted in the impairment of various immune responses (*32*). Gastric erosion is another reported complication of a daily dosage of 440 mg of zinc sulfate (*1*). Daily supplements of 80–150 mg of zinc caused a decline in high-density lipoprotein cholesterol levels in serum after several weeks (*1*), but this effect was not found in some other studies. In an Australian study, no detrimental effect of 150 mg of zinc per day on plasma copper levels was seen in healthy volunteers over a period of 6 weeks (*33*).

Acute toxic effects of inhaled zinc have been reported in industrial workers exposed to zinc fumes (*1*); the symptoms include pulmonary distress, fever, chills, and gastroeneritis.

In a small-scale study on zinc-refinery workers, no evidence was found of increased mortality from any type of cancer (*1*). In subjects with low baseline levels of serum zinc, no significant difference in the risk of death from cancer or cardiovascular diseases, as compared with those with high baseline levels, was observed (*34*).

## 13.36.7 Conclusions

In 1982, JECFA proposed a daily dietary requirement of zinc of 0.3 mg/kg of body weight and a provisional maximum tolerable daily intake (PMTDI) of 1.0 mg/kg of body weight (*35*). The daily requirement for adult humans is 15–22 mg/day. It was concluded that, in the light of recent studies on humans, the derivation of a health-based guideline value is not required at this time. However, drinking-water containing zinc at levels above 3 mg/litre tends to be opalescent, develops a greasy film when boiled, and has an undesirable astringent taste.

## References

1.   Elinder CG. Zinc. In: Friberg L, Nordberg GF, Vouk VB, eds. *Handbook on the toxicology of metals*, 2nd ed. Amsterdam, Elsevier Science Publishers, 1986:664-679.

2.   Nriagu JO, ed. *Zinc in the environment*, Part I, *Ecological cycling*. New York, NY, John Wiley, 1980.

3.   Cohen JM et al. Taste threshold concentrations of metals in drinking water. *Journal of the American Water Works Association*, 1960, 52:660.

4.   International Organization for Standardization. *Water quality – determination of cobalt, nickel, copper, zinc, cadmium and lead – flame atomic absorption spectrometric methods*. Geneva, 1986 (ISO 8288:1986).

5. *Deutsche Einheitsverfahren zur Wasser-, Abwasser- un Schlamm-Untersuchung.* [*German standard procedures for testing water, wastewater and sludge.*] Lieferung 22. Weinheim, Verlag Chemie, 1989.

6. Klemm RF, Gray JML. *A study of the chemical composition of particulate matter and aerosols over Edmonton.* Edmonton, Alberta Research Council, 1982 (Report RMD 82/9).

7. Mattsson R, Jaakkola T. An analysis of Helsinki air 1962 to 1977 based on trace metals and radionuclides. *Geophysica*, 1979, 16.

8. Hiisvirta L et al. [Metals in drinking water.] *Vatten*, 1986, 42:201 (in Swedish with English abstract).

9. Lahermo P et al. *The geochemical atlas of Finland*, Part 1. *The hydrogeochemical mapping of Finnish groundwater.* Espoo, Finland, Geological Survey of Finland, 1990.

10. Solomons NW. Zinc and copper. In: Shils ME, Young VR, eds. *Modern nutrition in health and disease.* Philadelphia, PA, Lea & Febiger, 1988.

11. Varo P, Koivistoinen P. Mineral element composition of Finnish foods. XII. General discussion and nutritional evaluation. *Acta agriculturae Scandinavica*, 1980, 22 (Suppl.): 165.

12. National Research Council. *Recommended dietary allowances*, 10th ed. Washington, DC, National Academy Press, 1989.

13. Cousins RJ, Hempe JM. Zinc. In: Brown ML, ed. *Present knowledge in nutrition.* Washington, DC, International Life Sciences Institute, 1990.

14. Gillies ME, Paulin HV. Estimations of daily mineral intakes from drinking water. *Human nutrition: applied nutrition*, 1982, 36:287-292.

15. O'Dell BL. History and status of zinc in nutrition. *Federation proceedings*, 1984, 43:2821-2822.

16. Sax NJ, Lewis RJ Jr. *Dangerous properties of industrial materials*, 7th ed. New York, NY, Van Nostrand Reinhold, 1989.

17. Torrance AG, Fulton RB Jr. Zinc-induced hemolytic anemia in a dog. *Journal of the American Veterinary Medical Association*, 1987, 191:443-444.

18. Graham TW et al. Economic losses from an episode of zinc toxicosis on a California veal calf operation using a zinc sulfate-supplemented milk replacer. *Journal of the American Veterinary Medical Association*, 1987, 190:668-671.

19. Yamaguchi M, Takahashi K, Okada S. Zinc-induced hypocalcemia and bone resorption in rats. *Toxicology and applied pharmacology*, 1983, 67:224-228.

20. Reddy CS et al. Mobilization of tissue cadmium in mice and calves and reversal of cadmium induced tissue damage in calves by zinc. *Bulletin of environmental contamination and toxicology*, 1987, 39:350-357.

21. Waalkes MP et al. Protective effects of zinc acetate toward the toxicity of nickelous acetate in rats. *Toxicology*, 1985, 34:29-41.

22. Hietanen E et al. Tissue concentrations and interaction of zinc with lead toxicity in rabbits. *Toxicology*, 1982, 25:113-127.

23. Rath FW et al. Zur Wirkung oral applizierten Zink auf die Metastasenbildung nach intravenoser Applikation von Zellen eines benzpyreninduzierten Rattensarkoms. [Effect of the oral administration of zinc on metastasis after intravenous application of benzpyrene-induced rat sarcoma.] *Acta histochemica*, 1990, 39(Suppl.):201-203.

24. Chen XC et al. Low levels of zinc in hair and blood, pica, anorexia and poor growth in Chinese preschool children. *American journal of clinical nutrition*, 1985, 42:694-700.

25. Smith RM et al. Growth-retarded aboriginal children with low plasma zinc levels do not show a growth response to supplementary zinc. *Lancet*, 1985, i(8434):923-924 (letter).

26. Cadvar AO et al. Zinc deficiency in geophagia in Turkish children and response to treatment with zinc sulfate. *Haematologica*, 1980, 65:403-408.

27. Jackson MJ et al. Stable isotope metabolic studies of zinc nutrition in slum-dwelling lactating women in the Amazon valley. *British journal of nutrition*, 1988, 59:193-203.

28. Porter KG et al. Anaemia and low serum-copper during zinc therapy. *Lancet*, 1977, ii(8041):774 (letter).

29. Prasad AS et al. Hypocupremia induced by zinc therapy in adults. *Journal of the American Medical Association*, 1978, 240:2166-2168.

30. Hoogenraad TU, Dekker AW, van den Hamer CJA. Copper responsive anaemia, induced by oral zinc therapy in a patient with acrodermatitis enteropathica. *Science of the total environment*, 1985, 42:37-43.

31. Festa MD et al. Effect of zinc intake on copper excretion and retention in man. *American journal of clinical nutrition*, 1985, 41:285-292.

32. Chandra RK. Excessive intake of zinc impairs immune responses. *Journal of the American Medical Association*, 1984, 252:1443-1446.

33. Samman S, Robert DCK. The effect of zinc supplements in plasma zinc and copper levels and the reported symptoms in healthy volunteers. *Medical journal of Australia*, 1987, 146:246-249.

34. Kok FJ et al. Serum copper and zinc and the risk of death from cancer and cardiovascular disease. *American journal of epidemiology*, 1988, 128:352-359.

35. Joint FAO/WHO Expert Committee on Food Additives. *Evaluation of certain food additives and contaminants*. Cambridge, Cambridge University Press, 1982 (WHO Food Additives Series, No. 17).

# 14.
# Organic constituents

## 14.1 Carbon tetrachloride

### 14.1.1 General description

**Identity**

CAS no.:                056-23-5
Molecular formula:  $CCl_4$

**Physicochemical properties** *(1, 2)*[1]

| Property | Value |
|---|---|
| *Melting point* | *-23 °C* |
| Boiling point | 76.5 °C |
| Density | 1.594 g/cm$^3$ at 25 °C |
| Vapour pressure | 15.36 kPa at 25 °C |
| Water solubility | 785 mg/litre at 20 °C |
| Log octanol–water partition coefficient | 2.64 |

**Organoleptic properties**

The odour thresholds for carbon tetrachloride in water and air are 0.52 mg/litre and < 64 mg/m$^3$, respectively *(3)*.

**Major uses**

Carbon tetrachloride is used mainly in the production of chlorofluorocarbon refrigerants, foam-blowing agents, and solvents. It is also used in the manufacture of paints and plastics, as a solvent in metal cleaning, and in fumigants *(4)*.

**Environmental fate**

Most carbon tetrachloride released to the environment reaches the atmosphere, where it is uniformly distributed. It does not react with photochemically pro-

---

[1] Conversion factor in air: 1 ppm = 6.4 mg/m$^3$.

duced hydroxyl radicals in the troposphere but may undergo photolysis in the stratosphere. It has an estimated half-life of 50 years in the atmosphere (*1, 5*).

Carbon tetrachloride readily migrates from surface water to the atmosphere in a matter of days or weeks; however, levels in anaerobic groundwater may remain elevated for months or even years (*5*). Carbon tetrachloride is capable of being adsorbed onto organic matter in soils (*1*). Migration to groundwater is possible (*6*). Bioaccumulation has not been observed.

## 14.1.2 Analytical methods

Carbon tetrachloride in drinking-water is determined by purge-and-trap gas chromatography (*7*). It is usually detected by mass spectrometry, the detection limit being about 0.3 µg/litre (*8*).

## 14.1.3 Environmental levels and human exposure

### *Air*

Most urban air concentrations of carbon tetrachloride are close to the background level of 0.8–0.9 µg/m$^3$ found in the continental air mass. Outdoor concentrations as high as 3.7 µg/m$^3$ have been reported near point sources. Indoor concentrations (1 µg/m$^3$) tend to be higher than outdoor levels (*1*).

### *Water*

Carbon tetrachloride was detected in the drinking-water of 30 of 945 cities in the USA at mean levels ranging from 0.3 to 0.7 µg/litre. Levels as high as 2–3 µg/litre have been measured (*1*). In Italy, carbon tetrachloride concentrations in drinking-water averaged 0.2 µg/litre (*9*). Carbon tetrachloride is an occasional contaminant of the chlorine used for drinking-water disinfection (*1*).

### *Food*

Carbon tetrachloride has been detected in a variety of foodstuffs at levels ranging from 0.1 to 20 µg/kg (*10*). Foods often become contaminated when they are fumigated with it. However, carbon tetrachloride is now seldom used for this purpose.

### *Estimated total exposure and relative contribution of drinking-water*

Although available data on concentrations in food are limited, the intake from air is expected to be much greater than that from food or drinking–water. At a typical carbon tetrachloride concentration of 1 µg/m$^3$ in air, the daily exposure by inhalation is estimated to be about 20 µg for an adult with an air intake of 20 m$^3$/day. At a typical concentration of 0.5 µg/litre in drinking-water, a daily exposure of 1 µg is estimated for an adult with an average consumption of 2 litres of water per day.

## 14.1.4 Kinetics and metabolism in laboratory animals and humans

Carbon tetrachloride is readily absorbed from the gastrointestinal tract, the respiratory tract, and the skin, the extent depending on the administration vehicle (*11–13*). It appears to be distributed to all major organs following absorption (*2*), the highest concentrations being in fat.

Carbon tetrachloride is thought to be metabolized by the hepatic cytochrome P-450 enzymes with the production of the highly toxic trichloromethyl radical, which binds to macromolecules, initiating lipid peroxidation and destroying cell membranes (*14*). The resulting metabolites depend on the aerobic state of the tissue in which metabolism occurs (*1*) and include chloroform, hexachloroethane, and possibly phosgene (*15, 16*). The trichloromethyl radical can also combine with oxygen to form peroxy free radicals capable of binding to cellular molecules (*17*). Carbon tetrachloride and its metabolites are excreted primarily in exhaled air and to a lesser extent in the urine and faeces (*2*).

## 14.1.5 Effects on laboratory animals and *in vitro* test systems

### Acute exposure

Oral $LD_{50}$ values ranging from 1000 to 12 800 mg/kg of body weight were reported in mice and rats (*2*).

### Short-term exposure

Hepatotoxic effects (increased serum enzymes and histopathology) were observed in rats given carbon tetrachloride in corn oil by gavage at daily doses of 20 mg/kg of body weight and above for 9 days. The same effects were observed in rats given daily oral doses of 10 mg/kg of body weight, 5 days per week for 12 weeks. No measurable adverse effects were observed in rats given 1 mg/kg of body weight per day for 12 weeks (*18*).

Hepatotoxicity (increased serum enzymes, increased organ weight, and pathological changes) was observed in male and female CD-1 mice given carbon tetrachloride in corn oil by gavage at doses of 625, 1250, or 2500 mg/kg of body weight for 14 consecutive days. After 90 days, hepatotoxic effects were observed in animals that had ingested 12, 120, 540, or 1200 mg/kg of body weight (*19*).

Male and female CD-1 mice were given carbon tetrachloride at 0, 1.2, 12, or 120 mg/kg of body weight per day for 90 days (5 days per week) by gavage in corn oil or as an aqueous suspension in 1% polysorbate 60 (*20*). A significant increase in serum enzyme activity was detected at 12 and 120 mg/kg of body weight per day in the corn oil groups as compared with the polysorbate 60 ones. Liver and liver-to-body-weight ratios were significantly greater at 120 mg/kg of body weight per day. Hepatocellular changes (e.g. necrosis, fat) occurred at 12 and 120 mg/kg of body weight per day and were more frequently observed in the corn oil groups. Use of a corn oil vehicle yielded a NOAEL that was an order of magnitude lower than that obtained when the polysorbate 60 suspension was used (12 v. 1.2 mg/kg of body weight per day).

### Long-term exposure

Carbon tetrachloride at doses of 0, 80, or 200 mg/kg of diet (high dose equivalent to about 10–18 mg/kg of body weight per day) was fed to rats (18 per sex, strain not given) until sacrifice at 2 years (21). Although no adverse effects were observed, tissues were not examined microscopically, liver weights were not measured, and survival was below 50% at 21 months.

### Reproductive toxicity, embryotoxicity, and teratogenicity

No reproductive effects were noted in rats fed diets containing carbon tetrachloride at 80 or 200 mg/kg for up to 2 years (22). Degeneration of testicular germinal epithelium has been reported in rats exposed to air concentrations of 1280 mg/m³ or above (23). An intraperitoneal dose of 2400 mg/kg of body weight resulted in adverse effects on testicular function in rats (24).

### Mutagenicity and related end-points

In general, carbon tetrachloride is not mutagenic in bacterial test systems or cultured liver cells (2). However, weakly positive results were reported at cytotoxic levels in an alkaline elution–rat hepatocyte assay that measures DNA single-strand breaks. It has caused point mutations and gene recombination in a eukaryotic (yeast) test system (25). Carbon tetrachloride induced cell transformation in Syrian hamster embryo cells (26). In an *in vivo–in vitro* hepatocyte DNA repair assay, carbon tetrachloride did not induce unscheduled DNA synthesis in male or female B6C3F₁ mice (27), although significant increases in hepatic cell proliferation were observed. This effect was also produced by carbon tetrachloride in male Fischer 344 rats.

### Carcinogenicity

In a number of studies, the development of liver tumours (primarily hepatomas and hepatocellular carcinomas) in several animal species, including hamsters, mice, and rats, has been reported following oral, subcutaneous, or inhalation exposure. In general, the first tumours appeared early, within 12–16 weeks in some experiments, and the incidence was high.

After inbred strain L mice were exposed to oral doses of 0.04 ml (approximately 64 mg) of carbon tetrachloride 2–3 times per week for 4 months, hepatomas developed in 47% of the treated animals, as compared with 1% of controls (28). In a study in which Syrian golden hamsters (10 per sex per group) were exposed to oral doses of carbon tetrachloride of 6.25–12.5 μl/day (approximately 10–20 mg/day) for 43 weeks, all animals that survived the treatment period (5 per sex) developed liver cell carcinomas (29).

Groups of B6C3F$_1$ mice (50 per sex) were given carbon tetrachloride at 0, 1250, or 2500 mg/kg of body weight five times per week for 78 weeks by corn oil gavage, and Osborne-Mendel rats were given 47 or 94 mg/kg of body weight (males) and 80 or 159 mg/kg of body weight (females) (30). The incidence of hepatocellular carcinomas was markedly increased in treated mice (96–100%) but only slightly in rats (2–8%) as compared with controls (0–6%).

## 14.1.6 Effects on humans

Single oral doses of 2.5–15 ml (57–343 mg/kg of body weight) do not usually produce serious effects, although changes may occur in liver and kidney tissue, including fat accumulation in the liver and renal swelling. Some adults suffer adverse effects (including death) from the ingestion of as little as 1.5 ml (34 mg/kg of body weight). A dose of 0.18–0.92 ml (29–150 mg/kg of body weight) may be fatal in children. Alcohol consumption potentiates carbon tetrachloride-induced hepatic and renal effects in humans (1, 2).

Occupational exposure to 128–512 mg/m$^3$ carbon tetrachloride for 2–3 months produced neurological effects (nausea, depression, dyspepsia, and narcosis) in workers. Hepatic and renal effects similar to those described for acute oral exposures have been reported after short-term exposures to 1280 mg/m$^3$ (1).

Although an epidemiological study of workers in the rubber industry suggested an association between exposure to carbon tetrachloride and lymphosarcoma and lymphatic leukaemia, the authors stressed that the results should be interpreted cautiously because of multiple exposure, possible bias, and small sample size (31). The development of liver cancer in humans exposed to carbon tetrachloride fumes has been reported only in a few cases, and the data are insufficient to establish a causal relationship (1).

### 14.1.7 Guideline value

IARC has concluded that there is sufficient evidence that carbon tetrachloride is carcinogenic in laboratory animals to assign it to group 2B as a possible human carcinogen (4).

As there is unequivocal evidence that carbon tetrachloride is carcinogenic in several species, and as it metabolizes to give the highly toxic trichloromethyl radical, the linearized multistage model was chosen for calculating concentrations of carbon tetrachloride in drinking-water associated with lifetime excess cancer risks of $10^{-4}$, $10^{-5}$, and $10^{-6}$. Based on the geometric means of risk estimates for liver cancer from four bioassays in laboratory rodents, the concentrations in drinking-water associated with lifetime excess cancer risks of $10^{-4}$, $10^{-5}$, and $10^{-6}$ are 600, 60, and 6 µg/litre, respectively.

Because carbon tetrachloride has not been shown to be genotoxic in most available studies, and because there is a possibility that it may act as a nongeno-toxic carcinogen, a guideline value has been derived based on the division of a NOAEL by an uncertainty factor. The NOAEL in a 12-week oral gavage study in rats was 1 mg/kg of body weight per day (*18*). A TDI of 0.71 µg/kg of body weight (allowing for dosing for 5 days per week) was calculated by applying an uncertainty factor of 1000 (100 for intra- and interspecies variation, and 10 for evidence of possible nongenotoxic carcinogenicity). No additional factor for the short duration of the study (12 weeks) was incorporated, as the compound was administered in corn oil in the critical study, and available data indicate that tox-icity following administration in water may be an order of magnitude less. The guideline value based on a 10% allocation to drinking-water is 2 µg/litre (round-ed figure). This value is lower than the range of values associated with lifetime ex-cess cancer risks of $10^{-4}$, $10^{-5}$, and $10^{-6}$ calculated by linear extrapolation.

## References

1. Agency for Toxic Substances and Disease Registry. *Toxicological profile for carbon tet-rachloride.* Atlanta, GA, US Department of Health and Human Services, 1989.

2. Office of Drinking Water. *Final draft criteria document for carbon tetrachloride.* Washington, DC, US Environmental Protection Agency, 1985 (TR-540-131A).

3. Amoore JE, Hautala E. Odor as an aid to chemical safety: odor thresholds compared with threshold limit values and volatilities for 214 industrial chemicals in air and water dilution. *Journal of applied toxicology,* 1983, 3:272-290.

4. International Agency for Research on Cancer. *Some halogenated hydrocarbons.* Lyon, 1979:371-399 (IARC Monographs on the Evaluation of the Carcinogenic Risk of Chemicals to Humans, Volume 20).

5. Environmental Criteria and Assessment Office. *Health assessment document for carbon tetrachloride.* Cincinnati, OH, US Environmental Protection Agency, 1984 (EPA-600/8-82-001F).

6. Office of Drinking Water. *Health advisory for carbon tetrachloride.* Washington, DC, US Environmental Protection Agency, 1987.

7. Environmental Monitoring and Support Laboratory. *Method 502.1. Volatile halogen-ated organic compounds in water by purge-and-trap gas chromatography.* Cincinnati, OH, US Environmental Protection Agency, 1985.

8. Environmental Monitoring and Support Laboratory. *Method 524.1. Volatile organic compounds in water by purge-and-trap gas chromatography/mass spectrometry*. Cincinnati, OH, US Environmental Protection Agency, 1985.

9. Aggazzotti G, Predieri G. Survey of volatile halogenated organics (VHO) in Italy. *Water research*, 1986, 20(8):959-963.

10. McConnell G, Ferguson DM, Pearson CR. Chlorinated hydrocarbons in the environment. *Endeavour*, 1975, 34:13-18.

11. Paul BP, Rubinstein D. Metabolism of carbon tetrachloride and chloroform by the rat. *Journal of pharmacology and experimental therapy*, 1963, 141:141-148.

12. McCollister DD et al. The absorption, distribution and elimination of radioactive carbon tetrachloride by monkeys upon exposure to low vapor concentrations. *Journal of pharmacology and experimental therapy*, 1951, 102:112-124.

13. Bruckner JV et al. Influence of route and pattern exposure on the pharmacokinetics and hepatotoxicity of carbon tetrachloride. In: Gerrity TR, Henry CJ, eds. *Principle of route to route extrapolation for risk assessment*. Amsterdam, Elsevier Science Publishing, 1990: 271-284.

14. Bini A et al. Detection of early metabolites in rat liver after administration of carbon tetrachloride and CBrCl$_3$. *Pharmacology research communications*, 1975, 7:143-149.

15. Fowler JSL. Carbon tetrachloride metabolism in the rabbit. *British journal of pharmacology*, 1969, 37:733-737.

16. Shah H, Hartman SP, Weinhouse S. Formation of carbonyl chloride in carbon tetrachloride metabolism by rat liver *in vitro. Cancer research*, 1979, 39:3942-3947.

17. Rao KS, Recknagel RO. Early incorporation of carbon-labeled carbon tetrachloride into rat liver particulate lipids and proteins. *Experimental molecular pathology*, 1969, 10:219-228.

18. Bruckner JV et al. Oral toxicity of carbon tetrachloride: acute, subacute and subchronic studies in rats. *Fundamental and applied toxicology*, 1986, 6:16-34.

19. Hayes JR, Condie LW Jr, Borzelleca JF. Acute, 14-day repeated dosing, and 90-day subchronic toxicity studies of carbon tetrachloride in CD-1 mice. *Fundamental and applied toxicology*, 1986, 7:454-463.

20. Condie LW et al. Effect of gavage vehicle on hepatotoxicity of carbon tetrachloride in CD-1 mice: corn oil versus Tween-60 aqueous emulsion. *Fundamental and applied toxicology*, 1985, 7:199-206.

21. Alumot E et al. Tolerance and acceptable daily intake of chlorinated fumigants in the rat diet. *Food and cosmetics toxicology*, 1976, 14:105-110.

22. Prendergast JA et al. Effects on experimental animals of long-term inhalation of trichloroethylene, carbon tetrachloride, 1,1,1-trichloroethane, dichlorodifluoro-methane, and 1,1-dichloroethylene. *Toxicology and applied pharmacology*, 1967, 10: 270-289.

23. Adams EM et al. Vapor toxicity of carbon tetrachloride determined by experiments on laboratory animals. *Archives of industrial hygiene and occupational medicine*, 1952, 6:50-66.

24. Chatterjee A. Testicular degeneration in rats by carbon tetrachloride intoxication. *Experientia*, 1966, 22:394-396.

25. Callen DF, Wolfe CR, Philpot RM. Cytochrome P-450 mediated genetic activity and cytotoxicity of seven halogenated aliphatic hydrocarbons in *Saccharomyces cerevisiae*. *Mutation research*, 1980, 77:55-63.

26. Amacher DE, Zelljadt I. The morphological transformation of Syrian hamster embryo cells by chemicals reportedly nonmutagenic to *Salmonella typhimurium*. *Carcinogenesis*, 1983, 4(3):291-296.

27. Mirsalis JC et al. Induction of hepatic cell proliferation and unscheduled DNA synthesis in mouse hepatocytes following *in vivo* treatment. *Carcinogenesis*, 1985, 6:1521-1524.

28. Edwards JE. Hepatomas in mice induced with carbon tetrachloride. *Journal of the National Cancer Institute*, 1941, 2:197-199.

29. Della Porta G, Terracini B, Shubik P. Induction with carbon tetrachloride of liver cell carcinomas in hamsters. *Journal of the National Cancer Institute*, 1961, 26:855-863.

30. Division of Cancer Cause and Prevention. *Report on carcinogenesis bioassay of chloroform*. Bethesda, MD, National Cancer Institute, 1976.

31. Wilkosky TC et al. Cancer mortality and solvent exposures in the rubber industry. *American Industrial Hygiene Association journal*, 1984, 45:809-811.

# 14.2 Dichloromethane

## 14.2.1 General description

### Identity

CAS no.:                75-09-2
Molecular formula:   $CH_2Cl_2$

Dichloromethane is also known as methylene chloride.

## Physicochemical properties *(1, 2)*[1]

| Property | Value |
|---|---|
| Melting point | -95.1 °C |
| Boiling point | 40 °C |
| Density | 1.3255 g/cm$^3$ at 20 °C |
| Vapour pressure | 46.53 kPa at 20 °C |
| Water solubility | 20 000 mg/litre at 20 °C |
| Log octanol–water partition coefficient | 1.3 |

## Organoleptic properties

The odour thresholds for dichloromethane in air and water are 530–2120 mg/m$^3$ and 9.1 mg/litre, respectively *(3, 4)*.

## Major uses

Dichloromethane is widely used as an organic solvent and is found in paints, insecticides, degreasing and cleaning fluids, and other products *(2, 5, 6)*.

## Environmental fate

Most dichloromethane released to water and soil will be vaporized. It can persist in air for up to 500 days, but is rapidly biodegraded in water. In soil, it undergoes only slight biodegradation and is highly mobile, being leached from subsurface soil into groundwater *(5, 6)*.

## 14.2.2 Analytical methods

Purge-and-trap gas chromatography is routinely used for the determination of dichloromethane and other volatile organohalides in drinking-water *(7)*. This method is suitable for use at concentrations of 1–1500 µg/litre, but there are difficulties at low concentrations because dichloromethane vapour readily penetrates tubing during the procedure. Mass spectrometry (detection limit 0.3 µg/litre) can be used to confirm the identity of the compound *(8)*.

---

[1] Conversion factor in air: 1 ppm = 3.53 mg/m$^3$.

## 14.2.3 Environmental levels and human exposure

### Air

Background levels in air are usually about 0.1 mg/m$^3$; average concentrations in urban air range between 1 and 7 µg/m$^3$ (2).

### Water

Dichloromethane has been found in surface water samples at concentrations ranging from 0.1 to 743 µg/litre. Levels are usually higher in groundwater because volatilization is restricted; concentrations as high as 3600 µg/litre have been reported (5). Mean concentrations in drinking-water were less than 1 µg/litre.

### Food

Food is not expected to be a significant source of exposure to dichloromethane, which is now rarely used in food-extraction processes (e.g. decaffeination of coffee); however, it is used as a post-harvest fumigant on some foods (e.g. strawberries and grains).

### Estimated total exposure and relative contribution of drinking-water

Inhalation is the major route of environmental exposure (2), the estimated average daily intake from urban air being 33–307 µg (5). Exposure to dichloromethane through food and drinking-water is insignificant.

## 14.2.4 Kinetics and metabolism in laboratory animals and humans

Dichloromethane appears to be readily absorbed from the gastrointestinal tract (2, 9). Distribution in rats after oral administration was primarily to liver (10). The cytochrome P-450 and glutathione S-transferase systems can both metabolize dichloromethane to carbon monoxide or carbon dioxide (5, 11). Animal data indicate that it is excreted primarily through the lungs, the excretion products depending on the dose (10).

## 14.2.5 Effects on laboratory animals and in vitro test systems

### Acute exposure

Dichloromethane has a low acute toxicity; LD$_{50}$ values of 2000 mg/kg of body weight for rats and mice have been reported (2, 12, 13). The primary effect associated with acute exposure is depression of the central nervous system.

### Short-term exposure

Fischer 344 rats (20 per sex per group) were given dichloromethane in drinking-water for 90 days (0, 166, 420, or 1200 mg/kg of body weight per day in males, and 0, 209, 607, or 1469 mg/kg of body weight per day in females) (14). Centrilobular necrosis and granulomatous foci were noted in mid- and high-dose animals, and changes in some clinical chemistry parameters were noted in mid- and high-dose females. An increased incidence of hepatocyte vacuolization (lipid accumulation) was found in all dose groups. The LOAELs were 166 and 209 mg/kg of body weight per day for male and female rats, respectively.

In a study in which B6C3F$_1$ mice (20 per sex per group) received dichloromethane in drinking-water for 90 days at doses of 0, 226, 587, or 1911 mg/kg of body weight per day (males) and 0, 231, 586, or 2030 mg/kg of body weight per day (females), subtle centrilobular fatty changes in liver and slight decreases in body weight were seen in the mid- and high-dose groups. The NOAELs were 226 and 231 mg/kg of body weight per day for male and female mice, respectively (14).

Dichloromethane administered to Wistar rats in drinking-water at 125 mg/litre (17.5 mg/kg of body weight per day) (15) for 13 weeks did not affect behaviour, body weight, blood and urine chemistries, organ-to-body-weight ratios, or histopathology, except that the urine albumin test was often positive (2, 16).

### Long-term exposure

Fischer 344 rats (85 per sex per group) received estimated mean doses of 6, 52, 125, or 235 mg/kg of body weight per day (males) and 6, 58, 136, or 263 mg/kg of body weight per day (females) for 104 weeks (17). Hepatic histological alterations (including an increased incidence of foci/areas of cellular alterations and fatty changes) were detected at 52 mg/kg of body weight per day and above. There were no other treatment-related effects (e.g. on survival, organ weight, or gross pathology) at any dose tested. The NOAEL for hepatic effects was 6 mg/kg of body weight per day.

When given to B6C3F$_1$ mice for 104 weeks at estimated mean doses of 0, 61, 124, 177, or 234 mg/kg of body weight per day for males (100–200 per dose) and 0, 59, 118, 172, or 238 mg/kg of body weight per day for females (50–100 per dose), dichloromethane did not affect body weight, water consumption, survival, clinical signs, haematological parameters, or gross pathology in any dose group. The histological alterations seen consisted of increased Oil Red O-positive material in both sexes at the highest dose tested. A NOAEL of 175 mg/kg of body weight per day (average for males and females) was identified (18).

### Reproductive toxicity, embryotoxicity, and teratogenicity

In a two-generation study in which Fischer 344 rats were exposed to dichloromethane via inhalation at levels up to 5.3 g/m³, no effects on fertility, litter size, neonatal growth and survival, or histopathology were observed (*19*). In a study in which mice and rats were exposed to dichloromethane at 4.4 or 15.9 g/m³ during gestation (*2, 20, 21*), fetal body weights were reduced in rats at 15.9 g/m³ (*21*), and minor skeletal variants (e.g. decreased incidence of lumbar spur in rats and increased incidence of a single extra sternal ossification centre in mice) were found at 4.4 g/m³ (*20*).

### Mutagenicity and related end-points

Dichloromethane was positive in the *Salmonella typhimurium* assay with and without activation (*22*). Test results in cultured mammalian cells are usually negative, but dichloromethane has been shown to transform rat embryo cells and to enhance the viral transformation of Syrian hamster embryo cells (*23, 24*). No DNA alkylation was detected in rats and mice after inhalation of dichloromethane (*25*).

### Carcinogenicity

Fischer 344 rats (85 per sex per group) received estimated mean doses of 6, 52, 125, or 235 mg/kg of body weight per day (males) and 6, 58, 136, or 263 mg/kg of body weight per day (females) in drinking-water for 104 weeks (*17*). Although the incidence of combined hepatocellular carcinomas and neoplastic nodules increased significantly in females in the groups receiving doses of 58 and 263 mg/kg of body weight per day (4/83, 6/85) as compared with controls (0/134), the number of tumours was similar to that for historical controls. No significant increase in liver tumours was evident in any of the male dose groups. The dose of 235 mg/kg of body weight per day was concluded to be borderline for carcinogenicity in Fischer 344 rats (*6*).

B6C3F₁ mice received dichloromethane in drinking-water for 104 weeks at estimated mean doses of 0, 61, 124, 177, or 234 mg/kg of body weight per day (males) and 0, 59, 118, 172, or 238 mg/kg of body weight per day (females) (*18*). There was a marginal increase in the incidence of combined hepatocellular adenomas/carcinomas in male mice in the groups receiving doses of 124, 177 and 234 mg/kg of body weight per day (30/100, 31/99, 35/125) as compared with controls (24/125) but the incidence rates were within the historical control range. Liver tumours were not observed in female mice. This study is regarded as providing suggestive but not conclusive evidence for the carcinogenicity of dichloromethane (*6*).

Groups of B6C3F₁ mice (50 per sex per dose) were exposed by inhalation to 0, 7.1 or 14.1 g/m³ dichloromethane for 102 weeks (*26*). The incidence of alveolar/bronchiolar carcinomas was increased in both dose groups in males (10/50,

28/50) and females (13/48, 29/48) as compared with controls (2/50 males, 1/50 females). The combined incidence of hepatocellular adenomas and hepato-cellular carcinomas was increased in high-dose males (33/49 v. 22/50 and 24/49 for the control and low-dose group) and high-dose females (40/48 vs. 3/50 and 16/48). This study was regarded as clear evidence of carcinogenicity in mice.

## 14.2.6 Effects on humans

Inhalation of a high concentration of dichloromethane has been associated with a variety of central nervous system effects, most notably narcosis. Acute exposure to levels of 1.06 g/m$^3$ in air can impair sensory and motor function (*2*, *27*). Epidemiological studies involving occupational exposure (*2*, *28–31*) have failed to show a positive correlation between inhalation exposure and increased cancer incidence.

## 14.2.7 Guideline value

Dichloromethane is of low acute toxicity. An inhalation study in mice provided conclusive evidence of carcinogenicity, whereas a drinking-water study provided only suggestive evidence. IARC has placed dichloromethane in group 2B (possible human carcinogen) (*32*); however, the evidence suggests that it is not a genotoxic carcinogen and that genotoxic metabolites are not formed in significant amounts *in vivo*.

A TDI of 6 µg/kg of body weight was calculated by applying an uncertainty factor of 1000 (100 for inter- and intraspecies variation and 10 reflecting concern about carcinogenic potential) to a NOAEL of 6 mg/kg of body weight per day for hepatotoxic effects in a 2-year drinking-water study in rats (*17*). This gives a guideline value of 20 µg/litre (rounded figure), based on the allocation of 10% of the TDI to drinking-water. It should be noted that widespread exposure from other sources is possible.

## References

1.  Verschueren K. *Handbook of environmental data on organic chemicals*, 2nd ed. New York, NY, Van Nostrand Reinhold, 1983:848-849.

2.  *Methylene chloride*. Geneva, World Health Organization, 1984 (Environmental Health Criteria, No. 32).

3.  Amoore JE, Hautala E. Odor as an aid to chemical safety: odor thresholds compared with threshold limit values and volatilities for 214 industrial chemicals in air and water dilution. *Journal of applied toxicology*, 1983, 3:272-290.

4.  Ruth JH. Odor thresholds and initiation levels of several chemical substances. A review. *American Industrial Hygiene Association journal*, 1986, 47:A142-151.

5.  Agency for Toxic Substances and Disease Registry. *Toxicological profile for methylene chloride.* Atlanta, GA, US Department of Health and Human Services, 1992.

6.  Office of Health and Environmental Assessment. *Health assessment document for dichloromethane (methylene chloride). Final report.* Washington, DC, US Environmental Protection Agency, 1985.

7.  Environmental Monitoring and Support Laboratory. *Method 502.1. Volatile halogenated organic compounds in water by purge-and-trap gas chromatography.* Cincinnati, OH, US Environmental Protection Agency, 1985.

8.  Environmental Monitoring and Support Laboratory. *Method 524.1. Volatile organic compounds in water by purge-and-trap gas chromatography/mass spectrometry.* Cincinnati, OH, US Environmental Protection Agency, 1985.

9.  Angelo MJ et al. The pharmacokinetics of dichloromethane. II. Disposition in Fischer 344 rats following intravenous and oral administration. *Food chemistry and toxicology,* 1986, 24(9):975-980.

10.  McKenna MJ, Zempel JA. The dose-dependent metabolism of $^{14}$C-methylene chloride following oral administration to rats. *Food and cosmetics toxicology,* 1981, 19:73-78.

11.  Gargas ML, Clewell HJ, Andersen ME. Metabolism of inhaled dihalomethanes *in vivo*: differentiation of kinetic constants for two independent pathways. *Toxicology and applied pharmacology,* 1986, 82:211-223.

12.  Kimura ET, Ebert DM, Dodge PW. Acute toxicity and limits of solvent residue for sixteen organic solvents. *Toxicology and applied pharmacology,* 1971, 19:699-704.

13.  Aviado DM, Zakhari S, Watanabe T. Methylene chloride. In: Golberg L, ed. *Non-fluorinated propellants and solvents for aerosols.* Cleveland, OH, CRC Press, 1977:19-45.

14.  Kirschman JC et al. Review of investigations of dichloromethane metabolism and subchronic oral toxicity as the basis for the design of chronic oral studies in rats and mice. *Food chemistry and toxicology,* 1986, 24:943-949.

15.  Environmental Criteria and Assessment Office. *Reference values for risk assessment.* Cincinnati, OH, US Environmental Protection Agency, 1986 (ECAO-CIN-477).

16.  Bornmann G, Loeser A. Zur Frage einer chronisch-toxischen Wirkung von Dichloromethan. [On the chronic toxic effect of dichloromethane.] *Zeitschrift für Lebensmittel-Untersuchung und -Forschung,* 1967, 136:14-18.

17.  Serota DG, Thakur AK, Ulland BM. A two-year drinking water study of dichloromethane in rodents. I. Rats. *Food chemistry and toxicology,* 1986, 24:951-958.

18. Serota DG, Thakur AK, Ulland BM. A two-year drinking water study of dichloro-methane in rodents. II. Mice. *Food chemistry and toxicology*, 1986, 24:959-963.

19. Nitschke KD et al. Methylene chloride: two-generation inhalation reproductive study in rats. *Fundamental and applied toxicology*, 1988, 11:60-67.

20. Schwetz BA, Leong BKJ, Gehring PJ. The effect of maternally inhaled trichloro-ethylene, perchloroethylene, methyl chloroform, and methylene chloride on embry-onal and fetal development in mice and rats. *Toxicology and applied pharmacology*, 1975, 32:84-96.

21. Hardin BD, Manson JM. Absence of dichloromethane teratogenicity with inhalation exposure in rats. *Toxicology and applied pharmacology*, 1980, 52:22-28.

22. Green T. The metabolic activation of dichloromethane and chlorofluoromethane in a bacterial mutation assay using *Salmonella typhimurium*. *Mutation research*, 1983, 118(4):277-288.

23. Price PJ, Hassett CM, Mansfield JI. Transforming activities of trichloroethylene and proposed industrial alternatives. *In vitro*, 1978, 14:290-293.

24. Hatch GG et al. Chemical enhancement of viral transformation in Syrian hamster embryo cells by gaseous and volatile chlorinated methanes and ethanes. *Cancer research*, 1983, 43:1945-1950.

25. Green T et al. Macromolecular interactions of inhaled methylene chloride in rats and mice. *Toxicology and applied pharmacology*, 1988, 93:1-10.

26. National Toxicology Program. *NTP technical report on the toxicology and carcinogen-esis studies of dichloromethane in F344/N rats and B6C3F$_1$ mice (inhalation studies)*. Research Triangle Park, NC, 1986 (NTP-TR-306).

27. Winneke G. Behavioral effects of methylene chloride and carbon monoxide as assessed by sensory and psychomotor performance. In: Xintras C, Johnson BL, deGroot I, eds. *Behavioral toxicology*. Washington, DC, US Government Printing Office, 1974:130-144.

28. Friedlander BR, Hearne FT, Hall S. Epidemiologic investigation of employees chronically exposed to methylene chloride. *Journal of occupational medicine*, 1978, 20:657-666.

29. Ott MG et al. Health evaluation of employees occupationally exposed to methylene chloride. *Scandinavian journal of work, environment and health*, 1983, 9(Suppl.1): 1-38.

30. Hearne FT et al. Methylene chloride mortality study: dose-response characterization and animal model comparison. *Journal of occupational medicine*, 1987, 29:217-228.

31. Hearne FT, Pifer JW, Grose F. Absence of adverse mortality effects in workers exposed to methylene chloride: an update. *Journal of occupational medicine*, 1990, 32:234-240.

32. International Agency for Research on Cancer. *Overall evaluations of carcinogenicity: an updating of IARC monographs volumes 1-42*. Lyon, 1987:194-195 (IARC Monographs on the Evaluation of Carcinogenic Risks to Humans, Suppl. 7).

## 14.3  1,1-Dichloroethane

### 14.3.1 General description

#### Identity

CAS no.:            75-34-3
Molecular formula:  $C_2H_4Cl_2$

#### Physicochemical properties (1, 2 )[1]

| Property | Value |
| --- | --- |
| Melting point | -97.4 °C |
| Boiling point | 57.3 °C |
| Density | 1.174 g/cm³ at 20 °C |
| Vapour pressure | 31.2 kPa at 20 °C |
| Water solubility | 5500 mg/litre at 20 °C |
| Log octanol–water partition coefficient | 61.7 |

#### Organoleptic properties

1,1-Dichloroethane has an aromatic, ethereal and chloroform-like odour. Its odour threshold in air is 486 or 810 mg/m³ (2).

#### Major uses

The major use of 1,1-dichloroethane is as an intermediate in the production of 1,1,1-trichloroethane, vinyl chloride, and other chemicals (3). It is also used as a solvent in paint and varnish removers, as a degreaser and cleaning agent, and in ore flotation. It was formerly used as an anaesthetic.

---

1 Conversion factor in air: 1 ppm = 4.05 mg/m³.

## Environmental fate

Most 1,1-dichloroethane released to the environment will be vaporized and enter the atmosphere, where photo-oxidation takes place; the estimated half-life is 44 days. Biodegradation is not expected to be significant in aquatic systems (3).

## 14.3.2 Analytical methods

A purge-and-trap gas chromatographic procedure is used for the determination of 1,1-dichloroethane and other volatile organohalides in drinking-water (4). This method is applicable to the measurement of 1,1-dichloroethane over a concentration range of 0.02–1500 µg/litre. Mass spectrometry (detection limit 0.17 µg/litre) can be used to confirm the identity of the compound (5).

## 14.3.3 Environmental levels and human exposure

### Air

1,1-Dichloroethane has been detected in urban air at concentrations ranging from 0.4 to 6.1 µg/m³. A median concentration of 0.22 µg/m³ was reported for urban, rural, and industrial sites across the United States. Concentrations in the vicinity of industrial sources ranged from 0.23 to 0.56 µg/m³, and a concentration of 22.5 µg/m³ was reported near a hazardous waste site. 1,1-Dichloroethane has also been detected in indoor air at a mean concentration of 12.8 µg/m³ (3).

### Water

1,1-Dichloroethane was detected in 4.3% of 945 public water supplies in the USA at levels of up to 4.2 µg/litre. It was also detected in private wells used for drinking-water and in surface water and groundwater supplies, generally at levels below 10 µg/litre, although concentrations up to 400 µg/litre have been reported (3).

### Estimated total exposure and relative contribution of drinking-water

Exposure to 1,1-dichloroethane may occur through drinking-water, but from the point of view of the general population the greatest exposure is usually from the inhalation of ambient air. Based on a median air level of 0.22 µg/m³, the average inhalation exposure to 1,1-dichloroethane is estimated at 4 µg/day (3).

## 14.3.4 Kinetics and metabolism in laboratory animals and humans

The detection of metabolites in the urine following oral exposure and its former use as an anaesthetic provide evidence for the absorption of 1,1-dichloroethane by the oral and inhalation routes (6). In general, chlorinated organic solvents are

405

distributed throughout the body following absorption into the blood but preferentially to adipose tissue (7). Following intraperitoneal administration of 1,1-dichloroethane to rats, the compound was detected in liver, kidney, lung, and stomach tissues (8).

Following oral administration of 1,1-dichloroethane to mice and rats, 29% and 7% was metabolized, respectively (6), the major metabolite in both species being carbon dioxide. *In vitro* studies suggest that the primary route of biotransformation involves the hepatic microsomal cytochrome P-450 system, the major metabolite being ethanoic acid (9,10). The metabolic capacity of the P-450 system may be exceeded at high oral doses (3). Absorbed 1,1-dichloroethane is excreted mainly in the urine and expired air (6, 7).

## 14.3.5 Effects on laboratory animals and *in vitro* test systems

### Acute exposure

Reported oral $LD_{50}$s in rats range from 0.7 to 14 g/kg of body weight (11,12).

### Short-term exposure

Groups of five male and five female Osborne-Mendel rats and $B6C3F_1$ mice received 1,1-dichloroethane in corn oil by gavage, 5 days per week for 6 weeks; this was followed by a 2-week observation period (13). Dose levels were 0, 562, 1000, 1780, 3160, or 5620 mg/kg of body weight per day for rats and 0, 1000, 1780, 3160, 5620, or 10 000 mg/kg of body weight per day for mice. Body weight was depressed in male rats at 562 and 1000 mg/kg of body weight per day and in female rats at 1780 and 3160 mg/kg of body weight per day. Two female rats in the group receiving 3160 mg/kg of body weight per day and two male and three female mice in that receiving 5620 mg/kg of body weight per day died.

Groups of 10 rats, 10 guinea pigs, four rabbits, and four cats were exposed to 2025 mg/m³ 1,1-dichloroethane by inhalation for 6 h per day, 5 days per week for 13 weeks (14). Because no effects were observed in these animals, the concentration was increased to 4050 mg/m³ for an additional 10–13 weeks. Elevated blood urea nitrogen values were observed in cats only. At termination, histopathological examination revealed renal tubular dilatation and degeneration.

### Long-term exposure

Groups of Osborne-Mendel rats and $B6C3F_1$ mice were given 1,1-dichloroethane by gavage in corn oil, 5 days per week for 78 weeks, at time-weighted average doses of 382 or 764 mg/kg of body weight per day (male rats), 475 or 950 mg/kg of body weight per day (female rats), 1442 or 2885 mg/kg of body weight per day (male mice), and 1665 or 3331 mg/kg of body weight per day (female mice) (13). High mortality was seen in both treated and control animals; mortality in male rats and mice showed a significant dose-related trend. The increased mortality was thought to be related to pneumonia, which was observed in about 80% of the rats.

Male B6C3F$_1$ mice were given 1,1-dichloroethane in drinking-water at concentrations of 835 or 2500 mg/litre (high dose equivalent to about 540 mg/kg of body weight per day) for 52 weeks (15). No histopathological changes were observed in the liver, kidneys, or lungs.

### Reproductive toxicity, embryotoxicity, and teratogenicity

1,1-Dichloroethane has been found to be embryotoxic but not teratogenic following inhalation exposure. Exposure of pregnant rats to 15.4 or 24.3 g/m$^3$ 1,1-dichloroethane in air 7 h per day on days 6–15 of gestation did not affect the incidence of fetal resorptions or gross or soft tissue anomalies, although a significantly increased incidence of delayed ossification of the sternebrae, reflecting retarded fetal development, was observed in offspring of the rats exposed at 24.3 g/m$^3$ (16).

### Mutagenicity and related end-points

1,1-Dichloroethane was found to be mutagenic in several strains of *Salmonella typhimurium* with or without metabolic activation (17) but not in others (3, 18). It was not mutagenic in *Saccharomyces cerevisiae* strains with or without metabolic activation (3, 18). 1,1-Dichloroethane increased the frequency of DNA viral transformations in Syrian hamster embryo cells (19) but did not increase cell transformations in BALB/c-3T3 mouse cells (20). 1,1-Dichloroethane was positive in DNA binding assays in mouse and rat organs *in vivo*. Following intraperitoneal injection, it was reported to be covalently bound to macromolecules (DNA, RNA, proteins) in liver, lung, stomach, and kidney tissues of both species (8).

### Carcinogenicity

Groups of Osborne-Mendel rats and B6C3F$_1$ mice were given 1,1-dichloroethane by gavage in corn oil, 5 days per week for 78 weeks, at time-weighted average doses of 382 or 764 mg/kg of body weight per day (male rats), 475 or 950 mg/kg of body weight per day (female rats), 1442 or 2885 mg/kg of body weight per day (male mice), and 1665 or 3331 mg/kg of body weight per day (female mice) (13). Marginally significant dose-related increases in mammary adenocarcinomas and haemangiosarcomas in female rats and a nonsignificant increase in hepatocellular carcinomas in male mice were observed. A statistically significant increase in uterine endometrial stromal polyps (benign tumours) was also observed. Lymphomas of the cervical lymph nodes were reported in 2 of 47 female mice in the high-dose group but not in other groups. The authors concluded that the high mortality in all the groups prevented the appearance of late-developing tumours. The results of this study suggest that 1,1-dichloroethane is carcinogenic in rats and mice, but the evidence is not considered conclusive.

1,1-Dichloroethane was administered in drinking-water to male B6C3F$_1$ mice at concentrations of 835 or 2500 mg/litre (the latter is equivalent to about 540 mg/kg of body weight per day) for 52 weeks, either alone or following initiation with diethylnitrosamine (15). Lung and liver tumours were found in all groups, but neither the incidence nor the number of tumours per animal was increased as compared with controls in any treatment group. This was not a lifetime study, and there was a high incidence of spontaneous tumours in the controls, so that its value is limited. The authors suggested that 1,1-dichloroethane may be more toxic by gavage than by drinking-water exposure.

## 14.3.6 Effects on humans

It can be assumed that inhalation exposures to high concentrations of 1,1-dichloroethane cause central nervous system depression, as the compound was used as an anaesthetic until its use was discontinued because of the occurrence of cardiac arrhythmias at the concentrations required for anaesthesia (>100 000 mg/m$^3$) (21).

## 14.3.7 Conclusions

The acute toxicity of 1,1-dichloroethane is relatively low, and only limited data on its toxicity are available from short- and long-term studies. There is limited *in vitro* evidence of genotoxicity. One carcinogenicity study by gavage in mice and rats provided no conclusive evidence of carcinogenicity, although there was some evidence of an increased incidence of mammary adenocarcinomas and haemangiosarcomas in treated animals (13).

In view of the very limited database on toxicity and carcinogenicity, it is concluded that no guideline value should be proposed.

## References

1.  Office of Health and Environmental Assessment. *Drinking water criteria document for 1,1-dichloroethane.* Cincinnati, OH, 1983.

2.  Verschueren K. *Handbook of environmental data on organic chemicals,* 2nd ed. New York, NY, Van Nostrand Reinhold, 1983:486-487.

3.  Agency for Toxic Substances and Disease Registry. *Toxicological profile for 1,1-dichloroethane.* Atlanta, GA, US Department of Health and Human Services, 1989.

4.  Environmental Monitoring and Support Laboratory. *Method 502.1. Volatile halogenated organic compounds in water by purge-and-trap gas chromatography.* Cincinnati, OH, US Environmental Protection Agency, 1985.

5.  Environmental Monitoring and Support Laboratory. *Method 524.1. Volatile organic compounds in water by purge-and-trap gas chromatography/mass spectrometry*. Cincinnati, OH, US Environmental Protection Agency, 1985.

6.  Mitoma C et al. Metabolic disposition study of chlorinated hydrocarbons in rats and mice. *Drug chemistry and toxicology*, 1985, 8:183-194.

7.  Sato A, Nakajima T. Pharmacokinetics of organic solvent vapors in relation to their toxicity. *Scandinavian journal of work, environment and health*, 1987, 13:81-93.

8.  Colacci A et al. Genotoxicity of 1,1-dichloroethane. *Research communications in chemical pathology and pharmacology*, 1985, 49:243-254.

9.  Loew G, Trudell J, Motulsky H. Quantum chemical studies of the metabolism of a series of chlorinated ethane anesthetics. *Molecular pharmacology*, 1973, 9(2):152-162.

10. McCall SN, Jurgens P, Ivanetich KM. Hepatic microsomal metabolism of the dichloroethanes. *Biochemical pharmacology*, 1983, 32(2):207-213.

11. *Registry of Toxic Effects of Chemical Substances (RTECS)*. Bethesda, MD, National Toxicology Information Program, 1988.

12. Smyth HF Jr. Improved communication: hygienic standards for daily inhalation. *American Industrial Hygiene Association quarterly*, 1956, 17:129-195.

13. National Cancer Institute. *Bioassay of 1,1-dichloroethane for possible carcinogenicity*. Bethesda, MD, 1978 (NCI/NTP TR 066; DHEW Publ. No. (NIH) 78-1316).

14. Hofmann HT, Birnstiel H, Jobst P. On the inhalation toxicity of 1,1- and 1,2-dichloroethane. *Archives of toxicology*, 1971, 27(3):248-265 (English translation).

15. Klaunig JE, Ruch RJ, Pereira MA. Carcinogenicity of chlorinated methane and ethane compounds administered in drinking water to mice. *Environmental health perspectives*, 1986, 69:89-95.

16. Schwetz BA, Leong BKJ, Gehring PJ. Embryo- and fetotoxicity of inhaled carbon tetrachloride, 1,1-dichloroethane, and methyl ethyl ketone in rats. *Toxicology and applied pharmacology*, 1974, 28(3):452-464.

17. Riccio E et al. A comparative mutagenicity study of volatile halogenated hydrocarbons using different metabolic activation systems. *Environmental mutagenesis*, 1983, 5:472 (abstract).

18. Simmon VF, Kauhanen A, Tardiff RG. Mutagenic activity of chemicals identified in drinking water. In: Scott D, Bridges BA, Sobels FH, eds., *Progress in genetic toxicology*. Vol. 2. *Developments in toxicology and environmental science*, 1977:249-258.

19. Hatch GG et al. Chemical enhancement of viral transformation in Syrian hamster embryo cells by gaseous and volatile chlorinated methanes and ethanes. *Cancer research*, 1983, 43(5):1945-1950.

20. Tu AS et al. *In vitro* transformation of BALB/c-3T3 cells by chlorinated ethanes and ethylenes. *Cancer letters*, 1985, 28:85-92.

21. Browning E. *Toxicity and metabolism of industrial solvents*. Amsterdam, Elsevier, 1965:247-252.

## 14.4 1,2-Dichloroethane

### 14.4.1 General description

#### Identity

CAS no.: 107-06-2
Molecular formula: $C_2H_4Cl_2$

1,2-Dichloroethane is also known as ethylene dichloride.

#### Physicochemical properties (1)[1]

| Property | Value |
|---|---|
| Melting point | -35 °C |
| Boiling point | 83 °C |
| Density | 1.23 g/cm$^3$ at 20 °C |
| Vapour pressure | 8.53 kPa at 20 °C |
| Water solubility | 8.69 g/litre at 20 °C |
| Log octanol–water partition coefficient | 1.48 |

#### Organoleptic properties

The odour thresholds for 1,2-dichloroethane in air and water are 356 mg/m$^3$ and 7 mg/litre, respectively (2).

#### Major uses

The major use of 1,2-dichloroethane is in the production of vinyl chloride (1). It is also used as a solvent, in the synthesis of other chlorinated solvents, and as a lead scavenger in leaded petrol.

---

[1] Conversion factor in air: 1 ppm = 4.05 mg/m$^3$.

## Environmental fate

Most 1,2-dichloroethane released to the environment volatilizes to the atmosphere, where it is photo-oxidized with a lifetime of up to 4 months. Biodegradation is not expected to be significant in aquatic systems (*3*). 1,2-Dichloroethane may persist for long periods in groundwater, where volatilization is restricted (*1*).

## 14.4.2 Analytical methods

A purge-and-trap gas chromatographic procedure is used for the determination of 1,2-dichloroethane and other volatile organohalides in drinking-water (*4*). This method is applicable to the measurement of 1,2-dichloroethane over a concentration range of 0.2–1500 µg/litre. Confirmatory analysis is by mass spectrometry, the detection limit being 0.3 µg/litre (*5*).

## 14.4.3 Environmental levels and human exposure

### Air

1,2-Dichloroethane has been detected in urban air at concentrations ranging from 0.04 to 38 µg/m$^3$ (*6*). Concentrations in the vicinity of industrial sources may be higher (*1, 7*).

### Water

1,2-Dichloroethane was detected in drinking-water in 26 of 80 cities in the USA at levels up to 6 µg/litre (*8*). It was not detected in the drinking-water of 100 cities in Germany, but was present at levels up to 61 µg/litre in tapwater in other areas of Europe (*7*).

### Food

1,2-Dichloroethane was detected in 11 of 17 spice samples at levels of 2–23 µg/g (*9*) and in milk products with added fruit at an average concentration of 0.8 µg/kg (*7*). There is no significant bioconcentration of 1,2-dichloroethane in fish (*9*).

### Estimated total exposure and relative contribution of drinking-water

The greatest exposure of the general population is usually from the inhalation of ambient air (*3*). Exposure from drinking-water may be important for about 5% of the population and may exceed exposure by inhalation in places where the water concentration is greater than 6 µg/litre (*3*). Volatilization of 1,2-dichloroethane from water during showering or other water uses and from consumer products (cleaning agents, wallpaper, and carpet glue) may also contribute to inhalation exposure.

## 14.4.4 Kinetics and metabolism in laboratory animals and humans

1,2-Dichloroethane is readily absorbed through the lungs, skin, and gastrointestinal tract by both humans and laboratory animals (1, 10–12). It appears to be readily distributed following oral or inhalation exposure, accumulating in the liver and kidneys (13). 1,2-Dichloroethane appears to cross the blood–brain barrier and the placenta (3), and it has been detected in human milk following occupational exposure (11).

1,2-Dichloroethane is readily metabolized following oral or inhalation exposure. The primary route of biotransformation appears to involve conjugation with glutathione in the liver to produce several urinary metabolites, including S-carboxymethylcysteine and thiodiacetic acid (3, 14, 15). Absorbed 1,2-dichloroethane is rapidly excreted, mainly in the urine and expired air (14, 15).

## 14.4.5 Effects on laboratory animals and *in vitro* test systems

### Acute exposure

Reported oral $LD_{50}$s are 670 mg/kg of body weight for rats, 489 mg/kg of body weight for mice, and 860 mg/kg of body weight for rabbits (1, 16).

### Short-term exposure

Mice exposed to 1,2-dichloroethane at 4.9 or 49 mg/kg of body weight per day for 14 days by gavage exhibited a significant depression of leukocyte counts at the higher dose, and a significant reduction in the number of antibody-forming cells and inhibition of cell-mediated immunity at both doses. No effects on other haematological parameters, body weights, or the hepatic, renal, or respiratory systems were observed. Mice exposed to 1,2-dichloroethane at time-weighted average doses of 3, 24, or 189 mg/kg of body weight per day for 90 days in drinking-water experienced no significant adverse effects on haematological, immunological, hepatic, renal, or respiratory parameters (17). Liver changes, including an increase in liver triglycerides and a 15% increase in fat accumulation in the liver, were observed in rats given 1,2-dichloroethane in the diet at 80 mg/kg of body weight per day for 5–7 weeks (12).

### Long-term exposure

Significantly increased mortality was reported in groups of rats and mice exposed to 1,2-dichloroethane by gavage in corn oil for 78 weeks at doses of 95 or 299 mg/kg of body weight per day, respectively (18). No treatment-related effects on growth or biochemical indices were observed in rats exposed to 1,2-dichloro-ethane at 250 or 500 mg/kg in the diet (the higher dose is equivalent to about 26–35 mg/kg of body weight per day) for 2 years (*12*).

### Reproductive toxicity, embryotoxicity, and teratogenicity

In rats exposed to 1,2-dichloroethane at 250 or 500 mg/kg in the diet for 2 years, no effect was seen on male fertility or on reproductive activity in either sex (*12*). No reproductive effects, as measured by fertility, gestation, viability or lactation indices, pup survival, or weight gain, were found in a multigeneration reproduction study using male and female ICR Swiss mice that received 0, 5, 15, or 50 mg/kg of body weight per day in drinking-water (*19*). In a study in which male and female mice were exposed to 1,2-dichloroethane in drinking-water at doses of 0, 5, 15, or 50 mg/kg of body weight per day, no statistically significant developmental effects, as indicated by the incidence of fetal visceral or skeletal anomalies, were observed (*19*).

### Mutagenicity and related end-points

1,2-Dichloroethane was mutagenic in several strains of *Salmonella typhimurium* and in *Escherichia coli* in some microsome assay test systems (*1, 3, 20, 21*) but not in others (*3, 22*). The mutagenic effects were enhanced by metabolic activation (*3, 21*). Sex-linked recessive lethal and somatic cell mutations were induced in *Drosophila melanogaster* (*3, 23, 24*). 1,2-Dichloroethane also induced mutations *in vitro* in human lymphoblasts and was positive in DNA-binding and DNA-damage assays in mice and rats *in vivo*. It did not induce micronucleus formation in mice (*3*).

### Carcinogenicity

1,2-Dichloroethane administered by gavage 5 days per week for 78 weeks to Osborne-Mendel rats (time-weighted average doses of 47 or 95 mg/kg of body weight per day) and B6C3F$_1$ mice (time-weighted average doses of 97 or 195 mg/kg of body weight per day (males) and 149 or 299 mg/kg of body weight per day (females)) was reportedly carcinogenic to both species (*1, 18*). Statistically significant increases in the incidence of squamous cell carcinomas of the fore-stomach and haemangiosarcomas of the circulatory system were observed in male rats, and female rats showed a statistically significant increased incidence in adenocarcinoma of the mammary glands. Statistically significant increases in the incidence of mammary adenocarcinomas and endometrial stromal polyps or sarcomas were seen in female mice, and the incidence of alveolar/bronchiolar adenomas was increased in male and female mice.

In a bioassay in which 1,2-dichloroethane was administered in drinking-water to male B6C3F$_1$ mice at concentrations of 835 or 2500 mg/litre (the higher dose is equivalent to about 470 mg/kg of body weight per day) for 52 weeks, either alone or following initiation with diethylnitrosamine (25), no increase was seen in the incidence of tumours as compared with controls. However, this was not a lifetime study, and there was a high incidence of spontaneous tumours in the controls. In addition, 1,2-dichloroethane appears to be more toxic by gavage than by exposure to drinking-water (3, 17).

## 14.4.6 Effects on humans

Acute oral exposure to 1,2-dichloroethane is reported to cause central nervous system, hepatic, gastrointestinal, respiratory, renal, and cardiovascular effects in humans (1, 3, 26–28). Death following acute intoxication is most often attributed to cardiovascular or respiratory failure (3, 28). Repeated inhalation exposures in the workplace result in anorexia, nausea, vomiting, weakness and fatigue, nervousness, epigastric pain, and irritation of the respiratory tract and eyes (1, 29).

## 14.4.7 Guideline value

IARC has classified 1,2-dichloroethane in Group 2B (possible human carcinogen) (30). It has been shown to produce statistically significant increases in a number of types of tumour in laboratory animals, including the relatively rare haemangiosarcoma, and the balance of evidence indicates that it is potentially genotoxic. There are no suitable long-term studies on which to base a TDI.

On the basis of haemangiosarcomas observed in male rats in a 78-week gavage study (18), and applying the linearized multistage model, concentrations in drinking-water of 300, 30, and 3 µg/litre, corresponding to excess cancer risks of $10^{-4}$, $10^{-5}$, and $10^{-6}$, respectively, were calculated.

## References

1.  *1,2-Dichloroethane.* Geneva, World Health Organization, 1987 (Environmental Health Criteria, No. 62).

2.  Amoore JE, Hautala E. Odor as an aid to chemical safety: odor thresholds compared with threshold limit values and volatilities for 214 industrial chemicals in air and water dilution. *Journal of applied toxicology,* 1983, 3:272-290.

3.  Agency for Toxic Substances and Disease Registry. *Toxicological profile for 1,2-dichloroethane.* Atlanta, GA, US Department of Health and Human Services, 1989 (NTIS No. PB90-171422).

4.  Environmental Monitoring and Support Laboratory. *Method 502.1. Volatile halogenated organic compounds in water by purge-and-trap gas chromatography.* Cincinnati, OH, US Environmental Protection Agency, 1985.

5.  Environmental Monitoring and Support Laboratory. *Method 524.1. Volatile organic compounds in water by purge-and-trap gas chromatography/mass spectrometry.* Cincinnati, OH, US Environmental Protection Agency, 1985.

6.  Okuno T et al. [Gas chromatography of chlorinated hydrocarbons in urban air.] *Hyogo ken kogai kenkyujo kenkyu hokoku,* 1974, 6:1-6 (in Japanese). (*Chemical abstracts,* 87.72564).

7.  Besemer AC et al. *Criteriadocument over 1,2-dichloorethaan.* [*Criteria document for 1,2-dichloroethane.*] Leidschendam, Netherlands, Ministerie van Volkshuisvesting, Ruimtelijke Ordening en Milieubeheer, 1984.

8.  Symons JM et al. National organics reconnaissance survey for halogenated organics. *Journal of the American Water Works Association,* 1975, 67:634-648.

9.  US Environmental Protection Agency. *Ambient water quality criteria for chlorinated ethanes.* Washington, DC, 1980 (EPA-44/5-80-029).

10. Spencer HD et al. Vapor toxicity of ethylene dichloride determined by experiments on laboratory animals. *Industrial hygiene and occupational medicine,* 1951, 4:482-493.

11. Urosova TP. [The possible presence of dichloroethane in human milk with exposure in industrial conditions.] *Gigiena i sanitarija,* 1953, 18:36-37 (in Russian).

12. Alumot E et al. Tolerance and acceptable daily intake of chlorinated fumigants in the rat diet. *Food and cosmetics toxicology,* 1976, 14:105-110.

13. Reitz RH et al. Pharmacokinetics and macromolecular interactions of ethylene dichloride: comparison of oral and molecular exposures. In: Ames B, Infante P, Reitz R, eds. *Ethylene dichloride: a potential health risk?* Cold Spring Harbor, NY, Cold Spring Harbor Laboratory, 1980:135-144 (Banbury Report 5).

14. Yllner S. Metabolism of [$^{14}$C]-1,2-dichloroethane in the mouse. *Acta pharmacologica et toxicologica,* 1971, 30:257-265.

15. Reitz RH et al. Pharmacokinetics and macromolecular interactions of ethylene dichloride in rats after inhalation or gavage. *Toxicology and applied pharmacology,* 1982, 62:190-204.

16. National Institute for Occupational Safety and Health. *Registry of Toxic Effects of Chemical Substances (RTECS), 1983 supplement.* Washington, DC, US Department of Health, Education, and Welfare, 1984:710-711.

17. Munson AE et al. *In vivo* assessment of immunotoxicity. *Environmental health perspectives,* 1982, 43:41-52.

18. National Cancer Institute. *Bioassay of 1,2-dichloroethane for possible carcinogenicity.* Washington, DC, US Department of Health, Education, and Welfare, 1978 (NCI-CG-TR-55).

19. Lane RW, Riddle BL, Borzelleca JF. Effects of 1,2-dichloroethane and 1,1,1-trichloroethane in drinking water on reproduction and development in mice. *Toxicology and applied pharmacology,* 1982, 63:409-421.

20. Brem H, Stein A, Rosenkrantz H. The mutagenicity and DNA-modifying effect of haloalkanes. *Cancer research,* 1974, 34:2576-2579.

21. Rannug U, Beije B. The mutagenic effect of 1,2-dichloroethane on *Salmonella typhimurium.* II. Activation by the isolated perfused rat liver. *Chemico-biological interactions,* 1979, 24(3):265-285.

22. McCann J et al. Mutagenicity of chloroacetaldehyde, a possible metabolic product of 1,2-dichloroethane (ethylene dichloride), chloroethanol (ethylene chlorohydrin), vinyl chloride and cyclophosphamide. *Proceedings of the National Academy of Sciences of the United States of America,* 1975, 72:3190-3193.

23. Rapoport IA. The reaction of genic proteins with 1,2-dichloroethane. *Doklady biological sciences (English translation),* 1960, 134:1214-1217.

24. Shakarnis V. Induction of X chromosome nondisjunctions and recessive sex-linked lethal mutations in females of *Drosophila melanogaster* by 1,2-dichloroethane. *Soviet genetics (English translation),* 1969, 5(12):89-95.

25. Klaunig JE, Ruch RJ, Pereira MA. Carcinogenicity of chlorinated methane and ethane compounds administered in drinking water to mice. *Environmental health perspectives,* 1986, 69:89-95.

26. Akimov GA et al. [Changes in the nervous system in acute dichloroethane poisoning.] *Voenno-medicinskij žurnal,* 1976, 5:35-37(in Russian).

27. Akimov GA et al. [Neurological disorders in acute dichloroethane poisoning.] *Žurnal nevropatologij i psihiatrij,* 1978, 78(5):687-692 (in Russian).

28. Yodaiken RE, Babcock JR. 1,2-Dichloroethane poisoning. *Archives of environmental health,* 1973, 26:281-284.

29. McNally WD, Fostvedt G. Ethylene dichloride poisoning. *Industrial medicine,* 1941, 10:373.

30. International Agency for Research on Cancer. *Overall evaluations of carcinogenicity: an updating of IARC monographs volumes 1-42.* Lyon, 1987:62 (IARC Monographs on the Evaluation of Carcinogenic Risks to Humans, Suppl. 7).

# 14.5 1,1,1-Trichloroethane

## 14.5.1 General description

### Identity

CAS no.:            71-55-6
Molecular formula:   $C_2H_3Cl_3$

### Physicochemical properties (1,2)[1]

| Property | Value |
|---|---|
| Melting point | -30.4 °C |
| Boiling point | 74.1 °C |
| Density | 1.339 g/cm$^3$ at 20 °C |
| Vapour pressure | 13.3 kPa at 25 °C |
| Water solubility | 0.3–0.5 g/litre at 25 °C |
| Log octanol–water partition coefficient | 2.49 |

### Organoleptic properties

1,1,1-Trichloroethane has a chloroform-like odour.

### Major uses

1,1,1-Trichloroethane is widely and increasingly used as a cleaning solvent for electrical equipment, motors, electronic instruments, and upholstery, as a solvent for adhesives, coatings, and textile dyes, as a coolant and lubricant in metal cutting oils, and as a component of inks and drain cleaners (1, 2).

### Environmental fate

1,1,1-Trichloroethane is found mainly in the atmosphere, where it has a half-life of approximately 2–6 years. It can be decomposed by photochemically produced hydroxyl radicals (1). In water, 1,1,1-trichloroethane is moderately soluble but can volatilize to air. It can be anaerobically dechlorinated by methane-producing bacteria to form 1,1-dichloroethane, and decomposed to give ethanoic acid and 1,1-dichloroethene by abiotic reactions, with a half-life of 200–300 days. 1,1,1-Trichloroethane is mobile in soils and readily migrates to groundwaters. Volatilization from surface soils is also likely. It does not bioaccumulate in animals (1).

---

[1] Conversion factor in air: 1 ppm = 5.4 mg/m$^3$.

## 14.5.2 Analytical methods

1,1,1-Trichloroethane in water is usually determined by a purge-and-trap gas chromatographic procedure (3). It can be detected by mass spectrometry, the detection limit being 0.3 µg/litre (4).

## 14.5.3 Environmental levels and human exposure

### Air

The median concentration of 1,1,1-trichloroethane in air was 0.6 µg/m$^3$ in rural and remote areas, 2.8 µg/m$^3$ in urban and suburban areas, and 6.5 µg/m$^3$ in source-dominated areas (5). Mean air levels in cities in the USA ranged from 0.001 to 60 µg/m$^3$ for urban air and from 0.36 to 1.08 µg/m$^3$ for rural air (1). Air concentrations are typically higher in the northern hemisphere (average 0.06–0.1 µg/m$^3$) than in the southern hemisphere (average 0.02 µg/m$^3$) (6).

### Water

Tributaries of the Rhine contained 1,1,1-trichloroethane at levels of 0.05–2.2 µg/litre. Surface waters in Switzerland contained an average of 0.06 µg/litre. In Europe, groundwater levels were in the range 0.04–130 µg/litre (6).

In the USA, the mean level of 1,1,1-trichloroethane in drinking-water was 0.02–0.6 µg/litre; in well-water, the corresponding level was 9–24 µg/litre (1). A mean concentration of 0.3 µg/litre was reported for drinking-water in Italy (7). Surface water samples from 20 of 106 drinking-water systems analysed for 1,1,1-trichloroethane in the USA between 1977 and 1981 contained detectable levels of this compound (0.1–3.3 µg/litre, mean 0.6 µg/litre; detection limit 0.1 µg/litre). Of 316 groundwater systems tested, 15 contained 1,1,1-trichloroethane at levels ranging from the detection limit (0.5 µg/litre) to 142 µg/litre (mean 13 µg/litre) (8).

### Food

Small amounts of 1,1,1-trichloroethane were found in various foodstuffs in the United Kingdom; it was present in meats, oils and fats, tea, and fruits and vegetables at levels ranging from 1 to 10 µg/kg (9). The highest levels of 1,1,1-trichloroethane found in a survey in the USA were in fatty foods (19 µg/kg) and margarine (45 µg/kg) (10).

### Estimated total exposure and relative contribution of drinking-water

Exposures to 1,1,1-trichloroethane are highly variable and should be evaluated on an individual basis. If an air concentration of 5 µg/m$^3$ is assumed, the daily intake will be 100 µg for an adult breathing 20 m$^3$ of air per day. On the assumption of a 1,1,1-trichloroethane level of 0.6 µg/litre in drinking-water, the daily intake will be 1.2 µg for an adult consuming 2 litres of drinking-water per day. If the average concentration in food is 5 µg/kg, the intake will be 10 µg/day for an adult consuming 2 kg of food.

### 14.5.4 Kinetics and metabolism in laboratory animals and humans

1,1,1-Trichloroethane appears to be absorbed rapidly and completely from the lungs of human subjects (*11*). After 4 h of continuous exposure to 378 or 756 mg/m$^3$, a steady-state lung retention of 30% was observed (*12,13*). The concentration of 1,1,1-trichloroethane in the expired air of humans after ingestion of 0.6 g/kg of body weight was equivalent to the expired air concentration following an inhalation exposure of 2700 mg/m$^3$ (*14*).

After inhalation by humans, blood levels of 1,1,1-trichloroethane were highly correlated with alveolar air levels. Within 2 h of exposure, 60–80% was eliminated from the blood (*12*). One day after intraperitoneal administration of 1,1,1-trichloroethane at 700 mg/kg of body weight, rats retained 0.9% (as the parent compound) in the skin, 0.02% in the blood, 0.02% in the fat, and 0.1% in other sites (*15*).

1,1,1-Trichloroethane is metabolized to a very limited extent in mammals (*12*); the proportion is probably less than 6% in humans. Metabolites include trichloroethanol, trichloroethane glucuronide, and trichloroethanoic acid. Less than 3% of a single intraperitoneal injection of 1,1,1-trichloroethane was metabolized by rats (*15*). The metabolic fate of inhaled 1,1,1-trichloroethane in rats and mice was not altered on repeated exposure (*16*).

1,1,1-Trichloroethane was detected in the expired air of human subjects exposed to oral doses (*14*). Metabolites were excreted primarily in urine; very small amounts of trichloroethanol (1%) were excreted by the lungs (*12*). Over 99% of intraperitoneally injected 1,1,1-trichloroethane was excreted by rats via the pulmonary route (98.7% unchanged); less than 1% was excreted via the urine, primarily as the trichloroethanol glucuronide (*15*). Rats and mice exposed via inhalation to radiolabelled 1,1,1-trichloroethane for 6 h excreted more than 96% of the administered radioactivity during the first 24 h, primarily via exhalation (*16*).

### 14.5.5 Effects on laboratory animals and *in vitro* test systems

#### *Acute exposure*

The acute oral LD$_{50}$ for 1,1,1-trichloroethane in several species ranged from 5.7 to 14.3 g/kg of body weight (*17*). A single oral dose of approximately 1.4 g/kg of body weight depressed the activities of hepatic cytochrome P-450 and epoxide hydratase in rats (*18*).

## Short-term exposure

1,1,1-Trichloroethane at doses of 5 or 10 g/kg of body weight per day for 9 days produced fatalities, transient hyperexcitability, and protracted narcosis in rats. There were no observed adverse effects at 0.5 g/kg of body weight per day. When 1,1,1-trichloroethane was administered to rats by gavage five times a week for up to 12 weeks at doses of 0, 0.5, 2.5, or 5.0 g/kg of body weight, the animals given 2.5 or 5.0 g/kg of body weight exhibited reduced body weight gain and central nervous system effects. Although 35% of these rats died during the first 50 days of the experiment, only the group receiving 5.0 g/kg of body weight showed an increase in serum enzyme levels indicative of toxicity. No adverse effects were observed following ingestion of 0.5 g/kg of body weight for 12 weeks (19).

Male mice were exposed continuously to 1,1,1-trichloroethane by inhalation at levels of 1365 or 5460 mg/m$^3$ for 14 weeks, while control mice were exposed to room air. Significant changes were observed in the centrilobular hepatocytes of mice in the high-dose group, namely vesiculation of the rough endoplasmic reticulum with loss of attached polyribosomes and increased smooth endoplasmic reticulum, microbodies, and triglyceride droplets. The NOAEL in this study was 1365 mg/m$^3$ (20).

## Long-term exposure

Decreases in survival and body weight gain were noted in mice and rats given 1,1,1-trichloroethane by gavage in corn oil, 5 days per week for 78 weeks. The rats were given doses of 750 or 1500 mg/kg of body weight per day, and the mice 2800 or 5600 mg/kg of body weight per day (21).

## Reproductive toxicity, embryotoxicity, and teratogenicity

In a multigenerational study, no dose-dependent effects on fertility, gestation, or viability indices were seen in mice exposed to 1,1,1-trichloroethane in their drinking-water at dose levels of 100, 300, or 1000 mg/kg of body weight from premating to lactation (22).

## Mutagenicity and related end-points

It was reported in several studies that 1,1,1-trichloroethane was not mutagenic in *Salmonella typhimurium* when tested with or without metabolic activation (1), but no attempt was made in the testing procedure used to prevent volatilization of the test compound. 1,1,1-Trichloroethane was mutagenic in various strains of *S. typhimurium* when tested with or without metabolic activation (1, 23), but not in *Saccharomyces cerevisiae* or *Schizosaccharomyces pombe* (24). In several mammalian cell lines, exposure to 1,1,1-trichloroethane led to an increased frequency of transformed cells (1).

### *Carcinogenicity*

Male and female rats (750 or 1500 mg/kg of body weight) and male and female mice (2800 or 5600 mg/kg of body weight) were given 1,1,1-trichloroethane in corn oil by gavage five times per week for 110 weeks (rats) and 78 weeks (mice). The incidence and types of tumours observed in treated animals were similar to those observed in controls. Because of the decreased survival time in both mice and rats, the authors concluded that this bioassay was not adequate to assess carcinogenicity in either species (*2, 21*).

Rats (375 or 750 mg/kg of body weight) and mice (1500 or 3000 mg/kg of body weight) were given 1,1,1-trichloroethane in corn oil by gavage five times per week for 103 weeks. No treatment-related tumours were observed in male rats, and the study was inadequate for the evaluation of female rats because of the high mortality rate. Although there was a significant dose–response trend and an increased incidence of hepatocellular carcinomas in male and high-dose female mice, the study was judged to be inadequate for assessment of carcinogenicity (*25*).

## 14.5.6 Effects on humans

Large oral doses of 1,1,1-trichloroethane have produced nausea, vomiting, and diarrhoea in humans. Acute inhalation exposures result in neurological effects (*1*). Impaired test performance occurs above 945 mg/m$^3$, while dizziness, light-headedness, and incoordination can occur above 2.7 g/m$^3$. Concentrations of 54 g/m$^3$ result in general anaesthesia. Acute pulmonary congestion and oedema were often found in fatalities resulting from inhalation (*26, 27*). Fatty vacuolization was also found in the liver of exposed subjects (*26*). High concentrations of 1,1,1-trichloroethane in air can produce respiratory failure and cardiac arrhythmia (*1*), while chronic exposure to low levels had no effect on parameters of serum and urine chemistry indicative of liver and kidney damage in humans (*1*).

## 14.5.7 Provisional guideline value

IARC has placed 1,1,1-trichloroethane in Group 3 (not classifiable as to its carcinogenicity to humans) (*28*). Available studies of oral administration were considered inadequate for calculation of a TDI. However, as there is an increasing need for guidance on this compound, a 14-week inhalation study in male mice was selected for use in calculating the guideline value (*20*). Based on a NOAEL of 1365 mg/m$^3$, a TDI of 580 µg/kg of body weight was calculated from a total absorbed dose of 580 mg/kg of body weight per day (assuming an average mouse body weight of 30 g, a breathing rate of 0.043 m$^3$/day, and absorption of 30% of the air concentration), applying an uncertainty factor of 1000 (100 for inter- and intraspecies variation and 10 for the short duration of the study). A provisional guideline value of 2000 µg/litre (rounded value) is proposed, if 10% of the TDI is allocated to drinking-water.

This value is provisional only because of the use of an inhalation rather than an oral study. It is strongly recommended that an adequate oral toxicity study be conducted to provide more acceptable data for the derivation of a guideline value.

## References

1. Agency for Toxic Substances and Disease Registry. *Toxicological profile for 1,1,1-trichloroethane*. Atlanta, GA, US Department of Health and Human Services, 1990.

2. *1,1,1-Trichloroethane*. Geneva, World Health Organization, 1992 (Environmental Health Criteria, No. 136).

3. Environmental Monitoring and Support Laboratory. *Method 502.1. Volatile halogenated organic compounds in water by purge-and-trap gas chromatography*. Cincinnati, OH, US Environmental Protection Agency, 1985.

4. Environmental Monitoring and Support Laboratory. *Method 524.1. Volatile organic compounds in water by purge-and-trap gas chromatography/mass spectrometry*. Cincinnati, OH, US Environmental Protection Agency, 1985.

5. Brodzinsky R, Singh HB. *Volatile organic chemicals in the atmosphere: an assessment of available data*. Menlo Park, CA, Atmospheric Service Center, SRI International, 1982 (contract no. 68-02-3452).

6. Herbert P et al. The occurrence of chlorinated solvents in the environment. *Chemistry and industry*, 1986, 15:861-869.

7. Aggazzotti G, Predieri G. Survey of volatile halogenated organics (VHO) in Italy. *Water research*, 1986, 20(8):959-963.

8. Office of Drinking Water. *1,1,1-Trichloroethane—occurrence in drinking water, food and air*. Washington, DC, US Environmental Protection Agency, 1982 (contract no. 68-01-6388).

9. US Environmental Protection Agency. *Ambient water quality criteria for chlorinated ethanes*. Washington, DC, 1980 (NTIS PB81-117400).

10. Pellizzari ED et al. *Total exposure assessment methodology (TEAM). Prepilot study—northern New Jersey*. Research Triangle Park, NC, US Environmental Protection Agency, Office of Research and Development, 1982 (contract no. 68-01-3849).

11. Stewart RD et al. Experimental human exposure to methyl chloroform vapor. *Archives of environmental health*, 1969, 19:467-472.

12. Monster AC, Boersma G, Steenweg M. Kinetics of 1,1,1-trichloroethane in volunteers: influence of exposure concentration and workload. *International archives of occupational and environmental health*, 1979, 42:293-301.

13. Humbert BE, Fernandez JG. [Exposure to 1,1,1-trichloroethane: contribution to the study of absorption, excretion and metabolism in human subjects.] *Archives des maladies professionelles*, 1977, 38:415-425 (in French).

14. Stewart RD, Andrews JT. Acute intoxication with methylchloroform. *Journal of the American Medical Association*, 1966, 195:904-906.

15. Hake CL et al. The metabolism of 1,1,1-trichloroethane by rats. *Archives of environmental health*, 1960, 1:101-105.

16. Schumann AM, Fox TR, Watanabe PG. A comparison of the fate of inhaled methyl chloroform (1,1,1-trichloroethane) following single or repeated exposure in rats and mice. *Fundamental and applied toxicology*, 1982, 2:27-32.

17. Torkelson TR et al. Toxicity of 1,1,1-trichloroethane as determined on laboratory animals and human subjects. *American Industrial Hygiene Association journal*, 1958, 19:353-362.

18. Vainio H, Parkki MG, Marniemi J. Effects of aliphatic chlorohydrocarbons on drug-metabolizing enzymes in rat liver *in vivo. Xenobiotica*, 1976, 6:599-604.

19. Bruckner JV et al. Acute and subacute oral toxicity studies of 1,1,1-trichloroethane (TRI) in rats. *Toxicologist*, 1985, 5(1):100.

20. McNutt NS et al. Hepatic lesions in mice after continuous inhalation exposure to 1,1,1-trichloroethane. *Laboratory investigations*, 1975, 32:642-654.

21. National Cancer Institute. *Bioassay of 1,1,1-trichloroethane for possible carcinogenicity*. Bethesda, MD, 1977 (Technical Report Series No. 3).

22. Lane RW, Riddle BL, Borzelleca JF. Effects of 1,2-dichloroethane and 1,1,1-trichloroethane in drinking water on reproduction and development in mice. *Toxicology and applied pharmacology*, 1982, 63:409-421.

23. Simmon VF, Kauhanen A, Tardiff RG. Mutagenic activity of chemicals identified in drinking water. In: Scott D, Bridges BA, Sobels FH, eds, *Progress in genetic toxicology*, Vol. 2, *Developments in toxicology and environmental science*. Amsterdam, Elsevier/North Holland, 1977:249-258.

24. Loprieno N et al. *In vivo mutagenicity studies with trichloroethylene and other solvents. Preliminary results*. Ivrea, Italy, Istituto di Ricerche biomediche, 1979.

25. National Toxicology Program. *Carcinogenesis bioassay of 1,1,1-trichloroethane in F344/N rats and B6C3F₁ mice*. Research Triangle Park, NC, 1983.

26. Caplan YH, Backer RC, Whitaker JQ. 1,1,1-Trichloroethane: report of a fatal intoxication. *Clinical toxicology*, 1976, 9:69-74.

27. Bonventure J et al. Two deaths following accidental inhalation of dichloromethane and 1,1,1-trichloroethane. *Journal of analytical toxicology*, 1977, 4:158-160.

28. International Agency for Research on Cancer. *Overall evaluations of carcinogenicity: an updating of IARC monographs volumes 1-42.* Lyon, 1987:73 (IARC Monographs on the Evaluation of Carcinogenic Risks to Humans, Suppl. 7).

# 14.6 Vinyl chloride

## 14.6.1 General description

### Identity

CAS no.:              75-01-4
Molecular formula:   $C_2H_3Cl$

The IUPAC name for vinyl chloride is chloroethene; it is also known as monochloroethylene.

### Physicochemical properties *(1-3 )*[1]

| Property | Value |
|---|---|
| Physical state | Colourless gas |
| Boiling point | -13.4 °C |
| Vapour density | 2.2 relative to air at 20 °C |
| Log octanol–water partition coefficient | 0.6 |
| Water solubility | Slightly soluble (1.1 g/litre) at 25 °C |

### Organoleptic properties

Vinyl chloride has a mild, sweetish odour at high concentrations. Odour thresholds in air range from 26–52 mg/m$^3$ in sensitive individuals to 10 000 mg/m$^3$ (*3, 4*). An odour threshold of 3.4 mg/litre in water has been reported (*5*).

### Major uses

Vinyl chloride is used primarily for the production of polyvinyl chloride (PVC). It is also used as a co-monomer with ethenyl ethanoate (vinyl acetate) or 1,1-dichloroethene (vinylidene chloride) and as a raw material in the manufacture of 1,1,1-trichloroethane and monochloracetaldehyde (*4*).

---

[1] Conversion factor in air: 1 ppm = 2.6 mg/m$^3$.

## Environmental fate

In the atmosphere, vinyl chloride reacts with hydroxyl radicals and ozone, ultimately forming formaldehyde, carbon monoxide, hydrochloric acid, and formic acid; its half-life is about 20 h. It is stable in the absence of sunlight or oxygen but polymerizes when exposed to air, light, or heat (3).

Vinyl chloride released to surface water migrates to the atmosphere in a few hours or days. When released to the ground, it is not adsorbed onto soil but migrates readily to groundwater, where it may be degraded to carbon dioxide and chloride ion or may remain unchanged for several months or even years. Vinyl chloride has been reported to be a degradation product of trichloroethene and tetrachloroethene in groundwater (6).

## 14.6.2 Analytical methods

Vinyl chloride in drinking-water can be determined by purge-and-trap gas chromatography over the concentration range 0.06–1500 µg/litre. Mass spectrometry is used for confirmation (detection limit 0.3 µg/litre) (6).

## 14.6.3 Environmental levels and human exposure

### Air

The background level of vinyl chloride in ambient air in western Europe is estimated to range from 0.1 to 0.5 µg/m$^3$ (3). Concentrations are higher close to industrial production sources. Vinyl chloride has been found in the smoke of cigarettes (1.3–16 ng per cigarette) and small cigars (14–27 ng) (2).

### Water

It was found in one survey that fewer than 2% of all groundwater-derived public water-supply systems contained vinyl chloride at levels of 1 µg/litre or higher. Those derived from surface water have also been found to contain vinyl chloride but at lower levels (6). The highest concentration of vinyl chloride detected in drinking-water in the USA was 10 µg/litre. In a five-city survey in that country, concentrations of vinyl chloride of up to 1.4 µg/litre were detected in drinking-water taken from distribution systems in which PVC pipe was used (7). Vinyl chloride has been detected only occasionally in samples of drinking-water from 100 cities in Germany. The highest level, 1.7 µg/litre, was ascribed to dissolution from PVC tubing (3).

### Food

With the implementation of stringent manufacturing specifications for PVC, residual levels of vinyl chloride in food and drinks have decreased from 20 mg/kg in the mid-1970s to well below 10 µg/kg (4). In a survey of 50 food samples in the United Kingdom, it was detected in only five of them, the highest levels being 0.04 µg/kg in sunflower oil and 0.74 µg/kg in orange drink (4).

### Estimated total exposure and relative contribution of drinking-water

If an ambient air concentration of 0.1–0.5 $\mu g/m^3$ and a daily inhalation of 20 $m^3$ of air are assumed, daily intake by the inhalation route would amount to 2–10 µg. Heavy smokers may inhale an additional 0.5 µg/day (2). At a concentration of 1–2 µg/litre in drinking-water, daily intake would be about 2–4 µg. Daily intake from food has been estimated to be about 0.02–0.025 µg (4). It appears that inhalation is the most important route of vinyl chloride intake, although drinking-water may contribute a substantial portion of daily intake where PVC piping with a high residual content of vinyl chloride monomer is used in the distribution network.

## 14.6.4 Kinetics and metabolism in laboratory animals and humans

Vinyl chloride is readily absorbed following oral administration or inhalation. Absorption through the skin is negligible (3). The highest concentrations of metabolites are found in the liver, kidneys, and spleen (2).

Vinyl chloride is metabolized via the microsomal mixed-function oxidase system, forming chloroethylene oxide, which can rearrange spontaneously to chloroacetaldehyde; both metabolites are highly reactive and mutagenic. Chloroacetaldehyde can be oxidized to chloroethanoic acid, and all three metabolites can be conjugated to glutathione or cysteine and excreted in the urine (3).

Vinyl chloride metabolism is dose-dependent and saturable. Low doses administered by gavage are metabolized and eliminated primarily in the urine, whereas with higher doses a substantial proportion is excreted unchanged via the lungs. Major urinary metabolites in rats include N-acetyl-S-2-hydroxyethyl cysteine and thiodiglycolic acid. These metabolites have also been found in the urine of humans following inhalation of vinyl chloride (3).

Vinyl chloride does not accumulate in the body to any significant extent. In rats, it is estimated to have a biological half-life of 20 min (2).

## 14.6.5 Effects on laboratory animals and in vitro test systems

### Acute exposure

The acute toxicity of vinyl chloride is low, 2-hour $LC_{50}$s ranging from 295 $g/m^3$ for mice to 595 $g/m^3$ for guinea-pigs and rabbits (3).

## Short-term exposure

Groups of 30 rats given vinyl chloride in soybean oil by gavage at 0, 30, 100, or 300 mg/kg of body weight, 6 days per week for 13 weeks, exhibited a dose-related increase in relative liver weight. A dose-related increase in adrenal gland weight (males only) was significant at the highest dose level. Histological changes in the liver and other organs were minimal. Hypertrophy of the endoplasmic reticulum was observed in hepatocytes of animals in the group given 300 mg/kg of body weight (8, 9).

## Long-term exposure

Groups of Wistar rats (60–80 per sex per dose) were fed diets containing PVC 7 days per week for 135–144 weeks (10). Oral exposure to vinyl chloride monomer during the period of feeding was 0, 1.7, 5.0, or 14.1 mg/kg of body weight per day. Another group of rats (80 per sex) received a 10% solution of vinyl chloride monomer in soybean oil by gavage, 5 days per week for 83 weeks, at a dose of approximately 300 mg/kg of body weight per day. There was a marked dose-related increase in mortality in the groups given 5.0 and 14.1 mg/kg of body weight per day. Rats in the groups given 14.1 and 300 mg/kg of body weight per day exhibited a significant decrease in blood clotting time, slightly increased levels of $\alpha$-fetoprotein in the blood serum, liver enlargement, and increased haematopoietic activity in the spleen. Liver-to-body-weight ratios were higher in the groups given 14.1 and 300 mg/kg of body weight per day than in controls, and the incidence of foci of cellular alteration was much higher in both of the treatment groups than in controls.

## Reproductive toxicity, embryotoxicity, and teratogenicity

No significant effects on malformations or anomaly rates were seen following the inhalation exposure of mice, rats, or rabbits to vinyl chloride during different periods of pregnancy. The results of other experiments, however, have suggested that it may be embryotoxic in rats and mice (2, 8).

## Mutagenicity and related end-points

Vinyl chloride induced sister chromatid exchange in human lymphocytes *in vitro*, mutations in Chinese hamster cells, unscheduled DNA synthesis in rat hepatocytes, and transformation of BALB/c 3T3 cells. It also caused sex-linked recessive lethal mutations but not aneuploidy, heritable translocations, or dominant lethal mutations in *Drosophila*. It was mutagenic to plants including the yeast *Schizosaccharomyces pombe*, but not to other fungi. It induced gene conversion in yeast, caused DNA damage and mutation in bacteria and, with metabolic activation, bound covalently to isolated DNA (11).

Vinyl chloride induced chromosomal aberrations, sister chromatid exchange, and micronuclei in rodents exposed *in vivo*, but did not induce mutation in the mouse spot test or dominant lethal mutations in rats or mice. It alkylated DNA in several tissues of mice and rats exposed *in vivo* (*11*).

## Carcinogenicity

There is sufficient evidence of the carcinogenicity of vinyl chloride to animals. When administered by inhalation, it induced angiosarcomas of the liver in rats, mice, and hamsters, Zymbal gland tumours in rats and hamsters, nephroblastomas in rats, pulmonary and mammary gland tumours in mice, and forestomach papillomas in hamsters. The minimum concentrations at which compound-related tumours were observed were 26, 130 and 1300 $mg/m^3$ in rats, mice, and hamsters, respectively (*4*).

In the study in which groups of Wistar rats were fed vinyl chloride monomer in the diet for 135–144 weeks (0, 1.7, 5.0, or 14.1 mg/kg of body weight per day) or a 10% solution of vinyl chloride monomer in soybean oil by gavage, 5 days per week for 83 weeks (300 mg/kg of body weight per day), angiosarcomas of the liver were observed in the three highest dose groups and there was a dose-related increase in hepatocellular carcinomas. Angiosarcomas were present in the lungs in the two highest dose groups, and the incidence of adenomas of the mammary glands was twice as high in the test groups as in the controls (*10*).

In extended studies carried out in the same laboratory using the same methods but lower doses (*12*), hepatocellular carcinomas and angiosarcomas were found at the highest dose (1.7 mg/kg of body weight per day), although in smaller numbers. A statistically significant increase in the incidence of liver nodules (presumed to be hepatomas) was the only neoplastic response at levels below 1.7 mg/kg of body weight per day.

In another study, groups of Sprague-Dawley rats (40 per sex per dose) and groups of DS rats (75 per sex per dose) were given vinyl chloride monomer in olive oil at dose levels equivalent to 0, 3.3, 16.6, or 50 mg/kg of body weight (Sprague-Dawley rats) and 0, 0.03, 0.3, or 1 mg/kg of body weight (DS rats), 5 times a week for 52 or 59 weeks; the study was terminated at 136 weeks. In the study on Sprague-Dawley rats, there was a dose-related increase in angiosarcomas: 18 at 50 mg/kg of body weight, nine at 16.6 mg/kg of body weight, and one at 3.3 mg/kg of body weight. In the study on DS rats, four angiosarcomas were found at 1 mg/kg of body weight, two at 0.3 mg/kg of body weight, and none at 0.03 mg/kg of body weight. Small numbers of other tumours were also found, including nephroblastomas, Zymbal gland carcinomas, and hepatomas (*13*).

In a study in which Wistar-derived rats (54 per sex per dose) were given vinyl chloride in drinking-water at concentrations of 0, 2.5, 25, or 250 mg/litre (equivalent to 0.12, 1.2, and 12 mg/kg of body weight per day for males, and 0.22, 2.2, and 22 mg/kg of body weight per day for females) for 101–152 weeks

(Evans et al., unpublished data, 1980, cited in references *4* and *8*), malignant tumours occurred with greater frequency in the highest dose groups, the increase being more pronounced in females. Liver angiosarcomas occurred only in the highest dose groups. In addition, five males in the group given 250 mg/litre developed angiosarcoma in the spleen, and a single subcutaneous angiosarcoma was present in a male in the group given 25 mg/litre.

## 14.6.6 Effects on humans

Vinyl chloride is a narcotic agent, and loss of consciousness can occur at 25 g/m$^3$. Effects of chronic inhalation exposure include Raynaud's phenomenon, a painful vasospastic disorder of the hands, and pseudoscleroderma (*2*).

There is sufficient evidence of the carcinogenicity of vinyl chloride in humans from studies of industrial populations exposed to high concentrations via the inhalation route, and IARC has classified vinyl chloride in Group 1 (*11*). The causal association between vinyl chloride exposure and angiosarcoma of the liver is commonly accepted. There are conflicting opinions, however, regarding the relationship between vinyl chloride exposure and hepatocellular carcinoma, brain tumours, lung tumours, and malignancies of the lymphatic and haematopoietic tissues (*4, 11*).

A number of cytogenetic studies have demonstrated an increased frequency of chromosomal aberrations in the peripheral lymphocytes of exposed workers, but negative studies have also been reported (*4*).

Although some studies suggest that paternal exposure to vinyl chloride may be associated with adverse reproductive outcomes, the available data cannot be considered conclusive, and no mechanism whereby the supposed reproductive effects could be produced is known (*4*).

## 14.6.7 Guideline value

There is sufficient evidence of the carcinogenicity of vinyl chloride in humans from industrial populations exposed to high concentrations via the inhalation route, and IARC has classified vinyl chloride in Group 1 (*11*). A causal association between vinyl chloride exposure and angiosarcoma of the liver is sufficiently proved, and some studies suggest that vinyl chloride is also associated with hepatocellular carcinoma, brain tumours, lung tumours, and malignancies of the lymphatic and haematopoietic tissues.

Animal data show vinyl chloride to be a multisite carcinogen. When administered orally or by inhalation to mice, rats, and hamsters it produced tumours in the mammary gland, lungs, Zymbal gland, and skin, as well as angiosarcomas of the liver and other sites.

Because there are no data on carcinogenic risk following oral exposure of humans to vinyl chloride, estimation of the risk of cancer in humans was based on animal carcinogenicity bioassays involving oral exposure. Using results from the rat bioassay, which yields the most protective value (*12*), and applying the linearized multistage model, the human lifetime exposure for a $10^{-5}$ excess risk of hepatic angiosarcoma was calculated to be 20 µg per day. It was also assumed that, in humans, the number of cancers at other sites may equal that of angiosarcoma of the liver, so that a correction (factor of 2) for cancers other than angiosarcoma is justified. Concentrations in drinking-water of 50, 5, and 0.5 µg/litre were calculated as being associated with excess risks of $10^{-4}$, $10^{-5}$, and $10^{-6}$, respectively.

## References

1.  International Agency for Research on Cancer. *Vinyl chloride, polyvinyl chloride and vinyl chloride–vinyl acetate copolymers.* Lyon, 1979:377-438 (IARC Monographs on the Evaluation of the Carcinogenic Risk of Chemicals to Humans, Volume 19).

2.  *Air quality guidelines for Europe.* Copenhagen, WHO Regional Office for Europe, 1987:158-169 (European Series, No. 23).

3.  Ministerie van Volkshuisvesting, Ruimtelijke Ordening en Milieubeheer. *Criteria-document over vinylchloride. [Vinyl chloride criteria document.]* The Hague, 1984 (Publikatiereeks Lucht, No. 34).

4.  European Chemical Industry Ecology and Toxicology Centre. *The mutagenicity and carcinogenicity of vinyl chloride: a historical review and assessment.* Brussels, 1988 (ECETOC Technical Report No. 31).

5.  Amoore JE, Hautala E. Odor as an aid to chemical safety: odor thresholds compared with threshold limit values and volatilities for 214 industrial chemicals in air and water dilution. *Journal of applied toxicology*, 1983, 3:272-290.

6.  Ware GW, ed. USEPA Office of Drinking Water health advisories: vinyl chloride. *Reviews of environmental contamination and toxicology*, 1989, 107:165-176.

7.  Dressman RC, McFarren EF. Determination of vinyl chloride migration from polyvinyl chloride pipe into water. *Journal of the American Water Works Association*, 1978, 70:29-30.

8.  Joint FAO/WHO Expert Committee on Food Additives. *Toxicological evaluation of certain food additives and contaminants.* Cambridge, Cambridge University Press, 1984:197-215 (WHO Food Additives Series, No. 19).

9.  Feron VJ et al. Observations on the oral administration and toxicity of vinyl chloride in rats. *Food and cosmetics toxicology*, 1975, 13:633-638.

10. Feron VJ et al. Lifespan oral toxicity study of vinyl chloride in rats. *Food and cosmetics toxicology*, 1981, 19:317-333.

11. International Agency for Research on Cancer. *Overall evaluations of carcinogenicity: an updating of IARC Monographs volumes 1-42*. Lyon, 1987:373-376 (IARC Monographs on the Evaluation of Carcinogenic Risks to Humans, Suppl. 7).

12. Til HP, Immel HP, Feron VJ. *Life-span oral carcinogenicity study of vinyl chloride in rats*. TNO-CIVO Report V 83.285/291099, September 1983, (cited in ref. *4*).

13. Maltoni C et al. Carcinogenicity bioassays of vinyl chloride monomer: a model of risk assessment on an experimental basis. *Environmental health perspectives*, 1981, 41:3-29.

# 14.7 1,1-Dichloroethene

## 14.7.1 General description

### Identity

CAS no.:            75-35-4
Molecular formula:   $C_2H_2Cl_2$

1,1-Dichloroethene is also known as vinylidene chloride.

### Physicochemical properties *(1, 2 )*[1]

| Property | Value |
|---|---|
| Melting point | -122.5 °C |
| Boiling point | 31.6 °C |
| Density | 1.21 g/cm$^3$ at 20 °C |
| Vapour pressure | 78.8 kPa at 25 °C |
| Water solubility | 2.5 g/litre at 25 °C |
| Log octanol–water partition coefficient | 1.66 |

### Organoleptic properties

1,1-Dichloroethene has a mild, sweet odour (*3*). Its odour thresholds in air and water are 760 mg/m$^3$ and 1.5 mg/litre, respectively (*4*).

### Major uses

1,1-Dichloroethene is used mainly as a monomer in the production of poly-vinylidene chloride co-polymers and as an intermediate in the synthesis of other organic chemicals, such as methyl chloroform and 1,1,1-trichloroethane (*1, 5, 6*).

---

[1] Conversion factor in air: 1 ppm = 4 mg/m$^3$.

### Environmental fate

Most 1,1-dichloroethene released to the environment volatilizes to the atmosphere, where it is oxidized by hydroxyl radicals with a lifetime of about 1–3 days (5, 7). Rapid photolysis is also expected to occur. Volatilization is the major removal mechanism in surface waters and soils, and anaerobic biotransformation to vinyl chloride is expected to be important in groundwater (5).

## 14.7.2 Analytical methods

The concentration of 1,1-dichloroethene is measured by a purge-and-trap gas chromatographic procedure used for the determination of volatile organohalides in drinking-water. This method is applicable to the measurement of 1,1-dichloroethene over a concentration range of 0.03–1500 µg/litre. Mass spectrometry is used for confirmation (detection limit of 0.2 µg/litre) (8).

## 14.7.3 Environmental levels and human exposure

### Air

1,1-Dichloroethene has been detected in urban air at mean concentrations of 19.6–120 ng/m$^3$ (7, 9). The median concentration in ambient air from all areas is less than 4 ng/m$^3$. Concentrations in the vicinity of industrial plants or hazardous waste sites may be higher. It has also been detected in indoor air at an average concentration of 78.8 µg/m$^3$ (5).

### Water

1,1-Dichloroethene was detected in 2.3% of 945 samples of finished drinking-water taken from groundwater sources in the USA at median concentrations of 0.28–1.2 µg/litre and in about 3% of public drinking-water supplies at concentrations ranging from 0.2 to 0.5 µg/litre. It was not detected in a survey of surface water in 105 cities (5).

### Food

1,1-Dichloroethene residues have been reported in foodstuffs wrapped with copolymer films at levels ranging from 0.005 to 0.01 mg/kg and in household food wraps at an average concentration of 8.8 mg/kg (5). Because of its high volatility, residual levels in food are expected to be low.

### Estimated total exposure and relative contribution of drinking-water

Estimated average exposure from drinking-water in the USA is less than 0.01 µg/day; the maximum is about 1 µg/day (10). At a mean concentration of 19.6–120 ng/m$^3$ in urban air, the estimated average inhalation exposure is 0.4–2.5 μg/day (7). Food is not expected to be a significant exposure source.

## 14.7.4 Kinetics and metabolism in laboratory animals and humans

1,1-Dichloroethene is rapidly and almost completely absorbed from the gastrointestinal tract following administration by gavage (1, 11, 12). It is also readily absorbed from the lungs (13), and dermal absorption is expected to occur (5). It is rapidly distributed following oral or inhalation exposure, accumulating preferentially in the liver, kidneys, and lungs (1, 11, 12).

Biotransformation of 1,1-dichloroethene involves the cytochrome P-450 system and pathways that include the formation of 1,1-dichloroethylene oxide and chloroacetyl chloride and detoxification via conjugation with glutathione. The major metabolites include thiodiglycolic acid and N-acetyl-S-(2-carboxymethyl)cysteine (1, 11, 12, 14). Mice metabolize more of an oral dose than rats (14), in which 1,1-dichloroethene metabolism may be a saturable process (12). Excretion occurs mainly via the urine and expired air (1, 11, 12, 14).

## 14.7.5 Effects on laboratory animals and in vitro test systems

### Acute exposure

Reported oral LD$_{50}$s for 1,1-dichloroethene are 1500 (15) and 1550 (14) mg/kg of body weight for rats and 194 and 217 mg/kg of body weight for female and male mice, respectively (14). Histopathological changes in the liver and kidneys (rats) and lungs (mice) were observed following administration of single oral doses of 200 mg/kg of body weight (16–18).

### Short-term exposure

Increased cytoplasmic vacuolation of hepatocytes was observed in rats exposed to 1,1-dichloroethene in drinking-water at doses of 19.3 or 25.6 mg/kg of body weight per day in males and females, respectively, for 90 days (19). Beagle dogs given 1,1-dichloroethene in gelatin capsules at doses of 6.2, 12.5, or 25 mg/kg of body weight per day for 97 days experienced no adverse effects on hepatic, haematological, renal, or neurological end-points (1, 20).

### Long-term exposure

No treatment-related adverse effects were observed in Sprague-Dawley rats dosed with 1,1-dichloroethene at 0.5, 5, 10, or 20 mg/kg of body weight per day by gavage in corn oil for 1 year (1, 21). Renal inflammation was observed in F344 rats receiving 5 mg/kg of body weight per day by gavage in corn oil for 2 years, but not in those receiving 1 mg/kg of body weight (22). In a study in which

B6C3F$_1$ mice were dosed by gavage at 2 or 10 mg/kg of body weight per day, liver necrosis was reported in male mice at the higher dose but not in female mice (1, 22).

Sprague-Dawley rats exposed to 1,1-dichloroethene in drinking-water for 2 years at doses of 7, 10, or 20 mg/kg of body weight per day (males) and 9, 14, or 30 mg/kg of body weight per day (females) experienced no treatment-related effects on mortality, body or organ weights, or haematological, urinary, or clinical chemistry end-points (1, 20). A statistically significant increase in the incidence of hepatic lesions (hepatocellular swelling and fatty changes) was observed in females at all dose levels and in males at the highest dose.

### Reproductive toxicity, embryotoxicity, and teratogenicity

Administration of 1,1-dichloroethene in drinking-water to rats at doses of up to 28 mg/kg of body weight per day for three generations produced no changes in reproductive outcome or neonatal development (1, 23). No evidence of toxicity to the dams or offspring was observed in rats exposed to drinking-water containing 1,1-dichloroethene at 200 mg/litre on days 6–15 of gestation (24).

### Mutagenicity and related end-points

1,1-Dichloroethene was mutagenic in several strains of *Salmonella typhimurium*, *Escherichia coli*, and *Saccharomyces cerevisiae* with metabolic activation but not without (1, 25–28). It increased the frequency of chromosomal aberrations and sister chromatid exchanges in Chinese hamster CHL cells (29), and was also positive in host-mediated gene mutation and conversion assays in yeast (28). Negative results were reported in assays for dominant lethal mutations in mice and rats (30, 31) and in a micronucleus test in mice (29).

### Carcinogenicity

In a study in which F344/N rats and B6C3F$_1$/N mice were given 1,1-dichloroethene by gavage for 104 weeks at 1 or 5 mg/kg of body weight per day (rats) and 2 or 10 mg/kg of body weight per day (mice), the only significant effect was an increase in the incidence of lymphomas or leukaemias in female mice in the low-dose group (22). Similarly, in a study in which Sprague-Dawley rats received 1,1-dichloroethene in drinking-water at 7, 10, or 20 mg/kg of body weight per day (male) or 9, 14, or 30 mg/kg of body weight per day (female) for 2 years, a significant increase in the incidence of combined mammary gland fibroadenomas and adenofibromas was observed only in the low-dose females (1, 20). Neither increase was considered to be treatment-related, because the effects were not seen in high-dose females or in male mice at either dose.

Swiss mice were exposed by inhalation to 1,1-dichloroethene for 4 h per day, 4–5 days per week for 1 year at 40 or 100 mg/m$^3$ (32). Carcinomas of the mammary gland were significantly increased in females at both doses, pulmonary adenomas were increased in males at 40 mg/m$^3$ and in both sexes at 100 mg/m$^3$, and renal adenocarcinomas were significantly increased in high-dose males.

## 14.7.6 Effects on humans

1,1-Dichloroethene reportedly induces central nervous system depression at high concentrations (16 g/m$^3$ in air) (5). A possible association of 1,1-dichloroethene with liver and kidney toxicity following exposure to lower concentrations has also been suggested (5).

## 14.7.7 Guideline value

IARC has placed 1,1-dichloroethene in Group 3 (33). It was found to be genotoxic in a number of test systems *in vitro* but was not active in the dominant lethal assay *in vivo*. It induced kidney tumours in mice in one inhalation study but was not carcinogenic in other studies, including several in which it was given in drinking-water.

A TDI of 9 μg/kg of body weight per day was calculated from a LOAEL of 9 mg/kg of body weight per day in a 2-year drinking-water study in rats (20), using an uncertainty factor of 1000 (100 for intra- and interspecies variation and 10 for the use of a LOAEL in place of a NOAEL and the potential for carcinogenicity). This gives a guideline value of 30 μg/litre (rounded figure) for a 10% contribution to the TDI from drinking-water.

## References

1. *Vinylidene chloride*. Geneva, World Health Organization, 1990 (Environmental Health Criteria, No. 100).

2. Torkelson TR, Rowe VK. Vinylidene chloride. In: Clayton GD, Clayton FE, eds. *Patty's industrial hygiene and toxicology*, Vol. 2B, 3rd ed. New York, NY, John Wiley, 1981:3545-3550.

3. American Conference of Governmental Industrial Hygienists. *Documentation of the threshold limit values and biological exposures indices*, 5th ed. Cincinnati, OH, 1986:184.

4. Amoore JE, Hautala E. Odor as an aid to chemical safety: odor thresholds compared with threshold limit values and volatilities for 214 industrial chemicals in air and water dilution. *Journal of applied toxicology*, 1983, 3:272-290.

5. Agency for Toxic Substances and Disease Registry. *Toxicological profile for 1,1-dichloroethene*. Atlanta, GA, US Department of Health and Human Services, 1989.

6. Gibbs DS, Wessling RA. Vinylidene chloride and polyvinylidene chloride. In: Mark HF et al., eds. *Kirk-Othmer encyclopedia of chemical technology*, Vol. 23, 3rd ed. New York, NY, John Wiley, 1983:764-798.

7. Singh HB et al. Measurements of some potentially hazardous organic chemicals in urban environments. *Atmospheric environment*, 1981, 15:601-612.

8. Environmental Monitoring and Support Laboratory. *Method 524.1. Volatile organic compounds in water by purge-and-trap gas chromatography/mass spectrometry.* Cincinnati, OII, US Environmental Protection Agency, 1985.

9. Singh HB, Salas LJ, Stiles RE. Distribution of selected gaseous organic mutagens and suspect carcinogens in ambient air. *Environmental science and technology*, 1982, 16:872-880.

10. US Environmental Protection Agency. *Health assessment document for vinylidene chloride.* Washington, DC, 1985.

11. Jones BK, Hathway DE. The biological fate of vinylidene chloride in rats. *Chemico-biological interactions*, 1978, 20:27-41.

12. McKenna MJ et al. Metabolism and pharmacokinetic profile of vinylidene chloride in rats following oral administration. *Toxicology and applied pharmacology*, 1978, 45:821-835.

13. Dallas CE et al. The uptake and disposition of 1,1-dichloroethylene in rats during inhalation exposure. *Toxicology and applied pharmacology*, 1983, 68:140-151.

14. Jones BK, Hathway DE. Differences in metabolism of vinylidene chloride between mice and rats. *British journal of cancer*, 1978, 37:411-417.

15. National Institute of Occupational Safety and Health. *Registry of Toxic Effects of Chemical Substances (RTECS), 1983 suppl.* Cincinnati, OH, 1983:740.

16. Chieco P, Moslen MT, Reynolds ES. Effect of administrative vehicle on oral 1,1-dichloroethylene toxicity. *Toxicology and applied pharmacology*, 1981, 57:146-155.

17. Andersen ME, Jenkins LJ Jr. Oral toxicity of 1,1-dichloroethylene in the rat: effects of sex, age and fasting. *Environmental health perspectives*, 1977, 21:157-163.

18. Forkert PG et al. Lung injury and repair: DNA synthesis following 1,1-dichloroethylene. *Toxicology*, 1985, 36:199-214.

19. Rampy LW et al. Interim results of two-year toxicological studies in rats of vinylidene chloride incorporated in the drinking water or administered by repeated inhalation. *Environmental health perspectives*, 1977, 21:33-43.

20. Quast JF et al. A chronic toxicity and oncogenicity study in rats and subchronic toxicity study in dogs on ingested vinylidene chloride. *Fundamental and applied toxicology*, 1983, 3:55-62.

21. Maltoni C, Cotti G, Chieco P. Chronic toxicity and carcinogenicity bioassays of vinylidene chloride. *Acta oncologica*, 1984, 5:91-146.

22. National Toxicology Program. *Carcinogenesis bioassay of vinylidene chloride in F344 rats and B6C3F₁ mice (gavage study)*. Research Triangle Park, NC, US Department of Health and Human Services, 1982 (NTP-80-2; NIH Publication No. 82-1784).

23. Nitschke KD et al. A three-generation rat reproductive toxicity study of vinylidene chloride in the drinking water. *Fundamental and applied toxicology*, 1983, 3:75-79.

24. Murray FJ et al. Embryotoxicity and fetotoxicity of inhaled or ingested vinylidene chloride in rats and rabbits. *Toxicology and applied pharmacology*, 1979, 49:189-202.

25. Bartsch H et al. Tissue-mediated mutagenicity of vinylidene chloride and 2-chlorobutadiene in *Salmonella typhimurium*. *Nature*, 1975, 155:641-643.

26. Greim H et al. Mutagenicity *in vitro* and potential carcinogenicity of chlorinated ethylenes as a function of metabolic oxiran formation. *Biochemical pharmacology*, 1975, 24:2013-2017.

27. Oesch F et al. Vinylidene chloride: changes in drug-metabolizing enzymes, mutagenicity and relation to its targets for carcinogenesis. *Carcinogenesis*, 1983, 4:1031-1038.

28. Bronzetti G et al. Genetic activity of vinylidene chloride in yeast. *Mutation research*, 1981, 89:179-185.

29. Sawada M, Sofuni T, Ishidate M Jr. Cytogenetic studies on 1,1-dichloroethylene and its two isomers in mammalian cells *in vitro* and *in vivo*. *Mutation research*, 1987, 187:157-163.

30. Anderson D et al. Dominant lethal studies with the halogenated olefins vinyl chloride and vinylidene dichloride in male CD-1 mice. *Environmental health perspectives*, 1977, 21:71-78.

31. Short RD et al. A dominant lethal study in male rats after repeated exposure to vinyl chloride or vinylidene chloride. *Journal of toxicology and environmental health*, 1977, 3:965-968.

32. Maltoni C et al. Experimental research on vinylidene chloride carcinogenesis. In: Maltoni C, Mahlman MA, eds. *Archives of research on industrial carcinogenesis*. Vol. III. Princeton, NJ, Princeton Scientific Publishers, 1985:1-229.

33. International Agency for Research on Cancer. *Overall evaluations of carcinogenicity: an updating of IARC Monographs volumes 1-42.* Lyon, 1987:376-377 (IARC Monographs on the Evaluation of Carcinogenic Risks to Humans, Suppl. 7).

## 14.8 1,2-Dichloroethene

### 14.8.1 General description

**Identity**

| Compound | CAS no. | Molecular formula |
|----------|---------|-------------------|
| *cis*-isomer | 156-59-2 | $C_2H_2Cl_2$ |
| *trans*-isomer | 156-60-5 | $C_2H_2Cl_2$ |

**Physicochemical properties** *(1, 2 )*[1]

| Property | cis-isomer | trans-isomer |
|----------|------------|--------------|
| Melting point (°C) | -80.5 | -50 |
| Boiling point (°C) | 60.3 | 47.5 |
| Density (g/cm³ at 20 °C) | 1.2837 | 1.2565 |
| Vapour pressure (kPa at 25 °C) | 27.7 | 35.3 |
| Water solubility (g/litre at 20 °C) | 3.5 | 6.3 |
| Log octanol–water partition coefficient | 1.86 | 2.09 |

**Organoleptic properties**

A mixture of 1,2-dichloroethene isomers has a pleasant odour (*3*). The odour thresholds for *trans*-1,2-dichloroethene in air and water are 68 mg/m³ and 0.26 mg/litre, respectively (*4*).

**Major uses**

1,2-Dichloroethene (*cis/trans* mixture) is used mainly as an intermediate in the synthesis of chlorinated solvents and compounds (*5*). It has also been used as an extraction solvent for organic materials.

**Environmental fate**

1,2-Dichloroethene is removed from the atmosphere mainly through reaction with photochemically generated hydroxyl radicals; the estimated half-lives for the *cis*- and *trans*-isomers are 8.3 and 3.6 days, respectively. Most 1,2-dichloroethene in surface water and surface soils is expected to be volatilized. The compound may be leached through subsurface soils to groundwater. Anaerobic biodegrada-

---

[1] Conversion factor in air: 1 ppm = 3.97 mg/m³.

tion may remove both isomers from groundwater, the half-life then being 13–48 weeks (5).

## 14.8.2 Analytical methods

The concentrations of *cis*- or *trans*-1,2-dichloroethene are measured by a purge-and-trap gas chromatographic procedure used for the determination of volatile organohalides in drinking-water (6). The method can differentiate between the *cis*- and *trans*-isomers at concentrations of 0.03–1500 µg/litre. Mass spectrometry is used for confirmation; the detection limit is 0.17 µg/litre (7).

## 14.8.3 Environmental levels and human exposure

### Air

1,2-Dichloroethene has been detected in the air of urban and industrial areas at concentrations in the range 0.04–0.3 µg/m³ (mean) for the *cis*-isomer to 10.3 µg/m³ (maximum) for a mixture of isomers. Mean concentrations up to 32.2 µg/m³ have been measured in indoor air (5).

### Water

1,2-Dichloroethene has been detected in industrial effluents, surface water, groundwater, and drinking-water supplies in the USA. It was detected in 16 of 466 randomly selected and 38 of 479 purposely selected drinking-water supplies derived from groundwater at levels of up to 2 and 120 µg/litre, respectively (5).

The *cis*-form of 1,2-dichloroethene is more frequently found as a water contaminant. The presence of the two isomers, which are metabolites of other unsaturated halogenated hydrocarbons in wastewater and anaerobic groundwater, may indicate the simultaneous presence of other more toxic organochlorine chemicals, such as vinyl chloride. Accordingly, more intensive monitoring is necessary if they are found to be present.

### Food

1,2-Dichloroethene was not detected in fish samples at 95 stations covered by the STORET database of the US Environmental Protection Agency, but was found in fish tissue samples from Commencement Bay, WA, at mean levels of 0.04 mg/kg (5).

### Estimated total exposure and relative contribution of drinking-water

Based on urban air levels of 0.04–0.3 µg/m³, the average inhalation exposure to 1,2-dichloroethene is about 1–6 µg/day (5). At a drinking-water concentration of 2 µg/litre, the daily intake by an adult would be about 4 µg.

## 14.8.4 Kinetics and metabolism in laboratory animals and humans

As the *cis-* and *trans-*isomers of 1,2-dichloroethene are lipid-soluble compounds of low relative molecular mass, they would be expected to be readily absorbed by the oral or dermal routes (*8*). In humans, about 75% of inhaled *trans-*1,2-dichloroethene is absorbed through the lungs (*9*). 1,2-Dichloroethene may be preferentially distributed to adipose tissue (*10*). On the basis of distribution data for 1,1-dichloroethene, the highest concentrations might be expected to occur in liver and kidney (*11*).

The first step in the metabolism of both isomers of 1,2-dichloroethene appears to be the formation of the chloroethylene epoxide, which undergoes rearrangement to form dichloroacetaldehyde and possibly monochloroacetic acid (*12, 13*). *In vitro* studies indicate that biotransformation involves the hepatic microsomal cytochrome P-450 system (*14, 15*). The *cis-*isomer is metabolized at a faster rate than the *trans-*isomer (*14*). High doses may saturate the P-450 system and exceed its metabolic capacity (*5*). If excretion is similar to that of 1,1-dichloroethene, elimination would be expected to be relatively rapid, so that most of a single dose would be excreted in the urine within 24–72 h (*15*).

## 14.8.5 Effects on laboratory animals and *in vitro* test systems
### Acute exposure

For a mixture of isomers, the reported oral $LD_{50}$ for rats is 770 mg/kg of body weight (*16*). Reported oral $LD_{50}$s for *trans-*1,2-dichloroethene are 1275 mg/kg of body weight for female rats, 7902 mg/kg of body weight for male rats, 2221 mg/kg of body weight for male mice, and 2391 mg/kg of body weight for female mice (*17–19*). Administration of single doses of *cis* -1,2-dichloroethene at 400 or 1500 mg/kg of body weight to rats caused significant elevations of liver alkaline phosphatase, whereas the same doses of *trans-*isomer did not (*20*).

### Short-term exposure

*trans-*1,2-Dichloroethene was administered by gavage to male CD-1 mice for 14 days at doses of 0, 21, or 210 mg/kg of body weight per day (*21*). No changes in body or organ weights, serum alanine aminotransferase, or blood urea nitrogen were reported at any dose level. However, fibrinogen levels, prothrombin times, and lactate dehydrogenase levels were significantly decreased at the highest dose. In a similar study, the *trans-*isomer, administered by gavage at doses equal to 1% and 10% of the $LD_{50}$ (22 or 222 mg/kg of body weight per day) to male mice for 14 days, caused no significant changes in body or organ weights, haematological or blood coagulation parameters, serum enzyme levels, or humoral immune response (*18*).

In a study on CD-1 mice (15–24 per sex per dose), male mice received *trans-*1,2-dichloroethene in doses of 17, 175, or 387 mg/kg of body weight per day and female mice received doses of 23, 224, or 452 mg/kg of body weight per day in drinking-water for 90 days (*21*). No changes in water consumption, body weight, or gross pathology were observed in any dose group. There were significant increases in serum alkaline phosphatase levels in male mice at the two highest doses, and liver glutathione concentrations were decreased at the highest dose. In females, thymus weight was significantly decreased at the two highest doses, and lung weight was depressed at the highest dose. A significant decrease in aniline hydroxylase activity was also observed in females exposed to the highest dose. In another phase of this study (*22*), dose-dependent effects were observed either in cell-mediated immunity in either sex or in the humoral immune status of female mice. However, a significant decrease in spleen antibody-forming cells was noted at all dose levels in male mice. Female mice exposed to the highest dose demonstrated an enhanced spleen cell response to lipopolysaccharide at some, but not all, concentrations.

CD rats were exposed to *trans*-1,2-dichloroethene at doses of 402, 1314, or 3114 mg/kg of body weight per day (males) and 353, 1257, or 2809 mg/kg of body weight per day (females) in drinking-water for 90 days (*19*). No compound-related effects on water consumption, body weight, serum chemistry, or urinary parameters were observed, nor were any effects on gross or histological pathology noted. However, a significant dose-dependent decrease in kidney weight was observed at the two highest doses in females.

### Mutagenicity and related end-points

*In vitro* investigations of the genotoxic potential of 1,2-dichloroethene yielded negative results for both isomers. 1,2-Dichloroethene was not found to be mutagenic in *Escherichia coli*, several strains of *Salmonella typhimurium*, or *Saccharomyces cerevisiae*, with or without metabolic activation (*23–26*). Neither isomer induced chromosomal aberrations or sister chromatid exchanges in Chinese hamster lung fibroblasts (*27*).

*In vivo* studies indicate that the *cis*-, and possibly the *trans*-, isomer may be genotoxic. The *cis*-isomer was found to be mutagenic in *S. typhimurium* and *S. cerevisiae* strains in two host-mediated assays in mice (*23, 24*). Repeated intraperitoneal injections of *cis*-1,2-dichloroethene induced chromosomal aberrations in mouse bone marrow cells (*24*). The *trans*-isomer gave negative results in these studies. However, an increase in the number of aneuploid V 79 Chinese hamster cells was reported following treatment with the *trans*-isomer (*28*).

## 14.8.6 Effects on humans

Inhalation of high concentrations (38 g/m$^3$ and above) of 1,2-dichloroethene in air causes central nervous system depression (*17*). Neurological effects, including nausea, drowsiness, fatigue, and vertigo, have been reported following exposure to lower levels (*9*). A burning sensation in the eyes was also reported. The *trans*-

isomer is reportedly about twice as potent a central nervous system depressant as the *cis*-isomer (*17*), which has been used as an anaesthetic.

## 14.8.7 Guideline value

In a 3-month study in mice given the *trans*-isomer in drinking-water, there was an increase in serum alkaline phosphatase and reduced thymus and lung weights, as well as transient immunological effects, the toxicological significance of which is unclear. Only one rat toxicity study is available for the *cis*-isomer. There are limited data to suggest that both isomers may possess some genotoxic activity. There is no information on carcinogenicity.

Data on the toxicity of the *trans*-isomer in mice (*21*) were used to calculate a joint guideline value for both isomers because of the lack of adequate toxicity data for the *cis*-isomer and because data suggest that the mouse is a more sensitive species than the rat. Accordingly, the NOAEL of 17 mg/kg of body weight per day from the *trans*-isomer toxicity study was used with an uncertainty factor of 1000 (100 for intra- and interspecies variation and 10 for the short duration of the study) to derive a TDI of 17 µg/kg of body weight. This gives a guideline value of 50 µg/litre (rounded figure) for an allocation of 10% of the TDI to drinking-water.

## References

1.  Weast RC. *CRC handbook of chemistry and physics*, 67th ed. Boca Raton, FL, CRC Press, 1986.

2.  Verschueren K. *Handbook of environmental data on organic chemicals*, 2nd ed. New York, NY, Van Nostrand Reinhold, 1983:488.

3.  American Conference of Governmental Industrial Hygienists. *Documentation of the threshold limit values and biological indices*, 5th ed. Cincinnati, OH, 1986:185.

4.  Amoore JE, Hautala E. Odor as an aid to chemical safety: odor thresholds compared with threshold limit values and volatilities for 214 industrial chemicals in air and water dilution. *Journal of applied toxicology*, 1983, 3:272-290.

5.  Agency for Toxic Substances and Disease Registry. *Toxicological profile for 1,2-dichloroethenes*. Atlanta, GA, US Department of Health and Human Services, 1990.

6.  Environmental Monitoring and Support Laboratory. *Method 502.1. Volatile halogenated organic compounds in water by purge-and-trap gas chromatography*. Cincinnati, OH, US Environmental Protection Agency, 1985.

7.  Environmental Monitoring and Support Laboratory. *Method 524.1. Volatile organic compounds in water by purge-and-trap gas chromatography/mass spectrometry*. Cincinnati, OH, US Environmental Protection Agency, 1985.

8.  Office of Drinking Water. *Draft health effects criteria document for the dichloroethy-lenes*. Washington, DC, US Environmental Protection Agency, 1988.

9.  Lehmann KB, Schmidt-Kehl L. [Study of the most important chlorohydrocarbons from the standpoint of industrial hygiene.] *Archiv für Hygiene und Bakteriologie*, 1936, 116:131-268 (in German).

10. Sato A, Nakajima T. Pharmacokinetics of organic solvent vapors in relation to their toxicity. *Scandinavian journal of work, environment and health*, 1987, 13:81-93.

11. McKenna MJ et al. The pharmacokinetics of [$^{14}$C]-vinylidene chloride in rats fol-lowing inhalation exposure. *Toxicology and applied pharmacology*, 1978, 45:599-610.

12. Henschler D. Metabolism and mutagenicity of halogenated olefins: a comparison of structure and activity. *Environmental health perspectives*, 1977, 21:61-64.

13. Leibman KC, Ortiz E. Metabolism of halogenated ethylenes. *Environmental health perspectives*, 1977, 21:91-97.

14. Costa AK. The chlorinated ethylenes: their hepatic metabolism and carcinogenicity. *Dissertation abstracts international, B*, 1983, 44(6):1797-B.

15. Costa AK, Ivanetich KM. The 1,2-dichloroethylenes: their metabolism by hepatic cytochrome P-450 *in vitro*. *Biochemical pharmacology*, 1982, 31:2093-2102.

16. National Institute of Occupational Safety and Health. *Registry of Toxic Effects of Chemical Substances (RTECS), 1983 suppl.* Cincinnati, OH, 1983:741.

17. Freundt KJ, Liebaldt GP, Lieberwirth E. Toxicity studies on *trans*-1,2-dichloroethy-lene. *Toxicology*, 1977, 7:141-153.

18. Munson AE et al. *In vivo* assessment of immunotoxicity. *Environmental health per-spectives*, 1982, 43:41-52.

19. Hayes JR et al. The acute and subchronic toxicity in rats of trans-1,2-dichloroethy-lene in drinking water. *Journal of the American College of Toxicologists*, 1987, 6:471-478.

20. Jenkins LJ Jr, Trabulus MJ, Murphy SD. Biochemical effects of 1,1-dichloroethylene in rats: comparison with carbon tetrachloride and 1,2-dichloroethylene. *Toxicology and applied pharmacology*, 1972, 23:501-510.

21. Barnes DW et al. Toxicology of *trans*-1,2-dichloroethylene in the mouse. *Drug chem-istry and toxicology*, 1985, 8:373-392.

22. Shopp GM et al. Humoral and cell-mediated immune status of mice exposed to trans-1,2-dichloroethylene. *Drug chemistry and toxicology*, 1985, 8:393-407.

23. Bronzetti G et al. Comparative genetic activity of *cis-* and *trans-*1,2-dichloroethylene in yeast. *Teratogenesis, carcinogenesis and mutagenesis*, 1984, 4:365-375.

24. Cerna M, Kypenova H. Mutagenic activity of chloroethylenes analyzed by screening tests. *Mutation research*, 1977, 46:214-215 (abstract).

25. Galli A et al. (a) Studio *in vitro*. Attività genetica dell' 1,2-dichloroetilene. [*In vitro* study. Genetic activity of 1,2-dichloroethylene.] *Bollettino della Società Italiana di Biologia Sperimentale*, 1982, 58:860-863.

26. Mortelmans K et al. *Salmonella* mutagenicity tests. II. Results from the testing of 270 chemicals. *Environmental mutagenesis*, 1986, 8(Suppl. 7):1-119.

27. Sawada M, Sofuni T, Ishidate M Jr. Cytogenetic studies on 1,1-dichloroethylene and its two isomers in mammalian cells *in vitro* and *in vivo*. *Mutation research*, 1987, 187:157-163.

28. Onfelt A. Spindle disturbances in mammalian cells. III. Toxicity, c-mitosis and aneuploidy with 22 different compounds. Specific and unspecific mechanisms. *Mutation research*, 1987, 182:135-154.

## 14.9 Trichloroethene

### 14.9.1 General description

#### Identity

CAS no.: 79-01-6
Molecular formula: $C_2HCl_3$

Trichloroethene is also known as trichloroethylene.

#### Physicochemical properties (1, 2)[1]

| Property | Value |
|---|---|
| Boiling point | 86.7 °C |
| Density | 1.4 g/cm$^3$ at 25 °C |
| Vapour pressure | 10.3 kPa at 25 °C |
| Water solubility | 1.07 g/litre at 20 °C |

#### Organoleptic properties

The odour thresholds for trichloroethene in air and water are 546–1092 mg/m$^3$ and 0.3 mg/litre, respectively (3, 4).

---

[1] Conversion factor in air: 1 ppm = 5.46 mg/m$^3$.

## Major uses

Trichloroethene is used mainly in dry cleaning, for the degreasing of fabricated metal parts, as a solvent for fats, waxes, resins, oils, rubber, paints, and varnishes, and as an inhalation analgesic and anaesthetic (1, 5).

## Environmental fate

Trichloroethene is readily released to the atmosphere, where it is highly reactive and does not persist for any significant length of time. In water, biodegradation occurs, possibly with some partitioning to sediment and suspended organic matter. Trichloroethene in anaerobic groundwater may be degraded to more toxic compounds, including vinyl chloride. It is highly mobile in soil and may be leached into groundwater supplies. Bioconcentration of trichloroethene in aquatic species is low to moderate (5).

## 14.9.2 Analytical methods

A purge-and-trap gas chromatographic procedure can be used to measure trichloroethene in drinking-water at concentrations of 0.01–1500 µg/litre (6). Mass spectrometry is used for confirmation (detection limit 0.2 µg/litre) (7).

## 14.9.3 Environmental levels and human exposure

### Air

Mean concentrations of 0.16 µg/m$^3$ and 2.5 µg/m$^3$ have been detected in the atmosphere of rural and urban areas, respectively (5).

### Water

Trichloroethene may be released directly into wastewater, deposited in water from the atmosphere, or formed as a by-product during water chlorination (5, 8). In a survey of drinking-water in the USA it was found at a mean concentration of 2.1 µg/litre in 28 of 113 cities in 1976–77 (9). It was present in 24% of 158 nonrandom samples collected in a groundwater supply survey in the USA; median levels of 1 µg/litre were reported and a maximum of 130 µg/litre was found in one sample (5).

### Food

Trichloroethene has been found at concentrations of up to 10 µg/kg in meat, up to 5 µg/kg in fruits and vegetables, and up to 60 µg/kg in tea in the United Kingdom (1, 10). It has also been detected in margarine samples in the USA at levels of 440–3600 µg/kg and in grain-based food at concentrations of up to 2.7 µg/kg (5).

### Estimated total exposure and relative contribution of drinking-water

Because of its high vapour pressure, potential human exposure to trichloroethene is greatest from the inhalation of contaminated air. Exposure from drinking-water or food is not expected to pose a significant health risk, as it volatilizes rapidly from water and does not bioaccumulate to any significant extent.

## 14.9.4 Kinetics and metabolism in laboratory animals and humans

Analysis of human blood and breath following inhalation of 546 mg/m³ trichloroethene showed that peak levels were reached within 1 h of exposure (*1, 5*). In rats, 72–85% of an orally administered dose was detected in expired air and 10–20% in urine (*11*), indicating that at least 80% of ingested trichloroethene is systemically absorbed. Transplacental diffusion has been demonstrated in humans following inhalation; the ratio of the concentrations in fetal and maternal blood ranged between 0.52 and 1.90 (*12*). Trichloroethene was widely distributed in rats given it by gavage (*13*), the highest concentration being in body fat.

Inhalation studies in humans show that 40–75% of the retained dose is metabolized (*5*). The principal urinary metabolites are trichloroacetaldehyde, trichloroethanol, trichloroethanoic acid, and trichloroethanol glucuronide (*14*). An important metabolic intermediate is the reactive epoxide, trichloroethene oxide, which can alkylate nucleic acids and proteins (*11*). Trichloroethene is eliminated with a half-time of about 1.5 h (*15*). Metabolites are excreted more slowly; the biological half-life measured in human urine is about 50 h for trichloroethanol and 36–73 h for trichloroethanoic acid (*16, 17*).

## 14.9.5 Effects on laboratory animals and *in vitro* test systems

### Acute exposure

The acute oral $LD_{50s}$ for trichloroethene in rats and mice are 4920 mg/kg of body weight and 2400 mg/kg of body weight, respectively (*1, 5, 18*).

### Short-term exposure

In a study in which groups of 12–24 male Swiss-Cox mice received trichloroethene by gavage in corn oil, 5 days per week for 6 weeks, at doses of 0, 100, 200, 400, 800, 1600, 2400, or 3200 mg/kg of body weight per day, dose-related increases in hepatic DNA, relative liver weight, and hypertrophy of the liver were apparent at 100 mg/kg of body weight per day and above, and glucose-6-phosphate levels were decreased by 30–40% at 800 mg/kg of body weight per day and above. The LOAEL was 100 mg/kg of body weight per day (*19*).

Fischer 344/N rats and B6C3F₁ mice (10 per sex per dose) were given trichloroethene at doses of up to 2000 (male rats), 1000 (female rats), or 6000 (mice) mg/kg of body weight per day in corn oil by gavage, 5 days per week for

13 weeks. Survival in mice was greatly decreased at 3000 and 6000 mg/kg of body weight per day. Body weight was decreased in male rats at 2000 mg/kg of body weight per day and in male mice at 750 mg/kg of body weight per day and above. Mild to moderate cytomegaly and enlarged cell nuclei of the renal tubular epithelial cells in the inner cortex were observed in both sexes of both species at 1000 and 2000 mg/kg of body weight per day (rats) and 3000 and 6000 mg/kg of body weight per day (mice) (20).

In rats exposed to air containing 300 mg/m$^3$ trichloroethene 5 days per week for 14 weeks, liver weights were elevated, possibly as the result of fatty accumulation. Haematological parameters, liver and renal function tests, blood glucose, and organ-to-body-weight ratios were the same as in controls (21).

## Long-term exposure

The toxicity of trichloroethene (epichlorohydrin-free) was investigated in F344 rats and B6C3F$_1$ mice (50 per sex per dose) given 0, 500, or 1000 mg/kg of body weight per day (rats) and 0 or 1000 mg/kg of body weight per day (mice) in corn oil, 5 days per week for 103 weeks. Survival was reduced in male rats and mice but not in females. Toxic nephrosis, characterized as cytomegaly, occurred in rats at 500 and 1000 mg/kg of body weight per day and in mice at 1000 mg/kg of body weight per day. LOAELs of 500 mg/kg of body weight per day for rats and 1000 mg/kg of body weight per day for mice were identified (20).

## Reproductive toxicity, embryotoxicity, and teratogenicity

No statistically significant effects on sperm count, motility, or morphology were detected in male Long-Evans rats (10 per dose) intubated with 1, 10, 100, or 1000 mg of trichloroethene per kg of body weight per day, 5 days a week for 6 weeks. Copulatory behaviour was impaired at 100 mg/kg of body weight per day during the initial 4 weeks of exposure but returned to normal by week 5 (13).

A continuous-breeding fertility study was conducted in which male and female Fischer 344 rats were fed diets containing microencapsulated trichloroethene at dose levels of approximately 0, 75, 150, or 300 mg/kg of body weight per day from 7 days before mating to the birth of the F$_2$ generation. Although testicular and epididymal weights decreased in the F$_1$ generation, no histopathological changes were observed (22). In a similar study in CD-1 mice given up to 750 mg of trichloroethene per kg of body weight per day, sperm motility was reduced by 45% in F$_0$ males and 18% in F$_1$ males. There were no treatment-related effects on mating, fertility, or reproductive performance in the F$_0$ or F$_1$ mice (23).

Mice and rats exposed to trichloroethene vapour at a concentration of 1600 mg/m$^3$ on days 6–15 of gestation for 7 h per day did not experience any teratogenic effects, although there was some evidence of haemorrhages in the cerebral ventricles and a few cases of undescended testicles (24).

### Mutagenicity and related end-points

There are numerous studies of the genotoxicity of trichloroethene, but the evidence is conflicting, in part because of impurities in the test material and the presence of stabilizers that are themselves mutagenic. In a range of *in vitro* assays, the data indicate that it is either negative or only weakly positive (*1, 25*). A dose-dependent increase in DNA single-strand breaks was observed in liver and kidney, but not lung, of male NMRI mice 1 h, but not 24 h, after intraperitoneal injection of 4–10 mmol of trichloroethene per kg of body weight (*26*).

### Carcinogenicity

There was a significant increase in hepatocellular tumours in both sexes of B6C3F$_1$ mice given trichloroethene by gavage in corn oil (*27*). However, in a similar study in a strain of mice with a low background incidence of liver tumours, there was no evidence of increased tumour incidence (*28*). There was some indication of a small increase in renal tumours in male rats given 250 mg of trichloroethene per kg of body weight by gavage in corn oil, but these tumours are of doubtful significance for humans (*1, 29*).

In an inhalation study, a dose-related increase in malignant lymphomas was reported in female HAN:NMRI mice exposed to 546 or 819 mg/m$^3$ trichloroethene vapour 6 h per day, 5 days per week for 18 months (*30*); this strain of mice has a high incidence of spontaneous lymphomas. An increased incidence of pulmonary adenocarcinomas was found in female ICR mice exposed to 820 or 2460 mg/m$^3$ trichloroethene vapour as compared with controls, but no such increase was found in female Sprague-Dawley rats (*31*).

### 14.9.6 Effects on humans

Acute exposure to high concentrations of trichloroethene causes central nervous system depression (*32*). Exposure to 147 mg/m$^3$ in air for 4 h caused drowsiness and mucous membrane irritation; at 442 mg/m$^3$, it caused headaches. Drowsiness, lethargy, and nausea were observed within 5 min at 10.9 g/m$^3$. Coma and respiratory depression may occur following prolonged exposure to levels above 10.9 g/m$^3$ (*5*). Hepatic failure and subsequent death were reported following the use of trichloroethene as an anaesthetic, generally in patients with complicating transfusions (*33*). Oral exposure of humans to 15–25 ml (21–35 g) resulted in vomiting and abdominal pain, followed by transient unconsciousness (*34*).

Humans exposed occupationally to trichloroethene had an increase in serum aminotransferases, indicating damage to the liver parenchyma (*35*). Neurological abnormalities were associated with occupational exposure to 76–464 mg/m$^3$ trichloroethene for between 1 month and 15 years, including decreased appetite, sleep disturbances, ataxia, vertigo, headache, and short-term memory loss (*5*).

## 14.9.7 Provisional guideline value

Trichloroethene has been classified by IARC in Group 3: not classifiable as to its carcinogenicity to humans (*35*). Although it induces lung and liver tumours in mice, there is no conclusive evidence that it causes cancer in other species. Trichloroethene is a weakly active mutagen in bacteria and yeast.

A TDI of 23.8 µg/kg of body weight has been calculated by applying an uncertainty factor of 3000 to a LOAEL of 100 mg/kg of body weight per day (normalized for 5 days per week exposure) for minor effects on relative liver weight in a 6-week study in mice (*19*). The uncertainty factor components are 100 for inter- and intraspecies variation, 10 for limited evidence of carcinogenicity, and an additional factor of 3 in view of the short duration of the study and the use of a LOAEL rather than a NOAEL. A provisional guideline value of 70 µg/litre (rounded figure) is derived by allocating 10% of the TDI to drinking-water.

## References

1.  *Trichloroethylene.* Geneva, World Health Organization, 1985 (Environmental Health Criteria, No. 50).

2.  Torkelson TR, Rowe VK. Halogenated aliphatic hydrocarbons. In: Clayton GD, Clayton FE, eds. *Patty's industrial hygiene and toxicology*, Vol. 2B, 3rd ed. New York, NY, John Wiley, 1981:3553-3560.

3.  Ruth JH. Odor threshold and irritation levels of several chemical substances. A review. *American Industrial Hygiene Association journal*, 1986, 47:A148-151.

4.  Amoore JE, Hautala E. Odor as an aid to chemical safety: odor thresholds compared with threshold limit values and volatilities for 214 industrial chemicals in air and water dilution. *Journal of applied toxicology*, 1983, 3:272-290.

5.  Agency for Toxic Substances and Disease Registry. *Toxicological profile for trichloroethylene. Update.* Atlanta, GA, US Department of Health and Human Services, 1993.

6.  Environmental Monitoring and Support Laboratory. *Method 502.1. Volatile halogenated organic compounds in water by purge-and-trap gas chromatography.* Cincinnati, OH, US Environmental Protection Agency, 1985.

7.  Environmental Monitoring and Support Laboratory. *Method 524.1. Volatile organic compounds in water by purge-and-trap gas chromatography/mass spectrometry.* Cincinnati, OH, US Environmental Protection Agency, 1985.

8.  Bellar TA, Lichtenberg JJ, Kroner RC. The occurrence of organohalides in chlorinated drinking waters. *Journal of the American Water Works Association*, 1974, 66: 703-706.

9.  Brass HJ et al. The national organic monitoring survey: sampling and analyses for purgeable organic compounds. In: Pojasek RB, ed. *Drinking water quality enhancement source protection*. Ann Arbor, MI, Ann Arbor Science, 1977:393-416.

10. McConnell G, Ferguson DM, Pearson CR. Chlorinated hydrocarbons and the environment. *Endeavour*, 1975, 34:13-18.

11. Daniel JW. The metabolism of Cl-labeled trichloroethylene and tetrachloroethylene in the rat. *Biochemical pharmacology*, 1963, 12:795-802.

12. Laham S. Studies on placental transfer: trichloroethylene. *Industrial medicine*, 1970, 39:46-49.

13. Zenick H et al. Effects of trichloroethylene exposure on male reproductive function in rats. *Toxicology*, 1984, 31:237-250.

14. Ikeda M et al. Urinary excretion of total trichloro-compounds, trichloroethanol, and trichloroacetic acid, as a measure of exposure to trichloroethylene and tetrachloroethylene. *British journal of industrial medicine*, 1972, 29:328-333.

15. Stewart RD et al. Observations on the concentrations of trichloroethylene in blood and expired air following exposure of humans. *American Industrial Hygiene Association journal*, 1962, 23:167-170.

16. Ertle T et al. Metabolism of trichloroethylene in man. I. The significance of trichloroethanol in long-term exposure conditions. *Archives of toxicology*, 1972, 19:171-188.

17. Ikeda M, Imanura T. Biological half-life of trichloroethylene and tetrachloroethylene in human subjects. *Internationales Archiv für Arbeitsmedizin*, 1973, 31:209-224.

18. National Institute for Occupational Safety and Health. *Registry of Toxic Effects of Chemical Substances (RTECS)*. Washington, DC, US Department of Health and Human Services, 1991 (DHHS [NIOSH] 91-101-2).

19. Buben JA, O'Flaherty EJ. Delineation of the role of metabolism in the hepatotoxicity of trichloroethylene and perchloroethylene: a dose-effect study. *Toxicology and applied pharmacology*, 1985, 78:105-122.

20. National Toxicology Program. *Carcinogenesis studies of trichloroethylene (without epichlorohydrin) in F344/N rats and B6C3F$_1$ mice (gavage studies)*. Research Triangle Park, NC, US Department of Health and Human Services, 1990 (NTP TR 90-1799).

21. Kimmerle G, Eben A. Metabolism, excretion and toxicology of trichloroethylene after inhalation. 1. Experimental exposure on rats. *Archives of toxicology*, 1973, 30:115-126.

22. National Toxicology Program. *Trichloroethylene: reproduction and fertility assessment in F344 rats when administered in the feed. Final report.* Research Triangle Park, NC, 1986 (NTP-86-085).

23. National Toxicology Program. *Trichloroethylene: reproduction and fertility assessment in CD-1 mice when administered in the feed. Final report.* Research Triangle Park, NC, 1985 (NTP-86-068).

24. Schwetz BA, Leong KJ, Gehring PJ. The effect of maternally-inhaled trichloroethylene, perchloroethylene, methylchloroform and methylene chloride on embryonal and fetal development in mice and rats. *Toxicology and applied pharmacology,* 1975, 32:84-96.

25. Crebelli R et al. Mutagenicity of trichloroethylene, trichloroethanol and chloral hydrate in *Aspergillus nidulans. Mutation research,* 1985, 155:105-111.

26. Walles SA. Induction of single-strand breaks in DNA of mice by trichloroethylene and tetrachloroethylene. *Toxicology letters,* 1986, 31:31-35.

27. National Cancer Institute. *Carcinogenesis bioassay of trichloroethylene.* Bethesda, MD, 1976 (Carcinogenesis Technical Report Series No. 2; DHEW Publication No. [NIH] 76-802).

28. Henschler D et al. Carcinogenicity study of trichloroethylene, with and without epoxide stabilizers, in mice. *Journal of cancer research and clinical oncology,* 1984, 107:149-156.

29. Dekant W, Metzler M, Henschler D. Identification of *S*-1,2-dichlorovinyl-*N*-acetylcysteine as a urinary metabolite of trichloroethylene: a possible explanation for its nephrocarcinogenicity in rats. *Biochemical pharmacology,* 1986, 35:2455-2458.

30. Henschler D et al. Carcinogenicity study of trichloroethylene by long-term inhalation in three animal species. *Archives of toxicology,* 1980, 43:237-248.

31. Fukuda K, Takemoto K, Tsuruta H. Inhalation carcinogenicity of trichloroethylene in mice and rats. *Industrial health,* 1983, 21:243-254.

32. Grandjean E et al. Investigations into the effects of exposure to trichloroethylene in mechanical engineering. *British journal of industrial medicine,* 1955, 12:131-142.

33. Defalque FJ. Pharmacology and toxicology of trichloroethylene. A critical review of world literature. *Clinical pharmacology and therapeutics,* 1961, 2:665-688.

34. Stephens CA. Poisoning by accidental drinking of trichloroethylene. *British medical journal,* 1945, 2:218-219.

35. International Agency for Research on Cancer. *Overall evaluations of carcinogenicity: an updating of IARC Monographs volumes 1-42.* Lyon, 1987:364-366 (IARC Monographs on the Evaluation of Carcinogenic Risks to Humans, Suppl. 7).

## 14.10 Tetrachloroethene

### 14.10.1 General description

#### *Identity*

CAS no.: 127-18-4
Molecular formula: $C_2Cl_4$

Tetrachloroethene is also known as tetrachloroethylene and perchloroethylene.

#### *Physicochemical properties* (1–3)[1]

| Property | Value |
|---|---|
| Melting point | -19 °C |
| Boiling point | 121 °C |
| Density | 1.623 g/ml at 25 °C |
| Vapour pressure | 2.53 kPa at 25 °C |
| Water solubility | 150 mg/litre at 25 °C |
| Log octanol–water partition coefficient | 2.86 |

#### *Organoleptic properties*

The odour thresholds for tetrachloroethene in water and air are 0.3 mg/litre and 7 mg/m$^3$, respectively (3).

#### *Major uses*

Tetrachloroethene is used primarily as a solvent in the dry-cleaning industry. It is also used as a degreasing solvent in metal industries, as a heat transfer medium, and in the manufacture of fluorohydrocarbons (1, 4).

#### *Environmental fate*

Most tetrachloroethene released to the environment is found in the atmosphere, where photochemically produced hydroxyl radicals degrade it to phosgene and chloroacetyl chlorides with a half-life of 96–251 days (3). In water, it does not readily undergo hydrolysis or photolysis but is biodegraded by microorganisms to

---

[1] Conversion factor in air: 1 ppm = 6.78 mg/m$^3$.

dichloroethene, vinyl chloride, and ethene. Tetrachloroethene can persist in waters where volatilization cannot occur. It volatilizes less readily from soil than from water and, with a soil adsorption coefficient of 72–534, is expected to be fairly mobile in soils. Degradation may occur in anaerobic soils. It does not appear to bioaccumulate in animals or food-chains (3).

## 14.10.2 Analytical methods

A purge-and-trap gas chromatographic procedure is used for the determination of tetrachloroethene in drinking-water (5). Mass spectrometry or electron capture, flame-ionization, and halide-sensitive detectors may be used for detection, the detection limits ranging from 0.1 to 1.9 µg/litre in water (3, 6).

## 14.10.3 Environmental levels and human exposure

### Air

Concentrations of tetrachloroethene in city air in the United Kingdom range from less than 0.7 to 70 µg/m³ (7). In Munich, suburban and urban air concentrations were 4 and 6 µg/m³, respectively (8). Surveys in the USA indicated concentrations of less than 0.01 µg/m³ in rural areas and up to 6.7 µg/m³ in urban areas (9).

### Water

A survey of drinking-water in the USA in 1976–77 detected tetrachloroethene in nine of 105 samples at levels ranging from 0.2 to 3.1 µg/litre (mean 0.8 µg/litre) (10). In other surveys of drinking-water supplies in the USA, it was found that 3% of all public water-supply systems that used well-water contained tetrachloroethene at concentrations of 0.5 µg/litre or higher, whereas those that used surface water contained lower levels (2). In the United Kingdom, it has been detected at levels of 0.4 µg/litre in municipal waters (1, 7) and, in Japan, in approximately 30% of all wells, at concentrations ranging from 0.2 to 23 000 µg/litre (3). In Switzerland, tetrachloroethene concentrations as high as 954 µg/litre have been found in contaminated groundwater (11). Tetrachloroethene in anaerobic groundwater may degrade to more toxic compounds, including vinyl chloride (3).

### Food

Tetrachloroethene concentrations in seafood in the United Kingdom ranged from 0.5 to 30 µg/kg (7, 12). Those in other foodstuffs ranged from almost undetectable (0.01 µg/kg) in orange juice to 13 µg/kg in butter (13). Some foods (particularly those with a high fat content) stored or sold near dry-cleaning facilities may contain considerably higher concentrations (14).

### *Estimated total exposure and relative contribution of drinking-water*

Based on a tetrachloroethene concentration in air of 6 μg/m³, estimated exposure would be about 120 μg/day for an adult with an air intake of 20 m³. If drinking-water contains 0.5 μg of tetrachloroethene per litre, the average daily exposure would be 1 μg for an adult consuming 2 litres of water per day. There are insufficient data on the levels of tetrachloroethene in foods to allow an average exposure to be determined.

## 14.10.4 Kinetics and metabolism in laboratory animals and humans

The results of animal studies indicate that tetrachloroethene is rapidly and completely absorbed from the gastrointestinal tract (*3, 15*). It reached near-steady-state levels in the blood of human volunteers after 2 h of continuous inhalation (*16*). Rats given a gavage dose of radiolabelled tetrachloroethene contained radioactivity in the liver, kidneys, and fat (*15*). Occupationally exposed subjects had whole-blood levels as high as 2500 μg/litre, as compared with 0.4 μg/litre in controls (*17*).

Metabolic products appear to be similar in humans and experimental animals (*1,18,19*). Tetrachloroethene is metabolized by a cytochrome P-450-mediated oxidation to tetrachloroethene oxide and trichloroacetyl chloride to form trichloroethanoic acid and trichloroethanol. In mice, trichloroethanoic acid is the major metabolite formed, whereas it is formed in relatively small amounts in rats (*20*). In humans, only 1.8% of the retained dose was converted into trichloroethanoic acid; 1.0% was converted into an unknown metabolite in 67 h (*21*).

Saturation of metabolism has been observed both in inhalation studies in rats (*22*) and in gavage studies in mice (*23*). After saturation of metabolism via the oxidative pathway, a second metabolic pathway through conjugation with glutathione to form a highly reactive trichlorovinylthiol compound has been shown to occur in rat kidney, activated by renal β-lyase enzyme. This metabolic pathway appears to be absent in humans (*22*) and to be significant only in male rats (*24*).

Tetrachloroethene is eliminated from the body primarily via the lungs; the half-life is about 65 h (*1, 25*). Trichloroethanoic acid is eliminated via the urine with a half-life of 144 h (*1, 26*).

## 14.10.5 Effects on laboratory animals and *in vitro* test systems

### *Acute exposure*

$LD_{50}$s of 3835 and 3005 mg/kg of body weight were found for male and female rats to which single doses of tetrachloroethene were administered by gavage. Acute effects were dominated by central nervous system depression (*27*).

### Short-term exposure

Groups of male Swiss-Cox mice were given oral doses of tetrachloroethene in corn oil at 0, 20, 100, 1000, or 2000 mg/kg of body weight, 5 days per week for 6 weeks (equivalent to 0, 14, 70, 700, or 1400 mg/kg of body weight per day). Mice treated with doses as low as 70 mg/kg of body weight per day exhibited significantly increased liver triglyceride levels and liver-to-body-weight ratios. At higher doses, hepatotoxic effects included decreased DNA content, increased serum alanine aminotransferase, decreased glucose-6-phosphatase serum levels, and hepatocellular necrosis, degeneration, and polyploidy. The NOAEL was 14 mg/kg of body weight per day (23).

Sprague-Dawley rats (20 per sex per dose) were given tetrachloroethene in drinking-water at doses of 14, 400, or 1400 mg/kg of body weight per day for 90 days. Males in the high-dose group and females in the mid- and high-dose groups exhibited depressed body weights. Increased liver- and kidney-to-body-weight ratios (equivocal evidence of hepatotoxicity) were also observed at the two highest doses (27).

There was moderate fatty degeneration of the liver in mice following a 4-h exposure to air containing 1340 mg of tetrachloroethene per m³ (28). Exposure to this level for 4 h per day, 6 days per week for up to 8 weeks increased the severity of the lesions (29).

### Long-term exposure

Male and female Osborne-Mendel rats and B6C3F$_1$ mice were exposed to tetrachloroethene by corn oil gavage for 78 weeks at doses ranging from 471 to 1072 mg/kg of body weight per day. Increased mortality and nephropathy, as shown by degenerative tubule changes, fatty changes, and cloudy swelling, were observed in all treated animals (30).

Exposure of F344 rats to tetrachloroethene administered by inhalation at doses of 0, 1.36, or 2.72 g/m³ for 103 weeks, 5 days per week, resulted in a significant reduction in survival, increased renal karyomegaly in both sexes, and renal tubular cell hyperplasia in males at both doses. Similar exposure of B6C3F$_1$ mice to 0, 1.36, or 2.72 g/m³ resulted in reduced survival and increased renal nephrosis, tubular cell karyomegaly, and renal casts, as well as hepatic degeneration and necrosis (31).

### Reproductive toxicity, embryotoxicity, and teratogenicity

Inhalation exposures to tetrachloroethene have resulted in maternal and fetal toxicity in mice, rats, and rabbits (3).

## *Mutagenicity and related end-points*

Short-term studies indicate that tetrachloroethene induces single-strand DNA breaks in the mouse but does not cause chromosomal aberrations in rat bone marrow or human lymphocytes (*1, 30, 32*). *In vitro* assays in *Salmonella typhimurium*, *Escherichia coli*, and *Saccharomyces cerevisiae* were negative both with and without microsomal activation.

## *Carcinogenicity*

The exposure by inhalation (6 h per day, 5 days per week for 103 weeks) of F344/N rats to 0, 1.36, or 2.72 g/m$^3$ tetrachloroethene produced a small (but not statistically significant) increase in the combined incidence of renal tubular-cell adenomas and adenocarcinomas in males but not in females. In both sexes, there was an increase in the incidence of mononuclear cell leukaemias at both doses, but the incidence was also unusually high in concurrent as compared with historical controls (*31*).

It has been suggested that the induction of kidney tumours in male rats is the combined result of the formation of a highly reactive metabolite and cell damage produced by renal accumulation of hyaline droplets (*33, 34*).

The exposure by inhalation (6 h per day, 5 days per week for 103 weeks) of B6C3F$_1$ mice at 0, 1.36, or 2.72 g/m$^3$ resulted in an increase in hepatocellular carcinomas in both males and females (*31*). In an earlier bioassay, in which tetrachloroethene was administered by gavage in corn oil, there was an increase in the incidence of hepatocellular carcinomas in both male and female mice but not in Osborne-Mendel rats. In this experiment, survival was reduced in both species as a result of pneumonia, and impurities later shown to be carcinogenic were present in the tetrachloroethene (*30*).

Hepatotoxic and related carcinogenic effects of tetrachloroethene in mice appear to be due to trichloroethanoic acid, which is formed in greater amounts by mice than by rats or humans (*19, 35*). In addition, mice are more sensitive than rats to trichloroethanoic acid, a peroxisome proliferator in mice (*36*).

## 14.10.6 Effects on humans

Oral doses of 4.2–6 g of tetrachloroethene administered to patients to control parasitic worm infections caused central nervous system effects, such as inebriation, perceptual distortion, and exhilaration (*37*). Several developmental effects, such as eye, ear, central nervous system, chromosomal, and oral cleft anomalies, were associated with exposure to tetrachloroethene and other solvents in contaminated drinking-water supplies (*38*). Inhalation exposures have been associated in female dry-cleaning workers with reproductive effects, including menstrual disorders and spontaneous abortions (*39, 40*).

A few case reports and small-scale epidemiological and clinical studies involving a group of men occupationally exposed to tetrachloroethene at levels of 1890-2600 mg/m³ suggest an association between such exposure and serious central nervous system problems (*1,41–43*). However, workers were often simultaneously exposed to several solvents (*44*). Evidence for the carcinogenicity of tetrachloroethene was obtained by observing laundry and dry-cleaning workers, but was rated as inadequate by IARC (*45*). Although an increased incidence of cancer was reported in several cohort and proportionate mortality studies (*1,46–48*) and increased risks of cancer in workers exposed to tetrachloroethene were found in case–control studies (*49, 50*), study limitations, such as concomitant exposures to other chemicals and small sample size, make it difficult to reach a definite conclusion.

## 14.10.7 Guideline value

IARC (*45*) has concluded that there is sufficient evidence of carcinogenicity in animals to classify tetrachloroethene in Group 2B: possible human carcinogen. It reportedly produces liver tumours in mice, with some evidence of mononuclear cell leukaemia in rats and kidney tumours in male rats. However, overall evidence indicates that this compound is not genotoxic.

In view of the overall evidence for nongenotoxicity and evidence for a saturable metabolic pathway leading to kidney tumours in rats, it is appropriate to use a NOAEL with a suitable uncertainty factor for calculation of the TDI. A 6-week gavage study in male mice and a 90-day drinking-water study in male and female rats both indicated a NOAEL for hepatotoxic effects of 14 mg/kg of body weight per day (*23, 27*). A TDI of 14 µg/kg of body weight was calculated by applying an uncertainty factor of 1000 (100 for intra- and interspecies variation and 10 for carcinogenic potential). In view of the database on tetrachloroethene and considerations regarding the application of the dose via drinking-water in one of the two critical studies, it was deemed unnecessary to include an additional uncertainty factor to reflect the length of the study. The guideline value is 40 µg/litre (rounded figure) for a drinking-water contribution of 10%.

## References

1. *Tetrachloroethylene.* Geneva, World Health Organization, 1984 (Environmental Health Criteria, No. 31).

2. Office of Drinking Water. *Health advisory for tetrachloroethylene.* Washington, DC, US Environmental Protection Agency, 1987.

3. Agency for Toxic Substances and Disease Registry. *Toxicological profile for tetrachloroethylene.* Atlanta, GA, US Department of Health and Human Services, 1993.

4. Condie LW. Target organ toxicology of halocarbons commonly found contaminating drinking water. *Science of the total environment*, 1985, 47:433-442.

5. Environmental Monitoring and Support Laboratory. *Method 502.1. Volatile halogenated organic compounds in water by purge-and-trap gas chromatography*. Cincinnati, OH, US Environmental Protection Agency, 1985.

6. Environmental Monitoring and Support Laboratory. *Method 524.1. Volatile organic compounds in water by purge-and-trap gas chromatography/mass spectrometry*. Cincinnati, OH, US Environmental Protection Agency, 1985.

7. Pearson CR, McConnell G. Chlorinated $C_1$ and $C_2$ hydrocarbons in the marine environment. *Proceedings of the Royal Society of London, Series B*, 1975, 189:305-332.

8. Lachner F. Perchloräthylen eine Bestandsaufnahme. [Perchloroethylene: an inventory.] *Umwelt*, 1976, 6:434.

9. Lillian D et al. Atmospheric fates of halogenated compounds. *Environmental science and technology*, 1975, 9:1042-1048.

10. Environmental Protection Agency. Water quality criteria documents. *Federal register*, 1980, 45:79318-79341.

11. Giger W, Molnar-Kubica E. Tetrachloroethylene in contaminated ground and drinking waters. *Bulletin of environmental contamination and toxicology*, 1978, 19(4):475-480.

12. Dickson AG, Riley JP. The distribution of short-chained halogenated aliphatic hydrocarbons in some marine organisms. *Marine pollution bulletin*, 1976, 7:167-169.

13. McConnell G, Ferguson DM, Pearson CR. Chlorinated hydrocarbons and the environment. *Endeavour*, 1975, 34:13-18.

14. Chutsch VM et al. Tetrachlorethen in Lebensmitteln. [Tetrachloroethene in foodstuffs.] *Bundesgesundheitsblatt*, 1990, 6:249-251.

15. Pegg DG et al. Disposition of [$^{14}$C]-tetrachloroethylene following oral and inhalation exposure in rats. *Toxicology and applied pharmacology*, 1979, 51:465-474.

16. Stewart RD et al. Human exposure to tetrachloroethylene vapor. *Archives of environmental health*, 1961, 2:516-522.

17. Hajimiragha H et al. Human exposure to volatile halogenated hydrocarbons from the general environment. *International archives of occupational and environmental health*, 1986, 58:141-150.

18. Ikeda M. Metabolism of trichloroethylene and tetrachloroethylene in human subjects. *Environmental health perspectives*, 1977, 21:239-245.

19. Ikeda M, Ohtsuji H. A comparative study of the excretion of Fujiwara reaction-positive substances in urine of humans and rodents given trichloro- or tetrachloro-derivatives of ethane and ethylene. *British journal of industrial medicine*, 1972, 29: 99-104.

20. Odum J et al. The role of trichloroacetic acid and peroxisome proliferation in the differences in carcinogenicity of perchloroethylene in the mouse and rat. *Toxicology and applied pharmacology*, 1988, 92:103-112.

21. Ogata M et al. Excretion of organic chlorine compounds in the urine of persons exposed to vapours of trichloroethylene and tetrachloroethylene. *British journal of industrial medicine*, 1971, 28:386-391.

22. Green T et al. Perchloroethylene-induced rat kidney tumours: an investigation of the mechanisms involved and their relevance to humans. *Toxicology and applied pharmacology*, 1990, 103:77-89.

23. Buben JA, O'Flaherty EJ. Delineation of the role of metabolism in the hepatotoxicity of trichloroethylene and perchloroethylene: a dose–effect study. *Toxicology and applied pharmacology*, 1985, 78:105-122.

24. Green T. Species differences in carcinogenicity: the role of metabolism in human risk evaluation. *Teratogenesis, carcinogenesis, and mutagenesis*, 1990, 10:103-113.

25. Stewart RD et al. Experimental human exposure to tetrachloroethylene. *Archives of environmental health*, 1970, 20:224-229.

26. Ikeda M, Imanura T. Biological half-life of trichloroethylene and tetrachloroethylene in human subjects. *Internationales Archiv für Arbeitsmedizin*, 1973, 31:209-224.

27. Hayes JR, Condie LW, Borzelleca JF. The subchronic toxicity of tetrachloroethylene (perchloroethylene) administered in the drinking water of rats. *Fundamental and applied toxicology*, 1986, 7:119-125.

28. Kylin B et al. Hepatotoxicity of inhaled trichloroethylene, tetrachloroethylene and chloroform. Single exposure. *Acta pharmacologica et toxicologica*, 1963, 20:16-26.

29. Kylin B, Sumegi I, Yllner S. Hepatotoxicity of inhaled trichloroethylene. Long-term exposure. *Acta pharmacologica et toxicologica*, 1965, 22:379-385.

30. National Cancer Institute. *Bioassay of tetrachloroethylene for possible carcinogenicity*. Washington, DC, US Department of Health, Education, and Welfare, 1977 (NCI-CG-TR-13; NIH 77-813).

31. National Toxicology Program. *Toxicology and carcinogenesis studies of tetrachloroethylene (perchloroethylene) (CAS no. 127-18-4) in F344/N rats and B6C3F₁ mice (inhalation studies)*. Research Triangle Park, NC, US Department of Health and Human Services, National Institutes of Health, 1986 (NTP TR 311).

32. Cherna M, Kypenova H. Mutagenic activity of chloroethylenes analyzed by screening system tests. *Mutation research*, 1977, 46:214-215.

33. Green T. Chloroethylenes: a mechanistic approach to human risk evaluation. *Annual review of pharmacology and toxicology*, 1990, 30:73-89.

34. Olson MJ, Johnson JT, Reidy CA. A comparison of male rat and human urinary proteins: implications for human resistance to hyaline droplet nephropathy. *Toxicology and applied pharmacology*, 1990, 102:524-536.

35. Schumann AM, Quast JF, Watanabe PG. The pharmacokinetics and macromolecular interactions of perchloroethylene in mice and rats as related to oncogenicity. *Toxicology and applied pharmacology*, 1980, 55:207-219.

36. Bull RJ et al. Liver tumor induction in B6C3F1 mice by dichloroacetate and trichloroacetate. *Toxicology*, 1990, 63:341-359.

37. Haerer AF, Udelman HD. Acute brain syndrome secondary to tetrachloroethylene ingestion. *American journal of psychiatry*, 1964, 12:78-79.

38. Lagakos SW, Wessen BJ, Zelen M. An analysis of contaminated well water and health effects in Woburn, Massachusetts. *Journal of the American Statistical Association*, 1986, 81:583-614.

39. Zielhuis GA, Gijsen R, Van Der Gulden JWJ. Menstrual disorders among dry-cleaning workers. *Scandinavian journal of work, environment and health*, 1989, 15:238 (letter).

40. Kyyronen P et al. Spontaneous abortions and congenital malformations among women exposed to tetrachloroethylene in dry cleaning. *Journal of epidemiology and community health*, 1989, 43:346-351.

41. Gold JH. Chronic perchloroethylene poisoning. *Canadian Psychiatric Association journal*, 1989, 14:627.

42. McMullen JK. Perchloroethylene intoxication. *British medical journal*, 1976, 2:1563-1564.

43. Coler HR, Rossmiller HR. Tetrachloroethylene exposure in a small industry. *Archives of industrial hygiene and occupational medicine*, 1953, 8:227-233.

44. Tuttle TC, Wood GD, Grether CB. *A behavioral and neurological evaluation of dry cleaners exposed to perchloroethylene*. Washington, DC, US Department of Health, Education, and Welfare, 1976 (NIOSH No. 77-214).

45. International Agency for Research on Cancer. *Overall evaluations of carcinogenicity: an updating of IARC Monographs volumes 1-42*. Lyon, 1987:355-356 (IARC Monographs on the Evaluation of Carcinogenic Risks to Humans, Suppl. 7).

46. Blair A, Decoufle P, Grauman D. Causes of death among laundry and dry cleaning workers. *American journal of public health*, 1979, 69:508-511.

47. Katz RM, Jowett D. Female laundry and dry cleaning workers in Wisconsin: a mortality analysis. *American journal of public health*, 1981, 71:305-307.

48. Lynge E, Thygesen L. Primary liver cancer among women in laundry and dry-cleaning work in Denmark. *Scandinavian journal of work, environment and health*, 1990, 16:108-112.

49. Lin RS, Kessler II. A multifactorial model for pancreatic cancer in man. Epidemiologic evidence. *Journal of the American Medical Association*, 1981, 245:147-152.

50. Stemhagen A et al. Occupational risk factors and liver cancer. A retrospective case–control study of primary liver cancer in New Jersey. *American journal of epidemiology*, 1983, 117:443-454.

## 14.11 Benzene

### 14.11.1 General description

#### *Identity*

CAS no.:            71-43-2
Molecular formula:   $C_6H_6$

#### *Physicochemical properties (1,2 )[1]*

| Property | Value |
|---|---|
| Physical state | Colourless liquid |
| Melting point | 5.5 °C |
| Boiling point | 80.1 °C |
| Density | 0.88 g/cm$^3$ at 20 °C |
| Vapour pressure | 13.3 kPa at 26.1 °C |
| Water solubility | 1.8 g/litre at 25 °C |
| Log octanol–water partition coefficient | 2.13 |

#### *Organoleptic properties*

Benzene has a characteristic odour. Its odour threshold in water is 10 mg/litre (*2*).

#### *Major uses*

Benzene is used in the chemical industry for the production of styrene/ethylben-

---

[1] Conversion factor in air: 1 ppm = 3.2 mg/m$^3$ at 20 °C and 101.3 kPa.

zene, cumene/phenol, and cyclohexane (*1*). Its use as a solvent has been greatly reduced in the last few years (*3*). Benzene is used as an additive in petrol to increase the octane number (*2*).

### Environmental fate

In soil, benzene biodegrades under aerobic conditions only. In surface water, it rapidly volatilizes to the air, biodegrades with a half-life of a few days to weeks, or reacts with hydroxyl radicals with a half-life of several weeks to months. In air, it reacts with hydroxyl radicals, with a half-life of about 5 days (*4*).

## 14.11.2 Analytical methods

Benzene can be determined by a purge-and-trap gas chromatographic procedure with photoionization detection, a method which is applicable over a concentration range of 0.02–1500 µg/litre. Confirmation is by mass spectrometry (detection limit 0.2 µg/litre) (*4*).

## 14.11.3 Environmental levels and human exposure

### Air

Rural background concentrations of benzene, which may originate from natural sources (forest fires and oil seeps), have been reported to range from 0.3 to 54 µg/m³. The general urban atmosphere reportedly contains 50 µg/m³. In several studies conducted since 1963, average concentrations in ambient air ranged from 5 to 112 µg/m³, mainly derived from vehicular emissions (*1*).

Exposure inside homes can occur from cigarette smoke or when houses are built on soil polluted with benzene. In one case, levels varying from 34 µg/m³ (in the living space) up to 230 µg/m³ (beneath the floor) were found. Benzene is found both in the main stream (0.01–0.1 mg/cigarette) and in the side stream (0.05-0.5 mg/cigarette) of cigarette smoke (*3*). In a study in three states of the USA, weighted median concentrations were 9.8–16 µg/m³ in indoor air and 0.4–7.2 µg/m³ in outdoor air (*5*).

### Water

The major sources of benzene in water are atmospheric deposition, spills of petrol and other petroleum products, and chemical plant effluents. Levels of up to 179 µg/litre have been reported in chemical plant effluents (*1*). In seawater, levels were reported to be in the range 5–20 ng/litre (coastal area) and 5 ng/litre (central part) (*3*). Levels between 0.2 and 0.8 µg/litre were reported in the Rhine in 1976 (*6*). Levels of 0.03–0.3 mg/litre were found in groundwater contaminated by point emissions (*7*).

Benzene was detected in 50–60% of potable water samples taken at 30 treatment facilities across Canada; mean concentrations ranged from 1 to 3 µg/litre (maximum 48 µg/litre) (8). Federal drinking-water surveys in the USA estimated that approximately 1.3% of all groundwater systems contained benzene at concentrations greater than 0.5 µg/litre (highest level reported 80 µg/litre) (4).

### Food

Benzene may occur in food naturally, through migration from metallic covering layers of packaging material, or through contamination from the environment. It has been reported in several foods (eggs: 500-1900 µg/kg; rum: 120 µg/kg; irradiated beef: 19 µg/kg; heat-treated or canned beef: 2 µg/kg), and has also been detected in such foodstuffs as haddock, cheese, cayenne pepper, pineapple, and blackcurrants (9).

### Estimated total exposure and relative contribution of drinking-water

Exposure to benzene may vary considerably. For nonsmokers, the estimated average daily intake is 200–450 µg/day. The estimated contribution from food is 180 µg/day but, as information on benzene levels in food is very scanty, this background level should be considered only as an approximate reference point. For smokers, the intake levels are increased by a factor of 2–3 (urban areas) or 2–6 (rural areas). The levels commonly found in drinking-water are minimal compared with the intake from food and air (3).

## 14.11.4 Kinetics and metabolism in laboratory animals and humans

Benzene is rapidly and efficiently (30–50%) absorbed following inhalation. Following ingestion, animal data suggest about 100% absorption from the gastrointestinal tract. Less than 1% is absorbed through the skin. After absorption, benzene is widely distributed throughout the body, independently of the route of administration. Levels fall rapidly once exposure stops. Following uptake, adipose tissues have been found to contain high levels of benzene metabolites.

The metabolism and elimination of absorbed benzene appear to follow similar pathways in laboratory animals and humans. Benzene is converted mainly to phenol by the mixed-function oxidase system, primarily in the liver, but also in bone marrow. A small amount of phenol is metabolized to hydroquinone and catechol, and an even smaller amount is transformed into phenylmercapturic or *trans*-muconic acid. Between 12% and 14% (up to 50% in laboratory animals) of the absorbed dose is excreted unchanged in expired air. The respiratory elimination of benzene in humans is triphasic. In the urine, a small part is excreted unchanged, the remainder being excreted as phenol conjugates (3, 9–11).

463

## 14.11.5 Effects on laboratory animals and *in vitro* test systems

### Acute exposure

Benzene has a low acute toxicity. The oral $LD_{50}$ in mice and rats is 1–10 g/kg of body weight; the 2.8-h $LC_{50}$ is 15-60 $g/m^3$ (3).

### Long-term exposure

Repeated exposure to low levels of benzene produces toxic effects principally in the blood and blood-forming tissues (3). Long-term exposure of mice to concentrations of 32–65 $mg/m^3$ results in inhibition of early differentiating blood cell elements (12).

In a study in which benzene was administered by gavage in corn oil 5 days per week for 103 weeks at doses of 0, 5, 100, or 200 mg/kg of body weight to F344/N rats or 0, 25, 50, or 100 mg/kg of body weight to B6C3F$_1$ mice, haematological effects, including lymphoid depletion of the splenic follicles (rats) and thymus (male rats), bone marrow haematopoietic hyperplasia (mice), lymphocytopenia, and associated leukocytopenia (rats and mice), were observed even at the lowest dose (13–15).

### Reproductive toxicity, embryotoxicity, and teratogenicity

Benzene is not teratogenic even at maternally toxic dose levels. However, embryotoxicity/fetotoxicity was observed in rats and mice at levels as low as 65 $mg/m^3$ (9).

### Mutagenicity and related end-points

Benzene was not mutagenic in several bacterial and yeast systems, in the sex-linked recessive lethal mutation assay with *Drosophila melanogaster*, or in the mouse lymphoma cell forward mutation assay. It can cause chromosome damage in plants and in mammalian somatic cells both *in vitro* and *in vivo*. Its clastogenic potential is partly due to its hydroxylated metabolites. Benzene and its metabolites may interfere with the formation of the mitotic spindle and perhaps do not interact directly with DNA. However, binding of benzene to nucleic acids has been reported (3, 10, 15).

### Carcinogenicity

Benzene is carcinogenic in rats and mice after oral and inhalation exposure, producing malignant tumours at many sites. In a study by the National Toxicology Program, it was administered by gavage in corn oil 5 days per week for 103 weeks at doses of 0, 5, 100, or 200 mg/kg of body weight to F344/N rats and 0, 25, 50, or 100 mg/kg of body weight to B6C3F$_1$ mice. Compound-related non-neoplastic or neoplastic effects on the haematopoietic system, Zymbal gland, forestomach, and adrenal gland were seen in both sexes of both species. In addition, the oral cavity was affected in rats, and the lung, liver, harderian gland, preputial gland, ovary, and mammary gland in mice (*13–15*).

## 14.11.6 Effects on humans

Acute exposure of humans to high concentrations of benzene primarily affects the central nervous system. Acute exposure to 65 g/m$^3$ may cause death. Extensive haemorrhages have been observed in fatal cases (*3*).

Occupational exposure to more than 162 mg/m$^3$ results in toxic effects on the haematopoietic system, including pancytopenia. The white blood cells are the most sensitive (*10*).

There is considerable evidence that exposure to high benzene concentrations ($\geqslant$325 mg/m$^3$) may eventually result in leukaemia, in many cases preceded by pancytopenia or aplastic anaemia. Both epidemiological studies (*16, 17*) and several case-studies showed that exposure to benzene was correlated with the occurrence of leukaemia (particularly acute myeloid leukaemia). Cytogenetic effects in peripheral lymphocytes were observed in human subjects with benzene haemopathy (*3, 9, 11, 18*).

## 14.11.7 Guideline value

Benzene is carcinogenic in mice and rats after both inhalation and oral exposure, producing malignant tumours at many sites. It is considered to be a human carcinogen and is classified by IARC in Group 1 (*18*). Although it does not induce mutations or DNA damage in standard bacterial assay systems, it has been shown to cause chromosomal aberrations in a variety of species *in vivo*.

Because of the unequivocal evidence of the carcinogenicity of benzene in humans and laboratory animals and its documented chromosomal effects, quantitative risk extrapolation was used to estimate lifetime cancer risks. Based on a risk estimate using data on leukaemia from epidemiological studies involving inhalation exposure, it was calculated that a drinking-water concentration of 1 µg/litre was associated with an excess lifetime cancer risk of 10$^{-6}$ (10 µg/litre is associated with an excess lifetime risk of 10$^{-5}$ and 100 µg/litre with an excess lifetime risk of 10$^{-4}$) (*15*).

As data on the carcinogenic risk to humans following the ingestion of benzene are not available, risk estimates were also carried out on the basis of a 2-year gavage study in rats and mice (*13*). The robust linear extrapolation model was used, as there was a statistical lack of fit of some of the data with the linearized multistage model. The estimated range of concentrations in drinking-water corresponding to excess lifetime cancer risks of 10$^{-4}$, 10$^{-5}$, and 10$^{-6}$, based on leukaemia and lymphomas in female mice and oral cavity squamous cell carcinomas in male rats, are 100–800, 10–80, and 1–8 µg/litre, respectively. These estimates are similar to those derived from epidemiological data, which formed the basis for the previous guideline value of 10 µg/litre associated with a $10^{-5}$ excess lifetime cancer risk.

Guideline values corresponding to excess lifetime cancer risks of $10^{-4}$, $10^{-5}$, and $10^{-6}$ are therefore 100, 10, and 1 µg/litre, respectively.

## References

1.  International Agency for Research on Cancer. *Some industrial chemicals and dyestuffs.* Lyon, 1982:93-148 (IARC Monographs on the Evaluation of the Carcinogenic Risk of Chemicals to Humans, Volume 29).

2.  Verschueren K. *Handbook of environmental data on organic chemicals.* New York, NY, Van Nostrand Reinhold, 1983.

3.  Slooff W, ed. *Integrated criteria document benzene.* Bilthoven, Netherlands, National Institute of Public Health and Environmental Protection, 1988 (Report no. 758476003).

4.  Office of Drinking Water. *Benzene. Health advisory.* Washington, DC, US Environmental Protection Agency, 1987.

5.  Wallace LA et al. The TEAM study: personal exposures to toxic substances in air, drinking water, and breath of 400 residents of New Jersey, North Carolina and North Dakota. *Environmental research,* 1987, 43:290-307.

6.  Merian E, Zander M. Volatile aromatics. In: Hutzinger O, ed. *The handbook of environmental chemistry,* Vol. 3, Part B: *Anthropogenic compounds.* Berlin, Heidelberg, New York, Springer-Verlag, 1982:117-161.

7.  Burmaster DE. The new pollution. Groundwater contamination. *Environment,* 1982, 24:33-36.

8.  Department of National Health and Welfare (Canada). *Guidelines for Canadian drinking water quality 1978. Supporting documentation.* Ottawa, 1978.

9.  Agency for Toxic Substances and Disease Registry. *Toxicological profile for benzene.* Atlanta, GA, US Department of Health and Human Services, 1993.

10. *Air quality criteria for benzene.* Berlin, Federal Office for the Environment, 1982 (Report 6/82).

11. Ware GW, ed. USEPA Office of Drinking Water health advisories. *Reviews of environmental contamination and toxicology,* 1988, 106:9-19.

12. *Air quality guidelines for Europe.* Copenhagen, WHO Regional Office for Europe, 1987:45-58 (European Series, No. 23).

13. National Toxicology Program. *Toxicology and carcinogenesis studies of benzene in F344/N rats and B6C3F₁ mice (gavage studies)*. Research Triangle Park, NC, US Department of Health and Human Services, 1986 (Technical Reports Series No. 289).

14. Huff JE et al. Multiple-site carcinogenicity of benzene in Fischer 344 rats and B6C3F1 mice. *Environmental health perspectives*, 1989, 82:125-163.

15. *Benzene*. Geneva, World Health Organization, 1993 (Environmental Health Criteria, No. 150).

16. Rinsky RA, Young RJ, Smith AB. Leukemia in benzene workers. *American journal of industrial medicine*, 1981, 2:217-245.

17. Rinsky RA. Benzene and leukemia: an epidemiologic risk assessment. *Environmental health perspectives*, 1989, 82:189-192.

18. International Agency for Research on Cancer. *Overall evaluations of carcinogenicity: an updating of IARC Monographs volumes 1-42*. Lyon, 1987:120-122 (IARC Monographs on the Evaluation of Carcinogenic Risks to Humans, Suppl. 7).

## 14.12 Toluene

### 14.12.1 General description

**Identity**

CAS no.: 105-88-3
Molecular formula: $C_7H_8$

The IUPAC name for toluene is methylbenzene.

**Physicochemical properties** *(1, 2 )*[1]

| Property | Value |
|---|---|
| Physical state | Clear, colourless liquid |
| Melting point | -95 °C |
| Boiling point | 110.6 °C |
| Vapour pressure | 3.78 kPa at 25 °C |
| Density | 0.8623 g/cm³ at 15.6 °C |
| Water solubility | 535 mg/litre |
| Log octanol–water partition coefficient | 2.69 |

[1] Conversion factor in air: 1 ppm = 3.75 mg/m³.

467

## *Organoleptic properties*

Toluene has a sweet, pungent, benzene-like odour. The lowest concentrations reported to be perceptible to humans on inhalation range from 0.64 to 139 mg/m$^3$ (*3*). The odour threshold in water is 0.024–0.17 mg/litre. The reported taste threshold ranges from 0.04 to 0.12 mg/litre (*2, 4, 5*).

## *Major uses*

Toluene is used as a solvent, especially for paints, coatings, gums, oils, and resins, and as raw material in the production of benzene, phenol, and other organic solvents. Most toluene (in the form of benzene-toluene-xylene mixtures) is used in the blending of petrol.

## *Environmental fate*

Toluene degrades readily in air. It is removed from the atmosphere mainly by reactions with atomic oxygen, peroxy- or hydroxyl radicals, and ozone. Its half-life in the atmosphere ranges between 13 h and 1 day (*1, 6*).

When toluene is released to surface water, it volatilizes to air very rapidly, the half-life being about 5 h at 25 °C and increasing with the depth of the water column. Biodegradation and sorption are less important for the removal of toluene from surface waters. The extent to which it is biodegraded in soil ranges from 63% to 86% after 20 days (*7*).

The amount of toluene in environmental compartments can be estimated with the aid of models (*8*) when emission data are known. In the Netherlands, for example, the estimated percentages of total toluene in air, water, and soil are 98.6%, 0.8%, and 0.6%, respectively (*6*).

## 14.12.2 Analytical methods

A purge-and-trap gas chromatographic procedure with photoionization detection can be used for the determination of toluene in water over a concentration range of 0.02–1500 µg/litre (*9*). Confirmation is by mass spectrometry (*10*). Methods for the determination of toluene in air, soil, and other matrices have been reviewed and compiled by Fishbein & O'Neill (*11*).

## 14.12.3 Environmental levels and human exposure

### *Air*

Mean atmospheric concentrations of toluene in urban areas around the world range from 2 to 200 µg/m$^3$; concentrations are higher in areas with high traffic density. Lower levels (0.2–4 µg/m$^3$) have been reported in rural areas. Indoor concentrations range from 17 to 1000 µg/m$^3$ and are related both to outdoor concentrations and to the presence of cigarette smoke (*1, 6*).

### Water

The concentration of toluene in rainwater in Germany has been reported to be 0.13–0.70 µg/litre (12). In the Netherlands, a median value of 0.04 µg/litre was found (6).

Toluene was found at concentrations of 1–5 µg/litre in water samples from a number of rivers in the USA (1). Concentrations of 0.8 µg/litre and 1.9 µg/litre have been reported in the Rhine in Germany and Switzerland, respectively (13). In coastal waters, levels of 0.01–1 µg/litre were found (14).

In groundwater contaminated by point emissions, toluene levels of 0.2–1.1 mg/litre were reported (15). The highest level reported in groundwater in the USA in 1983 was 1.4 µg/litre (2).

In approximately 1% of all groundwater-derived public drinking-water systems in the USA, toluene levels are above 0.5 µg/litre (2). In Canada, in a study of 30 water-treatment plants, drinking-water contained an average of 2 µg/litre (16). In a study of Ontario drinking-water, concentrations of up to 0.5 µg/litre were found (17). Toluene can be leached from synthetic coating materials commonly used to protect drinking-water storage tanks (18).

### Food

Toluene concentrations of 1 mg/kg have been reported in fish (19). In cyclodextrin flavour complexes, residual concentrations can be in the range 2.7–10.2 mg/kg (20).

### Estimated total exposure and relative contribution of drinking-water

Although information on the intake of toluene via food and drinking-water is limited, it can be expected that this intake will be low compared with that via air. Studies in the Netherlands suggest that the population is exposed to at least 30 µg/m$^3$. If a mean ventilation volume of 20 m$^3$/day and an absorption of 50% are assumed, the daily absorption ranges from 0.3 to 12 mg (6). Exposure is increased by traffic and cigarette smoking.

## 14.12.4 Kinetics and metabolism in laboratory animals and humans

In humans, toluene is probably completely absorbed from the gastrointestinal tract after oral uptake. The compound is rapidly distributed in animals, and tissue distribution is comparable after administration by inhalation and by mouth. After uptake, the compound is preferentially found in adipose tissue, followed in succession by the adrenal glands, kidneys, liver, and brain. It is rapidly converted into benzyl alcohol by the microsomal mixed-function oxidase system in the liver, then to benzoic acid, which is conjugated with either glycine or glucuronic acid and excreted in urine as hippuric acid or benzoyl glucuronide. Toluene is also metabolized to a small extent to *o*- and *p*-cresol. In the lungs, part of the absorbed toluene is excreted unchanged (*3*).

## 14.12.5 Effects on laboratory animals and *in vitro* test systems

### Acute exposure

Toluene has a low acute toxicity via the oral route; $LD_{50}$s in rats range from 2.6 to 7.5 g/kg of body weight.

### Short-term exposure

In most short-term studies, toluene was administered by inhalation; liver enzyme induction, liver weight increase, and neurophysiological changes are the main effects seen in these studies (*3*). Few oral studies are available, and only one is of value for assessment purposes. This study was carried out in rats and mice with doses of 0, 312, 625, 1250, 2500, or 5000 mg/kg of body weight administered 5 days per week for 13 weeks. In rats, increased liver and kidney weights (without concomitant histopathological changes) were the most sensitive effects, occurring at doses of 625 mg/kg of body weight and above; the NOAEL in this study was 312 mg/kg of body weight. In mice, an increased relative liver weight was the most sensitive effect, being present at 312 mg/kg of body weight in females (*21*).

### Long-term exposure

In the only adequate toxicity study, toluene was administered via the inhalation route in rats. In this study, the only significant difference between the treatment groups and the control group was a decrease in blood haematocrit (erythrocyte volume fraction), observed at 380 and 1100 mg/m$^3$ but not at 110 mg/m$^3$ (exposure 6 h per day, 5 days per week) (*3*).

### Reproductive toxicity, embryotoxicity, and teratogenicity

Toluene has been tested for teratogenicity via the inhalation route (in rats, mice, and rabbits) and via the oral route (mice only). In the inhalation studies, embryotoxicity and fetotoxicity, but not teratogenicity, were observed at high dose levels ($\geqslant$100 mg/m$^3$). In one of the two oral studies, a significant increase in embryonic deaths occurred at all dose levels ($\geqslant$260 mg/kg of body weight); a teratogenic effect (increased incidence of cleft palate) was observed at the highest dose level (870 mg/kg of body weight) only (*3,12*).

## Mutagenicity and related end-points

Toluene was found to be nongenotoxic in a number of *in vitro* systems (bacteria, yeasts, mammalian cells). *In vivo* studies on insects, rats, and mice have yielded conflicting results; chromosomal aberrations in rat bone marrow cells were observed in studies carried out in the former USSR but not in other countries, perhaps as a result of contamination with benzene in these studies. In mice, the induction of micronuclei in erythrocytes was observed, but not consistently. It has been concluded that toluene has not been demonstrated to be genotoxic (*3,12*).

## Carcinogenicity

In an inhalation study in rats exposed to 110, 380, or 1100 mg/m³, 6 h per day, 5 days per week, no clear evidence for the carcinogenicity of toluene was found; the same results were found in several special carcinogenicity studies, all of which, however, were very limited in design (*3*). In an adequate inhalation carcinogenicity study carried out in rats and mice, no evidence for a carcinogenic effect was found (*21*). IARC concluded that there is inadequate evidence for the carcinogenicity of toluene in both experimental animals and humans and classified it in Group 3 (not classifiable as to its carcinogenicity to humans) (*1*).

## 14.12.6 Effects on humans

Virtually all the available data relate to exposure to toluene by inhalation. For acute exposure, the predominant effects were impairment of the central nervous system and irritation of mucous membranes. Fatigue and drowsiness were the most sensitive effects, being present at 375 mg/m³ and absent at 150 mg/m³. The toxic effects of toluene after long-term exposure are basically the same. There have been few controlled long-term studies via the oral and inhalation routes (*3, 12, 22*).

Studies designed to detect a possible increase in the frequency of chromosomal aberrations or sister chromatid exchanges in the peripheral lymphocytes of people occupationally exposed to toluene have yielded inconclusive results (*1, 3, 12*). Epidemiological studies on the occurrence of cancer as a consequence of the exposure of human populations to toluene alone are not available (*3*).

## 14.12.7 Guideline value

The available evidence suggests that toluene should not be regarded as an initiating carcinogen; a TDI approach can therefore be used to derive the guideline value. The NOAEL from a 13-week gavage study in rats (*21*) was 312 mg/kg of body weight (administration 5 days per week); this dosage level had marginal effects in an identical study in mice. A TDI of 223 µg/kg of body weight can be derived using the LOAEL for marginal hepatotoxicity in mice of 312 mg/kg of body weight (equivalent to 223 mg/kg of body weight 7 days per week) and applying an uncertainty factor of 1000 (100 for inter- and intraspecies variation and 10 for the short duration of the study and use of a LOAEL instead of a NOAEL). This TDI yields a guideline value of 700 µg/litre (rounded figure), allocating 10% of the TDI to drinking-water. It should be noted, however, that this value exceeds the lowest reported odour threshold in water of 24 µg/litre.

## References

1.  International Agency for Research on Cancer. *Some organic solvents, resin monomers and related compounds, pigments and occupational exposures in paint manufacture and painting.* Lyon, 1990:79-123 (IARC Monographs on the Evaluation of Carcinogenic Risks to Humans, Volume 47).

2.  US Environmental Protection Agency. USEPA Office of Drinking Water health advisories. *Reviews of environmental contamination and toxicology,* 1988, 106:189-203.

3.  Van der Heijden CA et al. *Integrated criteria document toluene – effects. Appendix.* Bilthoven, Netherlands, National Institute of Public Health and Environmental Protection, 1988 (Report no. 75847310).

4.  Alexander HC et al. Aqueous odor and taste threshold values of industrial chemicals. *Journal of the American Water Works Association,* 1982, 74:595-599.

5.  Agency for Toxic Substances and Disease Registry. *Toxicological profile for toluene.* Atlanta, GA, Department of Health and Human Services, 1989.

6.  Slooff W, Blokzijl PJ, eds. *Integrated criteria document toluene.* Bilthoven, Netherlands, National Institute of Public Health and Environmental Protection, 1988 (Report no. 75847310).

7.  Wilson JT et al. Biotransformation of selected organic pollutants in groundwater. *Developments in industrial microbiology,* 1983, 24:225-233.

8.  Mackay D, Leinonen PJ. Rate of evaporation of low-solubility contaminants from water bodies to atmosphere. *Environmental science and technology,* 1975, 9:1178-1180.

9.  Environmental Monitoring and Support Laboratory. *Method 503.1. Volatile aromatics and unsaturated organic compounds in water by purge and trap gas chromatography.* Cincinnati, OH, US Environmental Protection Agency, 1985.

10. Environmental Monitoring and Support Laboratory. *Method 524.1. Volatile organic compounds in water by purge-and-trap gas chromatography/mass spectrometry.* Cincinnati, OH, US Environmental Protection Agency, 1985.

11. Fishbein L, O'Neill IK, eds. *Environmental carcinogens: methods of analysis and exposure measurement.* Vol. 10. *Benzene and alkylated benzenes.* Lyon, International Agency for Research on Cancer, 1988 (IARC Scientific Publications No. 85).

12. *Toluene.* Geneva, World Health Organization, 1985 (Environmental Health Criteria, No. 52).

13. Merian E, Zander M. Volatile aromatics. In: Hutzinger O, ed., *Handbook of environmental chemistry,* Vol. 3, Part B. *Anthropogenic compounds,* Berlin, Springer, 1982: 117-161.

14. Wakeham SG et al. The biochemistry of toluene in coastal seawater: radiotracer experiments in controlled ecosystems. *Biochemistry,* 1985, 1:307-328.

15. Loch JPG, van Dijk-Looijaard A, Zoeteman BCJ. Organics in groundwater. In: Wheeler D, Richardson ML, Bridges J, eds. *Watershed 89. The future for water quality in Europe.* Oxford, Pergamon, 1989: 39-55.

16. Otson R, Williams DT, Bothwell PD. Volatile organic compounds in water in thirty Canadian potable water treatment facilities. *Journal of the Association of Official Analytical Chemists,* 1982, 65:1370-1374.

17. Smillie RD, Sakuma T, Duholke WK. Low molecular weight aromatic hydrocarbons in drinking-water. *Journal of environmental science and health,* 1978, A13(2):187-191.

18. Bruchet A, Shipert E, Alben K. Investigation of organic coating material used in drinking-water distribution systems. *Journal français d'hydrologie,* 1988, 19:101-111.

19. US Environmental Protection Agency. *Health assessment document for toluene.* Washington, DC, 1983 (Publication No. PB84-100056).

20. Gerloczy A, Fonagy A, Szejtli J. Reduction of residual toluene content in beta-cyclodextrin through preparing inclusion complexes. *Starch,* 1983, 35:320-322.

21. National Toxicology Program. *Toxicology and carcinogenesis studies of toluene (CAS no. 108-88-3) in F344/N rats and B6C3F$_1$ mice (inhalation studies).* US Department of Health and Human Services, 1990 (NTP Technical Report Series No. 371; NIH Publication No. 90-2826).

22. Andersen I et al. Human response to controlled levels of toluene in six-hour exposures. *Scandinavian journal of work, environment and health,* 1983, 9:405-418.

## 14.13 Xylenes

### 14.13.1 General description

#### Identity

CAS no.:                1130-20-7
Molecular formula:  $C_8H_{10}$

The IUPAC name for xylene is dimethylbenzene. There are three possible xylene isomers: 1,2-, 1,3-, and 1,4-dimethylbenzene; these will be referred to as *o-* (ortho), *m-* (meta), and *p-* (para) xylene. The xylenes are for the most part manufactured and marketed as a mixture of the isomers, which will here be called xylene.

#### Physicochemical properties (1, 2 )[1]

| Property | o-Xylene | m-Xylene | p-Xylene |
|---|---|---|---|
| Melting point (°C) | -25 | -48 | 13 |
| Boiling point (°C) | 144.4 | 139.0 | 138.4 |
| Vapour pressure at 25 °C (kPa) | 0.906 | 1.11 | 1.17 |
| Density at 20 °C (g/cm³) | 0.88 | 0.86 | 0.86 |
| Water solubility at 20 °C (mg/litre) | 175 | 160 | 198 (25 °C) |
| Log octanol–water partition coefficient | 2.77–3.12 | 3.20 | 3.15 |

#### Organoleptic properties

The lowest xylene concentrations in air reported to be perceptible to humans range from 0.6 to 16 mg/m³ (3, 4). The odour threshold for xylene isomers in water is 0.02–1.8 mg/litre (4, 5). Concentrations of 0.3–1.0 mg/litre in water produce a detectable taste and odour (6).

#### Major uses

Xylene is used in the manufacture of insecticides and pharmaceuticals, as a component of detergents, and as a solvent for paints, inks, and adhesives. Xylene-containing petroleum distillates are used extensively and increasingly in blending petrol. The three isomers are used individually as starting materials in the manufacture of various chemicals (1, 2).

#### Environmental fate

Releases of xylene to the environment are largely to air because of its volatility; the calculated distribution of xylene is: air, 99.1%; water, 0.7%; soil, 0.1%; and

---

[1] Conversion factor in air: 1 ppm = 4.41 mg/m³.

sediment, 0.1% (7). Xylene degrades in air with a half-life of a few days. It is also readily biodegraded in soils and surface waters (2). Under aerobic conditions, it can be degraded in groundwater; half-lives of from 24 to over 161 days have been reported (8, 9). In anaerobic groundwater, no biotransformation is expected (10). When xylene is released to surface water, it volatilizes to air very rapidly.

## 14.13.2 Analytical methods

A purge-and-trap gas chromatographic procedure with photoionization detection can be used for the determination of xylene in water over a concentration range of 0.02–1500 µg/litre (11). Confirmation is by mass spectrometry (12). Methods for the determinaion of xylene in air, soil, and other matrices have been reviewed and compiled by Fishbein & O'Neill (13).

## 14.13.3 Environmental levels and human exposure

### Air

Mean atmospheric concentrations of xylene in urban areas around the world range from 3 to 390 µg/m$^3$ (1). Outdoor concentrations of 0.6–61 µg/m$^3$ have been reported in the USA (1,14). Concentrations of 100 µg/m$^3$ were found at cross-roads (1). Indoor air concentrations range from 5.2 to 29 µg/m$^3$ and are higher (200 µg/m$^3$) in the presence of cigarette smoke. The average ratio of indoor to outdoor air concentration is 1.2 for m-xylene and 4.0 for o-xylene (15).

### Water

Xylene has been found at levels of 2–8 µg/litre in the surface water of Florida Bay (16). In the Netherlands section of the Rhine, the average xylene concentration in 1987 was 0.3 µg/litre (0.1 µg/litre for each isomer); the maximum value was 1.2 µg/litre. In the surface water of Lake IJsselmeer, the average and maximum concentrations were 0.3 and 0.9 µg/litre, respectively (17).

In groundwater contaminated by point emissions, xylene levels of 0.3–5.4 mg/litre have been reported; levels in uncontaminated groundwater are low (<0.1 µg/litre) (18). The highest level in groundwater in the USA (1983) was 2.5 µg/litre (2). In the Netherlands, xylene was detected in 10.1% of 304 samples of groundwater used for potable water production; the maximum concentration found was 0.7 µg/litre (19).

Xylene levels in approximately 3% of all groundwater-derived public drinking-water systems and 6% of all surface-water-derived drinking-water systems in the USA were greater than 0.5 µg/litre, the maximum level being 5.2 µg/litre (2). In Canada, m-xylene was found in seven out of 30 potable water treatment plants at concentrations below 1 µg/litre (20). In Ontario, xylene was found in drinking-water at concentrations of less than 0.5 µg/litre (21). In drinking-water and tapwater in New Orleans, concentrations of 3–8 µg/litre were reported (16).

Concentrations in drinking-water can be increased by the leaching of xylene from the synthetic coating materials commonly used to protect the tanks used for its storage (22).

### Estimated total exposure and relative contribution of drinking-water

Because of the low levels of xylene reported in drinking-water, air is likely to be the major source of exposure. If a mean ventilation volume of 20 $m^3$/day (75% indoor air; 25% outdoor air) and an absorption of 65% are assumed, the daily exposure can be estimated to range from 0.05 to 0.5 mg. This exposure will be increased when air is polluted with cigarette smoke.

## 14.13.4 Kinetics and metabolism in laboratory animals and humans

Data on absorption after ingestion are not available. Xylene isomers are readily absorbed after inhalation, with retention percentages of 60–65% in humans. They are absorbed to some extent (exact percentages not known) via the skin; the few data available indicate rapid distribution of the compound after uptake. Xylenes can cross the placenta. They are stored in adipose tissue in both laboratory animals and humans. A small part (< 5%) of the absorbed amount is exhaled unchanged; the remainder is converted almost quantitatively into methyl benzoic acid, which is excreted in urine as methyl hippuric acid. Few data on rates of excretion are available; it is eliminated from subcutaneous fat in humans with a half-life ranging from 25 to 128 h (2, 7, 23).

## 14.13.5 Effects on laboratory animals and *in vitro* test systems

### Acute exposure

Xylene isomers have a low acute toxicity via the oral route; $LD_{50}$s in rats range from 3.6 to 5.8 g/kg of body weight (1).

### Short-term exposure

Available short-term oral studies are of limited design. The toxicological significance of the ultrastructural liver changes observed in rats (24) at the only dose level tested (200 mg of *o*-xylene per kg of feed) is questionable given the absence of any histopathological signs in the livers of rats tested at much higher dose levels in oral studies carried out under the US National Toxicology Program (25). In addition, the results of the single-dose study are presented only for the group of methylated benzenes tested; the results observed with the individual compounds are not reported. In inhalation studies in rats, liver enzyme induction was observed at concentrations of 217 $mg/m^3$ and above, 6 h per day (NOAEL not determined) (23, 26).

### Long-term exposure

A carcinogenicity study in rats and mice provided some relevant information on the toxic effects of xylenes after oral administration. In rats, 0, 250, or 500 mg/kg of body weight per day was administered by gavage in corn oil, 5 days per week for 103 weeks. Growth was decreased at 500 mg/kg of body weight per day; no compound-related histological lesions were observed. The NOAEL for rats was 250 mg/kg of body weight per day. In mice, the dose levels tested were 0, 500, and 1000 mg/kg of body weight per day. The only observed effect in this species was hyperactivity at 1000 mg/kg of body weight per day (*25*).

### Reproductive toxicity, embryotoxicity, and teratogenicity

Both of the oral studies carried out in mice showed maternal toxicity with concurrent embryotoxicity and teratogenicity (increased incidence of cleft palate) at the higher dose levels tested (LOAEL 640 mg/kg of body weight; NOAEL 255 mg/kg of body weight) (*27, 28*). Teratogenicity studies carried out in rats and mice by the inhalation route showed maternal toxicity at high dose levels but no teratogenicity (*7, 23*).

### Mutagenicity and related end-points

The mutagenic activity of xylenes was examined in bacteria and in mammalian cells (both *in vitro* and *in vivo*) with negative results. The significance of a weak positive effect observed with technical xylene in a *Drosophila* recessive lethal test is not clear, given the negative results in the same test system obtained with the individual components of the technical mixture (*7, 23, 29*).

### Carcinogenicity

An oral carcinogenicity study in rats (0, 250, or 500 mg/kg of body weight per day administered by gavage in corn oil, 5 days per week for 103 weeks) and mice (0, 500, or 1000 mg/kg of body weight per day) did not show xylenes to be carcinogenic (*25*).

## 14.13.6 Effects on humans

No oral data are available. In acute inhalation studies, irritation of eyes and throat was observed at concentrations of 480 mg/m$^3$ and above. After short-term exposure (6 h per day, 5 days per week), reaction time, manual coordination, body equilibrium, and electroencephalogram were affected at concentrations of 390 mg/m$^3$ and above (NOAEL not determined). Controlled studies of longer duration are not available (*7, 23*).

## 14.13.7 Guideline value

On the basis of the available evidence, xylenes should not be regarded as initiating carcinogens, so that a TDI approach may be used. A TDI of 179 µg/kg of body weight was derived using a NOAEL of 250 mg/kg of body weight per day based on decreased body weight in a 103-week gavage study in rats (25) with administration 5 days per week (equivalent to 179 mg/kg of body weight per day 7 days per week) and an uncertainty factor of 1000 (100 for intra- and interspecies variation and 10 for the limited toxicological end-point). This TDI yields a guideline value of 500 µg/litre (rounded figure), allocating 10% of the TDI to drinking-water. This value, however, exceeds the lowest reported odour threshold for xylenes in drinking-water of 20 µg/litre.

## References

1.  International Agency for Research on Cancer. *Some organic solvents, resin monomers and related compounds, pigments and occupational exposures in paint manufacture and painting.* Lyon, 1990:125-126 (IARC Monographs on the Evaluation of Carcinogenic Risks to Humans, Volume 47).

2.  US Environmental Protection Agency. USEPA Office of Drinking Water health advisories. *Reviews of environmental contamination and toxicology,* 1988, 106:189-203.

3.  Agency for Toxic Substances and Disease Registry. *Toxicological profile for xylenes.* Atlanta, GA, Department of Health and Human Services, 1990.

4.  Van Gemert LJ, Nettenbrijer AH, eds. *Compilation of odour threshold values in air and water.* Zeist, Netherlands, National Institute for Water Supply/Central Institute for Nutrition and Food Research TNO, 1977.

5.  Verschueren K. *Handbook of environmental data on organic chemicals,* 2nd ed. New York, NY, Van Nostrand Reinhold Company, 1983:1188-1195.

6.  Middleton FM, Rosen AA, Burtschell RH. Taste and odor research tools for water utilities. *Journal of the American Water Works Association,* 1958, 50:21-28.

7.  European Chemical Industry Ecology and Toxicology Centre. *Joint assessment of commodity chemicals No. 6: Xylenes CAS: 95-47-6(o), 108-38-3(m), 106-42-2(p), 1330-20-7(mixture).* Brussels, 1986.

8.  Barker JF et al. The organic geochemistry of a sanitary landfill leachate plume. *Journal of contaminant hydrology,* 1986, 1:171-189.

9.  Wilson JT et al. Relationship between the ATP content of subsurface material and the rate of biodegradation of alkylbenzenes and chlorobenzene. *Journal of contaminant hydrology,* 1986, 1:163-170.

10. Wilson JT et al. Biotransformation of selected organic pollutants in groundwater. *Developments in industrial microbiology*, 1983, 24:225-233.

11. Environmental Monitoring and Support Laboratory. *Method 503.1. Volatile aromatics and unsaturated organic compounds in water by purge and trap gas chromatography.* Cincinnati, OH, US Environmental Protection Agency, 1985.

12. Environmental Monitoring and Support Laboratory. *Method 524.1. Volatile organic compounds in water by purge-and-trap gas chromatography/mass spectrometry.* Cincinnati, OH, US Environmental Protection Agency, 1985.

13. Fishbein L, O'Neill IK, eds. *Environmental carcinogens: methods of analysis and exposure measurement.* Vol. 10. *Benzene and alkylated benzenes.* Lyon, International Agency for Research on Cancer, 1988 (IARC Scientific Publications No. 85).

14. Wallace LA. The TEAM Study: personal exposures to toxic substances in air, drinking-water, and breath of 400 residents of New Jersey, North Carolina, and North Dakota. *Environmental research*, 1987, 43:290-307.

15. Montgomery DD, Kalman DA. Indoor/outdoor air quality: reference pollutant concentrations in complaint-free residences. *Applied industrial hygiene*, 1989, 4:17-20.

16. Merian E, Zander M. Volatile aromatics. In: Hutzinger O, ed. *Handbook of environmental chemistry.* Vol. 3, Part B. *Anthropogenic compounds.* Berlin, Springer, 1982:117-161.

17. *De samenstelling van het Rijnwater in 1986 en 1987.* [*The composition of the water of the Rhine in 1986 and 1987.*] Amsterdam, Netherlands, RIWA (Rhine and Maas Waterworks Association), 1989.

18. Department of the Environment. *Environmental hazard assessment: xylenes.* Garston, Building Research Establishment, 1993.

19. Veenendaal G, van Beek CGEM, Puyker LM. *Het voorkomen van organische stoffen in het grondwater onttrokken door de Nederlandse Waterleidingbedrijven.* [*The occurrence of organic compounds in groundwater withdrawn by the Netherlands water-supply undertakings.*] Nieuwegein, KIWA (Netherlands Waterworks Testing and Research Institute), 1986 (KIWA Report No. 97).

20. Otson R, Williams DT, Bothwell PD. Volatile organic compounds in water in thirty Canadian potable water treatment facilities. *Journal of the Association of Official Analytical Chemists*, 1982, 65:1370-1374.

21. Smillie RD, Sakuma T, Duholke WK. Low molecular weight aromatic hydrocarbons in drinking water. *Journal of environmental science and health*, 1978, A13(2):187-191.

479

22. Bruchet A, Shipert E, Alben K. Investigation of organic coating material used in drinking water distribution systems. *Journal français d'hydrologie*, 1988, 19:101-111.

23. Janssen P, Van der Heijden CA, Knaap AGAC. [*Short summary and evaluation of toxicological data on xylene.*] Bilthoven, Netherlands, National Institute of Public Health and Environmental Protection, 1989 (in Dutch).

24. Bowers DE, Cannon MS, Jones DH. Ultrastructural changes in livers of young and aging rats exposed to methylated benzenes. *American journal of veterinary research*, 1982, 43:679-683.

25. National Toxicology Program. *Toxicology and carcinogenesis studies of xylenes (mixed) (60% m-xylene, 14% p-xylene, 9% o-xylene, 17% ethylbenzene) (CAS no. 1330-20-7) in F344/N rats and B6C3F₁ mice (gavage studies).* Research Triangle Park, NC, 1986 (NTP Technical Report Series No. 327).

26. US Environmental Protection Agency. USEPA Office of Drinking Water health advisories. *Reviews of environmental contamination and toxicology*, 1987, 106:213-222.

27. Marks TA, Ledoux TA, Moore JA. Teratogenicity of a commercial xylene mixture in the mouse. *Journal of toxicology and environmental health*, 1982, 9:97-105.

28. Nawrot PS, Staples RE. Embryofetal toxicity and teratogenicity of isomers of xylene in the mouse. *Toxicologist*, 1981, 1:A22.

29. Donner M et al. Genetic toxicology of xylenes. *Mutation research*, 1980, 74:171-172.

# 14.14 Ethylbenzene

## 14.14.1 General description

### Identity

CAS no.:           100-41-4
Molecular formula:  $C_8H_{10}$

### Physicochemical properties (1)[1]

| Property | Value |
|---|---|
| Physical state | Colourless liquid |
| Melting point | -95 °C |
| Boiling point | 136.2 °C |
| Vapour pressure | 0.933 kPa at 20 °C |
| Density | 0.86 g/cm³ at 20 °C |
| Water solubility | 152 mg/litre at 20 °C |
| Log octanol–water partition coefficient | 3.15 |

### Organoleptic properties

Ethylbenzene has an aromatic odour. The odour threshold is in the range 0.27–0.4 mg/m³ in air (1, 2) and 0.002–0.13 mg/litre in water (1, 3). The taste threshold ranges from 0.072 to 0.2 mg/litre (2, 3).

### Major uses

Ethylbenzene is present in xylene mixtures at levels up to 15–20% (4). This mixture is used in the paint industry, in insecticide sprays, and in petrol blends. Ethylbenzene is used primarily in the production of styrene and acetophenone, as a solvent, and as a constituent of asphalt and naphtha.

### Environmental fate

The primary source of ethylbenzene in the environment is the petroleum industry. Because of its high vapour pressure and low solubility, it will disperse into the atmosphere if released. More than 96% of ethylbenzene can be expected in the air compartment. It is phototransformed in the air by reaction with hydroxyl radicals; the half-life is approximately 1 day (5).

Biodegradation of ethylbenzene in soil under aerobic conditions with a half-life of 24.2 days has been reported. In activated sludge and water, it can be biodegraded under aerobic conditions (6).

---

[1] Conversion factor in air: 1 ppm = 4.35 mg/m³.

## 14.14.2 Analytical methods

A purge-and-trap gas chromatographic procedure with photoionization detection can be used for the determination of ethylbenzene in water over a concentration range of 0.02–1500 µg/litre (7). Confirmation is by mass spectrometry (8). Methods for the determination of ethylbenzene in air, soil, and other matrices have been reviewed and compiled by Fishbein & O'Neill (9). Continuous monitoring of ethylbenzene and other volatile hydrocarbons is possible at the microgram per litre level (10).

## 14.14.3 Environmental levels and human exposure

### Air

In Germany, average indoor and outdoor ethylbenzene concentrations of 13 µg/m$^3$ were found (11). In Italy, mean indoor and outdoor air concentrations of 27 and 7.4 µg/m$^3$ were reported (12).

The median daily concentrations of ethylbenzene in the urban air of nine major cities in the USA were 1.3–6.5 µg/m$^3$ (13). In the Netherlands, mean and maximum values of 0.9–2.8 and 10.0–25.7 µg/m$^3$, respectively, were reported (14).

### Water

The maximum ethylbenzene concentration in the Besós river in Spain was 15 µg/litre and in the Llobregat river 1.9 µg/litre (15). Levels of 0.03–0.3 mg/litre were reported in groundwater contaminated by point emissions (16).

In a survey of groundwater supplies (17), it was found that approximately 0.6% of 945 such supplies contained ethylbenzene; the median concentration was 0.87 µg/litre. In the Netherlands, ethylbenzene was detected in 1% of 304 samples of groundwater (18); the maximum concentration was 0.4 µg/litre. Concentrations of up to 0.07 µg/litre were found in aquifers in the United Kingdom (19). In Canada, in a study of 30 water-treatment plants, concentrations in drinking-water were below 1 µg/litre (20).

In Los Angeles, USA, an ethylbenzene concentration of 9 ng/litre was found in rainwater (21).

### Food

Ethylbenzene has been identified in volatiles of roasted hazelnuts. It can migrate from polystyrene food packaging into food. Concentrations of 2.5–21 µg/litre have been reported in milk and soup (5).

### Estimated total exposure and relative contribution of drinking-water

Although there is little information concerning the intake of ethylbenzene via food and drinking-water, it is expected to be low compared with that via air. In the Netherlands, the estimated daily exposure is 40 μg (*14*), based on a ventilation volume of 20 m³/day.

## 14.14.4 Kinetics and metabolism in laboratory animals and humans

Ethylbenzene in liquid form is easily absorbed by humans via both the skin and the intestinal tract (exact absorption percentages not reported); the vapour is readily absorbed when inhaled (reported absorption percentage 64% for humans, 44% for rats). Both distribution and excretion are rapid. In humans, storage of ethylbenzene in fat has been reported, and the compound has been observed to cross the placental barrier. Biotransformation in humans is almost completely to mandelic acid and phenylglyoxalic acid, both these metabolites being excreted in urine. Metabolism in experimental animals differs from that in humans in that benzoic acid is the major metabolite together with mandelic acid. Urinary excretion of metabolites is almost complete within 24 h (*1, 5*).

## 14.14.5 Effects on laboratory animals and *in vitro* test systems

### Acute exposure

Ethylbenzene has a low acute toxicity via the oral route; $LD_{50}$s in rats range from 3.5 to 4.7 g/kg of body weight (*22*).

### Short-term exposure

In a short-term oral study in rats, effects on liver and kidneys were observed at 400 mg/kg of body weight and higher dose levels (administered 5 days per week for 6 months); there were no such effects at 136 mg/kg of body weight (*23*). Liver effects were also found in a number of inhalation studies; the LOAEL for this type of effect was 1305 mg/m³, no effects being seen at 218 or 430 mg/m³ (concentrations administered for 6 h per day, 5 days per week) (*5, 24, 25*).

### Reproductive toxicity, embryotoxicity, and teratogenicity

In all the teratogenicity studies in rats and rabbits, dosing was via the inhalation route. No definite conclusions with regard to the observed effects (maternal toxicity, reduced fertility and, possibly, teratogenicity) can be drawn from the reports available (*5, 22*).

### Mutagenicity and related end-points

Studies were carried out in bacteria, yeasts, insects, mammalian cells (*in vitro*), and intact mammals; negative results were obtained in all test systems, showing ethylbenzene to be devoid of mutagenic activity (*1, 5, 22*).

## 14.14.6 Effects on humans

Relevant oral data are lacking. Data for the inhalation route are limited to acute studies considered to be insufficient as a basis for a guideline value (*1, 5, 22*).

## 14.14.7 Guideline value

No carcinogenicity data on ethylbenzene are available. The compound was shown to be nonmutagenic in a number of tests. Given these findings, a TDI approach may be applied.

The TDI is derived using a NOAEL of 136 mg/kg of body weight per day based on hepatotoxicity and nephrotoxicity observed in a limited 6-month study in rats (administration 5 days per week) (*23*); this dose level is equivalent to 97.1 mg/kg of body weight per day for dosing 7 days per week. After application of an uncertainty factor of 1000 (100 for intra- and interspecies variation and 10 for the limited database and short duration of the study), a TDI of 97.1 µg/kg of body weight results. This yields a guideline value of 300 µg/litre (rounded figure), allocating 10% of the TDI to drinking-water, which exceeds the lowest reported odour threshold in drinking-water (2.4 µg/litre).

## References

1.  US Environmental Protection Agency. USEPA Office of Drinking Water health advisories. *Reviews of environmental contamination and toxicology*, 1988, 106:189-203.

2.  Van Gemert LJ, Nettenbrijer AH, eds. *Compilation of odour threshold values in air and water.* Zeist, Netherlands, National Institute for Water Supply/Central Institute for Nutrition and Food Research TNO report, 1977.

3.  Alexander HC et al. Aqueous odor and taste threshold values of industrial chemicals. *Journal of the American Water Works Association*, 1982, 74:595-599.

4.  International Agency for Research on Cancer. *Some organic solvents, resin monomers and related compounds, pigments and occupational exposures in paint manufacture and painting.* Lyon, 1989:125-156 (IARC Monographs on the Evaluation of Carcinogenic Risk to Humans, Volume 47).

5.  European Chemical Industry Ecology and Toxicology Centre. *Joint assessment of commodity chemicals No. 7: Ethylbenzene CAS:100-41-4.* Brussels, 1986.

6.  Department of the Environment. *Environmental hazard assessment: ethylbenzene.* Garston, Building Research Establishment, 1992.

7.  Environmental Monitoring and Support Laboratory. *Method 503.1. Volatile aromatics and unsaturated organic compounds in water by purge and trap gas chromatography.* Cincinnati, OH, US Environmental Protection Agency, 1985.

8.  Environmental Monitoring and Support Laboratory. *Method 524.1. Volatile organic compounds in water by purge-and-trap gas chromatography/mass spectrometry.* Cincinnati, OH, US Environmental Protection Agency, 1985.

9.  Fishbein L, O'Neill IK, eds. *Environmental carcinogens: methods of analysis and exposure measurement.* Vol. 10. *Benzene and alkylated benzenes.* Lyon, International Agency for Research on Cancer, 1988 (IARC Scientific Publications No. 85).

10. Maitoza P, Valade JA, Madigan WT. Continuous monitoring of volatile hydrocarbons in water at the ppb level with a sparger and process chromatograph. *Hydrocarbons*, 1989, 1:23-28.

11. Seifert B, Abraham HJ. Indoor air concentrations of benzene and some other aromatic hydrocarbons. *Ecotoxicology and environmental safety*, 1982, 6:190-192.

12. De Bortoli M et al. Concentrations of selected organic pollutants in indoor and outdoor air in Northern Italy. *Environment international*, 1985, 12:343-350.

13. Edgerton SA et al. Inter-urban comparison of ambient volatile organic compound concentrations in U.S. cities. *Journal of the American Pollution Control Association*, 1989, 39:729-732.

14. Guicherit R, Schulting FJ. The occurrence of organic chemicals in the atmosphere of the Netherlands. *Science of the total environment*, 1985, 43:193-219.

15. Gomez-Belinchon JI, Grimalt JO, Abaigés J. Volatile compounds in two polluted rivers in Barcelona (Catalonia, Spain) *Water research*, 1991, 25:577-589.

16. Van Duijvenboden W, Kooper WF. Effects on groundwater flow and groundwater quality of a waste disposal site in Noordwijk, The Netherlands. *Science of the total environment*, 1981, 21:85-92.

17. Westrick JJ, Mello JW, Thomas RF. The groundwater supply survey. *Journal of the American Water Works Association*, 1984, 76(5):52-59.

18. Veenendaal G, Van Beek CGEM, Puyker LM. *Het voorkomen van organische stoffen in het grondwater onttrokken door de Nederlandse Waterleidingbedrijven.* [*The occurrence of organic compounds in groundwater withdrawn by the Netherlands water-supply undertakings.*] Nieuwegein, KIWA (Netherlands Waterworks Testing and Research Institute), 1986 (KIWA Report No. 97).

19. Kenrick MAP et al. *Trace organics in British aquifers – a baseline survey.* Medmenham, Water Research Centre, 1985 (Water Research Centre Report No. TR 223).

20. Otson R, Williams DT, Bothwell PD. Volatile organic compounds in water in thirty Canadian potable water treatment facilities. *Journal of the Association of Official Analytical Chemists*, 1982, 65:1370-1374.

21. Kawamura K, Kaplan IR. Organic compounds in the rain water of Los Angeles. *Environmental science and technology*, 1983, 17:497-502.

22. Janssen P, Van der Heijden CA. *Summary and evaluation of toxicological data on ethylbenzene.* Bilthoven, Netherlands, National Institute of Public Health and Environmental Protection, 1987.

23. Wolf MA et al. Toxicological studies of certain alkylated benzenes and benzene. *Archives of industrial health*, 1956, 14:387-398.

24. Elovaara E et al. Biochemical and morphological effect of long-term inhalation exposure of rats to ethyl benzene. *Xenobiotica*, 1985, 15:299-308.

25. Cragg ST et al. Subchronic inhalation toxicity of ethylbenzene in mice, rats and rabbits. *Fundamental and applied toxicology*, 1989, 13:399-408.

## 14.15 Styrene

### 14.15.1 General description

#### *Identity*

CAS no:        100-42-5
Molecular formula:  $C_8H_8$

The IUPAC name for styrene is phenylethene. It is also known as vinylbenzene, ethenylbenzene, and styrol.

#### *Physicochemical properties (1–3 )[1]*

| Property | Value |
|---|---|
| Physical state | Colourless, viscous liquid |
| Melting point | -30.6 °C |
| Boiling point | 145 °C |
| Vapour pressure | 0.6 kPa at 20 °C |
| Density | 0.91 g/cm$^3$ at 20 °C |
| Water solubility | 300 mg/litre at 20 °C |
| Log octanol–water partition coefficient | 2.95 |

---

[1] Conversion factor in air: 1 ppm = 4.2 mg/m$^3$.

## Organoleptic properties

The average taste threshold reported for styrene in water at 40 °C is 0.12 mg/litre (4). Styrene has a sweet odour, and odour thresholds for solutions in water range from 0.02 to 2.6 mg/litre (5). An odour threshold for solutions in water at 60 °C of 0.0036 mg/litre has also been reported (4). The estimated odour threshold for styrene in air is 0.1 mg/m$^3$ (6).

## Major uses

Styrene is used for the production of plastics and resins (1, 6).

## Environmental fate

Styrene in air is very reactive in the presence of hydroxyl radicals and ozone, having a half-life of about 2 h (7). In air, it is oxidized to aldehydes, ketones, and benzoic acid. High relative molecular mass peroxides can also be formed (6).

## 14.15.2 Analytical methods

The styrene content of water is determined by a purge-and-trap gas chromatographic procedure with photoionization detection, a method which is applicable over a concentration range of 0.05–1500 µg/litre. Confirmation is by mass spectrometry (detection limit 0.3 µg/litre) (2, 8).

## 14.15.3 Environmental levels and human exposure

### Air

Concentrations of styrene far from a source are negligible because of its high reactivity with ozone and hydroxyl radicals. In Munich, styrene was detected in the open air in industrial areas at a mean concentration of 0.5–5.9 µg/m$^3$. Near styrene production plants, concentrations were 0.3–3000 µg/m$^3$. Indoor air concentrations of styrene may be significantly higher in homes of smokers than nonsmokers (6). Reported median values for personal exposure are 1.3–1.9 µg/m$^3$ for indoor air and 0.1–0.7 µg/m$^3$ for outdoor air (9).

### Water

In 1985, styrene was detected in the Rhine at a maximum concentration of 0.1 µg/litre. In the Great Lakes, USA, it was detected at concentrations of 0.1–0.5 µg/litre. It was not detected in the raw water of groundwater pumping stations in Germany (6), but has been found in finished drinking-water in the USA at concentrations of less than 1 µg/litre and in commercial, charcoal-filtered drinking-water in New Orleans, USA (1).

## Food

Styrene has been found in food packaged in polystyrene containers, especially yoghurt (2.5–34.6 µg/kg). In other milk products and honey, some tens of micrograms were found up to 120 days after packaging (*1*). In east Australia, 146 food samples packaged in polystyrene, especially milk products, were analysed. About 85% of the yoghurt samples contained less than 50 µg/kg (maximum 100 µg/kg); the lowest concentrations were found in margarine (90% contained less than 10 µg/kg) (*10*). In a study on 133 different types of foodstuffs packaged in styrene-based materials (100–500 mg/kg), the concentration in the foodstuffs ranged from less than 1 to 200 µg/kg. In meat products, styrene was present in the outermost layers and was not detected after cooking (*11*).

## *Estimated total exposure and relative contribution of drinking-water*

The population exposure level for styrene is estimated to be approximately 40 µg per person per day for nonsmokers in nonindustrial areas. This figure is based on the levels in the open air (2 µg/day), traffic (mean of 10–50 µg/day), and food (5 µg derived from the consumption of 500 g of milk products in styrene-based packages). The most important exposure is active smoking (500 µg/day). Passive smoking accounts for only a few micrograms per day. In industrial areas, the exposure via open air is 400 µg/day. Exposure via drinking-water is negligible (*6*).

## 14.15.4 Kinetics and metabolism in laboratory animals and humans

After exposure by inhalation or administration by gavage, 60–90% of styrene is absorbed. Controlled laboratory studies in animals and humans have shown that uptake of styrene is rapid and that it is widely distributed to the whole body with a preference for lipids. Elimination from lipid depots is slower (half-life 2-4 days) than from other tissues. There is no tendency towards long-term accumulation.

Styrene is biotransformed mainly to styrene-7,8-oxide via the mixed function oxidase system. This occurs in the liver as well as in a number of other tissues and organs. The epoxide is further hydrolysed by the action of epoxide hydrolase to styrene glycol which, in turn, can be converted into mandelic acid, phenylglyoxylic acid, and hippuric acid, or conjugated to give glucuronic acid. Styrene-7,8-oxide can also be conjugated with glutathione to form mercapturic acid derivatives.

A small percentage of the dose absorbed is excreted unchanged in the expired air in both laboratory animals and humans after exposure via various routes. More than 90% of an oral dose is excreted rapidly as metabolites, mainly via the urine. In general, the metabolites in the urine of laboratory animals and humans are qualitatively the same, but the amounts are species-dependent. Major metabolites in humans are mandelic acid and phenylglyoxylic acid. Elimination of styrene and its metabolites can be described by a two-compartment kinetic model with an initial rapid phase and a slow terminal phase. At high exposure levels, elimination in animals appeared to be monophasic, suggesting a saturable metabolic pathway (2, 5, 12, 13).

## 14.15.5 Effects on laboratory animals and *in vitro* test systems

### Acute exposure

Styrene has a low acute toxicity. For the rat, the oral $LD_{50}$ is 5–8 g/kg of body weight, and the 4-h and 6-h $LC_{50}$s are 11 and 19 g/m$^3$ of air, respectively (5, 12). At lethal oral doses, rats became comatose before death. Autopsy revealed hepatic changes and incidental renal changes (5).

### Short-term exposure

The NOAEL in a 6-month oral toxicity study in the rat was 133 mg/kg of body weight (14). In rats given dose levels above 200 mg/kg of body weight, enhanced activities of drug-metabolizing enzymes and decreased glutathione-S-transferase activity in the liver were seen (5). An increased sensitivity of dopamine receptors was found at 200 and 400 mg/kg of body weight, suggesting involvement of neurotransmitter function in the central nervous system effects caused by styrene (15). At dose levels above 400 mg/kg of body weight, decreased body weight gain, increased liver and kidney weights, significantly reduced glutathione concentrations in liver, kidneys, and brain, significantly enhanced liver enzyme activities, and histopathological changes in the liver were observed (5). At doses above 500 mg/kg of body weight, irritation of the oesophagus and stomach and hyperkeratosis of the forestomach were observed and deaths occurred. No haematological changes were observed in short-term oral studies in the rat (5). In a 19-month oral study in dogs, a dose-related increased incidence in Heinz bodies in erythrocytes was observed down to the lowest dose tested (200 mg/kg of body weight) (16).

### Long-term exposure

In a study in which pregnant BDIV rats received a styrene dose of 1350 mg/kg of body weight in olive oil on day 17 of pregnancy and their offspring received 500 mg/kg of body weight in olive oil weekly from weaning for 120 weeks, congestion of lungs and kidneys and necrotic foci in liver parenchyma were seen in rats that died before 60 weeks. Rats dying after 80–90 weeks showed lesions of the forestomach (atrophy or local desquamation of epithelium, necrotic areas with inflammatory reactions of underlying tissues) and kidneys (hyperplasia of pelvis epithelium) (17).

In a study in which F344 rats were given styrene at 500, 1000, or 2000 mg/kg of body weight in corn oil, significantly increased mortality was seen in males at the highest dose level, probably due to hepatic necrosis. A dose-related growth depression in males was seen at all dose levels (18).

In a 2-year oral toxicity study, Charles River COBS CD (SD) rats received 0, 125, or 250 mg of styrene per litre of drinking-water. At 250 mg/litre, females showed a significantly lower terminal body weight than control females. No other treatment-related effects were seen. The parameters studied were clinical signs, mortality, growth, food and water intake, haemograms, clinical chemistry, urinalysis, gross necropsy, and histopathology. The NOAEL in this study was 125 mg/litre (corresponding to 7.7 mg/kg of body weight for males and 12 mg/kg of body weight for females) (19).

### Reproductive toxicity, embryotoxicity, and teratogenicity

In a three-generation reproductive study, Charles River COBS CD (SD) rats received 0, 125, or 250 mg of styrene per litre in drinking-water. No effect on reproductive parameters was observed (19). An oral teratogenicity study in rats did not reveal maternal toxicity, teratogenic effects, or embryotoxic effects at dose levels up to and including 300 mg/kg of body weight (20). In a study in which pregnant BDIV rats received styrene at 1350 mg/kg of body weight in olive oil on day 17 of pregnancy and their offspring received 500 mg/kg of body weight in olive oil weekly from weaning for 120 weeks, neonatal mortality in the test group was 10% compared with 2.5% in the control group (17).

Styrene was not teratogenic in studies on mice, rats, hamsters, and rabbits exposed by inhalation. Embryotoxic effects were seen at dose levels above 1050 $mg/m^3$. Styrene-7,8-oxide caused embryotoxic but not teratogenic effects in rats and rabbits exposed to concentrations above 73.5 $mg/m^3$ (5).

### Mutagenicity and related end-points

Styrene is mutagenic in a variety of test systems but only with metabolic activation. It induces gene mutations in both prokaryotic and eukaryotic microorganisms, *Drosophila*, and mammalian cells *in vitro*, as well as chromosomal abnormalities in mammalian cells *in vitro*. *In vivo* tests for chromosomal abnormalities gave contradictory results; positive results were observed mainly at high doses (3, 5).

Styrene-7,8-oxide, the main reactive intermediate of styrene biotransformation, is a direct-acting mutagen that induces gene mutations in microorganisms, *Drosophila*, and mammalian cells *in vitro* as well as chromosomal abnormalities in mammalian cells *in vitro*. *In vivo* studies of chromosomal aberrations, DNA breaks, and sister chromatid exchange gave contradictory results (3, 5).

### Carcinogenicity

Oral carcinogenicity studies were carried out with two strains of mice already exposed *in utero*. In the first study, with $O_{20}$ mice, a significantly increased incidence of lung tumours (adenomas and adenocarcinomas) was observed in the test group. However, only one extremely high dose level (1350 mg/kg of body weight in olive oil) was used in this study, and dosing was terminated at 16 weeks of age because of high mortality. The experiment was terminated at 100 weeks when all animals had died (*17*). In the second study, with C57B1 mice, no significantly increased tumour incidences were observed in the test group. Only one dose level of 300 mg/kg of body weight was tested (*17*).

In an oral carcinogenicity study with B6C3F$_1$ mice, a significantly increased incidence of lung tumours (adenomas and carcinomas) was seen in males at the highest dose level only (300 mg/kg of body weight in corn oil). However, the control group was rather small (*18*).

In a study on *in utero* exposure, pregnant BDIV rats received styrene at 1350 mg/kg of body weight in olive oil on day 17 of pregnancy. Their offspring received 500 mg of styrene per kg of body weight in olive oil weekly from weaning for 120 weeks. The incidence of tumours was not significantly increased (*17*). In a study with F344 rats dosed at 500, 1000, or 2000 mg/kg of body weight in corn oil, no significantly increased tumour incidences were observed (*18*). The same result was found both in a study, terminated after 140 weeks, in which Sprague-Dawley rats received 0, 50, or 250 mg of styrene per kg of body weight in olive oil, 4–5 days per week for 52 weeks (*21*), and in a study in which Charles River COBS CD (SD) rats received 0, 125, or 250 mg of styrene per litre in drinking-water (*19*).

In two long-term gavage studies in rats with styrene-7,8-oxide, significantly increased incidences of papillomas and carcinomas in the forestomach were observed. Dose levels were as high as 250 mg/kg of body weight (*22, 23*).

## 14.15.6 Effects on humans

Short-term controlled studies in volunteers exposed by inhalation showed that styrene at concentrations above 210 mg/m$^3$ in air can cause irritation of the mucous membranes of the eyes, nose, and respiratory tract and depression of the central nervous system, as indicated by listlessness, drowsiness, incoordination, increased simple reaction times, and changes in visual evoked response and EEG amplitude (*5, 12*).

In clinical studies in humans occupationally exposed for long periods, effects were generally observed at concentrations above 200 mg/m$^3$. Irritation of conjunctival and respiratory mucosa and prenarcotic symptoms were reported. Neurotoxicity involving the central as well as the peripheral nervous systems was seen in some cases. Effects were reported at dose levels of 100–200 mg/m$^3$. Some studies in workers suggested hepatotoxicity after long-term exposure to styrene, but no clear evidence for this effect could be found (*3, 5, 12*). In an extensive study in workers (*24*), 84 mg/m$^3$ caused only marginal effects. Because of the number of workers examined, the great number of parameters studied, and the absence of effects in other studies at concentrations below 100 mg/m³, 84 mg/m³ can be considered as the lowest observed marginal effect concentration in air for humans (5).

A few limited studies have reported on styrene-induced reproductive and teratogenic effects in occupationally exposed female workers. The results were contradictory, so that no definite conclusions could be drawn (3, 5, 12).

No chromosomal aberrations in peripheral lymphocytes could be detected in workers occupationally exposed to low concentrations of styrene, but significantly elevated frequencies of such chromosomal aberrations were observed in those occupationally exposed to much higher concentrations (5).

An association between the occurrence of leukaemia and lymphoma in humans and occupational exposure to styrene has been suggested. In the reinforced plastics industry, retrospective cohort mortality studies did not reveal any significantly increased mortality due to carcinogenicity. However, all the studies had serious defects, such as small or ill-defined cohorts and limited follow-up. In addition, mixed exposure to other compounds and/or past exposure to benzene had taken place (2, 5, 25).

## 14.15.7 Guideline value

On the basis of the available data, IARC classified styrene in Group 2B (25). It has been shown to be mutagenic in *in vitro* systems but only with metabolic activation. *In vivo* studies showed positive effects, but only at high doses. As the main metabolite, styrene-7,8-oxide, is a direct-acting mutagen, this compound is probably responsible for the positive effect of styrene after metabolic activation. Although carcinogenicity studies in mice and rats by various routes of administration did not provide evidence for the carcinogenicity of styrene, styrene-7,8-oxide was carcinogenic in long-term oral studies in rats. The available data therefore suggest that the carcinogenicity of styrene is due to the formation of the carcinogenic metabolite styrene-7,8-oxide as a consequence of the overloading of the detoxification mechanisms (e.g. glutathione conjugation and hydrolysis by epoxide hydrolase) after exposure to high styrene levels.

Based on the data given above, a TDI of 7.7 μg/kg of body weight can be derived from a NOAEL of 7.7 mg/kg of body weight per day for reduced body weight in the 2-year drinking-water study in rats (19), applying an uncertainty factor of 1000 (100 for intra- and interspecies variation and 10 for carcinogenicity and genotoxicity of the reactive intermediate styrene-7,8-oxide). If 10% of the TDI is allocated to drinking-water, a guideline value of 20 μg/litre (rounded figure) can be calculated. It should be noted that the lowest observed odour threshold for styrene in water is also 20 μg/litre.

# References

1. International Agency for Research on Cancer. *Some monomers, plastics and synthetic elastomers, and acrolein.* Lyon, 1979:231-274 (IARC Monographs on the Evaluation of the Carcinogenic Risk of Chemicals to Humans, Volume 19).

2. Ware GW, ed. USEPA Office of Drinking Water health advisories. *Reviews of environmental contamination and toxicology,* 1988, 107:131-145.

3. *Styrene.* Geneva, World Health Organization, 1983 (Environmental Health Criteria, No. 26).

4. Alexander HC, McCarty WM, Syverud AN. Aqueous odor and taste threshold values of industrial chemicals. *Journal of the American Water Works Association,* 1982, 74:595-599.

5. van Apeldoorn ME et al. *Integrated criteria document styrene – effects. Project No. 668310.* Bilthoven, Netherlands, National Institute of Public Health and Environmental Protection, 1985.

6. GDCh-Advisory Committee on Existing Chemicals of Environmental Relevance. *Styrene.* Weinheim, VCH, 1990 (BUA report 48).

7. Atkinson R et al. Rate constants for the gas-phase reactions of $O_3$ with selected organics at 296 K. *International journal of chemistry in the nineties,* 1982, 14:13-18.

8. Environmental Monitoring and Support Laboratory. *Method 524.1. Volatile organic compounds in water by purge-and-trap gas chromatography/mass spectrometry.* Cincinnati, OH, US Environmental Protection Agency, 1985.

9. Wallace LA et al. The TEAM Study: personal exposures to toxic substances in air, drinking water, and breath of 400 residents of New Jersey, North Carolina and North Dakota. *Environmental research,* 1987, 43:290-307.

10. Flanjak J, Sharrad J. Quantitative analysis of styrene monomer in foods. A limited East Australian survey. *Journal of the science of food and agriculture,* 1984, 35:457-462.

11. Gilbert J, Startin JR. A survey of styrene monomer levels in food and plastic packaging by coupled mass spectrometry–automatic headspace gas chromatography. *Journal of the science of food and agriculture,* 1983, 34:647-652.

12. Joint FAO/WHO Expert Committee on Food Additives. *Toxicological evaluation of certain food additives and food contaminants.* Cambridge, Cambridge University Press, 1984:171-196 (Food Additives Series No. 19).

13. Bond JA. Review of the toxicology of styrene. *CRC reviews in toxicology,* 1989, 19:227-249.

14. Wolf MA et al. Toxicological studies of certain alkylated benzenes and benzene. *Archives of industrial health*, 1956, 14:387-398.

15. Agrawal AK, Srivastava SP, Seth PK. Effect of styrene on dopamine receptors. *Bulletin of environmental contamination and toxicology*, 1982, 29:400-403.

16. Quast JF et al. Results of a toxicity study in dogs and teratogenicity studies in rabbits and rats administered monomeric styrene. *Toxicology and applied pharmacology*, 1978, 45:293-294.

17. Ponomarkov V, Tomatis L. Effects of long-term oral administration of styrene to mice and rats. *Scandinavian journal of work, environment and health*, 1978, 4:127-135.

18. National Cancer Institute. *National Cancer Institute bioassay of styrene for possible carcinogenicity*. Bethesda, MD, National Institutes of Health, 1979 (Technical Report Series No. 185; NIH Publication No. 79-1741).

19. Litton Bionetics. *Toxicological study on styrene incorporated in drinking water of rats for two years in conjunction with a three-generation reproduction study. Styrene. Revised final report, weeks 1-105. Vol. I.* Washington, DC, Chemical Manufacturers Association, 1980.

20. Murray FJ et al. Teratologic evaluation of styrene given to rats and rabbits by inhalation or by gavage. *Toxicology*, 1978, 11:335-343.

21. Maltoni C. *Study of the biological effects (carcinogenicity bio-assays) of styrene (St)*. Bologna, Bologna Tumour Centre Department of Experimental Oncology, 1978.

22. Maltoni C, Failla G, Kassapidis G. First experimental demonstration of the carcinogenic effects of styreneoxide. Long-term bioassays on Sprague-Dawley rats by oral administration. *Medicina del lavoro*, 1979, 70(5):358-362.

23. Ponomarkov V et al. A carcinogenicity study of styrene-7,8-oxide in rats. *Cancer letters*, 1984, 24:95-101.

24. Lorimer WV et al. Health status of styrene-polystyrene polymerization workers. *Scandinavian journal of work, environment and health*, 1978, 4:220-226.

25. International Agency for Research on Cancer. *Overall evaluations of carcinogenicity: an updating of IARC Monographs volumes 1-42*. Lyon, 1987:345-347 (IARC Monographs on the Evaluation of Carcinogenic Risk of Chemicals to Humans, Suppl. 7).

## 14.16 Polynuclear aromatic hydrocarbons

### 14.16.1 General description

Polynuclear aromatic hydrocarbons (PAHs) are a large group of substances with a molecular structure that includes two or more fused aromatic rings. Most of the available literature on PAHs is concerned with benzo[*a*]pyrene (BaP), on which this section will therefore be focused; information on other PAHs is included where appropriate.

### *Identity* (*1*)

Benzo[*a*]pyrene (BaP)
CAS no.:            50-32-8
Molecular formula:  $C_{20}H_{12}$

### *Physicochemical properties*

| *Property* | *Value* |
|---|---|
| Melting point | 179 °C |
| Boiling point | 495 °C |
| Vapour pressure | $7.47 \times 10^{-7}$ Pa at 25 °C |
| Water solubility | 3.8 µg/litre at 25 °C |
| Log octanol–water partition coefficient | 6.1 at 25 °C |

### *Major uses*

PAHs have no industrial uses but are produced primarily as a result of the incomplete combustion of organic material (*1*). The principal natural sources are forest fires and volcanic eruptions (*2*), while anthropogenic sources include the incomplete combustion of fossil fuels, coke oven emissions, aluminium smelters, and vehicle exhausts (*3, 4*).

### *Environmental fate*

PAHs are microbially biodegraded in the surface layers of soil (*5*). Biodegradation is faster in the presence of oxygen (*1*); the rate also depends on redox conditions, nitrate levels, and the presence of organic soil constituents and chemicals toxic to the degrading microorganisms (*5*). Half-lives for microbial degradation range from 5 to 240 days (*1*).

Direct atmospheric input appears to be the major source of BaP in surface waters (*6*). In water, most PAHs are adsorbed onto sediments and suspended solids. Volatilization may be important over periods exceeding 1 month. Most

PAHs are susceptible to aqueous photolysis under optimal conditions; they are biodegraded in water and taken up by aquatic organisms (*1*).

## 14.16.2 Analytical methods

Concentrations of BaP and other PAHs in water may be determined by gas chromatography in conjunction with mass spectrometry; the practical quantification limit is 0.01 µg/litre (Department of National Health and Welfare (Canada), unpublished data, 1988). High-pressure liquid chromatography with spectrofluorimetric detection (detection limit 0.1 ng/litre) can be used for the determination of BaP in drinking-water (*7*).

## 14.16.3 Environmental levels and human exposure

### *Air*

Mean levels of BaP in air are generally less than 1 ng/m$^3$ (*5, 8, 9*), although levels as high as 37.3 ng/m$^3$ have been measured (*10*); the levels tend to be higher in winter than in summer (*8, 9*). The mean level of total PAHs in Canadian cities sampled from 1984 to 1986 was 100 ng/m$^3$ (*8*).

Concentrations of PAHs in indoor air are likely to vary considerably depending on indoor sources, such as woodstoves and tobacco smoke. Levels of BaP in indoor air in New Jersey ranged from 0.1 to 8.1 ng/m$^3$ (*7*).

### *Water*

Water from 17 groundwater and 89 surface water systems was analysed for BaP, benzo[*b*]fluoranthene, and indeno[1, 2, 3-*c*,*d*]pyrene in 1976–77 in the USA; none of the systems sampled contained quantifiable levels of these PAHs (detection limits 0.03–0.1 µg/litre) (*1*).

The typical level of BaP in drinking-water in the USA is estimated to be 0.55 ng/litre (*11*). It was not detected (detection limit 1.0 µg/litre) in water from seven water-treatment plants in the area of Niagara Falls (*12*). The only PAH detected in treated drinking-water in Ontario (Canada) in surveys carried out in 1987 were benzo[*k*]fluoranthene (twice at 1 ng/litre), fluoranthene (20 and 30 ng/litre), and pyrene (twice at 40 ng/litre) (*13*). In 277 samples of municipal water supplies in the Atlantic provinces of Canada taken during 1985 and 1986, fluoranthene, benzo[*b*]fluoranthene, benzo[*k*]fluoranthene, BaP, indeno[1,2,3-*c*,*d*]pyrene, and benzo[*g*,*h*,*i*]perylene were detected in 58, 4, 1, 2, 0.4, and 0.7% of samples, respectively (detection limits 0.001–0.006 µg/litre; detected concentrations 0.001–0.024 µg/litre) (*14–17*).

## Food

BaP may be present in foodstuffs as a result of the absorption and deposition of particulates during processing (e.g. of smoked foods and leafy vegetables), the pyrolysis of fats, and the incomplete combustion of charcoal (18–20). Typical concentrations in food products range from nondetectable (<0.01 µg/kg) to 44 µg/kg.

## Estimated total exposure and relative contribution of drinking-water

Estimated daily intakes of total PAH in food range from 1.1 to 22.5 µg (11, 18); the corresponding figures for BaP range from 0.0014 to 1.6 µg (7, 11, 18, 21). Ranges for the estimated average daily intake of fluoranthene, benzo[k]fluoranthene, dibenzo[a,i]pyrene, 9,10-dimethylbenzanthracene, benzo[a]anthracene, benzo[b]fluoranthene, and dibenzo[a,h]anthracene in food by Canadians are 2.5–2.6, 0.026–0.030, 1.0–2.8, 0.046–0.12, 0.15–0.39, 0.082–0.12, and 0.061–0.10 µg/person, respectively (20, 22). Estimated daily intakes from water, food, and air are 20, 90–300, and 110 ng, respectively, for fluoranthene, and 0.4, 20–60, and 20 ng, respectively, for benzo[g,h,i]perylene (23, 24).

The mean total daily intake of BaP from air has been estimated to range from 0.025 µg/day (7) to 2.0 µg/day (1). The contribution of air to the daily intake is lower in rural areas than in urban areas (23, 24). Tobacco smoking is estimated to add a further 0.6 µg of BaP to daily intake (23, 24).

Daily intake of total PAHs from drinking-water is reported to be 0.027 µg (11). Daily intake of BaP in drinking-water is estimated to range from 0.1 to 1 ng (7, 11).

It would appear that food is the major and most variable source of daily exposure both to BaP and to PAHs in general; drinking-water makes only a minor contribution, probably no more than 1% of the total (1, 25).

## 14.16.4 Kinetics and metabolism in laboratory animals and humans

BaP is absorbed principally through the gastrointestinal tract and the lungs. Sprague-Dawley rats given BaP by duodenal infusion at 9.1–15.1 pmol/min absorbed approximately 40% of the dose from the duodenum (26). The rate of absorption of the different PAHs is influenced by their lipid solubilities (27) and by the content of polyunsaturated fatty acids in the diet (28). Absorbed BaP is rapidly distributed to the organs and tissues (29) and may be stored in mammary and adipose tissues (30). It crosses the placenta and is distributed in the developing fetus (31).

BaP is metabolized primarily in the liver, although significant metabolism can also occur in the tissues of the lung, gastrointestinal tract, placenta, skin, and kidney (32). It is metabolized in two steps, the first of which involves oxidation or hydroxylation via the cytochrome P-450-mediated mixed-function oxidase system, giving epoxides or phenols; the second step is detoxification of these metabolites to produce glucuronides, sulfates, or glutathione conjugates. Some of the epoxides may, however, be metabolized to dihydrodiols, which may undergo oxidation to diol-epoxides; these are thought to be responsible for carcinogenicity where this has been demonstrated. BaP metabolites are eliminated primarily in the faeces; only small amounts are excreted in the urine as water-soluble conjugates (25).

## 14.16.5 Effects on laboratory animals and *in vitro* test systems

The health effect of primary concern is carcinogenicity; doses of at least an order of magnitude greater than those that result in neoplastic lesions are required to induce other effects.

### Acute exposure

The oral $LD_{50}$s for various PAHs are reported to range between 490 and 18 000 mg/kg of body weight (33). Effects induced in animals following acute exposure include inflammation, hyperplasia, hyperkeratosis and ulceration of the skin, pneumonitis, damage to the haematopoietic and lymphoid systems, immunosuppression, adrenal necrosis, ovotoxicity, and antispermatogenic effects (11).

### Short-term exposure

No treatment-related effects were observed in groups of CD-1 mice given anthracene by gavage at doses of 0, 250, 500, or 1000 mg/kg of body weight per day for at least 90 days. Male and female CD-1 mice given 0, 125, 250, or 500 mg of fluoranthene per kg of body weight per day for 13 weeks by gavage exhibited increased alanine aminotransferase levels, kidney and liver changes, and clinical and haematological changes at 250 mg/kg of body weight per day. In a study in which CD-1 mice were exposed to fluorene suspended in corn oil at 0, 125, 250, or 500 mg/kg of body weight per day by gavage for 13 weeks, a significant decrease in red blood cell count and packed cell volume was observed in females treated with 250 mg/kg of body weight per day and in males and females treated with 500 mg/kg of body weight per day; decreased haemoglobin concentrations and increased total serum bilirubin levels were also observed in the group given 500 mg/kg of body weight per day. Male and female CD-1 mice gavaged with pyrene in corn oil at 0, 75, 125, or 250 mg/kg of body weight per day for 13 weeks exhibited kidney effects (renal tubular pathology, decreased kidney weights) at 125 mg/kg of body weight per day (34).

Other reported effects after short-term exposure to various PAHs include: hepatic changes in rats dosed orally with 1 g of naphthalene per kg of body weight per day for 10 days; decreased spleen weight in females and lowered hepatic aryl hydrocarbon hydroxylase activity in both sexes at the highest dose in

CD-1 mice given 5.3, 53, or 133 mg of naphthalene per kg of body weight per day for 90 days; loss of body weight and mild pathological changes in the liver and kidney in rats given oral doses of acenaphthene in olive oil at 2 g/kg of body weight per day for 32 days; and depression of body weight gain, elevated liver weight, and lowered spleen weight at the higher dose levels in rats fed diets containing 0.062–1.0% fluorene for 104 days (25).

### Reproductive toxicity, embryotoxicity, and teratogenicity

In the offspring of pregnant CD-1 mice given oral doses of 0, 10, 40, or 160 mg of BaP per kg of body weight per day on days 7–16 of gestation, total sterility was noted in 97% of the two highest dose groups, whereas 20% of males and 34% of females exposed *in utero* to 10 mg/kg of body weight per day were infertile; fertility was reduced in the remaining animals in the lowest dose group (35).

Topical administration of BaP to pregnant mice on days 13–17 of gestation resulted in the appearance of a highly mutagenic dihydrodiol epoxide attached to the haemoglobin in the newborn (36). Transplacental carcinogenesis has been observed following subcutaneous administration of large doses (37). However, little BaP was transferred to the fetus following the oral administration to mice of a single dose of 12 mg/kg of body weight on days 11–18 of gestation (38).

### Mutagenicity and related end-points

BaP was mutagenic in *Salmonella typhimurium* strain TA1538 after metabolic activation by a preparation of microsomal enzymes from a liver homogenate, fraction S9, obtained from rats (39); it has also induced mutations in cultured human lymphoblastoid cells (40). The diol-epoxide metabolites of BaP are considerably more mutagenic than the parent compound. Induction of sister chromatid exchanges in Chinese hamsters following intraperitoneal administration of BaP has been reported (41), and a correlation has been observed between sister chromatid exchange and the production of BaP metabolites in two variant mouse hepatoma cell lines (42).

### Carcinogenicity

Many PAH-containing mixtures have been associated with an increased incidence of cancer, but the contribution of each of the individual components to the overall carcinogenic potency is difficult to assess (43). The relative carcinogenic potencies of various PAHs, based on bioassays by several routes of administration and related toxicological data, have been ranked in decreasing order as follows: dibenz[a,h]anthracene, BaP, anthanthrene, indeno[1,2,3-cd]pyrene, benzo[a]anthracene, benzo[b]fluoranthene, pyrene, benzo[k]fluoranthene, benzo[j]fluoranthene, cyclopentadieno[c,d]pyrene, benzo[g,h,i]perylene, chrysene, and benzo[e]pyrene (44). The Environmental Protection Agency in the USA has determined that acenaphthene, anthracene, fluoranthene, fluorene, and pyrene are not classifiable as to human carcinogenicity because of the absence of human data and the inadequacy of the data from animal bioassays (*34*).

BaP is one of the most potent PAH carcinogens; primary tumours have been produced, both at the site of administration and in other tissues, in mice, rats, hamsters, guinea-pigs, rabbits, ducks, and monkeys following intragastric, subcutaneous, dermal, or intratracheal administration. The target sites appear to be proliferating tissues such as the intestinal epithelia, bone marrow, lymphoid organs, and testes, which interact with the active metabolites of BaP (*11*). There appear to be interspecies differences in the formation of DNA adducts, as the binding of anti-BaP 7,8-dihydrodiol-9,10-epoxide to endometrial DNA has been determined to be greatest in humans, followed by hamsters, mice, and rats (*45*).

Groups of CFW mice of varying ages (23–73 per dose; number per sex not specified) were fed BaP in the diet at concentrations of 0.001, 0.01, 0.02, 0.03, 0.04, 0.045, 0.05, 0.10, or 0.25 mg/g of food for periods of 98–197 days. The control group consisted of 171 males and 289 females. There was a significant dose-related increase in stomach tumours, mostly squamous cell papillomas and some carcinomas, in the treated animals as compared with the controls. The incidence of gastric tumours was 0 in the controls, and 0, 0, 5, 0, 2.5, 10, 70, 82, and 90% in the treatment groups in order of increasing dietary concentration (*46*).

In an additional study conducted by the same authors, groups of 9–26 CFW mice were fed diets containing 0.25 mg of BaP per g for periods ranging from 1 to 30 days, then observed for up to 105 days. The incidence of gastric tumours in these groups was 0, 11, 10, 44, 30, and 100% for periods of administration of 1, 2, 4, 5, 7, and 30 days, respectively (*46*).

A total of 63 male CF1 mice given BaP by forced drinking (0.003% solution in 95% ethanol), 5 days per week for up to 22 months developed 11 oesophageal tumours (10 papillomas and one carcinoma) and 15 forestomach tumours (13 papillomas and two carcinomas), as compared with no oesophageal tumours and five forestomach tumours (all papillomas) in the 67 controls (*47*).

Groups of 160 female albino mice fed diets containing 4 mg of BaP per kg or 3 mg of 9,10-dimethylbenzanthracene per kg for 14 months had an incidence of gastric tumours of 8.1 and 28% and an incidence of mesenteric tumours of 0 and 69%, respectively (*48*).

## 14.16.6 Effects on humans

There have been few studies on the human health effects of PAHs. Human subjects skin-painted with BaP developed skin lesions (*49, 50*). Cases of accidental poisoning by naphthalene, resulting in death by acute haemolytic anaemia, have been reported (*51*).

## 14.16.7 Guideline value

Available toxicological data are sufficient to serve as a basis for the derivation of a guideline value only for BaP, one of the most potent carcinogens among the PAHs tested to date. IARC has classified BaP in Group 2A (probably carcinogenic to humans) (52). The guideline value is therefore derived on the basis of the lifetime cancer risk estimated by extrapolation of the tumour incidence data observed in the most appropriate carcinogenicity bioassay in animals.

The only study by the most appropriate route of administration (i.e. the oral route) in which there was an increase of stomach tumours associated with an increase in the ingested concentration of BaP was that in which CFW mice were fed BaP in the diet at concentrations of 0.001, 0.01, 0.02, 0.03, 0.04, 0.045, 0.05, 0.10, or 0.25 mg/g of food for periods ranging from 98 to 197 days (46). Because of the variable dosing patterns and age of the animals at sacrifice, data on tumour incidence from this study cannot be confidently extrapolated by means of the models currently employed in quantitative risk assessment (i.e. model-free or linearized multistage extrapolation, which was used in deriving the previous BaP guideline), as they assume constant exposure and sacrifice at the median point of the life span. However, the tumour incidence data have been extrapolated using the two-stage birth–death mutation model, which can incorporate the variable exposure and sacrifice patterns (53). With this model, the estimate of the upper bound on the low-dose risk was 0.46 (mg/kg of body weight per day)$^{-1}$ without correction for differences in body surface area, as BaP is an indirect-acting carcinogen, i.e. the carcinogenicity appears to be attributable to a metabolite rather than to BaP itself. The resulting estimated concentrations of BaP in drinking-water corresponding to excess lifetime cancer risks of $10^{-4}$, $10^{-5}$, and $10^{-6}$ for stomach tumours are 7, 0.7, and 0.07 µg/litre.

There are insufficient data available to derive drinking-water guidelines for other PAHs. However, the following recommendations are made for the PAH group:

- Because of the close association of PAHs with suspended solids, the application of treatment, when necessary, to achieve the recommended level of turbidity will ensure that PAH levels are reduced to a minimum.
- Contamination of water with PAHs should not occur during water treatment or distribution. Therefore, the use of coal-tar-based and similar materials for pipe linings and coatings on storage tanks should be discontinued. It is recognized that it may be impracticable to remove coal-tar linings from existing pipes. Research is needed on methods of minimizing the leaching of PAHs from such lining materials.
- To monitor PAH levels, the use of several specific compounds as indicators for the group as a whole is recommended. The choice of indicator compounds will vary for each individual situation. PAH levels should be monitored regularly in order to determine the background levels against which any changes can be assessed so that remedial action can be taken, if necessary.

- In situations where drinking-water is known to have been contaminated by PAHs, the specific compounds present and the source of the contamination should be identified, as the carcinogenic potential of PAH compounds varies.

## References

1. Office of Drinking Water. *Estimated national occurrence and exposure to polycyclic aromatic hydrocarbons in public drinking water supplies.* Washington, DC, US Environmental Protection Agency, 1989.

2. Zedeck MS. Polycyclic aromatic hydrocarbons: a review. *Journal of environmental pathology and toxicology,* 1980, 3:537-567.

3. Lee ML et al. Source identification of urban airborne polycyclic aromatic hydrocarbons by gas chromatographic mass spectrometry and high resolution mass spectrometry. *Biomedical mass spectrometry,* 1977, 4:182-185.

4. Agency for Toxic Substances and Disease Registry. *Toxicological profile for benzo[a]pyrene.* Atlanta, GA, Department of Health and Human Services, 1990.

5. Sloof W et al., eds. *Integrated criteria document PAHs.* Bilthoven, Netherlands, National Institute of Public Health and Environmental Protection, 1989.

6. International Joint Commission. *Report on the Great Lakes water quality. Appendix, Report 66-81, Great Lakes surveillance.* Windsor, Canada, 1983.

7. Lioy PL et al. The total human environmental exposure study (THEES) to benzo(a)pyrene: comparison of the inhalation and food pathways. *Archives of environmental health,* 1988, 43:304-312.

8. Dann T. *Polycyclic aromatic hydrocarbons in the ambient air of Toronto, Ontario and Montreal, Quebec.* Ottawa, Canada, Environment Canada, Technology Development and Technical Services Branch, 1989.

9. Harkov R, Greenberg A. Benzo(a)pyrene in New Jersey – results from a twenty-seven-site study. *Journal of the Air Pollution Control Association,* 1985, 35:238-243.

10. Buck M. [Emission measurements of benzol and benzo[a]pyrene in areas affected by stationary and mobile sources of emissions.] *Schriftenreihe des Vereins für Wasser-, Boden-, und Lufthygiene,* 1986, 67:151-166 (in German).

11. Santodonato J, Howard P, Basu D. Health and ecological assessment of polynuclear aromatic hydrocarbons. *Journal of environmental pathology and toxicology,* 1981, 5: 1-364.

12. Ontario Ministry of the Environment. *Drinking water survey of selected municipalities in the Niagara area and Lake Ontario.* Toronto, 1984.

13. Ontario Ministry of the Environment. *Drinking Water Surveillance Program overview annual report 1987.* Toronto, 1989.

14. O'Neill HJ, MacKeigan KG. *Data summary report: federal–provincial drinking water sources toxic chemical study – Nova Scotia 1985–1986.* Moncton, Canada, Environment Canada, Water Quality Branch, Atlantic Region, 1987.

15. O'Neill HJ, MacKeigan KG. *Data summary report: federal–provincial drinking water sources toxic chemical study – Prince Edward Island 1986.* Moncton, Canada, Environment Canada, Water Quality Branch, Atlantic Region, 1987.

16. O'Neill HJ, MacKeigan KG. *Data summary report: federal–provincial drinking water sources toxic chemical study – Newfoundland 1985–1986.* Moncton, Canada, Environment Canada, Water Quality Branch, Atlantic Region, 1987.

17. O'Neill HJ, MacKeigan KG. *Data summary report: federal–provincial drinking water sources toxic chemical study – New Brunswick 1985–1986.* Moncton, Canada, Environment Canada, Water Quality Branch, Atlantic Region, 1987.

18. Vaessen HA, Jekel AA, Wilbers AAMM. Dietary intake of polycyclic aromatic hydrocarbons. *Toxicology and environmental chemistry,* 1988, 16:281.

19. International Agency for Research on Cancer. *Certain polycyclic aromatic hydrocarbons and heterocyclic compounds.* Lyon, 1973 (IARC Monographs on the Evaluation of the Carcinogenic Risk of Chemicals to Man, Volume 3).

20. Das BS. *Analysis of polycyclic aromatic hydrocarbons (PAH) in Canadian foods.* Ottawa, Agriculture Canada, Food Research Centre, Environmental and Chemical Engineering Division, 1987.

21. Larsson B. *Polycyclic aromatic hydrocarbons in Swedish foods: aspects on analysis, occurrence and intake.* Uppsala, Sweden, Swedish University of Agricultural Sciences, 1986 (dissertation).

22. Conacher HBS et al. The Health Protection Branch Total Diet Program. *Journal of the Institute of the Science and Technology of Alimentation,* 1989, 22(4):322.

23. US Environmental Protection Agency. *Exposure and risk assessment for benzo[a]pyrene and other polycyclic aromatic hydrocarbons.* Vol. 4. Washington, DC, 1982 (EPA-440/4-85-020).

24. US Environmental Protection Agency. *Exposure and risk assessment for benzo[a]pyrene and other polycyclic aromatic hydrocarbons.* Vol. 3. Washington, DC, 1982 (EPA-440/4-85-020).

25. Fawell JK, Hunt S. The polycyclic aromatic hydrocarbons. In: *Environmental toxicology: organic pollutants.* Chichester, Ellis Horwood, 1988:241-269.

26. Foth H, Kahl R, Kahl GF. Pharmacokinetics of low doses of benzo[*a*]pyrene in the rat. *Food chemistry and toxicology,* 1988, 26:45-51.

27. Vetter RD, Carey MC, Patton JS. Coassimilation of dietary fat and benzo[*a*]pyrene in the small intestine: an absorption model using the killifish. *Journal of lipid research,* 1985, 26:428-434.

28. Gower JD, Wills ED. The dependence of the rate of BP metabolism in the rat small intestinal mucosa on the composition of the dietary fat. *Nutrition and cancer,* 1986, 8:151-161.

29. Tyrer HW et al. Benzo[*a*]pyrene metabolism in mice exposed to diesel exhaust. *Environment international,* 1981, 5:307.

30. Weyand EH, Bevan DR. Species differences in disposition of benzo[*a*]pyrene. *Drug metabolism and disposition,* 1987, 15:442-448.

31. Tomatis L. Transplacental carcinogenesis. In: Raven RW, ed. *Modern trends in oncology.* Part I. *Research progress.* London, Butterworths, 1973:99.

32. Bakhe YS, Vane JR. *Metabolic function of the lung.* New York, NY, Marcel Dekker, 1977.

33. Montizaan GK et al. *Integrated criteria document. Polynuclear aromatic hydrocarbons (PAH): effects of 10 selected compounds.* Bilthoven, Netherlands, National Institute of Public Health and Environmental Protection, 1989.

34. US Environmental Protection Agency. *IRIS information on selected PAHs.* Cincinnati, OH, 1981.

35. Mackenzie KM, Angevine DM. Infertility in mice exposed *in utero* to benzo[*a*]pyrene. *Biology of reproduction,* 1981, 24:183-191.

36. Shugart L, Matsunami R. Adduct formation in hemoglobin of the newborn mouse exposed *in utero* to benzo[*a*]pyrene. *Toxicology,* 1985, 37:241-245.

37. Bulay OM, Wattenberg LW. Carcinogenic effects of subcutaneous administration of benzo[*a*]pyrene during pregnancy on the progeny. *Proceedings of the Society for Experimental Biology and Medicine,* 1970, 135:84-86.

38. Neubert D, Tapken S. Transfer of benzo(*a*)pyrene into mouse embryos and fetuses. *Archives of toxicology,* 1988, 62:236-239.

39. Teranishi K, Hamada K, Watanabe H. Quantitative relationship between carcinogenicity and mutagenicity of polyaromatic hydrocarbons in *Salmonella typhimurium* mutants. *Mutation research*, 1975, 31:97-102.

40. Danheiser SL, Liber HL, Thilly WG. Long-term, low-dose benzo[*a*]pyrene-induced mutation in human lymphoblasts competent in xenobiotic metabolism. *Mutation research*, 1989, 210:143-147.

41. Raszinsky K, Basler A, Rohrborn G. Mutagenicity of polycyclic hydrocarbons. V. Induction of sister-chromatid exchanges *in vivo*. *Mutation research*, 1979, 66:65-67.

42. Schaeffer EL, Au WW, Selkirk JK. Differential induction of sister-chromatid exchanges by benzo[*a*]pyrene in variant mouse hepatoma cells. *Mutation research*, 1985, 143:69-74.

43. US Environmental Protection Agency. *Health effects assessment for polycyclic aromatic hydrocarbons (PAH)*. Cincinnati, OH, 1984 (EPA 540/1-86/013).

44. Krewski D, Thorslund T, Withey J. Carcinogenic risk assessment of complex mixtures. *Toxicology and industrial health*, 1989, 5(5):851-867.

45. Kulkarni MS et al. Species differences in the formation of benzo(*a*)pyrene–DNA adducts in rodent and human endometrium. *Cancer research*, 1986, 46:2888-2891.

46. Neal J, Rigdon RH. Gastric tumours in mice fed benzo[*a*]pyrene: a quantitative study. *Texas reports on biology and medicine*, 1967, 25:553-557.

47. Horie A, Hohchi S, Kuratsune M. Carcinogenesis in the esophagus. II. Experimental production of esophageal cancer by administration of ethanolic solution of carcinogens. *Gann*, 1965, 56:429-441.

48. Chouroulinkov I, Gentil A, Guérin M. [Study of the carcinogenic action of orally administered 9,10-dimethyl-benzanthracene and 3,4-benzopyrene]. *Bulletin du cancer*, 1967, 54(1):67-78 (in French).

49. Cottini GB, Mazzone GB. The effects of 3,4-benzpyrene on human skin. *American journal of cancer*, 1939, 37:186.

50. Rhoades CP et al. Early changes in the skin of several species including man, after painting with carcinogenic materials. *Proceedings of the American Association of Cancer Research*, 1954, 1:40.

51. Clayton GD, Clayton FE. *Patty's industrial hygiene and toxicology*, 3rd rev. ed. New York, NY, John Wiley, 1981.

52. International Agency for Research on Cancer. *Overall evaluations of carcinogenicity: an updating of IARC Monographs volumes 1-42*. Lyon, 1987:58 (IARC Monographs on the Evaluation of Carcinogenic Risks to Humans, Suppl. 7).

53. Thorslund TW. *Ingestion dose–response model for benzo[a]pyrene.* Washington DC, US Environmental Protection Agency, 1990 (unpublished report prepared by Clement International Corporation).

## 14.17 Monochlorobenzene

### 14.17.1 General description

**Identity**

CAS no.:                108-90-7
Molecular formula:  $C_6H_5Cl$

**Physicochemical properties** *(1–3)*[1]

| Property | Value |
|---|---|
| *Property* | *Value* |
| Melting point | -45.6 °C |
| Boiling point | 132.0 °C |
| Density | 1.1058 g/cm$^3$ at 20 °C |
| Water solubility | 500 mg/litre at 20 °C |
| Log octanol–water partition coefficient | 2.84 |
| Vapour pressure | 1.18 kPa at 20 °C |

**Organoleptic properties**

Taste and odour thresholds of 10–20 µg/litre *(4)* and odour thresholds of 50, 40–120, and 100 µg/litre *(2, 5, 6)* have been reported for monochlorobenzene (MCB).

**Major uses**

MCB is used mainly as a solvent in pesticide formulations, as a degreasing agent, and as an intermediate in the synthesis of other halogenated organic compounds.

**Environmental fate**

The concentration of MCB released into water and onto land will decrease mainly because of volatilization into the atmosphere. In water, some biodegradation also occurs, proceeding more rapidly in fresh water than in estuarine and marine waters. The rate is also more rapid if there has been acclimatization of the degrading microorganisms. Some adsorption onto organic sediments occurs *(3)*. MCB is relatively mobile in sandy soil and aquifer material and biodegrades slowly in these soils; it may therefore leach into groundwater *(3)*. The octa-

---

[1]  Conversion factor in air: 1 ppm = 4.60 mg/m$^3$.

nol–water partition coefficient suggests that little or no bioconcentration of MCB will occur in aquatic species.

## 14.17.2 Analytical methods

A standard method for chlorobenzenes involves extraction with hexane followed by capillary column gas–liquid chromatography with electron-capture detection. The method is capable of achieving detection limits in tapwater and river water of about 0.1 µg/litre (7).

## 14.17.3 Environmental levels and human exposure

### Air

Because MCB is volatile and is used extensively as a solvent, large quantities are released to air. However, atmospheric concentrations are usually very low, often much less than 4.6 µg/m$^3$ (3, 8).

### Water

MCB has been detected in wastewaters, surface and groundwaters, and drinking-water. In some Canadian potable water sources, mean concentrations were less than 1 µg/litre; the maximum value recorded was 5 µg/litre (9).

### Food

Chlorobenzene has been found in edible freshwater and marine organisms, although levels are not significant. Human milk may be a source of exposure for infants; MCB was detected in five out of eight samples of human milk in a study in the USA (10).

### Estimated total exposure and relative contribution of drinking-water

Despite the low levels of MCB in air, inhalation is probably the major route of environmental exposure.

## 14.17.4 Kinetics and metabolism in laboratory animals and humans

MCB appears to be readily absorbed via the oral and inhalation routes and accumulates mainly in fatty tissue (11,12). The major metabolites of MCB in mammals are p-chlorophenol mercapturic acid, 4-chlorocatechol, and p-chlorophenol. In humans, the main metabolite is 4-chlorocatechol (13). The major route of MCB excretion is the urine; little is excreted in the faeces or retained in the body.

## 14.17.5 Effects on laboratory animals and *in vitro* test systems
### *Acute exposure*

MCB is of low acute toxicity to experimental animals via the oral and inhalation routes. Oral $LD_{50}$s in the grams per kilogram range have been reported for rodents. Major target organs of acute exposure are the liver and kidneys.

### *Short-term exposure*

In a 13-week study, groups of 10 Fischer 344 rats and 10 B6C3F$_1$ hybrid mice of each sex received MCB in corn oil at 0, 60, 125, 250, 500, or 750 mg/kg of body weight by gavage, for 5 days per week. Effects were seen mainly in the liver, kidney, and haematopoietic system. A NOAEL of 125 mg/kg of body weight was identified in the study. The LOAEL was 250 mg/kg of body weight, which caused a slight decrease in spleen weight and lymphoid or myeloid depletion of the thymus, spleen, or bone marrow (*14,15*).

### *Long-term exposure*

In a 2-year study, groups of 50 Fischer 344 rats and 50 B6C3F$_1$ mice of each sex received MCB in corn oil by gavage, 5 days per week for 103 weeks. The doses administered were 0, 60, or 120 mg/kg of body weight for female mice and rats of both sexes, and 0, 30, or 60 mg/kg of body weight for male mice. No evidence of MCB-related toxicity was reported. Although survival was reduced in male rats at 120 mg/kg of body weight and slightly reduced in male mice at 30 and 60 mg/kg of body weight, this was not thought to be compound-related, as body weight gains were unaffected and MCB-induced toxic lesions related to death were not observed. A NOAEL of 60 mg/kg of body weight was therefore identified for male mice and one of 120 mg/kg of body weight for female mice and male and female rats (*14,15*).

### *Reproductive toxicity, embryotoxicity, and teratogenicity*

Exposure of Fischer 344 rats and New Zealand white rabbits to 0, 75, 210, or 590 ppm MCB (0, 345, 966 or 2714 mg/m³) via inhalation for 6 h per day during the major period of organogenesis did not cause embryotoxicity or teratogenicity in the rats. Fetal effects in rats were limited to slight delays in skeletal development, which occurred only at concentrations causing maternal toxicity (2714 mg/m³). In rabbits, fetuses exhibited a low incidence of visceral malformations that were not dose-related (*16*). In a two-generation inhalation study, exposure levels of 50, 150, and 450 ppm (230, 690, and 2070 mg/m³) did not have any adverse effects on reproductive performance or fertility in male and female rats (*17*).

## Mutagenicity and related end-points

MCB was not mutagenic in *Salmonella typhimurium* strains TA98, TA100, TA1535, or TA1537, with or without activation with rat or hamster liver S9 enzymes (*18*). In one study, the intraperitoneal injection of MCB in corn oil (up to 70% of the $LD_{50}$) to groups of five mice led to a dose-related increase in the formation of micronucleated polychromatic erythrocytes. The authors considered that the effects were due to the clastogenic activity of MCB (*19*). However, similar results have not been reported by other workers (*20*). MCB appears to bind covalently to DNA in liver, kidney, and lung of rats and mice following intraperitoneal injection (*21*), but the level of binding was considered to be low (*20*).

## Carcinogenicity

In the 2-year study in which groups of 50 Fischer 344 rats and 50 $B6C3F_1$ mice of each sex received MCB in corn oil by gavage, 5 days per week for 103 weeks, doses of 60 or 120 mg/kg of body weight caused slight (statistically significant at 120 mg/kg of body weight) increases in the frequency of neoplastic nodules of the liver in male rats (*14,15*). Increased incidences of hepatocellular carcinomas were not observed in male or female rats. No increased tumour incidences were observed in female rats or in male or female mice. Rare tumours observed in three exposed animals were not statistically significant; they included one renal tubular-cell adenocarcinoma in a high-dose (120 mg/kg of body weight) female rat and transitional cell papillomas of the bladder in two male rats, one in the low-dose group (60 mg/kg of body weight) and one in the high-dose group (120 mg/kg of body weight). The frequency of pituitary tumours was reduced in rats receiving MCB; the significance of this finding is not known. The study provided some not altogether convincing evidence of carcinogenicity in male Fischer 344 rats, but none in female Fischer 344 rats or in male or female $B6C3F_1$ mice (*14, 15, 20*).

## 14.17.6 Effects on humans

MCB is toxic to humans; poisoning and occupational exposure caused central nervous system disturbances. In addition, subjects occupationally exposed to MCB for 2 years suffered from headaches, dizziness, and sleepiness (*22*).

## 14.17.7 Guideline value

Although there was a weak dose-related increase in neoplastic liver nodules in male rats, the weight of evidence suggests that MCB is not genotoxic; a TDI approach can therefore be adopted.

Based on the 2-year study with rats and mice in which a NOAEL of 60 mg/kg of body weight for neoplastic nodules was identified (*14,15*), a TDI of

85.7 µg/kg of body weight can be calculated by applying an uncertainty factor of 500 (100 for inter- and intraspecies variation and 5 for the limited evidence of carcinogenicity) to the NOAEL and allowing for dosing 5 days per week. This gives a guideline value of 300 µg/litre (rounded figure), based on an allocation of 10% of the TDI to drinking-water. However, this value far exceeds the lowest reported taste and odour threshold in water of 10 µg/litre.

## References

1. Weast RC, Astle MJ, Beyer WH, eds. *CRC handbook of chemistry and physics*, 67th ed. Boca Raton, FL, CRC Press, 1986.

2. Verschueren K. *Handbook of environmental data on organic chemicals*, 2nd ed. New York, Van Nostrand Reinhold Co., 1983.

3. Howard PH. *Handbook of environmental fate and exposure data for organic chemicals.* Vol. 1. *Large production and priority pollutants.* Chelsea, MI, Lewis Publishers, 1990.

4. Varšavskaja SP. [Comparative sanitary-toxicologic characteristics of chlorobenzene and dichlorobenzene (ortho- and para-isomers) from the viewpoint of the sanitary protection of water reservoirs.] *Gigiena i sanitarija*, 1968, 33(10):15-21 (in Russian) (*Chemical abstracts*, 1969, 70:22828y).

5. Alexander HC et al. Aqueous odour and taste values of industrial chemicals. *Journal of the American Water Works Association*, 1982, 74(11):595-599.

6. Zoeteman BCJ. *Sensory assessment of water quality.* Oxford, Pergamon Press, 1980.

7. Department of the Environment. *Methods for the examination of waters and associated materials – chlorobenzenes in water, organochlorine pesticides and PCBs in turbid waters, halogenated solvents and related compounds in sewage sludge and waters.* London, Her Majesty's Stationery Office, 1985.

8. US Environmental Protection Agency. Monochlorobenzene. *Reviews of environmental contamination and toxicology*, 1988, 106:37-50.

9. Otson R, Williams DT, Bothwell PD. Volatile organic compounds in water at thirty Canadian potable water treatment facilities. *Journal of the Association of Official Analytical Chemists*, 1982, 65:1370-1374.

10. Pellizzari ED et al. Purgeable organic compounds in mother's milk. *Bulletin of environmental contamination and toxicology*, 1982, 28:322-328.

11. Lindsay-Smith JR, Shaw BA, Foulkes DM. Mechanisms of mammalian hydroxylation: some novel metabolites of chlorobenzene. *Xenobiotica*, 1972, 2:215-226.

12. Sullivan TM, Born GS, Carlson GP. The pharmacokinetics of inhaled chlorobenzene in the rat. *Toxicology and applied pharmacology*, 1983, 71:194-203.

13. Ogata M, Shimada Y. Differences in urinary monochlorobenzene metabolites between rats and humans. *International archives of occupational and environmental health*, 1983, 51:51-57.

14. Kluwe WM et al. Toxic responses to acute, subchronic, and chronic oral administrations of monochlorobenzene to rodents. *Journal of toxicology and environmental health*, 1985, 15:745-767.

15. US Department of Health and Human Services. *National Toxicology Program technical report on the carcinogenesis studies of chlorobenzene (CAS no. 108-90-7) in F344/N rats and B6C3F1 mice (gavage studies)*. Research Triangle Park, NC, 1983:192 (NTP TR 255).

16. John JA et al. Inhalation teratology study of monochlorobenzene in rats and rabbits. *Toxicology and applied pharmacology*, 1984, 76:365-373.

17. Nair RS, Barter JA, Schroeder RE. A two-generation reproduction study with monochlorobenzene vapor in rats. *Fundamental and applied toxicology*, 1987, 9:678-686.

18. Haworth S et al. *Salmonella* mutagenicity test results for 250 chemicals. *Environmental mutagenesis*, 1983, 5 (Suppl. 1):3-142.

19. Mohtashamipur E et al. The bone marrow clastogenicity of eight halogenated benzenes in male NMRI mice. *Mutagenesis*, 1987, 2(2):111-113.

20. *Chlorobenzenes other than hexachlorobenzene*. Geneva, World Health Organization, 1991 (Environmental Health Criteria, No. 128).

21. Grilli S et al. *In vivo* and *in vitro* covalent binding of chlorobenzene to nucleic acids. *Japanese journal of cancer research*, 1985, 76:745-751.

22. Rozenbaum ND, Blekh RS, Kremneva SN. [Use of chlorobenzene as a solvent from the standpoint of industrial hygiene.] *Gigiena i sanitarija*, 1947, 12:21-24 (in Russian).

## 14.18 Dichlorobenzenes

### 14.18.1 General description

**Identity**

| Compound | CAS no. | Molecular formula |
|---|---|---|
| 1,2-Dichlorobenzene (1,2-DCB) | 95-50-1 | $C_6H_4Cl_2$ |
| 1,3-Dichlorobenzene (1,3-DCB) | 541-73-1 | $C_6H_4Cl_2$ |
| 1,4-Dichlorobenzene (1,4-DCB) | 106-46-7 | $C_6H_4Cl_2$ |

### Physicochemical properties (1–3)[1]

| Property | 1,2-DCB | 1,3-DCB | 1,4-DCB |
|---|---|---|---|
| Melting point (°C) | -17.0 | -24.7 | 53.1 |
| Boiling point (°C) | 180.5 | 173.0 | 174.0 |
| Water solubility at 25 °C (mg/litre) | 91 | 123 | 31 |
| Vapour pressure at 25 °C (kPa) | 0.2 | 0.31 | 0.226 |
| Density at 20 °C (g/cm$^3$) | 1.305 | 1.288 | 1.247 |
| Log octanol–water partition coefficient | 3.38 | 3.48 | 3.38 |

### Organoleptic properties

The organoleptic thresholds for all three isomers are low. Odour thresholds of 2–10, 20, and 0.3–30 µg/litre have been reported for 1,2-DCB, 1,3-DCB, and 1,4-DCB, respectively (4, 5). Taste thresholds of 1 and 6 µg/litre have been reported for 1,2-DCB and 1,4-DCB, respectively (4, 6).

### Major uses

The DCBs are widely used in industry and in domestic products such as odour-masking agents, dyestuffs, and pesticides. 1,2-DCB and 1,4-DCB are the most widely used (7).

### Environmental fate

The DCBs are expected to be adsorbed moderately to tightly onto soils of high organic content and are not expected to leach appreciably into groundwater. In soils, they are biodegraded slowly under aerobic conditions; volatilization may be important in surface soils. In water, the major DCB-removal processes are likely to be adsorption onto sediments and bioaccumulation in aquatic organisms. Evaporation from surface water may also be important, but not aquatic hydrolysis, oxidation, or direct photolysis. DCBs may biodegrade in aerobic water after microbial adaptation. However, they are not expected to biodegrade under the anaerobic conditions that may exist in lake sediments or various groundwaters (2).

## 14.18.2 Analytical methods

A standard method for chlorobenzenes involves extraction with hexane followed by capillary-column gas–liquid chromatography with electron-capture detection (detection limit in tapwater and river water approximately 0.01 µg/litre) (8).

---

[1] Conversion factor in air: 1ppm = 6.01 mg/m$^3$.

## 14.18.3 Environmental levels and human exposure

### *Air*

The DCBs have been detected in the atmosphere at extremely low levels. In the USA, mean 1,2-DCB concentrations of 1.2, 0.3 and 0.01 $\mu g/m^3$ have been measured in industrial, urban, and rural locations, respectively; the overall mean concentration was 0.54 $\mu g/m^3$. Similarly, mean 1,3-DCB concentrations of 0.9, 0.5 and 0.04 $\mu g/m^3$ have been reported for the same three locations, respectively; the overall mean concentration was 0.57 $\mu g/m^3$. Mean 1,2-DCB and 1,4-DCB concentrations of 0.06–0.18 $\mu g/m^3$ and 0.24–0.42 $\mu g/m^3$ were detected in the ambient air of three New Jersey (USA) cities in 1981 (*2*).

### *Water*

DCBs have been detected in wastewater, raw water, surface water, and drinking-water (*2*). Although all have been detected in drinking-water, 1,4-DCB is generally present in the greatest concentration. DCBs have been found in potable water sources before treatment at levels as high as 10 $\mu g/litre$ and in drinking-water at 0.01–3 $\mu g/litre$ (*7*). In a survey of the water supplies of three Canadian cities, total mean DCB concentrations ranged from 1.0 to 13 ng/litre, most of which was 1,4-DCB (*9*). In a study in the USA on the contamination of 685 groundwaters, 1,2-DCB, 1,3-DCB, and 1,4-DCB were detected in 20, 19, and 19 samples at maximum concentrations of 6800, 236 and 996 $\mu g/litre$, respectively (*2*).

### *Food*

DCBs tend to accumulate in biological materials rich in lipids, such as fatty tissue and milk. Mean levels of 1,2-DCB, 1,3-DCB, and 1,4-DCB of 2.6, 0.14, and 5.5 $\mu g/kg$, respectively, have been measured in milk (*2, 10*). Fish have also been shown to be a major source of DCBs; mean levels were 1, 0.3–3, and 1–4 $\mu g/kg$ for 1,2-DCB, 1,3-DCB, and 1,4-DCB, respectively (*2*).

### *Estimated total exposure and relative contribution of drinking-water*

General population exposure may occur through the inhalation of contaminated air, especially in areas where DCBs are manufactured, and from the ingestion of contaminated drinking-water and food, particularly contaminated fish.

## 14.18.4 Kinetics and metabolism in laboratory animals and humans

DCBs are almost completely absorbed from the gastrointestinal tract. Once absorbed, they are rapidly distributed, primarily to fat or adipose tissue because of their lipophilicity and to kidney, liver, and lungs. They are metabolized mainly by oxidation in the liver to the respective dichlorophenols and their glucuronide and sulfate conjugates, although other minor metabolites have been detected. The metabolites are excreted mainly via the kidneys, and excretion is relatively slow. In rats, almost 100% of an oral dose of 1,4-DCB was excreted within 5 days, mostly in the urine (7).

## 14.18.5 Effects on laboratory animals and *in vitro* test systems

### Acute exposure

The DCBs are of low acute oral toxicity in experimental animals. Oral $LD_{50}$s in rodents range from 500 to 3863 mg/kg of body weight. The major target organs are the liver and kidneys (7).

### Short-term exposure

F344/N rats and B6C3F$_1$ mice were given 1,2-DCB in corn oil at 0, 30, 60, 125, 250, or 500 mg/kg of body weight per day by gavage 5 days per week for 13 weeks. Decreased survival in male and female mice and female rats was seen at the highest dose level. Liver necrosis, hepatocellular degeneration, and depletion of lymphocytes were seen in the thymus and spleen of both sexes of rats and mice. At 250 mg/kg of body weight, necrosis of individual hepatocytes was observed in both sexes of rats and in male mice. Minimal hepatocellular necrosis was observed in a few rats at 125 mg/kg of body weight, but no hepatic alterations were observed in mice at this dose. A NOAEL of 125 mg/kg of body weight per day was identified (7).

### Long-term exposure

In a 2-year gavage study, B6C3F$_1$ female and male mice were given 0, 60, or 120 mg of 1,2-DCB per kg of body weight per day by gavage in corn oil, 5 days per week. The only evidence of toxicity was a dose-related trend towards tubular degeneration of the kidney in male mice, the incidence of which increased at the highest dose level. Otherwise, there was no evidence of non-neoplastic toxicity. NOAELs of 60 and 120 mg/kg of body weight per day were identified for male and female mice, respectively (7).

1,4-DCB was administered by gavage for 2 years, 5 days per week, to male and female Fischer 344 rats at dose levels of 0, 150, or 300, and 0, 300, or 600 mg/kg of body weight per day in corn oil. In males, reduced survival and body weight gain were observed at 300 mg/kg of body weight. Increased severity of nephropathy and hyperplasia of the parathyroid were observed at 150 mg/kg of body weight in males. In females, there was a dose-related increase in nephropathy at or above 300 mg/kg of body weight. LOAELs of 150 and 300 mg/kg of body weight per day were identified for male and female rats, respectively (7).

## Reproductive toxicity, embryotoxicity, and teratogenicity

All three isomers were reported to be non-teratogenic when Sprague-Dawley rats were given oral doses of 50, 100, or 200 mg/kg of body weight per day on days 6–15 of gestation (*11*). In another study, CD rats were given 1,4-DCB by gavage at doses of 0, 250, 500, 750, or 1000 mg/kg of body weight per day on days 6–15 of gestation. Reduction of fetal weight was seen at the highest dose, and an increase in skeletal variations was observed at or above 750 mg/kg of body weight per day. A dose-related increase in extra ribs was observed at doses at or above 500 mg/kg of body weight per day. A LOAEL and a NOAEL of 500 and 250 mg/kg of body weight per day were identified, respectively (*7*).

## Mutagenicity and related end-points

All three isomers were non-mutagenic in *Salmonella typhimurium* strains TA98, TA100, TA1535, or TA1537, both in the presence and in the absence of metabolic activation. A number of other *in vitro* tests, such as those for the induction of chromosomal aberrations in Chinese hamster ovary cells, forward mutations in mouse lymphoma cells, and unscheduled DNA synthesis in human lymphocytes, have also given negative results for 1,4-DCB. In all but one study, 1,4-DCB has not produced chromosome damage in bone marrow of mice when administered *in vivo*. Negative results have also been obtained for this isomer in an assay of DNA damage in liver of mice following oral exposure. Low-level covalent binding of 1,4-DCB to the liver, kidneys, and lungs of mice has been reported (*7*).

## Carcinogenicity

In the 2-year gavage study in which B6C3F$_1$ female and male mice were given 0, 60, or 120 mg of 1,2-DCB per kg of body weight in corn oil, 5 days per week, there was a dose-related trend in the incidence of malignant histiocytic lymphomas in both sexes; however, the authors concluded that there was no evidence for the carcinogenicity of 1,2-DCB in this study (*7*).

In the study in which 1,4-DCB was administered by gavage for 2 years, 5 days per week, to male and female Fischer 344 rats at dose levels of 0, 150, or 300, and 0, 300, or 600 mg/kg of body weight in corn oil, respectively, a dose-related increase in the incidence of tubular-cell adenocarcinomas of the kidney was observed in males only. A marginal increase in the incidence of mononuclear cell leukaemia was also noted in males when compared with the controls. It was concluded that the induction of kidney tumours in male rats was a species- and sex-specific response, probably a result of hyaline droplet formation. In the same study, 1,4-DCB increased the incidences of hepatocellular adenomas and carcinomas in mice dosed at 600 but not at 300 mg/kg of body weight (*7*).

## 14.18.6 Effects on humans

Data on the health effects of exposure to DCBs are restricted to case reports of accidental exposure to, or misuse of DCB products. Reported acute effects following short-term exposure (all of which are reversible) include acute haemolytic anaemia, respiratory irritation, glomerulonephritis, and allergic response of the skin. Prolonged exposure to 1,4-DCB has caused granulomatosis, anaemia, disturbances of the reticuloendothelial system, central nervous system effects, and liver damage. In workers exposed to 1,4-DCB, probably in combination with other chemicals, there have been case reports of haematological disorders, including anaemia, splenomegaly, and gastrointestinal and central nervous system effects. Two cases of acute myeloblastic anaemia were reported in females exposed mainly to 1,2-DCB over 1 year (7).

## 14.18.7 Guideline values

### 1,2-Dichlorobenzene

IARC has placed 1,2-DCB in Group 3 (12). This isomer is of low acute toxicity by the oral route of exposure. Oral exposure to high doses affects mainly the liver and kidneys. The balance of evidence suggests that 1,2-DCB is not genotoxic, and there is no evidence for its carcinogenicity in rodents. Using the NOAEL of 60 mg/kg of body weight per day for tubular degeneration of the kidney, identified in a 2-year mouse gavage study with administration 5 days per week (7), and applying an uncertainty factor of 100 (for inter- and intraspecies variation), a TDI of 429 µg/kg of body weight can be calculated. An allocation of 10% of the TDI to drinking-water gives a guideline value of 1000 µg/litre (rounded figure). This value far exceeds the lowest reported taste threshold in water of 1 µg/litre.

### 1,3-Dichlorobenzene

There are insufficient toxicological data on this compound to permit a guideline value to be proposed, but it should be noted that it is rarely found in drinking-water.

### 1,4-Dichlorobenzene

1,4-DCB is of low acute toxicity, but there is evidence that it increases the incidence of renal tumours in rats and hepatocellular adenomas and carcinomas in mice after long-term exposure. IARC has placed it in Group 2B (12).

1,4-DCB is not considered to be genotoxic, and the relevance for humans of the tumours observed in animals is doubtful. It is therefore valid to calculate a guideline value using the TDI approach. A TDI of 107 µg/kg of body weight has been calculated by applying an uncertainty factor of 1000 (100 for inter- and intraspecies variation and 10 for the use of a LOAEL instead of a NOAEL and because the toxic end-point is carcinogenicity) to a LOAEL of 150 mg/kg of body weight per day for kidney effects observed in a 2-year rat gavage study (administration 5 days per week) (7). A guideline value of 300 µg/litre (rounded figure) is proposed, based on an allocation of 10% of the TDI to drinking-water. This value far exceeds the lowest reported odour threshold in water of 0.3 µg/litre.

## References

1.  Weast R, Astle MJ, Beyer WH, eds. *CRC handbook of chemistry and physics*, 67th ed. Boca Raton, FL, CRC Press, 1986.

2.  Howard PH. *Handbook of environmental fate and exposure data for organic chemicals*. Vol. 1. *Large production and priority pollutants*. Chelsea, MI, Lewis Publishers, 1990.

3.  Verschueren K. *Handbook of environmental data on organic chemicals*, 2nd ed. New York, Van Nostrand Reinhold, 1983.

4.  Varsavskaja SP. [Comparative sanitary-toxicologic characteristics of chlorobenzene and dichlorobenzene (ortho- and para-isomers) from the viewpoint of the sanitary protection of water reservoirs.] *Gigiena i sanitarija*, 1968, 33(10):15-21 (in Russian) (*Chemical abstracts*, 1969, 70:22828y).

5.  Van Gemert LJ, Nettenbreijer AH, eds. *Compilation of odour threshold values in air and water*. Voorburg, Netherlands, National Institute for Water Supply, Central Institute for Nutrition and Food Research, 1977.

6.  Price GR, Wetzer A. *Handbook of ozone technology and applications*. Vol. III. *Ozone for drinking water*. London, Butterworths, 1984.

7.  *Chlorobenzenes other than hexachlorobenzene*. Geneva, World Health Organization, 1991 (Environmental Health Criteria, No. 128).

8.  Department of the Environment. *Methods for the examination of water and associated materials – chlorobenzenes in water, organochlorine pesticides and PCBs in turbid waters, halogenated solvents and related compounds in sewage sludge and waters*. London, Her Majesty's Stationery Office, 1985.

9.  Health Protection Branch. *Dichlorobenzenes. Canadian criteria document. Draft*. Ottawa, Canada, Department of National Health and Welfare, 1988.

10. Davies K. Concentrations and dietary intake of selected organochlorines, including PCBs, PCDDs and PCDFs in fresh food composites grown in Ontario, Canada. *Chemosphere*, 1988, 17(2):263-276.

11. Ruddick JA et al. A teratological evaluation following oral administration of trichloro- and dichlorobenzene isomers to the rat. *Teratology*, 1983, 27:73A-74A.

12. International Agency for Research on Cancer. *Overall evaluation of carcinogenicity: an updating of IARC Monographs volumes 1-42.* Lyon, 1987:192-193 (IARC Monographs on the Evaluation of Carcinogenic Risks to Humans, Suppl. 7).

## 14.19 Trichlorobenzenes

### 14.19.1 General description

#### Identity

| Compound | CAS no. | Molecular formula |
|---|---|---|
| 1,2,3-Trichlorobenzene (1,2,3-TCB) | 76-61-6 | $C_6H_3Cl_3$ |
| 1,2,4-Trichlorobenzene (1,2,4-TCB) | 120-82-1 | $C_6H_3Cl_3$ |
| 1,3,5-Trichlorobenzene (1,3,5-TCB) | 108-70-3 | $C_6H_3Cl_3$ |

#### Physicochemical properties (1–4)

| Property | 1,2,3-TCB | 1,2,4-TCB | 1,3,5-TCB |
|---|---|---|---|
| Melting point (°C) | 53–54 | 17 | 63–64 |
| Boiling point (°C) | 218–219 | 213.5 | 208 |
| Water solubility (mg/litre) | 12 (22 °C) | 19 (22 °C) | 5.8(20 °C) |
| Log octanol–water partition coefficient | 4.04 | 4.02 | 4.49 |
| Vapour pressure at 25 °C (kPa) | – | 0.04 | 0.08 |

#### Organoleptic properties

Odour thresholds of 10, 5–30, and 50 µg/litre have been reported for 1,2,3-TCB, 1,2,4-TCB, and 1,3,5-TCB, respectively (5, 6). A taste and odour threshold concentration of 30 µg/litre has been reported for 1,2,4-TCB (7).

#### Major uses

1,2,4-TCB is economically the most important isomer. Industrial-grade TCB, which consists of 93–98% 1,2,4-TCB and the remainder 1,2,3-TCB, is used as an intermediate in chemical synthesis, a solvent, a coolant, a lubricant, and a heat-transfer medium; it is also used in polyester dyeing, in termite-control preparations, and as an insecticide (8).

#### Environmental fate

The TCBs are expected to be adsorbed onto soils of high organic content, but not to leach appreciably into groundwater. They are not hydrolysed and are unlikely to biodegrade significantly. Some evaporation may occur from soil surfaces. In water, TCBs are likely to be adsorbed onto sediments and to bioconcentrate in aquatic organisms. Evaporation from water may be a significant removal process (3).

## 14.19.2 Analytical methods

A standard method for chlorobenzenes involves extraction with hexane followed by capillary column gas–liquid chromatography with electron-capture detection. Detection limits in tapwater and river water are about 0.1 µg/litre for TCBs (9).

## 14.19.3 Environmental levels and human exposure

### *Air*

Levels are likely to be significant only in areas where TCBs are produced. Mean levels of 22–51 ng/m$^3$ have been reported for three sites in California (10). An average of 181 ng/m$^3$ was reported in areas where they are produced in the USA (3).

### *Water*

TCBs have been detected in wastewater, surface and groundwater, and drinking-water (3). In a Canadian river, levels of 2, 7, and 2 µg/litre were reported for 1,2,3-TCB, 1,2,4-TCB, and 1,3,5-TCB, respectively (11). Tapwater concentrations were reported in the same study, the highest being for 1,2,4-TCB, for which the mean reported level was 2 ng/litre. The maximum value for all isomers found in a groundwater survey in the Netherlands was 1.2 µg/litre (12).

### *Food*

TCBs tend to accumulate in biological materials rich in lipids, such as fatty tissue and milk; residues at levels of 0.1–4 mg/kg on a fat basis were found in the liver of cod from areas polluted by industrial effluents (13). Mean levels reported in human milk were 1, 1, and 5 µg/kg for 1,3,5-TCB, 1,2,4-TCB, and 1,2,3-TCB, respectively (14).

### *Estimated total exposure and relative contribution of drinking-water*

General population exposure will occur mainly through the inhalation of contaminated air in areas where TCBs are manufactured and from the ingestion of contaminated food, especially fish.

## 14.19.4 Kinetics and metabolism in laboratory animals and humans

All three TCB isomers were readily absorbed following oral administration in rats. High concentrations of the parent compound were found in fat, skin, and liver, whereas high levels of metabolites were found in kidney and muscle (15). The major metabolic products are trichlorophenols (16). Species differences appear to exist in the metabolism of TCBs. Rats and rhesus monkeys given 1,2,4-TCB orally and intravenously excreted different urinary metabolites. Excretion was more rapid in rats than in monkeys; after 24 h, rats had excreted 84% of the oral dose in the urine and 11% in the faeces, as compared with 40% and <1%, respectively, in monkeys (17). There is also evidence that the TCBs are broad inducers of metabolizing enzymes (16).

## 14.19.5 Effects on laboratory animals and *in vitro* test systems

### Acute exposure

TCBs are of low to moderate acute toxicity. Oral $LD_{50}$s in rodents range from 300 to 800 mg/kg of body weight. Major target organs of acute exposure are the liver and kidneys (16).

### Short-term exposure

In a 13-week study, weanling Sprague-Dawley rats were fed diets containing TCB isomers at 1, 10, 100, or 1000 mg/kg. All three isomers at 1000 mg/kg caused increased relative liver and kidney weights and histological changes in the liver and thyroid of male rats. Males fed 1000 mg of 1,2,3-TCB per kg showed reduced weight gain; no other clinical signs of toxicity were observed. Only 1,2,4-TCB at 1000 mg/kg caused increases in hepatic aminopyrine methyl transferase and aniline hydroxylase activities in males and aminopyrine methyl transferase in females. The serum biochemical and haematological parameters measured were not affected. Only 1,3,5-TCB elicited moderate renal changes in male rats at 1000 mg/kg. Microscopic changes in females were milder than those in males. NOAELs were 100 mg/kg for all three isomers, equal to 7.8 mg/kg of body weight per day (1,2,4-TCB), 7.7 mg/kg of body weight per day (1,2,3-TCB), or 7.6 mg/kg of body weight per day (1,3,5-TCB) (18).

### Long-term exposure

Relevant chronic studies via the oral route have not been carried out. In a 2-year dermal study, S1c:ddy mice given 0.03 ml of a 30% or 60% solution of 1,2,4-TCB twice a week showed signs of clinical toxicity, decreased survival, and keratinization of the epidermis (19). The main causes of death were respiratory infection, amyloidosis, and tumours.

### Reproductive toxicity, embryotoxicity, and teratogenicity

No evidence of teratogenic effects was reported when Sprague-Dawley rats were given oral doses of 75, 150, or 300 mg/kg of body weight per day of 1,2,4-TCB or 150, 300, or 600 mg/kg of body weight per day of 1,2,3-TCB and 1,3,5-TCB on days 6–15 of gestation (20). Rats exposed to 0, 25, 100, or 400 mg/litre of

1,2,4-TCB in their drinking-water from the birth of the $F_0$ generation to the weaning of the $F_2$ generation did not show any effects on fertility (*21*).

### Mutagenicity and related end-points

None of the isomers of TCB was mutagenic in *Salmonella typhimurium* strains TA98, TA100, TA1535, and TA1537, with or without metabolic activation (*22, 23*). All three caused dose-related increases in the formation of micronucleated polychromatic erythrocytes in mice injected with TCBs in corn oil at doses up to 70% of the $LD_{50}$ (*24*). It was considered that the effects were due to the clastogenic activity of the TCBs; however, these results have not been confirmed by other workers (*16*).

### Carcinogenicity

Relevant carcinogenicity studies via the oral route have not been carried out. In the 2-year dermal study in which S1c:ddy mice were given 0.03 ml of a 30% or 60% solution of 1,2,4-TCB twice a week (*19*), tumours occurred in both experimental and control groups, suggesting that they were spontaneous in origin and not due to the carcinogenic effects of this compound.

## 14.19.6 Effects on humans

TCBs are moderately toxic when ingested or inhaled. They produce irritation of the skin, eyes, and respiratory tract (*8*). There has been one report of aplastic anaemia in a woman chronically exposed to 1,2,4-TCB from washing work clothes (*25*).

## 14.19.7 Guideline value

The TCBs are of moderate acute toxicity. After short-term oral exposure, all three isomers show similar toxic effects, predominantly on the liver. Long-term toxicity and carcinogenicity studies via the oral route have not been carried out, but the data available suggest that all three isomers are non-genotoxic.

A TDI of 7.7 µg/kg of body weight was calculated by applying an uncertainty factor of 1000 (100 for inter- and intraspecies variation and 10 for the short duration of the study) to the NOAEL of 7.7 mg/kg of body weight per day for liver toxicity identified in a 13-week rat study (*18*). The guideline value would be 20 µg/litre (rounded figure) for each isomer based on an allocation of 10% of the TDI to drinking-water; however, because of the similarity in the toxicity of the TCB isomers, the guideline value of 20 µg/litre is proposed for total TCBs. This value exceeds the lowest reported odour threshold in water of 5 µg/litre.

## References

1.  Weast RC, Astle MJ, Beyer WH, eds. *CRC handbook of chemistry and physics*, 67th ed. Boca Raton, FL, CRC Press, 1986.

2.  Verschueren K. *Handbook of environmental data on organic chemicals*, 2nd ed. New York, Van Nostrand Reinhold, 1983.

3.  Howard PH. *Handbook of environmental fate and exposure data for organic chemicals*. Vol. 1. *Large production and priority pollutants*. Chelsea, MI, Lewis Publishers, 1990.

4.  Miller MM et al. Aqueous solubilities, octanol/water partition coefficients, and entropies of melting of chlorinated benzenes and biphenyls. *Journal of chemical engineering data*, 1984, 29:184-190.

5.  Alexander HC et al. Aqueous odour and taste threshold values of industrial chemicals. *Journal of the American Water Works Association*, 1982, 574(11):595-599.

6.  Van Gemert LJ, Nettenbreijer AH, eds. *Compilation of odour threshold values in air and water*. Voorburg, Netherlands, National Institute for Water Supply, Central Institute for Nutrition and Food Research, 1972.

7.  Meleščenko KF. [Hygienic background for determining the maximum permissible concentration of trichlorobenzene in water basins.] *Gigiena i sanitarija*, 1969, 25(3):13-18 (in Russian with English summary).

8.  Slooff W et al. *Integrated criteria document chlorobenzenes*. Bilthoven, Netherlands, National Institute of Public Health and Environmental Protection, 1991.

9.  Department of the Environment. *Methods for the examination of waters and associated materials – chlorobenzenes in water, organochlorine pesticides and PCBs in turbid waters, halogenated solvents and related compounds in sewage sludge and waters*. London, Her Majesty's Stationery Office, 1985.

10. Singh HB et al. Measurement of some potentially hazardous organic chemicals in urban environments. *Atmospheric environment*, 1981, 15:601-612.

11. Oliver BG, Nicol KD. Chlorobenzenes in sediments, water and selected fish from Lakes Superior, Huron, Erie and Ontario. *Environmental science and technology*, 1982, 16:532-536.

12. Zoeteman BC et al. Persistent organic pollutants in river water and ground water of the Netherlands. *Chemosphere*, 1980, 9:231-249.

13. Ofstad EB, Lunde G, Martinsen K. Chlorinated aromatic hydrocarbons in fish from an area polluted by industrial effluents. *Science of the total environment*, 1978, 10:219-230.

14. Jan J. Chlorobenzene residues in human fat and milk. *Bulletin of environmental contamination and toxicology*, 1983, 30:595-599.

15. Chu I et al. Tissue distribution and elimination of trichlorobenzenes in the rat. *Journal of environmental science and health*, 1987, B22(4):439-453.

16. *Chlorobenzenes other than hexachlorobenzene.* Geneva, World Health Organization, 1991 (Environmental Health Criteria, No. 128).

17. Lingg RD et al. Comparative metabolism of 1,2,4-trichlorobenzene in the rat and rhesus monkey. *Drug metabolism and disposition*, 1982, 10:134-141.

18. Cote M et al. Trichlorobenzenes: results of a thirteen week feeding study in the rat. *Drug and chemical toxicology*, 1988, 11(1):11-28.

19. Yamaoto H et al. [Chronic toxicity and carcinogenicity test of 1,2,4-trichlorobenzene on mice by dermal painting.] *Nara igaku zasshi*, 1982, 33(2):132-145 (in Japanese).

20. Ruddick JA et al. A teratological evaluation following oral administration of trichloro- and dichlorobenzene isomers to the rat. *Teratology*, 1983, 27:73A-74A.

21. Robinson KS et al. Multigeneration study of 1,2,4-trichlorobenzene in rats. *Journal of toxicology and environmental health*, 1981, 8:489-500.

22. Schoeny RS, Smith CC, Loper JC. Non-mutagenicity for *Salmonella* of the chlorinated hydrocarbons Aroclor 1254, 1,2,4-trichlorobenzene, Mirex and kepone. *Mutation research*, 1979, 68:125-132.

23. Nohmi T et al. [Mutagenicity tests on organic chemical contaminants in city water and related compounds. I. Bacterial mutagenicity tests.] *Bulletin of the National Institute of Hygiene and Science, Tokyo*, 1985, 103:60-64 (in Japanese).

24. Mohtashamipur E et al. The bone marrow clastogenicity of eight halogenated benzenes in male NMRI mice. *Mutagenesis*, 1987, 2(2):111-113.

25. Girard R et al. [Severe hemopathy and exposure to chlorine derivatives of benzene.] *Journal de médecine de Lyon*, 1969, 50(164):771-773 (in French).

# 14.20 Di(2-ethylhexyl)adipate

## 14.20.1 General description

### *Identity*

CAS no.: 103-23-1

Molecular formula: $C_{22}H_{42}O_4$

This compound is also known as DEHA, bis(2-ethylhexyl)adipate (BEHA), and dioctyladipate (DOA).

### Physicochemical properties (1–3)

| Property | Value |
|---|---|
| Physical state | Light-coloured oily liquid |
| Melting point | -67.8 °C |
| Boiling point | 417 °C at 101.3 kPa |
| Density | 0.922 g/cm³ at 25 °C |
| Vapour pressure | < 0.00133 kPa at 20 °C |
| Water solubility | Insoluble (0.78 ± 0.16 mg/litre) |
| Log octanol–water partition coefficient | 6.3 |

### Major uses

DEHA is used mainly as a plasticizer for synthetic resins such as polyvinyl chloride (PVC), but significant amounts are also used as a lubricant and for hydraulic fluids (1).

### Environmental fate

Model experiments with activated sewage sludge systems have demonstrated the essentially complete biodegradation, measured as carbon dioxide evolution, of relatively high concentrations of DEHA in 35 days (3, 4). Because of its low water solubility, DEHA released into the environment would be expected to partition to solids (biota, sediment, soil). Under ideal equilibrium conditions, it would partition mainly to the atmosphere and to terrestrial soil, and less than 1% of environmental DEHA would be found in the aquatic environment (3).

## 14.20.2 Analytical methods

DEHA in tapwater and surface water has been determined by gas chromatography with flame ionization detection or identification by mass spectrometry. In surface water, the detection limit is stated to be 0.2 µg/litre (3), although lower levels have been reported for both surface water (5) and drinking-water (6).

## 14.20.3 Environmental levels and human exposure
### Water

DEHA was been found at microgram per litre levels in two out of five samples of finished water from a waste-treatment plant in the USA (6). A survey of 23 major rivers and lakes in the USA showed that 7% of the samples contained DEHA at levels ranging from 0.25 to 1.0 µg/litre (3). Water samples from the Great Lakes contained a maximum level of 7.0 µg/litre (5). In Europe, DEHA has been identified as a trace-level contaminant of the Rhine (7). Finished drinking-water in five cities in the USA had levels of about 0.001–0.1 µg/litre (6, 8, 9).

### Food

Food is the major source of exposure of the general population to DEHA because of its migration, particularly to fatty foods such as cheese and meat, from PVC films used for food packaging that have been plasticized with it. The estimated daily intake of DEHA through the diet in the United Kingdom is 16 mg (10); in the USA, it has been estimated to be as high as 20 mg (US Food and Drug Administration, personal communication, 1981).

### Estimated total exposure and relative contribution of drinking-water

Air and drinking-water are insignificant sources of human exposure to DEHA compared with the intake via food.

## 14.20.4 Kinetics and metabolism in laboratory animals and humans

DEHA appears to be readily absorbed when given orally to rats and mice. It is widely distributed in the body; the highest levels have been reported in adipose tissue, liver, and kidney (11, 12). Transplacental transport of DEHA has been noted (12).

DEHA is initially hydrolysed to mono(2-ethylhexyl)adipate (MEHA), adipic acid, and 2-ethylhexanol, which are excreted as such or further oxidized to several different compounds before being eliminated in the expired air, urine, and faeces of experimental animals. Major metabolites of DEHA are MEHA and its glucuronide (monkey), the glucuronide of 2-ethylhexanoic acid (mouse, rat), and adipic acid (mouse, rat). Single oral doses of DEHA seem to be completely excreted by rats, mice, and monkeys in 48 h (11, 13).

## 14.20.5 Effects on laboratory animals and *in vitro* test systems

### Acute exposure

The acute oral toxicity of DEHA is low. The oral $LD_{50}$ has been estimated to be 45 g/kg of body weight in male rats, 25 g/kg of body weight in female rats, 15 g/kg of body weight in male mice, and 25 g/kg of body weight in female mice (14).

## Short-term exposure

Short-term (3–4 weeks) mouse and rat toxicity studies have demonstrated that high dietary levels of DEHA ($\geqslant$6000 mg/kg) induce liver toxicity, including increased liver weights, histopathological liver changes, and proliferation of liver peroxisomes, accompanied by increased activities of catalase and of enzymes involved in the oxidation of fatty acids as well as hypolipidaemia. DEHA-induced peroxisomal proliferation with accompanying biochemical events was found to be a dose-dependent phenomenon. A NOAEL of 100 mg/kg of body weight per day can be identified from these studies (15–17).

A 13-week toxicity study was conducted in F344 rats and B6C3F$_1$ mice at dietary concentrations of up to 25 000 mg of DEHA per kg. At 25 000 mg/kg, decreased weight gain was observed in both species and sexes. At 12 500 mg/kg, male and female rats as well as male mice showed slightly reduced body weight gain. At 6300 mg/kg, body weight gain was decreased in female mice and male rats. No compound-related increased mortality, histopathological changes, or reduction in feed consumption were observed (14).

## Long-term exposure

In a 103-week study in which DEHA was administered to F344 rats and B6C3F$_1$ mice at dietary levels of 12 000 or 25 000 mg/kg, no dose-related effect on longevity was seen. A dose-related depression of growth rate was observed in mice. Except in the liver, where tumours developed, no histopathological changes were observed in the mouse. Growth rate was depressed in rats fed 25 000 mg of DEHA per kg. No DEHA-related histopathological changes were seen in rats (14).

## Reproductive toxicity, embryotoxicity, and teratogenicity

A fertility study was performed in which male and female Wistar rats were fed DEHA in the diet from 10 weeks before mating up to 36 days postpartum at levels of 300, 1800, or 12 000 mg/kg. At 12 000 mg/kg of diet, body weight gain was marginally reduced in females, and liver weights of both male and female parental animals were significantly increased. There were no effects on male or female fertility or on gestation length. At the highest dose level, total litter weights, body weight gain of pups, and mean litter size were reduced. No effect on pup survival was found at any treatment level. No treatment-related macroscopic abnormalities were found in the pups (18).

In a teratogenicity study, pregnant Wistar rats were fed DEHA in the diet at levels of 300, 1800, or 12 000 mg/kg, corresponding to daily doses of 28, 170, or 1080 mg/kg of body weight, on days 1–22 of gestation. Administration of 12 000 mg/kg resulted in slight maternal toxicity, expressed as a small reduction in body weight gain. There were no effects at any dietary level on fetal weight, litter weight, or number of intrauterine deaths. At the highest dose level, a small increase in pre-implantation loss as well as a minimal increase in post-implantation loss were noted. Incidences of major or minor external or visceral effects were low and were not increased by treatment with DEHA. However, two visceral variants (dilated and kinked ureter) were observed in increasing incidences in a dose-related manner at the two highest dose levels. Minor skeletal defects, indicating slightly poorer ossification, were also increased in a dose-related manner at the two highest dietary DEHA levels. No fetal effects were noted at 300 mg of DEHA per kg of diet. A NOAEL of 28 mg/kg of body weight can be identified from this study (19).

## Mutagenicity and related end-points

A large number of short-term tests have failed to demonstrate any mutagenic activity of DEHA (20–23). One *in vitro* test with Chinese hamster ovary cells demonstrated some capacity to induce chromosomal aberrations in the absence of activation by a rat liver homogenate (S9 fraction). Studies of sister chromatid exchange in the same *in vitro* system were negative without activation and equivocal with it (24). Orally administered DEHA does not bind covalently to mouse liver DNA (25).

## Carcinogenicity

In a 103-week carcinogenicity study, DEHA was administered to F344 rats and B6C3F$_1$ mice in the diet at levels of 12 000 or 25 000 mg/kg, equivalent to a daily intake of 600 or 1250 mg/kg of body weight in rats and 1715 or 3570 mg/kg of body weight in mice. No increased tumour incidences were noted in rats. An increased number of hepatocellular carcinomas was found in female mice at both doses. Hepatocellular adenomas and carcinomas combined occurred in high-dose mice of both sexes and in low-dose female mice at incidences that were dose-related and significantly higher than those in control mice. The association of liver tumours in male mice with the administration of DEHA was not considered to be conclusive because the increased number of liver tumours in males reflected only an increase in adenomas in the high-dose group and because the time to observation of tumours was not significantly different in dosed and control males (14).

As DEHA fails to elicit mutagenic or genotoxic responses in available test systems and does not form adducts with DNA, it may be an epigenetic carcinogen for which a dose threshold exists, probably related to its ability to induce peroxisomal proliferation. Liver tumours are likely to occur only at doses causing proliferation of peroxisomes and, as there is a dose threshold for such proliferation, there is probably also a dose threshold for tumour development. The available information suggests that primates are less sensitive than rodents to chemically induced peroxisomal proliferation (26).

## 14.20.6 Guideline value

IARC has concluded that there is limited evidence that DEHA is carcinogenic in mice (*1*). It is not classifiable as to its carcinogenicity in humans (*27*).

Although DEHA is carcinogenic in mice, its toxicity profile and lack of mutagenicity support the use of a TDI approach to setting a guideline value for DEHA in drinking-water. A TDI of 280 µg/kg of body weight can be calculated by applying an uncertainty factor of 100 (for inter- and intraspecies variation) to the lowest observed NOAEL for DEHA of 28 mg/kg of body weight in a fetotoxicity study in rats (*19*). This gives a guideline value of 80 µg/litre (rounded figure), based on an allocation of 1% of the TDI to drinking-water.

## References

1.   International Agency for Research on Cancer. *Some industrial chemicals and dyestuffs.* Lyon, 1982:257-267 (IARC Monographs on the Evaluation of the Carcinogenic Risk of Chemicals to Humans, Volume 29).

2.   British Industrial Biological Research Association. *Toxicity profile: di(2-ethylhexyl)-adipate.* Carshalton, 1986.

3.   Felder JD, Adams WJ, Saeger VW. Assessment of the safety of dioctyl adipate in freshwater environments. *Environmental toxicology and chemistry*, 1986, 5:777-784.

4.   Saeger VW et al. Activated sludge degradation of adipic acid esters. *Applied environmental microbiology*, 1976, 31:746-749.

5.   Sheldon LS, Hites RA. Organic compounds in the Delaware River. *Environmental science and technology*, 1978, 12:1188-1194.

6.   Lin DCK et al. Glass capillary gas chromatographic/mass spectrometric analysis of organic concentrates from drinking and advanced waste treatment waters. In: Keith LH, ed. *Advances in the identification and analysis of organic pollutants in water.* Vol. 2. Ann Arbor, MI, Ann Arbor Science Publishers, 1981:861-906.

7.   Güsten H, Schweer K-H, Stieglitz L. Identification of non-biodegradable organic pollutants in river water. *Arhiv za higijenu rada i toksikologiju*, 1974, 25:207-212.

8.   Sheldon LS, Hites RA. Sources and movement of organic chemicals in the Delaware River. *Environmental science and technology*, 1979, 13:574-579.

9.   Thruston AD Jr. High pressure liquid chromatography techniques for the isolation and identification of organics in drinking water extracts. *Journal of chromatographic science*, 1978, 16:254-259.

10. Ministry of Agriculture, Fisheries and Food. *Survey of plasticiser levels in food contact materials and in foods.* London, Her Majesty's Stationery Office, 1987 (Food Surveillance Paper No. 21).

11. Takahashi T, Tanaka A, Yamaha T. Elimination, distribution and metabolism of di(2-ethylhexyl)adipate (DEHA) in rats. *Toxicology,* 1981, 22:223-233.

12. Bergman K, Albanus L. Di(2-ethylhexyl)adipate: absorption, autoradiographic distribution and elimination in mice and rats. *Food chemistry and toxicology,* 1987, 25:309-316.

13. Woodward KN. *Phthalate esters: toxicity and metabolism.* Vol. II. Boca Raton, FL, CRC Press, 1988.

14. National Toxicology Program. *Carcinogenic bioassay of di(2-ethylhexyl)adipate (CAS No. 103-23-1) in F344 rats and B6C3F₁ mice (feed study).* Research Triangle Park, NC, 1982 (NTP Technical Report Series No. 212; NIH Publication No. 81-1768).

15. Midwest Research Institute. *Toxicological effects of diethylhexyladipate. Final report.* Washington, DC, Chemical Manufacturers Association, 1982 (MRI Project No. 7343-B; CMA Contract No. PE-14.0-BIO-MRI).

16. British Industrial Biological Research Association. *A 21-day feeding study of di(2-ethylhexyl)adipate to rats: effects on the liver and liver lipids.* Carshalton, 1986 (Report No. 0542/1/85).

17. Reddy JK et al. Comparison of hepatic peroxisome proliferative effect and its implication for hepatocarcinogenicity of phthalate esters, di(2-ethylhexyl)phthalate, and di(2-ethylhexyl)adipate with a hypolipidemic drug. *Environmental health perspectives,* 1986, 65:317-327.

18. Imperial Chemical Industries. *Di(2-ethylhexyl)adipate: fertility study in rats.* London, 1988 (ICI Report No. CTL/P.2229).

19. Imperial Chemical Industries. *Di(2-ethylhexyl)adipate: teratogenicity study in the rat.* London, 1988 (ICI Report No. CTL/P/2119).

20. Litton Bionetics. *Mutagenicity evaluation of di(2-ethylhexyl)adipate (DEHA) in the mouse micronucleus test. Final report.* Washington, DC, Chemical Manufacturers Association, 1982 (Contract No. PE-140-MUT-LB; LBI Project No. 20996).

21. Litton Bionetics. *Evaluation of di(2-ethylhexyl)adipate (DEHA) in the in vitro transformation of BALB/3T3 cell assay. Final report.* Washington, DC, Chemical Manufacturers Association, 1982 (Contract No. PE-140-MUT-LB; LBI Project No. 20992).

22. Litton Bionetics. *Evaluation of di(2-ethylhexyl)adipate (DEHA) in the in vitro trans-formation of BALB/3T3 cells with metabolic activation by primary rat hepatocytes. Final report.* Washington, DC, Chemical Manufacturers Association, 1982 (Contract No. PE-140-MUT-LB; LBI Project No. 20992).

23. Zeiger E et al. Mutagenicity testing of di(2-ethylhexyl)phthalate and related chemicals in *Salmonella. Environmental mutagenesis*, 1985, 7:213-232.

24. Galloway SM et al. Chromosomal aberrations and sister chromatid exchanges in Chinese hamster ovary cells: evaluations of 108 chemicals. *Environmental and molecular mutagenesis*, 1987, 10 (Suppl. 10):1-175.

25. von Däniken A et al. Investigation of the potential for binding of di(2-ethylhexyl)-phthalate (DEHP) and di(2-ethylhexyl)adipate (DEHA) to liver DNA *in vivo. Toxicology and applied pharmacology*, 1984, 73:373-387.

26. Reddy JK, Lalwani ND. Carcinogenesis by hepatic peroxisome proliferators: evaluation of the risk of hypolipidemic drugs and industrial plasticizers to humans. *CRC critical reviews in toxicology*, 1983, 12:1-58.

27. International Agency for Research on Cancer. *Overall evaluations of carcinogenicity: an updating of IARC Monographs volumes 1-42.* Lyon, 1987:62 (IARC Monographs on the Evaluation of Carcinogenic Risks to Humans, Suppl. 7).

## 14.21 Di(2-ethylhexyl)phthalate

### 14.21.1 General description

#### *Identity*

CAS no.:        117-81-7
Molecular formula:  $C_{24}H_{38}O_4$

Di(2-ethylhexyl)phthalate (DEHP) is also known as 1,2-benzenedicarboxylic acid bis(2-ethylhexyl)ester, bis(2-ethylhexyl) phthalate, and dioctyl phthalate (DOP).

## Physicochemical properties (1, 2 )[1]

Property | Value
--- | ---
Physical state | Light-coloured, viscous liquid
Melting point | -46 °C (pour-point)
Boiling point | 370 °C at 101.3 kPa
Density | 0.98 g/cm$^3$ at 20 °C
Vapour pressure | 0.056 x 10$^{-7}$ kPa at 20 °C
Water solubility | 23–340 µg/litre at 25 °C
Log octanol–water partition coefficient | 4.88

## Organoleptic properties

DEHP is odourless.

## Major uses

DEHP is used primarily as a plasticizer in many flexible polyvinyl chloride products and in vinyl chloride co-polymer resins. It is also used as a replacement for polychlorinated biphenyls in dielectric fluids for small (low-voltage) electrical capacitors (1, 2).

## Environmental fate

DEHP is insoluble in water (23–340 µg/litre) (2, 3). Because of the readiness with which it forms colloidal solutions, its "true" solubility in water is believed to be 25–50 µg/litre. DEHP has a very low volatilization rate. Photolysis in water is thought to be a very slow process (2). Hydrolysis half-lives of over 100 years at pH 8 and 30 °C have been found. DEHP biodegrades rapidly in water and sludges, especially under aerobic conditions; degradation of 40–90% in 10–35 days has been found. Biodegradation in sediment and water under anaerobic conditions is assumed to be very slow; however, the available information is contradictory (3).

## 14.21.2 Analytical methods

DEHP can be determined by gas chromatography with electron-capture detection; the method has a detection limit of 0.1 ng (4). The detection limit with flame ionization detection is 1 µg/litre. The identity of the compound can be confirmed by mass spectrometry with "single-ion" monitoring, especially when electron-capture detection is used (3, 5).

---

[1] Conversion factor in air: 1 ppm = 1.59 mg/m$^3$.

## 14.21.3 Environmental levels and human exposure

It should be noted that some reported occurrences of DEHP in certain matrices have been found to result from contamination of the latter by plasticizer extracted from plastic tubing or other equipment (1, 2).

### *Air*

DEHP has been detected in ocean air at levels ranging from 0.4 ng/m$^3$ over the Gulf of Mexico to 2.9 ng/m$^3$ over the North Atlantic (1, 2). Ambient air above the Great Lakes contains an average of 2 ng/m$^3$ (range 0.5–5 ng/m$^3$) (6). In the North Pacific, the average concentration in air was 1.4 ng/m$^3$ (range 0.3–2.7 ng/m$^3$) (3).

In city air, concentrations of phthalates in atmospheric particulate matter range from 5 to 132 ng/m$^3$ (7, 8), but a concentration of 300 ng/m$^3$ has been reported in the vicinity of a municipal incinerator (9). Where DEHP is used inside houses, the concentration increases with temperature but decreases with humidity; after 4 months, the concentration will be about 0.05 mg/m$^3$ (5).

### *Water*

In Japan, DEHP was detected in 71 out of 111 samples of rainwater; average concentrations were in the range 0.6–3.2 µg/litre, the highest average value being found in an industrial town (5). In the North Pacific, the average concentration in rainwater was 55 ng/litre (range 5.3–213 ng/litre) (3).

DEHP has been detected in water from several rivers at levels of up to 5 µg/litre (1, 2, 5). In the Netherlands, sediments of the Rhine and the Meuse contained 1–70 and 1–17 mg/kg, respectively (1). The average concentration in water from the Rhine in 1986 was 0.3 µg/litre (range 0.1–0.7 µg/litre) and in suspended particulate matter 20 mg/kg (range 10–36 mg/kg) (10). In surface water near industrial areas, levels of up to 300 µg/litre were found (1, 2).

In contaminated groundwater in the Netherlands, 20–45 µg of DEHP per litre was reported (11). A groundwater sample from New York State contained 170 µg/litre (12).

DEHP was detected in tapwater in two cities in the USA at an average level of 1 µg/litre and in Japan at levels in the range 1.2–1.8 µg/litre. In "finished" drinking-water in two cities in the USA, average concentrations were 0.05–11 µg/litre; in several major eastern cities in the USA, average levels were below 1 µg/litre. The highest concentrations in drinking-water (up to 30 µg/litre) were reported in older surveys (1975) (1, 2).

### *Food*

Levels of DEHP below 1 mg/kg were detected in fish in different parts of the USA; most fish contained less than 0.2 mg/kg. In a sampling of a wide variety of foods, the highest levels were found in milk (31.4 mg/litre, fat basis) and cheese (35 mg/kg, fat basis). In a study of the migration of DEHP from plastic packaging films, it was found in tempura (frying) powder (0.11–68 mg/kg), instant cream soup (0.04–3.1 mg/kg), fried potato cake (0.05–9.1 mg/kg), and orange juice (0.05 mg/kg) (1, 2).

Analysis of bottled beverages with polyvinyl chloride seals plasticized with DEHP demonstrated that very little migration occurs; all the concentrations reported were less than 0.1 mg/kg, the vast majority being below 0.02 mg/kg. Draught beer samples contained similar levels of DEHP (<0.01–0.04 mg/kg) (13).

### Estimated total exposure and relative contribution of drinking-water

Exposure among individuals may vary considerably because of the wide variety of products into which DEHP is incorporated. The estimated average daily adult dose from the consumption of commodities highly likely to be contaminated (such as milk, cheese, margarine) is about 200 μg (14). Levels in community drinking-water are generally thought to be negligible, although there may be individual instances of high levels of contamination. Exposure from air is negligible compared with that associated with food (e.g. when the concentration in city air is 50 ng/m³, the daily exposure will be less than 1 μg).

Patients undergoing kidney dialysis may be exposed to high levels of DEHP; it is estimated that each patient will receive up to 90 mg per treatment (15). Exposure also occurs during the transfusion of stored whole blood. Concentrations will be low in frozen plasma. The Netherlands standard for the migration of DEHP from blood containers is 10 mg of DEHP per 100 ml of ethanol (16).

### 14.21.4 Kinetics and metabolism in laboratory animals and humans

In rats, DEHP is readily absorbed from the gastrointestinal tract after oral administration. It is hydrolysed to a large extent to mono(2-ethylhexyl)phthalate (MEHP) with release of 2-ethylhexanol (EH) before intestinal absorption (17). Absorption is lower in primates (including humans). In rats, over 90% was excreted in urine after dietary administration, whereas only 0.9% was excreted in urine by marmosets (2,18). In humans, 11–25% of an ingested dose was found in urine (2,19).

DEHP undergoes further modification after hydrolysis to the monoester. Several species (primates, including humans, and some rodents) form glucuronide conjugates with the monoester, but rats appear unable to do so. In rats, the residual 2-ethylhexyl moiety is oxidized extensively (17). In mice and rats, urinary metabolites consist primarily of terminal oxidation products (diacids, ketoacids); in primates (monkeys, humans), they consist primarily of unoxidized or minimally oxidized products (MEHP, hydroxyacid) (18).

DEHP and its metabolites are extensively distributed throughout the body in rodents, the highest levels being found in the liver and adipose tissue. Little or no accumulation occurs in rats. Estimated half-lives for DEHP and its metabolites in rats are 3–5 days for fat and 1–2 days for other tissues (*20*).

## 14.21.5 Effects on laboratory animals and *in vitro* test systems

### Acute exposure

DEHP has a low acute oral toxicity in animals; the oral $LD_{50}$ for mice and rats is over 20 g/kg of body weight (*1*).

### Short-term exposure

Liver and testes appear to be the main target organs for DEHP toxicity. DEHP can cause functional hepatic damage, as reflected by morphological changes, alterations in energy-linked enzyme activity, and changes in lipid and carbohydrate metabolism. The most striking effect is the proliferation of hepatic peroxisomes (*21*).

In short-term oral studies in rats with dosing periods ranging from 3 days to 9 months and dose levels ranging from 50 to 25 000 mg/kg of diet (2.5–2500 mg/kg of body weight per day), doses greater than 50 mg/kg of body weight per day caused a significant dose-related increase in liver weight, a decrease in serum triglyceride and cholesterol levels, and microscopic changes in the liver, namely periportal accumulation of fat and mild centrilobular loss of glycogen. An initial burst of DNA synthesis in the liver (indicative of liver hyperplasia) followed by a decrease in liver DNA content (indicative of liver hypertrophy) was observed. Changes in peroxisomes, mitochondria, and endoplasmic reticulum in the liver were seen. Significant increases in hepatic peroxisomal enzyme activities and in the number of peroxisomes in the liver were found (*22–26*). NOAELs for changes in liver weight were 25 mg/kg of body weight per day by gavage (*23*) and 500 mg/kg of diet (25 mg/kg of body weight per day) (*22*). Morton (*22*) found significantly decreased serum triglyceride levels at 50, 100, and 500 mg/kg of diet, whereas Barber et al. (*25*) did not find this effect at 1000 and 100 mg/kg of diet.

NOAELs for peroxisomal proliferation (based on changes in peroxisome-related enzyme activities or ultramicroscopic changes) were 25 mg/kg of body weight per day (LOAEL 100 mg/kg of body weight per day) in a 14-day gavage study in Sprague-Dawley rats (*23*), 50 mg/kg of diet (2.5 mg/kg of body weight per day) in a 7-day study in Sprague-Dawley rats (*22*) (LOAEL 100 mg/kg of diet or 5 mg/kg of body weight per day), and 100 mg/kg of diet (10 mg/kg of body weight per day) in a 3-week study in F344 rats (LOAEL 1000 mg/kg of diet or 100 mg/kg of body weight) (*25*). Marked species differences in the occurrence of peroxisomal proliferation exist, the available information suggesting that primates, including humans, are less sensitive to this effect than rodents (*26*).

Changes in the kidneys and thyroid in Wistar rats have also been observed. The effects on the thyroid (increased activity accompanied by a decrease of plasma $T_4$) were observed at doses of 10 000 mg/kg of diet (1000 mg/kg of body weight per day) and higher (24).

## Long-term exposure

In 2-year oral toxicity studies in rats, doses of 100–200 mg/kg of body weight per day and higher caused growth depression, liver and kidney enlargement, microscopic changes in the liver, and testicular atrophy. The NOAEL was 50–65 mg/kg of body weight (2, 27, 28). Increased activities of peroxisome-associated enzymes were found in another study even at the lowest dose level of 200 mg/kg of diet (10 mg/kg of body weight per day) (26).

## Reproductive toxicity, embryotoxicity, and teratogenicity

Testicular effects, namely atrophy, tubular degeneration, and inhibition or cessation of spermatogenesis, were seen in mice, rats, guinea-pigs, and ferrets (29), supposedly caused by MEHP (2, 30). In rats, testicular changes were seen at oral doses above 100 mg/kg of body weight per day (31).

In a reproduction study in mice, complete suppression of fertility in both sexes was seen at 0.3% DEHP in the diet (430 mg/kg of body weight per day). At 0.1% in the diet (140 mg/kg of body weight), significantly reduced fertility indices, again in both sexes, were observed, but no effects on fertility were seen at 0.01% in the diet (15 mg/kg of body weight) (26).

In mice, fetal mortality, fetal resorption, decreased fetal weight, neural tube effects, and skeletal disorders (exencephaly, spina bifida, open eyelid, exophthalmia, major vessel malformations, club-foot, and delayed ossification) were seen in teratogenicity studies. The NOAEL for these effects was 0.025% in the diet (35 mg/kg of body weight per day) (32). The LOAELs were 0.05 mg/kg of body weight per day (33) and 0.05% in diet (70 mg/kg of body weight per day) (32). MEHP was more active than DEHP, which may, therefore, act as a result of conversion into MEHP. However, it was also hypothesized that 2-ethylhexanoic acid, the oxidation product of 2-ethylhexanol, was the proximate teratogen, as indicated in studies with rats (26).

Rats were less susceptible than mice to DEHP-related adverse effects on fetal development. At oral doses above 200 mg/kg of body weight per day, decreased fetal weights and an increased number of resorptions were observed (34, 35). Teratogenic effects were not observed in F344 rats at dose levels of 0.5–2.0% in the diet (250–1000 mg/kg of body weight per day). Embryofetal toxicity was seen at levels of 1.0% in the diet and higher ($\geqslant$500 mg/kg of body weight per day) (32).

## Mutagenicity and related end-points

DEHP showed negative results in most short-term mutagenicity studies *in vitro* and *in vivo* (i.e. it did not induce gene mutations in bacterial systems, eukaryotic systems, or mammalian systems *in vitro*, or chromosomal aberrations or sister chromatid exchange in mammalian cells *in vitro*, or chromosomal aberrations in somatic or germ cells *in vivo*). No evidence was found for a covalent interaction of DEHP with DNA, the induction of single-strand breaks in DNA, or unscheduled DNA repair. However, DEHP induced aneuploidy in eukaryotic cells *in vitro* and cell transformation in mammalian cells *in vivo* and *in vitro* (*20, 36*).

In general, MEHP and EH did not induce gene mutations in bacteria or mammalian cells *in vitro*. Contradictory results were reported for MEHP with respect to the induction of chromosomal aberrations and sister chromatid exchange in mammalian cells *in vitro*, but EH showed negative results in these test systems. In mammalian cells *in vivo*, MEHP and EH did not induce chromosomal aberrations (*36*).

## Carcinogenicity

In a 2-year oral study in mice, increased incidences of hepatocellular carcinomas were seen in males and females at 3000 and 6000 mg/kg of diet. Rats given 6000 or 12 000 mg of DEHP per kg of diet for 2 years showed increased incidences of hepatocellular carcinomas and hepatic neoplastic nodules (*2, 37*).

It has been suggested that the increased incidences of liver tumours in mice and rats in chronic bioassays are caused by the prolonged proliferation of hepatocellular peroxisomes and the enhanced production of the peroxisomal metabolic by-product, hydrogen peroxide. Primates, including humans, are far less sensitive to peroxisomal proliferation than mice and rats (*38*).

In *in vivo* studies with B6C3F$_1$ mice, DEHP had no tumour-initiating activity in the liver but, in the same strain, showed promoting activity, also in the liver, as indicated by an increase in focal hepatocellular proliferative lesions, including hyperplastic foci and neoplasms. In rats, *in vivo* studies showed neither tumour-initiating or promoting activity, nor sequential syncarcinogenic activity in the liver (*26*).

## 14.21.6 Effects on humans

Two male volunteers dosed with 10 g of DEHP experienced mild gastric disturbances and moderate catharsis; a 5-g dose had no effect (*1, 2*).

Dialysis patients receiving approximately 150 mg of DEHP intravenously per week were examined for liver changes. At 1 month, no morphological changes were observed by liver biopsy but, at 1 year, peroxisomes were reported to be "significantly higher in number" (*20*).

A high incidence of polyneuropathy was reported in studies on industrial workers exposed to different phthalic acid esters, including DEHP (*39*), but this was not confirmed in another study (*40*). In a small cohort study, eight deaths were observed among 221 workers exposed to DEHP for periods ranging from 3 months to 24 years. One carcinoma of the pancreas and one bladder papilloma were reported. The study was considered to be inadequate to provide proof of a causal association (*1, 2*).

Occupational exposure to 0.01–0.016 mg of DEHP per m$^3$ over 10–34 years did not cause an increase in the frequency of chromosomal aberrations in blood leukocytes (*1, 2*).

## 14.21.7 Guideline value

IARC has concluded that DEHP is possibly carcinogenic to humans (Group 2B) (*41*). Induction of liver tumours in rodents by DEHP was observed at high dietary dose levels. A relationship between the occurrence of hepatocellular carcinoma and prolonged induction of peroxisomal proliferation in the liver was suggested, although the mechanism of action is still unknown. On the basis of toxicity data in experimental animals, the induction of peroxisomal proliferation in the liver seems to be the most sensitive effect of DEHP, and the rat appears to be the most sensitive species. The available literature suggests that humans are less sensitive to chemically induced peroxisomal proliferation than rodents.

In 1988, JECFA evaluated DEHP and recommended that human exposure to this compound in food be reduced to the lowest level attainable. The Committee considered that this might be achieved by using alternative plasticizers or alternatives to plastic material containing DEHP (*26*).

In view of the absence of evidence for genotoxicity and the suggested relationship between the occurrence of hepatocellular carcinomas and prolonged proliferation of liver peroxisomes, a TDI was derived using the lowest observed NOAEL of 2.5 mg/kg of body weight per day based on peroxisomal proliferation in the liver in rats (*22*). Although the mechanism for hepatocellular tumour induction is not fully resolved, using a NOAEL derived from the species by far the most sensitive with respect to the particularly sensitive end-point of peroxisomal proliferation justifies the use of an uncertainty factor of 100 (for inter- and intraspecies variation). Consequently, the TDI is 25 µg/kg of body weight. This yields a guideline value of 8 µg/litre (rounded figure), allocating 1% of the TDI to drinking-water.

## References

1.  International Agency for Research on Cancer. *Some industrial chemicals and dyestuffs.* Lyon, 1982:269-294 (IARC Monographs on the Evaluation of the Carcinogenic Risk of Chemicals to Humans, Volume 29).

2. *Diethylhexyl phthalate*. Geneva, World Health Organization, 1992 (Environmental Health Criteria, No. 131).

3. European Chemical Industry Ecology and Toxicology Centre. *An assessment of the occurrence and effects of dialkyl ortho-phthalates in the environment*. Brussels, 1985 (Technical Report No. 19).

4. Thurén A. Determination of phthalates in aquatic environments. *Bulletin of environmental contamination and toxicology*, 1986, 36:33-40.

5. Beratergremium für umweltrelevante Altstoffe der Gesellschaft Deutscher Chemiker (BUA). *Di-(2-ethylhexyl)phthalat*, Weinham, 1986 (BUA-Stoffbericht 4).

6. Eisenreich SJ, Looney BB, Thornton JD. Airborne organic contaminants in the Great Lakes ecosystem. *Environmental science and technology*, 1981, 15:30-38.

7. Cautreels W, Van Cauwenberghe K. Comparison between the organic fraction of suspended matter at a background and an urban station. *Science of the total environment*, 1977, 8:79-88.

8. Bove JL, Dalvent L, Kukreja VP. Airborne di-butyl and di-(2-ethylhexyl)phthalate at three New York City air sampling stations. *International journal of environmental analytical chemistry*, 1977, 5:189-194.

9. Thomas GH. Quantitative determination and confirmation of identity of trace amounts of dialkyl phthalates in environmental samples. *Environmental health perspectives*, 1973, 3:23-28.

10. Ritsema R et al. Trace-level analysis of phthalate esters in surface waters and suspended particulate matter by means of capillary gas chromatography with electron-capture and mass-selective detection. *Chemosphere*, 1989, 18:2161-2175.

11. Wams TJ. Diethylhexylphthalate as an environmental contaminant – a review. *Science of the total environment*, 1987, 66:1-16.

12. Rao PSC, Hornsby AG, Jessup RE. Indices for ranking the potential for pesticide contamination of groundwater. *Soil and Crop Science Society proceedings*, 1985, 44:1-8.

13. Ministry of Agriculture, Fisheries and Food. *Survey of plasticiser levels in food contact materials and in foods*. London, Her Majesty's Stationery Office, 1987 (Food Surveillance Paper No. 21).

14. Directorate for Health Sciences. *Draft report to the U.S. Consumer Product Safety Commission by the Chronic Hazard Advisory Panel on di(ethylhexyl)phthalate (DEHP)*. Washington, DC, US Consumer Product Safety Commission, 1985.

15. Office of Toxic Substances. *Priority review level: 1-di-(2-ethylhexyl)phthalate (DEHP). Draft*. Washington, DC, US Environmental Protection Agency, 1980.

16. *De Nederlandse pharmocopee.* [*The Netherlands pharmacopoeia.*] 9th ed. The Hague, Netherlands, Staats Uitgeverij, 1983.

17. Kluwe WM. Overview of phthalate ester pharmacokinetics in mammalian species. *Environmental health perspectives*, 1982, 45:3-9.

18. Albro PW et al. Pharmacokinetics, interactions with macromolecules and species differences in metabolism of DEHP. *Environmental health perspectives*, 1982, 45:19-25.

19. Schmid P, Schlatter C. Excretion and metabolism of di(2-ethylhexyl)phthalate in man. *Xenobiotica*, 1985, 15:251-256.

20. National Research Council. *Drinking water and health*, Vol. 6. Washington, DC, National Academy Press, 1986:338-359.

21. Seth PK. Hepatic effects of phthalate esters. *Environmental health perspectives*, 1982, 45:27-34.

22. Morton SJ. *The hepatic effects of dietary di-2-ethylhexyl phthalate.* Ann Arbor, MI, John Hopkins University, 1979 (dissertation; abstract in *Dissertation abstracts international*, 1979, B 40(09):4236).

23. Lake BG et al. Comparative studies of the hepatic effects of di- and mono-n-octyl phthalates, di-(2-ethylhexyl)phthalate and clofibrate in the rat. *Acta pharmacologica et toxicologica*, 1986, 54:167-176.

24. Hinton RH et al. Effects of phthalic acid esters on the liver and thyroid. *Environmental health perspectives*, 1986, 70:195-210.

25. Barber ED et al. Peroxisome induction studies on seven phthalate esters. *Toxicology and industrial health*, 1987, 3:7-24.

26. Joint FAO/WHO Expert Committee on Food Additives. *Toxicological evaluation of certain food additives and contaminants.* Cambridge, Cambridge University Press, 1989:222-265 (WHO Food Additives Series 24).

27. Carpenter CP, Weil CS, Smyth HF Jr. Chronic oral toxicity of di-(2-ethylhexyl)-phthalate for rats, guinea-pigs and dogs. *Archives of industrial hygiene and occupational medicine*, 1953, 8:219-226.

28. Harris RS et al. Chronic oral toxicity of 2-ethylhexyl phthalate in rats and dogs. *American Medical Association archives of industrial health*, 1956, 13:259-264.

29. Gangolli SD. Testicular effects of phthalate esters. *Environmental health perspectives*, 1982, 45:77-84.

30. Albro PW et al. Mono-2-ethylhexyl phthalate, a metabolite of di-(2-ethylhexyl)-phthalate, causally linked to testicular atrophy in rats. *Toxicology and applied pharmacology*, 1989, 100:193-200.

31. Gray TJ et al. Short-term toxicity study of di(2-ethylhexyl)phthalate in rats. *Food and cosmetics toxicology*, 1977, 15:389-399.

32. Tyl RW et al. Developmental toxicity evaluation of dietary di(2-ethylhexyl)phthalate in Fischer 344 rats and CD-1 mice. *Fundamental and applied toxicology*, 1988, 10:395-412.

33. Nakamura Y et al. Teratogenicity of di-(2-ethylhexyl)phthalate in mice. *Toxicology letters*, 1979, 4:113-117.

34. Nikonorow M, Mazur H, Piekacz H. Effect of orally administered plasticizers and polyvinyl chloride stabilizers in the rat. *Toxicology and applied pharmacology*, 1973, 26:253-259.

35. Onda H et al. [Effect of phthalate ester on reproductive performance in rats.] *Japanese journal of hygiene*, 1976, 31:507-512 (in Japanese).

36. Turnbull D, Rodricks JV. Assessment of possible carcinogenic risk to humans resulting from exposure to di(2-ethylhexyl)phthalate (DEHP). *Journal of the American College of Toxicologists*, 1985, 4:111-145.

37. National Toxicology Program. *Carcinogenesis bioassay of di(2-ethylhexyl)phthalate (CAS no. 117-81-7) in F344 rats and B6C3F$_1$ mice (feed study)*. Research Triangle Park, NC, 1982.

38. Stott WT. Chemically induced proliferation of peroxisomes: implications for risk assessment. *Regulatory toxicology and pharmacology*, 1988, 8:125-159.

39. Burg RV. Toxicology update. Bis (2-ethylhexyl) phthalate. *Journal of applied toxicology*, 1988, 8:75-78.

40. Nielsen J, Akesson B, Skerfving S. Phthalate ester exposure – air levels and health of workers processing polyvinylchloride. *American Industrial Hygiene Association journal*, 1985, 46:643-647.

41. International Agency for Research on Cancer. *Overall evaluations of carcinogenicity: an updating of IARC Monographs volumes 1-42*. Lyon, 1987:62 (IARC Monographs on the Evaluation of Carcinogenic Risks to Humans, Suppl. 7).

## 14.22 Acrylamide

### 14.22.1 General description

**Identity**

CAS no.:            79-06-1
Molecular formula:  $C_3H_5NO$

**Physicochemical properties** *(1)*

| Property | Value |
|---|---|
| *Property* | *Value* |
| Physical state | White crystalline solid |
| Melting point | 84–85 °C |
| Boiling point | 125 °C at 3.33 kPa |
| Density | 1.122 g/cm$^3$ at 30 °C |
| Water solubility | 2150 g/l at 30 °C |
| Vapour pressure | 0.009 kPa at 25 °C |

**Major uses**

Most of the acrylamide produced is used as a chemical intermediate or as a monomer in the production of polyacrylamide. Both acrylamide and polyacrylamide are used mainly in the production of flocculants for the clarification of potable water and in the treatment of municipal and industrial effluents. They are also used as grouting agents in the construction of drinking-water reservoirs and wells (*1*).

**Environmental fate**

Acrylamide is highly mobile in aqueous environments and readily leachable in soil. As it has a higher mobility and lower rate of degradation in sandy soils than in clay soils (*2*), it may contaminate groundwater. However, its behaviour in subsurface soil, where most grouting takes place, has not been studied.

Acrylamide is susceptible to biodegradation in both soil and surface water. Its concentration decreased from 20 to 1 μg/litre in 24 h in the effluent from a sludge dewatering process (*3*). One of the most important mechanisms for the removal of acrylamide from soils is enzyme-catalysed hydrolysis; nonbiological hydrolysis may be important in natural water. Volatilization is not an important removal process. As acrylamide is both highly soluble in water and degraded by microorganisms, it is not likely to bioconcentrate significantly (*4*).

### 14.22.2 Analytical methods

The methods used for measuring acrylamide include polarography, electron-capture gas chromatography, and high-performance liquid chromatography.

A high-performance liquid chromatography/ultraviolet absorption detection procedure for the determination of acrylamide in water has a detection range of 0.2–100 µg/litre (5).

## 14.22.3 Environmental levels and human exposure

### Air

Because of its low vapour pressure and high water solubility, acrylamide is not expected to be a common contaminant in air. Available monitoring data are insufficient to confirm this.

### Water

The most important source of drinking-water contamination by acrylamide is the use of polyacrylamide flocculants containing residual levels of acrylamide monomer. Generally, the maximum authorized dose of polymer is 1 mg/litre. At a monomer content of 0.05%, this corresponds to a maximum theoretical concentration of 0.5 µg/litre monomer in water (6). In practice, concentrations may be lower by a factor of 2–3. This applies to both the anionic and nonionic polyacrylamides, but residual levels from cationic polyacrylamides may be higher.

Acrylamide was detected at levels of less than 5 µg/litre in both river water and tapwater in an area where polyacrylamides were used in the treatment of potable water. Samples from public drinking-water supply wells in West Virginia (USA) contained 0.024-0.041 µg of acrylamide per litre. In one study in the United Kingdom tapwater levels in the low microgram per litre range were reported (5).

### Food

No studies on the occurrence of acrylamide in foods were identified. However, polyacrylamide is used in the refining of sugar, and small amounts of acrylamide may remain in the final product.

## 14.22.4 Kinetics and metabolism in laboratory animals and humans

Acrylamide is readily absorbed by ingestion and inhalation, and through the skin (1), and is then widely distributed in body fluids. It can cross the placental barrier. The tissue distribution following intravenous injection of l-[$^{14}$C]acrylamide (100 mg/kg of body weight) into male Porton strain rats was highest (up to 1360 µmol per g of tissue) in blood; progressively lower amounts were present in kidney, liver, brain, spinal cord, sciatic nerve, and plasma (7).

In rats, biotransformation of acrylamide occurs through glutathione conjugation and decarboxylation. At least four urinary metabolites have been found in rat urine; N-acetyl-S-(3-amino-3-oxypropyl)cysteine accounted for 48% of the oral dose, and unmetabolized acrylamide (2%) and three non-sulfur-containing metabolites (total 14%) were also present. Acrylamide and its metabolites are accumulated (protein-bound) in both nervous system tissues and in blood, where it is bound to haemoglobin. Accumulation in the liver and kidney as well as in the male reproductive system has also been demonstrated (8).

The results of animal studies indicate that acrylamide is largely excreted as metabolites in urine and bile. Because of the enterohepatic circulation of biliary metabolites, faecal excretion is minimal. Two-thirds of the absorbed dose is excreted with a half-life of a few hours. However, protein-bound acrylamide or acrylamide metabolites in the blood, and possibly in the central nervous system, have a half-life of about 10 days. Acrylamide has been identified in rat milk during lactation (8).

There are no data indicating any major differences in acrylamide metabolism between humans and other mammals (1).

## 14.22.5 Effects on laboratory animals and *in vitro* test systems

### Acute exposure

Oral $LD_{50}$s for acrylamide were reported to range from 100 to 270 mg/kg of body weight in various strains of mice and rats. The dermal $LD_{50}$ in rats was reported to be 400 mg/kg of body weight (9–12).

### Short-term exposure

Studies have shown convincingly that acrylamide is a cumulative neurotoxin. Rats, cats, and dogs receiving 5–30 mg/kg of body weight per day in the diet exhibited weakness and ataxia in hind limbs for 14–21 days, which progressed to paralysis with continued exposure (13, 14). Other characteristic symptoms were testicular atrophy and degeneration of germinal epithelium (15).

### Long-term exposure

Signs of acrylamide toxicity in animals exposed for longer periods of time (several months to 1 year) are generally the same as those in animals exposed for short times, but average daily doses as low as 1 mg/kg of body weight per day sometimes produce effects. When male and female F344 rats were exposed to 0, 0.05, 0.2, 1.5, or 20 mg/kg of body weight per day in drinking-water for 90 days, definite peripheral nerve and spinal cord lesions and testicular atrophy were observed in the group receiving 20 mg/kg of body weight per day; although 1.5 mg/kg of body weight per day caused no external signs of toxicity, histological evidence of neuropathy was noted. The NOAEL was 0.2 mg/kg of body weight per day (16).

### Reproductive toxicity, embryotoxicity, and teratogenicity

Male Long-Evans rats exposed to acrylamide doses of up to 5.8 mg/kg of body weight per day for 10 weeks in their drinking-water experienced increased pre-implantation and post-implantation loss after mating (*17*). Another series of experiments carried out by the same authors suggested that acrylamide affected the spermatid–spermatozoa stages (*18*).

Acrylamide was administered to pregnant Porton rats either as a single intravenous dose (100 mg/kg of body weight) on day 9 of gestation or in the diet as a cumulative dose of either 200 or 400 mg/kg of body weight between days 0 and 20 of gestation. Apart from a slight decrease in the weight of individual fetuses from rats dosed with 400 mg/kg of body weight, no fetal abnormalities were seen, even at doses that induced neuropathy in the dams (*19*).

When fertilized chicken eggs were injected with 0.03–0.6 mg of acrylamide on days 5, 6, or 7 of incubation, embryonic mortality increased and leg deformities were observed in hatched chicks (*20*).

### Mutagenicity and related end-points

Acrylamide does not cause mutations in bacterial test systems but does cause chromosome damage to mammalian cells both *in vitro* and *in vivo* (*1, 21, 22*).

### Carcinogenicity

Recent results indicate that acrylamide may be a carcinogen. Male and female Fischer 344 rats were given 0, 0.01, 0.02, 0.5, or 2 mg/kg of body weight per day in drinking-water for 2 years. In male rats receiving doses of 0.5 and 2 mg/kg of body weight per day, there was an increase in the frequency of scrotal, thyroid, and adrenal tumours. In female rats receiving 2 mg/kg of body weight per day, there was an increased incidence of malignant tumours of the mammary gland, central nervous system, thyroid, and uterus (*23*).

Eight-week-old A/J male and female mice given oral doses of 6.3, 12.5, or 25.0 mg/kg of body weight three times per week for 3 weeks or intraperitoneal doses of 1, 3, 10, 30, or 60 mg/kg of body weight three times per week for 8 weeks showed a dose-dependent increased incidence of lung adenomas at 9 and 8 months of age, respectively (*22*).

## 14.22.6 Effects on humans

Subacute toxic effects were experienced by a family of five exposed through the ingestion and external use of well-water contaminated with 400 mg of acrylamide per litre as the result of a grouting operation (*24*). Symptoms of toxicity developed about a month later and included confusion, disorientation, memory disturbances, hallucinations, and truncal ataxia. The family recovered fully within 4 months.

Many other cases of human exposure to acrylamide have been reported, generally the result of the dermal or inhalation exposure of workers in grouting operations or factories manufacturing acrylamide-based flocculants (*25–28*). Typical clinical symptoms were skin irritation, generalized fatigue, foot weakness, and sensory changes, which reflect dysfunction of either the central or peripheral nervous system.

## 14.22.7 Guideline value

In mutagenicity assays, acrylamide does not cause mutations in bacterial test systems but does cause chromosome damage to mammalian cells *in vitro* and *in vivo*. In a long-term carcinogenicity study in rats exposed via drinking-water, it induced tumours at various sites (*23*). IARC has placed acrylamide in Group 2B (*29*).

On the basis of the available information, it was concluded that acrylamide is a genotoxic carcinogen. Therefore, the risk evaluation was carried out using a non-threshold approach. On the basis of combined mammary, thyroid, and uterine tumours observed in female rats in a drinking-water study (*23*) and using the linearized multistage model, guideline values associated with excess lifetime cancer risks of $10^{-4}$, $10^{-5}$, and $10^{-6}$ are estimated to be 5, 0.5, and 0.05 µg/litre, respectively.

The most important source of drinking-water contamination by acrylamide is the use of polyacrylamide flocculants that contain residual acrylamide monomer. Although the practical quantification level for acrylamide is generally of the order of 1 µg/litre, concentrations in drinking-water can be controlled by product and dose specification.

## References

1. *Acrylamide.* Geneva, World Health Organization, 1985 (Environmental Health Criteria, No. 49).

2. Lande SS, Bosch SJ, Howard PH. Degradation and leaching of acrylamide in soil. *Journal of environmental quality*, 1979, 8:133-137.

3. Arimitu H, Ikebukuro H, Seto I. The biological degradability of acrylamide monomer. *Journal of the Japan Water Works Association*, 1975, 487:31-39.

4. Neely WB, Baranson DR, Blau CE. Partition coefficient to measure bioconcentration potential of organic chemicals in fish. *Environmental science and technology*, 1974, 8:1113-1115.

5. Brown L, Rhead MM. Liquid chromatographic determination of acrylamide monomer in natural and polluted aqueous environments. *Analyst*, 1979, 104:391-399.

6.  National Sanitation Foundation. Drinking water treatment chemicals – health effects. Ann Arbor, MI, 1988 (Standard 60–1988).

7.  Hashimoto K, Aldridge WN. Biochemical studies on acrylamide, a neurotoxic agent. *Biochemical pharmacology*, 1970, 19:2591-2604.

8.  Miller MJ, Carter DE, Sipes IG. Pharmacokinetics of acrylamide in Fischer-344 rats. *Toxicology and applied pharmacology*, 1982, 63:36-44.

9.  Fullerton PM, Barnes JM. Peripheral neuropathy in rats produced by acrylamide. *British journal of industrial medicine*, 1966, 23:210-221.

10.  Paulet G, Vidal. [On the toxicity of some acrylic and methacrylic esters, acrylamide and polyacrylamides.] *Archives des maladies professionnelles, de médecine du travail et de sécurité sociale*, 1975, 36:58-60 (in French).

11.  Tilson HA, Cabe PA. The effects of acrylamide given acutely or in repeated doses on fore- and hindlimb function of rats. *Toxicology and applied pharmacology*, 1979, 47:253-260.

12.  Hashimoto K, Sakamoto J, Tanii H. Neurotoxicity of acrylamide and related compounds and their effects on male gonads in mice. *Archives of toxicology*, 1981, 47:179-189.

13.  Leswing RJ, Ribelin WE. Physiologic and pathologic changes in acrylamide neuropathy. *Archives of environmental health*, 1969, 18:23-29.

14.  Thomann P et al. The assessment of peripheral neurotoxicity in dogs: comparative studies with acrylamide and clioquinol. *Agents and actions*, 1974, 4:47-53.

15.  McCollister DD, Oyen F, Rowe VK. Toxicology of acrylamide. *Toxicology and applied pharmacology*, 1964, 6:172-181.

16.  Burek JD et al. Subchronic toxicity of acrylamide administered to rats in the drinking water followed by up to 144 days of recovery. *Journal of environmental pathology and toxicology*, 1980, 4:157-182.

17.  Smith MK et al. Dominant lethal effects of subchronic acrylamide administration in the male Long-Evans rat. *Mutation research*, 1986, 173:273-278.

18.  Sublet V et al. Spermatogenic stages associated with acrylamide (ACR) induced dominant lethality. *Toxicology*, 1986, 6:292 (abstract).

19.  Edwards PM. The insensitivity of the developing rat fetus to the toxic effects of acrylamide. *Chemico-biological interactions*, 1976, 12:13-l8.

20.  Parker RDR, Sharma RP, Obersteiner EJ. Acrylamide toxicity in developing chick embryo. *Pharmacologist*, 1978, 20:249 (Abstract No. 522).

21. Shiraishi Y. Chromosome aberrations induced by monomeric acrylamide in bone marrow and germ cells of mice. *Mutation research*, 1978, 57:313-324.

22. Bull RJ et al. Carcinogenic effects of acrylamide in Sencar and A/J mice. *Cancer research*, 1984, 44:107-111.

23. Johnson KA et al. Chronic toxicity and oncogenicity study on acrylamide incorporated in the drinking water of Fischer 344 rats. *Toxicology and applied pharmacology*, 1986, 85:154-168.

24. Igisu H et al. Acrylamide encephaloneuropathy due to well water pollution. *Journal of neurology, neurosurgery and psychiatry*, 1975, 38:581-584.

25. Auld RB, Bedwell SF. Peripheral neuropathy with sympathetic overactivity from industrial contact with acrylamide. *Canadian Medical Association journal*, 1967, 96:652-654.

26. Garland TO, Patterson MWH. Six cases of acrylamide poisoning. *British medical journal*, 1967, 4:134-138.

27. Fullerton PM. Electrophysiological and histological observations on peripheral nerves in acrylamide poisoning in man. *Journal of neurology, neurosurgery and psychiatry*, 1969, 32:186-192.

28. Davenport JG, Farrell DF, Sumi SM. Giant axonal neuropathy caused by industrial chemicals. *Neurology*, 1976, 26:919-923.

29. International Agency for Research on Cancer. *Overall evaluations of carcinogenicity: an updating of IARC Monographs volumes 1-42.* Lyon, 1987:56 (IARC Monographs on the Evaluation of Carcinogenic Risks to Humans, Suppl. 7).

## 14.23 Epichlorohydrin

14.23.1 General description

### *Identity*

CAS no.: 106-89-8
Molecular formula: $C_3H_5ClO$

Synonyms of epichlorohydrin (ECH) include 1-chloro-2,3-epoxypropane, 3-chloro-1,2-epoxypropane, 1-chloropropeneoxide, and 3-chloropropeneoxide.

### Physicochemical properties (1, 2 )[1]

| Property | Value |
|---|---|
| Physical state | Colourless liquid |
| Melting point | -25.6 °C |
| Boiling point | 116.2 °C |
| Vapour pressure | 1.60 kPa at 20 °C |
| Density | 1.18 g/cm$^3$ at 20 °C |
| Water solubility | 66 g/litre at 20 °C |
| Log octanol–water partition coefficient | 0.26 |

### Major uses

ECH is used mainly for the manufacture of glycerol and unmodified epoxy resins, and to a lesser extent in the manufacture of elastomers, water-treatment resins, surfactants, ion exchange resins, plasticizers, dyestuffs, pharmaceutical products, oil emulsifiers, lubricants, and adhesives (3).

### Environmental fate

ECH is released to the environment as a result of its manufacture, use, storage, transport, and disposal. Its half-lives in neutral, acidic, and alkaline solutions are 148, 79, and 62 h at room temperature, respectively. The rate of hydrolysis increases sevenfold when the temperature is raised to 40 °C (4).

## 14.23.2 Analytical methods

ECH in water can be determined by a purge-and-trap gas chromatographic/mass spectrometric procedure (GC-MS) (2), and by gas chromatography with flame-ionization (5) (detection limit 0.01 mg/litre), or electron-capture detection (6) (detection limit 0.05 µg/litre). A GC-MS method can also be used for the determination of ECH in ambient water and sediment (7) (detection limit 0.003 µg/litre).

## 14.23.3 Environmental levels and human exposure

### Air

Data on ambient air levels of ECH are extremely limited and relate mainly to occupational exposure. At 100–200 m from a factory discharging ECH into the atmosphere in the former USSR, the airborne ECH concentration ranged

---

[1] Conversion factor in air: 1 ppm = 3.78 mg/cm$^3$.

from 0.5 to 1.2 mg/m$^3$. At 400 m, 5 out of 29 samples had levels exceeding 0.2 mg/m$^3$, whereas no ECH was detected at 600 m (*3, 8*).

## Water

ECH can enter drinking-water supplies through the use of flocculating agents containing it and through leaching from epoxy resin coatings on pipes. No ECH residue was found in water kept in containers coated with epoxy resins (detection limit 3 µg/litre) (*9*).

## Food

Migration into food and drinking-water of ECH used as a cross-linking agent in packing materials and epoxy resins is possible but is expected to be low (*3*). No studies on its occurrence in food were identified. The compound has little potential for bioaccumulation in the food-chain (*10*).

## 14.23.4 Kinetics and metabolism in laboratory animals and humans

The pharmacokinetics of ECH have been reviewed by WHO (*3*) and the US Environmental Protection Agency (*2*). It is rapidly and extensively absorbed following oral administration and may be absorbed following both inhalation and dermal exposures (*11*).

Following oral administration of [$^{14}$C]-ECH to rats, peak tissue levels were reached after 2 h in males and 2–8 h in females, depending on the tissue. The tissues containing the highest levels of radioactivity were the kidneys, liver, pancreas, spleen, and adrenal glands. ECH is rapidly removed from blood and is therefore not likely to accumulate during chronic exposures. Metabolites of ECH, however, are much more persistent and may therefore accumulate to a small extent during chronic exposures (*11*).

ECH has two electrophilic centres, C1 and C3, and may thus bind to cellular nucleophiles such as glutathione. This binding is catalysed by glutathione-*S*-epoxide transferase, resulting in a considerable increase in reaction rate. The major metabolites in urine were identified as *N*-acetyl-*S*-(3-chloro-2-hydroxy-propyl)-L-cysteine, formed by conjugation with glutathione, and α-chloro-hydrin, accounting for about 36% and 4% of the administered dose, respectively (*11, 12*).

Following oral administration and inhalation, ECH metabolites are rapidly excreted in the urine and expired air. Urinary excretion is approximately twice that in expired air. Only minor amounts (4%) are excreted in the faeces. Unmetabolized ECH has not been detected in any excreta (*11*).

## 14.23.5 Effects on laboratory animals and *in vitro* test systems

### Acute exposure

ECH is a strong irritant and acutely toxic following oral, percutaneous, subcutaneous, or respiratory exposure. Death is due to effects on the central nervous system and the respiratory centre (*13*). Oral $LD_{50}$s were reported to range from 90 to 260 mg/kg of body weight in rats (*2*).

### Long-term exposure

There was a gradual increase in mortality following the oral administration of ECH in water by gavage to weanling Wistar rats of both sexes for 5 days per week for 2 years; clinical symptoms included dyspnoea, weight loss, a decrease in leukocytes, and hyperplasia in the forestomach at 2 and 10 mg/kg of body weight per day (*14*).

Lifetime inhalation of ECH by non-inbred male SD rats for 6 h per day, 5 days per week, caused weight loss, high mortality, severe inflammatory changes in the nasal cavity, lung congestion and pneumonia, tubular dilation, and dose-dependent tubular degeneration in the kidney at 38 and 114 mg/m$^3$ (*15*).

### Reproductive toxicity, embryotoxicity, and teratogenicity

The sperm of rats that had received an oral dose of 25 or 50 mg of ECH per kg of body weight showed an increased percentage of abnormal sperm heads at the higher dose and a reduced number of sperm heads at the lower dose; no microscopic changes in the testes or changes in their weight were observed (*16*). When male rabbits and male and female rats were exposed for 6 h per day, 5 days per week, to ECH vapour at concentrations of 0, 19.7, 93.4, or 189.0 mg/m$^3$ for 10 weeks, a dose-related transient infertility was induced at the two highest levels in male rats but not in female rats or male rabbits. Microscopic examination did not reveal any abnormalities in the reproductive organs. The sperm of the rabbits was investigated, but no adverse effects were found (*17*).

Female rats received oral doses of 0, 40, 80, or 160 mg of ECH per kg of body weight per day and female mice received 0, 80, 120, or 160 mg of ECH per kg of body weight per day in cottonseed oil between days 6 and 15 of pregnancy. Although the highest dose levels were toxic to the dams, no embryotoxic, fetotoxic, or teratogenic effects were observed (*18*). Similar negative results were obtained when female rats and rabbits inhaled vapours of ECH at concentrations of 0, 9.4, or 94.5 mg/m$^3$ for 7 h per day between days 6 and 15 or 18 of pregnancy (*19*).

## Mutagenicity and related end-points

ECH induced base-change-type mutations in *Salmonella typhimurium* and *Escherichia coli* in the absence of metabolic activation (*20*). It has been shown to cause chromosomal aberrations in mammalian cells *in vitro* (*3*) but was negative in the mouse micronucleus assay (*21*) and in the mouse dominant lethal assay (*22*).

## Carcinogenicity

Male Wistar rats that received 18, 39, or 89 mg of ECH per kg of body weight per day in drinking-water for 81 weeks developed forestomach tumours characterized as squamous cell papillomas and carcinomas at the two highest doses and hyperplasia at all three doses (*23*). Similar findings were reported in a 104-week study in which Wistar rats were given 0, 2, or 10 mg of ECH per kg of body weight by gavage in distilled water (*24*). Male SD rats exposed for 30 days to ECH at 378 mg/m$^3$ of air, 6 h per day, 5 days per week, developed squamous cell carcinomas in the nasal cavities during subsequent lifetime observation (*15*). In 100 rats, lifetime exposure to 113 mg/m$^3$ yielded only one malignant squamous cell carcinoma of the nasal cavity and one nasal papilloma. Subcutaneous injection of EHC in ICR/Ha Swiss mice induced local sarcomas and adenocarcinomas (*25*).

## 14.23.6 Effects on humans

Acute toxic responses following dermal exposure are characterized by an initial redness and itching or burning sensation. With time, the redness intensifies and the tissue becomes swollen and blistered. The initial symptoms following inhalation are local irritation, burning of the eyes and throat, swelling of the face, nausea, vomiting, and severe headache (*26*).

In a case study, long-term effects due primarily to damage to the liver and kidneys were still present 2 years after exposure (*26*). In workers occupationally exposed to ECH, increased incidences of chromatid and chromosomal breaks in peripheral lymphocytes and decreases in blood cell counts were observed (*27*).

An epidemiological study was undertaken on 863 workers with probable exposure to ECH at two chemical plants (*28*). All deaths due to cancer and leukaemia, and deaths from most other causes, were related to estimated levels of exposure to ECH. The most consistent relationship was between exposure level and heart disease.

The fertility status of 64 glycerol workers in the USA exposed to ECH, allyl chloride, and 1,3-dichloropropane was compared with that of a control group of 63 workers who had not handled chlorinated hydrocarbons for more than 5 years. No association was found between levels, duration, or intensity of exposure and sperm characteristics or hormone levels (*29*). A similar negative result for sperm count and hormone levels was obtained for a group of 128 workers from two plants compared with other chemical plant workers who had not been exposed to any chemical known to be toxic to the testes. In one of these plants, most of the employees were exposed to ECH concentrations below 3.8 mg/m³. The number of non-participating employees was high in both plants, namely 172 in total (*30*).

## 14.23.7 Provisional guideline value

The major toxic effects of ECH are local irritation and damage to the central nervous system. In rats, by the inhalation and oral routes, it induces squamous cell carcinomas in the nasal cavity and forestomach tumours, respectively. It has been shown to be genotoxic *in vitro* and *in vivo*. IARC has placed ECH in Group 2A (probably carcinogenic to humans) (*31*).

Although ECH is a genotoxic carcinogen, the use of the linearized multistage model for estimating cancer risk was considered inappropriate because tumours are seen only at the site of administration, where ECH is highly irritating. A TDI of 0.14 µg/kg of body weight was therefore calculated by applying an uncertainty factor of 10 000 (10 for the use of a LOAEL instead of a NOAEL, 100 for inter- and intraspecies variation, and 10 reflecting carcinogenicity) to a LOAEL of 2 mg/kg of body weight per day for forestomach hyperplasia in a 2-year study in rats by gavage (administration 5 days per week) (*14*). This gives a provisional guideline value of 0.4 µg/litre (rounded figure) based on an allocation of 10% of the TDI to drinking-water. A practical quantification level for ECH is of the order of 30 µg/litre, but concentrations in drinking-water can be controlled by specifying the ECH content of products coming into contact with water.

## References

1. International Agency for Research on Cancer. *Cadmium, nickel, some epoxides, miscellaneous industrial chemicals and general considerations on volatile anaesthetics.* Lyon, 1976:131-139 (IARC Monographs on the Evaluation of Carcinogenic Risk of Chemicals to Man, Volume 11).

2. Office of Health and Drinking Water. *Health advisory for epichlorohydrin.* Washington, DC, US Environmental Protection Agency, 1987.

3. *Epichlorohydrin.* Geneva, World Health Organization, 1984 (Environmental Health Criteria, No. 33).

4. von Piringer O. [Kinetics of the hydrolysis of epichlorohydrin in diluted aqueous solutions.] *Deutsche Lebensmittel-Rundschau,* 1980, 76:11-13 (in German).

5. Japan Water Works Association. [*Standard JWWA K 135: liquid epoxide resin coats for water supply facilities.*] Tokyo, 1989 (in Japanese).

6. Pesselman RL, Feit MJ. Determination of residual epichlorohydrin and 3-chloro-propanediol in water by gas chromatography with electron-capture detection. *Journal of chromatography*, 1988, 439(2):448-452.

7. Japan Environmental Agency. [*Annual report on developments and researches for chemical substances analysis.*] Tokyo, 1986 (in Japanese).

8. Fomin AP. [Biological action of epichlorohydrin and its hygienic significance as an atmospheric contamination factor.] *Gigiena i sanitarija*, 1966, 31:7-11 (in Russian).

9. van Lierop JBH. Simple and rapid determination of epichlorohydrin at the lower parts per billion level by gas chromatography–mass fragmentography. *Journal of chromatography*, 1978, 166:609-610.

10. Santodonato J et al. *Investigation of selected potential environmental contaminants: epichlorohydrin and epibromohydrin.* New York, Syracuse Research Corporation, New York Center for Chemical Hazard Assessment, 1980 (EPA-560/11-80-006).

11. Gingell R et al. Disposition and metabolism of 2-[14]C-epichlorohydrin after oral administration to rats. *Drug metabolism and disposition*, 1985, 13:333-341.

12. Gingell R et al. Evidence that epichlorohydrin is not a toxic metabolite of 1,2-dibromo-3-chloropropane. *Xenobiotica*, 1987, 17:229-240.

13. Freuder E, Leake CD. The toxicity of epichlorohydrin. *University of California, Berkeley, publications in pharmacology*, 1941, 2(5):69-78.

14. Wester PW, Van der Heijden CA, Van Esch GJ. Carcinogenicity study with epichlorohydrin (CEP) by gavage in rats. *Toxicology*, 1985, 36:325-339.

15. Laskin S, Sellakumar AR, Kuschner M. Inhalation carcinogenicity of epichlorohydrin in noninbred Sprague-Dawley rats. *Journal of the National Cancer Institute*, 1980, 65(4):751-758.

16. Cassidy SL, Dix KM, Jenkins T. Evaluation of a testicular sperm head counting technique using rats exposed to dimethoxyethyl phthalate (DMEP), glycerol α-monochlorohydrin (GMCH), epichlorohydrin (ECH), formaldehyde (FA), or methyl methanesulphonate (MMS). *Archives of toxicology*, 1983, 53:71-78.

17. John JA et al. Inhalation toxicity of epichlorohydrin: effects on fertility in rats and rabbits. *Toxicology and applied pharmacology*, 1983, 68:415-423.

18. Marks T, Gerling FS, Staples RE. Teratogenic evaluation of epichlorohydrin in the mouse and rat and glycidol in the mouse. *Journal of toxicology and environmental health*, 1982, 9:87-96.

19. John JA et al. Teratologic evaluation of inhaled epichlorohydrin and allyl chloride in rats and rabbits. *Fundamental and applied toxicology*, 1983, 3:437-442.

20. Bridges BA. On the detection of volatile liquid mutagens with bacteria: experiments with dichlorvos and epichlorohydrin. *Mutation research*, 1978, 54:367-371.

21. Kirkhart B. Micronucleus test on 21 compounds. In: deSerres FJ, Ashby J, eds. *Evaluation of short-term tests for carcinogens*. Amsterdam, Elsevier/North Holland, 1981: 698-704.

22. Epstein SS et al. Detection of chemical mutagens by the dominant lethal assay in the mouse. *Toxicology and applied pharmacology*, 1972, 23:288-325.

23. Konishi Y, Kawabata A, Denda A. Forestomach tumors induced by orally administered epichlorohydrin in male Wistar rats. *Gann*, 1980, 71:922-923.

24. Van Esch GJ, Wester PW. *Induction of preneoplastic lesions in the forestomach of rats after oral administration of 1-chloro-2,3-epoxypropane. II. Carcinogenicity study*. Bilthoven, Netherlands, National Institute of Public Health and Environmental Protection, 1982.

25. Van Duuren BL, Goldschmidt BM, Paul JS. Carcinogenic activity of alkylating agents. *Journal of the National Cancer Institute*, 1974, 53:695-700.

26. Schultz VC. Fettleber und chronisch-asthmoide Bronchitis nach Inhalation eines Farbenlösungsmittels (Epichlorohydrin). [Fatty liver and chronic asthmoid bronchitis following inhalation of a paint solvent (epichlorohydrin).] *Deutsche medizinische Wochenschrift*, 1964, 89:1342-1344.

27. Sram RJ, Zudova Z, Kuleshov NP. Cytogenetic analysis of peripheral lymphocytes in workers occupationally exposed to epichlorohydrin. *Mutation research*, 1980, 70:115-120.

28. Enterline PE, Henderson V, Marsh G. Mortality of workers potentially exposed to epichlorohydrin. *British journal of industrial medicine*, 1990, 47:269-276.

29. Venable JR et al. A fertility study of male employees engaged in the manufacture of glycerine. *Journal of occupational medicine*, 1980, 22:87-91.

30. Milby TH et al. Testicular function among epichlorohydrin workers. *British journal of industrial medicine*, 1981, 38:372-377.

31. International Agency for Research on Cancer. *Overall evaluations of carcinogenicity: an updating of IARC Monographs volumes 1-42*. Lyon, 1987:202-203 (IARC Monographs on the Evaluation of Carcinogenic Risks to Humans, Suppl. 7).

# 14.24 Hexachlorobutadiene

## 14.24.1 General description

### Identity

CAS no.:           87-68-3
Molecular formula:  $C_4Cl_6$

Synonyms of hexachlorobutadiene (HCBD) include perchlorobutadiene, 1,3-hexachlorobutadiene, and 1,1,2,3,4,4-hexachloro-1,3-butadiene.

### Physicochemical properties (1)

| Property | Value |
|---|---|
| Physical state | Clear, colourless liquid |
| Melting point | -19 to -22 °C |
| Boiling point | 210–220 °C |
| Density | 1.55 g/cm$^3$ at 20 °C |
| Vapour pressure | 0.02 kPa at 20 °C |
| Log octanol–water partition coefficient | 3.67 |
| Water solubility | 2.6 mg/litre |

### Organoleptic properties

The odour threshold for HCBD in air is 12 mg/m$^3$ (2).

### Major uses

HCBD is used as a solvent in chlorine gas production, an intermediate in the manufacture of rubber compounds, a lubricant, a gyroscopic fluid, a pesticide, and a fumigant in vineyards (1).

### Environmental fate

HCBD may not volatilize rapidly from water because of its low vapour pressure. Adsorption onto soil particles in water is important.

## 14.24.2 Analytical methods

HCBD can be determined by means of gas chromatography; the minimum detection limit is 0.34 µg/litre. The purge-and-trap gas chromatography/mass spectrometry (GC-MS) technique has a minimum detection limit of 0.4 µg/litre. Closed-loop stripping analysis with GC-MS can detect HCBD at nanogram per litre levels (3).

## 14.24.3 Environmental levels and human exposure

### *Air*

In a study of nine chemical plants, the highest levels of HCBD in air were found near those producing tetrachloroethene and trichloroethene (maximum 463 µg/m$^3$) (*1*).

### *Water*

In Europe, HCBD was detected in ambient water at 0.05–5 µg/litre, and in the USA at 0.9–1.9 µg/litre in Mississippi River water. It was also found in mud and soil at concentrations of up to 800 µg/kg in Louisiana (*1*). In the Rhine HCBD was found at concentrations of 0.1–5 µg/litre (*1*). HCBD was not detected in ambient water and mud in Japan (minimum detection limits: water 0.02 µg/litre; mud 2–200 µg/g) (*4*). It has been detected at 6.4 µg/litre in the effluent from a European chemical plant and at 0.27 µg/litre in European drinking-water (*1*).

### *Food*

HCBD residues have been found at levels of 4 µg/kg in evaporated milk, 42 µg/kg in egg yolk, and 33 µg/kg in margarine. They were found in the United Kingdom at levels of 0.08 µg/kg in fresh milk, 2 µg/kg in butter, 0.2 µg/kg in cooking oil, 0.2 µg/kg in light ale, 0.8 µg/kg in tomatoes, and 3.7 µg/kg in black grapes (*1*).

## 14.24.4 Kinetics and metabolism in laboratory animals and humans

In rats, about 95% of the ingested dose of HCBD is absorbed (*5*); it was found in the blood, liver, and brain 3 h after a single injection and in the kidney, spleen, and mesentery after 6 h (*6*). When a mixture of chlorinated hydrocarbons, including HCBD, was administered orally to rats at doses of 2 or 4 mg/kg of body weight per day for up to 12 weeks, less than 7 mg of HCBD per kg of body weight accumulated in adipose tissue (*7*).

HCBD is metabolized in rats and mice via conjugation with glutathione (GSH), followed by biliary excretion of *S*-(1,2,3,4,4-pentachloro-1,3-butadienyl)-GSH (PCBD-GSH) (*5, 8, 9*). The GSH conjugate of HCBD is further metabolized in the gastrointestinal tract and kidney to a number of water-soluble metabolites that are excreted mainly in the urine (*5, 9*). Experimental evidence suggests that the metabolism of PCBD-GSH involves, in part, degradation to PCBD-cysteine (PCBD-Cys), which is nephrotoxic via activation of the renal enzyme Cys conjugate β-lyase (*5, 9, 10*). PCBD-Cys is *N*-acetylated, presumably in a detoxification reaction, to give the mercapturic acid, *N*-acetyl-PCBD-Cys (*11*).

After a single oral administration of [$^{14}$C]-HCBD to rats, the principal route of excretion was in the bile; 17–20% of the initial dose was excreted on each of the first 2 days. Extensive enterohepatic circulation must have occurred, because faecal elimination amounted to only 5% of the total dose of radioactivity per day (5). In another study, 42–67% and 11-31% of the radioactivity was excreted in the faeces and urine by 72 h, respectively (9). Similar results were obtained in mice (67.5–76.7% in faeces, 6.6–7.6% in urine) (12).

## 14.24.5 Effects on laboratory animals and *in vitro* test systems

### Acute exposure

Oral LD$_{50}$s were reported to be 200–400 and 504–667 mg/kg of body weight, in adult female and male rats, respectively (13).

### Short-term exposure

Weanling Wistar rats given HCBD by gavage for 13 weeks at dose levels of 0, 0.4, 1, 2.5, 6.3, or 15.6 mg/kg of body weight per day exhibited an increase in relative kidney weight at the two highest doses and degeneration of the proximal renal tubules at and above 2.5 mg/kg of body weight per day (females) or 6.3 mg/kg of body weight per day (males). Increased cytoplasmic basophilia of hepatocytes associated with an increase in liver weight occurred in males at the two highest doses (14).

### Long-term exposure

The kidney was the primary target organ in a study in which Sprague-Dawley rats were given HCBD by feed for 2 years at dose levels of 0, 0.2, 2, or 20 mg/kg of body weight per day. Effects included a treatment-related increase in relative and absolute kidney weights in males at 20 mg/kg of body weight per day, an increased incidence of multifocal or disseminated renal tubular epithelial hyperplasia in rats at 20 and possibly at 2 mg/kg of body weight per day, and focal adenomatous proliferation of renal tubular epithelial cells in some males at 20 mg/kg of body weight per day and some females at 20 and 2 mg/kg of body weight per day. No discernible ill effects attributable to treatment were found at 0.2 mg/kg of body weight per day, which was the NOAEL in this study (15).

### Reproductive toxicity, embryotoxicity, and teratogenicity

In a 148-day study in which groups of 10–17 male and 20–34 female adult rats per group were fed diets containing HCBD at doses of 0, 0.2, 2.0, or 20 mg/kg of body weight per day for 90 days prior to mating, 15 days during mating, and subsequently throughout gestation (22 days) and lactation (21 days), there were no treatment-related effects on pregnancy or neonatal survival. The body weights of 21-day-old weanlings in the highest dose group were slightly but significantly lower than those of controls. No toxic effects were observed in neonates at doses of 0.2 or 2.0 mg/kg of body weight per day (13).

When oral doses of 8.1 mg of HCBD per kg of body weight per day were given to pregnant rats throughout gestation, ultrastructural changes in neurocytes and higher levels of free radicals in the brain and spinal cord were seen in the offspring, which also had lower body weights and shorter crown–rump lengths than controls (16).

Pups of rats injected intraperitoneally with 10 mg of HCBD per kg of body weight per day on days 1–15 of gestation experienced three times as many soft tissue anomalies as controls, although no particular type of anomaly was predominant (17).

### Mutagenicity and related end-points

Negative results have been reported in most (18,19) but not all (20) tests for the mutagenicity of HCBD in Ames test *Salmonella* strains. Metabolites and derivatives of HCBD were mutagenic to *Salmonella typhimurium* with metabolic activation (11, 21), and some putative metabolites were mutagenic in this organism without such activation (8).

### Carcinogenicity

Administration of HCBD in the diet at doses of 20 mg/kg of body weight per day for 2 years caused renal tubular adenomas and adenocarcinomas in SD rats. No renal tubular neoplasms were observed in rats ingesting 2.0 or 0.2 mg/kg of body weight per day. The authors concluded that HCBD-induced renal neoplasms developed only at doses higher than those causing discernible renal injury (15). Induction of lung adenomas was not observed in male strain A mice following intraperitoneal administration of HCBD (4 or 8 mg/kg of body weight) three times per week until a total of 52 or 96 mg had been administered (22). It did not act as an initiator in an initiation/promotion experiment in mouse skin, nor did it cause tumours in the skin or distant organs after repeated application to the skin (23).

## 14.24.6 Effects on humans

Farm workers exposed intermittently for 4 years to HCBD exhibited higher incidences of hypotension, myocardial dystrophy, nervous disorder, liver function disorders, and respiratory tract lesions (24).

## 14.24.7 Guideline value

Kidney tumours were observed in a long-term oral study in rats. HCBD has not been shown to be carcinogenic by other routes of exposure. IARC has placed HCBD in Group 3 (*25*). Both positive and negative results for HCBD have been obtained in bacterial assays for point mutation; however, several metabolites have given positive results.

On the basis of the available metabolic and toxicological information, it was considered that a TDI approach was most appropriate for derivation of a guideline value. A TDI of 0.2 µg/kg of body weight was therefore calculated by applying an uncertainty factor of 1000 (100 for inter- and intraspecies variation and 10 for limited evidence of carcinogenicity and the genotoxicity of some metabolites) to the NOAEL of 0.2 mg/kg of body weight per day for renal toxicity in a 2-year feeding study in rats (*15*). This gives a guideline value of 0.6 µg/litre, based on an allocation of 10% of the TDI to drinking-water. A practical quantification level for HCBD is of the order of 2 µg/litre, but concentrations in drinking-water can be controlled by specifying the HCBD content of products coming into contact with water.

## References

1.  International Agency for Research on Cancer. *Some halogenated hydrocarbons.* Lyon, 1979:179-193 (IARC Monographs on the Evaluation of the Carcinogenic Risk of Chemicals to Humans, Volume 20).

2.  Ruth JH. Odor thresholds and irritation levels of several chemical substances: A review. *Journal of the American Industrial Hygiene Association*, 1986, 47:A142-A151.

3.  Li RT, Going JE, Spigarelli JL. *Sampling and analysis of selected toxic substances, Task IB-Hexachlorobutadiene.* US Environmental Protection Agency, 1976 (Report No. EPA-560/6-76-015; available from National Technical Information Service, Springfield, VA, as report no. PB253491).

4.  Office of Health Studies. [*Chemicals in the environment.*] Tokyo, Japan Environment Agency, Environmental Health Department, 1982 (in Japanese).

5.  Nash JA et al. The metabolism and disposition of hexachloro-1,3-butadiene in the rat and its relevance to nephrotoxicity. *Toxicology and applied pharmacology*, 1984, 73:124-137.

6.  Gul'ko AG, Dranovskaja KM. [Distribution and excretion of hexachlorobutadiene from rats.] *Aktual'nye voprosy epidemiologij*, 1974, 1972:58-60 (in Russian) (*Chemical abstracts*, 1974, 81:346q).

7.  Jacobs A et al. [Accumulation of noxious chlorinated substances from Rhine River water in fatty tissue of rat.] *Vom Wasser*, 1974, 43:259 (in German).

8. Dekant W et al. Bacterial beta-lyase mediated cleavage and mutagenicity of cysteine conjugates derived from the nephrocarcinogenic alkenes, trichloroethylene, tetrachloroethylene and hexachlorobutadiene. *Chemico-biological interactions*, 1986, 60: 31-45.

9. Reichert D, Schutz S, Metzler M. Excretion pattern and metabolism of hexachlorobutadiene in rats. *Biochemical pharmacology*, 1985, 34:499-505.

10. Jaffe DR et al. *In vivo* and *in vitro* nephrotoxicity of the cysteine conjugate of hexachlorobutadiene. *Journal of toxicology and environmental health*, 1983, 11:857-867.

11. Reichert D, Schutz S. Mercapturic acid formation is an activation and intermediary step in the metabolism of hexachlorobutadiene. *Biochemical pharmacology*, 1986, 35:1271-1275.

12. Dekant W et al. Metabolism of hexachloro-1,3-butadiene in mice: *in vivo* and *in vitro* evidence for activation by glutathione conjugation. *Xenobiotica*, 1988, 18:803-816.

13. Schwetz BA et al. Results of a reproduction study in rats fed diets containing hexachlorobutadiene. *Toxicology and applied pharmacology*, 1977, 42:387-398.

14. Harleman JH, Seinen W. Short-term toxicity and reproduction studies in rats with hexachloro-(1,3)-butadiene. *Toxicology and applied pharmacology*, 1979, 47:1-14.

15. Kociba RJ et al. Results of a two-year chronic toxicity study with hexachlorobutadiene in rats. *Journal of the American Industrial Hygiene Association*, 1977, 38:589-602.

16. Badaeva LN, Ovsiannikova LM, Kiseleva NI. [Manifestation of the neurotoxic effect of the organochlorine pesticide hexachlorobutadiene in the postnatal period of ontogeny in the rat]. *Arkhiv anatomiĭ, gistologiĭ i embriologiĭ*, 1985, 89(8):44-49 (in Russian).

17. Harris SJ, Bond GP, Niemeier RW. The effect of 2-nitropropane, naphthalene and hexachlorobutadiene on fetal rat development. *Toxicology and applied pharmacology*, 1979, 48:A35 (Abstract).

18. Vamvakas S et al. Mutagenicity of hexachloro-1,3-butadiene and its S-conjugates in the Ames test—role of activation of the mercapturic acid pathway in its nephrocarcinogenicity. *Carcinogenesis*, 1988, 9:907-910.

19. Reichert D et al. Mutagenicity of dichloroacetylene and its degradation products trichloroacetyl chloride, trichloroacryloyl chloride and hexachlorobutadiene. *Mutation research*, 1983, 117:21-29.

20. Reichert D, Neudecker T, Schutz S. Mutagenicity of hexachlorobutadiene, perchlorobutenoic acid and perchlorobutenoic acid chloride. *Mutation research*, 1984, 137:89-93.

21. Wild D, Schutz S, Reichert D. Mutagenicity of the mercapturic acid and other S-containing derivatives of hexachloro-1,3-butadiene. *Carcinogenesis*, 1986, 7:431-434.

22. Theiss JC et al. Tests for carcinogenicity of organic contaminants of United States drinking waters by pulmonary tumor response in strain A mice. *Cancer research*, 1977, 37:2717-2720.

23. Van Duuren BL et al. Carcinogenicity of halogenated olefinic and aliphatic hydrocarbons in mice. *Journal of the National Cancer Institute*, 1979, 63:1433-1439.

24. Krasniuk EP et al. [Health condition of vine-growers in contact with fumigants hexachlorobutadiene and polychlorbutan-80.] *Vrachnoi Delo*, 1969, 7:111-115 (in Russian).

25. International Agency for Research on Cancer. *Overall evaluations of carcinogenicity: an updating of IARC Monographs volumes 1-42.* Lyon, 1987:64 (IARC Monographs on the Evaluation of Carcinogenic Risks to Humans, 1987, Suppl. 7).

# 14.25 Edetic acid

## 14.25.1 General description

### Identity

CAS no.:            60-00-4
Molecular formula:  $C_{10}H_{16}N_2O_8$

Edetic acid (ethylenediaminetetraacetic acid) and its salts are commonly referred to as EDTA. The IUPAC name for EDTA is (1,2-ethanediyldinitrilo)tetraacetic-acid.

### Physicochemical properties (1)

| Property | Value |
|---|---|
| Physical state | White crystalline solid |
| Melting point | Decomposes at 240 °C |
| Water solubility | 0.5 g/litre at 25 °C |

### Organoleptic properties

EDTA has a slight salty taste (1).

### Major uses

EDTA is widely used in many industrial processes, in agriculture, in domestic products, including food additives, and in drugs for chelation therapy; calcium EDTA is the drug of choice in the treatment of lead poisoning in humans and domestic animals. EDTA is also used in laundry detergents, cosmetics, photo-chemicals, pharmaceuticals, galvanizing, water softening, electroplating, polymerization, textile treatments, and paper production.

### Environmental fate

EDTA is only poorly degraded in the aquatic environment (2). It is present in the environment in the form of metal complexes (3). Although the mobilization of heavy metals by EDTA in water is a matter of some concern, it has been calculated that 40 µg of EDTA per litre—the maximum concentration observed in the Rhine and Meuse—would complex at most 4–15 µg of metals per litre. This would be likely to pose problems for drinking-water with regard to cadmium, but the effect on cadmium leaching would be limited because EDTA is primarily bound to other metals at these concentrations (2).

## 14.25.2 Analytical methods

EDTA can be determined by potentiometric stripping analysis, which has been used to measure EDTA in a wide variety of wastewater and natural water samples; it has a detection limit of 1 µg/litre (4).

## 14.25.3 Environmental levels and human exposure

### Water

EDTA is released to the aquatic environment in industrial emissions. It has been estimated that concentrations of 50–500 µg/litre are present in wastewaters (2).

Measured concentrations in natural waters have been reported to range from 10 to 70 µg/litre; the median value is 23 µg/litre (5). Annual average concentrations of EDTA in European surface waters ranged from 1 µg/litre to over 60 µg/litre; a concentration of 900 µg/litre was found in the Zerka river in Jordan (2).

### Food

EDTA is used as a food additive in a range of products, including canned shrimps and prawns, canned mushrooms, and frozen chips. Maximum levels of EDTA in these products have been limited by the Codex Alimentarius Commission to 250, 200, and 100 mg/kg, respectively (6).

## 14.25.4 Kinetics and metabolism in laboratory animals and humans

Calcium disodium edetate is poorly absorbed from the gut; it is metabolically inert, and does not accumulate in the body (7, 8).

## 14.25.5 Effects on laboratory animals and *in vitro* test systems

### Long-term exposure

The long-term toxicity of EDTA is complicated by its ability to chelate essential and toxic metals, both in water and in animals. Toxicity data are therefore equivocal and difficult to interpret.

In long-term feeding studies in rats and dogs, no evidence was found of interference with mineral metabolism in either species. Adverse effects on mineral metabolism and nephrotoxicity were seen only after parenteral administration of high doses (7, 8).

### Reproductive toxicity, embryotoxicity, and teratogenicity

The overall results of various studies indicate that EDTA and its salts have little or no propensity to teratogenicity in rats, when given orally (8–10).

### Carcinogenicity

High doses of EDTA tested on animals in the USA were not carcinogenic (7, 8).

## 14.25.6 Effects on humans

The vast clinical experience of the use of EDTA in the treatment of metal poisoning has demonstrated its safety in humans.

Calcium disodium edetate as a food additive was evaluated toxicologically in 1973 by JECFA (7). An ADI of 0–2.5 mg/kg of body weight was allocated to this compound (equivalent to 0–1.9 mg/kg as the free acid). However, JECFA recommended that no sodium edetate should remain in foods. There have been few new toxicological studies subsequent to this evaluation, and those that are available indicate that the apparent toxicological effects of EDTA have in fact been due to zinc deficiency as a consequence of complexation (9–11).

The view that the major problem for human health of oral exposure to EDTA is zinc complexation was reaffirmed by workers in the Netherlands in a recent review of EDTA toxicology (8); its possible effects on the metabolism of metal ions were not addressed in detail in the 1973 JECFA evaluation. It has also been suggested that EDTA may enter kidney cells and, by interfering with zinc metabolism, exacerbate the toxicity of cadmium (12). However, the very low absorption of EDTA from the gastrointestinal tract after oral intake would suggest that it will be the major site of any zinc complexation.

It has been concluded that the present levels of EDTA found in drinking-water do not present a significant risk to human health (2).

## 14.25.7 Provisional guideline value

JECFA proposed an ADI for calcium disodium edetate as a food additive of 2.5 mg/kg of body weight (equivalent to 1.9 mg/kg of body weight as the free acid) (7). However, JECFA recommended that no sodium edetate should remain in foods.

An extra uncertainty factor of 10 was introduced to reflect the fact that the JECFA ADI has not been considered since 1973 and concern over zinc complexation, giving a TDI of 190 µg/kg of body weight. In view of the possibility of zinc complexation a provisional guideline value was derived by assuming that a 10-kg child consumes 1 litre of water per day. The provisional guideline value is thus 200 µg/litre (rounded figure), allocating 10% of the TDI to drinking-water.

## References

1.  Dytlova NM et al. [*Complexones.*] Moscow, Medicina, 1970 (in Russian).

2.  Van Dijk-Looyard AM et al. *EDTA in drink- en oppervlaktwater.* [*EDTA in drinking-water and surface water.*] Bilthoven, Netherlands, National Institute of Public Health and Environmental Protection, 1990 (Report No. 718629006).

3.  Sillén LG, Martell AE. *Stability constants of metal-ion complexes.* London, The Chemical Society, 1964 (Special Publication No. 17).

4.  Fayyad M, Tutunji M, Taha Z. Indirect trace determination of EDTA in waters by potentiometric stripping analysis. *Analytical letters,* 1988, 21(8):1425-1432.

5.  Frank R, Rau H. Photochemical transformation in aqueous solution and possible environmental fate of ethylenediaminetetraacetic acid (EDTA). *Ecotoxicology and environmental safety,* 1990, 19(1):55-63.

6.  Smith LB, ed. *Codex Alimentarius, abridged version.* Rome, Codex Alimentarius Commission, 1990.

7.  *Toxicological evaluation of some food additives including anticaking agents, antimicrobials, antioxidants, emulsifiers and thickening agents.* Geneva, World Health Organization, 1974 (WHO Food Additives Series, No. 5).

8.  Janssen PJCM, Knaap AGAC, Taalman RDFM. *EDTA: Literatuuronderzoek naar de orale toxiciteit voor de mens.* [*EDTA: literature search on oral toxicity to humans.*] Bilthoven, Netherlands, National Institute of Public Health and Environmental Protection, 1990 (Report No. 718629008).

9.  Kimmel CA. Effect of route of administration on the toxicity and teratogenicity of EDTA in the rat. *Toxicology and applied pharmacology,* 1977, 40:299-306.

10. Schardein JL et al. Teratogenesis studies with EDTA and its salts in rats. *Toxicology and applied pharmacology*, 1981, 61:423-428.

11. Brownie CF et al. Teratogenic effects of calcium edetate (CaEDTA) in rats and the protective effects of zinc. *Toxicology and applied pharmacology*, 1986, 82:426-443.

12. Dieter HH. Implications of heavy metal toxicity related to EDTA exposure. *Toxicological and environmental chemistry*, 1990, 27:91-95.

## 14.26 Nitrilotriacetic acid

### 14.26.1 General description

#### *Identity*

CAS no:               139-13-9
Molecular formula:  $C_6H_9NO_6$

#### *Physicochemical properties (1)*

| Property | Value |
| --- | --- |
| Physical state | Needles or prismatic crystals in the undissociated acid form |
| Melting point | 241.5 °C |
| Water solubility | 1.28 g/l at 22.5 °C |
| pH of saturated solution | 2–3 |

#### *Major uses*

The trisodium salt of nitrilotriacetic acid (NTA) is used in laundry detergents as a "builder" to replace phosphates because of its ability to chelate calcium and magnesium ions (*1*). NTA is used extensively in the treatment of boiler water to prevent the accumulation of mineral scale and, to a lesser extent, in photography, textile manufacture, paper and cellulose production, and metal plating and cleaning operations. Its use as a therapeutic chelating agent for the treatment of manganese poisoning (*2*) and iron overloading has been suggested (*3*).

#### *Environmental fate*

NTA is degraded principally by microorganisms by carbon–nitrogen cleavage with the formation of such intermediates as iminodiacetate, glyoxylate, glycerate, glycine, and ammonia (*4–6*); the metabolic end-products are carbon dioxide, water, ammonia, and nitrate (*7*). NTA mobilizes heavy metals from aquatic sediments (*8*) and is present in water mainly in the form of metal complexes (*9*), most of which degrade rapidly. Under certain conditions, it is broken down by photochemical and chemical reactions (*7*).

The half-life for biodegradation of NTA in groundwater at 1–100 µg/litre is approximately 31 h (*10*). Concentrations of 5–50 mg/litre completely disappeared from river water containing acclimatized microorganisms in 2–6 days; concentrations below 5 mg/litre are expected to degrade within 1 day (*11,12*). Acclimatization of microorganisms in two lake waters resulted in the reduction of the disappearance time of up to 10 mg of NTA per litre from 6 and 11 days to 4 and 3 days, respectively (*13*). Sand-associated bacteria adapt more quickly to NTA and degrade it more actively than do plankton and algae (*14*).

## 14.26.2 Analytical methods

NTA concentrations in water may be determined by gas chromatography with a nitrogen-specific detector. This method is suitable for the detection of levels as low as 0.2 µg/litre (*15*).

## 14.26.3 Environmental levels and human exposure

### Water

NTA has been detected in both raw and treated water. In a national survey of 70 Canadian municipalities, the mean concentrations of NTA in drinking-water and raw water samples were 2.8 µg/litre (range < 0.2–30.4 µg/litre) and 3.9 µg/litre (range < 0.2–33.5 µg/litre), respectively. Concentrations exceeded 10 µg/litre in only 14% of the locations (*15*). In a survey of tapwater in eight cities in New York State, 68% of the samples contained no detectable levels of NTA (detection limit 1 µg/litre); the remaining samples contained an average of 2.1 µg/litre (*16*). Mean concentrations in surface water ranged from 0.3 to 4.7 µg/litre in Germany (*17*) and from 1.0 to 12.0 µg/litre in Switzerland (*18*).

### Other routes of exposure

No information on NTA concentrations in food or ambient air has been found. For a very small proportion of the population in households in which dishes are washed with detergents containing NTA, residues present on unrinsed dishes left to drip dry may be a source of exposure. Intake from this source may approximate 0.0025 mg/kg of body weight per day (0.15 mg for a 60-kg adult) (*19*).

### Estimated total exposure and relative contribution of drinking-water

The daily intake of NTA in drinking-water can be calculated to be 5.6 µg, using the mean concentration in drinking-water reported in the Canadian national survey (2.8 µg/litre) (*15*) and assuming an average daily water consumption of 2 litres.

### 14.26.4 Kinetics and metabolism in laboratory animals and humans

Absorption of NTA from the gastrointestinal tract is rapid; however, there is considerable variation among species in the proportion of NTA eliminated in the urine. It does not appear to be metabolized by mammals: this conclusion is based on studies in mice, rats, dogs, and humans in which unchanged NTA is excreted in the urine (20–23).

NTA accumulates in bone because it forms complexes with divalent cations such as calcium; its turnover time in bone is similar to that of calcium (7). Deposition of NTA in the kidney has also been reported, although this may be an artefact associated with the retention of urine in the kidney rather than uptake by renal tissue (7).

### 14.26.5 Effects on laboratory animals and *in vitro* test systems

#### Acute exposure

NTA does not appear to be highly acutely toxic to mammals. Oral $LD_{50}$s in rats and mice of 1470 mg/kg of body weight and 3160 mg/kg of body weight, respectively, have been reported (24). The oral $LD_{50}$ of $Na_3NTA \cdot H_2O$ in rodents is about 2000 mg/kg of body weight (7). The oral $LD_{50}$s in rats for the metal complexes of NTA commonly found in drinking-water range from 810 mg/kg of body weight for CuNaNTA to over 22 500 mg/kg of body weight for NiNaNTA (7).

#### Short-term exposure

Results of short-term studies in which NTA was administered orally indicate that the kidney is the target organ and that damage is dose-dependent and rapidly induced. In two studies in which male Sprague-Dawley rats and Charles River CD rats consumed drinking-water containing between 0.01 and 0.1% $Na_3NTA$ for 10 weeks, elevated blood glucose levels were observed at all dose levels. Six of the nine Sprague-Dawley rats in the high-dose group died by the fourth week; animals in this group showed marked vacuolization of renal tubules, and glycosuria was present in five rats (25). In a bioassay in which groups of weanling rats were fed diets containing 0, 2000, 7500, 10 000, or 20 000 mg of the trisodium salt per kg of diet for 90 days, hydronephrosis was observed in 63% of the animals in the group given 20 000 mg/kg; hydropic degeneration of the kidney tubular cells, tubular atrophy, and dilatation were reported in the groups given 7500 and 10 000 mg/kg; no adverse effects were observed at 2000 mg/kg (26). In a limited investigation in which two skeletally mature dogs were given 2.5 mg of trisodium salt per kg of body weight per day in their drinking-water for 7 months, radial closure rates and the percentage of osteoid seams taking a fluorescent label were decreased, suggesting interference with the mineralization process (27).

## Long-term exposure

Weanling Charles River CD rats (50 per sex per dose) were fed diets containing 0.03, 0.15, or 0.5% of the trisodium salt or 0.5% of the calcium chelate of NTA for 2 years. A dose-dependent increase in urinary zinc was reported in the groups receiving 0.15 and 0.5% $Na_3NTA$, accompanied by a dose-dependent increase in renal tubular cell toxicity. Mild nephrosis consisting of hydropic degeneration of tubular cells and the minor tubule was observed at 6 months at 0.15 and 0.5% $Na_3NTA$; its incidence and severity became more pronounced as the study continued. Renal effects at 0.5% for the trisodium salt and 0.5% for the calcium chelate were severe. The NOAEL for nephrosis or nephritis in rats was considered to be 0.03% for the trisodium salt, equivalent to 30 mg/kg of body weight per day in young rats and 15 mg/kg of body weight per day as they grew older (or 10 and 20 mg of NTA per kg of body weight per day, respectively) (19).

## Reproductive toxicity, embryotoxicity, and teratogenicity

NTA may be beneficial in neonatal development because it increases the bioavailability of essential elements (28).

NTA was not teratogenic or embryotoxic in studies with mice (0.2% NTA) (29), rats (0.1 or 0.5% trisodium salt), or rabbits (250 mg of trisodium salt per kg of body weight) (30).

## Mutagenicity and related end-points

The mutagenic and clastogenic potential of NTA has been investigated both *in vivo* and *in vitro*, but the results of the assays conducted to date have been largely negative (1, 7, 31, 32). It enhances the induction of sister chromatid exchange in Chinese hamster cells by insoluble salts of some heavy metals (33, 34), and some insoluble salts of chromium(VI) are mutagenic in the *Salmonella* microsome assay in the presence of NTA (35).

## Carcinogenicity

There was no evidence of carcinogenicity in studies in which weanling Charles River CD rats were fed diets containing 0.03, 0.15, or 0.5% of the trisodium salt or 0.5% of the calcium chelate of NTA for 2 years (19), groups of 80 Swiss mice were given drinking-water containing 5 g of NTA per litre or 5 g of NTA plus 1 g of sodium nitrite per litre for 26 weeks (36), or groups of 15 male and 15 female MRC rats were exposed to the same levels for 84 weeks (37).

In an experiment in which groups of 24 male and 24 female Fischer 344 rats were fed diets containing 200, 2000, or 20 000 mg of $Na_3NTA \cdot H_2O$ per kg of diet for 2 years, a significant increase in primary neoplasms of the urinary tract was reported in both males and females in the highest dose group; in addition, five males and five females in this group developed metastatic transitional cell carcinomas, which appeared most frequently in the lung and often in the lymph nodes, pancreas, adrenal gland, and seminal vesicle (*38*).

In an 18-month study, Fischer 344 rats were fed diets containing 7500 or 15 000 mg of NTA per kg of diet or 7500 or 15 000 mg of $Na_3NTA \cdot H_2O$ per kg of diet, and $B6C3F_1$ mice were fed diets containing 7500 or 15 000 mg of NTA per kg of diet or 2500 or 5000 mg of $Na_3NTA \cdot H_2O$ per kg of diet. Several carcinogenic effects were observed in both rats and mice. In rats, these included a significant increase in the incidence of a variety of neoplastic lesions of the urinary tract in those exposed to 15 000 mg of NTA per kg of diet, a slight increase in the incidence of neoplasms of the urinary system in those exposed to 7500 and 15 000 mg/kg of the trisodium salt, a positive dose–response relationship for the incidence of tumours of the endocrine system, and a dose-related increase in the incidence of neoplastic nodules of the liver in female rats consuming NTA. In mice, effects included a statistically significant increase in tumours of the kidney, especially tubular-cell adenocarcinomas, in males ingesting 15 000 mg of NTA per kg and a dose-related increase in the incidence of tumours of the haematopoietic system in males consuming $Na_3NTA \cdot H_2O$ (*38*).

In a study in which male Sprague-Dawley albino rats were exposed to drinking-water containing 1000 mg of trisodium salt per litre for 2 years, the incidence of renal tumours, including renal adenomas and adenocarcinomas, was significantly increased in the exposed animals (*39*).

The induction of tumours is considered to be due to cytotoxicity resulting from the chelation of divalent cations such as zinc and calcium in the urinary tract, leading to the development of hyperplasia and neoplasia. It has been observed, for example, that only NTA doses that increase urinary calcium are associated with transitional epithelial-cell tumours, leading to the hypothesis that uncomplexed NTA in urine extracts extracellular calcium from the transitional epithelial cells of the urinary tract faster than it can be replenished (*7*).

## 14.26.6 Effects on humans

There is little information on the toxicity of NTA in humans. On the basis of physical examination, blood chemistry analysis, and urinalysis, no adverse health effects were reported in a metabolism study in which volunteers ingested a single dose of 10 mg of NTA (*23*).

## 14.26.7 Guideline value

NTA is poorly absorbed in humans as compared with experimental animals and does not appear to be metabolized in mammals. It has not been shown to be teratogenic or genotoxic in the studies conducted to date but has induced urinary tract tumours in rats and mice at high doses (*38, 39*). IARC has placed NTA in Group 2B (*40*).

The reported induction of tumours in rodents is considered to be due to cytotoxicity resulting from the chelation of divalent cations such as zinc and calcium in the urinary tract, leading to the development of hyperplasia and subsequently neoplasia. In general, neoplasms have occurred only following long-term ingestion of NTA at concentrations greater than 100 mg/kg of body weight per day, whereas nephrotoxicity occurs at a lower level, between 10 and 60 mg/kg of body weight per day (*7*).

Because NTA is nongenotoxic and induces tumours only after prolonged exposure to doses higher than those that produce nephrotoxicity, the guideline value is derived on the basis of a NOAEL for nephrotoxic effects but incorporating a larger uncertainty factor to account for the evidence of urinary tumour induction at high doses. A TDI of 10 µg/kg of body weight was calculated by applying an uncertainty factor of 1000 (100 for inter- and intraspecies variation and 10 for carcinogenic potential at high doses) to the NOAEL of 10 mg/kg of body weight per day for nephritis and nephrosis in a 2-year study in rats (*19*). In view of the higher absorption of NTA in rats than in humans, it should be noted that this TDI is probably conservative. Because there is no substantial exposure from other sources, 50% of the TDI was allocated to drinking-water, resulting in a guideline value of 200 µg/litre (rounded figure).

## References

1.  International Joint Commission. *A report to the Great Lakes Research Advisory Board of the International Joint Commission on the health implications of NTA.* Windsor, Canada, 1977.

2.  Kaur G, Hasan SK, Srivastava RC. Effect of nitrilotriacetic acid (NTA) on the distribution of manganese-54 in rats. *Archives of toxicology,* 1980, 45:203-206.

3.  Pollack S, Ruocco S. Synergistic effect of nitrilotriacetate on iron mobilization by desferrioxamine *in vivo. Blood,* 1981, 57(6):1117-1118.

4.  Cripps RE, Noble AS. The metabolism of nitrilotriacetate by a pseudomonad. *Biochemistry journal,* 1973, 136:1059-1068.

5.  Tiedje JM et al. Metabolism of nitrilotriacetate by cells of *Pseudomonas* species. *Applied microbiology,* 1973, 25:811-818.

6.  Firestone MK, Tiedje JM. Pathway of degradation of nitrilotriacetate by a *Pseudomonas* species. *Applied environmental microbiology,* 1978, 35:955-961.

7.  Anderson RL, Bishop WE, Campbell RL. A review of the environmental and mammalian toxicology of nitrilotriacetic acid. *CRC critical reviews of toxicology,* 1985, 15(1):1-102

8. Samanidou V, Fytianos K. Mobilization of heavy metals from river sediments of Northern Greece by complexing agents. *Water, air, and soil pollution*, 1990, 52:217.

9. McFuff RE, Mord FM. Pasadena, CA, W.M. Keck Laboratory of Environmental Science, California Institute of Technology, 1973 (Technical Report EQ-73-02) (cited in reference 7).

10. Ventullo RM, Larson RJ. Metabolic diversity and activity of heterotrophic bacteria in ground water. *Environmental toxicology and chemistry*, 1985, 4:759.

11. Warren CB, Malec EJ. Biodegradation of nitrilotriacetic acid and related imino and amino acids in river water. *Science*, 1972, 176:277-279.

12. Thompson JE, Duthie JR. The biodegradability and treatability of NTA. *Journal of the Water Pollution Control Federation*, 1968, 40:303-319.

13. Chau YK, Shiomi MT. Complexing properties of nitrilotriacetic acid in the lake environment. *Water, air, and soil pollution*, 1972, 1(2):149.

14. McFeters GA et al. Activity and adaptation of nitrilotriacetate (NTA)-degrading bacteria: field and laboratory studies. *Water research*, 1990, 24(7):875.

15. Malaiyandi M, Williams DT, O'Grady R. A national survey of nitrilotriacetic acid in Canadian drinking water. *Environmental science and technology*, 1979, 13:59.

16. The Proctor and Gamble Company. *New York tap water monitoring for NTA, October 1981–June 1983*. Submission to the New York State Department of Environmental Conservation, Cincinnati, OH, 31 August 1983 (cited in reference 7).

17. Frimmel FH et al. Nitrilotriacetate (NTA) and ethylenedinitrilotetraacetate (EDTA) in rivers of the Federal Republic of Germany. *Vom Wasser*, 1989, 72:175.

18. Houriet J-P. Development of the concentration of the laundry detergent phosphate substitute "NTA" in Switzerland waters, situation 1990. *BUWAL-Bulletin*, 1990, 3/90:28.

19. Nixon GA, Buehler EV, Niewenhuis RJ. Two-year rat feeding study with trisodium nitrilotriacetate and its calcium chelate. *Toxicology and applied pharmacology*, 1972, 21:244-252.

20. Michael WR, Wakim JM. Metabolism of nitrilotriacetic acid (NTA). *Toxicology and applied pharmacology*, 1971, 18:407-416.

21. Chu I et al. Metabolism of nitrilotriacetic acid in the mouse. *Bulletin of environmental contamination and toxicology*, 1978, 19:417-422.

22. Budny JA. Metabolism and blood pressure effects of disodium nitrilotriacetate ($Na_2NTA$) in dogs. *Toxicology and applied pharmacology*, 1972, 22:655-660.

23. Budny JA, Arnold JD. Nitrilotriacetate (NTA): human metabolism and its impor-
    tance in the total safety evaluation program. *Toxicology and applied pharmacology*,
    1973, 15:48-53.

24. National Institute of Occupational Safety and Health. *Registry of Toxic Effects
    of Chemical Substances (RTECS), 1983–84 cumulative supplement to the 1981–82
    edition*. Cincinnati, OH, US Department of Health and Human Services, 1985.

25. Mahaffey DR, Goyer RA. Trisodium nitrilotriacetate in drinking water. Metabolic
    and renal effects in rats. *Archives of environmental health*, 1972, 25:271-275.

26. Nixon GA. Toxicity evaluation of trisodium nitrilotriacetate. *Toxicology and applied
    pharmacology*, 1971, 18:398-406.

27. Anderson C, Danylchuk KD. The effect of chronic administration of trisodium
    nitrilotriacetate ($Na_3NTA$) on the Haversian remodelling system in dogs. *Journal
    of environmental pathology and toxicology*, 1980, 3:413-420.

28. Keen CL et al. Effect of dietary iron, copper and zinc chelates of nitrilotriacetic acid
    (NTA) on trace metal concentrations in rat milk and maternal and pup tissues. *Jour-
    nal of nutrition*, 1980, 110:897-906.

29. Tjälve H. A study of the distribution and teratogenicity of nitrilotriacetic acid (NTA)
    in mice. *Toxicology and applied pharmacology*, 1972, 23:216-221.

30. Nolen GA et al. Reproduction and teratology studies of trisodium nitrilotriacetate in
    rats and rabbits. *Food and cosmetics toxicology*, 1971, 9:509-518.

31. Montaldi A et al. Nitrilotriacetic acid (NTA) does not induce chromosomal damage
    in mammalian cells either *in vitro* or *in vivo*. *Mutation research*, 1988, 208:95-100.

32. Ved Brat S, Williams GM. Nitrilotriacetic acid does not induce sister-chromatid ex-
    changes in hamster or human cells. *Food chemistry and toxicology*, 1984, 22(3):211-
    215.

33. Montaldi A et al. Interaction of nitrilotriacetic acid with heavy metals in the induc-
    tion of sister chromatid exchanges in cultured mammalian cells. *Environmental mu-
    tagenesis*, 1985, 7:381-390.

34. Nunziata A et al. Mutagenic activity of nitriloacetic acid. *Archives of toxicology*, 1984,
    Suppl. 7:407.

35. Loprieno N et al. Increased mutagenicity of chromium compounds by nitrilotri-
    acetic acid. *Environmental mutagenesis*, 1985, 7:185-200.

36. Greenblatt M, Lijinsky W. Carcinogenesis and chronic toxicity of nitrilotriacetic
    acid in Swiss mice. *Journal of the National Cancer Institute*, 1974, 52:1123-1126.

37. Lijinsky W, Greenblatt M, Kommineni C. Brief communication: feeding studies of nitrilotriacetic acid and derivatives in rats. *Journal of the National Cancer Institute,* 1973, 50:1061-1063.

38. National Cancer Institute. *Bioassays of nitrilotriacetic acid (NTA) and nitrilotriacetic acid, trisodium salt, monohydrate (Na₃NTA·H₂O) for possible carcinogenicity.* Bethesda, MD, 1977 (NCI-CG-TR-6; DHEW Publication No. [NIH] 77-806).

39. Goyer RA et al. Renal tumors in rats given trisodium nitrilotriacetic acid in drinking water for two years. *Journal of the National Cancer Institute,* 1981, 66:869-880.

40. International Agency for Research on Cancer. *Some flame retardants and textile chemicals, and exposures in the textile manufacturing industry.* Lyon, 1990:181-204 (IARC Monographs on the Evaluation of Carcinogenic Risks to Humans, Volume 48).

# 14.27 Organotins

## 14.27.1 General description

### Identity

The organotins are a large class of compounds which differ in their properties and applications. They can be divided into four groups of general formula $R_4Sn$, $R_3SnX$, $R_2SnX_2$, and $RSnX_3$, where R is usually an organic group and X an anion, e.g. chloride, fluoride, oxide, or hydroxide.

### Major uses

Of the various organotins, the disubstituted and trisubstituted compounds are the most widely used, the former being employed as stabilizers in plastics, including polyvinyl chloride (PVC) water pipes, and the latter in the preservation of materials (wood, stone, textiles), as fungicides, miticides, and disinfectants, as bactericides in cooling water, and in antifouling paints.

## 14.27.2 Analytical methods

Mono-, di-, and tributyltins can be determined by extraction followed by derivatization to form hexylbutyltins, which are measured by gas chromatography/mass spectrometry or gas chromatography with flame-photometric detection (GC-FPD). A detection limit of 2 ng/litre is reported (1). Similar detection limits are obtained when organotins are measured by preconcentration using a tropolene-loaded silica column, followed by ethylation, separation, and detection by capillary GC-FPD (2).

## 14.27.3 Environmental levels and human exposure

### Air

Unknown quantities of organotins may be released into air from factories that produce polyurethane or PVC resins in which they are used as stabilizers.

### Water

Tributyltins have been detected in raw water and sediment as a result of their use as antifouling agents (*3, 4*); levels of up to 2.6, 0.3, and 0.08 µg/litre have been found in marinas, estuaries, and the open sea, respectively. There is evidence that organotin stabilizers leach into water from plastic pipes; a dibutyltin sulfide concentration of 100 µg/litre was reported after a plastic pipe had been in contact with static water (*5*).

### Food

Tributyltin is thought to accumulate in aquatic food-chains incorporating crabs, mussels, or oysters (*6, 7*). In addition, the use of organotin compounds as miticides in agriculture and as PVC stabilizers may result in their presence in food. Triphenyltin residues in various foodstuffs, such as potatoes, carrots, and sugar-beet, rarely exceed 0.1 mg/kg and can be considerably reduced by washing (*8*).

## 14.27.4 Kinetics and metabolism in laboratory animals and humans

The available data suggest that organotins are poorly absorbed (*9*); for example, it was reported that only 20% of dioctyltin dichloride was absorbed in rats (*10*). Organotins tend to be primarily distributed in the liver and kidney following oral administration in rodents (*11,12*). Low levels of dioctyltin dichloride have been found in the adrenal, pituitary, and thyroid glands (*10*).

It appears that alkyltins are metabolized by dealkylation (*13*). *In vitro*, tributyltin was metabolized to dibutyltin, hydroxybutyltins, butanol, and butene (*14*), whereas di-, tri-, and tetraethyltin appeared to form ethene and ethane (*15*). Carbon dioxide and butene were detected as metabolites of both dibutyltin diethanoate and tributyltin ethanoate in mice *in vivo* (*14*).

After oral administration, it appears that the principal route of excretion of organotins is in the faeces (*11*). Bile is also a significant route for some compounds, such as tetraalkyltins (*13*). For others, significant amounts are expired as carbon dioxide (*14*).

## 14.27.5 Effects on laboratory animals and *in vitro* test systems

### *Dialkyltins*

Acute exposure

Acute oral $LD_{50}$s of dioctyltins in rodents range from 880 to 8500 mg/kg of body weight (*16, 17*). The acute oral $LD_{50}$ of dibutyltin dichloride in rats has been reported to be 100 mg/kg of body weight (*18*).

Short-term exposure

Rats were fed diets containing dioctyltin dichloride at 0, 50, or 150 mg/kg (equivalent to 0, 2.5, and 7.5 mg/kg of body weight) for 6 weeks. The principal effect was a reduction in thymus weight at both dose levels. Lymphocyte deple-tion was observed in the thymus and the thymus-dependent areas of the spleen and lymph nodes (*19*). A weekly oral dose of 500 mg/kg of body weight for 8 weeks reduced thymus weight and induced immunodeficiency in mice, whereas a dose of 100 mg/kg of body weight did not cause such effects (*20*).

Dibutyltin dichloride was fed to rats at 0, 10, 20, 40, or 80 mg/kg of diet (equivalent to 0, 0.5, 1, 2, or 4 mg/kg of body weight) for 90 days. Reduction in food intake, depressed growth, and mild anaemia were noted at the highest dose level, but no treatment-related effects were observed at lower doses (*21*). A re-duction in thymus weight and immunocompetence was observed in rats fed diets containing dioctyltin dichloride at 75 mg/kg (about 3.8 mg/kg of body weight per day) for 8 or 12 weeks (*22*).

Mutagenicity and related end-points

Dioctyltin dichloride gave negative results in the Ames test and in tests for the in-duction of unscheduled DNA synthesis in primary cultures of rat hepatocytes (*23*). No evidence of mutagenicity was found for dibutyltin diethanoate in the Ames test (*24*). Dibutyltin dichloride and dioctyltin dichloride have been report-ed to give positive results in mammalian cell mutation assays *in vitro* in the absence of metabolic activation (*23, 25*), and dibutyltin sulfide increased the in-cidence of chromosomal aberrations in rat bone marrow cells *in vivo* (*5*).

Carcinogenicity

F344 rats and B6C3F$_1$ mice were fed diets containing dibutyltin diethanoate at 66.5 or 133 mg/kg (rats) and 76 or 152 mg/kg (mice) for 78 weeks. Nonsignifi-cant increased incidences of hepatocellular adenomas in female mice and both hepatocellular adenomas and carcinomas in male mice were noted (*26*).

Rats were fed a mixture of octyltin trichloride and dioctyltin dichloride in the diet at doses equivalent to approximately 0.3, 0.7, 2.3, and 6.0 mg/kg of body weight for 2 years. A highly significant increased frequency of primary tumours of the thymus, especially thymic lymphomas, was noted in females in the highest dose group. The females also showed an increased incidence of generalized malig-nant lymphomas, as did the males in the two higher dose groups, although there seemed to be an unusually low incidence of such tumours in the control groups.

In animals treated at the lower dose levels, no increase in the incidence of primary thymic tumours or generalized malignant lymphomas was observed (*27*).

## Trimethyltins

### Acute exposure

An acute oral $LD_{50}$ of 12.6 mg/kg of body weight for trimethyltin chloride in rats has been reported (*28*).

### Short-term exposure

Trimethyltin is a potent neurotoxicant in rodents (*28, 29*). In a group of rats fed diets containing 15 mg of trimethyltin per kg (equivalent to 0.8 mg/kg of body weight per day) for 2 weeks, there were some deaths, relative thymus and spleen weights were decreased, and relative kidney, testes, and adrenal weights increased. Pathological changes indicative of severe neurotoxicity were observed in the brain. At 5 mg/kg, there was growth retardation but no effects on organ weights or brain (*30*).

### Mutagenicity and related end-points

Trimethyltin may have spindle-inhibiting properties. Human lymphocyte cultures treated with trimethyltin *in vitro* exhibited a reduction in average chromosome length (*31*).

## Triethyltins

### Short-term exposure

Triethyltin, like trimethyltin, is a potent neurotoxicant. Its effects tend to be more persistent than those of trimethyltin but can be reversible. The effects of triethyltin toxicity in rats are hind-limb weakness and cerebral oedema (*32*).

Rats fed diets containing 15 mg of triethyltin per kg (equivalent to 0.8 mg/kg of body weight per day) for 2 weeks exhibited growth retardation, a reduction in the relative weights of the thymus and spleen, and an increase in relative adrenal weight. At 50 mg/kg, 30% of animals died, and survivors exhibited brain oedema (*30*).

Groups of rats were fed diets containing triethyltin hydroxide at 0, 5, 10, or 20 mg/kg (equivalent to 0, 0.3, 0.5, and 1 mg/kg of body weight) for 90 days. All the rats given 20 mg/kg died during the experiment, as did 7 of 20 given 10 mg/kg. Brain weights were significantly increased in rats at 10 mg/kg, and the growth of animals was affected at 5 mg/kg. Interstitial oedema in the central nervous system was found in rats at all doses (*33*).

### Tributyltins

Acute exposure

Acute oral $LD_{50}$s of 46–114, 117–122, 85–197, and 10–234 mg/kg of body weight have been reported in rodents for tributyltin ethanoate, chloride, fluoride, and oxide, respectively (34).

Short-term exposure

Reductions in food consumption, weight gain, and absolute thymus weight were reported in rats fed tributyltin oxide (TBTO) at 100 mg/kg in the diet (about 5 mg/kg of body weight per day) for 4 weeks. No effects were observed at 4 or 20 mg/kg (0.2 or 1 mg/kg of body weight per day) (35).

Wistar rats fed diets containing 0, 5, 20, 80, or 320 mg of TBTO per kg (0, 0.3, 1, 4, and 16 mg/kg of body weight per day) for 4 weeks exhibited decreased mean relative weight of the thymus at 20 (males only), 80, and 320 mg/kg of diet. The only effect noted at 5 mg/kg of diet was some histopathological change in the spleen, which became more severe with increasing dose. Histopathological changes in the thymus, mesenteric lymph nodes and liver, and haematological and clinical chemistry effects were also evident in the higher dose groups (36). Using the same dose levels, Vos et al. (37) found effects on a number of immunological parameters at both 20 and 80 mg/kg of diet.

TBTO was fed to rats in their diet for 13–14 weeks. At 20 mg/kg (about 1 mg/kg of body weight per day), there was a slight increase in blood coagulation time in males and a slight decrease in food consumption without growth retardation in females. At 100 mg/kg, there were reductions in the weight of the thymus, lymph nodes, and thyroid, but an increase in adrenal weight. The NOAEL in this study was reported to be 4 mg/kg (about 0.2 mg/kg of body weight per day) (35).

Long-term exposure

TBTO was fed to male and female Wistar rats at 0, 0.5, 5, or 50 mg/kg in their diet for 106 weeks. At 50 mg/kg of diet, the ovaries, adrenals, spleen (females), heart (males), pituitary, liver, and kidneys were all increased in weight, but thyroid weight was decreased in females. Non-neoplastic alterations included a decrease in the cell weight of the thyroid follicles in all dose groups. In addition, vacuolation and pigmentation of the proximal tubular epithelium and nephrosis were enhanced at 50 mg/kg. On the basis of marginal effects at 5 mg/kg, a NOAEL of 0.5 mg of TBTO per kg can be established, equivalent to 0.025 mg/kg of body weight per day (38).

In a study in which weanling Wistar rats were fed diets containing 0, 0.5, 5, or 50 mg of TBTO per kg for up to 17 months, TBTO was found to alter both acquired and natural host resistance, particularly at the highest dose (39). In a similar experiment, Wistar rats given the same diets for 30 months exhibited changes, mostly at the highest dose level, that included a decrease in IgG and an increase in IgM in females, a decrease in lymphocyte numbers, elevated adrenal weight, reductions in liver glycogen and spleen iron, and bile duct hyperplasia (*40*).

Adverse effects on thymus-dependent immunity and nonspecific resistance in rats were reported following exposure to TBTO for 17 months. A dose-related suppression of resistance to the nematode *Trichinella spiralis* was reported at 5 and 50 mg/kg of diet. A NOAEL of 0.5 mg/kg of diet (equivalent to 0.025 mg/kg of body weight) was identified (*41*).

### Reproductive toxicity, embryotoxicity, and teratogenicity

Pregnant NMRI mice were given oral doses of 0, 1.2, 3.5, 5.8, 11.7, 23.4, or 35 mg of TBTO per kg of body weight per day on days 6–15 of gestation. At the highest dose, there was a significant increase in numbers of resorptions. A slight reduction in average fetal weight was noted at 23.4 mg/kg of body weight but was more pronounced at the highest dose. The frequency of cleft palate increased in a dose-dependent fashion, being statistically significant at 11.7 mg/kg of body weight. However, there was also evidence of maternal toxicity at this and higher dose levels (*42*).

Groups of pregnant Long-Evans rats were given oral doses of 0, 2.5, 5, 10, 12, or 16 mg of TBTO per kg of body weight per day on days 6–20 of gestation. Retarded fetal growth, a reduction in numbers of live births, and effects on post-natal growth and behaviour were observed at doses of 10 mg/kg of body weight per day and above. Maternal toxicity was also evident at these dose levels. At 12 mg/kg of body weight per day, two pups born dead exhibited cleft palate (*43*).

### Mutagenicity and related end-points

TBTO gave negative results in bacterial and yeast mutagenicity tests. In mammalian cells *in vitro*, it gave negative results for induction of point mutations and sister chromatid exchange, but chromosomal aberrations were induced in Chinese hamster ovary cells in the presence of the S9 fraction of a ratliver homogenate. Mice given oral doses failed to show an increased incidence of micronuclei in bone marrow polychromatic erythrocytes (*34, 35, 42*).

### Carcinogenicity

In a 106-week TBTO feeding study in rats, the incidence of benign tumours of the pituitary was significantly elevated at 0.5 and 50 mg/kg. At 50 mg/kg of diet (about 2.5 mg/kg of body weight per day), increases in phaeochromocytomas in the adrenal medulla and parathyroid adenomas were noted. There was also a low incidence of rare pancreatic adenocarcinomas. The incidence of tumours was not dose-related (*34, 38*).

### *Tricyclohexyltins*

#### Acute exposure

Acute oral $LD_{50}$s for tricyclohexyltin hydroxide in rodents range from 235 to 1070 mg/kg of body weight (*44*).

Long-term exposure
Groups of rats were fed diets containing tricyclohexyltin hydroxide at 0, 0.8, 3, 6, or 12 mg/kg of body weight per day for 2 years. At 12 mg/kg of body weight per day, there was reduced body weight gain and increased relative spleen and liver weights in females. Similar, but milder, effects were noted at 6 mg/kg of body weight per day, whereas no adverse effects were observed at 3 mg/kg of body weight per day. A NOAEL of 0.8 mg/kg of body weight per day was reported for dogs given the same doses for 2 years (8).

Reproductive toxicity, embryotoxicity, and teratogenicity
In a multigeneration study on rats, it was found that tricyclohexyltin hydroxide had no effects on reproduction at a dose of 4–6 mg/kg of body weight per day. Similarly, no evidence for teratogenicity was observed in rabbits receiving up to 3 mg/kg of body weight per day on days 8–16 of gestation (8).

Carcinogenicity
No evidence of carcinogenicity was found in a study of rats receiving tricyclohexyltin hydroxide at concentrations of up to 12 mg/kg of body weight per day for 2 years (8).

## Triphenyltins

Acute exposure
Acute oral $LD_{50}$s of 81–491, 80–135, 1170, and 108–500 mg/kg of body weight have been reported in rodents for triphenyltin ethanoate, chloride, fluoride, and hydroxide, respectively (44).

Short-term exposure
Weanling rats fed a diet containing 25 mg of triphenyltin hydroxide per kg for 3 or 4 weeks exhibited suppression of cell-mediated immunity but not humoral immunity (45). A reduction in relative thymus weight was observed in rats fed triphenyltin chloride at 15 mg/kg in the diet for 2 weeks. Relative spleen weight was reduced at a dietary concentration of 50 mg/kg (30).

Rats were fed diets containing up to 50 mg/kg (about 2.5 mg/kg of body weight per day) of either triphenyltin ethanoate or triphenyltin hydroxide for 90 days. Guinea-pigs received similar diets but only three times per week. Growth in rats and guinea-pigs was affected at 25 and 5 mg/kg for triphenyltin ethanoate and 50 and 20 mg/kg for triphenyltin hydroxide, respectively. Guinea-pigs given 5–20 mg of triphenyltin ethanoate per kg exhibited lymphocytopenia and histological changes in the lymphopoietic system and spleen (33).

Long-term exposure
In 2-year studies, the dietary NOAEL for triphenyltin hydroxide in rats was approximately 2 mg/kg (0.1 mg/kg of body weight); for triphenyltin ethanoate in guinea-pigs, it was 5 mg/kg (0.3 mg/kg of body weight) (8).

Reproductive toxicity, embryotoxicity, and teratogenicity

Groups of pregnant rats were given oral doses of triphenyltin ethanoate of 0, 5, 10, or 15 mg/kg of body weight on days 6–15 of gestation. A reduction in the body weight gain of dams and an increase in post-implantation loss were apparent at the highest dose. A reduction in fetal skeletal ossification was observed in all treated groups, but there was no evidence of teratogenicity (46).

Mutagenicity and related end-points

Triphenyltin hydroxide gave negative results for mutagenicity in bacteria but was positive for the induction of point mutations in mammalian cells in vitro (46) and in an early mouse dominant lethal assay (48).

Carcinogenicity

Groups of Fischer 344 rats and B6C3F$_1$ mice (50 per sex per dose) were fed triphenyltin hydroxide in their diet at 37.5 or 75 mg/kg for 78 weeks; they were then kept under observation for a further 26 weeks. There appeared to be no increase in tumour incidence as compared with controls (49).

## 14.27.6 Effects on humans

There is evidence that trimethyltin is neurotoxic in humans. Mental confusion and generalized epileptic seizures were noted in two chemists who had been exposed to trimethyltin in a pilot plant manufacturing dimethyltin dichloride. Both subjects recovered and regained apparently normal health (50). Severe neurological damage was reported in some workers exposed over 3 days to a mixture of trimethyltin and dimethyltin dichloride (51).

A drug containing triethyltin as an impurity produced neurological symptoms in 209 patients, 110 of whom died. Most symptoms were indicative of raised intracranial pressure as a consequence of cerebral oedema, but some patients developed paraplegia. For those patients that survived, the paraplegia was largely irreversible, but other neurotoxic effects were not (52).

## 14.27.7 Guideline values

### Dialkyltins

The disubstituted compounds that may leach from PVC water pipes for a short time after installation are primarily immunotoxins, although they appear to be of low general toxicity. The data available are insufficient to permit the proposal of guideline values for individual dialkyltins.

### Tributyltin oxide

TBTO is not genotoxic. Although one carcinogenicity study was reported in which neoplastic changes were observed in endocrine organs, the significance of these changes is considered questionable. The most sensitive end-point appears to be immunotoxicity, with a lowest NOAEL of 0.025 mg/kg of body weight per day in a 17-month feeding study in rats related to the suppression of resistance to the nematode *Trichinella spiralis* (*41*). The significance to humans of this finding is not completely clear, but this NOAEL is consistent, within an order of magnitude, with other NOAELs for long-term toxicity.

A TDI of 0.25 µg/kg of body weight was calculated by applying an uncertainty factor of 100 (for inter- and intraspecies variation) to the NOAEL of 0.025 mg/kg of body weight per day. The guideline value for TBTO is 2 µg/litre (rounded figure) based on an allocation of 20% of the TDI to drinking-water.

The database on the toxicity of the other trisubstituted organotin compounds is either limited or rather old. It was therefore not considered appropriate to propose guideline values for these compounds.

## References

1. Greaves J, Unger MA. A selective ion monitoring assay for tributyltin and its degradation products. *Biomedical and environmental mass spectrometry*, 1988, 15(10):565-569.

2. Mueller MD. Comprehensive trace level determination of organotin compounds in environmental samples using high resolution gas chromatography with flame photometric detection. *Analytical chemistry*, 1987, 59:617-623.

3. Maguire RJ et al. Occurrence of organotin compounds in water and sediment in Canada. *Chemosphere*, 1986, 15:253-274.

4. Waldock MJ, Waite ME, Thain JE. Changes in concentration of organotins in UK rivers and estuaries following legislation in 1986. In: *Proceedings of the Organotin Symposium, Oceans '87 Conference, Halifax, Nova Scotia, Canada, 28 September–1 October 1987*. New York, Institute of Electrical and Electronics Engineers, 1987, Vol. 4:1352-1356.

5. Mazaev VT, Slepnina TG. [Experimental data on hygienic standardization of dibutyltin sulfide in reservoir water.] *Gigiena i sanitarija*, 1973, 8:10-15 (in Russian).

6. Waldock MJ, Miller D. *The determination of total and tributyl tin in seawater and oysters in areas of high pleasure craft activity*. Copenhagen, International Council for the Exploration of the Sea (ICES), 1983 (Report No. C.M. 1983/E:12).

7. Evans DW, Laughlin RB Jr. Accumulation of bis(tributyltin) oxide by the mud crab, *Rhithropanopeus harrisii*. *Chemosphere*, 1984, 13:213-219.

8. *1970 evaluations of some pesticide residues in food*. Rome, Food and Agriculture Organization of the United Nations, 1971:327-366, 521-542.

9.  Duncan J. The toxicology of molluscicides: the organotins. *Pharmacology and thera-peutics*, 1980, 10:407-429.

10. Penninks AH, Hilgers L, Seinen W. The absorption, tissue distribution and excretion of di-*n*-octyltin dichloride in rats. *Toxicology*, 1987, 44:107-120.

11. Evans WH, Cardarelli NF, Smith DJ. Accumulation and excretion of [1-$^{14}$C]bis(tri-*n*-butyltin)oxide in mice. *Journal of toxicology and environmental health*, 1979, 5:871-877.

12. Mushak P, Krigman MR, Mailman RB. Comparative organotin toxicity in the developing rat: somatic and morphological changes and relationship to accumulation of total tin. *Neurobehavioral toxicology and teratology*, 1982, 4:209-215.

13. Iwai H et al. Intestinal uptake site, enterohepatic circulation, and excretion of tetra- and trialkyltin compounds in animals. *Journal of toxicology and environmental health*, 1982, 9:41-49.

14. Kimmel EC, Fish RH, Casida JE. Bioorganotin chemistry. Metabolism of organotin compounds in microsomal monooxygenase systems and in mammals. *Journal of agricultural and food chemistry*, 1977, 25:1-9.

15. Wiebkin P, Prough RA, Bridges JW. The metabolism and toxicity of some organotin compounds in isolated rat hepatocytes. *Toxicology and applied pharmacology*, 1982, 62:409-420.

16. Klimmer OR. Die Anwendung von Organozinn-verbindungen in experimentelltoxikologischer Sicht. [Use of organotin compounds from the experimental toxicological point of view.] *Arzneimittel-Forschung*, 1969, 19:934-939.

17. Pelikan Z, Cerny E, Polster M. Toxic effects of some di-*n*-octyltin compounds in white mice. *Food and cosmetics toxicology*, 1970, 8:655-658.

18. Klimmer OR, Nebel IU. Experimentelle Untersuchungen zur Frage der toxizität einiger Stabilisatoren in Kunststoffen aus Polyvinylchlorid. [Experimental investigations of the toxicity of some stabilizers in PVC plastics.] *Arzneimittel-Forschung*, 1960, 10:44-48.

19. Seinen W, Willems MI. Toxicity of organotin compounds. I. Atrophy of thymus and thymus-dependent lymphoid tissue in rats fed di-*n*-octyltin dichloride. *Toxicology and applied pharmacology*, 1976, 35:63-75.

20. Miller K, Maisey J, Nicklin S. Effect of orally administered dioctyltin dichloride on murine immunocompetence. *Environmental research*, 1986, 39:434-441.

21. Gaunt IF et al. Acute and short-term toxicity studies on di-*n*-butyltin dichloride in rats. *Food and cosmetics toxicology*, 1968, 6:599-608.

22. Miller K, Scott MP. Immunological consequences of dioctyltin dichloride (DOTC)-induced thymic injury. *Toxicology and applied pharmacology*, 1985, 78:395-403.

23. Westendorf J, Marquardt H, Marquardt H. DNA interaction and mutagenicity of the plastic stabilizer di-*n*-octyltin dichloride. *Arzneimittel-Forschung*, 1986, 36:1263-1264.

24. Tennant RW, Stasiewicz S, Spalding JW. Comparison of multiple parameters of rodent carcinogenicity and *in vitro* genetic toxicity. *Environmental mutagenesis*, 1986, 8:205-227.

25. Li AP, Dahl AR, Hill JO. *In vitro* cytotoxicity and genotoxicity of dibutyltin dichloride and dibutylgermanium dichloride. *Toxicology and applied pharmacology*, 1982, 64:482-485.

26. National Cancer Institute. *Bioassay of dibutyltin diacetate for possible carcinogenicity*. Washington, DC, 1979 (TR-183; DHEW Publication 79-1739).

27. US Environmental Protection Agency. *Report on 24 month carcinogenicity study in rats of DOTC 65*. Washington, DC, 1988 (EPA 88-8600000 90).

28. Brown AW et al. The behavioral and neuropathologic sequelae of intoxication by trimethyltin compounds in the rat. *American journal of pathology*, 1979, 97:59-82.

29. Dyer RS et al. The trimethyltin syndrome in rats. *Neurobehavioral toxicology and teratology*, 1982, 4:127-133.

30. Snoeij NJ et al. Toxicity of triorganotin compounds: comparative *in vivo* studies with a series of trialkyltin compounds and triphenyltin chloride in male rats. *Toxicology and applied pharmacology*, 1985, 81:274-286.

31. Jensen KG, Andersen O, Ronne M. Spindle-inhibiting effects of organotin compounds: effects of trimethyltin on chromosome length. *ATLA*, 1990, 17:195-198.

32. McMillan DE, Wenger GR. Neurobehavioral toxicology of trialkyltins. *Pharmacological reviews*, 1985, 37:365-379.

33. Verschuuren HG et al. Short-term toxicity studies with triphenyltin compounds in rats and guinea-pigs. *Food and cosmetics toxicology*, 1966, 4:35-45.

34. *Tributyltin compounds*. Geneva, World Health Organization, 1990 (Environmental Health Criteria, No. 116).

35. Schweinfurth H. Toxicology of tributyltin compounds. *Tin and its uses*, 1985, 143:9-12.

36. Krajnc EI et al. Toxicity of bis(tri-*n*-butyltin)oxide in the rat. I. Short-term effects on general parameters and on the endocrine and lymphoid systems. *Toxicology and applied pharmacology*, 1984, 75:363-386.

37. Vos JG et al. Toxicity of bis(tri-*n*-butyltin)oxide in the rat. II. Suppression of thy-mus-dependent immune responses and of parameters of nonspecific resistance after short-term exposure. *Toxicology and applied pharmacology*, 1984, 75:387-408.

38. Wester PW et al. Chronic toxicity and carcinogenicity of bis(tri-*n*-butyltin) oxide (TBTO) in the rat. *Food chemistry and toxicology*, 1990, 28(3):179-196.

39. Vos JG, Krajnc EI, Wester PW. Immunotoxicity of bis(tri-*n*-butyltin) oxide. In: Dean J, ed. *Immunotoxicology and immunopharmacology*, New York, Raven Press, 1985:327-340.

40. Wester PW et al. Chronic toxicity and carcinogenicity of bis(tri-*n*-butyltin)oxide (TBTO) in the rat. *Food chemistry and toxicology*, 1990, 28(3):179-196.

41. Vos JG et al. Immunotoxicity of bis(tri-*n*-butyltin)oxide in the rat: effects on thy-mus-dependent immunity and on nonspecific resistance following long-term exposure in young versus aged rats. *Toxicology and applied pharmacology*, 1990, 105:144-155.

42. Davis A et al. Evaluation of the genetic and embryotoxic effects of bis(tri-*n*-butyl-tin)oxide (TBTO), a broad spectrum pesticide, in multiple *in vivo* and *in vitro* short-term tests. *Mutation research*, 1987, 188:65-95.

43. Crofton KM et al. Prenatal or postnatal exposure to bis(tri-*n*-butyltin)oxide in the rat: postnatal evaluation of teratology and behavior. *Toxicology and applied pharma-cology*, 1989, 97:113-123..

44. Oakley SD, Fawell JK. *Toxicity of selected organotin compounds to mammalian species.* Medmenham, Water Research Centre, 1986 (Report ER 1307-M).

45. Vos JG et al. Effect of triphenyltin hydroxide on the immune system of the rat. *Toxi-cology*, 1984, 29:325-336.

46. Giavini E, Prati M, Vismara C. Effects of triphenyltin acetate on pregnancy in the rat. *Bulletin of environmental contamination and toxicology*, 1980, 24:936-939.

47. Shelby MD, Stasiewicz S. Chemicals showing no evidence of carcinogenicity in long-term, two-species rodent studies: the need for short-term test data. *Environmental mutagenesis*, 1984, 6:871-878.

48. Epstein SS et al. Detection of chemical mutagens by the dominant lethal assay in the mouse. *Toxicology and applied pharmacology*, 1972, 23:288-325.

49. National Cancer Institute. *Bioassay of triphenyltin hydroxide for possible carcino-genicity.* Bethesda, MD, US Department of Health, Education, and Welfare, 1978 (Technical Report 139).

50. Fortemps E et al. Trimethyltin poisoning. Report of two cases. *International archives of occupational and environmental health*, 1978, 41:1-6.

51. Rey CH, Reinecke HJ, Besser R. Methyltin intoxication in six men: toxicologic and clinical aspects. *Veterinary and human toxicology*, 1984, 26:121-122.

52. Alajouanine T, DeRobert L, Thieffry S. Étude clinique d'ensemble de 210 cas d'intoxication par les sels organiques de l'étain. *Revue neurologique*, 1958, 98:85-96.

# 15.
# Pesticides

## 15.1 Introduction

The evaluation of the health effects of pesticides was based on reviews of all available relevant information, including unpublished proprietary data developed by manufacturers of pesticides. The fact that pesticide manufacturers made available to the review groups their proprietary toxicological information on the products under discussion is gratefully acknowledged.

For the sake of completeness, these unpublished studies are included in the reference lists of the monographs as appropriate. Copies of the reports may be requested directly from the manufacturers; they are not available from WHO.

It should be noted that the recommended guideline values for pesticides in drinking-water are set at a level to protect human health; they may not be suitable for the protection of the environment or aquatic life.

It is recognized that the environmental degradation products of pesticides may be a problem in drinking-water. In most cases, however, the toxicities of these degradation products have not been taken into consideration in these guidelines, as data on their identity, presence, and biological activity are inadequate.

## 15.2 Alachlor

### 15.2.1 General description

#### Identity

CAS no.:                    15972-60-8
Molecular formula:       $C_{14}H_{20}ClNO_2$

Alachlor is the common name for 2-chloro-*N*-(2,6-diethylphenyl)-*N*-(methoxymethyl)acetamide.

#### Physicochemical properties *(1, 2)*

| Property | Value |
|---|---|
| Physical state | White crystalline solid at 23 °C |
| Water solubility | 242 mg/litre at 25 °C |
| Vapour pressure | $2.9 \times 10^{-3}$ Pa at 25 °C |
| Log octanol–water partition coefficient | 2.6–3.1 |

### Organoleptic properties

Taste and odour thresholds in water of 33 and 110 mg/litre, respectively, have been reported (*1*).

### Major uses

Alachlor is used pre- or early post-emergence to control annual grasses and many broad-leaved weeds mainly in maize, but also in cotton, brassicas, oilseed rape, peanuts, radish, soy beans, and sugar-cane (*2*).

### Environmental fate

Alachlor dissipates from soil mainly through volatilization, photodegradation, and biodegradation (*3–5*). Many metabolites have been identified; diethylaniline, detected in some soil studies, interacts rapidly with humic substances in the soil (*3*). A half-life in soil of 7–38 days has been reported (*6*). Under certain conditions, alachlor can leach beyond the root zone and migrate to groundwater (*1, 3*).

## 15.2.2 Analytical methods

Water samples are extracted with chloroform, and alachlor determined in the extracts by gas–liquid chromatography with electrolytic conductivity detection in the nitrogen mode or by capillary column gas chromatography with a nitrogen–phosphorus detector (*7*). The detection limit is about 0.1 µg/litre.

## 15.2.3 Environmental levels and human exposure

### Water

Alachlor was detected in the surface water and groundwater of 10 states of the USA between 1979 and 1987 (*3*). In two recent surveys in the USA, alachlor was detected in one of 750 and in 38 of 1430 private wells sampled (A.J. Klein, Monsanto Agricultural Company, personal communication). A review of monitoring data showed that alachlor was present in groundwaters in the USA at levels ranging from less than 0.1 to 16.6 µg/litre (*8*). In Italy, in a survey carried out in 1987–88, alachlor was detected in three out of 322 drinking-water supplies at a maximum level of 1.6 µg/litre (*9*).

### Food

Food does not appear to be a major route of exposure for the general population since residues of alachlor in food are usually below the detection limit. It is rapidly metabolized by crops after application and does not bioaccumulate (*1*). In tolerant plants, it is detoxified by rapid conjugation with glutathione (*10*).

## 15.2.4 Kinetics and metabolism in laboratory animals and humans

Alachlor is absorbed through the gastrointestinal tract of rats and distributed to the blood, spleen, liver, kidney, heart, and, to a lesser extent, eyes, brain, stomach, and ovaries (11). Rats, mice, and monkeys differ in the ways in which they metabolize, distribute and excrete it (12–14). 4-Amino-3,5-diethylphenol, which is suspected to be a key metabolite from the point of view of the carcinogenicity of alachlor has been found in much larger quantities in the urine of rats than in that of mice and monkeys. Alachlor and its metabolites in urine and faeces are excreted much more slowly in rats than in mice and monkeys. Mice excrete alachlor metabolites mainly via the faeces, rats in equal proportions in the urine and faeces, and monkeys mainly via urine (15, 16).

## 15.2.5 Effects on laboratory animals and *in vitro* test systems

### Acute exposure

Acute oral $LD_{50}$s of 930–1350 and 1100 mg/kg of body weight for rats and mice, respectively, have been reported (2).

### Short-term exposure

In a 6-month feeding study, dogs were given alachlor at 0, 5, 25, 50, or 75 mg/kg of body weight per day; dose-related hepatotoxicity was seen at all dose levels (17). In a subsequent 1-year feeding study in which dogs were given alachlor at 1, 3, or 10 mg/kg of body weight per day, the NOAEL was 1 mg/kg of body weight per day (18).

### Long-term exposure

A 2-year feeding study in Long-Evans rats showed alachlor to be toxic at all doses tested (14, 42, or 126 mg/kg of body weight per day). Effects observed included dose-related hepatotoxicity at all dose levels and highly significant levels of ocular lesions, identified as the uveal degeneration syndrome, in the mid- and high-dose groups (19). In another 2-year feeding study in which the same strain of rats was given alachlor at 0, 0.5, 2.5, or 15 mg/kg of body weight per day, 2.5 mg/kg of body weight per day was considered to be the NOAEL for uveal degeneration syndrome (20).

### Reproductive toxicity, embryotoxicity, and teratogenicity

In a three-generation study, 10 male and 20 female CD rats were fed a diet containing 0, 3, 10, or 30 mg of alachlor per kg. No effects were observed on the reproductive cycle or on postnatal development (21). After female CD rats were treated by gastric intubation with 0, 50, 150, or 400 mg of technical alachlor per kg of body weight per day on days 6 to 19 of gestation, no signs of embryotoxicity were observed at any of the doses tested (22).

Female Dutch Belted rabbits were exposed to alachlor by gavage on days 7–19 of gestation at 0, 10, 30, or 60 mg/kg of body weight per day. No signs of maternal toxicity or embryotoxicity were observed at these doses (23).

### Mutagenicity and related end-points

Alachlor does not induce gene mutations in bacteria or in mammalian cells *in vitro* (24), but does induce chromosomal aberrations in mammalian cells *in vitro* (25) and is weakly active in a gene conversion test in yeast (26) and in an *in vitro/in vivo* test of DNA repair in rat hepatocytes (27). Samples of varying purity gave contrasting results for chromosomal aberrations in *in vivo* tests in the rat (26, 28). A broad spectrum of genetic damage was observed in plant systems (29, 30). There are positive mutagenicity data for 2,6-diethylaniline, which is a known metabolite of alachlor in animals.

### Carcinogenicity

Doses of 0, 14, 42, or 126 mg/kg were administered in the diet to Long-Evans rats (50 of each sex) for 2 years. This study provided clear evidence of carcinogenicity based on a statistically significant increase in the incidence of adenomas of the nasal turbinate, malignant stomach tumours, and thyroid follicular tumours in high-dose males. This conclusion is also based on the incidence of adenocarcinomas of the nasal turbinate in mid-dose males and females and the observation of submucosal hyperplasia in nasal tissues, and was supported by a repeated study of the highest dose only (126 mg/kg), in which adenomas and adenocarcinomas of the nasal cavity and malignant stomach tumours were found (31).

A second study on the same rat strain at doses of 0, 0.5, 2.5, and 15 mg/kg for 2 years also provided clear evidence of carcinogenicity. A statistically significant increase in the incidence of adenomas of the nasal turbinate was observed at the highest dose. Submucosal gland hyperplasia of the nasal turbinate was also noted. The presence of stabilizers in the technical material is unlikely to have influenced the carcinogenic response observed in the rat (20).

CD-1 mice were fed technical-grade alachlor in the diet for 18 months at doses of 0, 26, 78, or 260 mg/kg of body weight per day. Statistically significant increases in lung bronchiolar tumours at the highest dose tested were seen in female mice (32). The increase of lung tumours in male mice was not significant at any dose. In the United States, the Environmental Protection Agency has concluded that this study provides inadequate evidence of carcinogenicity (A.J. Klein, Monsanto Agricultural Company, personal communication).

## 15.2.6 Effects on humans

The probable oral lethal dose in humans is 0.5–5 g/kg of body weight.[1]

## 15.2.7 Guideline value

IARC has not evaluated alachlor. On the basis of available experimental data, evidence for the genotoxicity of alachlor is considered to be equivocal. However, a metabolite of alachlor has been shown to be mutagenic. Available data from two studies in rats clearly indicate that this compound is carcinogenic, causing benign and malignant tumours of the nasal turbinate, malignant stomach tumours, and benign thyroid tumours.

In view of the data on carcinogenicity, guideline values were calculated by applying the linearized multistage model to data on the incidence of nasal tumours in rats (20). Concentrations of 200, 20, and 2 µg/litre in drinking-water are associated with excess lifetime cancer risks of $10^{-4}$, $10^{-5}$, and $10^{-6}$, respectively.

## References

1. US Environmental Protection Agency. Alachlor. *Reviews in environmental contamination and toxicology*, 1988, 104:9-20.

2. Worthing CR, ed. *The pesticide manual*, 9th ed. Farnham, British Crop Protection Council, 1991.

3. Chesters G et al. Environmental fate of alachlor and metolachlor. *Reviews in environmental contamination and toxicology*, 1989, 110:1-74.

4. Walker A, Brown PA. The relative persistence in soil of five acetanilide herbicides. *Bulletin of environmental contamination and toxicology*, 1985, 34:143-149.

5. Fang CH. [Effects of soils on the degradation of herbicide alachlor under the light.] *Journal of the Chinese Agricultural Chemists Society*, 1977, 15:53-59 (in Chinese).

6. Laskowsky DA et al. *Environmental risk analysis for chemicals*. New York, NY, Van Nostrand Reinhold, 1982.

7. Frank R et al. Survey of farm wells for pesticide residues, southern Ontario, Canada, 1981-1982, 1984. *Archives of environmental contamination and toxicology*, 1987, 16:1-8.

8. Ritter WF. Pesticide contamination of ground water in the United States—a review. *Environmental science and health*, 1990, B25(1):1-29.

[1] Source: Toxicology Data Bank, Bethesda, MD, National Library of Medicine.

9. Funari E et al. Erbicidi nelle acque destinate al consumo umano in Italia. [Herbicides in waters intended for human consumption in Italy.] *Acqua aria*, 1989, 9:1011-1024.

10. Breaux EJ et al. Flurazole mode of action studies. *Plant physiology*, 1986, Suppl. No. 690 (abstract).

11. Monsanto Agricultural Company. *Rat metabolism study*. Parts I and II. St Louis, MO, 1983 (unpublished study submitted to WHO).

12. Johnson DE. *Pharmacokinetic study of alachlor in Rhesus monkeys following intravenous administration*. Prepared by International Research and Development Corporation, 1984 (unpublished study submitted to WHO by Monsanto Agricultural Company, St Louis, MO).

13. Wilson AGE, Hall LJ. *Pharmacokinetic study of alachlor distribution and elimination in the Long-Evans rat. Part I. Absorption, distribution and excretion*. St Louis, MO, Monsanto Agricultural Company, 1986 (unpublished study submitted to WHO).

14. Wilson AGE, Reisch CM. *The study of alachlor metabolism and elimination in the mouse. Part I: Elimination*. St Louis, MO, Monsanto Agricultural Company, 1985 (unpublished study submitted to WHO).

15. *Monsanto alachlor technical seminar proceedings*. 1986 (unpublished study submitted to WHO by Monsanto Agricultural Company, St Louis, MO).

16. Mulder GJ et al. Reaction of mutagenic phenacetin metabolites with glutathione and DNA. Possible implications for toxicity. *Molecular pharmacology*, 1984, 26:342-347.

17. Ahmed FE et al. *Alachlor: six month study in the dog*. St Louis, MO, Monsanto Agricultural Company, 1981 (unpublished study submitted to the US Environmental Protection Agency).

18. Naylor MW et al. *Chronic study of alachlor administered by gelatin capsule to dogs*. St Louis, MO, Monsanto Agricultural Company, 1984 (unpublished study submitted to WHO).

19. Stout LD et al. *A chronic study of alachlor administered in feed to Long-Evans rats*. St Louis, MO, Monsanto Agricultural Company, 1983 (unpublished report no. CDL:252498, submitted to WHO).

20. Stout LD et al. *A chronic study of alachlor administered in feed to Long-Evans rats*, Vols. I and II. St Louis, MO, Monsanto Agricultural Company, 1983 (unpublished report no. CDL:252496 submitted to WHO).

21. Schroeder RD et al. *A three-generation reproduction study in rats with alachlor.* St Louis, MO, Monsanto Agricultural Company, 1981 (unpublished study submitted to WHO).

22. Rodwell DE, Tracher EJ. *Teratology study in rats.* St Louis, MO, Monsanto Agricultural Company, 1980 (unpublished study submitted to WHO).

23. Monsanto Agricultural Company. *Teratology study—rabbit.* St Louis, MO, 1984 (unpublished study submitted to WHO).

24. Shirasu S et al. *Microbial mutagenicity study.* St Louis, MO, Monsanto Agricultural Company, 1980 (unpublished study submitted to WHO).

25. Lin MF, Wu CL, Wang TC. Pesticide clastogenicity in Chinese hamster ovary cells. *Mutation research*, 1987, 188:241-250.

26. Georgian L et al. Cytogenetic effects of alachlor and mancozeb. *Mutation research*, 1983, 116:341-348.

27. Monsanto Agricultural Company. *Evaluation of the potential of alachlor to induce unscheduled DNA synthesis in the in vivo-in vitro hepatocyte DNA repair assay.* St Louis, MO, 1984 (unpublished study submitted to WHO).

28. Monsanto Agricultural Company. *In vivo bone marrow chromosome study in rats with alachlor.* St Louis, MO, 1984 (unpublished study submitted to WHO).

29. Singh HN, Singh HR, Vaishampayan A. Toxic and mutagenic action of the herbicide alachlor (lasso) on various strains of the nitrogen-fixing blue-green alga *Nostoc muscorum* and characterization of the herbicide-induced mutants resistant to methylanine-*dl*-sulfoximine. *Environmental experiments in botany*, 1978, 19:5-12.

30. Reddy SS, Rao GM. Cytogenetic effects of agricultural chemicals. II. Effect of herbicides 'Lasso and Basagran' on chromosomal mechanism in relation to yield and yield components in chili (*Capsicum annuum* L). *Cytologia*, 1982, 47:257-267.

31. Daly IW et al. *A chronic feeding study of alachlor in rats.* St Louis, MO, Monsanto Agricultural Company, 1981 (unpublished study submitted to WHO).

32. Daly IW et al. *An eighteen-month chronic feeding study of alachlor in mice.* St Louis, MO, Monsanto Agricultural Company, 1981 (unpublished study submitted to WHO).

## 15.3 Aldicarb

### 15.3.1 General description

#### *Identity*

CAS no.:                116-06-3
Molecular formula:      $C_7H_{14}N_2O_2S$

Aldicarb is the common name for 2-methyl-2(methylthio)propionaldehyde O-methylcarbamoyloxime.

#### *Physicochemical properties (1–3)*

| Property | Value |
|---|---|
| Vapour pressure | 13 Pa at 25 °C |
| Water solubility | 6 g/litre at 20 °C |
| Log octanol–water partition coefficient | 1.359 |

#### *Major uses*

Aldicarb is a systemic carbamate insecticide used to control nematodes in soil and insects and mites on a wide variety of crops, including citrus fruits, grain, peanuts, potatoes, soy beans, sugar-beet, and tobacco.

#### *Environmental fate*

Aldicarb is oxidized by microorganisms in soil to the sulfoxide and sulfone (4); its degradation half-life ranges from a few days to more than 2 months (5, 6). Aldicarb and its degradation products are generally mobile in soil (5, 6); leaching is most extensive in soils with a low content of organic matter (5).

Aldicarb is very persistent in groundwaters, particularly those that are acidic; the half-life for degradation to nontoxic products ranges from a few weeks to as long as several years (7). The primary mode of degradation is chemical hydrolysis, although there may also be some microbial decay in shallow groundwater (8).

### 15.3.2 Analytical methods

Aldicarb and its degradation products in water may be determined by high-performance liquid chromatography (3). When followed by post-column derivatization to form fluorescent compounds, this method has detection limits of about 1.3, 0.8, and 0.5 µg/litre for aldicarb, the sulfoxide, and the sulfone, respectively (9). Aldicarb and its oxidation products can also be determined as their nitrile derivatives by capillary gas chromatography with a nitrogen–phosphorus detector (10).

## 15.3.3 Environmental levels and human exposure

### *Water*

Aldicarb was detected in 111 of 1017 samples in surveys of private and municipal drinking-water supplies in Canada (detection limits 0.01–3.0 µg/litre); the maximum concentration was 28 µg/litre (*11*). It has been detected in well-water in the USA at concentrations ranging from less than 10 to 500 µg/litre (*7*). Neither aldicarb nor its metabolites were detected in over 700 community groundwater drinking supplies in Florida (detection limit 2–5 µg/litre for each compound) (*12*). Concentrations in groundwater near potato fields to which it had been applied were detectable (⩾1 µg/litre) in 31.3% of samples taken in Long Island, NY; 0.9% of samples contained aldicarb at concentrations above 100 µg/litre (*13*). Aldicarb sulfoxide and aldicarb sulfone residues are found in an approximately 1:1 ratio in groundwater (*5, 6*).

### *Food*

Aldicarb was detected in 94% of potatoes analysed in the USA in 1980 at concentrations ranging from 50 to 520 µg/kg (*14*). Aldicarb sulfoxide was found in 1981–1986 in seven of 6391 samples of domestic agricultural commodities at levels at or below 1.0 mg/kg (*15*).

### *Estimated total exposure and relative contribution of drinking-water*

Based on maximum residue limits for aldicarb established by the Codex Alimentarius Commission (*16*), the theoretical maximum daily intake of aldicarb from food is about 0.09 mg/day for a 60-kg adult (1.5 µg/kg of body weight per day). The average daily intake for a male aged 25–30 years has been estimated to be 0.2 µg/kg of body weight per day, based on residues in foods in the USA (*17*).

Based on a concentration of aldicarb in drinking-water of 5 µg/litre and consumption of 2 litres of drinking-water per day by a 60-kg adult, the daily intake by this route can be estimated to be 10 µg (0.2 µg/kg of body weight), which is about the same as that from food.

## 15.3.4 Kinetics and metabolism in laboratory animals and humans

Aldicarb is rapidly absorbed from the gastrointestinal tract, the respiratory tract, and the skin. It is rapidly oxidized to aldicarb sulfoxide, which is metabolized more slowly by oxidation and hydrolysis to aldicarb sulfone. Both metabolites and the parent compound are degraded to the corresponding oximes and nitriles, which are then broken down into aldehydes, acids, and alcohols (*1, 18*).

Elimination of aldicarb is rapid; in rats, 80% of an orally administered dose was eliminated in the urine within 24 h (*19*). It does not accumulate in tissues (*19*), but appears to cross the placental barrier (*20*).

Aldicarb forms a complex with acetylcholinesterase, thus inhibiting the enzyme's action. The complex can dissociate to form aldicarb and the enzyme or break down into the oxime plus a carbamylated enzyme, which is then hydrolysed into the free enzyme and methyl carbamic acid, thus detoxifying the insecticide (*18, 21*).

## 15.3.5 Effects on laboratory animals and *in vitro* test systems

### Acute exposure

Aldicarb is highly acutely toxic in animals; the oral $LD_{50}$ in rats ranges from 650 to 930 µg/kg of body weight (*22*), depending on the vehicle (*21*). The oral $LD_{50}$ in rats for aldicarb sulfoxide is similar to that of the parent compound, whereas the $LD_{50}$ for the sulfone is approximately 25 times higher (*18*).

### Short-term exposure

A 1:1 mixture of aldicarb sulfoxide and aldicarb sulfone was administered in drinking-water to Wistar rats (10 per sex per dose) at nominal concentrations of 0, 0.075, 0.3, 1.2, 4.8, or 19.2 mg/litre for 29 days. Mean plasma and erythrocyte cholinesterase activities were reduced by 54–77% in both males and females at 19.2 mg/litre at 8, 15, and 29 days. Although male rats exposed to 4.8 mg/litre experienced a 28% reduction in plasma cholinesterase activity at day 8 and a 25% reduction in erythrocyte cholinesterase activity at day 29, the authors considered these effects to be of questionable biological significance and determined the "no-ill-effect level" to be 4.8 mg/litre, equivalent to 0.5 mg/kg of body weight per day. Because the actual concentration in drinking-water was on average approximately 80% of the nominal concentration (*1, 23*), the NOAEL can be considered to be 0.4 mg/kg of body weight per day.

### Long-term exposure

Groups of rats (15 per sex per dose, strain unspecified) were fed diets containing concentrations of aldicarb sulfoxide equivalent to doses of 0, 0.125, 0.25, 0.5, or 1.0 mg/kg of body weight per day for 6 months. Plasma and erythrocyte cholinesterase activities were depressed in males consuming 0.25 mg/kg of body weight per day and above and in females consuming 0.5 mg/kg of body weight per day and above. No cholinesterase inhibition was observed in rats allowed to recover for 1 day before sacrifice. The NOAEL for cholinesterase inhibition was considered to be 0.125 mg/kg of body weight per day (*1, 24*).

In a 2-year study, groups of rats (20 per sex per dose) were fed diets containing aldicarb (0.3 mg/kg of body weight per day), aldicarb sulfoxide (0.3 or 0.6 mg/kg of body weight per day), aldicarb sulfone (0.6 or 2.4 mg/kg of body weight per day), or a 1:1 mixture of aldicarb sulfoxide and aldicarb sulfone (0.6 or 1.2 mg/kg of body weight per day). Plasma cholinesterase activity and body weight gain were depressed in males consuming 1.2 mg/kg of body weight per day of the aldicarb sulfoxide/sulfone mixture. Mortality was increased in male and female rats consuming 0.6 mg of aldicarb sulfoxide per kg of body weight per day. The authors considered the NOAELs to be 0.3 mg/kg of body weight per day for aldicarb and aldicarb sulfoxide, 2.4 mg/kg of body weight per day for aldicarb sulfone, and 0.6 mg/kg of body weight per day for the 1:1 mixture of aldicarb sulfoxide and sulfone (25).

No adverse effects were observed in two 2-year studies in which rats (26) and beagle dogs (27) were fed aldicarb in the diet at concentrations ranging from 0 to 0.1 mg/kg of body weight per day.

## Reproductive toxicity, embryotoxicity, and teratogenicity

No significant effects on fertility, gestation, viability of offspring, lactation, mean weights, or histological features in litters were observed in a three-generation reproduction study in CFE rats in which aldicarb was administered in the diet at doses of 0.05 or 0.1 mg/kg of body weight per day (28). In a three-generation study in Harlan-Wistar albino rats, there was a significant difference in the body weight of second-generation pups at 0.7 mg/kg of body weight per day (29), although no adverse effects on reproduction were observed when aldicarb sulfone was administered in the diet at doses of up to 9.6 mg/kg of body weight per day (30).

Single doses of 0.001, 0.01, or 0.1 mg of aldicarb per kg of body weight per day administered by gastric intubation to pregnant Sprague-Dawley rats on day 18 of gestation caused a significant inhibition of brain acetylcholinesterase activity, which was greater in fetal than in maternal tissues (20, 31).

No significant differences in fetal malformations or developmental variations were observed in the offspring of pregnant Dutch Belted rabbits given daily aldicarb doses of 0, 0.1, 0.25, or 0.50 mg/kg of body weight per day via gavage on days 7–27 of gestation (32). Similarly, teratogenic effects were not observed in a study in which pregnant CD rats were given up to 0.5 mg/kg of body weight per day orally for 10 days during gestation (1, 33).

## Mutagenicity and related end-points

Most *in vivo* and *in vitro* assays of aldicarb for mutagenicity have been negative (34, 35), although increases in both chromosomal aberrations in bone marrow cells (36) and sister chromatid exchange in cultured human lymphocytes (1, 37) have been observed.

## *Carcinogenicity*

No significant increases in the incidence of tumours of any type were reported in studies in rats (0–0.3 mg/kg of body weight per day) and mice (0–0.7 mg/kg of body weight per day) fed aldicarb in the diet for periods ranging from 18 months to 2 years (*25, 26, 38, 39*).

## 15.3.6 Effects on humans

Clinical symptoms of aldicarb intoxication include dizziness, weakness, diarrhoea, nausea, vomiting, abdominal pain, excessive perspiration, blurred vision, headache, muscular convulsions, temporary paralysis of the extremities, and dyspnoea. Recovery is rapid, usually within 6 h (*21*).

Aldicarb is one of the most acutely toxic pesticides. Poisoning has resulted from the ingestion of contaminated cucumbers at a dose ranging from 0.006 to 0.25 mg/kg of body weight (*40*) and contaminated melons at a dose as low as 0.0021 mg/kg of body weight (*41*).

Groups of four adult male volunteers ingested single doses of aqueous aldicarb of 0.025, 0.05, or 0.1 mg/kg of body weight. Cholinergic symptoms were observed at 0.1 mg/kg of body weight. A dose-related depression of acetylcholinesterase activity (47–73%), predominantly in the first 2 h following exposure, was observed in all subjects. It should be noted, however, that acetylcholinesterase levels in individuals varied considerably between 18 h and 1 h before dosing (*42*). In a study in which two volunteers ingested doses of aqueous aldicarb of 0.05 or 0.26 mg/kg of body weight, clinical signs of intoxication were observed only in the subject receiving 0.26 mg/kg of body weight (*43*).

The effects of chronic ingestion of aldicarb on human immune function were investigated in two limited cross-sectional epidemiological studies of women (*1, 44, 45*). In the first study, an association was found between the consumption of aldicarb in drinking-water (1–61 µg/litre) and abnormalities in various subsets of T-cell populations in women with otherwise intact immune systems (*44*). However, the study had several limitations, including the limited size of the exposed group, the failure to calculate aldicarb dose on a body weight basis, and the failure to match exposed and control groups with respect to water supply. In a follow-up study (*45*), which suffered from many of the same limitations as the first, the authors concluded that changes in the cellular distribution of immune system parameters occurred in women exposed to aldicarb in their drinking-water. The findings of these studies suggest that further research on the effects of aldicarb on the immune system is warranted.

A significant association between the age-adjusted rates for all neurological syndromes and increasing aldicarb concentration was found in a study on the relationship between levels of aldicarb in drinking-water and delayed neuropathy (*46* ). Information on somewhat subjective symptoms was obtained from individuals by self-administered questionnaire; no clinical examinations were conducted. It was not reported whether the subjects were classified blindly on the basis of the results of the questionnaire or whether the respondents were aware of their exposure status.

No relationship between aldicarb concentrations in drinking-water and food consumption or other reported symptoms or diagnosed illnesses was found in a survey of 1035 residents of 462 households in Long Island, NY (*47*).

## 15.3.7 Guideline value

IARC has concluded that aldicarb is not classifiable as to its carcinogenicity (Group 3) (*48*). The only consistently observed toxic effect with both long-term and single-dose administration of aldicarb in studies conducted to date is the rapidly reversible inhibition of acetylcholinesterase activity. The toxic effects of aldicarb appear to be dependent both on the method (i.e. single or repeated dosing) and the means of administration (e.g. by gavage, in the diet or in drinking-water), possibly because of reduced bioavailability of the compound or the bolus effect of certain forms of administration. The studies considered most appropriate for the derivation of the guideline, therefore, are those in which aldicarb was administered in the diet or drinking-water.

In 1992, the Joint FAO/WHO Meeting on Pesticide Residues (JMPR) recommended an ADI of 0.003 mg/kg of body weight, based on a single oral dose study in human volunteers with a NOAEL of 0.025 mg/kg of body weight per day and an uncertainty factor of 10 (*49*).

For the purposes of deriving a guideline value for drinking-water, the TDI is derived from a NOAEL of 0.4 mg/kg of body weight per day for acetylcholinesterase inhibition found in a 29-day study in rats given drinking-water containing a 1:1 mixture of aldicarb sulfoxide and aldicarb sulfone (*1, 23*). This study is considered to be the most relevant to the derivation of a drinking-water guideline because the rats were given water containing the two aldicarb metabolites in a ratio similar to that normally found in drinking-water. Based on an uncertainty factor of 100 (for inter- and intraspecies variation), the TDI is 4 µg/kg of body weight. No allowance was made for the short duration of the study in view of the extremely sensitive and rapidly reversible biological end-point used. The guideline value is 10 µg/litre (rounded figure), assuming an allocation of 10% of the TDI to drinking-water.

## References

1. *Aldicarb*. Geneva, World Health Organization, 1991 (Environmental Health Criteria, No. 121).

2. Suntio LR et al. Critical review of Henry's law constants for pesticides. *Reviews of environmental contamination and toxicology*, 1988, 103:1.

3. Moye HA, Miles CJ. Aldicarb contamination of groundwater. *Reviews of environmental contamination and toxicology*, 1988, 105:99-146.

4. Lightfoot EN, Thorne PS. Laboratory studies on mechanisms for the degradation of aldicarb, aldicarb sulfoxide, and aldicarb sulfone. *Environmental toxicology and chemistry*, 1987, 6:377-394.

5. US Environmental Protection Agency. EPA notice of preliminary determination regarding continued registrations of products containing aldicarb. *Federal register*, 1988, 53:24630.

6. Cohen SZ et al. Potential pesticide contamination of groundwater from agricultural uses. In: Krueger RF, Seiber JN, eds. *Treatment and disposal of pesticide wastes*. Washington, DC, American Chemical Society, 1984:297–325 (ACS Symposium Series, No. 259).

7. US Environmental Protection Agency. EPA notice initiating review of aldicarb pesticides. *Federal register*, 1984, 49:28320.

8. Jones RL. Field, laboratory and modelling studies on the degradation and transport of aldicarb residues in soil and groundwater. In: Garner WY, ed. *Evaluation of pesticides in groundwater*. Washington, DC, American Chemical Society, 1986:197-218 (ACS Symposium Series, No. 315).

9. Foerst DL, Moye HA. *Aldicarb and related compounds in drinking water via direct aqueous injection HPLC (high performance liquid chromatography) with post column derivatization*. Cincinnati, OH, US Environmental Protection Agency, Environmental Monitoring and Support Laboratory, 1985 (NTIS PB85-173144).

10. Zhong WZ, Lemley AT, Spalik J. Quantitative determination of ppb levels of carbamate pesticides in water by capillary gas chromatography. *Journal of chromatography*, 1984, 299:269-274

11. Hiebsch S. *The occurrence of thirty-five pesticides in Canadian drinking water and surface water*. Ottawa, Canada, Department of National Health and Welfare, Environmental Health Directorate, 1988.

12. Miller WL et al. Ground water monitoring for Temik (aldicarb) in Florida. *Water resources bulletin*, 1989, 25(1):79.

13. Jones RL, Marquardt TE. Monitoring of aldicarb residues in Long Island, New York potable wells. *Archives of environmental contamination and toxicology*, 1987, 16:643-647.

14. US Environmental Protection Agency. Proposed rules. *Federal register*, 1985, 50:219.

15. Hundley HK et al. Pesticide residue findings by the Luke method in domestic and imported foods and animal feeds for fiscal years 1982–1986. *Journal of the Association of Official Analytical Chemists,* 1988, 71(5):875-892.

16. Codex Alimentarius Commission. *Pesticide residues in food,* 2nd ed. Rome, Food and Agriculture Organization of the United Nations, 1993.

17. Gunderson EL. FDA Total Diet Study, April 1982–April 1984, dietary intakes of pesticides, selected elements, and other chemicals. *Journal of the Association of Official Analytical Chemists,* 1988, 71(6):1200-1209.

18. Baron RL, Merriam TL. Toxicology of aldicarb. *Reviews of environmental contamination and toxicology,* 1988, 105:1-70.

19. Andrawes NR, Dorough HW, Lindquist DA. Degradation and elimination of Temik in rats. *Journal of economic entomology,* 1967, 60:979-987.

20. Cambon C, Declume C, Derache R. Foetal and maternal rat brain acetylcholinesterase: isoenzyme changes following insecticidal carbamate derivatives poisoning. *Archives of toxicology,* 1980, 45:257-262.

21. Risher JF, Franklin LM, Stara JF. The toxicologic effects of the carbamate insecticide aldicarb in mammals: a review. *Environmental health perspectives,* 1987, 72:267-281.

22. National Institute of Occupational Safety and Health. *Registry of Toxic Effects of Chemical Substances (RTECS).* Washington, DC, US Department of Health and Human Services, 1989.

23. DePass LR, Weaver EV, Mirro EJ. Aldicarb sulfoxide/aldicarb sulfone mixture in drinking water of rats: effects on growth and acetylcholinesterase activity. *Journal of toxicology and environmental health,* 1985, 16:163-172.

24. Weil CS, Carpenter CP. *Temik sulfoxide. Results of feeding in the diet of rats for six months and dogs for three months.* Mellon Institute, 1968 (unpublished report no. 31-141, submitted to WHO by Union Carbide Corporation).

25. Weil CS, Carpenter CP. *Aldicarb (A), aldicarb sulfoxide (ASO), aldicarb sulfone (ASO₂) and a 1:1 mixture of ASO:ASO₂. Two year feeding in the diet of rats.* Mellon Institute, 1972 (unpublished report no. 35-82).

26. Weil CS, Carpenter CP. *Two-year feeding of compound 21149 in the diet of rats.* Mellon Institute, 1965 (unpublished report no. 28-123).

27. Weil CS, Carpenter CP. *Two-year feeding of compound 21149 in the diet of dogs.* Mellon Institute, 1966 (unpublished report no. 29-5).

28. Weil CS, Carpenter CP. *Results of a three generation reproduction study on rats fed compound 21149 in their diet.* Mellon Institute, 1974 (unpublished report no. 27-158, submitted to WHO by Union Carbide Corporation).

29. Weil CS, Carpenter CP. *Aldicarb. Inclusion in the diet of rats for three generations and a dominant lethal mutagenesis test.* Mellon Institute, 1974 (unpublished report no. 37-90, submitted to WHO by Union Carbide Corporation).

30. Woodside MD, Weil CS, Cox EF. *Aldicarb sulfone. Inclusion in the diet of rats for three generations, dominant lethal mutagenesis and teratology studies.* Carnegie-Mellon Institute, 1977 (unpublished report no. 40-1).

31. Cambon C, Declume C, Derache R. Effect of the insecticidal carbamate derivatives (carbofuran, pirimicarb, aldicarb) on the activity of acetylcholinesterase in tissues from pregnant rats and foetuses. *Toxicology and applied pharmacology,* 1979, 49:203-208.

32. International Research and Development Corporation. *Teratology study in rabbits.* West Virginia, Union Carbide Corporation, 1983 (unpublished report).

33. Tyl RW, Neeper-Bradley TL. *Developmental toxicity evaluation of aldicarb technical administered by gavage to CD (Sprague-Dawley) rats.* Lyon, Rhône-Poulenc 1988 (unpublished report).

34. Dunkel VC et al. Reproducibility of microbial mutagenicity assays: II. Testing of carcinogens and noncarcinogens in *Salmonella typhimurium* and *Escherichia coli. Environmental mutagenicity,* 1985, 7(Suppl. 5):1.

35. Ivett JL, Myhr BC, Lebowitz HD. *Mutagenicity evaluation of aldicarb technical 93.47% in the bone marrow cytogenetic assay.* Litton Bionetics Inc., 1984 (unpublished report no. 22202, submitted to WHO by Rhône-Poulenc).

36. Sharaf AA et al. Effect of aldicarb (Temik), a carbamate insecticide, on chromosomes of the laboratory rat. *Egyptian journal of genetics and cytology,* 1982, 11:143.

37. Cid MG, Matos E. Induction of sister-chromatid exchanges in cultured human lymphocytes by aldicarb, a carbamate pesticide. *Mutation research,* 1984, 138:175.

38. National Cancer Institute. *Bioassay of aldicarb for possible carcinogenicity.* Bethesda, MD, US Department of Health, Education and Welfare, 1979 (NCI-CG-TR-136).

39. Weil CS, Carpenter CP. *Aldicarb, 18-month feeding in the diet of mice, Study II.* Mellon Institute, 1974 (unpublished report no. 37-98).

40. Hirsch GH et al. Report of illnesses caused by aldicarb-contaminated cucumbers. *Food additives and contaminants,* 1987, 5(2):155.

601

41. Witt JM, Wagner SL. Aldicarb poisoning. *Journal of the American Medical Association*, 1986, 256(23):3218 (letter).

42. Haines RG. *Ingestion of aldicarb by human volunteers: a controlled study of the effects of aldicarb on man.* Terrytown, NY, Union Carbide Corporation, 1971 (unpublished study).

43. Cope OE, Romine RR. *Temik aldicarb pesticide. Results of aldicarb ingestion and exposure studies with humans and results of monitoring human exposure in working environments.* Union Carbide Agricultural Products Co., 1973 (unpublished study no. 18269).

44. Fiore MC et al. Chronic exposure to aldicarb-contaminated groundwater and human immune function. *Environmental research*, 1986, 41:633.

45. Mirkin IR et al. Changes in T-lymphocyte distribution associated with ingestion of aldicarb-contaminated drinking water: a follow-up study. *Environmental research*, 1990, 51:35-50.

46. Sterman AB, Varma A. Evaluating human neurotoxicity of the pesticide aldicarb: when man becomes the experimental animal. *Neurobehavioral toxicology and teratology*, 1983, 5:493-495.

47. Whitlock NH, Schuman SH, Loadholt CB. *Executive summary and epidemiologic survey of potential acute health effects of aldicarb in drinking water—Suffolk County, N.Y.* Charleston, South Carolina Pesticide Hazard Assessment Program Center, Medical University of South Carolina, 1982 (prepared for the Health Effects Branch, Hazard Evaluation Division, Office of Pesticide Programs, US Environmental Protection Agency).

48. International Agency for Research on Cancer. *Occupational exposures in insecticide applications, and some pesticides.* Lyon, 1991:93-113 (IARC Monographs on the Evaluation of Carcinogenic Risks to Humans, Volume 53).

49. *Pesticide residues in food—1992.* Rome, Food and Agriculture Organization of the United Nations, 1993 (Joint FAO/WHO Meeting on Pesticide Residues: report no. 116).

## 15.4 Aldrin and dieldrin

### 15.4.1 General description

#### *Identity*

| Compound | CAS no. | Molecular formula |
|----------|---------|-------------------|
| Aldrin | 309-00-2 | $C_{12}H_8Cl_6$ |
| Dieldrin | 60-57-1 | $C_{12}H_8Cl_6O$ |

The IUPAC name for aldrin is (1R,4S,4aS,5S,8R,8aR)-1,2,3,4,10,10-hexachloro-1,4,4a,5,8,8a-hexahydro-1,4:5,8-dimethanonaphthalene (HHDN). Aldrin is most commonly used to mean HHDN with a purity greater than 95%, except in Denmark and the countries of the former Soviet Union, where it is the name given to pure HHDN. Impurities include octachlorocyclopentene, hexachlorobutadiene, toluene, and polymerization products (1).

The IUPAC name for dieldrin is (1R,4S,4aS,5R,6R,7S,8S,8aR)-1,2,3,4,10,10-hexachloro-1,4,4a,5,6,7,8,8a-octahydro-6,7-epoxy-1,4:5,8-dimethanonaphthalene (HEOD). Dieldrin is most commonly used to mean HEOD with a purity greater than 85%, except in Denmark and the countries of the former Soviet Union, where it is the name given to pure HEOD. Impurities include other polychloroepoxyoctahydrodimethanonaphthalenes and endrin (1).

## Physicochemical properties (1, 2)

| Property | Technical aldrin (95% pure) | Technical dieldrin |
|---|---|---|
| Melting point (°C) | 49–60 | 175–176 |
| Density at 20 °C (g/cm³) | 1.54 | 1.62 |
| Water solubility at 20 °C (μg/litre) | 27 | 186 |
| Log octanol–water partition coefficient | 3.0 | 4.6 |
| Vapour pressure at 20 °C (Pa) | $8.6 \times 10^{-3}$ | $0.4 \times 10^{-3}$ |

## Organoleptic properties

Odour threshold values of 17 and 41 μg/litre have been reported for aldrin and dieldrin, respectively, in water (3, 4).

## Major uses

Aldrin and dieldrin are highly effective insecticides for soil-dwelling pests and for the protection of wooden structures against termites and wood borers. Dieldrin has also been used against insects of public health importance (1). Although the use of aldrin and dieldrin has been severely restricted or banned in many parts of the world since the early 1970s, they are still used in termite control in some countries (5).

## Environmental fate

In soil, aldrin is removed by oxidation to dieldrin and evaporation. In temperate climates, only 75% is oxidized within a year after application. The further disappearance of dieldrin is very slow under these conditions; the half-life is approximately 5 years. Under tropical conditions, both oxidation and further disappearance of dieldrin are rapid, 90% disappearing within 1 month, primarily by volatilization (*1*).

## 15.4.2 Analytical methods

Aldrin and dieldrin are determined by extraction with pentane followed by gas chromatography with electron-capture detection. The detection limits in tap-water and river water are about 0.001 µg/litre for aldrin and 0.002 µg/litre for dieldrin.

## 15.4.3 Environmental levels and human exposure

### *Air*

Dieldrin has been detected at very low concentrations in ambient air, on dust particles, and in rainwater. In nonagricultural areas, concentrations of 0.06–1.6 ng/m$^3$ have been reported; in agricultural areas, mean levels are in the range 1–2 ng/m$^3$, with a maximum of about 40 ng/m$^3$ (*1*).

Concentrations found in the air of houses treated for termites are much higher (40–7000 ng/m$^3$). The presence of aldrin/dieldrin-treated wood in houses results in indoor air concentrations of 10–500 ng/m$^3$ (1).

### *Water*

The concentrations of aldrin and dieldrin in aquatic environments and drinking-water are normally less than 10 ng/litre. Higher levels are attributed to contamination from industrial effluents and soil erosion during agricultural use. River sediments may contain higher amounts (up to 1 mg/kg). These pesticides are rarely present in groundwater, as little leaching from soils occurs (*1*).

### *Food*

Dieldrin is stored in the adipose tissue, liver, brain, and muscle of mammals, fish, birds, and other parts of the food-chain. The reduction in use since the 1970s has decreased the residues in food in many countries to well below the levels that may result in an intake of 0.1 µg/kg of body weight per day (the ADI established by the Joint FAO/WHO Meeting on Pesticide Residues) (*6*). The intake in 1980–82 was estimated to be 0–0.2 µg/kg of body weight per day in several countries (*1*).

Dieldrin has been detected in breast milk at a mean concentration of 0.5–11 µg/kg of milk in Europe and the USA. Breast-fed babies receive doses of approximately 1 µg/kg of body weight per day when mothers' milk contains 6 µg of dieldrin per litre (*1*). Although concentrations in breast milk decreased from an average of 1.33 µg/kg of milk in 1982 to 0.85 µg/kg of milk in 1986 (*7*), higher concentrations (mean 13 µg/litre) have been found in breast milk from women whose houses were treated annually with aldrin (*8*).

## 15.4.4 Kinetics and metabolism in laboratory animals and humans

Aldrin and dieldrin are absorbed by the oral, inhalation, and dermal routes. They tend to accumulate in adipose tissue. A steady state between intake, storage, and excretion is reached following repeated dosing. Aldrin and dieldrin can be mobilized from the adipose tissue compartment, causing an increase in blood level that results in toxic manifestations. Dieldrin is metabolized in the liver and is excreted, with its metabolites, primarily in the faeces via the bile in humans and in most animals tested (mouse, rat, monkey). The major metabolite is 9-hydroxy dieldrin. Small amounts of *trans*-6,7-hydroxy dieldrin, dicarboxylic acids, and bridged pentachloroketone are excreted, but only in laboratory animals. The ratios between the amounts of the various metabolites produced differ for different animals (*1*).

## 15.4.5 Effects on laboratory animals and *in vitro* test systems

### Acute exposure

Acute oral $LD_{50}$s of 33–65 mg/kg of body weight have been reported for aldrin and dieldrin for mice, rats, dogs, pigs, and rabbits. The reported value for dieldrin in monkeys is 3 mg/kg of body weight (*1*).

### Short-term exposure

Short-term studies on rodents have shown that the liver is the major target organ of aldrin and dieldrin exposure. The liver-to-body-weight ratio increases, and histopathological changes are observed, which have become known as "chlorinated hydrocarbon insecticide rodent liver". In rats, the changes were minimal at a dose of 0.025 mg/kg of body weight per day, and this value was selected as the LOAEL (*1*).

### Long-term exposure

Dogs seem more sensitive to aldrin and dieldrin than rats. In a 2-year study with beagle dogs receiving dieldrin in olive oil at doses of 0.005 or 0.05 mg/kg of body weight per day, female dogs given 0.05 mg/kg of body weight per day had an increased liver-to-body-weight ratio. The NOAEL was estimated to be 0.005 mg/kg of body weight per day (*1*).

### Reproductive toxicity, embryotoxicity, and teratogenicity

The results of a number of reproductive studies suggest that dieldrin at levels of 2 mg/kg in the rat diet and 3 mg/kg in the mouse diet has no effects on reproduction. At these levels, however, there may be biochemical and histopathological effects.

In a limited study with dogs fed aldrin or dieldrin, pup survival was generally lower. No effects were observed in dogs receiving 0.2 mg of dieldrin per kg in the diet (*1*).

### Mutagenicity and related end-points

The majority of studies on aldrin and dieldrin have not shown them to be mutagenic. In one study in which dieldrin was mutagenic in two out of three strains of *Salmonella typhimurium*, a dose–response relationship was not demonstrated (*1*).

### Carcinogenicity

A number of long-term studies have shown aldrin and dieldrin to produce benign and malignant tumours of the liver in various strains of mice but not in other species. This indicates that the effect of aldrin/dieldrin on the mouse liver is species-specific. Aldrin and dieldrin have also been tested for carcinogenicity by the oral route in hamsters, dogs, and monkeys (*1*). After assessing much of the available data, IARC concluded that the evidence for the carcinogenicity to animals of both aldrin and dieldrin is limited, and classified both chemicals in Group 3 (*9*).

## 15.4.6 Effects on humans

Both aldrin and dieldrin are highly toxic to humans, the target organs being the central nervous system and the liver. Severe cases of both accidental and occupational poisoning and a number of fatalities have been reported. The lethal dose of dieldrin is estimated to be approximately 10 mg/kg of body weight per day. The majority of those poisoned by aldrin or dieldrin recover, and irreversible effects have not been reported.

Male volunteers exposed to dieldrin doses of 0–3 µg/kg of body weight per day for 18 months showed no effects on health. The concentration of dieldrin in blood and adipose tissue was found to be proportional to the daily intake (*1*).

Effects on occupationally exposed workers have been studied in two epidemiological mortality studies. In one study (232 subjects), no indication of specific carcinogenic activity was found. In another study (1040 subjects), the mortality due to malignant neoplasms was lower than expected. There was a slight excess of cancers of the oesophagus, rectum, and liver, based on very small numbers. The only disease showing higher mortality rates than expected was nonmalignant respiratory system disease, specifically pneumonia (*1*).

Chromosome studies have been carried out on human peripheral lymphocytes from agricultural workers and workers engaged in the control of Chagas disease with at least 10 years of exposure to dieldrin. There were no differences between the control and exposure groups in structural chromosomal aberrations and sister chromatid exchange (*1*).

## 15.4.7 Guideline value

As already mentioned, IARC has classified aldrin and dieldrin in Group 3 (9). All the available information on aldrin and dieldrin taken together, including studies on humans, supports the view that these chemicals make very little contribution, if any, to the incidence of cancer in humans. Therefore, a TDI approach can be used to calculate a guideline value.

In 1977 JMPR recommended an ADI of 0.1 µg/kg of body weight (combined total for aldrin and dieldrin). This was based on NOAELs of 1 mg/kg of diet in the dog and 0.5 mg/kg of diet in the rat, which are equivalent to 0.025 mg/kg of body weight per day in both species. JMPR applied an uncertainty factor of 250 based on concern about carcinogenicity observed in mice (6).

This ADI is reaffirmed. Although levels of aldrin and dieldrin in food have been decreasing, dieldrin is highly persistent and bioaccumulates. There is also the potential for exposure in the atmosphere of houses where it is being used for termite control. The guideline value is therefore based on an allocation of 1% of the ADI to drinking-water, giving a value of 0.03 µg/litre.

## References

1. *Aldrin and dieldrin.* Geneva, World Health Organization, 1989 (Environmental Health Criteria, No. 91).

2. Worthing CR, ed. *The pesticide manual*, 9th ed. Farnham, British Crop Protection Council, 1991.

3. Office of Health and Environmental Assessment. *Carcinogenicity assessment of aldrin and dieldrin.* Washington, DC, US Environmental Protection Agency, 1987 (EPA/600/6-87-006).

4. Waggot A, Bell SM. *An inventory of organic compounds potentially causing taste and odour problems in water.* Medmenham, Water Research Centre, 1988.

5. Meister R, ed. *Farm chemicals handbook.* Willoughby, OH, Meister Publishing, 1989.

6. Food and Agriculture Organization of the United Nations. *Pesticide residues in food: 1977 evaluation.* Rome, 1978 (Joint FAO/WHO Meeting on Pesticide Residues: FAO Plant Production and Protection Paper 10, Suppl.).

7. National Board of Health (Denmark). *Dioxins in mothers milk.* Copenhagen, 1987 (Hygiejnemeddelelser 7).

8. Stacey CI, Tatum T. House treatment with organochlorine pesticides and their levels in human milk – Perth, Western Australia. *Bulletin of environmental contamination and toxicology*, 1985, 35:202-208.

9.  International Agency for Research on Cancer. *Overall evaluations of carcinogenicity: an updating of IARC Monographs volumes 1-42.* Lyon, 1987:88-89, 196-197 (IARC Monographs on the Evaluation of Carcinogenic Risks to Humans, Suppl. 7).

# 15.5 Atrazine

## 15.5.1 General description

### Identity

CAS no.:                    1912-24-9
Molecular formula:          $C_8H_{14}ClN_5$

The IUPAC name for atrazine is 6-chloro-*N*-ethyl-*N'*-isopropyl-1,3,5-triazine-2,4-diamine or 2-chloro-4-ethylamino-6-isopropylamino-1,3,5-triazine (*1*). Most commercial atrazine products are about 95% pure. Common impurities include sodium chloride and other symmetric triazines, such as simazine and propazine.

### Physicochemical properties (1–3)

| Property | Value |
| --- | --- |
| Melting point | 175–177 °C |
| Density | 1.187 g/cm³ at 20 °C |
| Water solubility | 30 mg/litre at 20 °C |
| Log octanol–water partition coefficient | 2.3 |
| Vapour pressure | 40 x 10⁻⁶ Pa at 20 °C |

### Major uses

Atrazine is used as a selective pre- and post-emergence herbicide for the control of weeds in asparagus, maize, sorghum, sugar-cane, and pineapple. It is also used in forestry and for non-selective weed control on non-crop areas (*1*). Several countries have restricted its use.

### Environmental fate

Atrazine can be degraded in surface water by photolysis and microorganisms via *N*-dealkylation and hydrolysis of the chloro substituent; the corresponding half-lives are greater than 100 days at 20 °C. Hydrolysis and microbial degradation also take place in soil, depending mainly on temperature, moisture, and pH. Half-lives of 20–50 days at 20–25 °C have been found under laboratory conditions, increasing at lower temperatures (*4*). These are similar to the half-lives found under natural conditions, but longer half-lives have been seen under special conditions (*5*). Degradation rates normally decrease with increasing depth, and atrazine can be fairly stable in groundwater (*6*).

Atrazine's degradation products in soil include 2-chloro-4-amino-6-isopropyl-amino-1,3,5-triazine, 2-chloro-4-ethylamino-6-amino-1,3,5-triazine, 2-chloro-4-amino-6-amino-1,3,5-triazine, 2-hydroxy-4-ethylamino-6-isopropylamino-1,3,5-triazine, and 2-hydroxy-4-amino-6-isopropylamino-1,3,5-triazine (the main metabolite) (7). Unsubstituted amino metabolites and triazine are formed later and may be mineralized completely. Atrazine and its dealkylated metabolites are moderately to very mobile in sandy, silt, and clay soils (8). Hydroxytriazines, however, are of low mobility (9) and persist for long periods in the soil (10).

## 15.5.2 Analytical methods

Atrazine is determined by extraction with pentane followed by gas chromatography with nitrogen–phosphorus detection. The detection limit in tapwater and river water is about 0.1 µg/litre (4).

## 15.5.3 Environmental levels and human exposure

### Air

Evaporation tests in fields treated with atrazine have shown a loss of about 0.2% of the dose per day. It is found in precipitation just after spraying (11) and may then also be expected to be found in air.

### Water

In many countries, after application in agricultural areas, atrazine has been found in groundwater at levels of 0.01–6 µg/litre. It has also been detected in drinking-water in several countries at levels of 0.01–5 µg/litre (11, 12).

### Food

Hydroxy metabolites of atrazine have been found in plants grown in soil treated with it (10), but atrazine itself has not been found on crops. When sprayed on maize, it is quickly transformed by the plant into its hydroxy metabolites (13).

## 15.5.4 Kinetics and metabolism in laboratory animals and humans

Atrazine appears to be readily absorbed from the gastrointestinal tract. In a study of rats given a single dose by gavage, at least 80% of the dose was absorbed. Within 3 days, 66% of the dose was excreted in the urine, 14% was retained in tissues, mainly the blood cells, and only 0.1% was found in the expired air (14). Doses given orally are retained mainly in erythrocytes, liver, spleen, and kidney. Most of the metabolites found in soil can also be found as degradation products in rats, 2-chloro-4,6-diamino-1,3,5-triazine being the major compound present in urine (*15*). Absorption through skin is limited, amounting to less than 2% after a 10-h exposure (*16*).

## 15.5.5 Effects on laboratory animals and *in vitro* test systems
### Acute exposure

When technical atrazine (97% active ingredient) was administered to very young rats (<7 weeks), $LD_{50}$s of 1900–2300 mg/kg of body weight were found, whereas $LD_{50}$s in the range 670–740 mg/kg of body weight were found for 3-month-old rats (*17*). $LD_{50}$s of 1750–4000 mg/kg of body weight were established in mice (*18*).

Atrazine causes moderate irritation to rabbit skin but is not appreciably irritating to the rabbit eye. It causes dermal sensitization in the guinea-pig. The dermal $LD_{50}$ was reported to be higher than 3100 mg/kg of body weight in the rat (*19*).

### Short-term exposure

A 2-week study on female rats on oral toxicity and hormonal effects showed that 100 mg/kg of body weight per day influenced the serum concentrations of estrogen, luteinizing hormone, prolactin, and progesterone. These effects may be important in the development of breast cancer in rats (*20*).

### Long-term exposure

In a 1-year oral study on beagle dogs with technical atrazine (97% active ingredient) at doses of 0, 0.5, 5, or 34 mg/kg of body weight per day, the heart was the main target organ. Dogs given 34 mg/kg of body weight per day showed ECG alterations and clinical signs referable to cardiac toxicity after only 17 weeks. Treatment-related changes in haematological values were also reported in males of this group. Slight decreases in total serum protein and albumin were reported for males at 34 mg/kg of body weight per day. The NOAEL in this study was 5 mg/kg of body weight per day (*21*).

Technical atrazine (98.9% active ingredient) was fed to Sprague-Dawley rats for 2 years at 0, 10, 70, 500, or 1000 mg/kg in the diet. At 500 and 1000 mg/kg, there was a significant decrease in mean body weights of both sexes and decreased food consumption. At 1000 mg/kg, females were found to have a consistent reduction in red blood cell count, haemoglobin and haematocrit, and glucose levels were depressed in both females and males during the first 12 months. The NOAEL in this study was 70 mg/kg (equivalent to 3.5 mg/kg of body weight per day) based on non-neoplastic effects as well as reduced body weight and food consumption (*22*).

## Reproductive toxicity, embryotoxicity, and teratogenicity

In a two-generation rat study utilizing technical atrazine (97% active ingredient) in doses of 0, 0.5, 2.5, or 25 mg/kg of body weight per day, pup weights in the second generation at the two highest doses were statistically significantly lower than those of the control group. Both parental animals had significant decreases in body weight, body weight gain, and food consumption at 25 mg/kg of body weight per day. In addition, a statistically significant increase in relative testis weight was seen in both generations at this dose level. Thus, the reproductive NOAEL was 0.5 mg/kg of body weight per day, and the parental NOAEL 2.5 mg/kg of body weight per day (23).

No teratogenic response was found in New Zealand white rabbits that received atrazine by gavage on days 7–19 of gestation at dose levels of 1, 5, or 75 mg/kg of body weight per day. Maternal toxicity, in the form of decreased body weight gain and food consumption, was seen in the mid- and high-dose groups. Fetotoxicity was demonstrated only at 75 mg/kg of body weight per day by an increased resorption rate, reduced fetal weights, and delay of ossification. The embryotoxic NOAEL appears to be 5 mg/kg of body weight per day, and the maternal NOAEL is 1 mg/kg of body weight per day (24).

## Mutagenicity and related end-points

Atrazine has been tested in several systems, but there is no convincing evidence that it has any significant genotoxic action. However, deficiencies exist with respect to certain of the tests performed, and some evidence of genotoxic effects *in vivo* needs confirmation (25–28).

## Carcinogenicity

In the study in which technical atrazine (98.9% active ingredient) was fed to Sprague-Dawley rats for 2 years at 0, 10, 70, 500, or 1000 mg/kg in the diet, a significant increase in the incidence of mammary tumours in females was seen at the three highest doses (22). The doses in the middle of the range (70 and 500 mg/kg) showed 95% significance for the occurrence of adenocarcinomas and carcinosarcomas, suggesting that atrazine interferes with hormonal regulation in male rats. The effect of atrazine on rat hormones confirms this hypothesis (20). The NOAEL in this study was 10 mg/kg, equivalent to 0.5 mg/kg of body weight per day. Studies on mice have not shown any signs of tumours (29).

## 15.5.6 Effects on humans

In an epidemiological study in northern Italy, an increased relative risk of ovarian neoplasia was found among women exposed to triazine herbicides (30). An 80% formulation of atrazine did not cause skin sensitization on repeated application to humans.

## 15.5.7 Guideline value

The weight of evidence from a wide variety of genotoxicity assays indicates that atrazine is not genotoxic. There is some evidence that it can induce mammary tumours in rats as a result of hormonal changes, but it is highly probable that the mechanism for this process is non-genotoxic. No significant increase in neoplasia has been observed in mice. IARC has concluded that there is inadequate evidence in humans and limited evidence in experimental animals for the carcinogenicity of atrazine (Group 2B) (*31*).

A TDI approach can therefore be used to calculate a guideline value. Based on a NOAEL of 0.5 mg/kg of body weight per day in a carcinogenicity study in the rat (*22*) and an uncertainty factor of 1000 (100 for inter- and intraspecies variation and 10 to reflect potential neoplasia), a TDI of 0.5 µg/kg of body weight can be calculated. With an allocation of 10% of the TDI to drinking-water, the guideline value is 2 µg/litre (rounded figure).

## References

1. Worthing CR, ed. *The pesticide manual*, 9th ed. Farnham, British Crop Protection Council, 1991.

2. Meister R, ed. *Farm chemicals handbook*. Willoughby, OH, Meister Publishing, 1989.

3. Royal Society of Chemistry. *The agrochemicals handbook*, 3rd ed. Cambridge, 1991.

4. US Environmental Protection Agency. Method 525. Determination of organic compounds in drinking water by liquid-solid extraction and capillary column gas chromatography/mass spectrometry. In: *Methods for the determination of organic compounds in drinking water*. Cincinnati, OH, Environmental Monitoring Systems Laboratory, 1988:325-356 (EPA Report No. EPA-600/4-88/039; US NTIS PB89-220461).

5. Schoen SR, Winterlin WR. The effects of various soil factors and amendments on the degradation of pesticide mixtures. *Journal of environmental science and health, Series B*, 1987, 22(3):347-377.

6. Burnside OC, Fenster CR, Wicks GA. Dissipation and leaching of monuron, simazine and atrazine in Nebraska soils. *Weeds*, 1963, 11:209-213 (cited in Roeth FW, Lavy TL, Burnside OC. Atrazine degradation in two soil profiles. *Weed science*, 1969, 17:202-205).

7. Keller A. *Degradation of atrazine (Gesaprim) in soil under aerobic/anaerobic conditions*. Basel, Ciba-Geigy, 1978 (unpublished report 25/78).

8. *Determination of the mobility of atrazine in selected soils by thin layer chromatography*. Basel, Ciba-Geigy, 1986 (Hazleton report, Study No. 6015-300).

9. Helling CS. Pesticide mobility in soil. II. Application of soil thin-layer chromatography. *Proceedings of the Soil Science Society of America*, 1971, 35:737-748.

10. Kahn SU, Saidak WJ. Residues of atrazine and its metabolites after prolonged usage. *Weed research*, 1981, 21:9-12.

11. Mair DCG, Yoo JY, Baker BE. Residues of atrazine and *N*-dealkylated atrazine in water from five agricultural watersheds in Quebec. *Archives of environmental contamination and toxicology*, 1978, 7:221-225.

12. Funari E et al. Preliminary report on the atrazine and molinate water supply contamination in Italy. *Chemosphere*, 1989, 18:2339-2343.

13. Shimabukuro RH. Atrazine metabolism in resistant corn and sorghum. *Plant physiology*, 1968, 43:1925-1930.

14. Bakke JE, Larson JD, Price CE. Metabolism of atrazine and 2-hydroxy-atrazine by the rat. *Journal of agricultural and food chemistry*, 1972, 20:602-607.

15. *Disposition of atrazine in the rat (general metabolism). Characterization and identification of atrazine metabolites from rat urine (general metabolism)* (addendum). Basel, Ciba-Geigy, 1987 (unpublished reports).

16. *Dermal absorption of $^{14}$C-atrazine in rats.* Basel, Ciba-Geigy, 1987 (unpublished report).

17. Gaines TB, Linder RE. Acute toxicity of pesticides in adult and weanling rats. *Fundamental and applied toxicology*, 1986, 7:299-308.

18. *Acute oral $LD_{50}$ of technical atrazine (G 30027) in the mouse.* Basel, Ciba-Geigy, 1975 (unpublished report).

19. *Dermal irritation study carried out by Hazleton Laboratories America, May 1975, and primary eye irritation study by Instituto Di Richerche, December 1976.* Basel, Ciba-Geigy, 1975-1976 (unpublished reports, reviewed by the Office of Pesticide Programs of the US Environmental Protection Agency, Toxicology Chapter of the Registration Standard for Atrazine, 1989).

20. Kniewald J, Mildner P, Kniewald Z. Effects of *s*-triazine herbicides on hormone-receptor complex formation, 5α-reductase and 3α-hydroxysteroid dehydrogenase activity at the anterior pituitary level. *Journal of steroid biochemistry*, 1979, 11:833-838.

21. *Atrazine technical—52 week oral feeding study in dogs.* Basel, Ciba-Geigy, 1987 (unpublished report).

22. *Twenty-four month combined oral toxicity and oncogenicity study in rats utilizing atrazine technical.* Basel, Ciba-Geigy, 1986 (unpublished report).

23. *2-Generation rat reproduction study.* Basel, Ciba-Geigy, 1987 (unpublished report).

24. *Rabbit teratology study.* Basel, Ciba-Geigy, 1984 (unpublished report).

25. *Ames' test.* Basel, Ciba-Geigy, 1986 (unpublished report).

26. *Mutagenicity studies conducted by the Nomura Research Institute (Japan).* Basel, Ciba-Geigy, 1979 (unpublished report).

27. Adler ID. A review of the coordinated research effort on the comparison of test systems for the detection of mutagenic effects, sponsored by the EEC. *Mutation research*, 1980, 74:77-93.

28. *Micronucleus assay in mice.* Basel, Ciba-Geigy, 1988 (unpublished report).

29. *Atrazine-technical: 91 week oral carcinogenicity study in mice.* Basel, Ciba-Geigy, 1986 (unpublished report).

30. Donna A et al. Triazine herbicides and ovarian epithelial neoplasms. *Scandinavian journal of work, environment and health*, 1989, 15(1):47-53.

31. International Agency for Research on Cancer. *Occupational exposures in insecticide application, and some pesticides.* Lyon, 1991:441-466 (IARC Monographs on the Evaluation of Carcinogenic Risks to Humans, Volume 53).

## 15.6 Bentazone

### 15.6.1 General description

**Identity**

CAS no.:                 50 723-80.3
Molecular formula:      $C_{10}H_{12}N_2O_3S$

The IUPAC name for bentazone is 3-isopropyl-(1H)-2,1,3-benzothiadiazin-4(3H)-one 2,2-dioxide. Technical bentazone is 92–96% pure. Its main impurities are *N*-isopropylsulfamoyl anthranilic acid (reactant; 2.4%), sodium chloride (raw material; 1.0%), and anthranilic acid (reactant; 0.6%). Some 50 other compounds have been found as impurities at very low concentrations (*1*).

### Physicochemical properties (1–3)

| Property | Value |
|---|---|
| Melting point | 137–139 °C |
| Density | 1.5 g/cm³ at 20 °C |
| Water solubility | 500 mg/litre at 20 °C |
| Log octanol–water partition coefficient | Low |
| Vapour pressure | $0.46 \times 10^{-3}$ Pa at 20 °C |

### Major uses

Bentazone is a contact herbicide used in winter and spring cereals, maize, peas, rice, and soy beans. It is absorbed by the leaves and has a short herbicidal effect (2).

### Environmental fate

The mechanism for degradation in soil is not known. The metabolite 2-amino-*N*-isopropyl benzamide (AIBA) has been found; two others, 6- and 8-hydroxy bentazone, may occur but are not extractable from soils after application and may be incorporated in the humic fraction. In a sandy soil assay, 80% of radioactively labelled bentazone was still present in the soil a year after application. The half-life of bentazone under optimal conditions is 1.5–15 weeks, depending on soil type. At temperatures below 10 °C, the half-life is longer than 20 weeks. In lysimeter and laboratory assays of mobility, 20–50% of bentazone and AIBA appears in the eluate (1).

## 15.6.2 Analytical methods

Bentazone may be determined by extraction with dichloromethane followed by gas chromatography with electron-capture detection. The detection limit in tap-water and river water is about 0.05 µg/litre (1).

## 15.6.3 Environmental levels and human exposure

### Air

Bentazone is unlikely to occur in air owing to its low vapour pressure.

### Water

Bentazone can be detected in groundwaters in cultivated areas where it is used. Surface waters can be polluted by effluents from production plants, drainage waters, and actual use in the water (rice fields). Concentrations range from <0.1 to 6 µg/litre in groundwater and from <0.1 to 2 µg/litre in surface water (4).

## Food

Bentazone may be present in crayfish farmed in rice fields where it is sprayed (*3*).

## 15.6.4 Kinetics and metabolism in laboratory animals and humans

In rats, [14]C-labelled bentazone was rapidly absorbed from the gastrointestinal tract and distributed via the bloodstream to various organs and tissues. Liver and kidneys exhibited the highest activity, but no penetration across the blood–brain barrier was observed. Of the dose administered, 90% was excreted in the urine within 24 h as unchanged bentazone. Little was recovered in the faeces (1%), and even less detected in exhaled air (<0.02%) (*5*). More than 80% of a single dose of bentazone administered to a rabbit in the feed was excreted in the urine un-metabolized. Two unidentified metabolites, accounting for about 3% of the dose, were detected, together with small quantities of 6- and 8-hydroxy bentazone (*6, 7*).

## 15.6.5 Effects on laboratory animals and *in vitro* test systems

### Acute exposure

The acute toxicity of bentazone appears to be moderate to low. For rats, the $LD_{50}$ for oral intake in carboxymethylcellulose gel was 1220 mg/kg of body weight, and for dermal exposure in water, greater than 2500 mg/litre. Poor muscle co-ordination, tremor, and breathing difficulties were noted, but no exposure-related pathological changes were discovered on necropsy (*8, 9*).

### Short-term exposure

Beagle dogs were given technical bentazone at 0, 2.5, 7.5, 25, or 75 mg/kg of body weight per day for 13 weeks (*10*). The highest dose level produced weight loss, reduced haemoglobin, and fatty degeneration of liver and heart muscle. One-third of males and two-thirds of females died. Effects at lower dose levels were much less marked or absent. Prostatitis was observed in all males at 75 mg/kg of body weight per day and in one male at 25 and another at 7.5 mg/kg of body weight per day. This suggests a compound-related dose-dependent effect, with 2.5 mg/kg of body weight per day as the NOAEL (*11*). Others have suggested that 7.5 mg/kg of body weight per day is the NOAEL (*12*).

### Long-term exposure

In a 2-year study, rats were fed bentazone in the diet at 10, 40, or 200 mg/kg of body weight per day. Decreased mean body weight gain, increased absolute and relative kidney weights, increased water consumption, and changes in urine and blood data were apparent in animals of both sexes at the highest dose level. In addition, males had depressed food consumption and an equivocal increase in eye lesions and cataracts. Less severe effects were seen in the group receiving 40 mg/kg of body weight per day, and no compound-related effects were observed at 10 mg/kg of body weight per day (13).

In a 52-week feeding study carried out in dogs at dose levels of 0, 100, 400, and 1600 mg/kg, the NOAEL was 400 mg/kg (13.1 mg/kg of body weight per day). At the highest dose, various clinical signs were observed in males, an increase in prothrombin time and in partial thromboplastin time was observed in both sexes, and two dogs showed reduced spermiogenesis (14).

In a long-term toxicity/carcinogenicity study in which mice were given bentazone at concentrations of 0, 100, 400, or 2000 mg/kg in the diet, the NOAEL was 100 mg/kg, equal to 12 mg/kg of body weight per day, based on increases in prothrombin time and changes in pituitary weights in males (15).

## Reproductive toxicity, embryotoxicity, and teratogenicity

Pregnant Sprague-Dawley rats were given technical bentazone by gavage at doses of 22.2, 66.7, or 200 mg/kg of body weight per day on days 6–15 after conception. At 200 mg/kg of body weight per day, a dose level not associated with maternal toxicity, signs of fetotoxicity and teratogenicity were observed, such as increased late resorptions, fetuses with thickened and/or shortened extremities, runting, and anasarca. The NOAELs for fetuses and dams were 66.7 and 200 mg/kg of body weight per day, respectively (16).

Pregnant Wistar rats were fed bentazone at 40, 100, or 250 mg/kg of body weight per day on days 6–15 after conception. At 250 mg/kg of body weight per day, the dams showed significantly decreased food intake but no weight decrease. Signs of fetotoxicity, such as increased resorption, smaller litter sizes, and lower mean pup weight, were also noticed. The NOAEL for both fetuses and dams was 100 mg/kg of body weight per day (17).

In a two-generation rat study at dose levels of 0, 200, 800, or 3200 mg/kg of feed, no reproductive or teratogenic effects were observed. The NOAELs for reduced body weight were 800 mg/kg (50 mg/kg of body weight per day) in parental animals and 200 mg/kg (15 mg/kg of body weight per day) in pups (18).

In a study in which pregnant Chinchilla rabbits were given 75, 150, or 375 mg of bentazone per kg of body weight per day by gavage on days 6–18 of gestation, maternal toxicity was observed at the highest dose level. There were no indications of teratogenicity or effects on fetal or embryonic development at any dose level. The NOAEL was 150 mg/kg of body weight per day (19).

## Mutagenicity and related end-points

Mutagenicity tests, Ames tests, and cytogenetic tests gave negative results, except for a mouse liver cell assay and a point mutation test carried out on CHO cells, in which bentazone gave a weak mutagenic response (20).

*Carcinogenicity*

No carcinogenic effects have been observed in the different studies carried out.

## 15.6.6 Effects on humans

No cases of human poisoning have been reported following bentazone exposure.

## 15.6.7 Guideline value

Long-term studies conducted in rats and mice have not indicated a carcinogenic potential, and a variety of *in vitro* and *in vivo* assays have indicated that bentazone is not genotoxic. The guideline value is therefore derived using a TDI approach.

JMPR evaluated bentazone in 1991 (*20*) and established an ADI of 0.1 mg/kg of body weight by applying an uncertainty factor of 100 to a NOAEL of 10 mg/kg of body weight per day, based on haematological effects at higher doses, derived from a 2-year dietary study in rats (*13*) and supported by NOAELs in dogs and mice (*14, 15*). To allow for uncertainties regarding dietary exposure, 1% of the ADI was allocated to drinking-water, resulting in a guideline value of 30 µg/litre.

## References

1.  *Pesticide residues in food—1991 evaluations. Part I. Residues.* Rome, Food and Agriculture Organization of the United Nations, 1991 (FAO Plant Production and Protection Paper, 113/1).

2.  Worthing CR, ed. *The pesticide manual*, 9th ed. Farnham, British Crop Protection Council, 1991.

3.  Office of Drinking Water. *Bentazon health advisory*. Washington, DC, US Environmental Protection Agency, 1987.

4.  KIWA (Netherlands Waterworks Testing and Research Institute). *Pesticides and the drinking water supply in the Netherlands.* Zeist, 1990 (Report No. 113).

5.  Chasseau LF et al. The metabolic fate of bentazon in the rat. *Xenobiotica*, 1972, 2:269-276.

6.  Otto S. *Investigations of rabbit urine and faeces after oral administration of* $^{14}C$-*bentazone.* 1974 (unpublished report of BASF Aktiengesellschaft, Agricultural Experimental Station, submitted to WHO by BASF, Limburgerhof, Germany).

7. Davis AL, Roger JC. *Metabolism and balance study of $^{14}$C-BAS351-H in rabbits.* Cannon Laboratories Inc., 1974 (unpublished report MRID 00039859, submitted to WHO by BASF, Limburgerhof, Germany).

8. Hofmann HT. *Acute oral toxicity of 3-isopropyl-1H-2,1,3-benzothiadiazin-4(3H)-one-2,2-dioxide to the rat.* BASF Medizinisch-Biologische Forschungslaboratorien Gewerbehygiene und Toxikologie, 1973 (unpublished report submitted to WHO by BASF, Limburgerhof, Germany).

9. Zeller H. *Acute dermal toxicity of 3-isopropyl-2,1,3-benzothiadiazon-(4)-2,2-dioxide on rats.* BASF Gewerbe-Hygienisch-Pharmakologisches Institute, 1970 (unpublished report submitted to WHO by BASF, Limburgerhof, Germany).

10. Leuschner F et al. *Thirteen week toxicity of 3-isopropyl-1H-2,1,3-benzothiadiazin-4(3H)-one 2,2-dioxide to beagles when administered with the food.* Hamburg, Pharmacology and Toxicology Laboratory, 1970 (unpublished report submitted to WHO by BASF, Limburgerhof, Germany).

11. Office of Pesticides and Toxic Substances. *Memorandum concerning the toxicology chapter for the bentazon registration standard.* Washington, DC, US Environmental Protection Agency, 1984.

12. *Drinking water quality: guidelines for selected herbicides.* Copenhagen, WHO Regional Office for Europe, 1987 (Environmental Health 27).

13. Takehara K, Tajima M, Shirasu Y. *Studies on the 24-month chronic toxicity of bentazone in rats.* Nippon Institute for Biological Science, 1984 (unpublished report submitted to WHO by BASF, Limburgerhof, Germany).

14. Allen TR et al. *Report on the 52-week oral toxicity (feeding) study with bentazone technical in the dog.* Research and Consulting Company AG, 1989 (unpublished report submitted to WHO by BASF, Limburgerhof, Germany).

15. Takehara K et al. *Studies on the 24-month chronic toxicity of bentazone reg. no. 51,929 (ZNT No. 81/273) in mice.* Nippon Institute for Biological Sciences and the Institute of Environmental Toxicology, 1985 (unpublished report submitted to WHO by BASF, Limburgerhof, Germany).

16. Hofmann HT, Merkle J. *Investigation to determine the pre-natal toxicity of 3-isopropyl-2,1,3-benzothiadiazin-4-one-2,2-dioxide on rats.* BASF Gewerbehygiene und Toxikologie, 1978 (unpublished report submitted to WHO by BASF, Limburgerhof, Germany).

17. Becker H et al. *Embryotoxicity (including teratogenicity) study with bentazone technical in the rat.* Research and Consulting Company AG, 1987 (unpublished report submitted to WHO by BASF, Limburgerhof, Germany).

18. Suter P et al. *Two generation reproduction study with bentazone technical (ZST No. 86/48) with rat.* Research and Consulting Company AG, 1989 (unpublished report submitted to WHO by BASF, Limburgerhof, Germany).

19. Becker H et al. *Embryotoxicity (including teratogenicity) study with bentazone technical in the rabbit.* Research and Consulting Company AG, 1987 (unpublished report submitted to WHO by BASF, Limburgerhof, Germany).

20. International Programme on Chemical Safety. *Pesticide residues in food —1991. Joint FAO/WHO Meeting on Pesticide Residues—Evaluations 1991. Part II. Toxicology.* Geneva, World Health Organization, 1992 (unpublished document, WHO/PCS/92.52).

## 15.7 Carbofuran

### 15.7.1 General description

#### *Identity*

CAS no.: 1563-66-2
Molecular formula: $C_{12}H_{15}NO_3$

Carbofuran is the common name for 2,3-dihydro-2,2-dimethylbenzofuran-7-yl-methylcarbamate.

#### *Physicochemical properties* (1, 2)

| *Property* | *Value* |
| --- | --- |
| Melting point | 153–154 °C |
| Water solubility | 320 mg/litre at 25 °C |
| Vapour pressure | $2.7 \times 10^{-3}$ Pa at 33 °C |
| Octanol–water partition coefficient | 17–26 at 20 °C |

#### *Major uses*

Carbofuran is a systemic acaricide, insecticide, and nematocide. It is used mainly on alfalfa, sugar-beet, cereals, citrus fruit, coffee, cotton, grapes, fruit trees, maize, potatoes, rice, soy beans, sugar-cane, tobacco, and vegetables (*2*).

#### *Environmental fate*

Carbofuran can dissipate from water by direct photolysis and photo-oxidation. In soil, photodecomposition is not an important degradation pathway. Volatilization from soil and water is not expected to be significant.[1]

---

[1] Source: Hazardous Substances Data Bank. Bethesda, MD, National Library of Medicine.

Carbofuran undergoes chemical and microbial degradation mainly through hydrolysis and hydroxylation (*3, 4*). Repeated applications do not result in an accumulation of residues. It does not bind to soil or sediments and has been shown to migrate extensively in soil (*1*). Its half-life in soil has been reported to be 1–37 weeks (*5*).

## 15.7.2 Analytical methods

Carbofuran is determined by a high-performance liquid chromatographic procedure used for the determination of *N*-methylcarbamoyloximes and *N*-methylcarbamates in drinking-water. The detection limit has been estimated to be approximately 0.9 µg/litre (*6*).

## 15.7.3 Environmental levels and human exposure

### Air

In a study designed to evaluate human exposures to carbofuran following aerial applications, it was estimated that maximum inhaled doses were in the range 0.7–2.0 mg/day (*7*).

### Water

In the USA, carbofuran has been detected in the groundwater of seven states (*8*), and in 30% of 5100 groundwater samples examined (*9*). In a field study, it was found in groundwater 12–16 months after application to potato and corn crops on sandy soil; maximum concentrations were 10 and 30 µg/litre, respectively (*9*). Typical levels of 1–5 µg/litre have been reported for groundwaters in areas with sandy soils (*5*).

### Food

Monitoring of carbofuran residues in or on foods has revealed only the occasional occurrence of low levels of the parent compound and its metabolites (*10*). There is no evidence for bioaccumulation or biomagnification in fish (*11*).

## 15.7.4 Kinetics and metabolism in laboratory animals and humans

Carbofuran administered to female mice by gavage was rapidly absorbed (*12*). Metabolism appears to involve hydroxylation and/or oxidation reactions that result in the formation of carbofuran phenols, 3-hydroxycarbofuran, 3-hydroxy-carbofuran-7-phenol, 3-ketofuran, and 3-ketofuran-7-phenol. Hydrolysis is a significant pathway for carbofuran metabolism in mammals (*13*).

621

Elimination of carbofuran is rapid in rats; approximately 72% of a single orally administered dose was excreted in the urine within 24 h, and 92% after 120 h, while total faecal excretion was about 3% (*13*). Some pulmonary excretion has been found in mice. After 60 min, 6% and 24% of an orally administered dose were recovered as exhaled carbon dioxide and in urine, respectively (*14*).

## 15.7.5 Effects on laboratory animals and *in vitro* test systems

### *Acute exposure*

Oral $LD_{50}$s have been reported to be 6–34 mg/kg of body weight for the rat (*15*), 2.0 mg/kg of body weight for the mouse (*16*), and 15–19 mg/kg of body weight for the dog (*15*). Acute toxicity effects, including death, resulting from exposure to carbofuran are attributed to rapid inhibition of acetylcholinesterase activity (*16*).

### *Short-term exposure*

In a 1-year feeding study in beagle dogs exposed to carbofuran at doses of 0, 0.25, 0.5, or 12.5 mg/kg of body weight per day, no biologically significant adverse effects on various biochemical, haematological, or clinical parameters were reported at 0.25 or 0.5 mg/kg of body weight per day. At 12.5 mg/kg of body weight per day, marked depression of plasma and erythrocyte cholinesterase levels was observed in both sexes, as well as testicular degeneration and some aspermia in males, and uterine hyperplasia and hydrometria in females. The NOAEL for dogs was 0.5 mg/kg of body weight per day, based on this study (*17*).

### *Long-term exposure*

In a 2-year study, rats were fed carbofuran in the diet at 0, 0.5, 1, or 5 mg/kg of body weight per day. At the highest dose, slight decreases in mean body weight were observed in males; there was also inhibition of plasma, red blood cells, and brain cholinesterase levels in both sexes. No adverse effects on body weight, food consumption, behaviour, ophthalmology, haematology, biochemistry, urinalysis, or histopathology were observed at the two lower doses. The NOAEL for this study was 1 mg/kg of body weight per day (*18*).

In a similar 2-year study in which mice were fed carbofuran in the diet at 3, 19, or 75 mg/kg of body weight per day, those receiving the highest dose showed a temporary decrease in body weight. At the two highest doses, a reduction in brain cholinesterase levels was observed. No adverse effects on food consumption, behaviour, haematology, biochemistry, urinalysis, or histopathology were observed at the lowest dose. This study supports a NOAEL of 3 mg/kg of body weight per day (*19*).

### Reproductive toxicity, embryotoxicity, and teratogenicity

In beagle dogs fed carbofuran for 1 year at 0.25, 0.5, or 12.5 mg/kg of body weight per day, aspermia in males was observed at the two highest doses. The highest dose resulted in testicular degeneration in males and uterine hyperplasia and hydrometria in females (17).

In a three-generation study in which rats were fed carbofuran at 1 or 5 mg/kg of body weight per day, no adverse effects on male or female fertility, length of gestation, litter size, or growth were observed. At the highest dose, however, the survival rate of the first litter in all three generations was slightly lower by day 4 of lactation. The NOAEL for reproductive effects was 1 mg/kg of body weight per day (20).

Dose-related inhibition of cholinesterase activity in the blood, liver, and brain of pregnant rats and their fetuses was found in a study in which carbofuran was administered orally at 0.05, 0.3, or 2.5 mg/kg of body weight on day 18 of gestation. In the high-dose group, toxic signs appeared within 5 min; 8 of 32 dams died within 30 min; and acetylcholinesterase activity was reduced in all maternal and fetal tissues sampled 1 h after dosing. At lower doses, inhibition was found in some tissues at 1 h. In this study, the LOAEL was 0.05 mg/kg of body weight for a single dose, based on the inhibition of maternal and fetal blood acetylcholinesterase and maternal liver acetylcholinesterase (21).

No teratogenic effects have been found in studies conducted on rats, mice, and rabbits (22–24). The NOAEL was 0.1 mg/kg of body weight per day in a teratology study in rats (24).

### Mutagenicity and related end-points

Carbofuran was negative in Ames bacterial tests except for one in which it was mutagenic in *Salmonella typhimurium* strains TA98 and TA1538 with activation by rat liver homogenate (S9 fraction) (1, 25). Mutagenicity tests in other organisms were negative, except that positive results were reported with Chinese hamster ovary V79 cells without, but not with, activation by rat liver homogenate (S9 fraction) (1, 26).

### Carcinogenicity

No evidence of carcinogenicity was found in the 2-year dietary studies on rats and mice mentioned above (18, 19).

## 15.7.6 Effects on humans

Carbofuran was administered orally to healthy males in a controlled experiment in which there were two subjects at each dose level. The subjects were observed for 24 h after dosing. At 0.1 mg/kg of body weight, symptoms of acetylcholinesterase depression were observed, including salivation, diaphoresis, abdominal pain, drowsiness, dizziness, anxiety, and vomiting. No symptoms were observed at 0.05 mg/kg of body weight, and this dose level was defined as the NOAEL in this study (27).

Several cases of adverse effects have been reported in individuals involved in the application and formulation of carbofuran. There were mild and reversible symptoms of acetylcholinesterase depression, such as malaise, hypersalivation, and vomiting. Following more severe poisoning, symptoms included chest tightness, muscular twitching, convulsions, and coma (28).

## 15.7.7 Guideline value

IARC has not evaluated carbofuran. On the basis of the available studies, this compound appears to be neither carcinogenic nor mutagenic.

While clinical signs of acetylcholinesterase inhibition were observed in humans at a single oral dose of 0.1 mg/kg of body weight, they were absent at 0.05 mg/kg of body weight, which can therefore be regarded as a NOAEL in humans (27).

A NOAEL of 0.5 mg/kg of body weight per day was derived from a 1-year study in dogs (17). The NOAEL for systemic effects in dams in a rat teratology study was 0.1 mg/kg of body weight per day (24).

A TDI of 1.67 µg/kg of body weight was calculated by applying an uncertainty factor of 30 (10 for intraspecies variation and 3 for the steep dose–response curve) to the NOAEL of 0.05 mg/kg of body weight in humans. This TDI is supported by observations in laboratory animals, giving an adequate margin of safety for the NOAELs in rats and dogs. An allocation of 10% of the TDI to drinking-water results in the guideline value of 5 µg/litre (rounded figure).

## References

1.  US Environmental Protection Agency. Carbofuran. *Reviews in environmental contamination and toxicology*, 1988, 104:35-45.

2.  Worthing CR, ed. *The pesticide manual*, 9th ed. Farnham, British Crop Protection Council, 1991.

3.  Caro JH et al. Dissipation of soil-incorporated carbofuran in the field. *Journal of agricultural and food chemistry*, 1973, 21:1010-1015.

4.  Seiber JN, Catahan MP, Barril CR. Loss of carbofuran from rice paddy water: chemical and physical factors. *Journal of environmental science and health*, 1978, B(13):131-148.

5. Cohen SZ et al. Potential for pesticide contamination of ground water from agricultural use. In: Kruger RF, Seiber JN, eds. *Treatment and disposal of pesticide wastes.* Washington, DC, American Chemical Society, 1984:297-325 (ACS Symposium Series No. 259).

6. Environmental Monitoring and Support Laboratory. *Method 531. Measurement of N-methyl carbamoyloximes and N-methylcarbamates in drinking water by direct aqueous injection HPLC with post column derivatization.* Cincinnati, OH, US Environmental Protection Agency, 1984.

7. Draper WM, Gibson RD, Street JC. Drift from and transport subsequent to a commercial, aerial application of carbofuran: an estimation of potential human exposure. *Bulletin of environmental contamination and toxicology,* 1981, 26:537-543.

8. Ritter WF. Pesticide contamination of ground water in the United States. A review. *Journal of environmental science and health,* 1990, B25(1):1-29.

9. Holden P. *Pesticides and ground water quality: issues and problems in four states.* Washington, DC, National Academy Press, 1986.

10. Bureau of Foods. *Surveillance index for pesticides.* Washington, DC, US Food and Drug Administration, 1984.

11. Jaraman J et al. Fate of carbofuran in rice–fish model ecosystem. An international study. *Water, air and soil pollution,* 1989, 45:371-375.

12. Ahdaya S, Guthrie FE. Stomach absorption of intubated insecticides in fasted mice. *Toxicology,* 1982, 22:311-317.

13. Dorough HW. Metabolism of Furadan (NIA-10242) in rats and houseflies. *Journal of agricultural and food chemistry,* 1968, 16:319-325.

14. Ahdaya S, Monroe FJ, Guthrie FE. Absorption and distribution of intubated insecticides in fasted mice. *Pesticide biochemistry and physiology,* 1981, 16:38-46.

15. Food and Agriculture Organization of the United Nations. *1976 Evaluations of some pesticide residues in food.* Rome, 1977 (unpublished document AGP:1976/M/14).

16. Fahmy MA et al. The selective toxicity of new N-phosphorothiol-carbamate esters. *Journal of agricultural and food chemistry,* 1970, 18:793-796.

17. Agricultural Chemical Group. *One-year chronic oral toxicity study in beagle dogs with carbofuran.* Middleport, NY, FMC Corporation, 1983 (unpublished study submitted to WHO).

18. Goldenthal EI. *A two-year dietary toxicity and carcinogenicity study in rats.* Middleport, NY, FMC Corporation, Agricultural Chemical Group, 1980 (unpublished study submitted to WHO).

19. Goldenthal EI. *Two-year dietary toxicity and carcinogenicity study in mice.* Middleport, NY, FMC Corporation, Agricultural Chemical Group, 1980 (unpublished study submitted to WHO).

20. Goldenthal EI. *Three-generation reproduction study in rats.* Middleport, NY, FMC Corporation, Agricultural Chemical Group, 1980 (unpublished study submitted to WHO).

21. Cambon C, Declume C, Derache R. Effect of the insecticidal carbamate derivates (carbofuran, pirimicarb, aldicarb) on the activity of acetylcholinesterase in tissues from pregnant rats and fetuses. *Toxicology and applied pharmacology*, 1979, 49:203-208.

22. Agricultural Chemical Group. *Pilot teratology study in the rat with carbofuran in the diet.* Middleport, NY, FMC Corporation, 1980 (unpublished study submitted to WHO).

23. Barnett JB et al. Immunocompetence over the lifespan of mice exposed *in utero* to carbofuran or diazinon: I. Changes in serum immunoglobulin concentrations. *Journal of environmental pathology and toxicology*, 1980, 4:53-63.

24. Barron P, Giesler P, Rao GN. *Teratogenicity of carbofuran in rats.* WARF Institute, 1978 (unpublished study submitted to WHO by FMC Corporation, Middleport, NY, USA).

25. Moriya M et al. Further mutagenicity studies on pesticides in bacterial reversion assay systems. *Mutation research*, 1983, 116(3-4):185-216.

26. Wojciechowski JP, Kaur P, Sabharwal PS. Induction of ouabain resistance in V-79 cells by four carbamate pesticides. *Environmental research*, 1982, 29:48-53.

27. Agricultural Chemical Group. *Industrial hygiene studies. Final report.* Middleport, NY, FMC Corporation, 1977 (unpublished study submitted to WHO).

28. Tobin JS. Carbofuran: a new carbamate insecticide. *Journal of occupational medicine*, 1970, 12:16-19.

## 15.8 Chlordane

### 15.8.1 General description

#### *Identity*

CAS no.: 57-47-9
Molecular formula: $C_{10}H_6Cl_8$

The IUPAC name for chlordane is 1,2,4,5,6,7,8-octachloro-2,3,3a,4,7,7a-hexahydro-4,7-methano-1H-indene. Chlordane is a mixture of isomers, mainly *cis-*

and *trans*-chlordane. Technical chlordane contains 60–75% chlordane isomers and at least 25 other compounds, including heptachlor ($C_{10}H_5Cl_7$) and nonachlor ($C_{10}H_5Cl_9$).

## Physicochemical properties (1, 2)

| Property | Value |
|---|---|
| Melting point | 106–107 °C (*cis*); 104–105 °C (*trans*) |
| Density | 1.59–1.63 g/cm$^3$ at 25 °C |
| Water solubility | 0.1 mg/litre at 25 °C |
| Log octanol–water partition coefficient | 5.5 (pure chlordane) |
| Vapour pressure | 61 x 10$^{-3}$ Pa at 25 °C (technical) |
| | 1.3 x 10$^{-3}$ Pa at 25 °C (refined) |

## Organoleptic properties

A taste threshold of 500 µg/litre[1] and an odour threshold of 0.5 µg/litre have been reported for chlordane in water (*3*).

## Major uses

Chlordane is a versatile, broad-spectrum contact insecticide used mainly for non-agricultural purposes (primarily for the protection of structures, but also on lawn and turf, ornamental trees, and drainage ditches). It is also used on corn, potatoes, and livestock. When used for termite control, it is applied to the soil by subsurface injection. Recently, the use of chlordane has been increasingly restricted in many countries (*1, 2, 4*).

## Environmental fate

Chlordane is very resistant to chemical and biological degradation. It is highly immobile and migrates very poorly. Dissipation of chlordane from soils is mainly due to volatilization. The soil half-life is about 4 years (*5*). In spite of its very low mobility in soil, chlordane may be a low-level source of contamination of groundwater when applied by subsurface injection. Once in water bodies, it is not removed by photodegradation, hydrolysis, or biodegradation. Chlordane can be dissipated from surface water by volatilization, sorption to bottom and suspended sediments and particulates, and uptake by aquatic organisms (*6, 7*).

---

[1] Source: Hazardous Substances Data Bank, Bethesda, MD, National Library of Medicine, 1985 (NIH/EPA:OHM/TADS).

## 15.8.2 Analytical methods

Chlordane can be determined by extraction with pentane followed by gas chromatography with electron-capture detection. The detection limit in tapwater and river water is about 0.01 µg/litre (8).

## 15.8.3 Environmental levels and human exposure

### *Air*

Chlordane levels range from less than 0.1 to 60 ng/m$^3$ in urban air and from 0.01 to 1 ng/m$^3$ in rural air. It is a contaminant of indoor air when used for termite control; levels exceeding 1 µg/m$^3$ have been measured (2).

### *Water*

In the USA, chlordane is rarely present in drinking-water; when found, it is mainly at levels below 0.1 µg/litre (6). Levels in drinking-water and groundwater higher than its solubility have been reported (4).

### *Food*

Chlordane has been found in meat, eggs, and milk. Some chlordane metabolites have been found in human milk. Food is considered to be the major source of exposure of the general population (7).

## 15.8.4 Kinetics and metabolism in laboratory animals and humans

When *cis*-chlordane was administered orally, at least 2–8% of the dose was absorbed by rats and at least 30% by rabbits (9). It is also absorbed by the pulmonary and dermal routes in rats (10). Chlordane and its metabolites, mainly oxychlordane, are quickly distributed throughout the body and stored at the highest levels in adipose tissue (9). Oxychlordane has been detected in adipose tissue in the general human population (11).

Various faecal metabolites of both *cis*- and *trans*-chlordane have been identified. A metabolic scheme involving dehydrogenation, epoxidation, hydroxylation, and dechlorination reactions has been presented. A glucuronide conjugate was found in urine (12). Lactation is a route of excretion of chlordane in females; chlordane is present in breast milk mainly as oxychlordane (13).

## 15.8.5 Effects on laboratory animals and *in vitro* test systems

### Acute exposure

Chlordane is moderately toxic in acute exposure. Oral $LD_{50}$s of 335–430 mg/kg of body weight have been found in rats and mice, whereas in hamsters the oral $LD_{50}$ was 1720 mg/kg of body weight. Cows seem to be more sensitive, with oral $LD_{50}$s of 25–90 mg/kg of body weight. Acute exposure to chlordane produces ataxia, convulsions, respiratory failure, and cyanosis (7).

### Long-term exposure

In a 2-year study, dogs fed chlordane at 0, 7.5, 75, 375, or 750 µg/kg of body weight per day showed altered liver enzyme activities and slightly increased relative liver weight at the two highest doses. The NOAEL in this study was 75 µg/kg of body weight per day (14).

F-344 rats (80 per sex per dose) were fed technical chlordane in the diet at 0, 1, 5, or 25 mg/kg for 130 weeks. Absolute and relative liver weights were increased in all treated groups as compared with controls. Serum bilirubin levels were increased in mid- and high-dose male rats. Histopathological examination revealed a significantly increased incidence of hepatocellular swelling in both sexes at the high dose and in some of the mid- and low-dose males. A NOAEL of 1 mg/kg of diet, or approximately 0.05 mg/kg of body weight per day, was indicated by this study (15).

### Reproductive toxicity, embryotoxicity, and teratogenicity

Male rats exposed for 90 days to 19.5 mg/kg of diet (about 1 mg/kg of body weight per day) showed changes in the ventral prostate (16). Chlordane reduced litter viability and delayed growth in multigenerational studies in rats and mice; in these studies, the NOAEL was 30 mg/kg of diet and the LOAEL 50 mg/kg of diet. At lower doses, significant effects appeared only in the third and fourth generations (17, 18). Effects were also seen in pups born to untreated dams but nursed by treated dams (17). Female mice exposed on days 1–19 of pregnancy to 8 mg/kg of body weight gave birth to apparently healthy progeny in which cell-mediated immunity was significantly reduced at adult age (19).

### Mutagenicity and related end-points

Chlordane was positive in *Saccharomyces cerevisiae* for mitotic gene conversion after metabolic activation (20) and in maize for reverse mutation (21). It was mutagenic to Chinese hamster V79 cells and induced sister chromatid exchange in intestinal cells of fish treated *in vivo* (22). Chlordane was negative in *Bacillus subtilis* and *Salmonella typhimurium* for reverse mutation (21, 23), in primary cultures of rat, mouse, and hamster hepatocytes for unscheduled DNA synthesis, and in mice for the dominant lethal assay (*23, 24*). It was not mutagenic to cultures of human fibroblasts, and studies on DNA damage in transformed human cells yielded conflicting results (*22*).

### Carcinogenicity

Chlordane gave positive results in carcinogenicity studies conducted in three strains of mice, one of which has a very low frequency of spontaneous liver lesions (*25–27*). In all of these studies, chlordane exposure resulted in very high incidences of hepatic carcinomas in both male and female mice. In carcinogenicity studies on three strains of rats, chlordane did not exhibit carcinogenic effects (*27–29*); however, it produced an increased incidence of hepatocellular adenomas in F-344 SPF male rats (*30*).

## 15.8.6 Effects on humans

Neurological symptoms, including headache, dizziness, vision problems, incoordination, irritability, excitability, weakness, muscle twitching, and convulsions, were consistently mentioned in a compilation of case reports and personal reports of people accidentally exposed by inhalation or ingestion to unquantified concentrations of chlordane. A woman died 9 days after ingestion of 104 mg/kg of body weight (*2*). Following ingestion of drinking-water contaminated with chlordane at concentrations of up to 1.2 g/litre, 13 persons showed gastrointestinal and/or neurological symptoms (*7*).

## 15.8.7 Guideline value

IARC re-evaluated chlordane in 1991 and concluded that there was inadequate evidence for its carcinogenicity in humans and sufficient evidence for its carcinogenicity in animals, classifying it in Group 2B (*22*).

JMPR re-evaluated chlordane in 1986 and established an ADI of 0.5 µg/kg of body weight by applying an uncertainty factor of 100 to the NOAEL of 50 µg/kg of body weight per day derived from a long-term dietary study in rats (*15*).

Although levels of chlordane in food have been decreasing, it is highly persistent and has a high bioaccumulation potential. An allocation of 1% of the JMPR ADI to drinking-water, gives a guideline value of 0.2 µg/litre (rounded figure).

## References

1. Worthing CR, ed. *The pesticide manual*, 9th ed. Farnham, British Crop Protection Council, 1991.

2. Agency for Toxic Substances and Disease Registry. *Toxicological profile for chlordane.* Atlanta, GA, US Public Health Service, 1989.

3. Sigworth EA. Identification and removal of herbicides and pesticides. *Journal of the American Water Works Association*, 1965, 57:1016.

4. Food and Agriculture Organization of the United Nations. *Pesticide residues in food—1984 evaluations*. Rome, 1985 (FAO Plant Production and Protection Paper 67).

5. Rao PSC, Davidson JM. *Retention and transformation of selected pesticides and phosphorus in soil systems: a critical review*. Athens, GA, US Environmental Protection Agency, 1982 (EPA-600/53-82-060).

6. Environmental Criteria and Assessment Office. *Drinking water criteria document for heptachlor epoxide and chlordane*. Cincinnati, OH, US Environmental Protection Agency, 1987 (Report No. ECAO-CIN-406).

7. *Chlordane*. Geneva, World Health Organization, 1984 (Environmental Health Criteria, No. 34).

8. Environmental Monitoring and Support Laboratory. *Test methods for organic chemical analysis of municipal and industrial wastewater. Method no. S. 608 and 625*. Cincinnati, OH, US Environmental Protection Agency, 1982.

9. Barnett JR, Dorough HW. Metabolism of chlordane in rats. *Journal of agricultural and food chemistry*, 1974, 22:612-619.

10. Nye DE, Dorough HW. Fate of insecticides administered endotracheally to rats. *Bulletin of environmental contamination and toxicology*, 1976, 15:291-296.

11. Barquet A, Morgade C, Pfaffenberger CD. Determination of organochlorine pesticides and metabolites in drinking water, human blood serum and adipose tissue. *Journal of toxicology and environmental health*, 1981, 7(3-4):469-479.

12. Tashiro S, Matsumura F. Metabolism of *trans*-nonachlor and related chlordane components in rat and man. *Archives of environmental contamination and toxicology*, 1978, 7(1):113-127.

13. Strassman SC, Kutz FW. Insecticide residues in human milk from Arkansas and Mississippi, 1973-1974. *Pesticides monitoring journal*, 1977, 10:130-133.

14. Wazeter FX. *Two year chronic feeding study in the beagle dog*. Mattawan, MI, International Research and Development Organization, 1967 (unpublished report for Velsicol Chemical Corporation, Chicago, IL).

15. Food and Agriculture Organization of the United Nations. *Pesticide residues in food—1986 evaluations*. Rome, 1987 (Joint FAO/WHO Meeting on Pesticide Residues: FAO Plant Production and Protection Paper 78/2).

16. Shain SA, Shaeffer JC, Boesel RW. The effect of chronic ingestion of selected pesticides upon rat ventral prostate homeostasis. *Toxicology and applied pharmacology*, 1977, 40(1):115-130.

17. Ambrose AM et al. Toxicological and pharmacological studies on chlordane. *Industrial hygiene and occupational medicine*, 1953, 7:197-210.

18. Keplinger ML, Deichmann WB, Sala F. Effects of combinations of pesticides on reproduction in mice. *Industrial medicine and surgery*, 1968, 37:525.

19. Spyker-Cranmer JM et al. Immunoteratology of chlordane: cell-mediated and humoral immune responses in adult mice exposed *in utero*. *Toxicology and applied pharmacology*, 1982, 62:402-408.

20. Blevins RD, Sholes TE. Response of HeLa cells to selected pesticides and hallucinogens. *Growth*, 1978, 42(4):478-485.

21. Gentile JM et al. An evaluation of the genotoxic properties of insecticides following plant and animal activation. *Mutation research*, 1982, 101(1):19-29.

22. International Agency for Research on Cancer. *Occupational exposures in insecticide application, and some pesticides*. Lyon, 1991:115-175 (IARC Monographs on the Evaluation of Carcinogenic Risks to Humans, Volume 53).

23. Probst GS et al. Chemically-induced unscheduled DNA synthesis in primary rat hepatocyte cultures: a comparison with bacterial mutagenicity using 218 compounds. *Environmental mutagenesis*, 1981, 3(1):11-32.

24. Maslansky CJ, Williams GM. Evidence for an epigenetic mode of action in organochlorine pesticides hepatocarcinogenicity: a lack of genotoxicity in rat, mouse and hamster hepatocytes. *Journal of toxicology and environmental health*, 1981, 8(1-2): 121-130.

25. Epstein SS. Carcinogenicity of heptachlor and chlordane. *Science of the total environment*, 1976, 6:103-154.

26. Becker FF, Sell S. Alpha-fetoprotein levels and hepatic alterations during chemical carcinogenesis in C57BL/6N mice. *Cancer research*, 1979, 39:3491-3494.

27. National Cancer Institute. *Bioassay of chlordane for possible carcinogenicity*. Bethesda, MD, 1977 (NCI Carcinogenesis Technical Report Series No. 8; US Department of Health, Education and Welfare Publication No. (NIH) 77-B08).

28. *Chlordane chronic feeding study in mice*. Research Institute for Animal Science in Biochemistry and Toxicology, 1983 (unpublished report for Velsicol Chemical Corporation, Chicago, IL).

29. Ingle L. Chronic oral toxicity of chlordane to rats. *Archives of industrial hygiene and occupational medicine*, 1952, 6:357-367.

30. Ihui S et al. *Thirty-month chronic toxicity and tumorigenicity test in rats with chlordane technical.* Research Institute for Animal Science in Biochemistry and Toxicology, 1983 (unpublished report submitted to WHO by Velsicol Chemical Corporation, Chicago, IL).

# 15.9 Chlorotoluron

## 15.9.1 General description

### Identity

CAS no.:                    15545-48-9
Molecular formula:     $C_{10}H_{13}ClN_2O$

The IUPAC name for chlorotoluron is 3-(3-chloro-*p*-tolyl)-1,1-dimethylurea.

### Physicochemical properties (1)

| Property | Value |
|---|---|
| Physical state | Colourless crystals |
| Melting point | 147–148 °C |
| Vapour pressure | $0.017 \times 10^{-3}$ Pa at 20 °C |
| Density | 1.4 g/cm³ at 20 °C |
| Water solubility | 70 mg/litre at 20 °C |
| Log octanol–water partition coefficient | 2.29 |

### Organoleptic properties

No odour was detected at a concentration of 9.0 mg/litre (99.3% purity, dissolved in still, bottled water, equilibrated to 40 °C, eight assessors) (Water Research Centre, unpublished data, 1990).

### Major uses

Chlorotoluron is a pre- or early post-emergence herbicide widely used to control annual grasses and broad-leaved weeds in winter cereals (*1*).

### Environmental fate

Chlorotoluron is slowly degraded in water and is quite persistent. Chemical hydrolysis is not a significant degradation mechanism. However, it is degraded by photolysis in water and under laboratory conditions; the half-lives at pH 5, 7, and 9 at 22 °C were over 200 days. In another study, half-lives of approximately

120 and 80 days were reported for river and pond water (containing 1% sediment), respectively. Degradation proceeded via N-demethylation, yielding 3-(3-chloro-p-tolyl)-1-methylurea as the major metabolite and some minor polar metabolites (Ciba-Geigy, unpublished data, 1989).

In laboratory studies, the rate of degradation of chlorotoluron in soil is slow and follows first-order kinetics. The estimated half-life in loamy sand and organic and peat soil is several months (2). Rates of degradation were nearly tripled by raising the temperature from 25 °C to 35 °C. Under field conditions, chlorotoluron appears to degrade at a higher rate. When applied in the spring on bare soil, it disappeared from the 0–5-cm soil layer with a half-life of 30–40 days; dissipation was slower in autumn (Ciba-Geigy, unpublished data, 1989).

## 15.9.2 Analytical methods

Chlorotoluron may be determined by separation by reverse-phase high-performance liquid chromatography followed by ultraviolet and electrochemical detection (3). Detection limits of 0.1 µg/litre have been reported (4). Gas chromatography/mass spectroscopy can also be used for the determination stage.

## 15.9.3 Environmental levels and human exposure

### Air

Because of its low vapour pressure, chlorotoluron is unlikely to be a major contaminant in air.

### Water

Chlorotoluron is slightly mobile in soil and likely to reach surface waters following agricultural application. It has occasionally been detected in waters in the United Kingdom at concentrations ranging from 0.4 to 0.6 µg/litre (5). In Germany, levels of up to 1.2 µg/litre have been detected in drainage water from fields soon after normal treatment (Ciba-Geigy, unpublished data, 1989). In another German study, chlorotoluron was frequently detected in raw waters, concentrations of 0.2 and 0.3 µg/litre were reported for surface water and groundwater, respectively (6).

### Food

It is generally considered that there is only limited exposure to chlorotoluron from food. In one study, residues of 0.04–0.08 and 0.06–0.35 mg/kg were detected in grain and straw samples, respectively (Ciba-Geigy, unpublished data, 1989). However, the majority of samples contained no measurable residues.

### *Estimated total exposure and relative contribution of drinking-water*

Based on exposure from food and water, the estimated daily intake was 4.2 µg/person in a German study (Ciba-Geigy, unpublished data, 1989).

## 15.9.4 Kinetics and metabolism in laboratory animals and humans

Chlorotoluron is readily and rapidly absorbed when given orally. No evidence of its accumulation in any particular organ or tissue has been reported. In the rat, it is metabolized mainly via *N*-demethylation and stepwise oxidation of the ring methyl group to hydroxymethyl and carboxymethyl derivatives. At doses above 50 mg/kg, the phenylmethyl group is transformed to a methylthiomethyl group. Chlorotoluron is rapidly excreted in the urine in the form of metabolites, a negligible amount being excreted in expired air (Ciba-Geigy, unpublished data, 1989).

## 15.9.5 Effects on laboratory animals and *in vitro* test systems

### *Acute exposure*

Chlorotoluron is of low acute oral toxicity in various species; oral $LD_{50}$s range from 2700 to more than 10 000 mg/kg of body weight. The rat dermal $LD_{50}$ was more than 2000 mg/kg of body weight. It caused no eye or skin irritation in the rabbit or skin sensitization in the guinea-pig (*7*; Ciba-Geigy, unpublished data, 1989).

### *Short-term exposure*

Short-term feeding studies in animals suggest that chlorotoluron is of low toxicity. Rats were fed chlorotoluron in the diet at doses of 0, 800, 3200, or 12 800 mg/kg for 3 months. At the highest dose, there was a slight decrease in body weight in both males and females and an increased incidence of splenic haemosiderosis and Kupffer's cell activity in the liver. There were slight reversible increases in haemoglobin concentration, erythrocyte counts, and haematocrit values in females at 12 800 mg/kg and transient increases in serum alkaline phosphatase activity at 3200 and 12 800 mg/kg. The NOAEL was 800 mg/kg, equal to 52 mg/kg of body weight per day (Ciba-Geigy, unpublished data, 1989).

In a 3-month study, dogs were fed diets containing 0, 600, 2400, or 9200 mg of chlorotoluron per kg. Animals in the highest dose group died after 10 weeks from severe cachexia, resulting from starvation. At the two highest doses, there were decreases in food intake and body weights, but the only histopathological changes that could be related to treatment were increased incidence of splenic and hepatic haemosiderosis (Ciba-Geigy, unpublished data, 1989).

## Long-term exposure

Mice were fed chlorotoluron in the diet at levels of 0, 100, 500, or 2500 mg/kg for 2 years. At 2500 mg/kg, there was a statistically significant reduction in body weight, a slight increase in white blood cell count, increased plasma urea levels, an increase in the activity of alkaline phosphatase in females, and a statistically significant reduction in the mean relative kidney weights in both sexes. There was a slightly increased concentration of albumin in males at 500 and 2500 mg/kg. The NOAEL for this study was 100 mg/kg, equal to 11.3 mg/kg of body weight per day (Ciba-Geigy, unpublished data, 1989).

In a 2-year study, rats were fed chlorotoluron in the diet at dose levels of 0, 100, 500, or 2500 mg/kg. Marked depression in body weight gain was observed at 2500 mg/kg, accompanied by a slight reduction in feed consumption. At the same dose level, slight increases in the incidence of spleen haemosiderosis in females and in aminotransferase activity in males were observed. The NOAEL for this study was 100 mg/kg, equivalent to a daily intake of 5 mg/kg of body weight (Ciba-Geigy, unpublished data, 1989).

## Reproductive toxicity, embryotoxicity, and teratogenicity

Chlorotoluron was not teratogenic in rats at doses of up to 1000 mg/kg of body weight per day when administered by gavage on days 6–15 of gestation (Ciba-Geigy, unpublished data, 1989). A mild retardation in the ossification rate of the hindlimb was seen in the 1000 and 500 mg/kg groups; this was considered to be related to maternal toxicity.

In a two-generation study, chlorotoluron was administered orally to rats at dietary doses of 0, 300, 1000, or 3000 mg/kg. At 3000 mg/kg, there was a significant reduction in body weight and food consumption of both parents and offspring, a significantly reduced mean number of implantation sites per dam, and depressed locomotor activity in some pups. The NOAEL in this study was 300 mg/kg (Ciba-Geigy, unpublished data, 1989).

No changes were observed in the testes and spermatozoa of male rats given chlorotoluron intragastrically at doses of 0.2 or 2.0 mg/kg of body weight per day, 5 days per week for 10 weeks, although the offspring had lower body weights and body lengths. When the doses were administered in the feed, no effects were observed in the fetuses, indicating that the toxicity is affected by the method of administration (8).

## Mutagenicity and related end-points

Chlorotoluron and its metabolites have shown no evidence of mutagenicity in a number of bacterial or *in vitro* and *in vivo* mammalian test systems (Ciba-Geigy, unpublished data, 1989).

### *Carcinogenicity*

No carcinogenic effects were reported in rats exposed to doses of 0, 100, 500, or 2500 mg/kg in the diet for 2 years. However, in a 2-year dietary study, an increased incidence of adenomas and carcinomas of the kidney was reported in male mice at 2500 mg/kg. The incidence of hepatocellular carcinomas was also increased in male mice receiving 2500 mg/kg and slightly increased at 500 mg/kg. When the incidences of hepatocellular carcinomas and adenomas were combined, the total number of tumours remained within the historical control ranges. No carcinogenic effects were reported at 100 mg/kg of diet (Ciba-Geigy, unpublished data, 1989). These studies suggest that chlorotoluron has a carcinogenic potential that is both species- and sex-specific.

## 15.9.6 Effects on humans

No cases of human poisoning have been reported following chlorotoluron exposure.

## 15.9.7 Guideline value

Chlorotoluron is of low toxicity in acute, short-term, and long-term exposures in animals, but has been shown to cause an increase in adenomas and carcinomas of the kidney in male mice given high doses for 2 years. Chlorotoluron and its metabolites have shown no evidence of genotoxicity. In view of this, the guideline value can be calculated using a TDI approach.

The NOAEL in a 2-year feeding study in mice was 11.3 mg/kg of body weight per day (Ciba-Geigy, unpublished data, 1989). A TDI of 11.3 µg/kg of body weight can be calculated by applying an uncertainty factor of 1000 (100 for inter- and intraspecies variation and 10 for evidence of carcinogenicity). An allocation of 10% of the TDI to drinking-water results in the guideline value of 30 µg/litre (rounded figure).

## References

1.  Royal Society of Chemistry. *The agrochemicals handbook*, 3rd ed. Cambridge, 1991.

2.  Madhun YA, Freed VH. Degradation of the herbicides bromacil, diuron and chlortoluron in soil. *Chemosphere*, 1987, 16(5):1003-1011.

3.  Department of the Environment. The determination of carbamates, thiocarbamates, related compounds and ureas in waters. In: *Methods for the examination of waters and associated materials*. London, Her Majesty's Stationery Office, 1987.

4.  Crathorne B, James CP, Stratford JA. *HPLC method for the analysis of chlortoluron, isoproturon and linuron in water.* Medmenham, Water Research Centre, 1987 (Water Research Centre Report PRU 1498-M).

5.  Lees A, McVeigh K. *An investigation on pesticide pollution in drinking water in England and Wales.* London, Friends of the Earth, 1988.

6.  Reupert R, Ploger E. The determination of *N*-herbicides in ground-, drinking and surface water: analytical method and results. *Vom Wasser,* 1989, 72:211-233.

7.  Zak F, Sachsse K. Oral toxicity of the herbicide chlortoluron [*N*-(3-chloro-4-methyl-phenyl)-*N,N'*-dimethylurea] in rats and dogs. *Proceedings of the European Society to Study Drug Toxicity,* 1971, 12:272-281 (*Chemical abstracts,* CA77(3):15229v).

8.  Šepel'skaja NR. [Gonadotoxic effect of dicurine after its intragastric administration by tube and with food.] *Gigiena i sanitarija,* 1988, 11:78-79 (in Russian) (*Chemical abstracts,* CA110(9):70782v).

## 15.10 DDT and its derivatives

### 15.10.1 General description

**Identity**

| | |
|---|---|
| CAS no.: | 107917-42-0 |
| Molecular formula: | $C_{14}H_9Cl_5$ |

The term DDT refers to *p,p'*-DDT, or *p,p'*-dichlorodiphenyl trichloroethane. The compound's structure permits several different isomeric forms, such as *o,p'*-DDT. The term DDT is also applied to commercial products consisting predominantly of *p,p'*-DDT, but also containing smaller amounts of other compounds, including *p,p'*- and *o,p'*-DDD (dichlorodiphenyl dichloroethane) and *p,p'*- and *o,p'*-DDE (dichlorodiphenyl dichloroethene) (*1*).

**Physicochemical properties** (1)

| | |
|---|---|
| Physical state | White, crystalline solid |
| Melting point | 108.5–109 °C |
| Vapour pressure | $2.53 \times 10^{-5}$ Pa at 20 °C |
| Water solubility | Highly insoluble (1 µg/litre) |
| Log octanol–water partition coefficient | 7.48 |

**Organoleptic properties**

All DDT isomers are tasteless, almost odourless solids. The odour threshold for DDT in water is 0.35 mg/litre (*2*).

## Major uses

DDT is a nonsystemic contact insecticide with a broad spectrum of activity (*3*). It was banned in several countries in the early 1970s, because of ecological considerations, and a number of developed countries have more recently restricted or banned its use except when it is needed for the protection of human health.

DDT is still used extensively for the control of yellow fever, sleeping sickness, typhus, malaria, and other insect-transmitted diseases. Without it, vast populations would suffer the ravages of endemic and epidemic malaria. Replacement of DDT by malathion or propoxur would increase the cost of malaria control considerably, forcing some countries to decrease the coverage of their control programmes (*4*).

## Environmental fate

DDT and its metabolites are persistent in the environment and resistant to complete degradation by microorganisms, although photochemical degradation does occur. The persistence of DDT is substantially lower in tropical climates than in temperate ones (a few months as compared with years) (*1*).

DDT and its metabolites are readily adsorbed on to sediments and soils, which can act both as sinks and as long-term sources of exposure. Because of its strong tendency to be adsorbed on to surfaces, most DDT that enters water is and remains firmly attached to soil particles. If it does find its way into water, it is gradually lost by adsorption on to surfaces (*1*).

The physical and chemical properties of DDT and its metabolites enable these compounds to be taken up readily by organisms from the surrounding medium and from food. In aquatic organisms, uptake from water is generally more important, whereas food is the major source for terrestrial fauna. High lipid solubility and low water solubility lead to the retention of DDT and its stable metabolites in fatty tissue. In general, organisms at higher trophic levels tend to contain more DDT-type compounds than those at lower ones. These compounds can be transported around the world in the bodies of animals, as well as in ocean and air currents (*1*).

## 15.10.2 Analytical methods

DDT and its metabolites may be determined in water by gas chromatography with electron-capture detection. The limits of detection are 60 ng/litre for *p,p'*-DDT, 10 ng/litre for *p,p'*-DDE, and 2.5 ng/litre for *p,p'*-DDD (*3*).

## 15.10.3 Environmental levels and human exposure
### Air

When DDT is sprayed, any that fails to adhere to its target drifts away; vaporization from treated fields can be detected for more than 6 months after application. Although most of it settles in the same area, some drifts over long distances. Traces of DDT have been found in dust known to have drifted over 1000 km and in water produced by melting Antarctic snow.

With rare exceptions, concentrations of DDT in air in nonagricultural areas have been in the range <1–2.36 ng/m$^3$. In agricultural communities, concentrations have ranged from 1 to 22 ng/m$^3$. In communities with antimosquito fogging programmes, concentrations may be much higher, 8.5 µg/m$^3$ being the highest level recorded (4).

### Water

In a study of surface waters in the USA during 1964–1968, the highest level recorded for a DDT-related compound was 0.84 µg/litre. Concentrations in Germany were even lower, averaging 10 ng/litre and never going as high as 1 µg/litre. The average concentrations of total DDT in drinking-water in Czechoslovakia were 11 and 15 ng/litre in 1972 and 1973, respectively. DDT was not detected (limit 0.01 ng/litre) in tapwater in a 1977 survey carried out in Ottawa (Canada) (4).

Within the Global Environment Monitoring System (GEMS) water network, DDT and its metabolites were found in some rivers during 1979–84. The following average concentrations were measured (5): India, 560 ng/litre; Italy, 3 ng/litre; Netherlands, <2 ng/litre; USA, 0.2 ng/litre; Canada and France, not detected.

### Food

Daily intake of DDT from food has been measured in several countries. During 1985–88, in Australia, Finland, Guatemala, Japan, Thailand, the United Kingdom, and the USA, the reported mean daily dietary intake by the average adult was less than 2 µg (6). In Egypt, in 1988, a mean daily intake of 960 µg was reported for the average adult (7).

Human milk may contain a higher concentration of DDT than cows' milk in the same country. So far, there is no evidence that this difference is of any significance for breast-fed babies, even where the concentration of DDT in human milk is comparatively high (4). The average concentration of total DDT in whole human milk in 15 countries between 1976 and 1986 ranged from 2 to 380 µg/litre (8). On the assumption that a 5-kg infant consumes 0.6 litres of milk per day, the intake at the highest concentration found would amount to about 200 µg/day, or 40 µg/kg of body weight per day. It should be remembered that such intake is limited to a few months in a lifetime. Furthermore, neonates are not at increased risk, as they are not particularly susceptible to DDT's adverse effects (9).

### Estimated total exposure and relative contribution of drinking-water

It has been estimated that over 90% of the DDT stored in the general population is derived from food (4). In 1965, intake in the USA was approximately 40 µg/day per person from food, less than 46 ng/day from water, less than 60 ng/day from urban air, and less than 0.5 µg/day from air in small agricultural communities. Other investigators have also concluded that food is the major source of intake of DDT and related compounds for the general population (4).

## 15.10.4 Kinetics and metabolism in laboratory animals and humans

DDT is absorbed after inhalation and ingestion, the latter being the more important route of absorption. Absorption of small doses, such as those found in food residues, is virtually complete and is facilitated by the presence of fat in food. Even in solution, DDT is poorly absorbed through the skin.

Most of the known facts concerning the distribution, storage, and excretion of DDT have been demonstrated in humans as well as in laboratory animals. The compound is stored preferentially in fat, and its storage in organs and other tissues following repeated intake is proportional to their neutral fat content. However, uptake of DDT by fat is slow; therefore, much more is distributed to other tissues following a single, large dose, and much more to adipose tissue following many small doses. In spite of the affinity of DDT for adipose tissues, most of the DDT-related compounds in blood are carried by proteins, less than 1% being carried in the tiny droplets of fat normally present in the blood.

Following repeated doses, storage in adipose tissue increases rapidly at first and then more gradually until a steady state is reached. Storage is relatively less at higher dosages because excretion is relatively greater. In humans, the time necessary to reach storage equilibrium is at least 1 year. There is a gradual reduction in the amount of DDT stored in the tissues if exposure to the compound is discontinued.

Like most species, humans convert some DDT to DDE, which is stored even more avidly than the parent compound. A small amount of DDD, an intermediate in the formation of the main excretory product 2,2-bis(4-chlorophenyl)-ethanoic acid (DDA), may also be found in tissues. A number of other metabolites have been detected in laboratory animals but not in humans. Technical DDT is more readily excreted and less readily stored than $p, p'$-DDT because it contains 15–20% of $o,p'$-DDT (4).

## 15.10.5 Effects on laboratory animals and *in vitro* test systems

### Acute exposure

The acute toxicity of DDT is high in insects (the $LD_{50}$ is 14 mg/kg of body weight) and lower in mammals (oral $LD_{50}$: 150–400 mg/kg of body weight). Acute intoxication with DDT elicits symptoms mainly from the central nervous system, and death is usually caused by respiratory arrest. Large doses cause focal necrosis of liver cells in several species (*3*).

### Long-term exposure

Long-term studies of oral administration have been performed in rats, mice, hamsters, dogs, and monkeys. The liver is one of the main target organs, and hepatic effects range from increased liver weights to cellular necrosis. The NOAEL for hepatic effects was 32 mg/kg of body weight per day for 78 weeks in rats and about 10 mg/kg of body weight per day when given to rhesus monkeys for 3.5–7.5 years (*3*).

Effects on the central nervous system, such as tremors and hyperactivity, are also associated with long-term exposure to DDT. Nervous symptoms were apparent at doses of 20 mg/kg of body weight per day in rats, whereas hamsters showed no clinical signs of neurotoxicity at doses of up to 40 mg/kg of body weight per day for life (*3, 9*).

### Reproductive toxicity, embryotoxicity, and teratogenicity

Levels of DDT as high as 200 mg/kg of food that do not produce any sign of poisoning have not produced any adverse effects in rats and mice on fertility, gestation, viability, lactation, and the health of the progeny. Reproduction was normal in dogs receiving a dose of 10 mg/kg of body weight per day, which is approximately equivalent to a dietary level of 500 mg/kg for this species (*4*).

Because of its estrogenic properties, DDT was considered as a possible cause of abortion in dairy cattle, but no evidence of a relationship was found. Except for the weak estrogenic properties of *o, p'*-DDT, the endocrine-related effects of DDT and its analogues are confined to the adrenal glands, and even these effects are now considered to be mainly secondary to microsomal enzyme induction in the liver (*4*).

No teratogenic effects of DDT have been observed in multigeneration studies of reproduction in several animal species (*4*).

### Mutagenicity and related end-points

In most studies, DDT did not induce genotoxic effects in rodent or human cell systems, nor was it mutagenic to fungi or bacteria (*3*).

## *Carcinogenicity*

DDT produces an increase in liver tumours in mice. However, the susceptibility of the mouse to the formation of liver tumours when exposed to it may be the consequence of major species differences in the metabolism of DDT and in the activation of chemical carcinogens by this species. Mice form more DDE than humans and other species; humans form more of the polar metabolite DDA. Indeed, DDE has been considered to be the metabolite responsible for carcinogenicity in mice (*9*).

Male and female Porton Wistar rats were fed 125, 250, or 500 mg of DDT per kg in the diet for life. No adverse effects were observed on body weight gain or growth or on the survival rate. The study showed slight increases in the incidence of hepatomas in females only at 250 and 500 mg/kg in the diet; the 125 mg/kg dose level was without effect, and no increase in the incidence of cancer was seen in males at any of these doses. No metastases of any kind were observed. JMPR concluded that the 125 mg/kg dose, equivalent to 6.25 mg/kg of body weight per day, was the NOAEL for tumorigenesis in the rat (*9*).

## 15.10.6 Effects on humans

Signs and symptoms reported following acute intoxication by DDT include nausea, vomiting, paraesthesia, dizziness, ataxia, confusion, tremor, and, in severe cases, convulsions (*3*).

Repeated exposure of workers for 25 years at an average dose of 0.25 mg/kg of body weight per day was without any adverse effect, and this may be taken as a no-effect level for humans (*9*). Epidemiological observations of humans have not provided firm evidence that DDT has any reproductive or teratogenic effects. All epidemiological studies in humans have indicated that DDT is not carcinogenic (*9*).

## 15.10.7 Guideline value

IARC has concluded that there is insufficient evidence in humans and sufficient evidence in experimental animals for the carcinogenicity of DDT (Group 2B) (*3*).

Based on NOAELs of 6.25 mg/kg of body weight per day in rats, 10 mg/kg of body weight per day in monkeys, and 0.25 mg/kg of body weight per day in humans, JMPR recommended an ADI for humans of 0.02 mg/kg of body weight (*9*). For adults, this ADI would provide a 500-fold margin of safety for the NOAEL of 10 mg/kg of body weight per day found in the study in monkeys. This ADI is used for the derivation of the guideline value.

Because infants and children may be exposed to greater amounts of chemicals in relation to their body weight and because of concern over the bioaccumulation of DDT, the guideline value was calculated on the basis of a 10-kg child drinking 1 litre of water per day. Moreover, because there is significant exposure to DDT by routes other than water a 1% allocation of the ADI to drinking-water was chosen. This leads to a guideline value for DDT and its metabolites in drinking-water of 2 µg/litre.

This guideline value exceeds the water solubility of DDT of 1 µg/litre. However, some DDT may be adsorbed on to the small amount of particulate matter present in drinking-water, so that the guideline value of 2 µg/litre could be reached under certain circumstances.

It should be emphasized that, as for all pesticides, the recommended guideline value for DDT in drinking-water is set at a level to protect human health; it may not be suitable for the protection of the environment or aquatic life. The benefits of DDT use in malaria and other vector-control programmes far outweigh any health risk from the presence of DDT in drinking-water.

## References

1.  *DDT and its derivatives—environmental aspects.* Geneva, World Health Organization, 1989 (Environmental Health Criteria, No. 83).

2.  Zoeteman BCJ. *Sensory assessment of water quality.* Oxford, Pergamon Press, 1980.

3.  International Agency for Research on Cancer. *Occupational exposures in insecticide application, and some pesticides.* Lyon, 1991:179-249 (IARC Monographs on the Evaluation of Carcinogenic Risks to Humans, Volume 53).

4.  *DDT and its derivatives.* Geneva, World Health Organization, 1979 (Environmental Health Criteria, No. 9).

5.  Meybeck M, Chapman D, Helmer R, eds. *Global freshwater quality: WHO/UNEP Global Environment Monitoring System.* Oxford, Alden Press, 1989.

6.  Galal-Gorchev H. Dietary intake of pesticide residues, cadmium, mercury, and lead. *Food additives and contaminants,* 1991, 8:793-806.

7.  Abdel-Gawaad AA, Shams El Dine A. Insecticide residues in total diet samples. *Journal of the Egyptian Society of Toxicology,* 1989, 4:79-89.

8.  United Nations Environment Programme. *Assessment of chemical contaminants in food: Global Environment Monitoring System.* Nairobi, 1988.

9.  Food and Agriculture Organization of the United Nations. *Pesticide residues in food—1984 evaluations.* Rome, 1985 (Joint FAO/WHO Meeting on Pesticide Residues: FAO Plant Production and Protection Paper 67).

# 15.11 1,2-Dibromo-3-chloropropane

## 15.11.1 General description

### Identity

CAS no.:               96-12-8
Molecular formula:     $C_3H_5Br_2Cl$

### Physicochemical properties (1)[1]

| Property | Value |
|---|---|
| Physical state | liquid |
| Boiling point | 196 °C |
| Vapour pressure | 0.1 kPa at 21 °C |
| Water solubility | 1230 mg/litre |
| Log octanol–water partition coefficient | 2.43 |

### Organoleptic properties

The odour and taste thresholds for 1,2-dibromo-3-chloropropane (DBCP) in water are both 0.01 mg/litre (1).

### Major uses

DBCP is used as a nematocidal fumigant (1).

### Environmental fate

DBCP is expected to volatilize from surface water. It is highly persistent in soil and has been shown to remain there for more than 2 years. It is mobile in soil and may migrate to groundwater (1).

## 15.11.2 Analytical methods

DBCP is determined by a purge-and-trap gas chromatographic procedure used for the determination of volatile organohalides in drinking-water (2). This method is applicable to the measurement of DBCP over a concentration range of 0.03–1500 µg/litre. Confirmation is by mass spectrometry (detection limit 0.2 µg/litre). A detection limit of 0.02 µg/litre is possible when gas chromatography and electron-capture detection are used (3).

---

[1] Conversion factor in air: 1 ppm = 9.67 mg/m$^3$.

## 15.11.3 Environmental levels and human exposure

### *Air*

DBCP is a low-level contaminant in air (*1*).

### *Water*

In a survey of drinking-water wells near locations where DBCP had been used within the previous 2 years, this compound was found at low (µg/litre) levels. In wells not used for drinking-water, it has been detected at levels of up to 20 µg/litre (*1*).

### *Food*

DBCP has been identified as a contaminant in vegetables grown in soils treated with it (*1*).

## 15.11.4 Kinetics and metabolism in laboratory animals and humans

On the basis of excretion studies, absorption is expected to be high by the oral route. Distribution is primarily to the liver and kidneys (*4*). Transplacental transfer also appears to occur (*5*).

Metabolic pathways for DBCP may involve epihalohydrin, other reactive epoxides, or 2-bromoacrolein as intermediates. Urinary metabolites in rats include mercapturic acid conjugates, β-chlorolactic acid, β-bromolactic acid, and 2-bromoacrylic acid (*1*). Most DBCP is excreted by the urinary and faecal routes; smaller amounts are excreted in expired air. The urine is the predominant route for the elimination of metabolites (*6*).

## 15.11.5 Effects on laboratory animals and *in vitro* test systems

### *Acute exposure*

Acute oral $LD_{50}$s of 170, 410, and 440 mg/kg of body weight were reported for rats, mice, and rabbits, respectively (*1*).

### *Short-term exposure*

Dietary administration of DBCP to rats for 90 days resulted in increased kidney weights at 2 mg/kg of body weight per day, reduced body weight gain at 15 mg/kg of body weight per day, increased liver weight at 45 mg/kg of body weight per day, and muscular weakness and increased mortality at 135 mg/kg of body weight per day. The NOAEL was 0.5 mg/kg of body weight per day (*7*).

In a study in which Sprague-Dawley rats were given DBCP in drinking-water at concentrations of 0, 5, 50, 100, or 200 mg/litre (approximately 0, 0.4, 3.2, 5.2, and 9.4 mg/kg of body weight) for 64 days, renal lesions, increased protein and glucose levels, and increased urinary specific gravity were apparent at the two highest doses (8).

## Long-term exposure

In a chronic study in which mice and rats received DBCP by gavage, a dose-related increase in mortality and a high incidence of toxic tubular nephropathy were reported at time-weighted average doses of 78.6–149.3 mg/kg of body weight per day in mice and 10.7 and 20.7 mg/kg of body weight per day in rats (9). Lifetime treatment of Charles River CD rats with doses of 0, 0.2, 0.7, or 2 mg/kg of body weight per day in the diet resulted in kidney lesions in female rats and reduced body weight and organ weight changes in male rats given 2 mg/kg of body weight per day (10).

## Reproductive toxicity, embryotoxicity, and teratogenicity

In a study in which male Dutch rabbits (6 per group) were given DBCP at 0, 0.9, 1.9, 3.7, 7.5, or 15 mg/kg of body weight in drinking-water 5 days per week for 10 weeks, testis weights and sperm production decreased and follicle stimulating hormone levels increased at 15 mg/kg of body weight, mean seminiferous tubular diameter decreased at 7.5 mg/kg of body weight, and abnormal sperm morphology was observed at 1.9 mg/kg of body weight. The NOAEL was 0.9 mg/kg of body weight (11, 12).

In a study in which DBCP was administered at 0.02, 0.2, 2, or 20 mg/kg of body weight per day in drinking-water to male and female Sprague-Dawley rats for 60 days before mating, throughout mating, during gestation, and during the first 5 days of lactation, fetal body weights, pup weights, and food and water intake were reduced at the highest dose (13).

Administration of DBCP at 0, 25, 50, or 100 mg/kg of body weight by gavage in corn oil to male and female CD-1 mice during the premating period (7 days), cohabitation (98 days) and segregation (21 days) was without effect on reproduction in the $F_0$ generation; however, when treatment at 100 mg/kg of body weight was administered to the offspring of $F_1$ mice, organ weights were reduced (14).

Male Sprague-Dawley rats given DBCP in corn oil by gavage at doses of 0, 0.9, 1.9, 3.7, 7.5, or 15 mg/kg of body weight for 77 days and mated with untreated females on days 65–71 had decreased body and testis weights at 3.7 but not at 7.5 mg/kg of body weight. Daily spermatozoa production was significantly lower in vehicle controls than in controls not given corn oil (15).

No teratogenic effects were found in fetuses of pregnant Wistar rats treated with DBCP by gavage at 12.5, 25, or 50 mg/kg of body weight per day on days

6–15 of gestation (5). The dose of 50 mg/kg of body weight per day was fatal to embryos, and those of 25 and 50 mg/kg of body weight per day reduced maternal body weights.

## Mutagenicity and related end-points

Technical-grade DBCP was mutagenic in *Salmonella typhimurium* strains TA1535, TA1530, TA100, and TA98 and in *Escherichia coli*, with and without metabolic activation (16–21). Results were negative with *S. typhimurium* strains A-98, TA1537, and TA1538 (16, 19, 20). DBCP was positive in the recessive lethal assay, in a genetic crossing-over assay, and for chromosome breakage in *Drosophila melanogaster* (22–24). Results of a dominant lethal assay were positive in rats (25) but negative in mice (26). Positive results were obtained in a study on sister chromatid exchange in cultured Chinese hamster cells, for chromosomal aberrations in rats treated *in vivo*, and for unscheduled DNA synthesis in germ cells of prepubertal mice treated *in vivo* (26–28). Results were negative in the mouse specific locus test (29).

## Carcinogenicity

In a chronic study in which Osborne-Mendel rats received time-weighted average doses by gavage of 10.7 and 20.7 mg/kg of body weight per day, highly significant dose-related increased incidences of squamous cell carcinoma of the forestomach in males and females and mammary adenocarcinoma in females were observed. Significant dose-related increased incidences of squamous cell carcinoma of the forestomach of male and female B6C3F$_1$ mice were found at time-weighted average doses of 78.6–149.3 mg/kg of body weight per day (9).

In a chronic dietary carcinogenicity bioassay in Charles River rats, high-dose (2.0 mg/kg of body weight per day) male and female rats had significantly increased incidences of carcinoma of the renal tubules and squamous cell carcinoma of the stomach. Male rats also showed an increase in liver tumours following exposure to DBCP for 104 weeks (10).

In a chronic inhalation study, dose-related increased incidences of nasal cavity tumours were found in male and female F344 rats and B6C3F$_1$ mice at DBCP concentrations of 5.8 or 29 mg/m$^3$, 6 h per day, 5 days per week. The mice also exhibited treatment-related increased incidences of pulmonary tumours (30).

DBCP was positive as a tumour initiator in the skin of Han/ICR Swiss mice but negative as a whole carcinogen for skin (31).

## 15.11.6 Effects on humans

Reduced spermatogenesis, which was reversible, was reported in chemical plant workers and agricultural workers exposed to DBCP (1). Possible permanent destruction of germinal epithelium was reported in a follow-up of exposed workers

(*32*). No chromosomal aberrations were identified in men in whom spermato-genesis was suppressed as a result of occupational exposure to DBCP, nor were there increases in abortions and malformations in offspring (*33*). Results were negative in an epidemiological study of the relationship between DBCP contamination of drinking-water and reproductive indices (e.g. birth rate, birth weight, birth defects) (*34*). Approximately 98% of 45 914 mothers were exposed to 3 µg/litre or less of DBCP.

No association was found between DBCP contamination of drinking-water (average levels 0.004–5.8 µg/litre) and incidences of gastric cancer and leukaemia (*35*); 14% of the areas concerned had levels greater than 1 µg/litre. These results differ from those of a similar earlier study that indicated a tentative association between DBCP exposure in drinking-water and gastric cancer and leukaemia (*36*). There was no association between cancer incidence and DBCP exposure in a cohort of 550 chemical workers potentially exposed to this compound during its production from 1957 to 1975 (*37*). Exposure levels were not estimated.

## 15.11.7 Guideline value

On the basis of data from studies on different strains of rats and mice, DBCP was determined to be carcinogenic in both sexes by the oral, inhalation, and dermal routes. It was also determined to be a reproductive toxicant in humans and several species of laboratory animals. IARC has classified DBCP in Group 2B (possible human carcinogen) based on sufficient evidence of carcinogenicity in animals (*38*). Recent epidemiological evidence suggests an increase in cancer mortality in individuals exposed to high levels of DBCP. It was found to be genotoxic in a majority of *in vitro* and *in vivo* assays.

The linearized multistage model was applied to the data on the incidence of stomach, kidney, and liver tumours in the male rat in a 104-week dietary study (*10*). The concentrations in drinking-water relating to excess lifetime cancer risks of $10^{-4}$, $10^{-5}$, and $10^{-6}$ are 10, 1, and 0.1 µg/litre, respectively. The guideline values associated with these excess lifetime cancer risks are therefore 10, 1, and 0.1 µg/litre, respectively. An adequate margin of safety exists at these concentrations for the reproductive toxicity of DBCP. For a contaminated water supply, extensive treatment (e.g. air stripping followed by adsorption to granular activated carbon) would be required to reduce the level of DBCP to the guideline values.

## References

1. Office of Drinking Water. *Drinking water criteria document for 1,2-dibromo-3-chloropropane (DBCP)*. Washington, DC, US Environmental Protection Agency, 1988 (ECAO-CIN-410).

2.  Environmental Monitoring and Support Laboratory. *Method 502.1. Volatile halogenated organic compounds in water by purge-and-trap gas chromatography*. Cincinnati, OH, US Environmental Protection Agency, 1985.

3.  Environmental Monitoring and Support Laboratory. *Method 524.1. Volatile organic compounds in water by purge-and-trap gas chromatography/mass spectrometry*. Cincinnati, OH, US Environmental Protection Agency, 1985.

4.  Kato Y et al. Metabolic fate of DBCP in rats. III. Correlation between macromolecular binding of DBCP-metabolite and pathogenicity of necrosis. *Journal of pesticide science*, 1980, 5(1):81-88.

5.  Ruddick JA, Newsome WH. A teratogenicity and tissue distribution study on dibromochloropropane in the rat. *Bulletin of environmental contamination and toxicology*, 1979, 21:483-487.

6.  Kato Y et al. Metabolic fate of 1,2-dibromo-3-chloropropane (DBCP) in rats. *Journal of pesticide science*, 1979, 4:195-203.

7.  Torkelson TR, Sadek SE, Rowe VK. Toxicologic investigations of 1,2-dibromo-3-chloropropane. *Toxicology and applied pharmacology*, 1961, 3:545-559.

8.  Heindel JJ, Bruckner JV, Steinberger E. *A protocol for the determination of the no-effect level of 1,2-dibromo-3-chloropropane (DBCP) on the qualitative morphological integrity of the testicular seminiferous epithelium*. Washington, DC, US Environmental Protection Agency, Office of Drinking Water, 1983.

9.  National Cancer Institute. *Bioassay of dibromochloropropane for possible carcinogenicity*. Bethesda, MD, 1977 (NCI Carcinogenesis Technical Report Serial No. 28; NTIS PB 277-472).

10. Hazleton Laboratories America, Inc. *104-week dietary study in rats: 1,2-dibromo-3-chloropropane (DBCP). Final report*. Midland, MI, Dow Chemical Co., 1977 (unpublished report, project no. 174-122).

11. Foote RH, Schermerhorn EC, Simkin ME. Measurement of semen quality, fertility, and reproductive hormones to assess dibromochloropropane (DBCP) effects in live rabbits. *Fundamental and applied toxicology*, 1986, 6:628-637.

12. Foote RH, Berndtson WE, Rounsaville TR. Use of quantitative testicular histology to assess the effect of dibromochloropropane (DBCP) on reproduction in rabbits. *Fundamental and applied toxicology*, 1986, 6:638-647.

13. Johnston RV et al. Single-generation drinking water reproduction study of 1,2-dibromo-3-chloropropane in Sprague-Dawley rats. *Bulletin of environmental contamination and toxicology*, 1986, 37(4):531-537.

14. Reel JR et al. *Dibromochloropropane: reproduction and fertility assessment in CD-1 mice when administered by gavage.* Research Triangle Park, NC, US Department of Health and Human Services, National Toxicology Program, 1984 (NTP-84-263).

15. Amann RP, Berndtsen WE. Assessment of procedures for screening agents for effects on male reproduction. Effects of dibromochloropropane (DBCP) in the rat. *Fundamental and applied toxicology,* 1986, 7(2):244-255.

16. Rosenkranz HS. Genetic activity of 1,2-dibromo-3-chloropropane, a widely used fumigant. *Bulletin of environmental contamination and toxicology,* 1975, 14(1):8-12.

17. Prival MJ et al. Tris(2,3-dibromopropylphosphate): mutagenicity of a widely used flame retardant. *Science,* 1977, 195:76-78.

18. Stolzenberg SJ, Hine CH. Mutagenicity of halogenated and oxygenated three-carbon compounds. *Journal of toxicology and environmental health,* 1979, 5(6):1149-1158.

19. McKee RH, Phillips RD, Traul KA. The genetic toxicity of 1,2-dibromo-3-chloropropane, 1,2-dibromo-3-chloro-2-methylpropane, and 1,2,2-tribromo-2-methylpropane. *Cell biology and toxicology,* 1987, 3(4):391-406.

20. Ratpan F, Plaumann H. Mutagenicity of halogenated propanes and their methylated derivatives. *Environmental and molecular mutagenesis,* 1988, 12(2):253-259.

21. Ohta T et al. The SOS function-inducing activity of chemical mutagens in *Escherichia coli. Mutation research,* 1984, 131:101-109.

22. Kale PG, Baum JW. Genetic effects of 1,2-dibromo-3-chloropropane (DBCP) in *Drosophila. Environmental mutagenesis,* 1982, 4(6):681-688.

23. Inoue T et al. Induction of sex-linked recessive lethal mutations in *Drosophila melanogaster* males by gaseous 1,2-dibromo-3-chloropropane (DBCP). *Mutation research,* 1982, 105:89-94.

24. Zimmering S. 1,2-Dibromo-3-chloropropane (DBCP) is positive for sex-linked recessive lethals, heritable translocations and chromosome loss in *Drosophila. Mutation research,* 1983, 119(3):287-288.

25. Teramoto S et al. Dominant lethal mutation induced in male rats by 1,2-dibromo-3-chloropropane (DBCP). *Mutation research,* 1980, 77(1):71-78.

26. Lee IP, Suzuki K. Induction of unscheduled DNA synthesis in mouse germ cells following 1,2-dibromo-3-chloropropane (DBCP) exposure. *Mutation research,* 1979, 68:169-173.

27. Tezuka H et al. Sister-chromatid exchanges and chromosomal aberrations in cultured Chinese hamster cells treated with pesticides positive in microbial reversion assays. *Mutation research,* 1980, 78(2):177-191.

28. Whorton M, Foliart D. Mutagenicity, carcinogenicity and reproductive effects of dibromochloropropane (DBCP). *Mutation research*, 1983, 123:13-30.

29. Russell LB, Hunsicker PR, Cacheiro NLA. Mouse specific-locus test for the induction of heritable gene mutations by dibromochloropropane (DBCP). *Mutation research*, 1986, 170:161-166.

30. National Toxicology Program. *Carcinogenesis bioassay of 1,2-dibromo-3-chloropropane in F344 rats and B6C3F₁ mice (inhalation study)*. Research Triangle Park, NC, US Department of Health and Human Services, 1982 (NTP Technical Report No. 81-21; DHHS [NIH] 82-1762).

31. Van Duuren BL et al. Carcinogenicity of halogenated olefinic and aliphatic hydrocarbons in mice. *Journal of the National Cancer Institute*, 1979, 63(6):1433-1439.

32. Eaton M et al. Seven-year follow-up of workers exposed to 1,2-dibromo-3-chloropropane. *Journal of occupational medicine*, 1986, 28:1145-1150.

33. Potashnik G, Abeliovich D. Chromosomal analysis and health status of children conceived to men during or following dibromochloropropane-induced spermatogenic suppression. *Andrologia*, 1985, 17:291-296.

34. Environmental Health Associates, Inc. *An epidemiologic investigation of the relationship between DBCP contamination in drinking water and reproductive effects in Fresno County, CA.* Houston, TX, Shell Oil Company, 1986 (unpublished report).

35. Environmental Health Associates, Inc. *Final report: examination of the possible relationship between DBCP water contamination and leukemia and gastric cancer in Fresno County, CA.* Houston, TX, Shell Oil Company, 1986 (unpublished report).

36. Jackson RJ et al. *Literature review on the toxicological aspects of DBCP and an epidemiological comparison of patterns of DBCP drinking water contamination with mortality rates from selected cancers in Fresno County, CA, 1970-1979.* California Department of Health Services, 1982 (unpublished report).

37. Hearn S et al. Mortality experience of employees with occupational exposure to DBCP. *Archives of environmental health*, 1984, 39:49-55.

38. International Agency for Research on Cancer. *Overall evaluations of carcinogenicity: an updating of IARC Monographs volumes 1-42.* Lyon, 1987:191-192 (IARC Monographs on the Evaluation of Carcinogenic Risks to Humans, Suppl. 7).

# 15.12 2,4-Dichlorophenoxyacetic acid (2,4-D)

## 15.12.1 General description

### Identity

CAS no.:                    94-75-7
Molecular formula:          $C_8H_6O_3Cl_2$

### Physicochemical properties (1, 2)

| Property | Value |
|---|---|
| Water solubility | 620 mg/litre at 20 °C |
| Vapour pressure | 1.4 Pa at 25 °C |
| Log octanol–water partition coefficient | 2.62 |

### Organoleptic properties

Some individuals may be able to detect 2,4-D in drinking-water by taste or odour at about 20 µg/litre (2).

### Major uses

2,4-D is a systemic chlorophenoxy herbicide widely used throughout the world in the control of broad-leaved weeds in cereal cropland and on lawns, turf and pastures. It is also used to control aquatic weeds. Commercial 2,4-D products are marketed as alkali salts, amine salts, and ester formulations. Impurities may be present in the technical product as a result of the manufacturing process (1).

### Environmental fate

2,4-D can enter the environment through effluents and spills arising from its manufacture and transport and through direct application as a weed-control agent. It is removed from the environment principally by biodegradation, the main degradation product being 2,4-dichlorophenol (3). The half-life of 2,4-D in soil is reported to range from 4–7 days in most soil types (4, 5) to up to 6 weeks in acidic soils (5, 7). It is rapidly biodegraded in water, although some may be degraded by photolysis near the surface. Half-lives in water range from one to several weeks under aerobic conditions and can exceed 120 days under anaerobic conditions (8). 2,4-D is not expected to accumulate in bottom sediments and muds. Except in some algae, it does not bioaccumulate in aquatic or terrestrial organisms because of its rapid degradation (9).

## 15.12.2 Analytical methods

Residues of 2,4-D in water are commonly measured by extraction, chemical derivatization, separation by gas–liquid chromatography, and electron-capture detection. This method is suitable for the detection of picogram levels (2). Electrolytic conductivity detection is also used; the detection limit is then 0.1 µg/litre (10).

## 15.12.3 Environmental levels and human exposure

### Air

Residues of 2,4-D in the atmosphere are predominantly in the form of the isopropyl and butyl esters (8). In areas of Saskatchewan, Canada, where the herbicide was heavily used, 30% of ambient air samples collected from 1966 to 1975 contained less than 0.01 µg/m³, while 10% contained more than 1 µg/m³ (11). Average concentrations in air surveyed in Washington State, USA, in 1973 and 1974 ranged from 0.10 to 1.41 µg/m³; at 85% of the locations surveyed, average concentrations were less than 1.0 µg/m³ (12).

### Water

2,4-D was detected, at a maximum concentration of 29 µg/litre in 52 of 805 samples of raw and treated drinking-water from municipal and private supplies in surveys conducted in six Canadian provinces from 1971 to 1986 (13). No residues were detected in drinking-water samples analysed routinely in market basket surveys (detection limit 5 µg/litre) in the USA (2). In Germany, 910 samples of raw and treated drinking-water contained no 2,4-D; 23 samples were above the detection limit (0.1 µg/litre) (Federal Environmental Office, unpublished data).

Of 447 samples of surface waters in three Canadian agricultural areas surveyed from 1981 to 1985, 78 had detectable 2,4-D concentrations; mean annual concentrations ranged from 0.01 to 0.7 µg/litre (10). 2,4-D was detected in 38.5% of 1386 surface water samples from the Canadian prairies tested between 1971 and 1977 (detection limit 0.004 µg/litre); mean levels were less than 0.3 µg/litre (14). Maximum concentrations of 0.3 µg/litre were measured in infiltrated river bank water in the Netherlands (15). Concentrations in groundwater in the range 0.4–0.7 µg/litre have been reported (16).

### Food

No residues of 2,4-D ester were detected in a total diet study conducted in Canada in 1976–78 (detection limit 0.5 mg/kg) (17). The rate of occurrence of detectable 2,4-D residues in food samples in the USA surveyed from 1965 to 1980 ranged from 0 to 4.2%; all levels were below 0.2 mg/kg (2).

### *Estimated total exposure and relative contribution of drinking-water*

Based on the maximum limits for pesticide residues established by the Codex Alimentarius Commission (*18*), the theoretical maximum daily intake of 2,4-D in food ranges from 0.03 to 0.4 mg/day for a 60-kg adult; the global mean is 0.1 mg/day (2 μg/kg of body weight per day). The intake found in a total diet study in the USA in 1987 was 0.1 ng/kg of body weight per day for females aged 60–65 years and less than 0.1 ng/kg of body weight per day for children aged 6–11 months and males aged 14–16 years (*19*).

## 15.12.4 Kinetics and metabolism in laboratory animals and humans

2,4-D administered orally as the free acid or salt is absorbed rapidly and almost completely in rats and humans (*20, 21*). The amine salt is also well absorbed in rats, calves, and pigs, but absorption is much slower and less complete for esters of 2,4-D, which are probably hydrolysed to the free acid before absorption (*22*).

After absorption in rats, 2,4-D is distributed throughout the body; peak concentrations are reached in blood after 3 h (*23*) and in kidney, liver, spleen, and lung after 6 h (*22*). In humans given an oral dose of 5 mg/kg of body weight, elimination was fairly rapid (half-time 17.7 h); 82% was excreted unchanged in urine, and 13% as a conjugate (*21*). Similar results were observed in rats (*24*).

## 15.12.5 Effects on laboratory animals and *in vitro* test systems

### *Acute exposure*

Oral LD$_{50}$s for 2,4-D, for the acid equivalent of the isooctyl, isobutyl, butyl, and butoxyethanol esters, and for the sodium and dimethylamine salts range from 420 to 840 mg/kg of body weight in F344 rats (*24*). Similar results have been obtained for other species (*2*).

### *Long-term exposure*

In a 2-year chronic toxicity study in Fischer 344 rats (60 per sex per dose), animals were fed 2,4-D in the diet at doses equivalent to 0, 1, 5, 15, or 45 mg/kg of body weight per day. Kidney weights were increased significantly in males and females at 45 mg/kg of body weight per day and in males at 15 mg/kg of body weight per day, and thyroid/parathyroid weights were increased significantly in males and females at 45 mg/kg of body weight per day and in females at 15 mg/kg of body weight per day. At doses of 5, 15, and 45 mg/kg of body weight per day, an increased incidence of brown pigment was observed in kidney tubular cells of both males and females, and renal transitional epithelial cell hyperplasia was observed in females at 45 mg/kg of body weight per day. An increased frequency of renal microcalculi was observed in males at 15 and 45 mg/kg of body weight per day and in females at 45 mg/kg of body weight per day. Vacuolization of the cytoplasm of the renal cortex was noted in females at 45 mg/kg of body weight per day. The NOAEL in this study was 1 mg/kg of body weight per day (25).

In a 2-year study in which B6C3F$_1$ mice (60 per sex per dose) were fed 2,4-D in the diet at doses equivalent to 0, 1, 5, 15, or 45 mg/kg of body weight per day, the only evidence of an effect was an increase in cytoplasmic homogeneity of renal tubular epithelium in male mice at 5 mg/kg of body weight per day and above. The NOAEL was 1 mg/kg of body weight per day (26).

## Reproductive toxicity, embryotoxicity, and teratogenicity

Fertility and litter size were not affected by doses of 2,4-D up to 1500 mg/kg of diet (about 75 mg/kg of body weight) in a three-generation study in rats, although pup survival was sharply reduced at this dose (27). In rats orally dosed with 2,4-D on days 6–15 of gestation, there were no effects on fertility, gestation, viability of pups, or neonatal growth at any dose up to 87.5 mg/kg of body weight, but administration of the isooctyl or propylene glycol butyl ethers at 75 or 87.5 mg/kg of body weight resulted in decreased viability of offspring (28). 2,4-D given to rats at 1000 mg/litre in drinking-water during and after pregnancy did not cause any effects on reproduction, but retarded growth and increased mortality were observed in the second generation given the same dose for 2 years (29). Abnormal spermatogenesis and reductions in testis and prostate weights were reported in rats given 87.5 mg/kg of body weight of 2,4-D butyl ether; no effects were seen at 37.5 mg/kg of body weight (30).

Administration of 2,4-D acid and its butyl, isooctyl, and butoxyethanol esters to rats on days 6–15 of gestation caused reduced fetal weights and increased the frequency of minor skeletal malformations at doses of 100 mg/kg of body weight or higher; this effect was noted only at 300 mg/kg of body weight for the dimethylamine salt (31). Embryotoxic and fetotoxic effects, including reduced fetal body weight, subcutaneous oedema, delayed ossification, and wavy ribs, were observed in rats given 2,4-D or its isooctyl and propylene glycol butyl ether esters at doses of 50–87.5 mg/kg of body weight on days 6–15 of gestation; neither 2,4-D nor its esters were teratogenic at any dose (28).

In mice, embryotoxicity, reduced fetal weight, and increased fetal mortality were observed at a dose of 221 mg/kg of body weight per day of 2,4-D, the isopropyl ester, and the isooctyl ester. Teratogenic effects (cleft palate) were observed at doses of 124 mg/kg of body weight or greater for 2,4-D but not for the esters (32).

## Mutagenicity and related end-points

The results of short-term genotoxicity studies conducted to date have been largely negative, and it is concluded that 2,4-D is non-genotoxic. It was not mutagenic in a number of microbial assays on *Salmonella typhimurium, Bacillus subtilis,* and *Escherichia coli* (*2, 33–35*). The unscheduled DNA synthesis test gave negative results in rat hepatocytes (*36*) and in one of two tests on human fibroblasts (*37, 38*). Sister chromatid exchange tests *in vitro* gave negative results in Chinese hamster ovary cells (*39*) and positive results in human lymphocytes (*40*); *in vivo* tests were negative in mice (*41*), rat lymphocytes (*39*), hamsters (*39*), and humans (*42*).

### Carcinogenicity

2,4-D did not exhibit any carcinogenicity in three long-term studies in rats and mice (*33, 34*); however, these studies were inadequate for the evaluation of carcinogenicity (*34, 43*). In a bioassay conducted in B6C3F$_1$ mice (*26*), there were no carcinogenic effects at any dose; however, the lack of toxic effects at all dose levels indicates that the maximum tolerated dose (MTD) was unlikely to have been reached, thus precluding an assessment of carcinogenicity. In a 2-year carcinogenicity bioassay in Fischer 344 rats (*25*), an increase in astrocytomas of the brain was observed in males at the highest dose (45 mg/kg of body weight per day), as well as a significant positive dose-related trend for this effect. Although the systemic toxicity noted in the study supports the conclusion that an MTD was reached, the US Environmental Protection Agency concluded that it had not, and requested that the studies in rats and in mice be repeated at the same and higher doses to clarify the status of 2,4-D with respect to its carcinogenicity to animals.

## 15.12.6 Effects on humans

### Acute exposure

Symptoms of acute exposure to high doses of 2,4-D include effects on the gastrointestinal tract, such as nausea, vomiting, and diarrhoea, direct myotoxic effects, such as muscular weakness, stiffness, muscular spasms, and partial paralysis, effects on the kidney, pulmonary oedema, and effects on the central and peripheral nervous systems, including central nervous system depression, lethargy, slowed respiration, coma, and death (*2*).

### Carcinogenicity

Most epidemiological studies conducted to date have dealt with multiple exposures to various chlorophenoxy herbicides.

In a series of case–referent studies conducted in Sweden in the late 1970s and early 1980s, strong associations were noted between soft-tissue sarcomas (STS) and multiple lymphomas, including Hodgkin disease (HD) and non-Hodgkin lymphoma (NHL), and the use of chlorophenoxy herbicides by agricultural or forestry workers (*44, 45*). These studies served to focus attention on STS, HD and NHL as the outcomes of interest in subsequent case–referent and cohort studies.

The association between STS and chlorophenoxy use was not confirmed in other case–referent studies, including one that involved primarily 2,4-D exposure (46). Negative results were also obtained in several cohort studies carried out to investigate STS in occupationally exposed workers (47–49). No cohort was exposed solely or principally to 2,4-D, including the "2,4-D cohort" of 878 chemical workers engaged in its manufacture at a chemical plant in the USA, 75% of whom had also been exposed to 2,4,5-T (47). Because of the small size of most of the cohorts, little reliance can be placed on these results.

A weak link between NHL and chlorophenoxy exposure was found in several case–referent studies, only one of which, however, was specifically concerned with 2,4-D. In this study, the relative risk was not significant for those who used 2,4-D more than 21 days per year, but the trend towards increasing risk with increasing number of days of use was marginally significant, and the risk was highly significant for those who did not take precautionary measures to reduce exposure by changing clothing soon afterwards or washing immediately after handling the pesticide (50, 51). In a second study (576 cases of NHL), the relative risk increased from 1.1 for subjects with any past occupational exposure to chlorophenoxy herbicides (primarily 2,4-D and 2, 4, 5-T) to 1.7 for people occupationally exposed to such herbicides for at least 15 years (the minimum latency period) (52). In another study (200 cases), the relative risk of NHL from farm herbicide use was 1.4, indicating only a marginal association, but rose to 2.2 for farmers who had used chlorophenoxy herbicides at any time (almost all 2,4-D) and to 6.0 for those who had used unspecified herbicides for more than 20 days per year. The trend towards increasing risk with increasing number of days of use per year was highly significant (46).

No excess risk was observed for NHL in any of the cohort studies on occupational exposure (47–49), although the cohorts were generally too small to provide any conclusive evidence, and all had been exposed to chlorophenoxy herbicides other than 2,4-D. In a recent cohort study on farmers in Saskatchewan (Canada), where 2,4-D is extensively used, it was found that the risk of NHL increased with the use of herbicides, as measured by the number of acres sprayed, but it was not possible to conclude that the association was with 2,4-D (53).

In a Swedish case–referent study on malignant lymphoma, the combined relative risk for HD and NHL was 4.8, rising to 7.0 for more than 90 days of total exposure to a mixture of chlorophenoxy herbicides (45). Apart from this study, there is little evidence of an increase in risk of HD as a result of exposure to chlorophenoxy herbicides, based on another case–referent study (46) and three cohort studies (47–49).

Chlorophenoxy herbicides as a group, including 2,4-D, have been classified by IARC in Group 2B (possibly carcinogenic to humans) (54). However, based on the studies considered here, it is not possible to determine the status of 2,4-D with respect to carcinogenicity, as almost all the populations studied were exposed to a mixture of chlorophenoxy herbicides. In the only study in which exposure was clearly to 2,4-D alone (*51*), the association was weak.

### Mutagenicity

No significant elevations were observed in sister chromatid exchanges in forestry workers before, during, and after spraying of 2,4-D and MCPA (*42*). Similar results were obtained for the frequency of chromosomal aberrations in workers exposed to 2,4-D and MCPA (*55*).

## 15.12.7 Guideline value

IARC has classified chorophenoxy herbicides in Group 2B (limited evidence for carcinogenicity in humans, inadequate evidence in animals) (*54*). However, it is not possible to evaluate the carcinogenic potential of 2,4-D on the basis of the available data; epidemiological studies provide limited evidence that occupational exposure to chlorophenoxy herbicides may cause cancer, and long-term studies in animals continue to show equivocal evidence for carcinogenicity, in one sex and species only. 2,4-D was found to be non-mutagenic in the limited number of studies conducted.

Because the data on the carcinogenic potential of 2,4-D are inadequate, and because 2,4-D has not been found to be genotoxic, the TDI approach can be used to calculate a guideline value for drinking-water. Based on a NOAEL of 1 mg/kg of body weight per day for effects on the kidney in 2-year studies in rats and mice (*25, 26*) and an uncertainty factor of 100 (for intra- and interspecies variation), a TDI of 10 µg/kg of body weight can be derived. The use of an additional uncertainty factor for carcinogenicity was considered unnecessary, as the NOAEL should provide a sufficient margin of safety with respect to the lowest dose that was associated with an increase in brain tumours in rats. The guideline value, based on an allocation of 10% of the TDI to drinking-water, is 30 µg/litre.

## References

1.  Royal Society of Chemistry. *The agrochemicals handbook*, 3rd ed. Cambridge, 1991.

2.  *2,4-Dichlorophenoxyacetic acid (2,4-D)*. Geneva, World Health Organization, 1984 (Environmental Health Criteria, No. 29).

3.  Loos MA. Phenoxyalkanoic acids. In: Kearney PC, Kaufman DD, eds. *Herbicides— chemistry, degradation, and mode of action*. New York, NY, Marcel Dekker, 1975: 1-128.

4.  Smith AE. The hydrolysis of herbicidal phenoxyalkanoic esters to phenoxyalkanoic acids in Saskatchewan soils. *Weed research*, 1976, 16:19-22.

5. Thompson DG et al. Persistence of (2,4-dichlorophenoxy) acetic acid and 2-(2,4-dichlorophenoxy) propionic acid in agricultural and forest soils of northern and southern Ontario. *Journal of agricultural and food chemistry*, 1984, 32:578-581.

6. Sattar MA, Paasivirta J. Fate of chlorophenoxyacetic acids in acid soil. *Chemosphere*, 1980, 9:745-752.

7. Torstensson NT. Degradation of 2,4-D and MCPA in soils of low pH. *Environmental quality and safety*, 1975, 3(Suppl.):262-265.

8. *Phenoxy herbicides—their effects on environmental quality.* Ottawa, National Research Council of Canada, Associate Committee on Scientific Criteria for Environmental Quality, 1978.

9. *2,4-Dichlorophenoxyacetic acid (2,4-D)—environmental aspects.* Geneva, World Health Organization, 1989 (Environmental Health Criteria, No. 84).

10. Frank R, Logan L. Pesticide and polychlorinated biphenyl residues at the mouth of the Grand, Saugeen and Thames rivers, Ontario, Canada, 1986–1990. *Archives of environmental contamination and toxicology*, 1991, 21:585-595.

11. Grover R et al. Residues of 2,4-D in air samples from Saskatchewan: 1966–1975. *Journal of environmental science and health*, 1976, B11(4):331-347.

12. Farwell SO et al. Survey of airborne 2,4-D in south-central Washington. *Journal of the Air Pollution Control Association*, 1976, 26:224-230.

13. Hiebsch SC. *The occurrence of thirty-five pesticides in Canadian drinking water and surface water.* Ottawa, Canada, Department of National Health and Welfare, Environmental Health Directorate, 1988.

14. Gummer WD. Pesticide monitoring in the prairies of western Canada. *Environmental science research*, 1980, 16:345-372.

15. KIWA (Netherlands Waterwork Testing and Research Institute). *Pesticides and the drinking water supply in the Netherlands.* Nieuwegein, 1990 (KIWA Report No. 113).

16. Lock JP, Verdam B. Pesticide residues in groundwater in the Netherlands: state of observations and future directions of research. *Schriftenreihe des Vereins für Wasser-, Boden-, und Lufthygiene*, 1989, 79:349-363.

17. McLeod HA, Smith DC, Bluman N. Pesticide residues in the total diet in Canada, V: 1976 to 1978. *Journal of food safety*, 1980, 2:141.

18. Codex Alimentarius Commission. *Volume 2. Pesticide residues in food.* Rome, Food and Agriculture Organization of the United Nations, 1993.

19. Food and Drug Administration Pesticide Program. Residues in foods—1987. *Journal of the Association of Official Analytical Chemists*, 1988, 71(6):156A-174A.

20. Khanna S, Fang SC. Metabolism of C-14 labeled 2,4-dichlorophenoxyacetic acid in rats. *Journal of agricultural and food chemistry*, 1966, 14:500-503.

21. Sauerhoff MW et al. The fate of 2,4-dichlorophenoxyacetic acid (2,4-D) following oral administration to man. *Toxicology*, 1977, 8:3-11.

22. *Pesticide residues in food: report of the 1970 Joint FAO/WHO Meeting.* Geneva, World Health Organization, 1971 (WHO Technical Report Series, No. 474).

23. *Evaluations of some pesticide residues in food 1975.* Geneva, World Health Organization, 1976 (WHO Pesticide Residues Series, No. 5).

24. Gorzinski SJ et al. Acute, pharmacokinetic, and subchronic toxicological studies of 2,4-dichlorophenoxyacetic acid. *Fundamental and applied toxicology*, 1987, 9:423-435.

25. Industry Task Force on 2,4-D Research Data. *Combined toxicity and oncogenicity study in rats—2,4-dichlorophenoxy acetic acid.* Kensington, MD, Hazleton Laboratories America, Inc., 1986 (Project No. 2184-103).

26. Industry Task Force on 2,4-D Research Data. *Summary of preliminary pathology report, oncogenicity study in mice with 2,4-dichlorophenoxyacetic acid.* Kensington, MD, Hazleton Laboratories America, Inc., 1986 (Project No. 2184-105).

27. Hansen WH et al. Chronic toxicity of 2,4-dichlorophenoxyacetic acid in rats and dogs. *Toxicology and applied pharmacology*, 1971, 20:122-129.

28. Schwetz BA, Sparschu GL, Gehring PJ. The effect of 2,4-dichlorophenoxyacetic acid (2,4-D) and esters of 2,4-D on rat embryonal, foetal and neonatal growth and development. *Food and cosmetics toxicology*, 1971, 9:801-817.

29. Bjorklund N-E, Erne K. Toxicological studies of phenoxyacetic herbicides in animals. *Acta veterinaria scandinavica*, 1966, 7:364-390.

30. Schillinger JE. Hygienische Wertung von landwirtschaftlichen Erzeugnissen, angebaut unter Anwendung von Herbiziden. [Hygienic evaluation of agricultural products cultivated with the use of herbicides.] *Journal of hygiene and epidemiology (Praha)*, 1960, 4:243-252.

31. Khera KS, McKinley WP. Pre- and postnatal studies on 2,4,5-trichlorophenoxyacetic acid, 2,4-dichlorophenoxyacetic acid and their derivatives in rats. *Toxicology and applied pharmacology*, 1972, 22:14-28.

32. Courtney KD. Prenatal effects of herbicides: evaluation by the prenatal development index. *Archives of environmental contamination and toxicology,* 1977, 6:33-46.

33. International Agency for Research on Cancer. *Some fumigants, the herbicides 2,4-D and 2,4,5-T, chlorinated dibenzodioxins and miscellaneous industrial chemicals.* Lyon, 1977:111-147 (IARC Monographs on the Evaluation of the Carcinogenic Risk of Chemicals to Man, Volume 15).

34. International Agency for Research on Cancer. *Chemicals, industrial processes and industries associated with cancer in humans.* Lyon, 1982:101-103 (IARC Monographs on the Evaluation of the Carcinogenic Risk of Chemicals to Humans, Suppl. 4).

35. International Agency for Research on Cancer. *Genetic and related effects: an updating of selected IARC Monographs from volumes 1–42.* Lyon, 1987:233-236 (IARC Monographs on the Evaluation of Carcinogenic Risks to Humans, Suppl. 6).

36. Probst GS et al. Chemically-induced unscheduled DNA synthesis in primary rat hepatocyte cultures: a comparison with bacterial mutagenicity using 218 compounds. *Environmental mutagenesis,* 1981, 3:11-32.

37. Simmon VF. *In vitro microbiological mutagenicity and unscheduled DNA synthesis of eighteen pesticides.* Washington, DC, US Environmental Protection Agency, 1979 (No. 600/1-19-041).

38. Ahmed FE, Hart RW, Lewis NJ. Pesticide induced DNA damage and its repair in cultured human cells. *Mutation research,* 1977, 42:161-174.

39. Linnainmaa K. Induction of sister chromatid exchanges by the peroxisome proliferators 2,4-D, MCPA, and clofibrate *in vivo* and *in vitro. Carcinogenesis,* 1984, 5:703-707.

40. Korte C, Jalal SM. 2,4-D induced clastogenicity and elevated rates of sister chromatid exchanges in cultured human lymphocytes. *Journal of heredity,* 1984, 73:224-226.

41. Lamb JC et al. Male fertility, sister chromatid exchange, and germ cell toxicity following exposure to mixtures of chlorinated phenoxy acids containing 2,3,7,8-tetra-chlorodibenzo-*p*-dioxin. *Journal of toxicology and environmental health,* 1981, 8:825-834.

42. Linnainmaa K. Sister chromatid exchanges among workers occupationally exposed to phenoxy acid herbicides 2,4-D and MCPA. *Teratogenesis, carcinogenesis, and mutagenesis,* 1983, 3:269-279.

43. International Agency for Research on Cancer. *Occupational exposures to chlorophenoxy herbicides.* Lyon, 1986:357-407 (IARC Monographs on the Evaluation of the Carcinogenic Risk of Chemicals to Humans, Volume 41).

44. Hardell L et al. Malignant lymphoma and exposure to chemicals, especially organic solvents, chlorophenols and phenoxy acids: a case–control study. *British journal of cancer*, 1981, 43:169-176.

45. Eriksson M et al. Soft-tissue sarcomas and exposure to chemical substances: a case–referent study. *British journal of industrial medicine*, 1981, 38:27-33.

46. Hoar SK et al. Agricultural herbicide use and risk of lymphoma and soft-tissue sarcoma. *Journal of the American Medical Association*, 1986, 256(9):1141-1147.

47. Bond GG et al. Cause specific mortality among employees engaged in the manufacture, formulation, or packaging of 2,4-dichlorophenoxyacetic acid and related salts. *British journal of industrial medicine*, 1988, 45:98-105.

48. Wiklund K, Dich J, Holm L-E. Risk of soft tissue sarcoma, Hodgkin's disease and non-Hodgkin lymphoma among Swedish licensed pesticide applicators. *Chemosphere*, 1989, 18(1-6):395.

49. Lynge E. A follow-up study of cancer incidence among workers in manufacture of phenoxy herbicides in Denmark. *British journal of cancer*, 1985, 52:259-270.

50. Weisenburger DD. Environmental epidemiology of non-Hodgkin's lymphoma in eastern Nebraska. *American journal of industrial medicine*, 1990, 18(3):303-305.

51. Zahm SH et al. A case–control study of non-Hodgkin's lymphoma and the herbicide 2,4-dichlorophenoxyacetic acid (2,4-D) in eastern Nebraska. *Epidemiology*, 1990, 1:349-356.

52. Woods JS et al. Soft tissue sarcoma and non-Hodgkin's lymphoma in relation to phenoxy herbicide and chlorinated phenol exposure in Western Washington. *Journal of the National Cancer Institute*, 1987, 78:899-910.

53. Wigle DT, Semenciw RM, Wilkins K. Mortality study of Canadian male farm operators: non-Hodgkin's lymphoma mortality and agricultural practices in Saskatchewan. *Journal of the National Cancer Institute*, 1990, 82:575-582.

54. International Agency for Research on Cancer. *Overall evaluation of carcinogenicity: an updating of IARC Monographs volumes 1-42*. Lyon, 1987:156-160 (IARC Monographs on the Evaluation of the Carcinogenic Risk of Chemicals to Humans, Suppl. 7).

55. Mustonen R et al. Effects of phenoxyacetic acids on the induction of chromosome aberrations *in vitro* and *in vivo*. *Mutagenesis*, 1986, 1:241-245.

# 15.13 1,2-Dichloropropane

## 15.13.1 General description

### Identity

CAS no.: 78-87-5
Molecular formula: $C_3H_6Cl_2$

### Physicochemical properties (1, 2)[1]

| Property | Value |
|---|---|
| Boiling point | 96.8 °C |
| Melting point | -100 °C |
| Density | 1.1560 g/cm³ at 20 °C |
| Vapour pressure | 5.60 kPa at 20 °C |
| Water solubility | 2700 mg/litre at 20 °C |
| Log octanol–water partition coefficient | 1.99 |

### Organoleptic properties

1,2-Dichloropropane has a chloroform-like odour. The odour threshold in water is 10 µg/litre (2).

### Major uses

1,2-Dichloropropane, or propylene dichloride, is used primarily as a chemical intermediate, lead scavenger for antiknock fluids, dry-cleaning solvent, soil fumigant, scouring compound, spotting agent, and metal-degreasing agent (1).

### Environmental fate

1,2-Dichloropropane is degraded in air by photochemically produced hydroxyl radicals; the half-life is 23 days or more. Direct photolysis probably does not occur. In water, it is relatively resistant to hydrolysis and has a half-life of 25–200 weeks. It volatilizes from surface waters. Its relatively low soil adsorption coefficient and high water solubility suggest that it is not appreciably adsorbed on to soil but migrates from it to groundwater. Little or no degradation in soil has been reported. Bioconcentration in animals or food-chains is unlikely to occur (2).

---

[1] Conversion factor in air: 1 ppm = 4.76 mg/m³.

## 15.13.2 Analytical methods

1,2-Dichloropropane is usually determined by a purge-and-trap gas chromato-graphic procedure used for the determination of volatile organohalides in drinking-water (*3, 4*). Confirmatory analysis is by mass spectrometry or halide-specific detectors (detection limit 0.03–0.2 µg/litre) (*2*).

## 15.13.3 Environmental levels and human exposure

### Air

Median concentrations of 1,2-dichloropropane were reported to be 0.0 µg/m$^3$ in rural/remote areas, 0.26 µg/m$^3$ in urban/suburban areas, and 0.55 µg/m$^3$ in source-dominated areas (*5*).

### Water

1,2-Dichloropropane was detected in samples from six of 466 randomly selected US groundwater supply systems in the USA from 1980 to 1981; levels ranged from 0.48 to 21 µg/litre (mean 0.86 µg/litre). It was also detected in seven of 479 systems with a high potential for contamination, at concentrations ranging from 0.21 to 18 µg/litre (mean 0.84 µg/litre; the detection limit was 0.2 µg/litre) (*6*).[1] Most samples of raw, treated, and tapwater from the Great Lakes collected from the mid-1970s to early 1985 contained levels of 1,2-dichloropropane near or below the detection limit (*7*).

### Estimated total exposure and relative contribution of drinking-water

At an air concentration of 0.26 µg/m$^3$, the exposure will be 5.2 µg/day for an adult with an air intake of 20 m$^3$/day. At a concentration of 0.86 µg/litre in drinking-water, the daily exposure for an adult consuming 2 litres of water per day is 1.7 µg.

## 15.13.4 Kinetics and metabolism in laboratory animals and humans

Studies in rats indicate that 1,2-dichloropropane is readily absorbed from the gastrointestinal tract (*8, 9*). Two days after the administration of [$^{14}$C]1,2-di-chloropropane to rats by gavage, the highest concentrations of the radiolabel were detected in the liver, kidney, and blood (*10*).

---

[1] Includes data from: Groundwater supply survey. Computer data file. Cincinnati, OH, US Environmental Protection Agency, Office of Drinking Water, Technical Support Division, 1983.

It has been suggested that, in rats, 1,2-dichloropropane is dechlorinated and oxidized to epoxide intermediates, which are then hydrolysed and conjugated to form *N*-acetyl-*S*-(2-hydroxypropyl) cysteine. β-Chloroacetate, lactate, carbon dioxide, and oxalate have been identified as other metabolites (*10*). 1,2-Dichloropropane and its metabolites were eliminated by orally dosed rats in the urine (50%), faeces (5%), and expired air (30%) in the first 24 h after dosing (*8*).

## 15.13.5 Effects on laboratory animals and *in vitro* test systems

### Acute exposure

$LD_{50}$s for 1,2-dichloropropane were reported to be 1000–2200 mg/kg of body weight in rats (oral), 500 mg/kg of body weight in mice (oral), 9224 mg/m³ in rats (inhalation), and 10 200 mg/kg of body weight in rabbits (dermal) (*11–13*). In dogs, oral doses of 250 or 350 mg/kg of body weight produced gastrointestinal irritation, 580 mg/kg of body weight produced swelling of the epithelial cells of the kidney tubules and fatty infiltration in the convoluted tubules, and 5800 mg/kg of body weight resulted in incoordination and partial narcosis (*14*).

### Short-term exposure

1,2-Dichloropropane doses of 0, 100, 250, 500, or 1000 mg/kg of body weight per day were administered to rats for 1, 5, or 10 days. Mild anaemia, liver necrosis, and decreased body weight gain were reported at 250 mg/kg of body weight per day, more severe anaemia at 500 mg/kg of body weight per day, and elevated blood urea levels at 1000 mg/kg of body weight per day. No effects were observed at 100 mg/kg of body weight per day (*15*).

When rats were given oral doses of 1,2-dichloropropane at 14.5 or 360 mg/kg of body weight per day for 30 days, levels of serum cholesterol, betalipoprotein, and gamma-globulin were increased, serum cholinesterase activity was inhibited, and the activities of fructose-1-monophosphate aldolase, alanine aminotransferase, and aspartate aminotransferase were increased (*16*). Rats given 1,2-dichloropropane orally at 8.8, 44, or 220 mg/kg of body weight per day for 20 days showed disturbances in protein formation, hepatic enzyme levels, and lipid metabolism (*11*).

In a 13-week study, 1,2-dichloropropane was administered by gavage in corn oil to mice at 0, 30, 60, 125, 250, or 500 mg/kg of body weight per day and to rats at 0, 60, 125, 250, 500, or 1000 mg/kg of body weight per day for 5 days per week (*12*). Increased mortality was observed in both species at doses of 500 mg/kg of body weight per day or more. Decreased body weight gain and anaemia were observed in rats given 125 mg/kg of body weight per day or more. Centrilobular congestion of the liver was noted in rats at the highest dose.

Male rats were gavaged with 1,2-dichloropropane 5 times per week for up to 13 weeks at 0, 100, 250, 500, or 750 mg/kg of body weight per day. More than 50% of the highest dose animals died within 10 days; the survivors exhibited histopathological changes in the liver (mild hepatitis and splenic haemosiderosis) and adrenals (medullary vacuolization and cortical lipidosis). More than 50% of the animals receiving 500 mg/kg of body weight per day died by 13 weeks. Dose-dependent elevations in serum bilirubin became significant at 10–12 weeks in animals receiving 100 mg/kg of body weight per day. Haemosiderosis and hyperplasia of erythropoietic elements of the spleen were present at all exposure levels. The LOAEL was 100 mg/kg of body weight per day (*15*).

### Long-term exposure

Groups of F344 rats were dosed by gavage with 1,2-dichloropropane in corn oil at 0, 125, or 250 mg/kg of body weight per day (females) and 0, 62, or 125 mg/kg of body weight per day (males), 5 days per week for 103 weeks. Females in the highest dose group showed decreased survival, increased incidence of liver lesions (focal and centrilobular necrosis), and decreased mean body weight. Rats exposed to 125 mg/kg of body weight per day showed decreased mean body weight (males) and an increased incidence of mammary gland hyperplasia (females). The NOAEL was 62 mg/kg of body weight per day in male rats, and the LOAEL was 125 mg/kg of body weight per day for both sexes (*12*).

In the same study, groups of $B6C3F_1$ male and female mice were exposed to 1,2-dichloropropane at 0, 125, or 250 mg/kg of body weight per day. The decrease in survival rate in treated females was attributed in part to a high incidence of severe respiratory tract infection. The only other non-neoplastic effect observed was an increased incidence of liver lesions (hepatomegaly, focal and centrilobular necrosis) in treated males. The LOAEL was 125 mg/kg of body weight per day (*12*).

### Reproductive toxicity, embryotoxicity, and teratogenicity

In a 13-week study in which rats were given 1,2-dichloropropane at 0, 100, 250, 500, or 750 mg/kg of body weight per day by gavage 5 times per week, rats exposed at the two highest dose levels showed testicular degeneration and an increased number of degenerate spermatogonia in the epididymis (*15*). Doses of 0, 30, or 125 mg/kg of body weight per day administered to pregnant rats on days 6–21 of gestation did not affect the number of implantation sites, pregnancies, resorptions, or fetuses. However, an increased incidence of delayed ossification of the skull was observed in the fetuses of the highest dose group (*17*).

### Mutagenicity and related end-points

When tested with and without metabolic activation, 1,2-dichloropropane was mutagenic in *Salmonella typhimurium* (*12, 18, 19*). It was also mutagenic in *Aspergillus nidulans* when tested with activation by a rat liver homogenate (S9 fraction) but did not cause forward mutation in *Salmonella coelicolor* when

667

tested without activation (*18, 19*). Sister chromatid exchanges and chromosomal aberrations were induced in Chinese hamster ovary cells exposed to 1,2-dichloropropane *in vitro* with or without metabolic activation (*12*).

### Carcinogenicity

1,2-Dichloropropane induced a significant increase in the incidence of hepatocellular neoplasms, primarily adenomas, in male and female $B6C3F_1$ mice given doses of 125 or 250 mg/kg of body weight per day. There was no statistically significant increase in the incidence of any specific tumour type in F344 rats; however, there was a marginal but statistically significant increased incidence of mammary adenocarcinomas in female rats given 250 mg/kg of body weight per day. This was considered to be equivocal evidence for carcinogenicity in the female rat (*12*).

## 15.13.6 Effects on humans

Clinical signs following the ingestion of 1,2-dichloropropane typically involve effects on the gastrointestinal system (nausea, burning, and vomiting), central nervous system (dizziness, disorientation, headache, and coma), kidney failure, and liver necrosis. Effects on the respiratory system, heart, and blood have also been described (*2*).

## 15.13.7 Provisional guideline value

IARC has classified 1,2-dichloropropane in Group 3 (not classifiable as to its carcinogenicity in humans), as there are no human data and only limited data from animal studies (*20*).

A LOAEL of 100 mg/kg of body weight per day was identified on the basis of a variety of systemic effects in a 13-week oral study in rats (administration 5 days per week) (*15*). Use of an uncertainty factor of 10 000 (100 for intra- and interspecies variation, 10 for use of a LOAEL instead of a NOAEL, and 10 to reflect the limited evidence of carcinogenicity in animals and a limited toxicity database, particularly for reproductive effects) gives a TDI of 7.14 µg/kg of body weight. With an allocation of 10% of the TDI to drinking-water, the provisional guideline value is 20 µg/litre (rounded figure).

## References

1. Office of Drinking Water. *Drinking water criteria document of 1,2-dichloropropane. Draft.* Washington, DC, US Environmental Protection Agency, 1987.

2. Agency for Toxic Substances and Disease Registry. *Toxicological profile for 1,2-dichloropropane.* Atlanta, GA, US Department of Health and Human Services, 1989.

3.  Environmental Monitoring and Support Laboratory. *Method 502.1. Volatile halogenated organic compounds in water by purge-and-trap gas chromatography.* Cincinnati, OH, US Environmental Protection Agency, 1985.

4.  Environmental Monitoring and Support Laboratory. *Method 524.1. Volatile organic compounds in water by purge-and-trap gas chromatography/mass spectrometry.* Cincinnati, OH, US Environmental Protection Agency, 1985.

5.  Brodzinsky R, Singh HB. *Volatile organic chemicals in the atmosphere: an assessment of available data.* Research Triangle Park, NC, Environmental Science Research Laboratory, Office of Research and Development, US Environmental Protection Agency, 1982 (Contract No. 68-02-3452).

6.  Westrick JJ, Mellow JW, Thomas RF. The groundwater supply survey. *Journal of the American Water Works Association*, 1984, 76:52-59.

7.  Canadian Public Health Association. *Comprehensive survey of the status of Great Lakes drinking water.* Ottawa, Canada, 1986.

8.  Hutson DH, Moss JA, Pickering BA. The excretion and retention of components of the soil fumigant D-D and their metabolites in the rat. *Food and cosmetics toxicology*, 1971, 9(5):677-680.

9.  Timchalk C et al. Disposition and metabolism of [$^{14}$C]-1,2-dichloropropane following oral and inhalation exposure in Fischer 344 rats. *Toxicology*, 1991, 68:291-306.

10. Jones AR, Gibson J. 1,2-Dichloropropane: metabolism and fate in the rat. *Xenobiotica*, 1980, 10:835-846.

11. Ekštat BJ et al. [Study of the cumulative properties of substances at different levels of activity]. *Učenye zapiski Moskovskij Naučno-Issledovatel'skij Institut Gigieny*, 1975, 22:46-48 (in Russian).

12. National Toxicology Program. *Toxicology and carcinogenesis studies of 1,2-dichloropropane (propylene dichloride) in F344/N rats and B6C3F$_1$ mice (gavage study).* Research Triangle Park, NC, US Department of Health and Human Services, 1986.

13. Smyth HF Jr et al. Range-finding toxicity data. List VII. *American Industrial Hygiene Association journal*, 1969, 30(5):470-476.

14. Wright WH, Schaffer JM. Critical antihelminthic tests of chlorinated alkyl hydrocarbons and a correlation between the antihelminthic efficacy, chemical structure and physical properties. *American journal of hygiene*, 1932, 16:325-428.

15. Bruckner JV et al. Oral toxicity of 1,2-dichloropropane: acute, short-term and long-term studies in rats. *Fundamental and applied toxicology*, 1989, 12:713-730.

16. Kuryševa NG, Ekštat BJ. Effect of 1,3-dichloropropylene and 1,2-dichloropropane on the functional state of the liver in animal experiments.] *Učenye zapiski Moskovskij Naučno-Issledovatel'skij Institut Gigieny*, 1975, 22:89-92 (in Russian) (*Chemical abstracts*, 86:115725).

17. Kirk HD et al. *Propylene dichloride: oral teratology study in Sprague-Dawley rats.* Midland, MI, Dow Chemical Company, Mammalian and Environmental Toxicology Research Laboratory, 1989.

18. Carere A, Morpurgo G. Comparison of the mutagenic activity of pesticides *in vitro* in various short-term assays. *Progress in mutation research*, 1981, 2:87-104.

19. Principe P et al. Mutagenicity of chemicals of industrial and agricultural relevance in *Salmonella, Streptomyces* and *Aspergillus. Journal of the science of food and agriculture*, 1981, 32:826-832.

20. International Agency for Research on Cancer. *Overall evaluations of carcinogenicity: an updating of IARC Monographs volumes 1-42.* Lyon, 1987 (IARC Monographs on the Evaluation of Carcinogenic Risks to Humans, Suppl. 7).

# 15.14 1,3-Dichloropropane

## 15.14.1 General description

### Identity

CAS no.:            142-28-9
Molecular formula:  $C_3H_6Cl_2$

### Physicochemical properties (1)[1]

| Property | Value |
|---|---|
| Melting point | -99.5 °C |
| Boiling point | 120.4 °C |
| Density | 1.1876 g/cm³ at 25 °C |
| Water solubility | 2800 mg/litre at 25 °C |

### Major uses

1,3-Dichloropropane is used as an alkylating agent, ring-forming agent, and polymerization catalyst or promoter in the synthesis of organic chemicals (2). It may be found as a contaminant of soil fumigants containing 1,3-dichloropropene.

---

[1] Conversion factor in air: 1 ppm = 4.62 mg/m³.

## 15.14.2 Analytical methods

1,3-Dichloropropane is determined by a purge-and-trap gas chromatographic procedure used for the determination of volatile organohalides in drinking-water (*3*). Mass spectrometry is used for confirmation; the detection limit is 0.10 µg/litre (*4*).

## 15.14.3 Environmental levels and human exposure

### Water

In the Ohio River and its tributaries, 1,3-dichloropropane was detected at levels below 0.8 µg/litre (*2*). No data on levels in drinking-water were found in the available literature.

## 15.14.4 Effects on laboratory animals and *in vitro* test systems

### Acute exposure

An oral $LD_{50}$ of 3.0 g/kg of body weight for 1,3-dichloropropane was reported in dogs (*5*). An $LD_{50}$ of 3.6 g/kg of body weight was reported in mice for an unspecified route of exposure; the slight inflammation of the digestive tract noted suggests that it may have been oral (*6*).

### Short-term exposure

1,3-Dichloropropane induced mild dermatitis on the shaved dorsal skin of mice. Peripheral blood changes, including an increased number of leukocytes and reticulocytes, were observed in dermally exposed animals (*7*).

### Mutagenicity and related end-points

1,3-Dichloropropane was mutagenic in *Salmonella typhimurium* strain TA100 with and without metabolic activation at concentrations of 10 µmol per plate or more (*8*). It was also mutagenic in *S. typhimurium* strain TA1535 with but not without metabolic activation. The compound was not mutagenic with or without metabolic activation in *S. typhimurium* strains TA98, TA100, TA1537, and TA1538; *Escherichia coli* strains $WP_2$ and $WP_2$ uvr A; or *Saccharomyces cerevisiae* strain $JD_L$ (*9*).

## 15.14.5 Conclusions

There is some indication that 1,3-dichloropropane may be genotoxic in bacterial systems. However, no short-term, long-term, reproductive, or developmental toxicity data pertinent to exposure via drinking-water could be located for this compound. The available data were considered to be insufficient to permit recommendation of a guideline value.

## References

1.  Weast RC, ed. *CRC handbook of chemistry and physics*, 67th ed. Boca Raton, FL, CRC Press, 1986.

2.  Office of Health and Environmental Assessment. *Health and environmental effects profile on dichloropropanes*. Cincinnati, OH, US Environmental Protection Agency, 1985.

3.  Environmental Monitoring and Support Laboratory. *Method 502.1. Volatile organic compounds in water by purge-and-trap gas chromatography*. Cincinnati, OH, US Environmental Protection Agency, 1985.

4.  Environmental Monitoring and Support Laboratory. *Method 524.1. Volatile organic compounds in water by purge-and-trap gas chromatography/mass spectrometry*. Cincinnati, OH, US Environmental Protection Agency, 1985.

5.  Sax NI. *Dangerous properties of industrial materials*, 6th ed. New York, NY, Van Nostrand Reinhold, 1984:962.

6.  Matsumoto T et al. Acute toxicity testing of some chlorinated lower hydrocarbons: dichloromethane, 1,2-dichloropropane and 1,3-dichloropropane. *Eisei kagaku*, 1981:28-31.

7.  Kudo Y et al. [A fluorescent microscopic observation of changes in mice blood cells after individual administration of several industrial chemicals.] *Sei marianna ika daigaku zasshi*, 1983, 11(4):409-415 (in Japanese) (*Chemical abstracts,* 101:185534X).

8.  Stolzenberg SJ, Hine CH. Mutagenicity of 2- and 3-carbon halogenated compounds in the *Salmonella*/mammalian microsome test. *Environmental mutagenesis*, 1980, 2(1):59-66.

9.  Dean BJ et al. Genetic toxicology testing of 41 industrial chemicals. *Mutation research*, 1985, 153(1):57-77.

## 15.15 1,3-Dichloropropene

### 15.15.1 General description

**Identity**

| Compound | CAS no. |
|---|---|
| Isomer mixture | 542-75-6 |
| *cis*-Isomer | 10061-01-5 |
| *trans*-Isomer | 10061-02-6 |

The molecular formula is $C_3H_4Cl_2$.

**Physicochemical properties (1–2)[1]**

| Property | cis-Isomer | trans-Isomer |
|---|---|---|
| Boiling point (°C) | 104 | 112 |
| Density at 25 °C (g/cm³) | 1.22 | 1.22 |
| Vapour pressure at 25 °C (kPa) | 5.7 | 4.5 |
| Water solubility at 25 °C (g/litre) | 2.7 | 2.8 |
| Log octanol–water partition coefficient | 1.6 | 1.6 |

**Major uses**

1,3-Dichloropropene is a broad-spectrum soil fumigant used primarily for nematode control on crops grown in sandy soils.

**Environmental fate**

1,3-Dichloropropene is released to the environment when used as a fumigant. It volatilizes from both soil and surface waters to the atmosphere, where it can be photolytically degraded. Hydrolysis and microbial biodegradation also remove it from the environment (2).

### 15.15.2 Analytical methods

EPA Methods 524.2 (3) and 502.2 (4), which are standard purge-and-trap capillary-column gas chromatographic techniques for volatile organic compounds in water, should be suitable for the analysis of 1,3-dichloropropene. The detection limits for the compound are believed to range from 0.02 to 0.05 µg/litre.

---

[1] Data also from Dow Chemical Company. Conversion factor in air: 1 ppm = 4.54 mg/m³.

### 15.15.3 Environmental levels and human exposure

**Water**

1,3-Dichloropropene was found in 41 of 1088 surface water samples and in 10 of 3949 groundwater samples in the USA. The 85th percentile values for all samples containing detectable levels of 1,3-dichloropropene were 1.3 µg/litre in surface water and 3.4 µg/litre in groundwater.[1] These data have not been validated and must therefore be accepted with caution.

### 15.15.4 Kinetics and metabolism in laboratory animals and humans

1,3-Dichloropropene is absorbed through the skin and the respiratory and gastrointestinal systems (*1*). Oral administration in rats resulted in approximately 90% absorption of the administered dose (*5*). Both *cis*- and *trans*-1,3-dichloropropene administered orally in rats were excreted primarily in the urine in 24–48 h (*5, 6*). *cis*-1,3-Dichloropropene is probably biotransformed into an intermediate glutathione conjugate, and then follows the mercapturic acid pathway, and is excreted in the urine as a cysteine derivative. The main urinary metabolite (92%) of *cis*-1,3-dichloropropene was *N*-acetyl-*S*-[(*cis*)-3-chloroprop-2-enyl]cysteine (*6*).

### 15.15.5 Effects on laboratory animals and *in vitro* test systems

**Acute exposure**

The acute oral $LD_{50}$s of 1,3-dichloropropene in male and female rats are 713 and 740 mg/kg of body weight, respectively (*7*). In mice, the oral $LD_{50}$ is 640 mg/kg of body weight. The dermal $LD_{50}$ in rabbits ranges from 504 to 2100 mg/kg of body weight (*8*).

**Short-term exposure**

Exposure of rats to 1,3-dichloropropene by gavage (10 or 30 mg/kg, 6 days per week, for 13 weeks) resulted in increased kidney weight (*9*). Exposure by inhalation to 13.6 mg/m³, 7 h per day, 5 days per week, for 6 months, resulted in discoloration of kidney and swelling of renal tubular epithelium (*7*).

---

[1] STORET water quality file. US Environmental Protection Agency, Office of Water (data file search conducted in May 1988).

## Long-term exposure

Hyperplasia of the urinary bladder epithelium was observed as a result of inhalation exposure of B6C3F$_1$ mice to 1,3-dichloropropene at doses of 91 or 270 mg/m$^3$, 6 h per day, 5 days per week for 24 months (*10*). Hyperplasia of the urinary bladder epithelium and kidney hydronephrosis were seen in B6C3F$_1$ mice after gavage exposure to Telone II (in which 1,3-dichloropropene is the active ingredient) in corn oil at doses of 0, 50, or 100 mg/kg of body weight, 3 times per week for 104 weeks (*11*).

## Reproductive toxicity, embryotoxicity, and teratogenicity

No studies on the reproductive toxicity of 1,3-dichloropropene by the oral route of administration are available. In a study in which male and female Wistar rats were exposed to technical D-D (28% *cis* isomer, 27% *trans* isomer) by inhalation at 0, 64, 145, or 443 mg/m$^3$ for 10 weeks, male and female mating, fertility, and reproductive indices were unaffected, litter sizes and weights were normal, and pup survival over 4 days was not affected (*12*). In a study of the effects of inhalation exposure to 1,3-dichloropropene on fetal development, pregnant Fischer 344 rats were exposed to 0, 91, 270, or 540 mg/m$^3$ 1,3-dichloropropene for 6 h per day on gestation days 6–15. Effects included dose-related depression of maternal body weight gain, significant depression of feed consumption, decreases in water consumption at 540 mg/m$^3$, and significant increases in relative kidney weights and decreases in absolute liver weights at 270 mg/m$^3$ (*13*).

## Mutagenicity and related end-points

Tests of commercial formulations containing 1,3-dichloropropene or a mixture of pure *cis*- and *trans*-1,3-dichloropropene (*14*), and pure *cis*-1,3-dichloropropene (*15*) were positive in *Salmonella typhimurium* strains TA1535 and TA100 with and without metabolic activation, indicating that 1,3-dichloropropene is a direct-acting mutagen. Positive results have also been reported in TA1978 (with and without metabolic activation) for a commercial mixture of 1,3-dichloropropene and a mixture of the pure isomers (*14*). 1,3-Dichloropropene was negative in a reverse-mutation assay with *Escherichia coli* B/r Wp2 and in the mouse host-mediated test with *S. typhimurium* G46 (*16*).

## Carcinogenicity

F344 rats were gavaged 3 times per week with Telone II in corn oil at doses of 0, 25, or 50 mg/kg of body weight (77 per sex per dose: 52 per sex per dose gavaged for 104 weeks in the main carcinogenicity study, plus 5 per sex per dose sacrificed after 9, 16, 21, 24, and 27 months of exposure to 1,3-dichloropropene in an ancillary study). There was no increase in mortality in treated animals. Neoplastic lesions included squamous cell papillomas of the forestomach (male rats: 1/52;

675

1/52; 9/52; female rats: 0/52; 2/52; 3/52), squamous cell carcinomas of the forestomach (male rats: 0/52; 0/52; 4/52), and neoplastic nodules of the liver (male rats: 1/52; 6/52; 7/52). The increased incidence of forestomach tumours was accompanied by a positive trend for forestomach basal cell hyperplasia in male and female rats of both treated groups. The highest dose level tested in rats (50 mg/kg of body weight) was approximately the maximum tolerated dose level (11).

B6C3F$_1$ mice (50 per sex per dose) were gavaged with Telone II in corn oil at doses of 0, 50, or 100 mg/kg of body weight, three times per week for 104 weeks. Because of excessive mortality from myocardial inflammation in control male mice approximately 1 year after the initiation of the study, conclusions concerning carcinogenicity were based on concurrent and National Toxicology Program (NTP) historical control data. Neoplastic lesions in female mice included squamous cell papillomas of the forestomach (0/50; 1/50; 2/50), squamous cell carcinomas of the forestomach (0/50; 0/50; 2/50), transitional-cell carcinomas of the urinary bladder (0/50; 8/50; 21/48), and alveolar/bronchiolar adenomas (0/50; 3/50; 8/50). The increased incidence of forestomach tumours was accompanied by an increased incidence of stomach epithelial cell hyperplasia in males and females at 100 mg/kg of body weight, and the increased incidence of transitional-cell carcinoma of the urinary bladder was accompanied by a positive trend for bladder hyperplasia in male and female mice of both treated groups. Incidences of neoplasms were not significantly increased in male mice (11).

In the NTP gavage studies (11), epichlorohydrin (1%), which can cause papillomas, carcinomas, and hyperplasia of the forestomach (17), was added as a stabilizer. It is possible that the gavage dosing procedure adopted in the NTP study produced epichlorohydrin concentrations at the site of application similar to those in the drinking-water study (17), albeit for much shorter periods. If this is true, it is possible that epichlorohydrin was involved in the development of the papillomas and carcinomas of the forestomach during the NTP study.

Exposure of Fischer 344 rats for 2 years to vapours of Telone II (0, 23, 91, and 270 mg/m$^3$) did not result in increases in tumour incidence (18). The only tumorigenic effect of a similar exposure of B6C3F$_1$ mice was an increased incidence in benign lung tumours (bronchioloalveolar adenomas) in males exposed to 270 mg/m$^3$ (10).

## 15.15.6 Effects on humans

The only known human fatality occurred a few hours after the accidental ingestion of a D-D mixture at an unknown dosage. The symptoms were abdominal pain, vomiting, muscle twitching, and pulmonary oedema. Treatment by gastric lavage failed. Inhalation of 1,3-dichloropropene at concentrations above 6.8 g/m$^3$ resulted in gasping, coughing, substernal pain, and extreme respiratory distress (19).

A total of 64 male workers exposed to three compounds, including 1,3-dichloropropene, were evaluated to determine whether fertility was adversely affected. The exposed study population was divided into groups with up to 5 and more than 5 years of exposure. Sperm counts and percentage of normal sperm forms were the major variables evaluated. No adverse effects on fertility were observed (*20*), but the study participation rate for the exposed group was only 64%.

## 15.15.7 Guideline value

IARC concluded that there was sufficient evidence for the carcinogenicity of 1,3-dichloropropene in experimental animals to classify it in Group 2B (possible human carcinogen) (*21*). It is also a direct-acting mutagen. Based on observation of lung and bladder tumours in female mice in a 2-year NTP gavage study (*11*) and using the linearized multistage model, the drinking-water concentrations (and hence the guideline values) associated with excess lifetime cancer risks of $10^{-4}$, $10^{-5}$, and $10^{-6}$ are estimated to be 200, 20, and 2 µg/litre, respectively.

## References[1]

1. Clayton GD, Clayton FE. *Patty's industrial hygiene and toxicology*, 3rd ed., Vol. 2B. New York, NY, John Wiley, 1981:3573-3577.

2. Agency for Toxic Substances and Disease Registry. *Toxicological profile for 1,3-dichloropropene*. Atlanta, GA, US Department of Health and Human Services, 1992.

3. Office of Drinking Water. *Volatile organic compounds in water by purge and trap capillary column gas chromatography/mass spectrometry*. Washington, DC, US Environmental Protection Agency, 1986.

4. Office Of Drinking Water. *Volatile organic compounds in water by purge and trap capillary column gas chromatography with photoionization and electrolytic conductivity detectors in series*. Washington, DC, US Environmental Protection Agency, 1986.

5. Hutson DH, Moss JA, Pickering BA. The excretion and retention of components of the soil fumigant D-D and their metabolites in the rat. *Food and cosmetics toxicology*, 1971, 9:677-680.

6. Climie IJG, Morrison BJ. *Metabolism studies on (Z)1,3-dichloropropene in the rat: group research report*. Shell Research Ltd, 1978 (unpublished study TLGR.010178 submitted by Dow Chemical Company, Midland, MI;(MRID 32984).*

7. Torkelson TR, Oyen F. The toxicity of 1,3-dichloropropene as determined by repeated exposure of laboratory animals. *American Industrial Hygiene Association journal*, 1977, 38:217-223.

---

[1] References marked with an asterisk are confidential business information submitted to the Office of Pesticide Programs of the US Environmental Protection Agency.

8.  Office of Drinking Water. *Health advisory for 1,3-dichloropropene.* Washington, DC, US Environmental Protection Agency, 1987.

9.  Til HP et al. *Subchronic (90-day) toxicity study with Telone in albino rats. Final report.* Central Institute for Nutrition and Food Research, 1973 (unpublished report submitted by Dow Chemical Company, Midland, MI; MRID 39684, 67977).*

10. Scott WT et al. *Telone II soil fumigant: 2-year inhalation chronic toxicity-oncogenicity study in mice.* Health and Environmental Sciences, 1987 (unpublished report submitted by Dow Chemical Company, Midland, MI; MRID 403123).*

11. National Toxicology Program. *NTP technical report on the toxicology and carcinogenesis studies of Telone II in F344/N rats and B6C3F$_1$ mice (gavage studies).* Research Triangle Park, NC, Department of Health and Human Services, 1985 (NTP TR 269; NIH Publ. No. 85-2525).

12. Clark D, Blair D, Cassidy S. *A 10-week inhalation study of mating behaviour, fertility and toxicity in male and female rats: group research report.* Shell Research Ltd, 1980 (unpublished report TLGR.80.023, submitted by Dow Chemical Company, Midland, MI; MRID 117055, 103280, 39691).*

13. Hanley TR et al. Evaluation of the effects of inhalation exposure to 1,3-dichloropropene on fetal development in rats and rabbits. *Fundamental and applied toxicology,* 1987, 8:562-570.

14. DeLorenzo F, Degl Innocenti S, Ruocco A. *Mutagenicity of pesticides containing 1,3-dichloropropene: University of Naples, Italy.* Midland, MI, Dow Chemical USA, 1975 (unpublished report MRID 119179).*

15. Brooks TM, Dean BJ, Wright AS. *Toxicity studies with dichloropropenes: mutation studies with 1,3-D and cis-1,3-dichloropropene and the influence of glutathione on the mutagenicity of cis-1,3-dichloropropene in Salmonella typhimurium: group research report.* Shell Research Ltd, 1978 (unpublished study TLGR.0081 78, by Shell Chemical Co., Washington, DC; MRID 61059).*

16. Sudo S et al. *The mutagenicity test on 1,3-dichloropropene in bacteria test systems.* Nomura Sogo Research Institute, 1978 (unpublished report submitted by Dow Chemical, Midland, MI; MRID 39688).

17. Konishi Y et al. Forestomach tumors induced by orally administered epichlorohydrin in male Wistar rats. *Gann,* 1980, 71:922-923.

18. Lomax LG et al. *Telone II soil fumigant: 2-year inhalation chronic toxicity-oncogenicity study in rats.* Health and Environmental Sciences, 1989 (unpublished report submitted by Dow Chemical Company, Midland, MI; MRID 403122).

19. Gosselin RE et al. *Clinical toxicology of commercial products,* 5th ed. Baltimore, MD, Williams and Wilkins Co, 1984:141-143.

20. Venable JR et al. A fertility study of male employees engaged in the manufacture of glycerine. *Journal of occupational medicine*, 1980, 22(2):87-91.

21. International Agency for Research on Cancer. *Overall evaluations of carcinogenicity: an updating of IARC Monographs volumes 1-42.* Lyon, 1987 (IARC Monographs on the Evaluation of Carcinogenic Risks to Humans, Suppl. 7).

## 15.16 Ethylene dibromide

### 15.16.1 General description

#### Identity

CAS no.:                    106-93-4
Molecular formula:          $C_2H_4Br_2$

The IUPAC name for ethylene dibromide (EDB) is 1,2-dibromoethane.

#### Physicochemical properties (1)

| Property | Value |
| --- | --- |
| Melting point | 9.3 °C |
| Boiling point | 131.5 °C |
| Density | 2.17 g/cm³ at 20 °C |
| Water solubility | 4.3 g/litre at 20 °C |
| Octanol–water partition coefficient | 86 |
| Vapour pressure | 1.5 kPa at 20 °C |

#### Major uses

EDB is used as a fumigant against pests, certain insects, and nematodes (*1*), although its use for this purpose has been restricted or prohibited in several countries. Its main use is in leaded petrol, but it is also used to a lesser extent in solvents, waterproofing preparations, and medicine (*2*).

#### Environmental fate

Evaporated EDB in the atmosphere reacts with photochemically produced hydroxyl radicals; the half-life is 32 days (*3*).

In surface water, evaporation plays an important role in the removal of EDB; the half-life is in the range 1–5 days. It is very stable in groundwater, especially under anaerobic conditions, with an estimated half-life of about 20 years at 10 °C. Hydrolysis of EDB to bromide, ethylene, ethylene glycol, and carbon dioxide takes place in soil. Formation of vinyl bromide has so far been seen only under laboratory conditions (*2, 3*).

## 15.16.2 Analytical methods

Gas-phase extraction followed by gas chromatography with electron-capture detection is used for the determination of EDB. The method is capable of achieving a detection limit in tapwater and river water of about 0.01 µg/litre (*4*).

## 15.16.3 Environmental levels and human exposure

### *Air*

In the USA, concentrations of EDB in air of less than 0.6 ng/m$^3$ in rural areas and 80–460 ng/m$^3$ (mean 200 ng/m$^3$) in urban and suburban areas were reported (*4*).

### *Water*

EDB is found mainly in groundwater as a result of petrol spills and agricultural use. In groundwater in agricultural areas, levels of 0.01–15 µg/litre have been reported (*2*).

### *Food*

EDB may be present in treated foods depending on the treatment and storage conditions. It is found in grain, oats, and fruits at mg/kg levels and in white and wholemeal bread at µg/kg levels (*3*).

## 15.16.4 Kinetics and metabolism in laboratory animals and humans

EDB is readily absorbed following oral, dermal, and inhalation exposure in rats and pigs (*5, 6*). After ingestion, the concentration of metabolites is highest in the liver and kidney (*6*).

In the rat, two main metabolic pathways lead to the formation of the metabolites that seem to be responsible for the biological effects of EDB. 2-Bromoacetaldehyde, which is formed via the oxidative pathway, is associated with some histopathological changes, such as liver damage (*6, 7*). Another metabolite is formed via the conjugative pathway and is believed to be responsible for binding to DNA and, hence, mutagenesis. Four times as much EDB in metabolized via the oxidative pathway as by the conjugative one (*6*). In pigs, rats and mice, the metabolites are excreted mainly in the urine (*6*).

## 15.16.5 Effects on laboratory animals and *in vitro* test systems

### Acute exposure

When EDB was administered orally, acute $LD_{50}$s were found to be 117–146 mg/kg of body weight for rats, 110 mg/kg of body weight for guinea-pigs, and 55 mg/kg of body weight for female rabbits (*6*).

### Long-term exposure

In a 2-year gavage study in rats and mice, non-neoplastic effects were found in the forestomach (hyperkeratosis) and testes (atrophy) of both species and in the liver (hepatitis) and renal cortex (degeneration) of rats (*8*). In chronic inhalation studies in F344 rats and B6C3F₁ mice, EDB administration was associated with increased mortality and non-cancerous lesions of the respiratory system (inflammation, epithelial hyperplasia, squamous metaplasia) in both species and liver necrosis, kidney nephropathy, and degeneration of the testes, adrenal cortex, and retina in rats (*9*).

### Reproductive toxicity, embryotoxicity, and teratogenicity

Oral administration of EDB to bulls at doses of 4 mg/kg of body weight per day for 2–3 weeks resulted in the formation of abnormal spermatozoa. Doses of 2 mg/kg of body weight per day had no effect on the reproductive capacity of cows and ewes (*6*). Hens given feed containing 50–320 mg of EDB per kg laid smaller eggs; egg-laying ceased irreversibly after 6 weeks at the highest dose (*10*).

### Mutagenicity and related end-points

EDB induced sister chromatid exchange, mutations, and unscheduled DNA synthesis in both human and rodent cells *in vivo*. In rodents, DNA strand breaks were found *in vitro* and *in vivo* (*11*).

### Carcinogenicity

EDB has been demonstrated to be carcinogenic in rodents after administration by all three routes of exposure. It was administered by gavage in corn oil 5 times per week to Osborne-Mendel rats (50 per sex per dose for the test compound, 20 per sex per dose for controls) at time-weighted average doses of 38 or 41 mg/kg of body weight per day to males and 37 or 39 mg/kg of body weight per day to females. Because of high toxicity and premature deaths during the course of the study, the high dose was readjusted and the study was terminated early, after 49 weeks for males and 61 weeks for females. Early developing squamous cell carcinoma of the forestomach, a contact-site cancer preceded by tissue damage, was observed in both sexes; incidences were 0/20, 45/50, and 33/50 in males and 0/20, 40/50, and 29/50 in females. Liver cancers were observed in females, and haemangiosarcomas of the spleen, a relatively rare tumour at a site remote from the site of administration, were seen in males at incidences of 0/20, 11/50, and 4/50 in controls, low-, and high-dose groups, respectively (8).

A similar protocol was followed with B6C3F$_1$ mice given 0, 62, or 107 mg/kg of body weight per day (time-weighted average doses) for 78 weeks, except for low-dose females, in which the study was terminated at 90 weeks. EDB produced squamous cell carcinomas of the forestomach and alveolar/bronchiolar lung tumours in both sexes (8).

In long-term inhalation studies in mice and rats, EDB produced adenomas and carcinomas of the nasal cavity, haemangiosarcomas of the spleen, and mammary tumours in both species. An increased incidence of tunica vaginalis mesotheliomas in male rats and lung tumours in both sexes of mice was also observed (9). EDB also induced skin and lung tumours in mice after skin application (12).

## 15.16.6 Effects on humans

One lethal case of poisoning has been reported in an adult female who ingested 65 mg of EDB per kg of body weight (6). Prolonged contact with EDB has caused skin irritation (13). Long-term occupational exposure affects semen quality. Statistically significant decreases in sperm count, the percentage of viable and motile sperm, and increases in the proportion of sperm with specific morphological abnormalities (tapered heads, absent heads, and abnormal tails) were observed among exposed men as compared with controls (3). No sister chromatid exchanges have been seen in humans occupationally exposed during spraying and fruit packing (11).

In 1987, IARC found the evidence for carcinogenicity to humans to be inadequate (14), on the basis of three studies. The first study looked at the mortality of 161 men exposed to EDB in two factories since the mid-1920s and 1942, respectively. By 1 January 1976, 36 workers had died, seven of them from cancer (5.8 expected) (15). In the second study, the mortality of 2510 male workers employed at a chemical plant was investigated. EDB was one of several chemicals used and was apparently a minor component of the mixed exposure. No statistically significant excess of cancer was found at any site (16). Finally an excess of lymphoma was detected in a mortality study of grain workers in the USA who might have been exposed to EDB, among other compounds (17).

## 15.16.7 Conclusions

In 1987, IARC concluded that the evidence for carcinogenicity to humans was inadequate but that the animal data were sufficient to establish carcinogenicity, assigning EDB to Group 2A (14). EDB has been found to be genotoxic in both *in vitro* and *in vivo* assays.

Although EDB appears to be a genotoxic carcinogen, the studies to date are inadequate for mathematical risk extrapolation. Therefore, a guideline value for EDB has not been derived. EDB should be re-evaluated as soon as new data become available.

## References

1.  Worthing CR, ed. *The pesticide manual*, 9th ed. Farnham, British Crop Protection Council, 1991.

2.  Pignatello JJ, Cohen SZ. Environmental chemistry of ethylene dibromide in soil and groundwater. *Reviews of environmental contamination and toxicology*, 1990, 112:1-47.

3.  Hill DL et al. Macromolecular binding and metabolism of the carcinogen 1,2-dibromoethane. *Cancer research*, 1978, 38(3):2438-2442.

4.  US Environmental Protection Agency. National primary drinking water regulations; synthetic organic chemicals, inorganic chemicals and microorganisms; proposed rules. 40 CFR Part 141. *Federal register*, 1985, 50(219):46995-46996.

5.  Watanabe PG et al. Fate of inhaled ethylene dibromide in rats. *Toxicology and applied pharmacology*, 1978, 45:224 (abstract).

6.  Alexeeff GV, Kilgore WW, Li MY. Ethylene dibromide: toxicology and risk assessment. *Reviews of environmental contamination and toxicology*, 1990, 112:49-122.

7.  Nachtomi E. Role of diethyldithiocarbamate in ethylene dibromide metabolism and covalent binding. *Toxicology and applied pharmacology*, 1981, 57(2):247-253.

8.  National Cancer Institute. *Bioassay of 1,2-dibromoethane for possible carcinogenicity.* Bethesda, MD, National Cancer Institute, 1978 (NCI Carcinogenesis Technical Report Series No. 86).

9.  National Toxicology Program. *Carcinogenesis bioassay of 1,2-dibromoethane in F344 rats and B6C3F1 mice (inhalation study).* Research Triangle Park, NC, Department of Health and Human Services, 1982 (NTP Technical Report Series No. 210; NTP-80-28).

10. Alumot E. The mechanism of ethylene dibromide action on laying hens. *Residue reviews*, 1972, 41:1-11.

11. International Agency for Research on Cancer. *Genetic and related effects: an updating of selected IARC Monographs from volumes 1 to 42.* Lyon, 1987:296-299 (IARC Monographs on the Evaluation of Carcinogenic Risks to Humans, Suppl. 6).

12. Van Duuren BL et al. Carcinogenicity of halogenated olefinic and aliphatic hydrocarbons in mice. *Journal of the National Cancer Institute*, 1979, 63:1433-1439.

13. International Labour Office. *Encyclopedia of occupational health and safety*, Vol. 1. Geneva, 1971:384-385.

14. International Agency for Research on Cancer. *Overall evaluations of carcinogenicity: an updating of IARC Monographs volumes 1-42*. Lyon, 1987:204-205 (IARC Monographs on the Evaluation of Carcinogenic Risks to Humans, Suppl. 7).

15. Ott MG, Scharnweber HC, Langner RR. Mortality experience of 161 employees exposed to ethylene dibromide in two production units. *British journal of industrial medicine*, 1980, 37:163-168.

16. Sweeney MH et al. An investigation of mortality from cancer and other causes of death among workers employed at an East Texas chemical plant. *Archives of environmental health*, 1986, 41:23-28.

17. Alavanja MCR et al. Proportionate mortality study of workers in the grain industry. *Journal of the National Cancer Institute*, 1987, 78:247-252.

# 15.17 Heptachlor and heptachlor epoxide

## 15.17.1 General description

### Identity

| Compound | CAS no. | Molecular formula |
|---|---|---|
| Heptachlor | 76-44-8 | $C_{10}H_5Cl_7$ |
| Heptachlor epoxide | 1024-57-3 | $C_{10}H_5Cl_7O$ |

Heptachlor is the common name for 1, 4, 5, 6, 7, 8, 8-heptachlor-3a, 4, 7, 7a-tetrahydro-4, 7-methano-1H-indene. Heptachlor epoxide is the common name for 2, 3, 4, 5, 6, 7, 7-heptachloro-1a, 1b, 5, 5a, 6, 6a-hexahydro-2,5-methano-2H-indene(1,2b)oxirene (*1*).

### Physicochemical properties (1–7)

| Property | Heptachlor | Heptachlor epoxide |
|---|---|---|
| Melting point (°C) | 93 | 160–161.5 (99.5% pure) |
| Specific gravity | 1.57–1.59 | - |
| Vapour pressure at 25 °C (kPa) | $53 \times 10^{-6}$ | $53 \times 10^{-6}$ |
| Log octanol–water partition coefficient | 3.87–5.44 | 4.43–5.40 |
| Water solubility at 25 °C (mg/litre) | 0.056 | 0.35 |

### Organoleptic properties

Pure heptachlor is a white crystalline solid with a camphor-like odour.

## Major uses

Heptachlor is applied as a soil treatment, a seed treatment (maize, small grains, and sorghum), or directly to foliage. It is used to control ants, cutworms, maggots, termites, thrips, weevils, wireworms, and many other insect pests in both cultivated and uncultivated soils. It also controls household insects and pests of humans and domestic animals (5). In many countries, heptachlor is banned or may be applied only by subsurface injection.

Heptachlor epoxide is not commercially available but is an oxidation product of heptachlor (1).

## Environmental fate

Heptachlor is moderately persistent in soil, where it is mainly transformed into its epoxide. It may undergo significant photolysis, oxidation, and volatilization (6, 8, 9). It binds to soil particles and migrates slowly (10). The soil half-life of heptachlor under certain conditions may be as long as 2 years (11). Heptachlor epoxide is very resistant to further chemical or biological changes in soil. It binds to soil particles and migrates slowly (10). Its half-life in various soils has been reported to be as long as several years (12).

Photolysis, oxidation, hydrolysis, and biotic reactions do not appear to be important in reducing heptachlor epoxide levels in aquatic media (6, 8), whereas volatilization seems to be significant (13).

## 15.17.2 Analytical methods

Heptachlor may be determined in water samples by liquid–liquid extraction followed by gas chromatography. Detection and measurement may be accomplished by electron-capture or electrolytic conductivity gas chromatography. The sensitivity of the method is 1–10 ng/litre (14).

## 15.17.3 Environmental levels and human exposure

### Air

In a survey carried out in the USA in 1971, heptachlor was found in samples from two of nine cities at a maximum level of 19.2 ng/m$^3$ (15). In air samples taken from 1972 to 1974 in a cotton-growing area of the USA, the maximum heptachlor level was 0.8 ng/m$^3$ (16).

### Water

Heptachlor and heptachlor epoxide have been found in drinking-water at ng per litre levels (17–19). Heptachlor epoxide has been found in drinking-water, groundwater, land run-off, and river water at seven locations in the USA and

Europe and in sediments, lakes, rivers, tapwater, and effluent from a biological sewage treatment plant at 28 such locations (*19, 20*).

### Food

Heptachlor and heptachlor epoxide have been found in many food classes (*21, 22*). Human milk can be contaminated with heptachlor epoxide (*23*). Based on a total diet study conducted by the US Food and Drug Administration, estimated daily intakes of heptachlor and heptachlor epoxide for men aged 25–30 were 0.007 µg and 0.184 µg, respectively (*24*).

### Estimated total exposure and relative contribution of drinking-water

Diet is likely to be the greatest source of exposure to heptachlor epoxide.

## 15.17.4  Kinetics and metabolism in laboratory animals and humans

Heptachlor is rapidly absorbed from the gastrointestinal tract of rats following intragastric administration (*25*). Heptachlor epoxide is distributed throughout the body of rats and dogs (*25, 26*). Heptachlor is metabolized by rats to heptachlor epoxide, 1-hydroxychlordene, and 1-hydroxy-2,3-epoxychlordene, which are the major faecal metabolites. *In vitro* studies have shown that heptachlor epoxide formation is greater in rats than in humans, and that metabolism is, in general, comparable in the two species. Faeces represent the major route of heptachlor elimination by rats (*27*).

## 15.17.5  Effects on laboratory animals and *in vitro* test systems

### Acute exposure

In the rat, mouse, rabbit, guinea-pig, hamster, and chicken, oral $LD_{50}$s for heptachlor range from 40 to 260 mg/kg of body weight (*28*).

### Short-term exposure

Evidence of significant liver damage and altered liver function was reported in rats maintained on diets containing heptachlor at 7–12 mg/kg of body weight per day for up to 14 days and 1 mg/kg of body weight per day for 5–7 days (*29, 30*).

## Long-term exposure

Male and female rats were fed diets containing heptachlor epoxide at 0, 5, 10, 20, 40, 80, 160, or 300 mg/kg for 2 years. Concentrations of 80 mg/kg or higher resulted in 100% mortality in 2–20 weeks. At 40 mg/kg, all the females died within 54 weeks, but there was no effect on male mortality up to 104 weeks. Diets containing 20 mg/kg or less did not produce any sign of illness in male or female rats, but an increase in liver weight was observed in male rats dosed with more than 10 mg/kg and females given 5 mg/kg (*31*).

Diets containing 0, 0.5, 2.5, 5.0, or 7.5 mg of heptachlor epoxide per kg were given to groups of five dogs for 60 weeks. No deaths attributed to heptachlor epoxide occurred. The weights of the male dogs increased in inverse proportion to the concentration of the compound in the diet, whereas those of the females were normal. Liver weights increased at 5.0 mg/kg and above. Degenerative liver changes were seen in only one dog at 7.5 mg/kg. From this study, a NOAEL of 2.5 mg/kg of diet, equivalent to 0.06 mg/kg of body weight per day, can be derived (*31*).

In a 2-year study, dogs fed heptachlor epoxide in the diet at concentrations of 0, 1, 3, 5, 7, or 10 mg/kg, exhibited an increase in liver weight at the highest concentration and an increase in the incidence of histopathological changes in the liver (enlargement and vacuolation of centrilobular or scattered hepatocytes) at all but the lowest concentration. Similar histopathological changes persisted during 6 months of the recovery period. The NOAEL was 1 mg/kg of diet, equivalent to 0.025 mg/kg of body weight per day (*32*).

## Reproductive toxicity, embryotoxicity, and teratogenicity

According to a poorly documented multigenerational study in rats fed heptachlor, litter size and viability were reduced and cataracts occurred in pups (*33*). No indications of teratogenicity have been found in rats, rabbits, chickens, or beagle dogs exposed to heptachlor (*28*). Rats fed 19.5 mg of heptachlor per kg of diet for 90 days showed a decrease in androgen receptor sites, nucleic acids, and proteins in the ventral prostate (*34*).

Fertility was inhibited in female mice by three heptachlor injections of 25 mg/kg of body weight given at the rate of one per week. There was also an increase in estrogen metabolism and a decrease in the uterotropic activity of estrogen. Inhibition of the response of rat uterus to estrogen was seen; the LOAEL was 5 mg/kg of body weight for 7 days (*35*).

In a two-generation reproduction study in dogs fed heptachlor epoxide in the diet at concentrations of 1, 3, 5, 7, or 10 mg/kg, there was an increase in the mortality of $F_2$ pups at all but the lowest concentration. The NOAEL based on this finding was 1 mg/kg, equivalent to 0.025 mg/kg of body weight per day (*32*).

### Mutagenicity and related end-points

Heptachlor did not induce dominant lethal mutations in mice. In one study, it induced unscheduled DNA synthesis in human fibroblast cultures but not repair synthesis in cultured rodent cells. It inhibited intercellular communication in rodent cell systems but was not mutagenic in cultured rat liver cells. It did not induce sex-linked recessive mutations in *Drosophila* or gene conversion in yeast. It was mutagenic in plants but not in bacteria. In one study, positive results were reported for technical-grade but not commercial-grade heptachlor. It did not produce plasmid DNA breakage (*36*).

### Carcinogenicity

Heptachlor containing about 20% chlordane produced neoplasms in mice following oral administration; the results of studies on rats were inconclusive. Oral administration of heptachlor increased the incidence of liver tumours induced in mice by the oral administration of *N*-nitrosodiethylamine (*36*).

## 15.17.6 Effects on humans

Clinical case-studies of acute exposure (via ingestion, or the dermal or inhalation routes) to chlordane-containing heptachlor document a pattern of central nervous system effects similar to that found in animals (e.g. irritability, salivation, laboured respiration, muscle tremors, convulsions) (*37, 38*). Heptachlor does not appear to be carcinogenic in humans (*39–42*).

## 15.17.7 Guideline value

IARC reviewed the data on heptachlor in 1991 and concluded that the evidence for carcinogenicity was sufficient in animals and inadequate in humans, classifying it in Group 2B (*43*).

JMPR has evaluated heptachlor on several occasions and in 1991 established an ADI of 0.1 µg/kg of body weight on the basis of a NOAEL of 0.025 mg/kg of body weight per day from two studies in the dog, incorporating an uncertainty factor of 200 (100 for inter- and intraspecies variation and 2 for the inadequacy of the database) (*32*). With an allocation of 1% of the ADI to drinking-water, because the main source of exposure seems to be food, the guideline value is 0.03 µg/litre.

## References

1. International Agency for Research on Cancer. *Some halogenated hydrocarbons.* Lyon, 1979:129-154 (IARC Monographs on the Evaluation of the Carcinogenic Risk of Chemicals to Humans, Volume 20).

2. Deichmann WB. Halogenated cyclic hydrocarbons. In: Clayton GD, Clayton FE, eds. *Patty's industrial hygiene and toxicity*. Vol. 2B, 3rd rev. ed. New York, NY, John Wiley, 1981:3603-3669.

3. Rao PSC, Davidson JM. *Retention and transformation of selected pesticides and phosphorus in soil–water systems: a critical review*. Athens, GA, US Environmental Protection Agency, 1982 (EPA-600/53-82-060).

4. Mackay D. Correlation of bioconcentration factors. *Environmental science and technology*, 1982, 16:274-278.

5. Worthing CR, ed. *The pesticide manual*, 9th ed. Farnham, British Crop Protection Council, 1991.

6. Mabey WR et al. *Aquatic fate process data for organic priority pollutants*. Washington, DC, US Environmental Protection Agency, Monitoring Data Support Division, 1981 (EPA 440/4-81-014).

7. Geyer H et al. Prediction of ecotoxicological behavior of chemicals: relationship between physicochemical properties and bioaccumulation of organic chemicals in the mussel *Mytilus edulis*. *Chemosphere*, 1982, 11:1121-1134.

8. Callahan MA et al. *Water-related environmental fate of 129 priority pollutants*. Vol. II. Washington, DC, US Environmental Protection Agency, Office of Water Planning and Standards, Office of Water Waste Management, 1979 (EPA 440/4-79-029b).

9. Mill T et al. *Laboratory protocols for evaluating the fate of organic chemicals in air and water*. Athens, GA, US Environmental Protection Agency, Environmental Research Laboratory, 1982 (EPA-600/3-82-022a).

10. Tzapko VV, Rogovsky GF, Kurinov VN. [On the possibility of hexachlordane and heptachlor penetrating into subsoil water.] In: [*Hygiene of settlements*.] Kiev, Zdorovie Publishers, 1967:93-95 (in Russian).

11. Vročinsky KK, Gemetčenko MM, Merežko AI. [*Hydrobiological migration of pesticides*.] Moscow, Moscow University Press, 1980:8-14, 33-37, 59-63, 87-94, 119-120 (in Russian).

12. US Environmental Protection Agency. Heptachlor and heptachlor epoxide. *Reviews of environmental contamination and toxicology*, 1988, 104:131-145.

13. Huang JC. Fate of organic pesticides in the aquatic system. *Engineering bulletin of Purdue University, engineering extension series*, 1970:449-457.

14. Environmental Monitoring and Support Laboratory. *Method for organochlorine pesticides in drinking water. Methods for organochlorine pesticides and chlorophenoxy acid herbicides in drinking water and raw source water. Interim report July 1978*. Cincinnati, OH, US Environmental Protection Agency, 1978.

15. Stanley CW et al. Measurement of atmospheric levels of pesticides. *Environmental science and technology*, 1971, 5:430-435.

16. Arthur RD, Cain JD, Barrentine BF. The effect of atmospheric levels of pesticides on pesticide residues in rabbit adipose tissue and blood sera. *Bulletin of environmental contamination and toxicology*, 1975, 14:760-764.

17. Williams DT et al. Organochlorine pesticide levels in Ottawa drinking water, 1976. *Pesticides monitoring journal*, 1978, 12:163.

18. Sandhu SS, Warren WJ, Nelson P. Pesticidal residue in rural potable water. *Journal of the American Water Works Association*, 1978, 70:41-45.

19. Shackleford WM, Keith LH. *Frequency of organic compounds identified in water.* Athens, GA, US Environmental Protection Agency, 1976 (EPA-600/4-76-062).

20. Eurocop-Cost. *A comprehensive list of polluting substances which have been identified in various fresh waters, effluent discharges, aquatic animals and plants, and bottom sediments.* Luxembourg, Commission of the European Communities, 1976.

21. Johnson RD, Manske DD. Pesticide and other chemical residues in total diet samples (XI). *Pesticides monitoring journal*, 1977, 11:116-131.

22. Henderson C, Johnson WL, Inglis A. Organochlorine insecticide residues in fish. *Pesticides monitoring journal*, 1969, 3:145-171.

23. Savage EP. *National study to determine levels of chlorinated hydrocarbon insecticides in human milk.* Washington, DC, US Environmental Protection Agency, 1976 (EPA-540/9-78-005).

24. Gunderson EL. FDA total diet study, April 1982-April 1984, dietary intakes of pesticides, selected elements and other chemicals. *Journal of the Association of Official Analytical Chemists*, 1988, 71:1200-1209.

25. Mizjukova IG, Kurčatov GV. [Metabolism of heptachlor.] *Farmakologija i toksikologija*, 1970, 4:496-499 (in Russian).

26. Radomski JL, Davidow B. The metabolite of heptachlor, its estimation, storage and toxicity. *Journal of pharmacology and experimental therapeutics*, 1953, 107:266-272.

27. Tashiro S, Matsumura F. Metabolism of *trans*-nonachlor and related chlordane components in rat and man. *Archives of environmental contamination and toxicology*, 1978, 7:113-127.

28. *Heptachlor.* Geneva, World Health Organization, 1984 (Environmental Health Criteria, No. 38).

29. Krampl V. Relationship between serum enzymes and histological changes in liver after administration of heptachlor in the rat. *Bulletin of environmental contamination and toxicology*, 1971, 5:529-536.

30. Enan EE, El-Sebae AH, Enan OH. Effect of some chlorinated hydrocarbon insecticides on liver function in white rats. *Mededelingen van de Faculteit Landbouwwetenschappen, Rijksuniversiteit Gent*, 1982, 47:447-457.

31. Witherup S, Cleveland FP, Stemmer K. *The physiological effects of the introduction of heptachlor epoxide in varying levels of concentration into the diet of CFN rats.* Cincinnati, OH, Kettering Laboratory, University of Cincinnati, 1959 (unpublished report submitted to WHO by Velsicol Chemical Corp., Rosemont, IL, USA).

32. International Programme on Chemical Safety. *Pesticide residues in food—1991: Joint FAO/WHO Meeting on Pesticide Residues—Evaluations 1991. Part II. Toxicology.* Geneva, World Health Organization, 1992 (unpublished document WHO/PCS/92.52).

33. Mestitzova M. On reproduction studies on the occurrence of cataracts in rats after long-term feeding of the insecticide heptachlor. *Experientia*, 1967, 23:42-43.

34. Shain SA, Shaeffer JC, Boesel RW. The effect of chronic ingestion of selected pesticides upon rat ventral prostate homeostasis. *Toxicology and applied pharmacology*, 1977, 40:115-130.

35. Welch RM et al. Effects of halogenated hydrocarbon insecticides on the metabolism and uterotropic action of estrogens in rats and mice. *Toxicology and applied pharmacology*, 1971, 19:234-246.

36. International Agency for Research on Cancer. *Overall evaluations of carcinogenicity: an updating of IARC Monographs volumes 1-42.* Lyon, 1987:146-148 (IARC Monographs on the Evaluation of Carcinogenic Risks to Humans, Suppl. 7).

37. Dadey JL, Kammer AG. Chlordane intoxication. *Journal of the American Medical Association*, 1953, 153:723.

38. Derbes VJ et al. Fatal chlordane poisoning. *Journal of the American Medical Association*, 1955, 158:1367-1369.

39. Blair A et al. Lung cancer and other causes of death among licensed pesticide applicators. *Journal of the National Cancer Institute*, 1983, 71:31-37.

40. Wang HH, Macmahon B. Mortality of workers employed in the manufacture of chlordane and heptachlor. *Journal of occupational medicine*, 1979, 21:745-748.

41. Wang HH, Macmahon B. Mortality of pesticide applicators. *Journal of occupational medicine*, 1979, 21:741-744.

42. Ditraglia D et al. Mortality study of workers employed at organochlorine pesticide manufacturing plants. *Scandinavian journal of work, environment and health*, 1981, 7:140-146.

43. International Agency for Research on Cancer. *Occupational exposures in insecticide application, and some pesticides.* Lyon, 1991:115-175 (IARC Monographs on the Evaluation of Carcinogenic Risks to Humans, Volume 53).

# 15.18 Hexachlorobenzene

## 15.18.1 General description

### Identity

CAS no.:                          118-74-1
Molecular formula:           $C_6Cl_6$

### Physicochemical properties (1–4)

| | |
|---|---|
| Melting point | 230 °C |
| Boiling point | Sublimes at 322 °C |
| Vapour pressure | $1.45 \times 10^{-3}$ Pa at 20 °C |
| Water solubility | 5 µg/litre |
| Log octanol–water partition coefficient | 5.2 |

### Major uses

Hexachlorobenzene (HCB) is a selective fungicide used to control dwarf bunt of wheat, a soil- and seed-borne disease caused by *Tilletia contraversa*. In many countries, its production and use as a fungicide have ceased. At present, its main importance appears to be as a by-product of several chemical processes or an impurity in some pesticides (*2, 5*).

### Environmental fate

HCB is a widespread contaminant. It photolyses slowly in the atmosphere, where it has a half-life of about 80 days (*6*). It has a very low solubility in water but, despite its relatively low vapour pressure, volatilizes from water at a significant rate (*4, 7*). The main chemical reaction in water is slow photolysis, whereas hydrolysis and oxidation appear to be unimportant (*6*). Biotransformation of HCB in surface water, sludge, or soil suspensions is extremely low: <0.1% is converted into carbon dioxide in 5–7 days (*8*). HCB is strongly adsorbed by soil and sediments. Because of its resistance to abiotic and biotic degradation and very high octanol–water partition coefficient, it can bioaccumulate in aquatic organisms (*9*).

## 15.18.2 Analytical methods

HCB in water can be extracted with hexane and then determined by gas chromatography using an electron-capture detector. The detection limit of this method is 5 ng/litre (*10*).

## 15.18.3 Environmental levels and human exposure

### *Air*

Atmospheric concentrations of HCB have rarely been measured and are hardly quantifiable. Levels of 1–24 and 0.1 µg/m³ have been reported in the USA and Scandinavia, respectively (*11, 12*).

### *Water*

HCB was not found (detection limit of 0.1 µg/litre) in 104 surface waters and 12 groundwater supplies examined in the USA in 1984 (*13*). From 1970 to 1983, HCB concentrations of up to 0.12 µg/litre were present in the Rhine; after 1983, they decreased significantly. Concentrations in sediments were about 1000 times higher than those in the corresponding surface waters (*14*).

### *Food*

HCB can be taken up by crops if used as a fungicide or if present as a soil contaminant. Carrots show a particular affinity for HCB (*14*). In agricultural areas of the former Czechoslovakia, HCB was found at nearly all links in the food-chain in 1975–1983; the highest levels were found in wheat, milk fat from cows, and human milk (*15*). It has been found in many fish taken from surface waters; levels higher than 0.3 mg/kg have been found in fish from the river Rhine (*16*). Freshwater fish contain more HCB than saltwater fish (*17*).

### *Estimated total exposure and relative contribution of drinking-water*

Diet is probably the major route of exposure to HCB (*13*), through fish contaminated by industrial emissions, animal products contaminated by HCB-treated animal feed, and crops contaminated by soils and pesticides (*14*). In the Netherlands in 1978, daily HCB intake was in the range <1–12 µg, the median was 1 µg (*14*). The estimated dietary intake in the USA was 2 µg/kg of body weight per day in 1981–1982 (*18*).

## 15.18.4 Kinetics and metabolism in laboratory animals and humans

More HCB is absorbed when administered in olive oil than as an aqueous suspension or the solid crystalline form (80% v. 20%) (*19*). Following administration to male rats, the highest concentrations were detected in adipose tissue, bone marrow, skin, the Harderian gland, nasal mucosa, and the preputial gland (*20*).

HCB is metabolized slowly to give lower chlorinated benzenes, chlorinated phenols, and other lower metabolites; glucuronide and glutathione conjugates have also been detected (*21*). Most is excreted in faeces as the parent compound, a small fraction, about 5%, being excreted in the urine as polar metabolites (*22*). Lactation is an effective method of HCB elimination for the cow and mouse but not for humans (*23*).

## 15.18.5 Effects on laboratory animals and *in vitro* test systems

### Acute exposure

LD$_{50}$s varying from less than 1000 to over 10 000 mg/kg of body weight have been reported for different animal species. The symptoms observed were convulsions, tremors, weakness, ataxia, paralysis, and pathological changes in organs (*24*).

### Short-term exposure

HCB was fed in the diets to Swiss mice (0, 100, or 200 mg/kg), Sprague-Dawley rats, and Syrian golden hamsters (0, 200, or 400 mg/kg) for 90 days. It induced severe hyperplasia of lymphohaematopoietic centres, with frequent lymphocytic infiltrations into the liver and kidneys, as well as severe haemosiderosis in the spleen and liver. Toxic liver lesions, including severe degenerations, peliosis, necroses leading to toxic hepatitis, and cirrhosis that developed into neoplastic growths, were most severe in male hamsters and rats but were seldom seen in mice. The kidneys were also affected, showing toxic tubular nephrosis and nephritis (*25*).

### Reproductive toxicity, embryotoxicity, and teratogenicity

In a four-generation test with Sprague-Dawley rats, the NOAEL was 20 mg/kg in the diet (*26*). Some teratogenic effects of HCB were observed in Wistar rats at doses of up to 120 mg/kg of body weight administered during organogenesis, but could not be reproduced (*27*). HCB was found to cause developmental effects in fetal CD-1 mice whose mothers ingested 100 mg per kg of body weight per day on days 7–16 of gestation (*28*). HCB did not produce developmental effects in New Zealand rabbits (*29*).

### Mutagenicity and related end-points

HCB was not found to be mutagenic in five strains of *Salmonella typhimurium*, with or without metabolic activation (*30*). It was negative in dominant lethal mutation studies with rats (27), but was shown to be mutagenic in *Saccharomyces cerevisiae* (*31*). HCB gave negative results in the Ames test and sister chromatid exchange (*32*).

### Carcinogenicity

Groups of Swiss mice were fed diets containing HCB (>99.5% pure) at 0, 50, 100, or 200 mg/kg. Liver cell tumours were found in the two highest dose groups but not in controls or in the group receiving 50 mg/kg (*33*). In Syrian golden hamsters fed diets containing HCB (99.5% pure) at 0, 50, 100, or 200 mg/kg throughout their life, hepatomas, liver haemangioendotheliomas, and thyroid adenomas developed in both sexes (*34*).

Sprague-Dawley rats were fed diets containing 0, 75, or 150 mg of HCB per kg for 2 years (*25*). Hepatomas, bile duct adenomas, and hepatocellular carcinomas were seen in very high incidences in female rats; renal adenomas were observed in male rats.

In a two-generation feeding study in Sprague-Dawley rats, increased incidences of parathyroid adenomas and adrenal phaeochromocytomas were observed in animals of both sexes, and neoplastic nodules in females of the $F_1$ generation (*35*). HCB also induced liver neoplastic nodules and hepatocellular carcinomas in F334 rats, females yielding many more tumours than males (*36*).

## 15.18.6 Effects on humans

IARC has found the evidence for carcinogenicity of HCB in humans to be inadequate, as no report of a direct association between HCB and human cancer is available. Hepatocellular carcinoma has been associated with porphyria; however, although abnormal porphyrin metabolism persisted at least 20 years after an epidemic of porphyria cutanea tarda in Turkey, caused by the consumption of grain treated with HCB, no excess cancer occurrence was reported in this population 25 years after the accident (*37*).

## 15.18.7 Guideline value

IARC has evaluated the evidence for carcinogenicity of HCB in animals and humans and assigned it to Group 2B (*37*). Because HCB has been shown to induce tumours in three animal species and at a variety of sites, a linearized low-dose extrapolation model was used to calculate concentrations in drinking-water associated with excess lifetime cancer risks of $10^{-4}$, $10^{-5}$, and $10^{-6}$. On the basis of liver tumours observed in female rats in a 2-year dietary study (*25*) and applying the linearized multistage model, concentrations of 10, 1, and 0.1 µg/litre in drinking-water correspond to excess lifetime cancer risks of $10^{-4}$, $10^{-5}$, and $10^{-6}$, respectively.

## References

1. Weast RC, ed. *Handbook of chemistry and physics*, 67th ed. Boca Raton, FL, CRC Press, 1986.

2. Mumma CE, Lawless EW. *Survey of industrial processing data, Task 1—hexachlorobenzene and hexachlorobutadiene pollution from chlorocarbon processing.* Washington, DC, US Environmental Protection Agency, 1975 (EPA 560/3-75-003; Report No. PB-243641, available from National Technical Information Service, Springfield, VA, USA).

3. Lu PY, Metcalf RL. Environmental fate and biodegradability of benzene derivatives as studied in a model aquatic ecosystem. *Environmental health perspectives*, 1975, 10:269-284.

4. Korte F, Greim H. [*Feasibility of test guidelines and evidence of base-set testing according to the chemicals legislation, Environmental Research Plan of the Ministry of the Interior.*] Berlin, Federal Environmental Agency, 1981 (Research Report 10704006/1 [Ger.]) (in German).

5. Tobin P. Known and potential sources of hexachlorobenzene. In: Morris CR, Cabral JRP, eds. *Hexachlorobenzene: proceedings of an international symposium.* Lyon, International Agency for Research on Cancer, 1986:3-11 (IARC Scientific Publications No. 77).

6. Mill T, Haag W. The environmental fate of hexachlorobenzene. In: Morris CR, Cabral JRP, eds. *Hexachlorobenzene: proceedings of an international symposium.* Lyon, International Agency for Research on Cancer, 1986:61-66 (IARC Scientific Publications No. 77).

7. Smith JH, Bomberger DC, Haynes DL. Volatilization of intermediate and low volatility chemicals. *Chemosphere*, 1981, 10:281-289.

8. Mansour M et al. Assessment of the persistence of hexachlorobenzene in the ecosphere. In: Morris CR, Cabral JRP, eds. *Hexachlorobenzene: proceedings of an international symposium.* Lyon, International Agency for Research on Cancer, 1986:53-59 (IARC Scientific Publications No. 77).

9. Oliver BG, Niimi AJ. Bioconcentration of chlorobenzenes from water by rainbow trout: correlations with partition coefficients and environmental residues. *Environmental Science and Technology*, 1983, 17:287-291.

10. Ang C, Meleady K, Wallace L. Pesticide residues in drinking water in the north coast region of New South Wales, Australia, 1986-87. *Bulletin of environmental toxicology,* 1989, 42:595-602.

11. Landuer L, Skoglund PO. *Hexachlorobenzen (HCB), oktaklorstyren (OCS) och hexa-klorcyclohexan-lindan i vattenmiljö. [Hexachlorobenzene (HCB), octachlorostyrene (OCS) and hexachlorocyclohexane-lindane in the water environment.]* Stockholm, Swedish Environmental Protection Board, 1978 (NL Publication No. 13401).

12. Burton MA, Bennett BG. Exposure of man to environmental hexachlorobenzene (HCB)—an exposure commitment assessment. *Science of the total environment,* 1987, 66:137-146.

13. Office of Drinking Water. *Miscellaneous synthetic organic chemicals; occurrence in drinking water, food and air.* Washington, DC, US Environmental Protection Agency, 1984.

14. Greve PA. Environmental and human exposure to hexachlorobenzene in the Netherlands. In: Morris CR, Cabral JRP, eds. *Hexachlorobenzene: proceedings of an international symposium.* Lyon, International Agency for Research on Cancer, 1986:87-97 (IARC Scientific Publications No. 77).

15. Uhnak J et al. Dynamics of hexachlorobenzene residues in the food chain. In: Morris CR, Cabral JRP, eds. *Hexachlorobenzene: proceedings of an international symposium.* Lyon, International Agency for Research on Cancer, 1986:109-113 (IARC Scientific Publications No. 77).

16. Rijksinstituut voor Visserijonderzoek. *Jaarverslagen. [Annual reports.]* Ijmuiden, 1983-1984.

17. *Contaminantenboekje [List of contaminants.]* The Hague, Staatsuitgeverij, 1984:61-62.

18. Carey AE, Dixon TE, Yang HS. Environmental exposure to hexachlorobenzene in the USA. In: Morris CR, Cabral JRP, eds. *Hexachlorobenzene: proceedings of an international symposium.* Lyon, International Agency for Research on Cancer, 1986:115-120 (IARC Scientific Publications No. 77).

19. US Environmental Protection Agency. Hexachlorobenzene. USEPA Office of Drinking Water health advisories. *Reviews in environmental contamination and toxicology,* 1988, 106:143-154.

20. Ingebrigtsen K. Comparative studies on the distribution and excretion of $^{14}$C-hexachlorobenzene by whole-body autoradiography. In: Morris CR, Cabral JRP, eds. *Hexachlorobenzene: proceedings of an international symposium.* Lyon, International Agency for Research on Cancer, 1986:277-285 (IARC Scientific Publications No. 77).

21. Renner G. Biotransformation of the fungicides hexachlorobenzene and pentachloronitrobenzene. *Xenobiotica,* 1981, 11:435-446.

22. Koss G, Koransky W. Studies on the toxicology of hexachlorobenzene. I. Pharmacokinetics. *Archives of toxicology,* 1975, 34:203-212.

23. Matthews HB. Factors determining hexachlorobenzene distribution and persistence in higher animals. In: Morris CR, Cabral JRP, eds. *Hexachlorobenzene: proceedings of an international symposium.* Lyon, International Agency for Research on Cancer, 1986:253-260 (IARC Scientific Publications No. 77).

24. Strik JJ. Subacute toxicity of hexachlorobenzene. In: Morris CR, Cabral JRP, eds. *Hexachlorobenzene: proceedings of an international symposium.* Lyon, International Agency for Research on Cancer, 1986:335-342 (IARC Scientific Publications No. 77).

25. Erturk E et al. Oncogenicity of hexachlorobenzene. In: Morris CR, Cabral JRP, eds. *Hexachlorobenzene: proceedings of an international symposium.* Lyon, International Agency for Research on Cancer, 1986:417-423 (IARC Scientific Publications No. 77).

26. Grant DL, Phillips WEJ, Hatina GV. Effect of hexachlorobenzene on reproduction in the rat. *Archives of environmental contamination and toxicology,* 1977, 5:207-216.

27. Khera KS. Teratogenicity and dominant lethal studies on hexachlorobenzene in rats. *Food and cosmetics toxicology,* 1974, 12:471-477.

28. Courtney KD, Andrews JE. Neonatal and maternal body burdens of hexachlorobenzene in mice: gestational exposure and lactational transfer. *Fundamental and applied toxicology,* 1985, 5:265-277.

29. Villeneuve DC, Panopio LG, Grant DL. Placental transfer of hexachlorobenzene in the rabbit. *Environmental physiology and biochemistry,* 1974, 4:112-115.

30. Lawlor T, Haworth SR, Voytek P. Evaluation of the genetic activity of nine chlorinated phenols, seven chlorinated benzenes, and three chlorinated hexanes. *Environmental mutagenesis,* 1979, 1:143 (abstract).

31. Guerzoni ME, Del Cupolo L, Ponti I. [Mutagenic activity of pesticides.] *Rivista di scienza e tecnologia degli alimenti e di nutrizione umana,* 1976, 6:161-165 (in Italian).

32. Gorski T et al. Hexachlorobenzene is non-genotoxic in short-term test. In: Morris CR, Cabral JRP, eds. *Hexachlorobenzene: proceedings of an international symposium.* Lyon, International Agency for Research on Cancer, 1986:399-401 (IARC Scientific Publications No. 77).

33. Cabral JR et al. Carcinogenesis of hexachlorobenzene in mice. *International journal of cancer,* 1979, 23:47-51.

34. Cabral JR, Shubik P. Carcinogenic activity of hexachlorobenzene in mice and hamsters. In: Morris CR, Cabral JR, eds. *Hexachlorobenzene: proceedings of an international symposium.* Lyon, International Agency for Research on Cancer, 1986:411-416 (IARC Scientific Publications No. 77).

35. Arnold DL et al. Long-term toxicity of hexachlorobenzene in the rat and the effect of dietary vitamin A. *Food chemistry and toxicology,* 1985, 23:779-793.

36. Smith AG et al. Hepatocarcinogenicity of hexachlorobenzene in rats and the sex difference in hepatic iron status and development of porphyria. *Carcinogenesis,* 1985, 6:631-636.

37. International Agency for Research on Cancer. *Overall evaluations of carcinogenicity: an updating of IARC Monographs volumes 1-42.* Lyon, 1987:219-220 (IARC Monographs on the Evaluation of Carcinogenic Risks to Humans, Suppl. 7).

# 15.19 Isoproturon

## 15.19.1 General description

### Identity

CAS no.:                34123-59-6
Molecular formula:      $C_{12}H_{18}N_2O$

The IUPAC name for isoproturon is 3-(4-isopropylphenyl)-1,1-dimethylurea or 3-*p*-cumenyl-1,1-dimethylurea.

### Physicochemical properties *(1)*

| Property | Value |
|---|---|
| Physical state | Colourless crystals |
| Melting point | 155–156 °C |
| Vapour pressure | 0.003 x $10^{-3}$ Pa at 20 °C |
| Water solubility | 72 mg/litre at 20 °C |

### Organoleptic properties

No odour was detected at a concentration of 8.0 mg/litre (99% purity, dissolved in still, bottled water, equilibrated to 40 °C, eight assessors) (Water Research Centre, unpublished data, 1990).

### Major uses

Isoproturon is a selective, systemic herbicide used in the control of annual grasses and broad-leaved weeds in cereals (*1, 2*).

### Environmental fate

Isoproturon is mobile in soil and has been detected in both surface water and groundwater. In water, it is quite persistent and hydrolyses slowly; the half-life is about 30 days (3). In soil, isoproturon undergoes enzymatic and microbial de-methylation at the urea nitrogen and hydrolysis of the phenylurea to form 4-(2-hydroxyisopropyl)aniline. It also undergoes some photochemical degradation; photometabolites identified include 3-(4-isopropylphenyl)-1-methylurea, 3-(4-isopropylphenyl)urea, 4,4'-diisopropylazobenzene, and 4,4'-diisopropylazoxy-benzene. Under field conditions, its half-life is about 40 days in temperate climates and 15 days in tropical climates (4).

## 15.19.2 Analytical methods

Isoproturon may be determined by separation by reverse-phase high-performance liquid chromatography followed by ultraviolet or electrochemical detection. High levels of phenoxyacidic herbicides may interfere with the determination (5). Detection limits between 10 and 100 ng/litre have been reported (6, 7).

## 15.19.3 Environmental levels and human exposure

### Air

Because of isoproturon's low vapour pressure and short half-life in soil, it is un-likely that there is significant human exposure from air.

### Water

Raw waters may become contaminated with isoproturon from production plant discharges and diffuse agricultural sources. In Germany, concentrations of be-tween 0.1 and 0.125 µg/litre have been recorded in surface water (8). In ground-water, it has been detected at concentrations of between 0.05 and 0.1 µg/litre (8, 9). Levels above 0.1 µg/litre have occasionally been detected in drinking-water (3).

### Food

It is generally considered that diet is not a major source of exposure to isoprotu-ron for the general population. No measurable residues of isoproturon or any metabolites containing the isopropylaniline moiety were detected in grain sam-ples, where the detection limit ranged from 0.1 to 0.01 mg/kg (10).

*Estimated total exposure and relative contribution of drinking-water*

The data on environmental levels of isoproturon are limited. However, results suggest that exposure of the general population to this compound is not significant.

## 15.19.4 Kinetics and metabolism in laboratory animals and humans

Isoproturon is readily and rapidly absorbed when given orally. Distribution is rapid, and no accumulation in any particular organ or tissue has been reported (*11*). It is rapidly metabolized by the rat, the major routes being *N*-demethylation and oxidation of the *N*-methyl groups and isopropyl moiety followed by conjugation reactions. The *N*-hydroxymethyl derivative of substituted urea has not been detected, although this compound may be formed at a low concentration as a short-term intermediate. In the rat, isoproturon metabolites are rapidly excreted in the urine (*10, 11*).

## 15.19.5 Effects on laboratory animals and *in vitro* test systems

### *Acute exposure*

Isoproturon is of low acute oral toxicity in mammals, although the $LD_{50}$ varies considerably according to the vehicle used (*11*). Oral $LD_{50}$s range from 1826 to 3600 mg/kg of body weight for a number of species (*11, 12*). It does not cause skin or eye irritation or sensitization after repeated dermal exposure (*11*).

### *Short-term exposure*

In a 90-day dietary study in rats, animals receiving 400 mg/kg and higher showed a dose-dependent and reversible increase in liver weight, proliferation of the smooth endoplasmic reticulum in hepatocytes, and induction of several hepatic enzymes. Reversible haemolytic anaemia was also observed at 2000 mg/kg. The NOAEL was 80 mg/kg, equal to a daily dose of 7 mg/kg of body weight (*11*).

In a 90-day study, beagle dogs fed isoproturon at dose levels of 0, 50, 100, or 500 (which was increased to 800) mg/kg of diet showed a dose-dependent increase in liver weight. Toxic haemolytic anaemia and Heinz body formation were seen at the highest dose. Haematological abnormalities were also present in the 100 mg/kg group. The NOAEL for this study was 50 mg/kg, equal to a daily intake of 3.2 mg/kg of body weight (*11*).

Liver damage was not observed in a 30-day dietary study in mice, suggesting that isoproturon metabolism may be different in this species. The NOAEL was 2000 mg/kg, equal to a daily intake of 307 and 378 mg/kg of body weight in male and female mice, respectively (*11*).

## Long-term exposure

Rats (80 per sex per dose, strain not specified) were given isoproturon in the daily diet at concentrations of 0, 80, 400, or 2000 mg/kg for 104 or 115 weeks. At the highest dose, serum enzyme activities and cholesterol values were increased, indicative of hepatic enzyme induction. At the two highest doses, there was a marginal reduction in all red blood cell parameters, liver weights were increased, and acidophilic foci (areas of hepatocellular change) were noted on histopathological examination. The NOAEL was 80 mg/kg, equal to a daily intake of 3.1 and 3.8 mg/kg of body weight in males and females, respectively (*11*).

## Reproductive toxicity, embryotoxicity, and teratogenicity

Isoproturon was not teratogenic in rats or rabbits given doses of up to 25 or 100 mg/kg of body weight per day by gavage, respectively. In a two-generation study, rats were fed isoproturon at concentrations of 0, 80, 400, or 2000 mg/kg of diet per day. Marked indications of toxicity to the parents and pups were observed at the highest dose. Litter sizes and numbers of implantations were reduced as a result of maternal toxicity. A slight inhibition of body weight gain was also found in the group receiving 400 mg/kg of diet. No effects on reproduction, fertility, or sexual maturation were reported, and a NOAEL of 80 mg/kg of diet was identified (*11*).

## Mutagenicity and related end-points

Isoproturon has been tested in a number of *in vitro* and *in vivo* short-term assays for mutagenicity. The majority of the evidence, particularly in recent years, indicates that it is not mutagenic in bacterial, eukaryotic, or *in vitro* and *in vivo* mammalian test systems (*11*).

## Carcinogenicity

In a 2-year study in CD-1 mice, no evidence was found to show that isoproturon was carcinogenic. In addition, no evidence of hepatic enzyme induction or increased liver weights was seen. In a 2-year dietary study in Sprague-Dawley rats, isoproturon caused an increase in hepatocellular tumours, but only at doses that also caused liver toxicity. No liver toxicity was apparent at 80 mg/kg of diet, nor was there an increase in the incidence of tumours. From these studies, it appears that isoproturon may be a tumour promoter (*11*).

This was confirmed in a promoter study in male rats in which animals were pretreated with nitrosodiethylamine (NDEA) for 14 days followed by a treatment-free week. One group of animals was subsequently treated for 31 weeks with isoproturon and another group with NDEA only. In isoproturon-treated animals, there was a marked increase in the incidence of preneoplastic and neoplastic lesions in the liver as compared with the NDEA-treated group (*11*).

## 15.19.6 Effects on humans

Isoproturon has been in commercial use for a relatively short period, and so far no cases of human poisoning have been reported. Data on human health effects are limited to studies involving occupational exposures. One 3-year study was carried out on a group of workers employed in various parts of the manufacturing process. Urine and blood analysis failed to show any pathological abnormalities in the peripheral blood count or any indication of haemolytic anaemia (*11*).

## 15.19.7 Guideline value

The NOAELs in a 90-day study in dogs and a 2-year feeding study in rats were approximately 3 mg/kg of body weight per day (*11*). A TDI of 3 μg/kg of body weight can be calculated by applying an uncertainty factor of 1000 (100 for inter- and intraspecies variation and 10 because there is evidence of non-genotoxic carcinogenicity in rats). With an allocation of 10% of the TDI to drinking-water, a guideline value of 9 μg/litre was calculated.

## References

1.  Royal Society of Chemistry. *The agrochemicals handbook*, 3rd ed. Cambridge, 1991.

2.  Worthing CR, ed. *The pesticide manual*, 9th ed. Farnham, British Crop Protection Council, 1991.

3.  Department of the Environment. *Pesticides in water supplies*. London, 1989 (DoE Reference: WS/45/1/1).

4.  Kulshrestha G, Muckerjee SK. The photochemical decomposition of the herbicide isoproturon. *Pesticide science*, 1986, 17:289-494.

5.  Department of the Environment. The determination of carbamates, thiocarbamates, related compounds and ureas in waters 1987. In: *Methods for the examination of waters and associated materials*. London, Her Majesty's Stationery Office, 1987.

6.  Crathorne B, James CP, Stratford JA. *HPLC method for the analysis of chlortoluron, isoproturon, and linuron in water*. Medmenham, Water Research Centre, 1987 (Water Research Centre Report PRU 1498-M UK).

7.  Schussler W. Automatic measurement of some common herbicides by LC using simultaneous UV detection and electrochemical detection in series. *Chromatographia*, 1989, 27(9/10):431-435.

8.  Reupert R, Ploeger E. Determination of *N*-herbicides in groundwater, drinking-water and surface water: analytical method and results. *Vom Wasser*, 1989, 72:211-233.

9. Johnen BG, Iwan J. Results and implications from monitoring German raw water for residues of a wide range of pesticides. *Brighton Crop Protection Conference, Pesticide Discussion*, 1988, 1:319-328.

10. *Re-evaluation of the toxicological properties of isoproturon and its safety in use.* (unpublished report A 27779, submitted to WHO by Ciba-Geigy, Hoechst, Rhône-Poulenc).

11. *Isoproturon—Summary and evaluation of the toxicological data for isoproturon—active ingredient technical.* 1989 (unpublished report A 40025, submitted to WHO by Hoechst).

12. Mihailov G, Borisov I, Nikiforov I. [Clinico-experimental research on acute isoproturon poisoning in sheep.] *Veterinarno-medicinski nauki*, 1987, 24(2):30-35 (in Bulgarian).

## 15.20 Lindane

### 15.20.1 General description

#### *Identity*

CAS no.:           58-89-9
Molecular formula:     $C_6H_6Cl_6$

In the production of hexachlorocyclohexane, a mixture of isomers is formed, consisting mainly of the $\alpha$-, $\beta$-, and $\gamma$-isomers. Lindane is the name given to 99% pure $\gamma$-hexachlorocyclohexane ($\gamma$-HCH).

#### *Physicochemical properties of $\gamma$-HCH* (1-3)

| Property | Value |
|---|---|
| Melting point | 112.8 °C |
| Boiling point | 288 °C |
| Density | 1.85 g/cm³ at 20 °C |
| Water solubility | 7–17 mg/litre at 20 °C |
| Log octanol–water partition coefficient | 3.2–3.7 |
| Vapour pressure | 0.434 x $10^{-2}$ Pa at 20 °C |

#### *Organoleptic properties*

Odour thresholds of 12 mg/litre for lindane and 0.3 µg/litre for $\beta$-HCH have been reported (2).

## Major uses

Lindane is used as an insecticide on fruit and vegetable crops (including green-house vegetables and tobacco), for seed treatment, and in forestry. It is also used as a therapeutic pesticide (e.g. in the treatment of scabies) in humans and animals (*1, 2*). Several countries have restricted the use of lindane.

## Environmental fate

In soil, lindane can be degraded under aerobic conditions; the half-life ranges from 88 to 1146 days. γ-Pentachlorocyclohexene, hexa-, penta-, tetra-, and tri-chlorobenzenes, and penta- and tetrachlorophenols are the degradation products most commonly found. Anaerobic degradation is more rapid than aerobic degradation under laboratory conditions (half-life 12–174 days). Under anaerobic conditions, the same chlorinated benzenes and hexenes are found, but not the phenols. Leaching of lindane to groundwater rarely occurs. In surface waters, it can be removed by evaporation. Ultraviolet light seems to transform γ-HCH into α-HCH to some extent. Bacteria also influence the isomerization of γ-HCH to α-HCH. The degradation products found in soils have also been found in water (*1, 3*).

## 15.20.2 Analytical methods

Lindane in water can be determined by extraction with petroleum ether followed by gas chromatography. The limit of detection is 0.01 µg/litre (*1*).

## 15.20.3 Environmental levels and human exposure

### Air

Background levels of lindane in the range 0.01–0.7 ng/m$^3$ have been found in "unpolluted" remote areas, whereas levels in urban and agricultural areas range from 0.1 to 2 ng/m$^3$ (*2–4*). α-HCH is present together with γ-HCH, often in higher concentrations (*1, 3, 4*). In indoor air, levels range from 6 ng/m$^3$ (average for homes built on waste dumps) to 40–60 µg/m$^3$ after treatment for insect control (*1, 3*). Lindane can also be present in cigarette smoke (*2*).

### Water

Lindane enters water from direct application for the control of mosquitos, from use in agriculture and forestry, from precipitation and, to a lesser extent, from occasional contamination of wastewater from manufacturing plants. Normal levels in precipitation are 0.4–155 ng/litre, but levels up to 43 µg/litre have been measured in India (*4*).

In surface waters, levels of 0.01–0.1 µg/litre have been reported (*1–3*). Particularly high concentrations, up to 12 µg/litre, are found in wastewater-contaminated rivers (*4*). Concentrations in groundwaters have been reported to range from 3 to 163 ng/litre (*2, 4*).

### Food

HCH isomers are found in dairy products, meat, fish, poultry, garden fruits, oils and fats, leafy and root vegetables, and sugar. Spices and herbs contain the highest levels of α- and β-HCH, whereas pork and beef fat contain the highest levels of γ-HCH (up to 3200 and 1700 µg/kg of fat, respectively). Most animal fats and eggs contain less than 10 µg of γ-HCH per kg (*1, 3*). Breast milk contains β- and occasionally γ-HCH at mean levels of 3 and 6 µg/kg of milk, respectively (*2, 5*).

### Estimated total exposure and relative contribution of drinking-water

Daily intake of HCH isomers in adult diets in the USA in 1981–82 was reported to be 10 ng/kg of body weight for total HCH (8 ng of α-HCH and 2 ng of γ-HCH per kg of body weight) (*2*). In the Netherlands, the daily intake from food has been calculated to be 1 µg for the α-, β-, and γ-isomers, or approximately 15 ng/kg of body weight (*1, 3*). Intake from air may be considerable in people living in houses treated for pest-control purposes.

### 15.20.4 Kinetics and metabolism in laboratory animals and humans

After oral administration of lindane, absorption is almost complete. Dermal absorption also appears to be considerable. Absorption is enhanced in the presence of lipids. In rats, lindane is stored in fat to some extent, but elimination via urine is fairly rapid. In cattle, γ-HCH levels were found to be 10 times higher in adipose tissues than in feed (*2*).

In humans, γ-HCH content seems to increase with age, but is not correlated with levels or duration of exposure. Higher levels of the β-isomer are found in over 80% of postmortem human adipose tissue samples (*2*). Lindane crosses the placenta and can also be present in human milk (*2, 3*).

In general, lindane in animals and humans is metabolized via dehydrochlorination, dechlorination, dehydrogenation, and oxidation, yielding hexachlorocyclohexene, pentachlorocyclohexene, tetrachlorocyclohexene, and hexachlorocyclohexenol, respectively, as intermediates. The final metabolites are isomers of dichlorophenol, trichlorophenol, and tetrachlorophenol (*6*).

## 15.20.5 Effects on laboratory animals and *in vitro* test systems

### *Acute exposure*

The oral $LD_{50}$s of γ-HCH in mice and rats ranged from 70 to 480 and from 90 to 300 mg/kg of body weight, respectively. Dermal $LD_{50}$s in rats and rabbits ranged from 50 to 500 mg/kg of body weight. An inhalation test in rats gave an $LC_{50}$ of 1600 mg/m³ (*2*).

Neurotoxic effects have been reported in several species of animals. Convulsions and seizures were reported following a single intragastric dose of approximately 60–150 mg/kg of body weight in rats, and avoidance response latency was statistically increased in rats given a single dose of 15 mg/kg of body weight by gavage (*2*).

### *Short-term exposure*

Two 90-day studies in rats showed the same type of effects in liver and kidneys. Effects in kidneys were found only in males. In the first study, in which doses of 0.2, 0.8, 4, 20, or 100 mg/kg of feed were administered, the two highest dose levels resulted in liver enlargement, signs of liver enzyme induction, hypertrophy of the liver, renal tubular changes, and hyaline droplets in the kidneys. The dose level of 4 mg/kg, equal to 0.3 mg/kg of body weight per day, was considered as the NOAEL (*1, 7*).

In the second study (dose levels of 2, 10, 50, or 250 mg/kg in the diet), liver effects and kidney changes occurred at 10 mg/kg and higher, but not at 2 mg/kg (*8*). Because the effects at 10 mg/kg were minimal, this dose level was chosen by JMPR as the NOAEL in 1989 (*9*), to be used as the basis for the ADI. However, the reviewer of the study calculated the compound intake as 0.75 mg/kg of body weight on the basis of the food intake, which was measured only in weeks 1, 2, 3, 6, 9, and 13. This calculation is considered inappropriate, because food intake was measured only approximately as an indicator of toxicity and for the calculation of food efficiency, to determine whether any effect on body weight might have been caused by a decrease in food intake. Therefore, use of the normal factor of 20 for conversion of mg/kg in food to mg/kg of body weight per day is considered more appropriate. The NOAEL then becomes equivalent to 0.5 mg/kg of body weight per day.

### *Long-term exposure*

Beagle dogs (4 per sex per dose) were fed lindane in the diet at 0, 25, 50, or 100 mg/kg for 2 years. At 100 mg/kg, SAP activity was slightly increased and somewhat darker coloration and a friable consistency of the liver were observed. Liver function tests (BSP retention) showed no functional disturbance, and histological examination showed no morphological irregularity corresponding to the gross observations (*10*). The NOAEL, based on gross morphological changes in the liver and SAP elevations, was 50 mg/kg, which corresponds to 1.6 mg/kg of body weight per day, based on actual food consumption data (*1, 9*).

### Reproductive toxicity, embryotoxicity, and teratogenicity

No teratogenic effects of γ-HCH were observed in studies on mice, rats, rabbits, or hamsters; embryotoxicity (at maternally toxic doses) was observed in rats only (*6, 11*). In several reproduction studies on rats and in one study on rabbits, reproductive parameters were not affected. A marginal effect on liver weight was seen in a rat study at 25 mg/kg of feed, the lowest dose tested (*1, 6, 11*).

In a 13-week study on β-HCH in rats, pup viability was decreased at 0.5 mg/kg of body weight per day. In the dams, dose-related changes in ovaries and uterus epithelium were noticed even at the lowest dose tested (0.1 mg/kg of body weight per day) (*12*).

### Mutagenicity and related end-points

The mutagenic activity of lindane was examined in plants, bacteria, yeast, *Drosophila*, and mammalian and human cells *in vitro* as well as in live mammals. Lindane did not induce mutations in any of the systems examined; some cytogenetic damage, however, was observed in mammalian and human cells *in vitro*. Mitotic disturbances, polyploidy, and chromosomal aberrations have been observed (*6*).

### Carcinogenicity

α-HCH or γ-HCH administered in the diet to rats was not carcinogenic. Mice sometimes developed liver tumours when exposed to high doses of γ-HCH, whereas they always did so when fed high doses of α-HCH (*6*).

## 15.20.6 Effects on humans

Deaths of humans (usually children) have been reported following ingestion of lindane. A single dose of 840 mg/kg of body weight in adults and 180 mg/kg of body weight in children was lethal (*11*). An 18-h whole-body dermal application of 1% lindane lotion to a 2-month-old baby for the treatment of scabies resulted in death. γ-HCH concentrations of 110 and 33 µg/kg were found in the brain and heart blood, respectively (*13*).

The most commonly reported effects associated with oral or occupational exposure to γ-HCH are neurophysiological and neuropsychological disorders and gastrointestinal disturbances. In an occupational study on the neurological effects of HCH, no pathological signs were recorded (*14*). Total HCH levels found in serum were 10–72 µg/litre.

In a study conducted in an Indian pesticide factory, serum levels in handlers directly exposed to HCH for 7–30 years were 195–1152 µg/litre, in non-handlers exposed to HCH in air and dust 83–656 µg/litre, and in the control group (employed in the factory but not in contact with HCH) 0–370 µg/litre. Most of the HCH in the serum was in the form of β-HCH (70%), followed by α-HCH and γ-HCH. The main effects seen were paraesthesia of the face and extremities (94% of handlers and 69% of non-handlers). Headache and giddiness occurred in over 70% of the handlers and in about 40% of the non-handlers, as compared with 7% of the control group (15).

## 15.20.7  Guideline value

Lindane causes liver tumours in mice given very high doses, but there is evidence that this is a result of tumour promotion. In 1987, IARC classified lindane in Group 2B (16). Moreover, in 1989, after reviewing all available *in vitro* and *in vivo* short-term tests, JMPR concluded that there was no evidence of genotoxicity and established an ADI of 8 µg/kg of body weight based on liver and kidney toxicity observed in a short-term study in the rat (9).

On the basis of the same study, but using a compound intake estimate considered to be more appropriate in the light of additional data, a TDI of 5 µg/kg of body weight was derived from a NOAEL of 0.5 mg/kg of body weight per day by applying an uncertainty factor of 100 (for inter- and intraspecies variation). It was not considered necessary to include an additional uncertainty factor to allow for the tumour-promoting potential of lindane in view of the substantial database and numerous international evaluations of this compound supporting the TDI.

Although exposure from food is decreasing, there may be substantial exposure from its use in public health and as a wood preservative. Therefore, only 1% of the TDI was allocated to drinking-water. The guideline value is thus 2 µg/litre (rounded figure).

## References

1.  *Lindane.* Geneva, World Health Organization, 1991 (Environmental Health Criteria, No. 124).

2.  Agency for Toxic Substances and Disease Registry. *Toxicological profile for alpha-, beta-, gamma- and delta-hexachlorocyclohexane.* Atlanta, GA, US Public Health Service, 1989.

3.  Slooff W, Matthijsen ACJM, eds. *Integrated criteria document hexachlorocyclohexanes.* Bilthoven, Netherlands, National Institute of Public Health and Environmental Protection, 1988 (RIVM Report No. 758473011).

4. Gustavson K, Hilbert G, Jørgensen NS. *Occurrence, spreading and effects of pesticides in environment: studies on phenoxy acids and hexachlorocyclohexane.* Copenhagen, Ministry of Environment, National Agency of Environmental Protection and National Environmental Research Institute, 1990.

5. National Board of Health. *Dioxins in mothers milk.* Copenhagen, 1987 (Hygiejnemeddelelser 7).

6. Janssen PJCM et al. *Integrated criteria document hexachlorocyclohexanes, effects. Appendix to RIVM Report No. 758473011.* Bilthoven, Netherlands, National Institute of Public Health and Environmental Protection, 1988.

7. Suter P et al. *3-months toxicity study in rats with lindane.* Itingen, Switzerland, Research and Consulting Company Ltd, 1983 (unpublished report to Celamerck).

8. Van Velsen FL et al. *Semichronisch oraal toxiciteitsonderzoek van γ-HCH in de rat. [Semichronic oral toxicity study of γ-HCH in the rat.]* Bilthoven, Netherlands, National Institute of Public Health and Environmental Protection, 1984 (RIVM Report No. 618209001).

9. Food and Agriculture Organization of the United Nations. *Pesticide residues in food–1989.* Rome, 1990 (Joint FAO/WHO Meeting on Pesticide Residues: FAO Plant Production and Protection Paper 100/2).

10. Rivett KF et al. Effects of feeding lindane to dogs for periods of up to 2 years. *Toxicology*, 1978, 9:237-289.

11. Ware GW, ed. USEPA Office of Drinking Water health advisories. *Reviews of environmental contamination and toxicology*, 1988, 104:147-160.

12. Van Velsen FL et al. The subchronic oral toxicity of the beta-isomer of hexachlorocyclohexane in rats. *Fundamental and applied toxicology*, 1986, 6:697-712.

13. Davies JE et al. Lindane poisonings. *Archives of dermatology*, 1983, 119:142-144.

14. Baumann K et al. Occupational exposure to hexachlorocyclohexane. III. Neurophysiological findings and neuromuscular function in chronically exposed workers. *International archives of occupational and environmental health*, 1981, 48:165-172.

15. Kashyap SK. Health surveillance and biological monitoring of pesticide formulators in India. *Toxicology letters*, 1986, 3:107-114.

16. International Agency for Research on Cancer. *Genetic and related effects: an updating of selected IARC Monographs from volumes 1-42.* Lyon, 1987:33-34 ( IARC Monographs on the Evaluation of Carcinogenic Risks to Humans, Suppl. 6).

# 15.21 MCPA

## 15.21.1 General description

### Identity

CAS no.:                     94-74-6
Molecular formula:           $C_9H_9ClO_3$

MCPA is the common name for 4-chloro-2-methylphenoxyacetic acid.

### Physicochemical properties (1–4)

| Property | Value |
|---|---|
| Melting point | 118–119 °C |
| Water solubility | 825 mg/litre at room temperature |
| Vapour pressure | 0.2 x 10⁻³ Pa at 21 °C |
| Octanol–water partition coefficient | 26 |
| Organic carbon–water partition coefficient | 110 |
| Density | 1.56 g/cm³ at 25 °C |
| $pK_a$ | 3.07 |

### Major uses

MCPA is a systemic hormone-type selective herbicide, readily absorbed by leaves and roots. Its uses include the control of annual and perennial weeds in cereals, grassland, and turf (1).

### Environmental fate

MCPA did not volatilize from an aqueous solution (pH 7.0) heated for 13 days at 34–35 °C, nor was it hydrolysed at neutral pH (5). In aqueous solution at pH 8.3, MCPA had a photolytic half-life of 20–24 days in sunlight. In rice paddy water in the dark, it was totally degraded by aquatic microorganisms in 13 days (6). It undergoes various metabolic reactions.[1]

MCPA can be expected to leach readily in most soils (7). Mobility increases as organic matter content decreases. Its half-life in soil was 15–50 days (5, 6). It degrades twice as quickly (6–12 days) when applied a second time to soil than after one application (15–28 days) (8).

---

[1] Source: Hazardous Substances Data Bank. Bethesda, MD, National Library of Medicine.

## 15.21.2 Analytical methods

MCPA in water can be determined by a gas chromatographic method, after extraction with dichloromethane and esterification with diazomethane. The method sensitivity is about 0.1 µg/litre (9).

## 15.21.3 Environmental levels and human exposure

### Water

In the USA, MCPA was found at levels of 0.04–0.54 µg/litre in four of 18 surface water samples analysed, but in none of 118 groundwater samples (4). It was detected in some groundwaters in Montana (maximum level 5.5 µg/litre) (4) and in two of 237 wells in Ontario (10).

### Food

In surveys conducted during 1965–68 in the USA, MCPA was detected in food composites at a maximum concentration of less than 0.4 mg/kg. It was not detected in food composites of adult total diet samples during 1971–76 or in infant or toddler diet samples during 1974–75 (11).

## 15.21.4 Kinetics and metabolism in laboratory animals and humans

MCPA is readily absorbed from the gut of mice. After rats were exposed to MCPA, it was detected in all the organs tested (12). It is metabolized by the liver (13), 5-chloromethyl-catechol being one of its metabolites (14). Induction of microsomal oxidation by phenobarbital increases the rate of breakdown (13). Rats treated orally with MCPA excreted nearly all of it during the first 24 h after intake (90% in urine, 7% in faeces) (12). In rabbits and cattle, it is excreted rapidly, largely unchanged (15, 16). In humans, 50% of the total dose was detected in the urine within 48 h (17).

## 15.21.5 Effects on laboratory animals and in vitro test systems

### Acute exposure

Acute oral $LD_{50}$s for MCPA of 550 and 700 mg/kg of body weight have been reported in mice and rats, respectively (1).

### Short-term exposure

After administration of MCPA (80.6% active ingredient) in the diet for 90 days to SPF weanling rats at doses of about 0, 2.5, 20, or 160 mg/kg of body weight per day, no compound-related effects were reported except for growth retardation and elevated relative kidney weights at the two highest doses. A NOAEL of 2.5 mg/kg of body weight per day was identified (*18*).

MCPA administered in the diet of CD rats for 3 months at doses of 0, 4, 8, or 16 mg/kg of body weight per day did not cause any adverse effects, except for increases in kidney weight in males at 16 mg/kg of body weight per day. A NOAEL of 8 mg/kg of body weight per day was identified from this study (*19*).

MCPA (94% a.i.) was administered orally to beagle dogs in two separate 13-week studies at dosing regimens of 0, 3, 12, or 48 mg/kg of body weight per day and 0, 0.3, 1, or 12 mg/kg of body weight per day. Decreased kidney and liver function, characterized by increases in blood urea, SGPT, and creatinine, were observed at doses as low as 3 mg/kg of body weight per day. Low prostatic weight and mucopurulent conjunctivitis were observed at higher doses. A NOAEL of 1 mg/kg of body weight per day was identified from these studies (*20*).

Beagle dogs were given oral doses of MCPA (95% a.i.) of 0, 0.15, 0.75, or 1.5 mg/kg of body weight per day for 1 year. Kidney toxicity was observed at the two highest doses. A NOAEL of 0.15 mg/kg of body weight per day was identified (*21*).

## Long-term exposure

In a study in which Wistar rats (50 per sex per dose) were given MCPA (purity 84.8%) in their food at levels of 0, 20, 80, or 320 mg/kg for 2 years, a decrease in body weight gain, alterations of chemical and clinical parameters, and nephropathy were observed at the highest dose (*22*). In a study in which B6C21BRF$_1$ mice (50 per sex per dose) were given MCPA orally at levels of 0, 20, 100, or 500 mg/kg for 2 years, a greater frequency of renal lesions as a result of chronic nephropathy was observed at the highest dose (*23*).

## Reproductive toxicity, embryotoxicity, and teratogenicity

No effects on reproduction were found in rats exposed to MCPA (95% a.i.) at 0, 3.3, 10, or 30 mg/kg of body weight per day in the diet over two generations (*24*). After oral administration of MCPA (75% a.i.) at 0, 5, 25, or 100 mg/kg of body weight per day to mice on days 6–15 of gestation, significantly reduced fetal weights and delayed skeletal ossification were observed at the highest dose (*25*).

MCPA (purity not specified) was administered (0, 20, 50, or 125 mg/kg of body weight per day) by gavage to pregnant CD rats (16–38 per dose) on days 6–15 of gestation. No maternal or fetal toxicity or teratogenic effects were observed (*26*). The intragastric administration of technical MCPA (700 mg/kg) on days 9 or 10 of gestation to female Wistar rats caused an increase in the frequency of resorption, a reduction in fetal weight, and the appearance of major malformations (*13*).

After MCPA was administered (0, 5, 12, 30, or 75 mg/kg of body weight per day) by gavage to rabbits on days 6–18 of gestation, no fetotoxicity or teratogenicity was observed at any of the dose levels tested. Body weights of the does were markedly reduced in the group given 75 mg/kg of body weight per day. A fetal NOAEL of 75 mg/kg of body weight per day and a maternal NOAEL of 30 mg/kg of body weight per day were identified (27).

### Mutagenicity and related end-points

MCPA is slightly mutagenic at the gene level in yeast and *Drosophila* (28, 29). It induces sister chromatid exchange in *in vitro* tests but has given contradictory results *in vivo* (30). It is inactive in gene mutation tests on bacteria and in *in vivo* cytogenetic tests (micronucleus and chromosomal aberrations) (31–34).

### Carcinogenicity

MCPA (purity 84.8%) was administered to Wistar rats (50 per sex per dose) in their food at levels of 0, 20, 80, or 320 mg/kg for 2 years. No significant differences in the distribution of the various types of tumours in treated as compared with control animals were evident (22). Similarly, the oral administration of MCPA to B6C21BRF$_1$ mice (50 per sex per dose) at levels of 0, 20, 100, or 500 mg/kg for 2 years did not cause any significant differences in the distribution of the various types of tumours as between the treated and control groups (23).

## 15.21.6 Effects on humans

Epidemiological investigations on MCPA have involved both the producers and users of chlorophenoxyacetic weedkillers, so that exposure to this product is generally accompanied by exposure to 2,4-D, 2,4,5-T, mecoprop, and dichlorprop. IARC carried out a comprehensive evaluation related to occupational exposures to chlorophenoxy herbicides, which were considered to show "limited evidence" of carcinogenicity (35).

## 15.21.7 Guideline value

There are only limited and inconclusive data on the genotoxicity of MCPA. IARC evaluated MCPA in 1983 and concluded that the available data on humans and experimental animals were inadequate for an evaluation of carcinogenicity (11). In further evaluations by IARC on chlorophenoxy herbicides in 1986 and 1987 it was concluded that evidence for their carcinogenicity was limited in humans and inadequate in animals (Group 2B) (35, 36). No adequate epidemiological data on exposure to MCPA alone are available. Recent carcinogenicity studies on rats and mice (22, 23) did not indicate that MCPA was carcinogenic.

A 1-year feeding study in dogs indicated a NOAEL of 0.15 mg/kg of body weight per day, based on the renal and liver toxicity observed at higher dose levels (*21*). Using this value and applying an uncertainty factor of 300 (100 for inter- and intraspecies variation and 3 for the inadequacy of the database), a TDI of 0.5 µg/kg of body weight can be calculated. An allocation of 10% of the TDI to drinking-water gives a guideline value of 2 µg/litre (rounded figure).

## References

1.  Worthing CR, ed. *The pesticide manual*, 9th ed. Farnham, British Crop Protection Council, 1991.

2.  Gerstl Z, Helling CS. Evaluation of molecular connectivity as a predictive method for the adsorption of pesticides by soil. *Journal of environmental science and health*, 1987, B22(1):55-69.

3.  Kenaga EE. Predicted bioconcentration factors and soil sorption coefficients of pesticides and other chemicals. *Ecotoxicology and environmental safety*, 1980, 4:26-38.

4.  Office of Drinking Water. *MCPA. Health advisory*. Washington, DC, US Environmental Protection Agency, 1988.

5.  Sattar MA, Paasivirta J. Fate of the herbicide MCPA in soil. Analysis of the residue of MCPA by an internal standard method. *Chemosphere*, 1980, 9:365-375.

6.  Soderquist CJ, Crosby DG. Dissipation of 4-chloro-2-methylphenoxyacetic acid (MCPA) in a rice field. *Pesticide science*, 1975, 6:17-33.

7.  Herzel F, Schmidt G. [Testing the leaching behaviour of herbicides on lysimeters and small columns.] *WaBoLu-Berichte*, 1979, 3:1-16 (in German).

8.  Loos MA, Schlosser IF, Mapham WR. Phenoxy herbicide degradation in soils: quantitative studies of 2,4-D- and MCPA-degrading microbial populations. *Soil biology and biochemistry*, 1979, 11:377-385.

9.  Frank R, Sirons GJ. Chlorophenoxy and chlorobenzoic acid herbicides: their use in eleven agricultural watersheds and their loss to stream waters in southern Ontario, Canada, 1975-1977. *Science of the total environment*, 1980, 15:149-167.

10. Frank R, Sirons GJ, Ripley BD. Herbicide contamination and decontamination of well waters in Ontario, Canada, 1969-78. *Pesticides monitoring journal*, 1979, 13:120-127.

11. International Agency for Research on Cancer. *Miscellaneous pesticides*. Lyon, 1983:255-269 (IARC Monographs on the Evaluation of the Carcinogenic Risk of Chemicals to Humans, Volume 30).

12. Elo HA. Distribution and elimination of 2-methyl-4-chlorophenoxyacetic acid (MCPA) in male rats. *Scandinavian journal of work, environment and health*, 1976, 3:100-103.

13. Buslovich SY, Aleksashina ZA, Kolosovskaya VM. [Effect of phenobarbital on the embryotoxic action of 2-methyl-4-chlorophenoxyacetic acid (a herbicide).] *Russian pharmacology and toxicology*, 1979, 42:167-170 (in Russian).

14. Hattula MI. et al. Toxicity of 5 chloro-3-methyl-catechol to rat: chemical observation and light microscopy of the tissue. *Bulletin of environmental contamination and toxicology*, 1979, 22:457-461.

15. Verschueren K. *Handbook of environmental data on organic chemicals*, 2nd ed. New York, NY, Van Nostrand Reinhold, 1983:840-841.

16. Bache CA et al. Elimination of 2-methyl-4-chlorophenoxyacetic acid and 4-(2-methyl-4-chlorophenoxybutyric)acid in the urine from cows. *Journal of dairy science*, 1964, 47:93-95.

17. Fjeldstad P, Wannag A. Human urinary excretion of the herbicide 2-methyl-4-chlorophenoxyacetic acid. *Scandinavian journal of work, environment and health*, 1977, 3:100-103.

18. Verschueren HG, Kroes R, den Tonkelaar EM. Short-term oral and dermal toxicity of MCPA and MCPP. *Toxicology*, 1975, 3:349-359.

19. Holsing GC, Kundzin M. *Final report: three-month dietary administration—rats.* Ludwigshafen, BASF, 1970 (unpublished study submitted to WHO).

20. Reuzel PGJ, Hendriksen CFM. *Subchronic (13-week) oral toxicity study of MCPA in beagle dogs: final report.* Ludwigshafen, BASF, 1980 (unpublished study submitted to WHO).

21. Hellwing J. *Report on the study of the toxicity of MCPA in beagle dogs after 12-month administration in the diet.* Ludwigshafen, BASF, 1986 (unpublished study submitted to WHO).

22. *24-Month feeding study in rats.* Ludwigshafen, BASF, 1988 (unpublished study submitted to WHO).

23. *24-Month feeding study on mice.* Ludwigshafen, BASF, 1988 (unpublished study submitted to WHO).

24. Hazleton Laboratories. *Two-generation reproductive study with MCPA in rats.* Ludwigshafen, BASF, 1986 (unpublished study submitted to WHO).

25. Palmer AK, Lovell MR. *Effect of MCPA on pregnancy of the mouse.* Ludwigshafen, BASF, 1971 (unpublished study submitted to WHO).

26. Irvine L. *MCPA oral teratogenicity study in the rat.* Ludwigshafen, BASF, 1980 (unpublished study submitted to WHO).

27. Irvine L et al. *MCPA oral teratogenicity study in the Dutch belted rabbit.* Ludwigshafen, BASF, 1980 (unpublished study submitted to WHO).

28. Zetterberg G. Mechanism of the lethal and mutagenic effects of phenoxyacetic acids in *Saccharomyces cerevisiae. Mutation research*, 1979, 60:291-300.

29. Vogel C, Chandler JLR. Mutagenicity testing of cyclamate and some pesticides in *Drosophila melanogaster. Experientia*, 1974, 30:621-623.

30. Linnainmaa K. Induction of sister chromatid exchanges by the peroxisome proliferators 2,4-D, MCPA, and clofibrate *in vivo* and *in vitro. Carcinogenesis*, 1984, 5:703-707.

31. Kappas A. On the mutagenic and recombinogenic activity of certain herbicides in *Salmonella typhimurium* and in *Aspergillus nidulans. Mutation research*, 1988, 204:615-621.

32. Buselmaier W, Rohrborn G, Propping P. [Mutagenicity investigations with pesticides in the host-mediated assay and the dominant lethal test in mice.] *Biologisches Zentralblatt*, 1972, 91:311-325 (in German).

33. Fahrig R. Comparative mutagenicity studies with pesticides. In: Montesano R, Tomatis L, eds. *Chemical carcinogenesis essays.* Lyon, International Agency for Research on Cancer, 1974:161-181 (IARC Scientific Publications No. 10).

34. Mustonen R et al. Effects of phenoxyacetic acids on the induction of chromosome aberrations *in vitro* and *in vivo. Mutagenesis*, 1986, 1:241-245.

35. International Agency for Research on Cancer. *Some halogenated hydrocarbons and pesticide exposures.* Lyon, 1986:357-407 (IARC Monographs on the Evaluation of the Carcinogenic Risk of Chemicals to Humans, Volume 41).

36. International Agency for Research on Cancer. *Overall evaluations of carcinogenicity: an updating of IARC Monographs volumes 1-42.* Lyon, 1987:156-160 (IARC Monographs on the Evaluation of Carcinogenic Risks to Humans, Suppl. 7).

## 15.22 Methoxychlor

### 15.22.1 General description

**Identity**

CAS no.:                72-43-5
Molecular formula:      $C_{16}H_{15}Cl_3O_2$

Methoxychlor is the common name for 1,1,1-trichloro-2,2-bis(4-methoxyphenyl) ethane; other names include methoxy-DDT and DMDT. Technical methoxychlor contains about 88% of the *p,p'*-isomer together with more than 50 structurally related contaminants, including 1,1,1,2-tetrachloro-2-*p*-(4-methoxyphenyl)ethane, *o,p'*-dimethoxydiphenyltrichloroethane, *o,o'*-dimethoxydiphenyltrichloroethane, 1,1-*bis*(4-methoxyphenyl)-2,2-dichloroethene (DMDE), and *o,p'*-dimethoxydiphenyldichloroethene (*1, 2*).

## Physicochemical properties (1)

| Property | Value |
|---|---|
| Physical state | Light yellow crystals |
| Melting point | 78 °C or 86–88 °C (dimorphisms) |
| Boiling point | Decomposes |
| Water solubility | 0.1 mg/litre at 25 °C |
| Log octanol–water partition coefficient | 3.05–4.30 |
| Density | 1.41 g/cm³ at 25 °C |

## Organoleptic properties

Methoxychlor has a light fruity smell (*1*). Its odour threshold in water is 4.7 mg/litre.[1]

## Major uses

Methoxychlor is used as an insecticide to protect vegetables, fruit, trees, fodder cereals, farm animals, and pets against a variety of pests (*3*).

## Environmental fate

Methoxychlor residues may persist in top soil for up to 14 months. Anaerobic biodegradation results mainly in dimethoxydiphenyldichloroethane (DMDD) and the mono- and dihydroxy (demethylated) derivatives of methoxychlor and DMDD. Half-lives range from 1 week to 2 months. Aerobic degradation is much slower; half-lives are longer than 3 months. Methoxychlor may undergo indirect photolysis on the soil surface. The half-life for chemical hydrolysis in humid soils is about 1 year.[1]

In water, methoxychlor can be degraded to DMDE by ultraviolet light (*4*). The main route of disappearance from the water phase is volatilization; the half-life for volatilization from shallow waters is 4.5 days.[1] Methoxychlor is adsorbed onto suspended solids or sediment. In sediments, the same biodegradation products form under anaerobic conditions as in soil. Methoxychlor may be ingested

---

[1] Source: Hazardous Substances Data Bank. Bethesda, MD, National Library of Medicine.

by some aquatic organisms and bioaccumulated, except in fish, which quickly metabolize it (*4*).

## 15.22.2 Analytical methods

Methoxychlor is determined by a liquid–liquid extraction/gas chromatographic procedure. The sensitivity is 0.001–0.01 µg of methoxychlor per litre for single-component pesticides and 0.05–1.0 µg of methoxychlor per litre for multiple-component pesticides for a 1-litre sample and electron-capture detection (*5*).

## 15.22.3 Environmental levels and human exposure

### Air

Methoxychlor has been detected at a concentration of 254 ng/m$^3$ in the ambient air near a pesticide plant in southern California (USA).[1]

### Water

Although methoxychlor is poorly soluble in water, it has been found in surface water, groundwater, and drinking-water. Only one out of 71 groundwater samples from rural areas contained methoxychlor at 0.09 µg/litre, but concentrations of up to 50 µg/litre were detected in both surface water and groundwater close to agricultural areas where it was applied (*5*). Drinking-water in two rural areas in the USA was reported to contain methoxychlor at concentrations of up to 312 µg/litre (mean 33 ng/litre) and 100 µg/litre (mean 23 ng/litre), respectively.[1]

### Food

In studies performed in the USA from 1982 to 1985, the estimated daily intake of methoxychlor from food was 99 ng for men aged 25–30 years (*1*).

### Estimated total exposure and relative contribution of drinking-water

The estimated total exposure will generally be less than 1 µg/person per day. Significant contributions may be made by drinking-water, but this is rare.

## 15.22.4 Kinetics and metabolism in laboratory animals and humans

Although methoxychlor is absorbed from the gastrointestinal tract, it does not accumulate in mammalian tissues (*6*). Body stores built up during periods of continuous exposure are cleared within a few weeks after cessation of exposure.[1] Excretion in faeces exceeds that in urine (*7*).

---

[1] Source: Hazardous Substances Data Bank. Bethesda, MD, National Library of Medicine.

In the presence of liver microsomes and NADPH, methoxychlor is oxidatively demethylated to form formaldehyde and phenolic metabolites (8–10). This reaction is not a precondition for the covalent binding of methoxychlor to the microsomal cytochrome P-450 (9). The phenolic metabolites competitively inhibit the binding of estradiol to its receptor; methoxychlor, like most of its technical impurities, is considered to be a proestrogen (1).

## 15.22.5 Effects on laboratory animals and *in vitro* test systems

### Acute exposure

Reported $LD_{50}$s for mammals are generally higher than 2 g/kg of body weight (1). The main effects of single high exposures are disturbances of glycogen metabolism (11) and fatty degeneration of organs (12).

### Short-term exposure

A NOAEL of 140 mg/kg of body weight per day for testicular atrophy was reported in a 30–45-day study in rats (13). In a 56-day study, a LOAEL of 25 mg of methoxychlor per kg of body weight per day increased pituitary prolactin levels in rats, an early effect of methoxychlor on the reproductive system (14).[1]

### Long-term exposure

Chronic toxicity tests on rats and mice exposed to technical grade methoxychlor during a 78-week period revealed NOAELs of 70 and 450 mg/kg of body weight per day, respectively (15). In rats fed methoxychlor at up to 80 mg/kg of body weight per day for 2 years, tumours occurred at a similar frequency as in controls. The main effect observed at higher doses was growth retardation (16). Pigs and dogs seemed to be less sensitive than rats and mice (17).

### Reproductive toxicity, embryotoxicity, and teratogenicity

Methoxychlor reduced the weight of testicles, prostate, and seminal vesicles in rats (18) and disturbed spermatogenesis in sheep and rats (19, 20). In a two-generation study with rats, maternal toxicity and various effects on reproductive functions were seen after repeated exposure of dams to 50 mg of methoxychlor per kg of body weight per day (LOAEL) (21). Fetal effects (deformed ribs) occurred only at higher doses (22).

---

[1] Also based on data from Integrated Risk Information System (IRIS) data file, Cincinnati, OH, US Environmental Protection Agency.

Methoxychlor accelerates the displacement of developed embryos from the ovaries to the uterus (*23*). This can occur in rats at exposures as low as 25 mg/kg of body weight per day (LOAEL) (*24*).

A tentative maternal NOAEL of 5 mg of methoxychlor per kg of body weight per day was established in pregnant rabbits that lost their litters and exhibited reduced weight gain at or above 35 mg/kg of body weight (*25*). The high incidence of lung agenesis in all fetuses of all dose groups was unusual.[1]

### Mutagenicity and related end-points

Negative results were reported in various mutagenicity assays with or without metabolic activation.[1] A weakly positive cell transformation response was obtained only with BALB/3T3-cells (*1*).

### Carcinogenicity

Although increases in adenomas in rats (AA Nelson, OG Fitzburgh, personal communication, 1951) and in total tumour numbers in rats (*16, 26*) have been reported, they were considered to be insignificant.[1] A significant increase in hepatocellular carcinomas in male and female rats together with a significant increase in ovarian carcinomas was reported (*27*), but there is some doubt regarding the statistical evaluation (*1*). Studies on Osborne-Mendel rats and B6C3F$_1$ mice may indicate the potential carcinogenicity of methoxychlor (*15*) but are inadequate because of the lack of satisfactory histopathological investigations.

Some positive evidence is provided by a 2-year study in which mice were given 750 mg of technical methoxychlor per kg of feed (*27*; KJ Davis, personal communication, 1969). Higher incidences of liver tumours occurred as compared with control animals. The males exhibited more testicle tumours and tumours of higher malignancy than the respective control animals.

Methoxychlor is likely to be a tumour promoter because it disturbs the metabolic cooperation between 6-thioguanidine-sensitive and -resistant V79-cells (*28*).

## 15.22.6 Effects on humans

A single dose of 2 mg/kg of body weight was without effect on liver, testicles, or small intestine (*29*). Doses of 0.5, 1.0, or 2.0 mg/kg of body weight per day administered orally to men and women over periods of 4–6 weeks (*30*) and 6–8 weeks (*17*) were without effect on body weight and several biochemical parameters. Tissue damage did not occur. The menstrual cycle and the volume of ejacu-

---

[1] Source: Integrated Risk Information System (IRIS) data file, Cincinnati, OH, US Environmental Protection Agency.

lation were not affected, although a shortening of the neck of spermatozoa was observed in the first study (*30*).

## 15.22.7 Guideline value

In 1979, IARC assigned methoxychlor to Group 3 (*31*). Subsequent data suggest a carcinogenic potential of methoxychlor for liver and testes in mice, which may be due to the hormonal activity of proestrogenic metabolites of methoxychlor and may therefore have a threshold. The study, however, was inadequate because only one dose was used and because this dose may have been above the maximum tolerated dose (*27*). The genotoxic potential of methoxychlor appears to be negligible. It may be a tumour promoter.

The database for studies on long-term, short-term, and reproductive toxicity is inadequate. A teratology study in rabbits reported a systemic NOAEL of 5 mg/kg of body weight per day (*25*),[1] which is lower than the NOAELs and LOAELs from other studies. This NOAEL was therefore selected for use in the derivation of a TDI. Using this NOAEL and applying an uncertainty factor of 1000 (100 for intra- and interspecies variation and 10 for concern for threshold carcinogenicity and the limited database), a TDI of 5 µg/kg of body weight can be calculated. Allocation of 10% of the TDI to drinking-water results in a guideline value of 20 µg/litre (rounded figure).

## References

1. US Environmental Protection Agency. *Drinking water criteria document for methoxychlor (final)*. Cincinnati, OH, 1987 (PB89-192215).

2. West PR et al. High performance liquid chromatographic analysis of impurities and degradation products of methoxychlor. *Journal of the Association of Official Analytical Chemists*, 1982, 65(6):1457-1470.

3. US Environmental Protection Agency. *Methoxychlor*. Washington, DC, 1988 (Pesticide Fact Sheet No. 187; PB89-138531).

4. Menzie CM. *Metabolism of pesticides, update II*. Washington, DC, US Government Printing Office, 1978 (US Fish and Wildlife Service Special Scientific Report, Wildlife No. 2L2).

5. Office of Drinking Water. *Methoxychlor, health advisory*. Washington, DC, US Environmental Protection Agency, 1987.

---

[1] Also based on data from Integrated Risk Information System (IRIS) data file, Cincinnati, OH, US Environmental Protection Agency.

6. Villeneuve DC, Grant DL, Phillips WE. Modification of pentobarbital sleeping times in rats following chronic PCB ingestion. *Bulletin of environmental contamination and toxicology*, 1972, 7:264-269.

7. Kapoor IP et al. Comparative metabolism of methoxychlor, methiochlor and DDT in mouse, insects and in a model ecosystem. *Journal of agricultural and food chemistry*, 1970, 18:1145-1152.

8. Donovan MP, Schein LG, Thomas JA. Effects of pesticides on metabolism of steroid hormone by rodent liver microsomes. *Journal of environmental pathology and toxicology*, 1978, 2(2):447-454.

9. Bulger WH, Kupfer D. Studies on the formation of methoxychlor-protein adduct in rat and human liver microsomes. Is demethylation of methoxychlor essential for cytochrome P-450 catalyzed covalent binding? *Biochemical pharmacology*, 1990, 40(5):937-946.

10. Bulger WH, Muccitelli RM, Kupfer D. Studies on the *in vivo* and *in vitro* estrogenic activities of methoxychlor and its metabolites. Role of hepatic mono-oxygenase in methoxychlor activation. *Biochemical pharmacology*, 1978, 27:2417-2424.

11. Morgan JM, Hickenbottom JP. Comparison of selected parameters for monitoring methoxychlor-induced hepatotoxicity. *Bulletin of environmental contamination and toxicology*, 1979, 23:275-280.

12. Lillie RD, Smith MI, Stohlman EF. Pathological action of DDT and certain of its analogs and derivatives. *Archives of pathology*, 1947, 43:127-142.

13. Hodge HC et al. Short-term oral toxicity tests of methoxychlor (2,2-di-(*p*-methoxyphenyl)-1,1,1-trichloroethane) in rats and dogs. *Journal of pharmacology and experimental therapeutics,* 1950, 99:140-148.

14. Goldman JM et al. Effects of low subchronic doses of methoxychlor on the rat hypothalamic-pituitary reproductive axis. *Toxicology and applied pharmacology*, 1986, 86(3):474-483.

15. National Cancer Institute. *Bioassay of methoxychlor for possible carcinogenicity*. Bethesda, MD, 1978 (Technical Report Series, No. 35).

16. Hodge HC, Maynard EA, Blanchet HJ Jr. Chronic oral toxicity tests of methoxychlor (2,2-di-(*p*-methoxyphenyl)-1,1,1-trichloroethane) in rats and dogs. *Journal of pharmacology and experimental therapeutics*, 1952, 104:60-66.

17. Stein AA. Comparative methoxychlor toxicity in dogs, swine, rats, monkeys and man. *Industrial medicine and surgery*, 1968, 37:540-541.

18. Tullner WW, Edgcomb JH. Cystic tubular nephropathy and decrease in testicular weight in rats following oral methoxychlor treatment. *Journal of pharmacology and experimental therapeutics*, 1962, 138:126-130.

19. Bal HS. Effect of methoxychlor on reproductive systems of the rat. *Proceedings of the Society of Experimental Biology and Medicine*, 1984, 176:187-196.

20. Jackson C Jr et al. Effects of methoxychlor and malathion on semen characteristics of rams. *Journal of animal science*, 1975, 40(3):514-517.

21. Harris JS, Cecil HC, Bitman J. Effect of several dietary levels of technical methoxychlor on reproduction in rats. *Journal of agricultural and food chemistry*, 1974, 22:969-973.

22. Khera KS, Whalen C, Trivett G. Teratogenicity studies on linuron, malathion and methoxychlor in rats. *Toxicology and applied pharmacology*, 1978, 45:435-444.

23. Cummings AM, Perreault SD. Methoxychlor accelerates embryo transport through the rat reproductive tract. *Toxicology and applied pharmacology*, 1990, 102(1):110-116.

24. Gray LE Jr et al. A dose–response analysis of methoxychlor-induced alterations of reproductive development and function in the rat. *Fundamental and applied toxicology*, 1989, 12:92-108.

25. Hazleton Laboratories Inc., Kincaid Enterprises Inc. *Rabbit teratology study with methoxychlor, technical grade.* 1986; MRID No. 00159929 available from US Environmental Protection Agency, Washington, DC 20460.

26. Deichmann WB et al. Synergism among oral carcinogens. IV. The simultaneous feeding of four tumorigens to rats. *Toxicology and applied pharmacology*, 1967, 11:88-103.

27. Reuber MD. Carcinogenicity and toxicity of methoxychlor. *Environmental health perspectives*, 1980, 36:205-219.

28. Kurata M, Hirose K, Umeda M. Inhibition of metabolic cooperation in Chinese hamster cells by organochlorine pesticides. *Gann*, 1982, 73(2):217-221.

29. Coulston F, Serrone DM. The comparative approach to the role of nonhuman primates in evaluation of drug toxicity in man: a review. *Annals of the New York Academy of Sciences*, 1969, 162:681-704.

30. Wills JH. In: Miller MW, Berg GG, eds. Effects of chlorinated hydrocarbons on smaller animals as guides in the design of experiments with human volunteers. *Current research on persistent pesticides chemical fallout.* 1969:461-467.

31. International Agency for Research on Cancer. *Some halogenated hydrocarbons*. Lyon, 1979:259-281 (IARC Monographs on the Evaluation of the Carcinogenic Risk of Chemicals to Humans, Volume 20).

## 15.23 Metolachlor

### 15.23.1 General description

#### *Identity*

CAS no.:                    51218-45-2
Molecular formula:          $C_{15}H_{22}ClNO_2$

Metolachlor is the common name for 2-chloro-*6'*-ethyl-*N*-(2-methoxy-1-methyl-ethyl) acet-*o*-toluidine.

#### *Physicochemical properties (1)*

| Property | Value |
|---|---|
| Physical state | White to tan liquid |
| Vapour pressure | $1.7 \times 10^{-3}$ Pa at 20 °C |
| Water solubility | 530 mg/litre at 20 °C |
| Octanol–water partition coefficient | 2820 |

#### *Organoleptic properties*

Metolachlor is odourless.

#### *Major uses*

Metolachlor is a selective herbicide for pre-emergence and preplant weed control in corn, soy beans, peanuts, sorghum, pod crops, potatoes, cotton, safflower and woody ornamentals (*2*).

#### *Environmental fate*

Metolachlor photodegrades slowly in aqueous solution when exposed to sunlight (*3*). Its hydrolysis half-life is over 200 days at 20 °C (*1*). Volatilization from silty loam and sand has been observed (*4*). Metolachlor leaching is affected by adsorption onto soil organic matter, soil texture, precipitation, and water application. It can leach beyond the root zone in detectable amounts. The half-life in soil has been reported to range from 47 to 107 days (*5*). It can be metabolized by micro-organisms (*6*).

## 15.23.2 Analytical methods

Metolachlor may be determined by gas chromatographic methods applicable to the determination of certain nitrogen/phosphorus-containing pesticides in water samples. The estimated detection limit ranges from 0.75 to 0.01 µg/litre (7).

## 15.23.3 Environmental levels and human exposure

### Water

Metolachlor was found in 2091 of 4161 surface water samples and in 13 of 596 groundwater samples in the USA in 1988 (8). The 85th percentile of all non-zero samples was 12 µg/litre in surface water and 0.25 µg/litre in groundwater. In another survey in the same country, metolachlor residues from agricultural use were detected in groundwater at levels ranging from 0.1 to 0.4 µg/litre. In a survey of 160 water bodies in Italy, metolachlor was found, if at all, at levels of less than 0.1 µg/litre (9).

## 15.23.4 Kinetics and metabolism in laboratory animals and humans

Metolachlor is readily absorbed and excreted in the rat, male rats excreting 21.5% and 51.4% of the dose administered in the urine and faeces, respectively, within 48 h. It is metabolized via dechlorination, $O$-methylation, $N$-dealkylation, and side-chain oxidation. Urinary and faecal metabolites include 2-ethyl-6-methylhydroxyacetanilide and $N$-(2-ethyl-6-methylphenyl)-$N$-(hydroxyacetyl)DL-alanine. No unchanged chemical was isolated (10).

## 15.23.5 Effects on laboratory animals and in vitro test systems

### Acute exposure

Metolachlor has a low oral acute toxicity. Oral $LD_{50}$s in the rat are over 2000 mg/kg of body weight. The dermal $LD_{50}$ is over 10 000 mg/kg of body weight.[1]

### Short-term exposure

Beagle dogs given metolachlor at dose levels of 0, 50 (switched to 1000 mg/kg after 8 weeks), 150, or 500 mg/kg of diet for up to 15 weeks showed signs of toxicity only at the highest dose level (11).

In a 1-year study in beagle dogs, administration of metolachlor resulted in decreased kidney weight at the two highest dose levels. The NOAEL was determined to be 3.5 mg/kg of body weight per day (12).

---

[1] Source: Registry of Toxic Effects of Chemical Substances (RTECS) file on line. Bethesda, MD, National Library of Medicine, National Institute for Occupational Safety and Health, 1977.

## Long-term exposure

In a 2-year study with albino mice fed diets containing metolachlor at levels of 0, 100, 300, or 1000 mg/kg, the only toxicological effects observed were decreased body weight gain and decreased survival in females at the highest dose level (*13*).

Albino Sprague-Dawley CD rats fed metolachlor for two years at dose levels of 0, 30, 300, or 3000 mg/kg showed decreased body weight gain and food consumption at the highest dose level (*14*).

## Reproductive toxicity, embryotoxicity, and teratogenicity

Metolachlor was not teratogenic in gavage studies at daily dose levels up to and including 60 mg/kg of body weight in rats (*15*) and 360 mg/kg of body weight in rabbits (*16*). In a two-generation reproduction study, it decreased weight gain during lactation in pups at the highest dose level (equivalent to 14.7 mg/kg of body weight per day). The NOAEL in this study was 5 mg/kg of body weight per day (*17*).

## Mutagenicity and related end-points

Metolachlor does not induce gene mutations in bacterial or mammalian cells and is negative in the dominant lethal assay and for unscheduled DNA synthesis *in vivo* and *in vitro* in rat hepatocytes and human fibroblasts (*18*).

## Carcinogenicity

No evidence of carcinogenicity was found in a long-term dietary feeding study in albino mice at dose levels up to and including 3000 mg/kg (*19*). One study in rats showed an increase in the incidence of hepatocellular neoplasia in females receiving 3000 mg/kg in the diet for 2 years. One adenosarcoma and one fibrosarcoma were found in the nasal tissues of males at the highest dose only. No increase in tumour incidence was found in males or in females exposed to levels less than 3000 mg/kg. The increase in neoplasia in females was primarily due to an increased incidence of neoplastic nodules (*14*).

## 15.23.6 Effects on humans

Signs of intoxication by metolachlor include abdominal cramps, anaemia, ataxia, dark urine, methaemoglobinaemia, cyanosis, hypothermia, collapse, convulsions, diarrhoea, jaundice, weakness, nausea, shock, sweating, vomiting, central nervous system depression, dizziness, dyspnoea, liver damage, nephritis, cardiovascular failure, dermatitis, sensitization, eye and mucous membrane irritation, corneal opacity, and reproductive effects.[1]

[1] Source: HAZARDLINE. Bethesda, MD, National Library of Medicine, National Institutes of Health, 1985.

## 15.23.7 Guideline value

There is no evidence from available studies that metolachlor is carcinogenic in mice. In rats, an increase in liver tumours in females and a few nasal tumours in males have been observed. Metolachlor is not genotoxic.

Toxicity data are available from long-term studies in rodents and from a 1-year study in dogs. An apparent decrease in kidney weight was observed at the two highest dose levels in the 1-year dog study, giving a NOAEL of 3.5 mg/kg of body weight per day (*12*). An uncertainty factor of 1000 (100 for inter- and intraspecies variation and 10 because of some concern regarding carcinogenicity) was applied to this NOAEL to give a TDI of 3.5 µg/kg of body weight. A 10% allocation of the TDI to drinking-water results in a guideline value of 10 µg/litre (rounded figure).

## References

1. Worthing CR, ed. *The pesticide manual*, 9th ed. Farnham, British Crop Protection Council, 1991.

2. Meister R, ed. *Farm chemicals handbook*. Willoughby, OH, Meister Publishing Co., 1989.

3. US Environmental Protection Agency. *Metolachlor: pesticide registration standard.* Washington, DC, 1980:183 (NTIS No. PB81-123820).

4. Burkhard N, Guth JA. Rate of volatilization of pesticides from soil surfaces: comparison of calculated results with those determined in laboratory model system. *Pesticide science*, 1981, 12:37-44.

5. Walker A, Brown PA. The relative persistence in soil of five acetanilide herbicides. *Bulletin of environmental contamination and toxicology*, 1985, 34:143-149.

6. Saxena A, Zhang RW, Bollag JM. Microorganisms capable of metabolizing the herbicide metolachlor. *Applied environmental microbiology*, 1987, 53:390-396.

7. Environmental Monitoring and Support Laboratory. US EPA Method 507— *Determination of nitrogen and phosphorus containing pesticides in water by GC/NPD.* Cincinnati, OH, US Environmental Protection Agency, 1988.

8. Office of Drinking Water. *Metolachlor health advisory.* Washington, DC, US Environmental Protection Agency, 1988.

9. Funari E, Sampaolo A. Erbicidi nelle acque potabili. [Herbicides in drinking-water.] *Annali dell'Istituto Superiore di Sanità*, 1989, 25(2):353-362.

10. Hambock H. *Project 12/74: metabolism of CGA 24705 in the rat.* Basel, Switzerland, Ciba-Geigy Ltd, 1974 (report MRID 15425).

11. International Research and Development Corporation. *CGA 24705 Technical 6 month chronic oral toxicity study on Beagle dogs.* Basel, Ciba-Geigy Ltd, 1980.

12. Hazelette JR, Arthur AT. *Metolachlor technical 13/52-week oral toxicity study in dogs.* Summit, NJ, Ciba-Geigy Corporation, Pharmaceuticals Division, 1989 (Toxicology/Pathology Report 88086; MIN 862253).

13. Industrial Biotest Laboratories Inc. *Carcinogenicity study with CGA 24705 technical in albino mice.* Basel, Ciba-Geigy Ltd, 1977 (IBT 622-07925).

14. Hazleton-Raltech Inc. *Two-year chronic oral toxicity and oncogenicity study with metolachlor technical in albino rats.* Basel, Ciba-Geigy Ltd, 1983.

15. Argus Research Laboratory. *Teratogenicity study in rats.* Basel, Ciba-Geigy Ltd, 1985 (report no. 203-004).

16. Argus Research Laboratory, *Teratogenicity study in rabbits.* Basel, Ciba-Geigy Ltd, 1980 (report no. 203-001).

17. Ciba-Geigy. *Two-generation reproduction study in albino rats with metolachlor technical.* Basel, 1981 (report no. 450-0272).

18. Istituto Superiore della Sanità. Ministero della Sanità, Centro Studi Commissione Consultiva Tossicologica Nazionale. *Valutazione di un primo elenco di pesticidi (erbicidi).* [*Assessment of a first list of pesticides (herbicides).*] Rome, 1990:92-97 (Metolachlor Rapporti ISTISAN 90/12).

19. Hazleton-Raltech Inc. *Carcinogenicity study in mice.* Basel, Ciba-Geigy Ltd, 1982 (report no. 79020).

## 15.24 Molinate

### 15.24.1 General description

#### *Identity*

CAS no.:               2212-67-1
Molecular formula:     $C_9H_{17}NOS$

Molinate is the common name for *S*-ethylazepane-1-carbothiate.

## Physicochemical properties (1)

| Property | Value |
|---|---|
| Physical state | Clear liquid |
| Boiling point | 202 °C at 1.33 kPa |
| Vapour pressure | 0.746 Pa at 25 °C |
| Water solubility | 880 mg/litre at 20 °C |
| Octanol–water partition coefficient | 760 |

## Organoleptic properties

Molinate has an aromatic odour (1).

## Major uses

Molinate is used to control germinating broad-leaved and grassy weeds. It is applied either before planting to water-seeded or shallow soil-seeded rice or post-flood, post-emergence in other types of rice culture (1).

## Environmental fate

Volatilization is the main route of loss of molinate (active ingredient) from soil, taking place more easily on moist than on dry soils (2). Volatilization is also important in rice fields, increasing with temperature; the half-life is about 2 days at 28 °C. Photochemical degradation occurs to a lesser extent, and chemical hydrolysis and microbial degradation are negligible (3). Molinate is of low persistence in water and soil, with a half-life of about 5 days (4). In aerobic and flooded soils, the half-lives were 8–25 and 40–160 days, respectively (1).

## 15.24.2 Analytical methods

Capillary gas chromatography with a selective nitrogen–phosphorus detector may be used for the determination of molinate, following extraction with methylene chloride. A detection limit of 0.03 µg/litre is possible (1).

## 15.24.3 Environmental levels and human exposure

### Water

In 1987-88, water from 1288 drinking-water wells in the Lombardy region of Italy was analysed for molinate; it was detected in 27 wells at levels above 1 µg/litre and in 220 wells at levels between 0.1 and 1 µg/litre. In the Piedmont region, molinate was detected in 25 wells used as a source of drinking-water; in five of them, levels were above 1 µg/litre (5).

## 15.24.4 Kinetics and metabolism in laboratory animals and humans

Molinate is not absorbed percutaneously. In rats, it is metabolized primarily to the sulfoxide, then to mercapturic acid. Ring hydroxylation, mainly at the 3- and 4- positions, followed by glucuronidation and cleavage of the C–N bond to yield the imide, were also observed.[1] The active ingredient is quickly metabolized to carbon dioxide (18%) and eliminated through the urine (25%) and faeces (7–20%) within 3 days.[2]

## 15.24.5 Effects on laboratory animals and *in vitro* test systems

### Acute exposure

Acute oral $LD_{50}$s of 369 and 450 mg/kg of body weight have been reported for male and female rats, respectively (*1*).

### Short-term exposure

Rats (15 per sex per dose) were given oral doses of technical active ingredient at 0, 35, 70, or 140 mg/kg of body weight per day in the diet for 90 days. Effects at 140 mg/kg of body weight per day included increased body weight, markedly decreased food intake, marked decrease in haemoglobin and haematocrit, increased relative weights of liver, kidney, adrenals, and thyroid, and histopathological changes in liver, kidney, adrenals, testes, and ovaries. Similar but less marked changes occurred at 70 mg/kg of body weight per day. There was also a slight increase in the lipoid content of the adrenals at 35 mg/kg of body weight per day.[3]

In a study in which rats (15 per sex per dose) were fed technical active ingredient in their diets at 0, 8, 16, or 32 mg/kg of body weight per day for 90 days, effects observed at the highest dose included reduced food intake and weight gain, increased adrenal weight (females), and slight increases in relative weights for adrenals, thyroids, and testes in males and kidneys and adrenals in females. At the two highest doses, there were some cases of decreased differential leukocyte count (females), vacuolation of ovary stromal cells (females), and vacuolation of adrenocortical cells (both sexes). An increase in the content of lipoid bodies in the ovary and adrenal vacuolation were observed for all the treated groups.[3]

Dogs were given oral doses of technical active ingredient at 0, 15, 30, or 60 mg/kg of body weight for 90 days. There were no clear signs of toxicity or modification of haematological and clinical parameters at the two lowest doses, but a slight increase in thyroid weight was observed at the highest dose. No treatment-related histopathological changes were observed.[3]

---

[1] Source: Hazardous Substances Data Bank. Bethesda, MD, National Library of Medicine.
[2] Source: Toxicology Data Bank. Bethesda, MD, National Library of Medicine.
[3] US Environmental Protection Agency, Office of Pesticide Programs, reserved documentation.

### Reproductive toxicity, embryotoxicity, and teratogenicity

Fischer rats (60 per sex per dose) were fed technical molinate in the diet for 104 weeks. Initial concentrations corresponded to daily intakes of 0, 8, 16, or 32 mg/kg of body weight, which were reduced after 18 weeks (following a failed attempt to produce the $F_1$ generation) to 0, 0.6, 2.0, or 6.3 mg/kg of body weight per day. Rats were mated at 8–10 weeks from the beginning of the study. Administration of the diet was suspended 3 weeks before, and resumed 10–12 days after signs of mating were observed. Only one litter was born. At 21 weeks from the beginning of the study (3 weeks after reducing the diet concentration), all animals were mated again. Groups treated with 0, 0.6, 2.0, and 6.3 mg/kg of body weight per day generated 43, 18, 16, and 10 litters, respectively, of which 35, 8, 5, and 3 were alive at the age of 21 days; corresponding numbers of weanlings were 300, 37, 21, and 16, respectively (2).

Six groups of Sprague-Dawley rats were given technical molinate by gavage in corn oil at 0, 0.2, 4, 13, 30, or 60 mg/kg of body weight per day. There were no significant reductions in fertility parameters at 0.2 mg/kg of body weight per day, but they were considerably reduced in both sexes at 4 mg/kg of body weight per day. Dose-related alterations in sperm morphology were also noted at this level. The necropsy data for pregnant females indicated a significant reduction in the number of viable fetuses per litter as a result of mating in the group given 4 mg/kg of body weight per day. An increase in the number of resorptions per litter as a result of matings with males in this group was also observed (2).

### Mutagenicity and related end-points

Molinate did not show any significant mutagenic effect in the Ames test with five strains of *Salmonella typhimurium* with or without metabolic activation. It was also negative in assays for the induction of gene mutations in mouse lymphoma cells with and without metabolic activation, induction of micronuclei in CD-1 mice *in vivo*, induction of sister chromatid exchange in Chinese hamster ovary cells with and without metabolic activation, and induction of unscheduled DNA synthesis in human HeLa cells with and without metabolic activation.[1]

### Carcinogenicity

Fischer rats (60 per sex per dose) were fed technical molinate in the diet for 104 weeks at initial concentrations corresponding to daily intakes of 0, 8, 16, or 32 mg/kg of body weight, reduced after 18 weeks to 0, 0.6, 2.0, or 6.3 mg/kg of body weight per day. A greater than 90% incidence of interstitial-cell tumours of the testes was recorded in all groups (2).

---

[1] US Environmental Protection Agency, Office of Pesticide Programs, reserved documentation.

Groups of 20 CAF$_1$ mice (BALBcj x A/J) were given a molinate compound of unspecified composition for 99–101 weeks. Concentrations corresponded to intakes of 0, 3.6, 7.2, or 14.4 mg/kg of body weight per day. Adenomas, carcinomas, and lymphosarcomas of lungs, liver, kidney, spleen, and other organs were observed; there were no significant differences between the different dose groups (2). When BALB/cj females received doses of molinate up to 14 mg/kg of body weight per day, 10–12 days after mating with A/J males, and the F$_1$ mice (64–67 per dose) were fed the same diet for 76–78 weeks, tumour incidence was the same in all the groups (2).

## 15.24.6 Effects on humans

A review of epidemiological data based on the examination of workers involved in molinate production did not indicate any effect on fertility (4).

## 15.24.7 Guideline value

On the basis of the limited information available, molinate does not seem to be carcinogenic or mutagenic in animals. Evidence suggests that impairment of the reproductive performance of the male rat represents the most sensitive indicator of molinate exposure. However, epidemiological data based on the examination of workers involved in molinate production do not indicate any effect on human fertility.

The NOAEL for reproductive toxicity in the rat was 0.2 mg/kg of body weight per day (2), and this value was chosen as the basis for calculating a TDI for molinate. Using an uncertainty factor of 100 (for inter- and intraspecies variation), a TDI of 2 µg/kg of body weight was derived. An allocation of 10% of the TDI to drinking-water results in a guideline value of 6 µg/litre.

## References

1. Worthing CR, ed. *The pesticide manual*, 9th ed. Farnham, British Crop Protection Council, 1991.

2. ICI Americas Inc. Study No. 000792a09. Wilmington, DE, 1981 (available from US Environmental Protection Agency, Office of Pesticide Programs, Washington, DC, USA).

3. Soderquist CJ, Bowers JB, Crosby DG. Dissipation of molinate in a rice field. *Journal of agricultural and food chemistry*, 1977, 25:940.

4. *Drinking water quality: guidelines for selected herbicides.* Copenhagen, WHO Regional Office for Europe, 1987 (Environmental Health, 27).

5. Funari E et al. Erbicidi nelle acque destinate al consumo umano in Italia. [Herbicides in water intended for human consumption in Italy.] *Acqua aria*, 1989, 9:1011-1024.

# 15.25 Pendimethalin

## 15.25.1 General description

### Identity

CAS no.:     40487-42-1
Molecular formula:  $C_{13}H_{19}N_3O_4$

Pendimethalin is the common name for *N*-(1-ethylpropyl)-2,6-dinitro-3,4-xylidine.

### Physicochemical properties *(1)*

| Property | Value |
|---|---|
| Physical state | Orange-yellow crystals |
| Melting point | 54–58 °C |
| Vapour pressure | $4.0 \times 10^{-3}$ Pa at 25 °C |
| Water solubility | 0.3 mg/litre at 20 °C |
| Log octanol–water partition coefficient | 5.2 |

### Major uses

Pendimethalin is a selective herbicide, applied before emergence to cereals, maize, and rice, and with shallow soil incorporation before seeding bean, cotton, soy beans, and groundnuts. In vegetable crops, it is applied before emergence or transplanting, and is also used to control suckers on tobacco *(1)*.

### Environmental fate

Pendimethalin is stable under both alkaline and acidic conditions *(1)*. It is a moderately persistent herbicide that can give rise to long-lasting metabolites, mainly by photodegradation *(2)*. Three by-products of soil fungal degradation have been identified as the result of ring hydroxylation, nitro group reduction, and complete *N*-dealkylation *(3)*. Both pendimethalin and its metabolites bind tightly to soil particles, and the leaching potential is negligible *(2)*. A half-life in soil of 30–90 days has been estimated *(1)*. Pendimethalin has a low affinity for the water compartment. However, under anaerobic conditions, more polar metabolites of greater mobility are formed, and these can potentially contaminate both groundwater and surface waters *(2)*.

## 15.25.2 Analytical methods

Pendimethalin can be determined by capillary gas chromatography with a selective nitrogen–phosphorus detector following extraction with methylene chloride. Confirmation by a second capillary column of different polarity is recommended.

## 15.25.3 Environmental levels and human exposure

### Water

Pendimethalin was found at a concentration below 0.1 µg/litre in one of 76 drinking-water supplies examined in the Veneto Region in Italy in 1987–88 (4).

## 15.25.4 Kinetics and metabolism in laboratory animals and humans

Pendimethalin appears to be both poorly absorbed and rapidly excreted. About 95% is excreted within 24 h after oral administration, 75% being found in the faeces and 20% in the urine. Maximum tissue concentrations were found in the liver and kidney. Although most parent compound is excreted unchanged, the metabolites identified suggest that oxidation of the 4-methyl group on the phenyl moiety and the N-alkyl side chain of the dinitro-substituted aniline are the predominant metabolic pathways (5).

## 15.25.5 Effects on laboratory animals and *in vitro* test systems

### Acute exposure

Pendimethalin is of low acute toxicity. $LD_{50}$s of 1050–1250 mg/kg of body weight in albino rats, 1340–1620 mg/kg of body weight in albino mice, and over 5000 mg/kg of body weight in beagle dogs have been reported (1).

### Short-term exposure

In a study in which Charles River CD rats received pendimethalin in the diet at concentrations of 0, 100, 500, or 5000 mg/kg for 13 weeks, food intake and body weight gain were decreased only at 5000 mg/kg. A variety of indications of hepatotoxicity were also observed at this dose level. Absolute and relative kidney weights increased in males at 5000 mg/kg, and absolute and relative uterus and ovary weights decreased in females at 500 mg/kg (6).

### Long-term exposure

CD-1 mice (75 per sex per dose) were given a diet containing the technical-grade compound at 0, 100, 500, or 2500 mg/kg for 18 months (dose doubled after 8 weeks) (*7*), and Long-Evans rats (60 per sex per dose) were fed a diet containing 0, 100, 500, or 2500 mg/kg for 2 years (highest dose doubled after 6 weeks) (*8*). At the highest doses, general toxic effects were observed both in the mouse (hyperglycaemia and increased thyroid and adrenal gland weights) and in the rat (increase in alkaline phosphatase levels, increased thyroid and kidney weights, hepatomegaly). Some toxic effects (hyperglycaemia in the mouse and hepatotoxicity in the rat) were present even at the lowest dose level of 100 mg/kg of diet (equivalent to 5 mg/kg of body weight per day). It was therefore not possible to establish a NOAEL.

### Reproductive toxicity, embryotoxicity, and teratogenicity

Teratogenicity was not observed at the highest dose tested in rats (1000 mg/kg of body weight per day) (*9,10*) or rabbits (60 mg/kg of body weight per day) (*11*). In rats gavaged with pendimethalin on days 6–15 of gestation, embryotoxicity in the form of minor anomalies and reduced fetal weight was observed at 1000 mg/kg of body weight (*9*), and reduced ossification of the extremities was present at 250 and 500 mg/kg of body weight (*10*). Reproductive toxicity was not observed in a three-generation reproduction study in Long-Evans rats given pendimethalin in the diet at levels as high as 1000 mg/kg (*12*).

### Mutagenicity and related end-points

Although genetic mutations were induced by pendimethalin with metabolic activation in *Salmonella typhimurium*, higher-purity technical material did not induce mutations in the same test system. Pendimethalin did not induce chromosomal aberrations, unscheduled DNA synthesis, or dominant lethal mutations (*13–17*).

### Carcinogenicity

Neither CD-1 mice fed doses of pendimethalin up to 2500 mg/kg for 18 months (*7*) nor rats fed diets containing pendimethalin at up to 2500 mg/kg for 2 years showed evidence of carcinogenicity (*8*). However, these studies had important methodological limitations, including inadequate numbers of animals subjected to histological examinations.

## 15.25.6 Guideline value

Pendimethalin does not appear to have significant mutagenic activity. Long-term studies in mice and rats have not provided evidence of carcinogenicity; however, these studies have some important limitations.

The guideline value is based on the LOAEL for liver toxicity (5 mg/kg of body weight per day) observed in the 2-year rat study (8). An uncertainty factor of 1000 (100 for intra- and interspecies variation and 10 for the use of a LOAEL instead of a NOAEL and for the limitations of the database) is used, giving a TDI of 5 µg/kg of body weight per day. An allocation of 10% of the TDI to drinking-water results in a guideline value of 20 µg/litre (rounded figure).

## References

1.  Worthing CR, ed. *The pesticide manual*, 9th ed. Farnham, British Crop Protection Council, 1991.

2.  *Drinking-water quality: guidelines for selected herbicides.* Copenhagen, WHO Regional Office for Europe, 1987 (Environmental Health 27).

3.  Barua AS et al. Degradation of pendimethalin by soil fungi. *Pesticide science*, 1990, 29:419-425.

4.  Funari E, Sampaolo A. Erbicidi nelle acque potabili. [Herbicides in drinking water.] *Annali dell'Istituto Superiore di Sanità*, 1989, 25:353-362.

5.  American Cyanamid Co. *Toxicology report AX86-1, Doc. 13.* Wayne, NJ, 1986 (confidential information submitted to the Italian Ministry of Health).

6.  American Cyanamid Co. *Toxicology report AX86-1 experiment L-2190. AC 92,553: A 13 week rat feeding study.* Wayne, NJ, 1986 (confidential information submitted to the Italian Ministry of Health).

7.  Biodynamics Inc. *Report on project no. 72R-747.* Wayne, NJ, American Cyanamid, 1974 (confidential information submitted to the Italian Ministry of Health).

8.  Biodynamics Inc. *Report on project no. 72R-746.* Wayne, NJ, American Cyanamid, 1974 (confidential information submitted to the Italian Ministry of Health).

9.  American Cyanamid Co. *Report of December 12, 1972.* Wayne, NJ (confidential information submitted to the Italian Ministry of Health).

10. American Cyanamid Co. *Teratology study in rats.* Wayne, NJ, 1979 (confidential information submitted to the Italian Ministry of Health).

11. American Cyanamid Co. *Teratology study in rabbits. AC 92,553. Technical. Hazleton 362-164.* Wayne, NJ, 1986 (confidential information submitted to the Italian Ministry of Health).

12. Biodynamics Inc. *3 generation reproduction study in AC 92,553 in rats. Project 72R-748.* Wayne, NJ, American Cyanamid, 1974 (confidential information submitted to the Italian Ministry of Health).

13. American Cyanamid Co. *Project No. 0166.* Wayne, NJ, 1985 (confidential information submitted to the Italian Ministry of Health).

14. American Cyanamid Co. *Project No. S-0329.* Wayne, NJ, 1985 (confidential information submitted to the Italian Ministry of Health).

15. Pharmakon Research International Inc. *Study no. PH 320-AC-001-85.* Wayne, NJ, American Cyanamid, 1985 (confidential information submitted to the Italian Ministry of Health).

16. Pharmakon Research International Inc. *Study no. PH 311-AC-002-85.* Wayne, NJ, American Cyanamid, 1985 (confidential information submitted to the Italian Ministry of Health).

17. American Cyanamid Co. *Report of October 5, 1973.* Wayne, NJ (confidential information submitted to the Italian Ministry of Health).

## 15.26 Permethrin

### 15.26.1 General description

#### *Identity*

CAS no:              52645-53-1
Molecular formula:   $C_{21}H_{20}Cl_2O_3$

Permethrin is the common name for 3-phenoxybenzyl (1RS)-*cis, trans*-3-(2,2-dichlorovinyl)-2,2-dimethylcyclopropanecarboxylate. It is a mixture of four stereoisomers of the (1R, *trans*), (1R, *cis*), (1S, *trans*), and (1S, *cis*) configurations. In most technical products, the *cis:trans* ratio is about 2:3, and the 1R:1S ratio is 1:1 (racemic). The composition ratio of the above isomers is about 3:2:3:2 (*1*). Of the four isomers, the (1R, *cis*)- and the (1R, *trans*)-isomers are the two esters primarily responsible for insecticidal activity. The term permethrin is used here to refer to material with a *cis:trans* ratio of 2:3, unless otherwise stated.

## Physicochemical properties (1)

| Property | Value |
|---|---|
| Physical state | Crystal or viscous liquid |
| Melting point | 34–39 °C |
| Boiling point | 220 °C |
| Water solubility | 0.2 mg/litre at 30 °C |
| Log octanol–water partition coefficient | 6.5 |

## Organoleptic properties

An organoleptic threshold in water of 0.2 mg/litre was reported in one study (2).

## Major uses

Permethrin is a contact insecticide effective against a broad range of pests in agriculture, forestry, and public health. It is also used to control aquatic invertebrates, such as *Asellus aquaticus*, in water mains (3).

## Environmental fate

Permethrin is photodegraded both in water and on soil surfaces. Ester cleavage and *cis–trans* interconversion are the major reactions. At equilibrium, the *trans*-isomer constitutes 65–70% of the mixture. The major products of the ester cleavage of permethrin include 3-phenoxybenzaldehyde, 3-phenoxybenzoic acid, 3-phenoxybenzyl-3,3-dimethylacrylate, and benzyl alcohols, as well as the corresponding acids (1).

In soil, permethrin is rapidly degraded by hydrolysis and microbial action under aerobic conditions. Similar degradation processes seem to occur under anaerobic conditions but at slower rates. In laboratory studies, the soil half-life was approximately 28 days. The *trans*-isomer was more rapidly degraded than the *cis*-isomer, and ester cleavage was the major initial degradative reaction. In plants, permethrin degrades with a half-life of approximately 10 days (1, 4).

## 15.26.2 Analytical methods

Permethrin may be determined by gas–liquid chromatography with an electron-capture or flame-ionization detector. The minimum detectable concentration is about 0.05 µg/litre (1).

## 15.26.3 Environmental levels and human exposure

### Water

Surface waters may become contaminated by permethrin applied directly to water for mosquito control purposes, in discharges from production plants, and from agricultural sources. Concentrations as high as 0.8 mg/litre have been recorded in surface water. Levels in drinking-water have not been reported, but it is generally considered that permethrin is readily removed by conventional treatment methods and that neither *cis-* nor *trans-*permethrin reacts with chlorine under normal disinfection conditions (*5*). When permethrin is used to control aquatic invertebrates in water mains, concentrations of about 10 µg/litre will be present in the water for short periods (*3*).

### Food

Exposure of the general population to permethrin is mainly via the diet. Residue levels in crops grown according to good agricultural practice are generally low. The resulting exposure is expected to be low, but precise data from total diet studies are lacking (1).

## 15.26.4 Kinetics and metabolism in laboratory animals and humans

Permethrin is readily absorbed when given orally. Distribution occurs rapidly in the body, mostly to adipose tissue, followed by liver, kidney, and brain.

Metabolism appears to be similar in all mammals, including humans (*6, 7*). The main routes of metabolism for both the *trans-* and *cis-*isomers are ester cleavage and oxidation of the 4'-position of the terminal aromatic ring. Major metabolites formed include 3-(2,2-dichlorovinyl)-2,2-dimethylcyclopropane carboxylic acid ($Cl_2CA$), in free and glucuronide form, and hydroxymethyl-$Cl_2CA$ as a glucuronide conjugate (*1*).

Permethrin administered to mammals is almost completely eliminated from the body within several days. The *trans-*isomer is eliminated more quickly than the *cis-*isomer and is excreted mainly in the urine, whereas the *cis-*isomer is excreted in both the urine and faeces. Expiration as carbon dioxide plays a minor role in mammals. The very small amounts of unmetabolized permethrin found in fat and milk consist predominantly of the *cis-*isomer. Less than 0.7% of the administered dose was detected in the milk of goats or cows (*1*).

## 15.26.5 Effects on laboratory animals and *in vitro* systems

### *Acute exposure*

Permethrin has a low acute oral toxicity in mammals, although the $LD_{50}$ varies considerably according to the administration vehicle used and the *cis:trans* isomeric ratio. The *cis*-isomer is the more toxic form. When corn oil is used as the vehicle, oral $LD_{50}$s are in the 0.5 g/kg of body weight range. Aqueous suspensions are the least toxic; $LD_{50}$s range from 3 to over 4 g/kg of body weight. The oral toxicities of the major metabolites of permethrin are lower than those of the parent compound. The major signs of acute intoxication are effects on the central nervous system, namely uncoordinated movements, whole-body tremors, and loss of balance. Overt signs of toxicity do not appear until near-lethal doses (*1, 8*).

### *Short-term exposure*

No beagle dogs died when fed permethrin in gelatin capsules daily for 3 months at doses of up to 500 mg/kg of body weight per day. Growth, food consumption, clinical chemistry, haematology, and urological parameters were all normal, but doses of 50 mg/kg of body weight per day or higher resulted in significant increases in liver-to-body-weight ratios (*9*). No signs of toxicity were reported when beagle dogs received encapsulated doses of up to 250 mg/kg of body weight per day for 6 months (*10*).

### *Long-term exposure*

In a 2-year study on Wistar rats fed permethrin at 0, 25, 40, or 125 mg/kg of body weight per day, tremors and hypersensitivity to noise were noted in rats at the highest dose. Significant increases in endoplasmic reticulum were detected only at this dose, although nonsignificant increases were noted at all levels in both sexes. The liver weights and liver-to-body-weight ratios were higher in all permethrin-treated males, but in females only in those that received 40 mg/kg of body weight per day. Kidney weights in males were increased at all dose levels (*11*).

In a 2-year study on Long-Evans rats fed permethrin in the diet at dose levels of 0, 20, 100, or 500 mg/kg (0, 1, 5, or 25 mg/kg of body weight per day), the estimated NOAEL was 5 mg/kg of body weight per day (*12*).

A lifetime (80% mortality) feeding study was carried out on Swiss-derived mice (70 per sex per dose) fed permethrin (*cis* 35–45%:*trans* 55–65%) at dose levels of 0, 250, 1000, or 2500 mg/kg of diet for 2 years. The mortality rate was normal, and growth was only slightly decreased at the two highest dose levels. There was a significant dose-dependent increase in liver-to-body-weight ratios in females at the two highest dose levels and in males at the highest dose level (*11*).

### Reproductive toxicity, embryotoxicity, and teratogenicity

Dietary permethrin does not appear to adversely affect reproduction in rats or mice. Permethrin is not teratogenic to rats, mice, or rabbits at dose levels up to 225, 125, and 1800 mg/kg of body weight, respectively (*1*).

### Mutagenicity

Both 2:3 and 1:3 permethrin have been tested in a number of *in vitro* and *in vivo* short-term assays for mutagenicity, all of which have given negative results (*1*).

### Carcinogenicity

Studies carried out with both 2:3 and 1:3 permethrin have shown no evidence of carcinogenicity in rats (*11, 13*). There is limited evidence of a weak carcinogenic potential in one strain of mice in which the incidence of pulmonary adenoma was increased in female mice at a dose of 250 mg/kg of body weight per day; however, it remained within historical control ranges for this strain (*14*). Moreover, the absence of positive mutagenic results suggests that this is probably an epigenetic mechanism. It has been concluded that the results of this study do not indicate that permethrin has any carcinogenic potential (*15*).

## 15.26.6 Effects on humans

Six forestry workers using permethrin exhibited symptoms such as itching and burning of the skin and itching and irritation of the eyes. Only one of them excreted urine containing detectable amounts (0.26 µg/ml) of permethrin metabolite (*16*).

Paraesthesia was induced in volunteers approximately 30 min after the application of permethrin solution (total 0.5 mg permethrin) to the earlobe (*17*); it peaked by 8 h and abated by 24 h. Of 10 volunteers treated with 15–40 ml of permethrin (1:3) (1%) head louse solution, which was allowed to dry and then washed out, three developed mild, patchy erythema, which faded 4–7 days later (*1*).

## 15.26.7 Guideline value

IARC has classified permethrin in Group 3, as there are no human data and only limited data from animal studies (*18*). Permethrin is not genotoxic.

Using a NOAEL of 100 mg/kg in the diet (equivalent to 5 mg/kg of body weight per day) obtained in a rat study (*12*) and an uncertainty factor of 100, JMPR recommended an ADI for 2:3 and 1:3 *cis:trans*-permethrin of 0.05 mg/kg of body weight (*15*).

Because there is significant exposure to permethrin from the environment, only 1% of the ADI is allocated to drinking-water. The guideline value is therefore 20 µg/litre (rounded figure). However, if permethrin is to be used for short periods as a larvicide for the control of mosquitos and other insects of health significance in drinking-water sources, the share of the ADI allocated to drinking-water may be increased.

## References

1.  *Permethrin.* Geneva, World Health Organization, 1990 (Environmental Health Criteria, No. 94).

2.  Musamuhamedov SR. [Hygienic substantiation of the maximum permissible level of Ambuš in reservoir water.] *Gigiena i sanitarija,* 1988, 9:69-70 (in Russian).

3.  Fawell JK. *An assessment of the safety in use of permethrin for disinfection of water mains.* Medmenham, Water Research Centre, 1987 (WRC Report PRU 1412-M/l).

4.  Kaufman DD et al. Permethrin degradation in soil and microbial cultures. *American Chemical Society symposium series,* 1977, 42:147-161.

5.  Fielding M, Haley J. Aqueous chlorination of permethrin. *Water research,* 1989, 23(4):523-524.

6.  Food and Agriculture Organization of the United Nations. *Pesticide residues in food: 1979 evaluations.* Rome, 1980 (Joint FAO/WHO Meeting on Pesticide Residues: FAO Plant Production and Protection Paper 20, Supp.).

7.  Food and Agriculture Organization of the United Nations. *Pesticide residues in food: 1981 evaluations.* Rome, 1982 (Joint FAO/WHO Meeting on Pesticide Residues: FAO Plant Production and Protection Paper 42).

8.  International Programme on Chemical Safety. *The WHO recommended classification of pesticides by hazard and guidelines to classification 1992-1993.* Geneva, World Health Organization, 1992 (unpublished document WHO/PCS/92.14).

9.  Killeen JC, Rapp WR. *A three month oral toxicity study of FMC 33927 in beagle dogs.* Bio-Dynamics Inc., 1976 (unpublished report submitted to WHO by FMC Corporation, Philadelphia, PA, USA).

10. Reynolds J et al. *Permethrin oral administration to dogs for 6 months.* Berkhamstead Hill, Wellcome Research Laboratories, 1978 (unpublished report no. HEFG 78-14).

11. Ishmael J, Lithfield MH. Chronic toxicity and carcinogenic evaluation of permethrin in rats and mice. *Fundamental and applied toxicology,* 1988, 11:308-322.

12. Braun WG, Rinehart WE. *A twenty-four month oral toxicity/carcinogenicity study of FMC33297 in rats.* Bio-Dynamics Inc., 1977 (unpublished report submitted to WHO by FMC Corporation, Philadelphia, PA, USA).

13. McSheehy TW, Finn JP. *21Z: potential toxicity and oncogenicity in dietary administration to rats for a period of 104 weeks.* London, Wellcome Research Laboratory, 1980 (unpublished report from document HEFG 80-33, submitted to WHO by Wellcome Foundation Ltd; Life Science Research Stock Report No. 80/WRL003/283).

14. James JA, Taylor PE, Roe FJC. *Carcinogenicity study in mice with permethrin.* London, Wellcome Research Laboratories, 1980 (unpublished report from Bechenham doc. no. HEFG 80-29, submitted to WHO by Wellcome Foundation Ltd).

15. Food and Agriculture Organization of the United Nations. *Pesticide residues in food. Evaluations—1987.* Part II. *Toxicology.* Rome, 1988:101-110 (Joint Meeting on Pesticide Residues: FAO Plant Production and Protection Paper 86/2).

16. Kolmodin-Hedman B, Swensson A, Akerblom M. Occupational exposure to some synthetic pyrethroids (permethrin and fenvalerate). *Archives of toxicology*, 1982, 50:27-33.

17. Flannigan SA, Tucker SB. Variation in cutaneous sensation between synthetic pyrethroid insecticides. *Contact dermatitis*, 1985, 13:140-147.

18. International Agency for Research on Cancer. *Occupational exposure in insecticide application, and some pesticides.* Lyon, 1991:329-349 (IARC Monographs on the Evaluation of Carcinogenic Risks to Humans, Volume 53).

## 15.27 Propanil

### 15.27.1 General description

#### *Identity*

| | |
|---|---|
| CAS no.: | 709-98-8 |
| Molecular formula: | $C_9H_9Cl_2NO$ |

Propanil is the common name for 3′,4′-dichloropropionanilide.

#### *Physicochemical properties* (1)

| Property | Value |
|---|---|
| Physical state | Colourless solid |
| Melting point | 91.5 °C |
| Vapour pressure | $0.026 \times 10^{-3}$ Pa at 20 °C |
| Water solubility | 130 mg/litre at 20 °C |

## Major uses

Propanil is a contact post-emergence herbicide used mainly in rice to control broad-leaved and grass weeds. It is also used mixed with MCPA in wheat (*1*).

## Environmental fate

Propanil is hydrolysed in acidic and alkaline media to 3,4-dichloroaniline and propionic acid. In water, propanil and 3,4-dichloroaniline are rapidly degraded by sunlight to phenolic compounds, which then polymerize (*1*). Propanil is bio degraded in soil to various metabolites, including 3,4-dichloroaniline, which rapidly binds to soil, propionic acid, which is further metabolized to carbon dioxide, 3,3′,4,4′-tetrachloroazoxybenzene, and two isomeric forms of tetrachloroazobenzene (*1*).[1] Propanil's half-life in soil is less than 5 days (*1*).

## 15.27.2 Analytical methods

Capillary gas chromatography with a selective nitrogen–phosphorus detector may be used for the determination of propanil, following extraction with methylene chloride. Confirmation by a second capillary column of different polarity is strongly recommended.

## 15.27.3 Environmental levels and human exposure

### Water

Residues of less than 0.03 mg/litre were detected in 162 water samples collected from 16 rice fields treated with 0.4–2.8 kg of propanil per hectare, 1–120 days after application (*2*). It has only occasionally been detected in groundwater.

## 15.27.4 Kinetics and metabolism in laboratory animals and humans

Propanil and its metabolites do not appear to accumulate in tissues. It is hydrolysed by hepatic acylamidase, forming 3,4-dichloroaniline and propionic acid. Six metabolites have been detected in urine (*3*). When propanil was fed to a cow, 1.4% of the total dose was recovered in the faeces, but none was detected in urine or milk.[1]

---

[1] Source: Hazardous Substances Data Bank. Bethesda, MD, National Library of Medicine.

## 15.27.5 Effects on laboratory animals and *in vitro* test systems
### Acute exposure

Propanil is of moderate acute toxicity; the oral $LD_{50}$ is over 2500 mg/kg of body weight in the rat (*1*).

### Short-term exposure

Groups of albino rats (10 per sex per dose) were given the technical product in doses of 100, 330, 1000, 3300, 10 000, or 50 000 mg/kg in the diet (equivalent to 5, 17, 50, 165, 500, or 2500 mg/kg of body weight per day) for 3 months. All the animals in the highest dose group died. There was an increase in polychromatophilia at dose levels of 330 mg/kg and higher as well as evidence of haemolytic anaemia at 3300 and 10 000 mg/kg. From this study, a NOAEL of 100 mg/kg (equivalent to 5 mg/kg of body weight per day) was identified (*4*).

### Long-term exposure

Propanil was administered at concentrations of 0, 100, 400, or 1600 mg/kg in the diet to albino Wistar rats (25 per sex per dose) for 2 years. At 1600 mg/kg, rats exhibited increased mortality (males only), significant decreases in body weight, slightly lower haematocrit and haemoglobin values, and changes in spleen-to-body-weight ratio (females only). The NOAEL in this study was 400 mg/kg, equivalent to 20 mg/kg of body weight per day (*4*).

In a 2-year study, beagle dogs were given propanil at concentrations of 0, 100, 600, or 3000 (raised to 4000 at the start of the 5th week) mg/kg in the diet. Significantly decreased body weight gains were evident at the highest dose level. No other effects attributable to propanil were observed (*4*).

### Reproductive toxicity, embryotoxicity, and teratogenicity

Wistar rats fed technical-grade propanil in the diet (0, 100, 300, or 1000 mg/kg) for 11 weeks before mating and pregnancy did not exhibit any alterations in reproductive parameters (*3*).

### Mutagenicity and related end-points

Propanil was inactive in *in vitro* tests on gene mutation, mitotic recombination, and repair and damage of DNA in prokaryotic and eukaryotic cells (*4, 5*). It gave results that were essentially negative in the cytogenetic test on mice (induction of structural chromosomal aberrations) (*4, 6*) and positive in radical apex barley cells (*7*). Its metabolite 3,3',4,4'-tetrachloroazobenzene induces gene mutations in bacteria and fungal cells, as well as DNA repair synthesis in hepatic cultures in the rat (*4, 5, 8*).

### Carcinogenicity

In a study in which groups of 50 Wistar rats were given oral propanil doses of 100, 400, or 1600 mg/kg for 24 months, histopathological tests did not reveal any carcinogenic effects. However, this study was limited and does not allow the evaluation of the carcinogenic potential of propanil (4).

## 15.27.6 Effects on humans

The probable oral lethal dose is 0.5–5 g/kg of body weight. Exposure produces local irritation and central nervous system depression. Ingestion causes local irritation with a burning sensation in the mouth, oesophagus, and stomach, gagging, coughing, nausea, and vomiting followed by headache, dizziness, drowsiness, and confusion.[1]

Workers from a pesticide plant who were exposed to the propanil metabolite 3,4-dichloroaniline showed signs of methaemoglobinaemia. Of the 28 workers exposed to 3,4-dichloroaniline and propanil, 17 showed signs of chloracne, which is attributed to the presence of the contaminants 3,3′,4,4′-tetrachloroazobenzene or 3,3′,4,4′-tetrachloroazoxybenzene (9).

## 15.27.7 Guideline value

Propanil is not considered to be genotoxic. However, at least one of its environmental metabolites (tetrachloroazobenzene) is genotoxic. Data from a limited study in rats do not provide evidence of carcinogenicity.

Long-term exposure to propanil results in red blood cell toxicity. A TDI of 5 µg/kg of body weight was established, based on the NOAEL of 5 mg/kg of body weight per day from the 3-month rat feeding study (4) and applying an uncertainty factor of 1000 (100 for intra- and interspecies variation and 10 for the short duration of the study and the limitations of the database).

Based on an allocation of 10% of the TDI to drinking-water, the guideline value is 20 µg/litre (rounded figure). In applying this guideline, authorities should consider the possible presence in water of more toxic environmental metabolites.

## References

1. Worthing CR, ed. *The pesticide manual*, 9th ed. Farnham, British Crop Protection Council, 1991.

2. Cabras P et al. Herbicide residues in waste waters from ricefields. *Pesticide science*, 1983, 14:130-134.

---

[1] Source: Hazardous Substances Data Bank. Bethesda, MD, National Library of Medicine.

3.  US National Research Council. *Drinking water and health.* Washington, DC, 1977.

4.  *Project Summary 600/53-83-097.* Philadelphia, PA, Rohm and Haas Co., 1983-84 (registration documents submitted to the Italian Ministry of Health).

5.  Waters MD et al. Study of pesticide genotoxicity. *Basic life science,* 1982, 21:275-326.

6.  Pilinskaja MA et al. Pervičnaja ocenka citogenetičeskoj aktivnosti i potencial'noj mutagennoj opasnosti 22 pesticidov. [Primary evaluation of the cytogenetic activity and potential mutagenic hazard of 22 pesticides.] *Citologija i genetika,* 1980, 14(6):41-47 (English abstract).

7.  Das K et al. Cytological aberrations induced by Lasso, Machete & Stam F-34 in barley *Hordeum vulgare. Indian journal of experimental biology,* 1978, 16:446-449.

8.  Gilbert P et al. Genetic effects of chlorinated anilines and azobenzenes on *Salmonella typhimurium. Archives of environmental contamination and toxicology,* 1980, 9(5):533-541.

9.  Morse DL et al. Propanil-chloracne and methomyl toxicity in workers of a pesticide manufacturing plant. *Clinical toxicology,* 1979, 15(1):13-21.

# 15.28 Pyridate

## 15.28.1 General description

### *Identity*

CAS no.:                   55512-33-9
Molecular formula:         $C_{19}H_{23}O_2N_2SCl$

Pyridate is the common name for *O*-(6-chloro-3-phenyl-4-pyridazinyl) *S*-octyl carbonothioate.

### *Physicochemical properties (1)*

| Property | Value |
|---|---|
| Physical state | Colourless crystalline solid |
| Melting point | 27 °C |
| Boiling point | 220 °C |
| Vapour pressure | $1.33 \times 10^{-7}$ Pa at 25 °C |
| Water solubility | 1.5 mg/litre at 20 °C |

## Major uses

Pyridate is a foliar-acting contact herbicide used for the control of annual dicoty-ledonous plants and some grassy weeds. It controls weeds selectively in cereals, maize, rice, and other crops (*1*).

## Environmental fate

Pyridate has low water solubility and relatively low mobility. It is not persistent and is rapidly hydrolysed, photodegraded, and biodegraded. Its primary environmental metabolite (6-chloro-4-hydroxy-3-phenylpyridazine) is also not persistent but is more mobile. Under favourable conditions, the environmental half-life is of the order of a few days (*2*). Pyridate is rapidly metabolized and inactivated in plants that have a high tolerance for the active ingredient (*3*).

## 15.28.2 Analytical methods

The main pyridate metabolite, 6-chloro-4-hydroxy-3-phenylpyridazine, may be determined by high-performance liquid chromatography followed by ultraviolet absorption at 254 or 280 nm (*4*).

## 15.28.3 Environmental levels and human exposure

### Water

This compound has rarely been found in water supplies (*2*).

## 15.28.4 Kinetics and metabolism in laboratory animals and humans

After oral administration to rats, pyridate is rapidly absorbed by the gut and distributed to the organs. It is quickly excreted, mainly in the urine (*5, 6*). Three metabolites have been identified in the urine of rats, the most important being the hydrolysis product 6-chloro-4-hydroxy-3-phenylpyridazine (*7*). Pyridate is hydrolysed in the blood and in artificially prepared intestinal juices of rats (*8, 9*).

## 15.28.5 Effects on laboratory animals and *in vitro* test systems

### Acute exposure

The acute $LD_{50}$ for rats was reported to be 2000 mg/kg of body weight (*1*).

## Short-term exposure

The technical product (purity 90.3%) was administered in the diet to pure-bred beagle dogs for 1 year at doses of 0, 60, 240, or 2000 mg/kg, corresponding to about 0, 2, 8, and 77 mg/kg of body weight per day, without causing death. Dose-related vomiting and diarrhoea were observed in all groups; erythemas and alopecia were observed in some animals. At the highest dose, decreased adrenal weight, increased thyroid weight, decreased alpha-globulin, albumin, and lactate dehydrogenase, and increased platelet number were observed. From this study, a NOAEL of 8 mg/kg of body weight per day has been identified (*10*).

## Long-term exposure

The technical product (90.3% purity) was administered to Wistar SPF rats for 2 years in the diet at doses of 0, 80, 400, or 2500 mg/kg, corresponding to about 0, 3.5, 18, or 114 mg/kg of body weight per day. At the highest dose, the product caused reduced body growth, reduced food consumption, decreased trans-aminases of lacticodehydrogenasis and alkaline phosphatase, as well as increased kidney weight. At the middle dose, increased kidney weight was observed. From this study, a NOAEL of 3.5 mg/kg of body weight per day has been derived (*11*).

In a 2-year study, the product was administered to Swiss mice in the diet at doses of 0, 200, 1000, or 5000 mg/kg, corresponding to about 0, 24, 120, and 600 mg/kg of body weight per day. Mortality ranged from 24% to 52% and was lower in animals receiving the highest dose. The product caused decreased body growth in both sexes at the highest dose, as well as an increased relative weight of the liver in males at the middle and high doses. From this study, a NOAEL of 24 mg/kg of body weight per day was identified (*12*).

## Reproductive toxicity, embryotoxicity, and teratogenicity

In a three-generation study, Wistar rats were fed technical pyridate in their diets at doses of 0, 80, 400, or 2500 mg/kg. No changes in the reproductive cycle were observed (*13*). In two studies conducted on rats and rabbits, pyridate was found not to possess teratogenic potential (*14, 15*).

## Mutagenicity and related end-points

Pyridate does not induce gene mutations in bacteria, somatic mutation in mice, DNA repair synthesis in rat hepatocyte cultures, loss of X and Y chromosomes in *Drosophila*, micronuclei in mice, or transformation *in vitro* (*16–21*).

## Carcinogenicity

In a study in which the technical product (90.3% purity) was administered to Wistar SPF rats in the diet for 2 years at doses of 0, 80, 400, or 2500 mg/kg (0,

3.5, 18, or 114 mg/kg of body weight per day), non-dose-related excesses of benign and malignant phaeochromocytomas in males, mammary fibroadenomas in females, and thyroid adenomas in both sexes were observed (*11*). No excesses of tumours of any type were observed when the product was administered to Swiss mice at doses of 0, 200, 1000, or 5000 mg/kg in the diet (0, 24, 120, or 600 mg/kg of body weight per day) (*12*).

## 15.28.6 Guideline value

IARC has not evaluated pyridate. It has been tested in long-term feeding studies in rats and mice; no evidence of carcinogenicity was noted in either species. The available evidence indicates that it is not genotoxic.

A NOAEL of 3.5 mg/kg of body weight per day was established based on increased kidney weight in a 2-year study on rats (*11*). A TDI of 35 µg/kg of body weight was calculated by applying an uncertainty factor of 100 (for intra- and interspecies variation) to this NOAEL. An allocation of 10% of the TDI to drinking-water gives a guideline value of 100 µg/litre (rounded figure).

## References

1.  Worthing CR, ed. *The pesticide manual*, 9th ed. Farnham, British Crop Protection Council, 1991.

2.  *Drinking water quality: guidelines for selected herbicides.* Copenhagen, WHO Regional Office for Europe, 1987 (Environmental Health 27).

3.  *The agrochemicals handbook*, 3rd ed. Cambridge, Royal Society of Chemistry, 1991.

4.  *Method of analysis for determination of 6-chloro-4-hydroxy-3-phenylpyridazine in leaching water.* Linz, Chemie Linz, 1981 (unpublished study submitted to WHO).

5.  Österreichische Studiengesellschaft für Atomenergie, Institute of Biology, Seibersdorf Research Centre. *Orientating kinetic trials with $^{14}C$-pyridate.* Linz, Chemie Linz, 1978 (unpublished study submitted to WHO).

6.  Österreichische Studiengesellschaft für Atomenergie, Institute of Biology, Seibersdorf Research Centre. *Distribution of $^{14}C$-pyridate after single oral application in rats.* Linz, Chemie Linz, 1979 (unpublished study submitted to WHO).

7.  *Excretion of $^{14}C$-metabolites in urine of rats after repeated oral administration of $^{14}C$-pyridate.* Linz, Chemie Linz, 1980 (unpublished study submitted to WHO).

8.  *Life time of $^{14}C$-pyridate in blood of rats.* Linz, Chemie Linz, 1980 (unpublished study submitted to WHO).

9. *Investigation of the enzymatic decomposition of pyridate in artificial gastric and intestinal juice with* [14]*C-labelled pyridate.* Linz, Chemie Linz, 1979 (unpublished study submitted to WHO).

10. *12 months oral (feeding) toxicity study with pyridate in dogs.* Linz, Chemie Linz, 1982 (unpublished study submitted to WHO).

11. TNO. *Chronic/carcinogenicity study (I-II). Rats (pb: WU Wistar).* Linz, Chemie Linz, 1983 (unpublished study submitted to WHO).

12. TNO. *Carcinogenicity study. Mice (Cpb-Swiss random).* Linz, Chemie Linz, 1983 (unpublished study submitted to WHO).

13. TNO. *Multigeneration study with pyridate in rats.* Linz, Chemie Linz, 1982 (unpublished study submitted to WHO).

14. Institute of Biology, Seibersdorf Research Centre. *Teratological investigations of pyridate on rats.* Linz, Chemie Linz, 1978 (unpublished study submitted to WHO).

15. Institute of Biology, Seibersdorf Research Centre. *Teratological investigations of pyridate on rabbits.* Linz, Chemie Linz, 1978 (unpublished study submitted to WHO).

16. Huntington Research Centre. *Ames metabolic activation test to assess the potential mutagenic effects of pyridate.* Linz, Chemie Linz, 1978 (unpublished study submitted to WHO).

17. Litton Bionetics Inc. *Mutagenicity evaluation of pyridate in the somatic cell mutation assay (spot-test).* Linz, Chemie Linz, 1980 (unpublished study submitted to WHO).

18. Litton Bionetics Inc. *Evaluation of pyridate in the primary rat hepatocyte unscheduled DNA synthesis assay.* Linz, Chemie Linz, 1981 (unpublished study submitted to WHO).

19. Litton Bionetics Inc. *Mutagenicity evaluation of pyridate in the test for losses of X- or Y-chromosomes in Drosophila melanogaster.* Linz, Chemie Linz, 1980 (unpublished study submitted to WHO).

20. Huntington Research Centre. *Micronucleus test on pyridate.* Linz, Chemie Linz, 1978 (unpublished study submitted to WHO).

21. Huntington Research Centre. *Pyridate cell transformation test.* Linz, Chemie Linz, 1978 (unpublished study submitted to WHO).

## 15.29 Simazine

### 15.29.1 General description

#### *Identity*

CAS no.:            122-34-9
Molecular formula:   $C_7H_{12}ClN_5$

Simazine is the common name for 6-chloro-$N,N'$-diethyl-1,3,5-triazine-2,4-di-ylamine.

#### *Physicochemical properties* (1–3)

| | |
|---|---|
| Melting point | 225–227 °C (decomposes) |
| Density | 1.302 g/cm³ at 20 °C |
| Water solubility | 5 mg/litre at 20 °C |
| Vapour pressure | 8.1 x 10⁻⁴ Pa at 20 °C |
| Log octanol–water partition coefficient | 2.1 |

#### *Major uses*

Simazine is a pre-emergence herbicide used to control broad-leaved and grass weeds in artichokes, asparagus, berries, broad beans, citrus fruits, coffee, cocoa, hops, maize, oil palms, olives, orchards, ornamentals, sugar-cane, tea, tree nurseries, turf, and vineyards, as well as in non-crop areas (1).

#### *Environmental fate*

Under normal climatic conditions, volatilization and photodegradation are not expected to be important processes in the dissipation of simazine from soil (2).[1] Its half-life in soil has been reported as 46–174 days (3). Simazine can be degraded through hydrolysis and N-dealkylation (4, 5). It is mineralized slowly.[1] Even though it has a low solubility in water, it has been classified as a leacher (6).

### 15.29.2 Analytical methods

Simazine can be determined by a capillary column gas chromatographic method applicable to the determination of certain nitrogen/phosphorus-containing pesticides in water. In this method, the sample is extracted with methylene chloride, the extract is concentrated, and the compounds are separated by capillary-column gas chromatography, after which they are measured by means of a nitrogen–phosphorus detector. The estimated detection limit is 75 ng/litre (7).

---

[1] Source: Hazardous Substances Data Bank. Bethesda, MD, National Library of Medicine.

### 15.29.3 Environmental levels and human exposure

**Water**

Typical levels of 1–2 µg/litre have been reported in groundwater in the USA (8). Contamination of groundwater by simazine has also been reported in Italy and Germany (9, 10).

### 15.29.4 Kinetics and metabolism in laboratory animals and humans

Simazine is absorbed by the gut of rats and mice and distributed to various tissues; the highest concentrations are found in the spleen, liver, and kidney (11). In 24-h urine samples from female rats given simazine orally, conjugated mercapturates of hydroxysimazine, 2-hydroxy-4-amino-6-ethylamino-s-triazine, and 2-hydroxy-4,6-diamino-s-triazine were found, accounting for 6.8%, 6.1%, and 14% of the administered dose, respectively (12). In 24-h urine samples from male rats that had received simazine by gavage, the di-*N*-dealkylated metabolites were present at higher levels than the mono-*N*-dealkylated ones (13). Following oral administration in rats, most simazine was excreted within 7 days, mainly in the urine (11).

### 15.29.5 Effects on laboratory animals and *in vitro* test systems

**Acute exposure**

Oral $LD_{50}$s for simazine have been reported to be greater than 5000 mg/kg of body weight in the rat, mouse, and rabbit (1, 2).

**Long-term exposure**

Dogs (2 per sex per dose) were treated orally for 105 weeks with 0, 15, 150, or 1500 mg of simazine per kg of feed. No deaths or evident toxic effects were caused by the treatment, apart from a transitory increase in aspartate aminotransferase in two out of four animals at the highest dose. The NOAEL was 150 mg/kg, corresponding to 5 mg/kg of body weight per day (14).

Dogs (4 per sex per dose) were treated for 2 years with doses of 0, 20, 100, or 1250 mg/kg in the diet. At the highest dose, the treatment caused cachexia in one animal of each sex, as well as reduced weight gain in one female, accompanied by a transitory reduction in food consumption. There was also a reduction in erythrocyte parameters in both males and females and an increase in thrombocytes in males. At 100 mg/kg, there were both reduced weight gain and reduced erythrocyte parameters in females. From this study, a NOAEL of 20 mg/kg, corresponding to 0.8 mg/kg of body weight per day, can be derived (15).

Technical simazine (purity not specified) was administered orally for 2 years at doses of 0, 10, 100, or 1000 mg/kg of feed to Sprague-Dawley rats (70 per sex per dose; satellite groups were used in order to study chronic toxicity). The NOAEL for this study was 10 mg/kg (0.52 mg/kg of body weight per day), based on weight changes and haematological parameters (16).

## Reproductive toxicity, embryotoxicity, and teratogenicity

No reproductive effects were observed in a three generation study in which technical simazine was administered to rats at doses up to 100 mg/kg of feed (17). In studies on rats and rabbits, the compound was not embryotoxic or teratogenic when administered at doses that were not maternally toxic (18, 21).

## Mutagenicity and related end-points

Simazine did not induce micronuclei in mice. It induced a small increase in the frequency of sister chromatid exchange in human cells *in vitro* but not in Chinese hamster cells. It also induced chromosomal aberrations in plants and dominant lethal mutations in *Drosophila*, but not aneuploidy in yeast or gene conversion or mitotic recombination in bacteria (22).

## Carcinogenicity

Technical simazine (purity not specified) was administered orally for 2 years at doses of 0, 10, 100, or 1000 mg/kg of feed to Sprague-Dawley rats (70 per sex per dose). At the end of the experiment, the numbers surviving were, in order of increasing dose, 27, 24, 31, and 42 in males and 24, 23, 17, and 14 in females. Mortality was frequently related to tumours of the hypophysis, which were observed more often in the females; there were no significant differences between the various treated groups and the controls. In the females treated at 100 and 1000 mg/kg, there was an increase in mammary tumours with, in order of increasing dose: adenomas and fibroadenomas, 24/70, 31/70, 70/70, 45/70; and carcinomas, 14/70, 13/70, 19/70, 35/70. In the group receiving 1000 mg/kg, an increase in cystic glandular hyperplasia was observed. In the males, there was an increase in adenomas and carcinomas of the liver: 1/70, 3/70, 4/70, 6/70; a decrease in pancreatic tumours: 4/70, 14/70, 1/70, 0/70; and a decrease in benign phaeochromocytomas: 12/70, 14/70, 10/70, 3/70. The NOAEL from this study was 10 mg/kg (0.52 mg/kg of body weight per day) (16).

The same technical simazine was administered orally for 95 weeks at doses of 0, 40, 1000, or 4000 mg/kg to groups of Swiss CD-1 mice (60 per sex per dose) (23). At the end of the experiment, the numbers surviving were, in order of decreasing dose, 19, 15, 13, and 15 in males and 26, 26, 35, and 25 in females. There were no significant differences between the treated groups and the controls for the various types of tumours observed.

## 15.29.6 Effects on humans

A total of 124 cases of contact dermatitis were noted in the former USSR among workers manufacturing simazine and propazine. Serious cases lasting 7–10 days involved erythema, oedema and a vesiculopapular reaction that sometimes progressed to the formation of bullae (*24*). One study showed an association between ovarian tumours and exposure to triazine herbicides (*25*), but the number of subjects was small. IARC evaluated the carcinogenicity of simazine in humans and concluded that adequate data were not available (*22*).

## 15.29.7 Guideline value

Simazine does not appear to be genotoxic in mammalian systems. Recent studies have shown an increase in mammary tumours in the female rat but no effects in the mouse. IARC has classified simazine in Group 3 (*22*).

Based on a study in the rat, a NOAEL of 0.52 mg/kg of body weight per day has been established for carcinogenicity and long-term toxicity (*16*). By applying an uncertainty factor of 1000 (100 for intra- and interspecies variation and 10 for possible carcinogenicity), a TDI of 0.52 µg/kg of body weight was derived. An allocation of 10% of the TDI to drinking-water gives a guideline value of 2 µg/litre (rounded figure).

## References

1. Worthing CR, ed. *The pesticide manual,* 9th ed. Farnham, British Crop Protection Council, 1991.

2. *The agrochemical handbook,* 3rd ed. Cambridge, Royal Society of Chemistry, 1991.

3. Mauck WL, Mayer FL, Holz D. Simazine residue dynamics in small ponds. *Bulletin of environmental contamination and toxicology,* 1976, 16:1-8.

4. Sax IN, ed. *Dangerous properties of industrial materials.* New York, NY, Van Nostrand Reinhold, 1987.

5. Erickson LE, Lee KH. Degradation of atrazine and related S-triazine. *Critical reviews in environmental control,* 1989, 19:1-14.

6. Gustafson DI. Groundwater ubiquity score: a simple method for assessing pesticide leachability. *Environmental toxicology and chemistry,* 1989, 8:339-357.

7. Environmental Monitoring and Support Laboratory. *Method 507. Determination of nitrogen- and phosphorus-containing pesticides in water by gas chromatography with a nitrogen-phosphorus detector.* Cincinnati, OH, US Environmental Protection Agency, 1989.

8.  Cohen SZ et al. Potential for pesticide contamination of groundwater resulting from agricultural uses. In: Kruger RF, Seiber JN, eds. *Treatment and disposal of pesticide wastes*. Washington, DC, American Chemical Society, 1984:297-325 (ACS Symposium Series No. 259).

9.  Leistra M, Boesten JJ. Pesticide contamination in Western Europe. *Agriculture, ecosystems and environment*, 1989, 26:369-389.

10. Funari E et al. Erbicidi nelle acque destinate al consumo umano in Italia. [Herbicides in water intended for human consumption in Italy.] *Acqua aria*, 1989, 9:1011-1024.

11. Orr GR, Simoneaux BJ. *Disposition of simazine in rats*. Basle, Ciba-Geigy, 1986 (unpublished study submitted to WHO).

12. Simoneaux BJ, Sy A. *Metabolism of simazine and its metabolites in female rats*. Basle, Ciba-Geigy, 1971 (unpublished study submitted to the US Environmental Protection Agency, Washington, DC).

13. Bradway DE, Moseman RF. Determination of urinary residue levels of the *N*-dealkyl metabolites of triazine herbicides. *Journal of agricultural and food chemistry*, 1982, 30:244-247.

14. *Simazine 80 W; safety evaluation by oral administration to dogs for 104 weeks*. Basle, Ciba-Geigy, 1964 (unpublished study submitted to WHO).

15. *Chronic toxicity study in dogs*. Basle, Ciba-Geigy, 1988 (unpublished study submitted to WHO).

16. *Combined chronic toxicity/oncogenicity study in rats*. Basle, Ciba-Geigy, 1988 (unpublished study submitted to WHO).

17. *Three generation reproductive study in rats*. Basle, Ciba-Geigy, 1965 (unpublished study submitted to WHO).

18. *Reproductive study. Rat Seg. II (test for teratogenic or embryotoxic effects)*. Basle, Ciba-Geigy, 1976 (unpublished study submitted to WHO).

19. *Reproduction study. Rat Seg. II (test for teratogenic or embryotoxic effects)*. Basle, Ciba-Geigy, 1977 (unpublished study submitted to WHO).

20. *A teratology study in rats*. Basle, Ciba-Geigy, 1986 (unpublished study submitted to WHO).

21. *A teratology study of technical simazine in New Zealand white rabbits*. Basle, Ciba-Geigy, 1984 (unpublished study submitted to WHO).

22. International Agency for Research on Cancer. *Occupational exposures in insecticide application, and some pesticides.* Lyon, 1991:495-513 (IARC Monographs on the Evaluation of Carcinogenic Risks to Humans, Volume 53).

23. *Combined chronic toxicity/oncogenicity study in mice.* Basle, Ciba-Geigy, 1988 (unpublished study submitted to WHO).

24. Elizarov GP. [Occupational skin diseases caused by simazine and propazine.] *Vestnik dermatologij i venerologij*, 1972, 46(2):27-29 (in Russian).

25. Donna A et al. Triazine herbicides and ovarian epithelial neoplasms. *Scandinavian journal of work, environment and health*, 1989, 15:47-53.

# 15.30 Trifluralin

## 15.30.1 General description

### *Identity*

CAS no.: 1582-09-8
Molecular formula: $C_{13}H_{16}F_3N_3O_4$

Trifluralin is the common name for α,α,α-trifluoro-2,6-dinitro-$N$,$N$-dipropyl-$p$-toluidine.

### *Physicochemical properties* (1)

| Property | Value |
|---|---|
| Melting point | 48.5–49 °C |
| Water solubility | <1 mg/litre at 27 °C |
| Vapour pressure | $1.37 \times 10^{-2}$ Pa at 25 °C |
| Log octanol–water partition coefficient | 4.69 |

### *Major uses*

Trifluralin is a pre-emergence herbicide used for the control of annual grasses and broad-leaved weeds in beans, brassicas, cotton, groundnuts, forage legumes, orchards, ornamentals, transplanted peppers, soy beans, sugar-beet, sunflowers, tomatoes, and vineyards (*1*).

### *Environmental fate*

Trifluralin has low water solubility. It is dissipated by photodecomposition, volatilization, and biodegradation (*2–4*). Trifluralin has a high affinity for soil and is relatively immobile (*5*); the half-life is 3–18 weeks, depending on soil type and geographical location (*2*). Its degradation in soil involves a series of oxidative dealkylation steps, the reduction of the nitro group, and oxidative cyclization (*6*), resulting in the formation of small quantities of several transformation products as well as significant amounts of nonextractable soil-bound compounds that reside in the fulvic and humic acid fractions of soils (*7*).

## 15.30.2  Analytical methods

Trifluralin may be extracted with dichloromethane and determined by capillary gas chromatography with a nitrogen–phosphorus detector). The method sensitivity is 0.05 µg/litre (*8*).

## 15.30.3  Environmental levels and human exposure

### *Water*

In the USA, trifluralin was found in 172 of 2047 surface water samples and in one of 507 groundwater samples analysed. The 85th percentile of the levels in all non-zero surface water samples was 0.54 µg/litre (*9*). It was not found in 229 drinking-water supplies (mainly groundwater) analysed in Italy (*10*).

## 15.30.4  Kinetics and metabolism in laboratory animals and humans

Oral doses of trifluralin were not readily absorbed by the gastrointestinal tract of the rat. About 80% of the dose was found in the faeces, the remainder appearing in the urine. Even though unchanged trifluralin was isolated from the faeces (<8% of the administered dose), the absorbed fraction was extensively metabolized. *N*-dealkylation and nitro reduction were two of the principal metabolic pathways. The metabolic fate of trifluralin was similar in the rat and in the dog (*11*). Following intraperitoneal administration to rats, it was detected at higher concentrations in the fat than in the liver (*12*).

## 15.30.5  Effects on laboratory animals and *in vitro* test systems

### *Acute exposure*

Oral $LD_{50}$s of over 10 g/kg of body weight for rats, 0.5 g/kg of body weight for mice, and over 2 g/kg of body weight for rabbits and dogs have been reported (*1*).

### *Short-term exposure*

Beagle dogs were fed trifluralin at doses of 30, 150, or 750 mg/kg in the diet for 12 months. Effects at the highest doses included slightly decreased mean body weight gain, slight changes in plasma lipids, and a statistically significant increase in liver weight. A NOAEL of 30 mg/kg, equivalent to an average daily intake of 0.75 mg/kg of body weight, was derived, based on mild hepatic effects (*13*).

## Long-term exposure

The effects of trifluralin were studied in Fischer rats at doses of 813, 3250, or 6500 mg/kg in the diet for 24 months (*14*); in Wistar rats at doses of 200, 800, or 3200 mg/kg in the diet for 24 and 28 months (*15*); in NMRI mice at doses of 50, 200, or 800 mg/kg in the diet for 104 weeks (*16*); and in beagle dogs at doses of 400 or 1000 mg/kg in the diet for 3 years (*17*). These tests were not adequate by today's standards because of methodological limitations and contamination problems.

## Reproductive toxicity, embryotoxicity, and teratogenicity

Trifluralin is embryotoxic in the rat (*18,19*) and the rabbit (*21, 22*) at dose levels that are clearly maternally toxic; however, it is not teratogenic in these species.

## Mutagenicity and related end-points

Studies on the mutagenicity of trifluralin show that low-purity technical trifluralin may contain nitroso contaminants and is mutagenic. High-purity trifluralin, in contrast, is not (*20*).

## Carcinogenicity

Trifluralin containing the impurity nitrosodipropylamine was assayed for carcinogenicity in oral experiments on the rat and mouse (*15, 16, 23, 24*). For each species, the first experiment was carried out with trifluralin that contained large amounts of the impurity. Carcinogenic effects on the liver, lungs, and stomach in female mice were observed, as well as equivocal indications of carcinogenicity in the rat thyroid. In the second experiment in each species, the trifluralin used contained the impurity at 0.4 mg/kg, two orders of magnitude less than in the previous studies. No carcinogenic effects were found in mice. In rats, however, there was an excess, limited to males treated with high doses, of granular cellular meningiomas (a rare benign tumour whose normal occurrence in rats is unknown). The incidence of thyroid tumours was not statistically significant and was not dose-related.

On the basis of a recent evaluation, IARC concluded that there is limited evidence in experimental animals for the carcinogenicity of technical-grade trifluralin (*20*).

## 15.30.6 Effects on humans

In a study in the USA, the use of trifluralin was associated with an increased risk for non-Hodgkin lymphoma. In contrast, a study of ovarian cancer in Italy did not suggest an association with trifluralin exposure. In both studies, the numbers of exposed subjects were smaller. A larger study in the USA showed no association with leukaemia (*20*). IARC concluded that there is inadequate evidence in humans for the carcinogenicity of trifluralin (*20*).

## 15.30.7 Guideline value

IARC recently evaluated technical-grade trifluralin and assigned it to Group 3 (*27*). No evidence of carcinogenicity was found in a number of long-term toxicity/carcinogenicity studies with pure (>99%) test material. Trifluralin of high purity does not possess mutagenic properties. Technical trifluralin of low purity may contain nitroso contaminants and has been found to be mutagenic.

A NOAEL of 0.75 mg/kg of body weight per day was selected based on a 1-year feeding study in dogs (*13*). This species is the most sensitive for the mild hepatic effects on which the NOAEL was based. Using this NOAEL and an uncertainty factor of 100 (for inter- and intraspecies variation), a TDI of 7.5 µg/kg of body weight was derived. A guideline value of 20 µg/litre (rounded figure) is recommended, based on an allocation of 10% of the TDI to drinking-water.

Authorities should note that some impure technical grades of trifluralin could contain potent carcinogenic compounds and therefore should not be used.

## References

1. Worthing CR, ed. *The pesticide manual,* 9th ed. Farnham, British Crop Protection Council, 1991.

2. Sanders PF, Seiber JN. A chamber for measuring volatilization of pesticides for model soil and water disposal system. *Chemosphere,* 1983, 12:999-1012.

3. Helling CS. Dinitroaniline herbicides in soils. *Journal of environmental quality,* 1976, 5:1-15.

4. Parr JF, Smith S. Degradation of trifluralin under laboratory conditions and soil anaerobiosis. *Soil science,* 1973, 115(1):55-63.

5. *The agrochemicals handbook,* 3rd ed. Cambridge, Royal Society of Chemistry, 1991.

6. Wheeler WB et al. Trifluralin degradation and binding in soil. *Journal of agricultural and food chemistry,* 1979, 27:702-706.

7. Golab T, Occolowitz JL. Soil degradation of trifluralin; mass spectrometry of products and potential products. *Biomedical mass spectrometry*, 1979, 6:1-9.

8. Frank R et al. Survey of farm wells for pesticide residues, southern Ontario, Canada, 1981-1982, 1984. *Archives of environmental contamination and toxicology*, 1987, 16:1-8.

9. Office of Drinking Water. *Trifluralin. Health advisory.* Washington, DC, US Environmental Protection Agency, 1989.

10. Funari E, Sampaolo A. Erbicidi nelle acque potabili. [Herbicides in drinking water.] *Annali dell'Istituto Superiore di Sanità*, 1989, 25:353-362.

11. Emmerson JL, Anderson RC. Metabolism of trifluralin in the rat and dog. *Toxicology and applied pharmacology*, 1966, 9:84-97.

12. Heck HA et al. Determination and disposition of trifluralin in the rat. Separation by sequential high-pressure liquid chromatography and quantitation by field ionization mass spectrometry. *Journal of agricultural and food chemistry*, 1977, 25:901-908.

13. *12 Months oral toxicity (feeding) study in Beagle dogs.* Indianapolis, IN, Eli Lilly, 1984 (unpublished study submitted to WHO).

14. *The chronic toxicity of compound trifluralin given as a component of the diet to Fischer 344 rats for two years.* Indianapolis, IN, Eli Lilly, 1980 (unpublished study submitted to WHO).

15. *Combined chronic toxicity and carcinogenicity study in rats (24/28 months feeding study).* Frankfurt, Hoechst, 1985 (unpublished study submitted to WHO).

16. *Oncogenicity study with trifluralin in mice.* Frankfurt, Hoechst, 1986 (unpublished study submitted to WHO).

17. Worth HM et al. *Effects of trifluralin treatment on reproduction in rats and dogs.* Indianapolis, IN, Eli Lilly, 1966 (unpublished study submitted to WHO).

18. *Multiple generation study in the rat.* Indianapolis, IN, Eli Lilly, 1984 (unpublished study submitted to WHO).

19. *Testing for embryotoxicity in Wistar rats following oral administration.* Indianapolis, IN, Eli Lilly (unpublished study submitted to WHO).

20. International Agency for Research on Cancer. *Occupational exposures in insecticide application, and some pesticides.* Lyon, 1991:515-534 (IARC Monographs on the Evaluation of Carcinogenic Risks to Humans, Volume 53).

21. *Embryotoxicity study in the rabbit (oral administration).* Indianapolis, IN, Eli Lilly, 1984 (unpublished study submitted to WHO).

22. Elanco Product Company. *Teratology study in rabbits.* Indianapolis, IN, Eli Lilly, 1984 (unpublished study submitted to WHO).

23. National Cancer Institute. *Bioassay of trifluralin for possible carcinogenicity.* Bethesda, MD, 1978 (NCI Carcinogenesis Technical Report Series No. 34).

24. Donna A et al. Preliminary experimental contribution to the study of possible carcinogenic activity of two herbicides containing atrazine-simazine and trifluralin as active principles. *Pathologica*, 1981, 73:707-721.

# 15.31 Chlorophenoxy herbicides (excluding 2,4-D and MCPA)

## 15.31.1 General description

### Identity

Although many chlorophenoxy compounds are used in weed control, only dichlorprop, 2,4-DB, 2,4,5-T, fenoprop, mecoprop, and MCPB will be considered here.

| Compound | CAS no. | Molecular formula | Other names |
|---|---|---|---|
| Dichlorprop | 120-36-5 | $C_9H_8Cl_2O_3$ | 2,4-dichlorophenoxypropionic acid; 2,4-DP |
| 2,4-DB | 94-82-6 | $C_{10}H_{10}Cl_2O_3$ | 4-(2,4-dichlorophenoxy)butyric acid |
| 2,4,5-T | 93-76-5 | $C_8H_5Cl_3O_3$ | 2,4,5-trichlorophenoxyacetic acid |
| Fenoprop | 93-72-1 | $C_9H_7Cl_3O_3$ | 2,4,5-trichlorophenoxypropionic acid; 2,4,5-TP; silvex |
| Mecoprop | 93-65-2; 7085-19-0 (racemic mixture) | $C_{10}H_{11}ClO_3$ | 2(2-methyl-4-chlorophenoxy)propionic acid; MCPP |
| MCPB | 94-81-5 | $C_{11}H_{13}ClO_3$ | 4(2-methyl-4-chlorophenoxy)butyric acid |

## Physicochemical properties (1)

| Compound | Melting point (°C) | Water solubility (mg/litre) | Vapour pressure |
|---|---|---|---|
| Dichlorprop | 116–118 | 350 at 20 °C | Negligible |
| 2,4-DB | 117–119 | 46 at 25 °C | Negligible |
| 2,4,5-T | 153 | 150 at 25 °C | $1 \times 10^{-5}$ Pa at 25 °C |
| Fenoprop | 179–181.6 | 140 at 25 °C | Practically nonvolatile |
| Mecoprop | 94–95 | 620 at 20 °C | $<1 \times 10^{-5}$ Pa at 20 °C |
| MCPB | 100 | 44 at 20 °C | $<1 \times 10^{-5}$ Pa at 20 °C |

## Major uses

Chlorophenoxy herbicides are used extensively throughout the world for the control of broad-leaved annual and perennial weeds in a variety of agricultural crops. They are also used in brush control in non-agricultural areas, to control broad-leaved aquatic weeds, and as a pre-harvest treatment to reduce early drop in apple orchards. Chlorophenoxy herbicides are usually applied post-emergence, often in combination with other herbicides.

Chlorophenoxy compounds are derived from chlorophenols, which may be contaminated by dioxins; the herbicide preparations, especially those containing the trichlorophenoxy acids, may therefore also be contaminated by dioxins.

## Environmental fate

Residues of chlorophenoxy herbicides in the environment are the consequence of the direct application of these compounds to agricultural and non-agricultural areas. Biodegradation is the primary route of elimination from the environment; photolysis and hydrolysis also contribute to their removal.

The half-life for the degradation of dichlorprop to 2,4-dichlorophenol in soil is estimated to be 8–12 days (2–4); disappearance is essentially complete in 14 days (5). The degradation half-life of 2,4,5-T in soil is 12–59 days (2, 4); residues do not usually persist beyond one growing season (3). Reported half-lives of fenoprop are in the range 8–17 days (2, 3, 6) to 3–4 months (7). The primary degradation product of 2,4,5-T and fenoprop is 2,4,5-trichlorophenol (1, 8). Mecoprop is broken down in soil to 4-chloro-2-methylphenol (1), with a half-life of 7–9 days (9); residues of mecoprop have been reported to persist in soil for up to 2 months following application (10). The half-life of MCPB in soil is 4–6 days (3, 9), unless the soil microorganisms have been acclimatized to the herbicide, in which case its half-life is less than 1 day (3). MCPB degrades in soil to MCPA (9) and 4-chloro-2-methylphenol (1). The half-life of 2,4-DB in soil is less than 7 days (1).

The chlorophenoxy herbicides are considered to have only marginal potential for leaching to groundwater (11). In basic waters, phenoxy herbicide esters are hydrolysed to the anionic forms; in acidic waters, photodegradation or vaporization predominates, depending on the ester. The photolytic half-life of 2,4,5-T in near-surface waters has been calculated to be 15 days (*12*). Fenoprop was essentially cleared from three Louisiana ponds within 5 weeks of treatment (*13*).

## 15.31.2 Analytical methods

Common methods for the determination of chlorophenoxy herbicides in water include solvent extraction, separation by gas chromatography, gas–liquid chromatography, thin-layer chromatography, or high-performance liquid chromatography, with electron capture or ultraviolet detection. Detection limits range from 1 µg/litre to 1 mg/litre (*8, 14*). Specific ion monitoring mass spectroscopy can be used for confirmation (*8*). Chemical derivatization of chlorophenoxy acids and salts is often necessary, as they are practically nonvolatile and too polar to chromatograph directly (*15*).

## 15.31.3 Environmental levels and human exposure

### *Air*

Chlorophenoxy herbicides may be transported in the atmosphere in the form of droplets, vapour, or powder following application by spraying. Concentrations of particles of 2,4,5-T of up to approximately 0.045 µg/m$^3$ in air have been found in Pullman, Washington, whereas up to 0.04 mg/kg 2,4,5-T was present in a dust sample collected in Cincinnati, OH (*16*).

### *Water*

Mecoprop was not detected in a survey of 91 farm wells in Ontario (Canada) during 1984 (detection limit 0.1 µg/litre) (*17*). 2,4,5-T was not detected in 602 samples of private and municipal drinking-water supplies in 90 communities in three Canadian provinces surveyed from 1978 to 1986 (detection limits 0.005–0.05 µg/litre) (*18*). Fenoprop was detected in only a small number of drinking-water supplies in several national and regional surveys in the USA (detection limits not specified) (*7*).

In 1984, 2,4,5-T was detected in groundwater near a dump in New Brunswick (Canada) at a concentration of 3.7 µg/litre (*18*). In other studies, 2,4,5-T concentrations as high as 17 µg/litre have been reported in groundwater (*19*). Groundwater in the Netherlands was found to contain a maximum concentration of 2 µg of mecoprop per litre (*20*). Most groundwaters surveyed in the USA contained less than 0.1 µg of fenoprop per litre (*7*).

In a survey of three Canadian agricultural river basins, dichlorprop, mecoprop, 2,4-DB, and MCPB were found in 4%, 3%, 0.5%, and 0%, respectively, of 447 surface water samples at mean concentrations of 0.1–3.1 µg/litre (detection limits 0.1–0.5 µg/litre) (*21*). Concentrations of 2,4,5-T in 1548 samples of

Canadian surface waters surveyed from 1980 to 1985 ranged from not detectable to 0.04 µg/litre (detection limit 0.01 µg/litre); concentrations of fenoprop in 1339 surface water samples from western Canada were less than 4 ng/litre (22). Surface water in the Netherlands has been found to contain maximum mecoprop and MCPB concentrations of 1–10 µg/litre; a maximum concentration of 0.1 µg of mecoprop per litre was found in infiltrated river bank water (20).

### Food

Chlorophenoxy herbicides may be present in food as a result of their direct application to crops; however, concentrations are normally low (16). In a Canadian total diet study conducted from 1976 to 1978, MCPB, 2,4,5-T, and fenoprop were not detected (detection limits 300, 100, and 50 µg/kg, respectively) (23). Neither 2, 4, 5-T nor 2, 4-DB was detected in a survey of 14 492 domestic and imported foods in the USA in 1987 (24). Dichlorprop was present at levels of up to 0.1 mg/kg in cereal grains at harvest time (25).

### Estimated total exposure and relative contribution of drinking-water

Based on maximum residue limits for 2,4,5-T established by the Codex Alimentarius Commission (26), the theoretical maximum daily intake of 2,4,5-T from food ranges from 10.8 to 68.8 µg/day, with a global mean of 24.6 µg/day for a 60-kg adult. The average daily intake of 2,4,5-T in food is estimated to be 0.2 ng/kg of body weight per day for a male or female aged 25–30, based on the concentrations found in foods in the USA (27).

## 15.31.4 Kinetics and metabolism in laboratory animals and humans

In general, chlorophenoxy herbicides are rapidly absorbed from the gastrointestinal tract (28) and evenly distributed throughout the body; accumulation in human tissues is not expected (6). A steady-state level in the human body will be achieved within 3–5 days of exposure (6). The herbicides are eliminated mainly in the urine, mostly unchanged, although fenoprop may be conjugated to a significant extent (29). Biological half-lives of chlorophenoxy herbicides in mammals range from 10 to 33 h; between 75% and 95% of the ingested amount is excreted within 96 h (28). Dogs appear to retain chlorophenoxy acids longer than other species as a result of relatively poor urinary clearance and thus may be more susceptible to their toxic effects (29). Metabolic conversions occur only at high doses. The salt and ester forms are rapidly hydrolysed and follow the same pharmacokinetic pathways as the free acids (28).

## 15.31.5 Effects on laboratory animals and *in vitro* test systems

### *Dichlorprop*

*Acute exposure*

The oral $LD_{50}s$ of dichlorprop in rats and mice are 800 and 309 mg/kg of body weight, respectively (*30*).

*Short-term exposure*

Slight liver hypertrophy was seen in rats receiving a dietary dose of 50 mg of dichlorprop per kg of body weight per day for 3 months; no adverse effects were noted in rats consuming 12.4 mg/kg of body weight per day (*1*).

*Long-term exposure*

In a 2-year study in Fischer 344 rats (80 per sex per dose), animals were fed diets containing 0, 100, 300, 1000, or 3000 mg of dichlorprop per kg. At 3000 mg/kg, survival was slightly reduced in females; body weight was depressed by 10% in both males and females; there was diffuse hepatocellular swelling and deposition of brown pigment in liver cells; and rats exhibited mild anaemia, as indicated by decreased haematocrit, erythrocyte count, and haemoglobin. The incidence of brown pigment in the kidneys was increased in both sexes in the 1000 and 3000 mg/kg groups, possibly indicative of slight degeneration of the tubular epithelium. Urinary specific gravity and protein were decreased in males exposed to 300 mg/kg and in females exposed to 1000 mg/kg. The authors considered the NOAEL for renal toxicity to be 100 mg/kg (3.64 mg/kg of body weight per day) in males and 300 mg/kg (13.1 mg/kg of body weight per day) in females (*31*).

*Reproductive toxicity, embryotoxicity, and teratogenicity*

No adverse effects on reproduction or fertility were reported in a three-generation reproduction study in which groups of rats were fed diets containing 125, 500, or 2000 mg of dichlorprop per kg (*32*). In a study in which doses of 0, 100, 200, 300, 400, or 500 mg of dichlorprop per kg of body weight were orally administered to pregnant mice on days 6–15 of pregnancy, embryotoxic effects were observed at 300 mg/kg of body weight, and skeletal malformations occurred at 400 mg/kg of body weight (*33*). No toxic effects were reported in a summary of a study in which pregnant rats were given doses of 0, 5, 30, 100, or 200 mg of dichlorprop per kg of body weight by gavage on days 4, 10, 13, and 18, although it was shown to cross the placental barrier (*34*).

*Mutagenicity and related end-points*

Dichlorprop was not mutagenic in eight strains of *Salmonella typhimurium* in the absence of mammalian metabolic activation (*35*). However, it induced respiration-defective mutant cells of *Saccharomyces cerevisiae* (*36*) and caused mitotic gene conversion and gene mutation in *S. cerevisiae* (*37, 38*) and DNA damage in

*Escherichia coli* (*39*) at concentrations of 4.0 mg/ml or greater. Dichlorprop did not significantly influence testicular DNA synthesis in male mice following a single intraperitoneal dose of 200 mg/kg of body weight (*40*).

### Carcinogenicity

In an 18-month carcinogenicity study, Charles River CD-1 mice were fed diets containing 0, 25, 100, or 300 mg of dichlorprop per kg. The incidence of benign hepatomas was increased in males in the highest dose group, but the authors speculated that this was due to an increased metabolic burden on the liver, which impaired the metabolic process necessary for the suppression of neoplastic development; they concluded that dichlorprop was not carcinogenic at the doses administered (*41*).

## 2,4-DB

### Acute exposure

The oral $LD_{50}$ of 2,4-DB in rats is 700 mg/kg of body weight (*30*).

### Short-term exposure

Beagle dogs (4 per sex per dose) were fed diets containing 0, 316, 1000, or 3160 mg of 2,4-DB per kg for 2 weeks, then given the compound in capsules daily for 7 weeks at doses equivalent to 0, 8, 25, or 80 mg/kg of body weight per day. An additional group of 4 males and 4 females were given capsules containing the equivalent of 2.5 mg/kg of body weight per day for 13 weeks. At 25 and 80 mg/kg of body weight per day, effects on animals included diarrhoea, inactivity, depression, weakness, cysts, increased mortality, reduced body weight and food consumption, haematological effects, abnormal blood chemistry and urinalysis, jaundice, increased relative thyroid, liver, spleen, and kidney weights, and decreased relative testes weight. At 8 mg/kg of body weight per day, serum alanine aminotransferase was elevated and nodular lymphoid hyperplasia of the gastric mucosa occurred in one of four males and one of four females (both with gross lesions). The NOAEL was considered to be 2.5 mg/kg of body weight per day (Department of National Health and Welfare, Canada, unpublished data, 1973).

In a study in which groups of Charles River rats were fed diets containing 0, 100, 316, 1000, or 3160 mg of 2,4-DB per kg for 3 months, relative liver and kidney weights were significantly elevated in males in the 3160 mg/kg group and in females in the 1000 and 3160 mg/kg groups; a significant decrease in the relative adrenal weight in females at 3160 mg/kg was also noted. All animals consuming 1000 mg of 2,4-DB per kg and above had hepatocytic hypertrophy, as did one male and one female exposed to 316 mg/kg. The NOAEL for hepatocytic hypertrophy was considered to be 100 mg/kg, equivalent to 5 mg/kg of body weight per day (Department of National Health and Welfare, Canada, unpublished data, 1973).

*Long-term exposure*

Groups of Charles River Crl:CD (SD)BR rats were fed diets containing 0, 60, 600, or 1800 mg of 2,4-DB per kg (equivalent to doses of 0, 3, 30, or 90 mg/kg of body weight per day) for 2 years. Rats in the highest dose group exhibited adverse effects such as decreased body weight gain, lower spleen and liver weights, higher relative kidney weights, and altered blood chemistry and haematological parameters. Rats consuming 30 mg of 2,4-DB per kg of body weight per day had decreased mean body weight gain, lower mean body weights (females only), altered blood chemistry and haematological parameters (although to a lesser extent than in the highest dose group), and slightly but not significantly lower mean heart weight (males only). The NOAEL was considered to be 3 mg/kg of body weight per day (*42*).

*Reproductive toxicity, embryotoxicity, and teratogenicity*

In a two-generation reproduction study in which rats were fed diets containing 0, 60, 300, or 1500 mg of 2,4-DB per kg (equivalent to doses of 0, 3, 15, or 75 mg/kg of body weight per day), effects noted in the highest dose group included reduced ovarian weight, lower mean birth weights, slightly longer gestation periods, fewer total pups per litter at birth, greater numbers of dead pups at birth, and extremely high mortality during the lactation period. No effects on reproduction were reported in the 300 mg/kg group, although offspring had increased mean liver, spleen, and kidney weights and decreased mean thymus, heart, lung, and adrenal weights (*43*).

In a teratological study in New Zealand white rabbits, groups of pregnant does were given doses of 2.5, 12, or 60 mg of 2,4-DB per kg of body weight per day in capsules on days 5–15 or 5–20 of gestation. In the highest dose group, many rabbits lost weight, three rabbits aborted their litters before day 29, and three others resorbed their litters. No adverse effects were noted in the does in the low or intermediate dose groups. The mean body weight of live fetuses was significantly reduced in the group receiving 12 mg/kg of body weight per day. The authors concluded that 2,4-DB was not teratogenic in rabbits but had an indirect embryotoxic effect at 12 mg/kg of body weight per day (May and Baker Ltd, unpublished data, 1974).

In a study in which groups of pregnant Charles River mice were fed diets containing 0, 400, or 2000 mg of 2,4-DB per kg on days 6–15 of gestation, the number of resorption sites per dam was increased in the mice consuming 2000 mg/kg, as were the mean number of dead fetuses per female and the number of females with dead fetuses; the mean number of live fetuses per female was reduced in this group. The NOAEL for fetotoxic effects in this study has been considered to be 400 mg/kg (Department of National Health and Welfare, Canada, unpublished data, 1973), equivalent to 60 mg/kg of body weight per day (*44*).

*Mutagenicity and related end-points*
2,4-DB did not induce point mutations in *Salmonella typhimurium* (*35*) but was weakly mutagenic in the CHO/HGPRT forward mutation assay (*45*). It caused a significant increase in chromosomal aberrations in Chinese hamster ovary cells, but only in the absence of metabolic activation (*46*). No unscheduled DNA synthesis was induced in rat hepatocytes (*47*).

*Carcinogenicity*
Tumour incidence was not increased in a 2-year study in which groups of rats were fed 0, 3, 30, or 90 mg of 2,4-DB per kg of body weight per day in the diet (*42*). Except in the highest dose group, in which survival was significantly reduced, a possible dose–response relationship in the incidence of hepatocellular carcinomas was reported in male mice fed 0, 25, 250, or 750 mg of 2,4-DB per kg of diet (equivalent to doses of 0, 3.75, 37.5, and 112.5 mg/kg of body weight per day) for 78 weeks. Tumour incidence was not increased in females (*48*).

## 2,4,5-T

*Acute exposure*
The oral $LD_{50}$s for 2,4,5-T range from 100 mg/kg of body weight in the dog to 300 mg/kg of body weight in the rat and 425 mg/kg of body weight in the hamster (*30*).

*Long-term exposure*
Sprague-Dawley rats (50 per sex per dose in treated groups, 86 per sex in the control group) were fed 2,4,5-T (practically free from dioxin contamination) at doses equivalent to 0, 3, 10, or 30 mg/kg of body weight per day in the diet for 2 years. Rats of both sexes in the highest dose group had reduced body weight gain, elevated urinary excretion of porphyrins, and hepatocellular swelling and paleness. Animals in the groups receiving 10 and 30 mg/kg of body weight per day had increased relative kidney and liver weights. Dose-related increases in mineralization in the renal pelvis were noted in the kidneys of female rats fed diets containing 10 and 30 mg/kg of body weight per day. The NOAEL for reduced body weight gain, increased liver and kidney weights, and renal toxicity was considered to be 3 mg/kg of body weight per day (*49*).

*Reproductive toxicity, embryotoxicity, and teratogenicity*
In a three-generation reproduction study, Sprague-Dawley rats were fed dietary doses of dioxin-free (< 0.03 µg/kg) 2,4,5-T equivalent to 0, 3, 10, or 30 mg/kg of body weight per day. Reductions were seen in neonatal survival in the $F_2$ generation and decreases in fertility in the $F_{3b}$ litter in the group consuming 10 mg/kg of body weight per day; postnatal survival, relative liver weights, and thymus weights were reduced in several litters in the highest dose group. The NOAEL for reproductive effects was 3 mg/kg of body weight per day (*50*).

770

Results of various reproductive studies indicate that 2,4,5-T not appreciably contaminated with dioxin caused teratogenic effects (cleft palate and kidney malformations) only in mice at doses above 20 mg/kg of body weight (51,52). Some skeletal anomalies (delayed ossification) were observed in rats exposed to fetotoxic doses in excess of 50 or 100 mg/kg of body weight (53, 54). There was no teratogenic response in other studies in rats, rabbits, or monkeys (55).

*Mutagenicity and related end-points*
The results of several short-term genotoxicity tests on 2,4,5-T have been reviewed by IARC (55, 56). Negative results were obtained for several species of bacteria and yeast, but mutagenicity was observed in the yeast *Saccharomyces cerevisiae*. 2,4,5-T was not mutagenic in several *in vivo* tests in mammalian cells, including a mouse micronucleus test and dominant lethal tests in mice and rats. Chromosomal aberrations were induced in *in vitro* tests in bone marrow cells of gerbils but not in spermatogonia of Chinese hamsters. Aneuploidy was not induced in *Drosophila* or in oocytes of rats treated *in vivo*.

*Carcinogenicity*
No compound-related increase in the incidence of tumours was reported in a study in which Sprague-Dawley rats were fed doses equivalent to 0, 3, 10, or 30 mg of 2,4,5-T per kg of body weight per day in the diet for 2 years (51). 2,4,5-T was not carcinogenic when administered orally or subcutaneously in mice (55, 57). Although a significant increase in the incidence of total tumours was reported in female C3Hf mice given approximately 12 mg/kg of body weight per day for life (58), the small number of animals employed in the tests and the high incidence of spontaneous tumours in the controls suggest that the evidence for carcinogenicity in animals is inadequate (56).

## Fenoprop

*Acute exposure*
The oral $LD_{50}$ of fenoprop in rats is 650 mg/kg of body weight (30).

*Short-term exposure*
In a 90-day study in which rats were fed concentrations of 100, 300, 1000, 3000, or 10 000 mg of the sodium salt of fenoprop per kg in the diet, body weight gain was depressed at 300 mg/kg and above and liver weight was increased at 100 mg/kg; animals in all treatment groups, except females in the lowest dose group, had liver and kidney damage (59). In a study in which beagle dogs were fed doses equivalent to 53, 160, or 530 mg of fenoprop per kg of body weight for 89 days, no adverse effects were reported except for a decrease in body weight gain in females in the highest dose group (59).

771

*Long-term exposure*

In an 18-month study, rats were fed diets containing a potassium salt of fenoprop at concentrations equivalent to doses of 0, 0.26, 0.8, 2.6, or 7.9 mg/kg of body weight per day. Males in the highest dose group had reduced body weight and increased relative kidney weight. The NOAEL was considered to be 2.6 mg/kg of body weight per day (*29*). In a similar study in which male and female rats were fed the potassium salt of fenoprop in the diet at concentrations equivalent to 5.3, 16, 53, or 160 mg of fenoprop per kg of diet for 2 years, increased kidney weight was observed in males in the 160 mg/kg group. The authors concluded that the NOAEL was 53 mg/kg, equal to 3.18 mg/kg of body weight per day (*59*).

In a study in which beagle dogs were fed concentrations of 30, 101, or 300 mg of fenoprop per kg of diet as the potassium salt for 2 years, severe liver pathology was reported in both sexes in the highest dose group after 1 year and in males consuming 101 mg of fenoprop per kg of diet after 2 years. The NOAELs were considered to be 30 mg/kg in male dogs and 101 mg/kg in females, equivalent to 0.75 and 2.5 mg/kg of body weight per day, respectively (*59*).

In a 2-year study in beagle dogs, animals (4 per sex per dose) were fed diets containing the potassium salt of fenoprop at concentrations equivalent to doses of 0.9, 2.6, and 8.2 (males) or 9.9 (females) mg of fenoprop per kg of body weight per day. Adverse effects on the liver (mild degeneration and necrosis of the hepatocytes and fibroblastic proliferation) were reported in both males and females receiving the highest dose and in males receiving the intermediate dose. Females in the highest dose group had altered serum enzyme levels. The NOAEL was considered to be 0.9 mg/kg of body weight per day for males and 2.6 mg/kg of body weight per day for females (*29*).

*Reproductive toxicity, embryotoxicity, and teratogenicity*

A decrease in fetal body weight and an increase in maternal weight (probably due to increased liver weight) were observed when pregnant CD-1 mice were given 400 mg of fenoprop per kg of body weight per day by gavage or subcutaneously on days 12–15 of gestation; toxic effects appeared to be dependent on the vehicle and route of administration (*60*).

No teratogenic effects were reported in a study in which pregnant rats were given 100, 150, 200, or 300 mg of fenoprop per kg of body weight per day by gavage on days 6–15 of gestation, based on gross examination of the fetuses (Dow Chemical Company, unpublished data, 1970; cited in reference *16*). Fenoprop increased the incidence of cleft palate by 7% and 3%, respectively, for oral and subcutaneous administration (*60*). It was reported to be nonteratogenic in both the CD rat and the CD-1 mouse (dose not specified) (*61*). Significant effects on fetal mortality and birth weight were observed in litters of pregnant Sprague-Dawley rats given fenoprop (containing <0.05 mg/kg dioxin) at doses of 25–100 mg/kg of body weight per day on days 6–15 of gestation (*62*). It caused teratogenic effects on the fetuses (dose levels not specified), including skeletal anomalies such as cleft palate, retarded ossification and extra cervical ribs, microphthalmia, and cardiovascular abnormalities. Similar effects were observed in animals treated with the propylene glycol butyl ether ester of fenoprop (*62*).

*Mutagenicity and related end-points*
Fenoprop was not mutagenic in the *Salmonella typhimurium* assay (*35*).

*Carcinogenicity*
No increase in the incidence of tumours was reported in a 2-year study in which beagle dogs were fed doses of fenoprop ranging from 0.9 to 9.9 mg/kg of body weight per day in the diet (*29*). No significant increase in the incidence of tumours was noted in mice given 46.4 mg of fenoprop per kg of body weight per day initially by gavage (28 days) and subsequently in the diet for 76–77 weeks (*57*).

## Mecoprop

*Acute exposure*
The oral $LD_{50}$s for rats and mice are 650 and 369 mg/kg of body weight, respectively (*30*).

*Short-term exposure*
Weanling SPF-Wistar rats were fed diets containing 0, 50, 400, or 3200 mg of mecoprop per kg for 90 days; effects experienced at the highest dose included significantly decreased blood haemoglobin content and erythrocyte counts, a decrease in neutrophils (females only), a significant increase in alkaline phosphatase activity, and decreased relative kidney weights. Effects at 400 mg/kg included decreased relative kidney weights and significantly decreased numbers of erythrocytes. The NOAEL for effects on the kidney and blood parameters was considered to be 50 mg/kg, equivalent to 3 mg/kg of body weight per day (*63*).

Beagle dogs were fed diets containing mecoprop at concentrations equivalent to doses of 0, 4, 16, or 64 mg/kg of body weight per day for 13 weeks; effects experienced at the highest dose included depressed body weight gain, increased relative weights of heart, liver, kidney, brain, and lungs, increased blood urea levels, decreased blood haemoglobin levels (weeks 6 and 13), decreased packed cell volume and red blood cells (week 13), and decreased lymphocyte and increased neutrophil counts (week 6). Effects at 16 mg/kg of body weight per day included depressed body weight gain and a decrease in packed cell volume and red blood cell values (week 6). The NOAEL for blood parameters and body weight gain is considered to be 4 mg/kg of body weight per day (Department of National Health and Welfare, Canada, unpublished data, 1980).

In a study in which rats were fed diets containing 0, 100, 400, 1000, or 2500 mg of the diethanolamine salt of mecoprop per kg of feed for 7 months, animals consuming 400 mg/kg and above showed reduced erythrocyte counts, haemoglobin, and packed cell volume. Relative liver weight was increased in females in the 400 mg/kg group and in males in the 2500 mg/kg group. Relative kidney weights were increased in rats in all treatment groups. The NOAEL for effects on blood parameters and organ weights was 100 mg/kg of diet for the diethanolamine salt, equal to a dose of 67 mg of mecoprop per kg of diet, and equivalent to 4 mg/kg of body weight per day (*64*).

*Long-term exposure*

Male Wistar rats fed mecoprop over a period of 52 weeks at doses of 20, 100, or 400 mg/kg in the diet experienced an increase in relative kidney weights at the two highest doses. When the rats were fed the same doses for 24 months, there was a statistically significant increase in the absolute kidney weights of the males dosed at 100 and 400 mg/kg and in the relative kidney weights of those dosed at 400 mg/kg. No treatment-related effects were reported in female rats. The NOAEL of 20 mg/kg is equivalent to 1 mg/kg of body weight per day (*65*).

*Reproductive toxicity, embryotoxicity, and teratogenicity*

Groups of pregnant rats were given doses of 20, 50, or 125 mg of mecoprop per kg of body weight per day on days 6–15 of gestation. Increased intrauterine deaths, decreased crown–rump lengths, and an increased incidence of delayed or absent ossification of the sternebrae were reported in the highest dose group, although no toxic effects were noted in the dams (*66*). There were no teratogenic or fetotoxic effects in the offspring of groups of 15 pregnant rabbits receiving doses of 12, 30, or 75 mg of mecoprop per kg of body weight per day on days 6–18 of gestation (*66*). In a study in which mice were given doses of 0, 100, 200, 300, 400, 500, or 700 mg of mecoprop per kg of body weight per day by the oral route on days 6–15 of pregnancy, doses of 300 mg/kg of body weight per day and above were embryotoxic, and skeletal malformations were observed at doses of 400 mg/kg of body weight per day and above (*33*). In a summary of a study in which pregnant rats and mice were given the potassium salt of mecoprop (0–330 mg/kg of body weight per day for rats and 0–150 mg/kg of body weight per day for mice) by gavage on days 4, 10, 13, and 18, a significant increase in the number of fetuses with hydroureter was induced by the highest dose. Mecoprop was found to readily cross the placental barrier (*34*).

*Mutagenicity and related end-points*

Mecoprop was not mutagenic in reverse-mutation assays with *Salmonella typhimurium* (*35, 67*) and *Escherichia coli* (*67*). It was not mutagenic in *Streptomyces coelicolor* in the forward-mutation test (*68*), nor did it induce point mutation, nondisjunction, or mitotic crossing-over in *Aspergillus nidulans* (*69, 70*). It did induce mitotic gene conversion in yeast cultures heteroallelic at two loci (*71*).

*Carcinogenicity*
No significant increase in the incidence of tumours was reported in Wistar rats fed mecoprop in the diet at concentrations of 0, 20, 100, or 400 mg/kg for 2 years (*65*).

## MCPB

*Acute exposure*
The oral LD$_{50}$s of MCPB in rats and mice are 680 and 800 mg/kg of body weight, respectively (*30*).

*Short-term exposure*
In a 13-week study, rats were fed diets containing 0, 4, 12, or 40 mg of MCPB per kg of body weight per day. No effects on mortality, food intake, body weight gain, haematology, clinical chemistry, urinalysis, organ weights, gross pathology, or histopathology were reported. The NOAEL was considered to be 40 mg/kg of body weight per day (Department of National Health and Welfare, Canada, unpublished data, 1988). It should be noted, however, that the doses administered did not approach the maximum tolerated dose; thus, the potential short-term effects of MCPB were not fully assessed.

In a study in which beagle dogs were fed dietary concentrations of MCPB of 0, 160, 480, or 1600 mg/kg of diet for 13 weeks, no compound-related effects were reported on mortality, appearance, behaviour, food intake, body weight, haematology, clinical chemistry, urinalysis, or gross pathology. Weights of testes were depressed in males in the highest dose group; spermatogenesis was absent; the seminiferous tubules, which appeared atrophic, and the epididymis contained spermatozoal precursors and/or giant cells; and the prostate was not fully developed and appeared atrophic. The NOAEL for testicular effects was 480 mg/kg of diet, equivalent to 12 mg/kg of body weight per day (Department of National Health and Welfare, Canada, unpublished data, 1988).

*Mutagenicity and related end-points*
MCPB was not mutagenic in bacterial reverse-mutation assay systems in five strains of *Salmonella typhimurium* and one strain of *Escherichia coli* (*35, 67*). MCPB administered subcutaneously at doses of 200 mg/kg enhanced the mutation frequency of *S. typhimurium* in NMRI mice (*72*). It did not produce any deviation from normality when tested for chromosome loss, nondisjunction, or induced X–Y recombination in male *Drosophila* (*73*).

## 15.31.6 Effects on humans

### Acute exposure

Dichlorprop is rated as moderately to highly acutely toxic to humans (*74*). 2,4,5-T is considered to be moderately acutely toxic; the symptoms produced by high oral doses include nausea, vomiting, drowsiness, fever, increases in pulse and respiration rates, shock, coma, and death (75). No adverse effects were reported following the ingestion of a single dose of 1 mg of fenoprop per kg of body weight by eight human volunteers (76). The symptoms described in case histories of acute poisoning by weedkiller solutions containing mecoprop include coma, fever, respiratory problems, myotonia, muscle cramps, skeletal muscle damage, electrocardiographic changes, decreased blood pressure, distended abdomen, and rhabdomyolysis with renal failure (77–79).

## Carcinogenicity

Until recently, most epidemiological studies of the effects of chlorophenoxy herbicides dealt with populations exposed in the 1950s and 1960s, when the trichlorophenol-based herbicides 2,4,5-T and fenoprop were contaminated with polychlorinated dioxins and furans, including 2,3,7,8-tetrachlorodibenzodioxin (TCDD); the effects observed may therefore have been a consequence of the presence of the dioxin contaminants. In addition, most epidemiological studies on chlorophenoxy herbicides conducted to date have involved multiple exposures to chemical agents, including other pesticides and synthetic organic compounds.

In a series of case–referent studies conducted in Sweden in the late 1970s and early 1980s, strong associations were noted between soft tissue sarcomas (STS) and multiple lymphomas (including Hodgkin disease (HD) and non-Hodgkin lymphoma (NHL)) and the use of chlorophenoxy herbicides by agricultural or forestry workers (80–82). Although the methodology employed has been extensively criticized, these studies served to focus attention on STS, NHL, and HD as the outcomes of interest in subsequent case–referent and cohort studies.

The association between STS and chlorophenoxy herbicide use observed in the Swedish studies has not been confirmed in other case–referent studies (83–87). Although a number of cohort studies of occupationally exposed workers have been conducted, the small size of many of them limits their usefulness in assessing the relationship between STS and the herbicides.

The risk for malignant lymphoma (HD + NHL) was almost five times greater for agricultural and forestry workers exposed to a mixture of chlorophenoxy herbicides than for controls in the case–referent study in Sweden (81,88) but was not significantly elevated in a Danish cohort study of 3390 workers in a chemical plant manufacturing MCPA, dichlorprop, mecoprop, and 2,4-D, as well as other industrial chemicals and dyes (89).

Several case–referent studies suggest a weak link between chlorophenoxy herbicide use and NHL; however, concurrent exposure to other chemicals used in agriculture may contribute to this risk. In a study in Washington (576 cases of NHL), the relative risk increased from 1.1 for subjects with any past occupational exposure to chlorophenoxy herbicides, primarily 2,4-D and 2,4,5-T, to 1.7 for people occupationally exposed to such herbicides for at least 15 years (the minimum latency period) (87). In a case–referent study in Kansas (200 cases), farm herbicide use was marginally associated with NHL, with a relative risk of 1.4, which rose to 2.2 for farmers who had used chlorophenoxy herbicides at any time (almost all 2,4-D) and to 6.0 for those who had used unspecified herbicides for more than 20 days per year. The trend towards increasing risk with increasing number of days of use per year was highly significant (86). The risk for NHL (27 cases) was not elevated in a cohort of more than 20 000 Swedish pesticide applicators who applied MCPA, mecoprop, dichlorprop, and smaller amounts of 2,4-D (90). There was a slight nonsignificant trend towards a small increase in risk with increased number of years of exposure.

A nonsignificant excess in the relative risk for HD was seen in a cohort of 20 245 licensed pesticide applicators in Sweden who were exposed to MCPA, dichlorprop, mecoprop, and 2,4-D. There was a nonsignificant trend towards an increase in risk with the number of years since first licensing, with the risk increasing from 0.93 for those with 4 or fewer years to onset of disease to 2.2 for those with 10 or more years. The average follow-up time in this study was 13.9 years, a little less than the 15–20-year latency period reported for malignant lymphoma (90). In a study in Kansas, the relative risk for HD in people using herbicides (including chlorophenoxy compounds) was not elevated, nor was there evidence of a trend towards elevation of risk with increasing years of use of herbicides or frequency of use in days per year (86).

For the three end-points examined, the studies reviewed provide limited evidence that exposure to chlorophenoxy herbicides is associated with NHL rather than with HD or STS. With the exception of the early studies in Sweden (81, 88), the associations seen in most studies were weak; there was usually a less than two-fold increase in relative risk for all three outcomes.

### Reproductive effects

In cross-sectional epidemiological studies (91, 92), long-term maternal exposure to low doses of 2,4,5-T were suspected of causing miscarriages and birth defects, particularly cleft palate and neural tube defects. In similar cross-sectional studies (93–95) and a cohort study on chemical workers (96), there was no correlation between exposure of either parent to 2,4,5-T and these effects (97, 98).

## 15.31.7 Guideline values

Chlorophenoxy herbicides as a group, including 2,4-D and MCPA, have been classified by IARC in Group 2B (possibly carcinogenic to humans). However, the available data from studies in exposed populations and animals do not permit assessment of the carcinogenic potential to humans of any specific chlorophenoxy herbicide. Therefore, drinking-water guidelines for these compounds are based on a threshold approach for other toxic effects.

## Dichlorprop

Based on the 2-year study in rats (*31*), the NOAEL for renal toxicity is 100 mg/kg of diet, equal to 3.64 mg/kg of body weight per day. The TDI for dichlorprop was calculated to be 36.4 µg/kg of body weight by applying an uncertainty factor of 100 (for intra- and interspecies variation) to this NOAEL. With the allocation of 10% of the TDI to drinking-water, the guideline value is 100 µg/litre (rounded figure).

## 2,4-DB

In a 2-year study in rats, the NOAEL for effects on body and organ weights, blood chemistry, and haematological parameters was determined to be 3 mg/kg of body weight per day (*42*). This value is similar to the NOAEL of 2.5 mg/kg of body weight per day obtained in the short-term study in beagle dogs and the NOAEL for hepatocytic hypertrophy of 5 mg/kg of body weight per day obtained in a 3-month study in rats (Department of National Health and Welfare, Canada, unpublished data, 1973). A TDI of 30 µg/kg of body weight was derived using an uncertainty factor of 100 (for intra- and interspecies variation). With the allocation of 10% of the TDI to drinking-water, the guideline value is 90 µg/litre.

## 2,4,5-T

The NOAEL for reduced body weight gain, increased liver and kidney weights, and renal toxicity in a 2-year study in rats was 3 mg/kg of body weight per day (*49*). A NOAEL of 3 mg/kg of body weight per day for reproductive effects was also obtained in a three-generation study in rats (*50*). A TDI of 3 µg/kg of body weight was derived using the NOAEL from the 2-year rat study and an uncertainty factor of 1000 (100 for intra- and interspecies variation and 10 for the suggested association between 2,4,5-T and soft-tissue sarcoma and non-Hodgkin lymphoma in epidemiological studies). With the allocation of 10% of the TDI to drinking-water, the guideline value for 2,4,5-T is 9 µg/litre.

## Fenoprop

A NOAEL of 0.9 mg/kg of body weight per day for adverse effects on the liver was reported in a study in which beagle dogs were administered fenoprop in the diet for 2 years (*29*). A TDI of 3 µg/kg of body weight was derived using an uncertainty factor of 300 (100 for intra- and interspecies variation and 3 for limitations of the database). With an allocation of 10% of the TDI to drinking-water, the guideline value for fenoprop is 9 µg/litre.

## Mecoprop

A NOAEL of 1 mg/kg of body weight per day for effects on kidney weight in 1- and 2-year studies in rats (*65*) was used with an uncertainty factor of 300 (100 for intra- and interspecies variation and 3 for limitations of the database) to derive a TDI of 3.33 µg/kg of body weight. With the allocation of 10% of the TDI to drinking-water, the guideline value for mecoprop is 10 µg/litre (rounded figure).

## MCPB

Currently available toxicological data are insufficient to be used as the basis for a guideline value for MCPB in drinking-water.

## References

1. *The agrochemicals handbook*, 3rd ed. Cambridge, Royal Society of Chemistry, 1991.

2. Smith AE. Relative persistence of di- and tri-chlorophenoxyalkanoic herbicides in Saskatchewan soils. *Weed research*, 1978, 18:275.

3. Kirkland K, Fryer JD. Degradation of several herbicides in a soil previously treated with MCPA. *Weed research*, 1972, 12:90.

4. Altom JD, Stritzke JF. Degradation of dicamba, picloram and four phenoxy herbicides in soils. *Weed science*, 1973, 21:556.

5. Hance RJ. Effect of pH on the degradation of atrazine, dichlorprop, linuron and propyzamide in soil. *Pesticide science*, 1979, 10:89.

6. Associate Committee on Scientific Criteria for Environmental Quality. *Phenoxy herbicides. Their effects on environmental quality, with accompanying scientific criteria for 2,3,7,8-tetrachlorodibenzo-p-dioxin (TCDD)*. Ottawa, National Research Council of Canada, 1978.

7. US Environmental Protection Agency. Health advisory—Silvex. *Reviews of environmental contamination and toxicology*, 1988, 104:195.

8. Que Hee SS, Sutherland RG. *The phenoxyalkanoic herbicides*, Vol. I. *Chemistry, analysis, and environmental pollution*. Boca Raton, FL, CRC Press, 1981 (Chemical Rubber Company Series in Pesticide Chemistry).

9. Smith AE, Hayden BJ. Relative persistence of MCPA, MCPB and mecoprop in Saskatchewan soils, and the identification of MCPA in MCPB-treated soils. *Weed research*, 1981, 21:179.

10. Bovey RW, Young AL. *The science of 2,4,5-T and associated phenoxy herbicides.* New York, NY, John Wiley, 1980.

11. US Environmental Protection Agency. EPA draft final list of recommendations for chemicals in the national survey for pesticides in groundwater (August 1985). *Chemical regulations reporter*, 1985, 9(34):988.

12. Skurlatov YI, Zepp RJ, Baughnan GL. Photolysis rate of 2,4,5-trichlorophenoxy-acetic acid and 4-amino-3,4,6-trichloropicolinic acid in natural waters. *Journal of agricultural and food chemistry*, 1983, 31(5):1065.

13. Bailey GW et al. The degradation kinetics of an ester of silvex and the persistence of silvex in water and sediment. *Weed science*, 1970, 18:413-419.

14. Hamman R, Kettrup A. Determination of phenoxy acid herbicides in water samples. *Chemosphere*, 1987, 16(2-3):527.

15. Crompton TR. *Determination of organic substances in water*, Vol. I. Toronto, Canada, John Wiley, 1985.

16. Johnson JE. The public health implications of widespread use of the phenoxy herbicides and picloram. *Bioscience*, 1971, 21:899-905.

17. Frank R et al. Investigation of pesticide contaminations in rural wells, 1979-1984, Ontario, Canada. *Archives of environmental contamination and toxicology*, 1987, 16:9.

18. Hiebsch SC. *The occurrence of thirty-five pesticides in Canadian drinking water and surface water.* Ottawa, Department of National Health and Welfare, Environmental Health Directorate, 1988.

19. Loch JPG et al. In: Wheeler D, Richardson ML, Bridges J eds. *Watershed 89, the future for water quality in Europe*, Vol. 1. Pergamon Press, 1989:48.

20. KIWA (Netherlands Waterworks Testing and Research Institute). *Pesticides and the drinking water supply in the Netherlands.* Nieuwegein, 1990 (KIWA Report No. 113).

21. Frank R, Logan L. Pesticide and industrial chemical residues at the mouth of the Grand, Saugeen and Thames rivers, Ontario, Canada, 1981-85. *Archives of environmental contamination and toxicology*, 1988, 17:741.

22. Canadian Council of Ministers of the Environment. *Canadian water quality guidelines.* Ottawa, Environment Canada, Inland Waters Directorate, 1987.

23. McLeod HA, Smith DC, Bluman N. Pesticide residues in the total diet in Canada, V: 1976 to 1978. *Journal of food safety*, 1980, 2:141.

24. US Food and Drug Administration Pesticide Program. Residues in foods—1987. *Journal of the Association of Official Analytical Chemists*, 1988, 71(6):156A-174A

25. Goedicke HJ, Banasiak U. Fate and metabolism of dichlorprop in cereals and field grass. *Archives of environmental contamination and toxicology*, 1988, 17:81-85.

26. Codex Alimentarius Commission. *Pesticide residues in food.* Volume 2. Rome, Food and Agriculture Organization of the United Nations, 1993.

27. Gunderson EL. FDA total diet study, April 1982-April 1984, dietary intakes of pesticides, selected elements, and other chemicals. *Journal of the Association of Official Analytical Chemists*, 1988, 71(6):1200-1209.

28. Seiler JP. The genetic toxicology of phenoxy acids other than 2,4,5-T. *Mutation research*, 1978, 55:197-226.

29. Gehring PJ, Betso JE. Phenoxy acids: effects and fate in mammals. *Ecological bulletin (Stockholm)*, 1978, 27:122-133.

30. National Institute of Occupational Safety and Health. *Registry of Toxic Effects of Chemical Substances (RTECS).* Cincinnati, OH, US Department of Health and Human Services, 1978.

31. Institute of Environmental Toxicology. *2,4-DP acid 24-month oral chronic dietary study in rats.* Union Carbide, 1984 (unpublished report).

32. Calkins J, Anderson M, McElroy K. *A three generation study of 2,4-DP technical acid in rats:* HRC No. 1-361. Huntingdon Research Center, 1979 (unpublished study submitted by Union Carbide Agricultural Products Co. Inc., Research Triangle Park, NC; cited in: US Environmental Protection Agency. *Guidance for the reregistration of pesticide products containing 2,4-DP as the active ingredient.* Washington, DC, 1988).

33. Roll R, Matthiaschk G. [Comparative studies on the embryotoxicity of 2-methyl-4-chlorophenoxyacetic acid, mecoprop and dichlorprop in NMRI mice.] *Arzneimittel-Forschung*, 1983, 33:1479-1483 (in German).

34. Buschmann J et al. Comparative prenatal toxicity of phenoxyalkanoic herbicides: transplacental movement and effects on prenatal development. *Teratology*, 1986, 33:11A.

35. Anderson KJ, Leighty EG, Takahashi MT. Evaluation of herbicides for possible mutagenic properties. *Journal of agricultural and food chemistry*, 1972, 20:649-656.

36. Schubert A. Untersuchungen über die Induktion atmungsdefekter Hefemutanten durch chemische Pflanzenschutzmittel. II. [Studies on the induction of respiration-defective yeast mutants by plant protection products.] *Zeitschrift für allgemeine Mikrobiologie*, 1984, 9(6):483.

37. Naismith R, Matthews R, Godek E. *Summary data: mitotic gene conversion—Saccharomyces cerevisiae:* study no. PH-304-AM-179-2,4-DP. Pharmakon Laboratories, 1979 (unpublished study submitted by Union Carbide Agricultural Products Co. Inc., Research Triangle Park, NC; cited in: US Environmental Protection Agency. *Guidance for the reregistration of pesticide products containing 2,4-DP as the active ingredient.* Washington, DC, 1988).

38. Naismith R, Matthews R, Godek E. *Summary data: reverse mutation assay—Saccharomyces cerevisiae:* Pharmakon Laboratories, 1979 (unpublished study no. PH-303-AM-179-2,4-DP, submitted by Union Carbide Agricultural Products Co. Inc., Research Triangle Park, NC; cited in: US Environmental Protection Agency. *Guidance for the reregistration of pesticide products containing 2,4-DP as the active ingredient.* Washington, DC, 1988).

39. Naismith R, Matthews R, Godek E. Summary data: primary DNA damage: *Escherichia coli plate test.* Pharmakon Laboratories, 1979 (unpublished study submitted by Union Carbide Agricultural Products Co. Inc., Research Triangle Park, NC; cited in: US Environmental Protection Agency. *Guidance for the reregistration of pesticide products containing 2,4-DP as the active ingredient.* Washington, DC, 1988).

40. Seiler JP. Phenoxyacids as inhibitors of testicular DNA synthesis in male mice. *Bulletin of environmental contamination and toxicology,* 1979, 21(1-2):89-92.

41. CDC Research Incorporated. *Oncogenicity study in mice with 2,4-DP acid.* 1986 (unpublished study no. CDC-AM-002-77, submitted to Union Carbide, Agricultural Products Company, Research and Development Center).

42. MacKenzie KM. *Final report: lifetime dietary combined chronic toxicity and oncogenicity study in albino rats with 2,4-DB:* project no. HLA 6158-103. Hazleton Laboratories America Inc., 1987 (unpublished study submitted by 2,4-DB task force as monitored by Union Carbide Agricultural Products Co. Inc., Research Triangle Park, NC; cited in: US Environmental Protection Agency. *Guidance for the reregistration of pesticide products containing 2,4-DB as the active ingredient.* Washington, DC, 1988).

43. Bottomley AM et al. *2,4-DB effect on two generations of the rat: laboratory project ID UNC/138-R.* Hazleton Laboratories America Inc., 1987 (unpublished study submitted by Union Carbide Agricultural Products Co., Research Triangle Park, NC; cited in: US Environmental Protection Agency. *Guidance for the reregistration of pesticide products containing 2,4-DB as the active ingredient.* Washington, DC, 1988).

44. US Environmental Protection Agency. Pesticide tolerance for 4-(2,4-dichlorophenoxy)butyric acid. *Federal register,* 1986, 51(112):21188.

45. Young RR. *Final report: mutagenicity test on 2,4-DB, technical lot number RTC 5838AA in the CHO/HGPRT forward mutation assay:* HLA study no. 9360-0-435. Hazleton Laboratories America Inc., 1987 (unpublished study submitted by Union Carbide Agricultural Products Co. Inc., Research Triangle Park, NC; cited in: US Environmental Protection Agency. *Guidance for the reregistration of pesticide products containing 2,4-DB as the active ingredient.* Washington, DC, 1988).

46. Ivett JL. *Final report: mutagenicity test on 2,4-DB Tech 98.03% in an in vitro cytogenetic assay measuring chromosomal aberration frequencies in Chinese hamster ovary (CHO) cells.* Hazleton Laboratories America Inc., 1987 (unpublished study submitted by Union Carbide Agricultural Products Co. Inc., Research Triangle Park, NC; cited in: US Environmental Protection Agency. *Guidance for the reregistration of pesticide products containing 2,4-DB as the active ingredient.* Washington, DC, 1988).

47. Cifone MA. *Amended final report: mutagenicity test on 2,4-DB Technical 98.03% in the rat primary hepatocyte unscheduled DNA synthesis assay.* Hazleton Laboratories America Inc., 1987 (unpublished study submitted by Union Carbide Agricultural Products Co. Inc., Research Triangle Park, NC; cited in: US Environmental Protection Agency. *Guidance for the reregistration of pesticide products containing 2,4-DB as the active ingredient.* Washington, DC, 1988).

48. MacKenzie KM. *Final report: lifetime dietary oncogenicity study in albino mice with 2,4-DB:* project no. HLA 6158-104. Hazleton Laboratories America Inc., 1987 (unpublished study submitted by 2,4-DB task force as monitored by Union Carbide Agricultural Products Co. Inc., Research Triangle Park, NC; cited in: US Environmental Protection Agency. *Guidance for the reregistration of pesticide products containing 2,4-DB as the active ingredient.* Washington, DC, 1988).

49. Kociba RJ et al. Results of a two-year chronic toxicity and oncogenic study of rats ingesting diets containing 2,4,5-trichlorophenoxyacetic acid (2,4,5-T). *Food and cosmetics toxicology,* 1979, 17:205-221.

50. Smith FA et al. Three-generation reproduction study of rats ingesting 2,4,5-trichlorophenoxyacetic acid in the diet. *Food and cosmetics toxicology,* 1981, 19:41-45.

51. Courtney K et al. Teratogenic evaluation of 2,4,5-T. *Science,* 1970, 168:864-866.

52. Neubert D, Dillmann I. Embryotoxic effects in mice treated with 2,4,5-trichlorophenoxyacetic acid and 2,3,7,8-tetrachlorodibenzo-*p*-dioxin. *Naunyn-Schmiedeberg's archives of pharmacology,* 1972, 272:243-264.

53. Khera KS, McKinley WP. Pre- and postnatal studies on 2,4,5-trichlorophenoxyacetic acid, 2,4-dichlorophenoxyacetic acid and their derivatives in rats. *Toxicology and applied pharmacology,* 1972, 22:14-28.

54. Sparschu GL et al. Study of the effects of high levels of 2,4,5-trichlorophenoxyacetic acid on fetal development in the rat. *Food and cosmetics toxicology,* 1971, 9:527-530.

55. International Agency for Research on Cancer. *Some fumigants, the herbicides 2,4-D and 2,4,5-T, chlorinated dibenzodioxins and miscellaneous industrial chemicals.* Lyon, 1977:273-299 (IARC Monographs on the Evaluation of the Carcinogenic Risk of Chemicals to Man, Volume 15).

56. International Agency for Research on Cancer. *Overall evaluations of carcinogenicity: an updating of IARC Monographs volumes 1-42.* Lyon, 1987:156-160 (IARC Monographs on the Evaluation of Carcinogenic Risks to Humans, Suppl. 7).

57. Inne JR et al. Bioassay of pesticides and industrial chemicals for tumorigenicity in mice: a preliminary note. *Journal of the National Cancer Institute,* 1969, 42:1101-1114.

58. Muranyi-Kovacs I, Rudali G, Imbert J. Bioassay of 2,4,5-trichlorophenoxyacetic acid for carcinogenicity in mice. *British journal of cancer,* 1976, 33:626-633.

59. Mullison WR. Some toxicological aspects of silvex. In: *Proceedings of the Southern Weed Conference, 19th annual meeting.* Jackonsville, FL, 1966:420-435: (cited in: National Academy of Sciences. *Drinking water and health,* Vol. I. Washington, DC, National Research Council, 1977).

60. Courtney KD. Prenatal effects of herbicides: evaluation by the Prenatal Development Index. *Archives of environmental contamination and toxicology,* 1977, 6:33-46.

61. Moore JA, Courtney KD. Teratology studies with 2,4,5-trichlorophenoxyacetic acid and 2,3,7,8-tetrachlorodibenzo-*p*-dioxin. *Toxicology and applied pharmacology,* 1971, 20:396-403.

62. US Environmental Protection Agency. *Drinking water criteria document for 2(2,4,5-trichlorophenoxy)propionic acid (2,4,5-TP).* Washington, DC, 1987.

63. Verschuuren HG, Kroes R, Den Tonkelaar EM. Short-term oral and dermal toxicity of MCPA and MCPP. *Toxicology,* 1975, 3(3):349-359.

64. Gurd MR, Harmer GLM, Lessel B. Summary of toxicological data—acute toxicity and 7-month feeding studies with mecoprop and MCPA. *Food and cosmetics toxicology,* 1965, 3:883.

65. *Pathology report. Study on the chronic toxicity and oncogenic potential of MCPP in rats. Administration in the diet over 24 months.* Ludwigshafen/Rhein, Department of Toxicology, BASF Aktiengesselschaft, 1988 (project no. 7150047/8352).

66. US Environmental Protection Agency. *Guidance for the reregistration of pesticide products containing mecoprop (MCPP) as the active ingredient.* Washington, DC, 1988.

67. Moriya M et al. Further mutagenicity studies on pesticides in bacterial reversion assay system. *Mutation research,* 1983, 116(3-4):185-216.

68. Carere A et al. Microbial mutagenicity studies of pesticides *in vitro*. *Mutation research*, 1978, 57:277-286.

69. Bignami M et al. Mutagenic and recombinogenic action of pesticides in *Aspergillus nidulans*. *Mutation research*, 1977, 46:395-402.

70. Aulicino F et al. Mutational studies with some pesticides in *Aspergillus nidulans*. *Mutation research*, 1976, 38:138.

71. Parry JM. The induction of gene conversion in yeast by herbicide preparations. *Mutation research*, 1973, 21:83-91.

72. Buselmaier W, Rohrborn G, Propping P. [Mutagenicity studies with pesticides in the host-mediated assay and with the dominant lethal test in the mouse.] *Biologisches Zentralblatt*, 1972, 91:311-325 (in German).

73. Ramel C. The effect of phenoxyacetic acids in animals. In: *Conference on chlorinated phenoxy acids and their dioxins. Mode of action, health risks and environmental effects.* Stockholm, Royal Swedish Academy of Sciences, 1977 (cited in *28*).

74. Gosselin RE, Smith RP, Hodge HC. *Clinical toxicology of commercial products*, 5th ed. Baltimore, MD, Williams and Wilkins, 1984:II-324.

75. Hayes WJ, Jr. *Pesticides studied in man*. Baltimore, MD, Williams and Wilkins, 1982:520-577

76. Sauerhoff MW et al. Fate of silvex following oral administration to humans. *Journal of toxicology and environmental health*, 1977, 3:941-952.

77. Prescott LF, Park J, Darrien I. Treatment of severe 2,4-D and mecoprop intoxication with alkaline diuresis. *British journal of clinical pharmacology*, 1979, 7:111-116.

78. Fraser AD, Isner AF, Perry RA. Toxicologic studies in a fatal overdose of 2,4-D, mecoprop, and dicamba. *Journal of forensic science*, 1984, 29(4):1237-1241.

79. Meulenbelt J et al. Acute MCPP intoxication: report of two cases. *Human toxicology*, 1988, 7:289-292.

80. Hardell L, Sandstrom A. Case-control study: soft-tissue sarcomas and exposure to phenoxyacetic acids or chlorophenols. *British journal of cancer*, 1979, 39:711-717.

81. Hardell L et al. Malignant lymphoma and exposure to chemicals, especially organic solvents, chlorophenols and phenoxy acids: a case-control study. *British journal of cancer*, 1981, 43:169-176.

82. Eriksson M et al. Soft-tissue sarcomas and exposure to chemical substances: a case-referent study. *British journal of industrial medicine*, 1981, 38:27-33.

83. Smith AH et al. Soft tissue sarcoma and exposure to phenoxyherbicides and chloro-phenols in New Zealand. *Journal of the National Cancer Institute*, 1984, 75(5):1111-1117.

84. Smith AH, Pearce NE. Update on soft tissue sarcoma and phenoxyherbicides in New Zealand. *Chemosphere*, 1986, 15(9-12):1795.

85. Vineis P et al. Phenoxy herbicides and soft-tissue sarcomas in female rice weeders. A population-based case-referent study. *Scandinavian journal of work, environment and health*, 1987, 13:9-17.

86. Hoar SK et al. Agricultural herbicide use and risk of lymphoma and soft-tissue sarco-ma. *Journal of the American Medical Association*, 1986, 256(9):1141-1147.

87. Woods JS et al. Soft tissue sarcoma and non-Hodgkin's lymphoma in relation to phenoxyherbicide and chlorinated phenol exposure in Western Washington. *Journal of the National Cancer Institute*, 1987, 78(5):899-910.

88. Hardell L. Relation of soft-tissue sarcoma, malignant lymphoma and colon cancer to phenoxy acids, chlorophenols and other agents. *Scandinavian journal of work, envi-ronment and health*, 1981, 7:119-130.

89. Lynge E. A follow-up study of cancer incidence among workers in manufacture of phenoxy herbicides in Denmark. *British journal of cancer*, 1985, 52:259-270.

90. Wirklund K, Holm LE. Dich J. Risk of soft tissue sarcoma, Hodgkin's disease and non-Hodgkin lymphoma among Swedish licensed pesticide applicators. *Chemo-sphere*, 1989, 18(1-6):395.

91. Field B, Kerr C. Herbicide use and incidence of neural-tube defects. *Lancet*, 1979, i:1341-1342 (letter).

92. US Environmental Protection Agency. *Report of assessment of a field investigation of six-year spontaneous abortion rates in three Oregon areas in relation to forest 2,4,5-T spray practices*. Washington, DC, 1979 (Alsea 11 report).

93. Thomas HF. 2,4,5-T use and congenital malformation rates in Hungary. *Lancet*, 1980, ii:214-215 (letter).

94. Nelson CJ et al. Retrospective study of the relationship between agricultural use of 2,4,5-T and cleft palate occurrence in Arkansas. *Teratology*, 1979, 19:377-383.

95. Hanify JA et al. Aerial spraying of 2,4,5-T and human birth malformations: an epidemiological investigation. *Science*, 1981, 212:349-351.

96. Townsend JC et al. Survey of reproductive events of wives of employees exposed to chlorinated dioxins. *American journal of epidemiology*, 1982, 115(5):695-713.

97. Food and Agriculture Organization of the United Nations. *Pesticide residues in food—1981 evaluations.* Rome, 1982 (Joint FAO/WHO Meeting on Pesticide Residues; (FAO Plant Production and Protection Paper No. 42).

98. International Agency for Research on Cancer. *Some halogenated hydrocarbons and pesticide exposures.* Lyon, 1986:357-406 (IARC Monographs on the Evaluation of the Carcinogenic Risk of Chemicals to Humans, Volume 41).

# 16.
# Disinfectants and disinfectant by-products

## 16.1 Introduction

Disinfection is unquestionably the most important step in the treatment of water for public supply. The destruction of microbiological pathogens is essential and almost invariably involves the use of reactive chemical agents such as chlorine, which are not only powerful biocides but also capable of reacting with other water constituents to form new compounds with potentially harmful long-term health effects. Thus, an overall assessment of the impact of disinfection on public health must consider not only the microbiological quality of the treated water, but also the toxicity of the disinfectants and their reaction products.

The paramount importance of microbiological quality requires some flexibility in the derivation of guideline values for these substances. Fortunately this is possible because of the substantial margin of safety incorporated into these values. Guideline values for carcinogenic disinfectant by-products are presented here for an excess lifetime cancer risk of $10^{-5}$. The conditions specified for disinfection vary not only according to water composition and temperature but also with available technology and socioeconomic factors in different parts of the world. Where local circumstances require that a choice must be made between meeting either microbiological guidelines or guidelines for disinfectants or disinfectant by-products, the microbiological quality must always take precedence, and where necessary, a chemical guideline value can be adopted corresponding to a higher level of risk. Efficient disinfection must never be compromised.

Although not addressed with respect to the individual parameters presented below, it is noted that, in a number of epidemiological studies, positive associations between the ingestion of chlorinated drinking-water and mortality rates from cancer, particularly of the bladder, have been reported. The degree of evidence for this association is considered inadequate by IARC (1).

The level of disinfection by-products can be reduced by optimizing the treatment process (see Volume 1, section 6.3). Removal of organic substances prior to disinfection reduces the formation of potentially harmful by-products.

The following guidance is provided to help authorities decide which guideline values may be of greater or lesser importance for setting national standards: guideline values for chemicals of greater importance generally include those for chloramines and chlorine (when used as disinfectants); followed by those for bromoform, dibromochloromethane, bromodichloromethane, chloroform, and chloral hydrate; and chlorite, bromate, dichloroacetic acid, and trichloroacetic acid (provisional guideline values have been established for this last group). Guideline values for chemicals of lesser importance generally include those for 2,4,6-trichlorophenol, formaldehyde, dichloroacetonitrile, dibromoacetonitrile, trichloroacetonitrile, and cyanogen chloride. Although given less importance, it may be appropriate to measure their levels at least once. It should also be noted that a number of non-volatile, poorly characterized by-products may be formed as well, including those derived from humic substances. These recommendations are general, and local monitoring and surveillance capabilities must be considered in the setting of national standards.

## Reference

1. International Agency for Research on Cancer. *Chlorinated drinking-water; chlorination by-products; some other halogenated compounds; cobalt and cobalt compounds.* Lyon, 1991:45-359 (IARC Monographs on the Evaluation of Carcinogenic Risks to Humans, Volume 52).

# Disinfectants

## 16.2 Chloramines

### 16.2.1 General description

#### *Identity*

CAS no.:                    10599-90-3
Molecular formula:          $NH_2Cl$

Mono-, di-, and trichloramines are formed when water containing ammonia is chlorinated. Only monochloramine, the most abundant chloramine, will be considered here, as it has been the most extensively studied.

#### *Physicochemical properties (1–3)[1]*

| Property | Value |
|---|---|
| Melting point | - 66 °C |
| Water solubility | Soluble |

#### *Organoleptic properties*

Most individuals are able to taste chlorine and its by-products, including chloramines, at concentrations below 5 mg/litre, and some at levels as low as 0.3 mg/litre (*1*).

---

[1] Conversion factor in air: 1 ppm = 2.1 mg/m³.

### Major uses

The chloramines are used as intermediates in the manufacture of hydrazine; when formed *in situ* from ammonia and chlorine, they are also disinfectants for drinking-water (4).

### Environmental fate

Monochloramine is persistent in the environment. Its rate of disappearance is primarily a function of pH and salinity: its half-life increases with increasing pH and decreases with increasing salinity. It decomposes more quickly if discharged into receiving waters containing bromide, presumably as a result of the formation of bromochloramine and the decomposition of the dihalamine. Monochloramine is expected to decompose via chlorine transfer to give organic nitrogen-containing compounds in receiving waters (5).

## 16.2.2 Analytical methods

Chloramines can be determined by colorimetric methods; the detection limit is about 10 μg/litre (6, 7).

## 16.2.3 Environmental levels and human exposure

### Water

Inorganic chloramines are found as by-products of the chlorination of water. In one survey, mono- and dichloramines were found in secondary sewage effluents and cooling water at levels in the range of 0.03–1.0 and 0.002–0.70 mg/litre, respectively (8). Many water companies have begun to use chloramines for disinfection instead of chlorine to prevent the formation of trihalomethanes. Typical chloramine concentrations of 0.5–2 mg/litre are found in drinking-water supplies where chloramine is used as a primary disinfectant or to provide a chlorine residual in the distribution system (9).

## 16.2.4 Kinetics and metabolism in laboratory animals and humans

Monochloramine administered by the oral route in the rat is readily absorbed from the gastrointestinal tract, the highest concentration 5 days after administration being found in plasma followed by whole blood, skin, testes, packed cells, bone marrow, kidney, lung, stomach, thyroid and thymus, carcass, liver, ileum, and fat. Monochloramine is metabolized to the chloride ion, which is excreted mainly in the urine and to a lesser extent in the faeces (10).

## 16.2.5 Effects on laboratory animals and *in vitro* test systems

### Short-term exposure

Male A/JAX mice (12 per dose) were exposed to monochloramine at concentrations of 0, 2.5, 25, 50, 100, or 200 mg/litre (approximately 0, 0.4, 4, 8, 15, or 30 mg/kg of body weight per day) for 30 days. No significant adverse effects on various haematological parameters, including blood cell counts, haemoglobin, GSH levels, and glucose-6-phosphate dehydrogenase activity, were reported at any dose level tested. The NOAEL in this study was 30 mg/kg of body weight per day (*11*).

Monochloramine was administered to Fischer 344 rats and B6C3F$_1$ mice in drinking-water at concentrations of 0, 25, 50, 100, 200, or 400 mg/litre (approximately 0, 2.5, 5, 10, 20, or 40 mg/kg of body weight per day in rats and 0, 4, 8, 15, 30, or 60 mg/kg of body weight per day in mice) for 13 weeks. Decreased body weight gain and liver damage (e.g. cellular hypertrophy) were reported in mice exposed at concentrations of 100, 200, and 400 mg/litre. The authors also reported decreased body weight gain and decreased relative liver weight in male and female rats and increased protein excretion in male rats given 200 and 400 mg/litre. The NOAELs in this study were 50 mg/litre (8 mg/kg of body weight per day) for mice and 100 mg/litre (10 mg/kg of body weight per day) for rats (*12*).

Monochloramine at 0, 25, 50, 100, or 200 mg/litre was administered in drinking-water to male and female Sprague-Dawley rats for 90 days, corresponding to 0, 1.8, 3.4, 5.8, and 9.0 mg/kg of body weight per day for males and 0, 2.6, 4.3, 7.7, and 12.1 mg/kg of body weight per day for females. The authors considered the highest dose a LOAEL for both sexes, based on the respective reductions in liver and spleen weights. In addition, overall reductions in body weight gain were observed at 50 mg/litre and higher, but significant reductions only at 200 mg/litre. The authors concluded that 100 mg/litre (7.7 and 5.8 mg/kg of body weight per day for female and male rats, respectively) can be considered a NOAEL (*13*).

### Long-term exposure

Monochloramine was administered for 2 years to male and female F344/N rats at 0, 50, 100, or 200 mg/litre in the drinking-water, corresponding to average doses of 2.9, 5.2, and 9.4 mg/kg of body weight per day in males and 3.1, 5.7, and 10.2 mg/kg of body weight per day in females. The authors failed to find any clinical changes attributable to the consumption of chloraminated water. Mean body weights of rats given the highest dose were lower than those of their respective control groups. Significant decreases in liver and kidney weights in high-dose males and increases in brain- and kidney-weight-to-body-weight ratios in high-dose rats of both sexes were related to the lower body weights in these groups. Based on these considerations, the authors considered the NOAELs for this study

791

to be 5.2 and 5.7 mg/kg of body weight per day for male and female rats, respectively. However, it is probable that the observed weight decreases were a direct result of the unpalatability of the drinking-water (*14*).

In a second bioassay, B6C3F$_1$ mice were exposed for 2 years to monochloramine in their drinking-water at levels of 0, 50, 100, or 200 mg/litre, corresponding to average doses of 0, 5.4, 9.8, and 17.0 mg/kg of body weight per day for males and 0, 5.8, 10.6, and 19.0 mg/kg of body weight per day for females. The authors reported that there were no clinical changes attributable to the consumption of chloraminated water. Based on changes in body weight at the highest dose, the NOAELs were 9.8 and 10.6 mg/kg of body weight per day for male and female mice, respectively (*14*).

## Reproductive toxicity, embryotoxicity, and teratogenicity

Chloramine was administered by gavage at doses of 0, 2.5, 5.0, or 10 mg/kg of body weight per day to male and female Long-Evans rats for 66–76 days before and during mating and throughout gestation and lactation. No significant differences were observed between controls and exposed rats in fertility, viability, litter size, mean weight of pups, or day of eye opening. There were no alterations in sperm count, direct progressive sperm movement, percentage mobility, or sperm morphological characteristics in adult males. The weights of male and female reproductive organs were not significantly different between the test and control groups, and no significant anatomical changes were seen on tissue examination. A NOAEL of 10 mg/kg of body weight per day was identified (*15*).

In a study in which monochloramine was administered to female Sprague-Dawley rats (6 per dose) at 0, 1, 10, or 100 mg/litre daily (approximately 0, 0.1, 1, or 10 mg/kg of body weight per day) in drinking-water before mating and throughout gestation, it was found not to be teratogenic or embryotoxic. The reliability of these findings is reduced because of the small number of dams exposed and the lack of data on maternal toxicity (*16*).

## Mutagenicity and related end-points

Monochloramine was reported to be weakly mutagenic at the *trpC* locus of *Bacillus subtilis* (*17*). It did not increase the number of revertant colonies above the levels in untreated controls in assays employing *Salmonella typhimurium* strains TA97, TA100, and TA102 (*18*), nor did it significantly increase bone marrow chromosomal aberrations or micronuclei in CD-1 mice, or cause sperm-head abnormalities in B6C3F$_1$ mice (*19*).

## Carcinogenicity

In 2-year bioassays, mice and rats were exposed to chloramine at 0, 50, 100, or 200 mg/litre in drinking-water, the highest doses being equivalent to 9.4 and

10.2 mg/kg of body weight per day for male and female rats, respectively, and 17.0 and 19.0 mg/kg of body weight per day for male and female mice, respectively. The studies provided equivocal evidence of the carcinogenic activity of chloraminated drinking-water in female F344/N rats, as indicated by an increase in comparison with concurrent controls, in the incidence of mononuclear-cell leukaemia. This increase, however, was within the range observed in historical controls. There was no evidence of carcinogenic activity in male rats or male and female mice (*14*).

## 16.2.6 Effects on humans

Chloramine was administered at increasing doses (approximately 0.0001, 0.01, 0.11, 0.26, or 0.34 mg/kg of body weight per day) to five groups of 10 human subjects each, over a 16-day period. There were no adverse effects on clinical signs, urinalysis, haematology, and clinical chemistry in comparison with controls. In a second phase of the study, 10 healthy adult males were given a chloramine solution of concentration 5 mg/litre (0.04 mg/kg of body weight per day). There were no adverse effects on physical condition, urinalysis, or clinical chemistry and no serious objections to the taste of chloramine at the dose tested (*20*).

Acute haemolytic anaemia, characterized by the denaturation of haemoglobin and the lysis of red blood cells, was reported in haemodialysis patients when tapwater containing chloramines was used for dialysis (*21*).

In epidemiological studies, no association was found between the ingestion of chloraminated drinking-water and increased mortality rates for bladder cancer (*22, 23*).

## 16.2.7 Guideline value

IARC has not evaluated the carcinogenic potential of inorganic chloramines. In the National Toxicology Program (NTP) bioassay in two species (*14*), the incidence of mononuclear cell leukaemias in female F344/N rats was increased, but no other increases in tumour incidence were observed. Although monochloramine has been shown to be mutagenic in some *in vitro* studies, it has not been found to be genotoxic *in vivo*.

The guideline value for monochloramine is 3 mg/litre (rounded figure), based on a TDI of 94 µg/kg of body weight, calculated from a NOAEL of 9.4 mg/kg of body weight per day (the highest dose administered to males in the 2-year NTP rat drinking-water study, chosen because of the probability that the lower body weights were caused by the unpalatability of the drinking-water) (*14*). An uncertainty factor of 100 (for intra- and interspecies variation) is incorporated, and 100% of the TDI is allocated to drinking-water. An additional uncertainty factor for possible carcinogenicity was not applied because equivocal cancer effects reported in the NTP study in only one species and in only one sex were within the range observed in historical controls.

Available data are insufficient for the establishment of guideline values for dichloramine and trichloramine. The odour thresholds of dichloramine and trichloramine are much lower than that for monochloramine.

## References

1. National Institute for Occupational Safety and Health. *Registry of Toxic Effects of Chemical Substances (RTECS)*. Cincinnati, OH, US Department of Health and Human Services, 1985-86.

2. Weast RC, ed. *CRC handbook of chemistry and physics*, 67th ed. Boca Raton, FL, CRC Press, 1986.

3. Hawley GG. *The condensed chemical dictionary*, 10th ed. New York, Van Nostrand Reinhold, 1981:228.

4. Moore GS, Calabrese EJ. The health effects of chloramines in potable water supplies: a literature review. *Journal of environmental pathology and toxicology*, 1980, 4(1):257-263.

5. Jolley RL, Carpenter JH. A review of the chemistry and environmental fate of reactive oxidants in chlorinated water. In: Jolley RL et al., eds. *Water chlorination: environmental impact and health effects*. Vol. 4. Ann Arbor, MI, Ann Arbor Science, 1983:3-47.

6. International Organization for Standardization. *Water quality. Determination of free chlorine and total chlorine*. Geneva, 1985 (ISO7393/1,2:1985).

7. International Organization for Standardization. *Water quality. Determination of free chlorine and total chlorine*. Geneva, 1990(ISO7393/3:1990).

8. Jolley RL et al. Chlorination of organics in cooling waters and process effluents. In: Jolley RL, ed. *Water chlorination: environmental impact and health effects*, Vol. 1. Ann Arbor, MI, Ann Arbor Science, 1978:105-138.

9. Bull RJ et al. *Health effects of disinfectants and disinfection by-products*. Denver, CO, American Water Works Association, 1991.

10. Abdel-Rahman MS, Waldron DM, Bull RJ. A comparative kinetics study of monochloramine and hypochlorous acid in rat. *Journal of applied toxicology*, 1983, 3(4):175-179.

11. Moore GS, Calabrese EJ, McGee M. Health effects of monochloramines in drinking water. *Journal of environmental science and health*, 1980, A15(3):239-258.

12. Gulf South Research Institute. *A subchronic study of chloramine generated in-situ in the drinking water of F344 rats and B6C3F₁ mice.* Rockville, MD, Tracor-Jitco, 1981 (unpublished report).

13. Daniel FB et al. Comparative subchronic toxicity studies of three disinfectants. *Journal of the American Water Works Association*, 1990, 82:61-69.

14. National Toxicology Program. *NTP technical report on the toxicology and carcinogenicity studies of chlorinated and chloraminated water in F344/N rats and B6C3F₁ mice.* Research Triangle Park, NC, 1990.

15. Bull RJ et al. Use of biological assay systems to assess the relative carcinogenic hazards of disinfection by-products. *Environmental health perspectives*, 1982, 46:215-227.

16. Abdel-Rahman MS, Berardi MR, Bull RJ. Effect of chlorine and monochloramine in drinking water on the developing rat fetus. *Journal of applied toxicology*, 1982, 2(3):156-159.

17. Shih KL, Lederberg J. Chloramine mutagenesis in *Bacillus subtilis*. *Science*, 1976, 192:1141-1143.

18. Thomas EL et al. Mutagenic activity of chloramines. *Mutation research*, 1987, 188:35-43.

19. Meier JR et al. Evaluation of chemicals used for drinking water disinfection for production of chromosomal damage and sperm-head abnormalities in mice. *Environmental mutagenesis*, 1985, 7:201-211.

20. Lubbers JR, Chauhan S, Bianchine JR. Controlled clinical evaluations of chlorine dioxide, chlorite and chlorate in man. *Fundamental and applied toxicology*, 1981, 1:334-338.

21. Kjellstrand CM et al. Hemolysis in dialyzed patients caused by chloramines. *Nephron*, 1974, 13:427-433.

22. Zierler S, Danley RA, Feingold L. Type of disinfectant in drinking water and pattern of mortality in Massachusetts. *Environmental health perspectives*, 1986, 69:275-279.

23. Zierler S et al. Bladder cancer in Massachusetts related to chlorinated and chloraminated drinking water: a case control study. *Archives of environmental health*, 1988, 43(2):195-200.

## 16.3 Chlorine

### 16.3.1 General description

**Identity**

| Element or compound | CAS no. | Molecular formula |
|---|---|---|
| Chlorine | 7782-50-5 | $Cl_2$ |
| Hypochlorous acid | 7790-92-3 | HOCl |
| Sodium hypochlorite | 7681-52-9 | NaOCl |

**Physicochemical properties of chlorine (1, 2) [1]**

| Property | Value |
|---|---|
| Boiling point | -34.6 °C |
| Melting point | -101 °C |
| Density | 3.214 g/litre at 0 °C and 101.3 kPa |
| Vapour pressure | 480 Pa at 0 °C |
| Water solubility | 14.6 g/litre at 0 °C |

**Organoleptic properties**

The taste and odour thresholds for chlorine in distilled water are 5 and 2 mg/litre, respectively. In air, chlorine has a pungent and disagreeable odour (2).

**Major uses**

Large amounts of chlorine are produced for use as disinfectants and bleach for both domestic and industrial purposes, and it is also widely used to disinfect drinking-water and swimming-pool water and to control bacteria and odours in the food industry (3, 4).

**Environmental fate**

In water, chlorine reacts to form hypochlorous acid and hypochlorites. All three species exist in equilibrium with each other, the relative amounts varying with the pH. In dilute solutions and at pH levels above 4.0, very little molecular chlorine exists in solution. The concentrations of hypochlorous acid and the hypochlorite ion are approximately equal at pH 7.5 and 25 °C. Chlorine can react with ammonia or amines in water to form chloramines (4, 5).

---

[1] Conversion factor in air: 1 ppm = 2.9 mg/m³.

## 16.3.2 Analytical methods

A colorimetric method can be used to determine free chlorine in water at concentrations of 0.1–10 mg/litre. Other methods allow for the determination of free chlorine, chloramines, other chlorine species, and total available chlorine, and are suitable for total chlorine concentrations up to 5 mg/litre. The minimum detectable concentration of chlorine is about 0.02 mg/litre (6).

## 16.3.3 Environmental levels and human exposure

### Air

A mean ambient air level of 1 mg/m$^3$ was reported for chlorine (7).

### Water

Chlorine is present in most disinfected drinking-water at concentrations of 0.2–1 mg/litre (3).

### Food

Cake flour bleached with chlorine contains chloride at levels in the range 1.3–1.9 g/kg. Unbleached flour may contain small amounts of chlorite (400–500 mg/kg) (8).

### Estimated total exposure and relative contribution of drinking-water

The major routes of exposure to chlorine are through drinking-water, food, and contact with items either bleached or disinfected with it.

## 16.3.4 Kinetics and metabolism in laboratory animals and humans

Most studies on the pharmacokinetics of chlorine, hypochlorous acid, or hypochlorites employ reactive $^{36}$Cl-labelled compounds and probably reflect the fate of the chloride ion or other reaction products generated from the parent molecules. In rats, hypochlorous acid was readily absorbed through the gastrointestinal tract, distribution being highest in the plasma; smaller amounts were found in bone marrow, kidney, testes, lung, skin, duodenum, spleen, liver, and bone (9, 10). *In vivo*, sodium hypochlorite was metabolized to trichloroethanoic acid, dichloroethanoic acid, chloroform, and dichloroacetonitrile (11). Hypochlorous acid administered to rats was excreted primarily in the urine and faeces, mostly in the form of chloride ion (10). None was excreted in expired air (9).

## 16.3.5 Effects on laboratory animals and *in vitro* test systems

### Acute exposure

Calcium hypochlorite has an oral $LD_{50}$ in the rat of 850 mg/kg of body weight (2).

### Short-term exposure

No consistent effects on organ weights or histopathology of tissues were noted in Sprague-Dawley rats (10 per sex per dose) given chlorine in drinking-water at 0, 25, 50, 100, 175, or 200 mg/litre (males: 0, 2, 7.5, 12.8, or 16.7 mg/kg of body weight per day; females: 0, 3.5, 12.6, 19.5, or 24.9 mg/kg of body weight per day) for 90 days (12) or in rats fed flour containing 1257 or 2506 mg of chlorine per kg (63 or 125 mg/kg of body weight per day) for 28 days (13).

Enhanced weight gain was observed in all male rats (10 per dose) given drinking-water containing chlorine at 0, 20, 40, or 80 mg/litre (0, 4.1, 8.1, or 15.7 mg/kg of body weight per day) for 6 weeks (14). The results of a 4-week study in which female C57BL/6N mice were given hyperchlorinated tapwater (4.8–5.8 mg/kg of body weight per day) suggested an adverse effect on the macrophage defence mechanisms of mice. The LOAEL in this study was 4.8 mg/kg of body weight per day (15).

In a study in which male CR-1:CD-1 mice (30 per dose) received chlorinated drinking-water (0.02, 0.2, 2.9, or 5.8 mg/kg of body weight per day) for 120 days, none of the mice showed evidence of a statistically significant change in humoral or cell-mediated immune response. A NOAEL of 5.8 mg/kg of body weight per day was identified (16).

### Long-term exposure

F344 rats (50 per sex per dose) were given sodium hypochlorite in drinking-water (males: 0.05% or 0.1%, 75 or 150 mg/kg of body weight per day; females: 0.1% or 0.2%, 150 or 300 mg/kg of body weight per day) for 2 years. Effects included a dose-related depression in body weight gain in all groups, depressed liver, brain, and heart weights in males given a 0.05% dose, decreased salivary gland weights in both female groups, and decreased kidney weights in females given 0.2% (17).

In a 2-year bioassay, F344 rats and B6C3F$_1$ mice were given chlorine in drinking-water at levels of up to 275 mg/litre (up to 24 mg/kg of body weight per day for male rats and male mice, 15 mg/kg of body weight per day for female rats, and 22 mg/kg of body weight per day for female mice). There was a dose-related decrease in water consumption for both mice and rats. No effects on body weight or survival were observed in any of the treated animals (18).

Wistar rats were fed cake prepared from flour treated with 1250 or 2500 mg of chlorine per kg (males: 12.8 or 25.3 mg/kg of body weight per day; females: 17.0 or 35.0 mg/kg of body weight per day) for 104 weeks. A dose-related reduction in spleen weight was seen in females, and dose-related haematological effects were observed in both sexes. A LOAEL of 12.8 mg/kg of body weight per day was identified in this study (*19*).

### Reproductive effects, embryotoxicity, and teratogenicity

C3H/HeJ and C57BL/6J mice given drinking-water containing 10 mg of residual chlorine per litre (1.9 mg/kg of body weight per day) for 6 months showed no adverse reproductive effects (*20*). In a seven-generation study in which rats were given drinking-water chlorinated at 100 mg/litre (10 mg/kg of body weight per day), no treatment-related effects on fertility were found (*21*).

Oral administration of hypochlorite ion or hypochlorous acid at 100, 200, or 400 mg of chlorine per litre (1.6, 4.0, or 8.0 mg/kg of body weight per day) resulted, in the case of hypochlorite, in dose-related increases in the number of sperm-head abnormalities in male B6C3F$_1$ mice. A NOAEL of 8.0 mg/kg of body weight per day was identified for hypochlorous acid and a LOAEL of 1.6 mg/kg of body weight per day for hypochlorite ion (*22*).

### Mutagenicity and related end-points

Sodium hypochlorite has been found to be mutagenic in *Salmonella typhimurium* TA1530 and TA100 but not TA1538 (*23, 24*). Calcium and sodium hypochlorite both produced chromosomal aberrations in Chinese hamster fibroblast cells without metabolic activation (*24*). Hypochlorite ion and hypochlorous acid were negative in the *in vivo* erythrocyte micronucleus assay and in bone marrow aberration studies (*22*).

### Carcinogenicity

F344 rats (50 per sex per dose) were given sodium hypochlorite in drinking-water (males: 0.05% or 0.1%, 75 or 150 mg/kg of body weight per day; females: 0.1% or 0.2%, 150 or 300 mg/kg of body weight per day) for 2 years. Experimental groups did not differ from controls with respect to total tumour incidences or mean survival times, and most of the tumours found were of types that commonly occur spontaneously in F344 rats. The authors concluded that sodium hypochlorite was not carcinogenic in rats (*16*).

In a seven-generation toxicity study, the incidence of malignant tumours in rats consuming drinking-water with a free chlorine level of 100 mg/litre (10 mg/kg of body weight per day) did not differ from that in controls (*21*). The incidence of tumours in treated animals was not significantly elevated in F344 rats and B6C3F$_1$ mice (50 per sex per dose) given solutions of sodium hypochlorite (70 or 140 mg/kg of body weight per day for male rats, 95 or 190 mg/kg of body weight per day for female rats, 84 or 140 mg/kg of body weight per day for male and female mice) in their drinking-water for 103–104 weeks (*25*).

In a 2-year bioassay, F344 rats and B6C3F$_1$ mice were given chlorine in drinking-water at levels of 0, 70, 140, or 275 mg/litre (8, 13, or 24 mg/kg of body weight per day for male rats; 5, 7, or 15 mg/kg of body weight per day for female rats; 8, 15, or 24 mg/kg of body weight per day for male mice; and 1, 13, or 22 mg/kg of body weight per day for female mice). Although there was a marginal increase in mononuclear-cell leukaemia in the groups of female rats given 140 and 275 mg/litre, it was considered to be equivocal evidence of carcinogenic activity because the incidence was significantly elevated compared with controls only for the middle dose and the incidence of leukaemia in the concurrent controls was lower than the mean in historical controls (*18*).

## 16.3.6 Effects on humans

Exposure to chlorine, hypochlorous acid, and hypochlorite ion through ingestion of household bleach occurs most commonly in children. Intake of a small quantity of bleach generally results in irritation of the oesophagus, a burning sensation in the mouth and throat, and spontaneous vomiting. In these cases, it is not clear whether it is the sodium hypochlorite or the extremely caustic nature of the bleach that causes the tissue injury.

The effects of heavily chlorinated water on human populations exposed for varying periods were summarized in a report that was essentially anecdotal in character and did not describe in detail the health effects observed (*26*). In a study on the effects of progressively increasing chlorine doses (0, 0.001, 0.014, 0.071, 0.14, 0.26, or 0.34 mg/kg of body weight) on healthy male volunteers (10 per dose), there was an absence of adverse, physiologically significant toxicological effects in all of the study groups (*27*). It has been reported that asthma can be triggered by exposure to chlorinated water (*28*). Episodes of dermatitis have also been associated with exposure to chlorine and hypochlorite (*29, 30*).

In a study of 46 communities in central Wisconsin where chlorine levels in water ranged from 0.2 to 1 mg/litre, serum cholesterol and low-density lipoprotein levels were higher in communities using chlorinated water. Levels of high-density lipoprotein (HDL) and the cholesterol:HDL ratio were significantly elevated in relation to the level of calcium in the drinking-water, but only in communities using chlorinated water. The authors speculated that chlorine and calcium in drinking-water may interact in some way that affects lipid levels (*31*).

An increased risk of bladder cancer appeared to be associated with the consumption of chlorinated tapwater in a population-based, case–control study of adults consuming chlorinated or non-chlorinated water for half of their lifetimes (*32*).

## 16.3.7 Guideline value

In humans and animals exposed to chlorine in drinking-water, specific adverse treatment-related effects have not been observed. IARC has concluded that hypochlorites are not classifiable as to their carcinogenicity to humans (Group 3) (*17*).

The guideline value for free chlorine in drinking-water is derived from a NOAEL of 15 mg/kg of body weight per day, based on the absence of toxicity in rodents that received chlorine as hypochlorite in drinking-water for up to 2 years (*18*). Application of an uncertainty factor of 100 (for inter- and intraspecies variation) to this NOAEL gives a TDI of 150 µg/kg of body weight. With an allocation of 100% of the TDI to drinking-water, the guideline value is 5 mg/litre (rounded figure). It should be noted, however, that this value is conservative, as no adverse effect level was identified in this study. Most individuals are able to taste chlorine or its by-products (e.g. chloramines) at concentrations below 5 mg/litre, and some at levels as low as 0.3 mg/litre.

## References

1. Sconce JS, ed. *Chlorine: its manufacture, properties and uses.* New York, Reinhold Publishing Corporation, 1962:1-45.

2. National Institute for Occupational Safety and Health. *Criteria for a recommended standard for occupational exposure to chlorine.* Cincinnati, OH, US Department of Health, Education, and Welfare, 1976 (NIOSH Publication No. 760170; NTIS PB-266367/2).

3. White GC. Current chlorination and dechlorination practices in the treatment of potable water, wastewater and cooling water. In: Jolley RL, ed. *Water chlorination: environmental impact and health effects.* Vol. 1. Ann Arbor, MI, Ann Arbor Science, 1978:1-18.

4. Dychdala GR. Chlorine and chlorine compounds. In: Black SS, ed. *Disinfection, sterilization and preservation,* 2nd ed. Philadelphia, PA, Lea and Febiger, 1977:167-195.

5. *Chlorine and hydrogen chloride.* Geneva, World Health Organization, 1982:1-95 (Environmental Health Criteria, No. 21).

6. American Public Health Association. *Standard methods for the examination of water and waste water,* 17th ed. Washington, DC, 1989:4-45–4-67.

7. National Academy of Sciences. *Drinking water and health: disinfectants and disinfectant by-products.* Vol. 7. Washington, DC, National Academy Press, 1987.

8. Sollars WF. Chloride content of cake flours and flour fractions. *Cereal chemistry,* 1961, 38:487-500.

9. Abdel-Rahman MS, Couri D, Bull RJ. Metabolism and pharmacokinetics of alternate drinking water disinfectants. *Environmental health perspectives,* 1982, 46:19-23.

10. Abdel-Rahman MS, Waldron DM, Bull RJ. A comparative kinetics study of monochloramine and hypochlorous acid in rat. *Journal of applied toxicology,* 1983, 3:175-179.

11. Mink FL et al. *In vivo* formation of halogenated reaction products following peroral sodium hypochlorite. *Bulletin of environmental contamination and toxicology*, 1983, 30:394-399.

12. Daniel FB et al. Comparative subchronic toxicity studies of three disinfectants. *Journal of the American Water Works Association*, 1990, 82:61-69.

13. Lehman A. Appraisal of the safety of chemicals in foods, drugs and cosmetics. *Association of Food and Drug Officials of the United States, quarterly bulletin*, 1959.

14. Cunningham HM. Effect of sodium hypochlorite on the growth of rats and guinea pigs. *American journal of veterinary research*, 1980, 41:295-297.

15. Fidler IJ. Depression of macrophages in mice drinking hyperchlorinated water. *Nature*, 1977, 270:735-736.

16. Hermann LM, White WJ, Lang CM. Prolonged exposure to acid, chlorine, or tetracycline in drinking water: effects on delayed-type hypersensitivity, hemagglutination titers, and reticuloendothelial clearance rates in mice. *Laboratory animal science*, 1982, 32:603-608.

17. International Agency for Research on Cancer. *Chlorinated drinking-water; chlorination by-products; some other halogenated compounds; cobalt and cobalt compounds.* Lyon, 1991:45-359 (IARC Monographs on the Evaluation of Carcinogenic Risks to Humans, Volume 52).

18. National Toxicology Program. *Report on the toxicology and carcinogenesis studies of chlorinated and chloraminated water in F344/N rats and B6C3F$_1$ mice (drinking water studies).* Research Triangle Park, NC, US Department of Health and Human Services, 1992 (NTP TR 392).

19. Fisher N et al. Long-term toxicity and carcinogenicity studies of cake made from chlorinated flour. 1. Studies in rats. *Food chemistry and toxicology*, 1983, 21:427-434.

20. Les EP. Effect of acidified-chlorinated water on reproduction in C3H/HeJ and C57BL/5J mice. *Laboratory animal care*, 1968, 18:210-213.

21. Druckrey H. Chlorinated drinking water toxicity tests involving seven generations of rats. *Food and cosmetics toxicology*, 1968, 6:147-154.

22. Meier JR et al. Evaluation of chemicals used for drinking water disinfection for production of chromosomal damage and sperm-head abnormalities in mice. *Environmental mutagenesis*, 1985, 7:201-211.

23. Wlodkowski TJ, Rosenkranz HS. Mutagenicity of sodium hypochlorite for *Salmonella typhimurium*. *Mutation research*, 1975, 31:39-42.

24. Ishidate M et al. Primary mutagenicity screening of food additives currently used in Japan. *Food chemistry and toxicology*, 1984, 22:623-636.

25. Kurokawa Y et al. Long-term *in vivo* carcinogenicity tests of potassium bromate, sodium hypochlorite, and sodium chlorite conducted in Japan. *Environmental health perspectives*, 1986, 69:221-235.

26. Muegge OJ. Physiological effects of heavily chlorinated drinking water. *Journal of the American Water Works Association*, 1956, 48:1507-1509.

27. Lubbers JR, Chauan S, Bianchine JR. Controlled clinical evaluations of chlorine dioxide, chlorite and chlorate in man. *Environmental health perspectives*, 1982, 46:57-62.

28. Watson SH, Kibler CS. Drinking water as a cause of asthma. *Journal of allergies*, 1933, 5:197-198.

29. Environmental Criteria and Assessment Office. *Ambient water quality criterion for the protection of human health: chlorine*. Washington, DC, Office of Water Regulations and Standards, US Environmental Protection Agency, 1981.

30. Eun HC, Lee AY, Lee YS. Sodium hypochlorite dermatitis. *Contact dermatitis*, 1984, 11:45.

31. Zeighami EA, Watson AP, Craun GF. Serum lipid levels in neighboring communities with chlorinated and nonchlorinated drinking water. *Fundamental and applied toxicology*, 1990, 6:421-432.

32. Cantor KP et al. Bladder cancer, drinking water source and tap water consumption: a case-control study. *Journal of the National Cancer Institute*, 1987, 79:1269-1279.

## 16.4 Chlorine dioxide, chlorite, and chlorate

### 16.4.1 General description

**Identity**

| Compound | CAS no. | Molecular formula |
|---|---|---|
| Chlorine dioxide | 10049-04-4 | $ClO_2$ |
| Chlorite (sodium salt) | 7758-19-2 | $NaClO_2$ |
| Chlorate (sodium salt) | 7775-09-0 | $NaClO_3$ |

## Physicochemical properties *(1–3)*

| Property | Chlorine dioxide[1] | Sodium chlorite | Sodium chlorate |
|---|---|---|---|
| Boiling point (°C) | 11 | – | >300 (decomposes) |
| Melting point (°C) | -59 | 180–200 (decomposes) | 248 |
| Density at 0 °C (g/cm$^3$) | 1.64 (liquid) | – | 2.5 |
| Vapour pressure at 25 °C | – | Negligible | – |
| Water solubility (g/litre) | 3.0 (25 °C) | 390 (17 °C) | – |

## Organoleptic properties

The taste and odour threshold for chlorine dioxide in water is 0.4 mg/litre *(3)*.

## Major uses

Chlorine dioxide is used for disinfection and odour/taste control of water; as a bleaching agent for cellulose, paper pulp, flour, and oils; and for cleaning and de-tanning leather. Sodium chlorite is used in on-site production of chlorine dioxide; as a bleaching agent in production of paper, textiles, and straw products; and in the manufacture of waxes, shellacs, and varnishes. Sodium chlorate is used in the preparation of chlorine dioxide; in the manufacture of dyes, matches, and explosives; for tanning and finishing leather; and in herbicides and defoliants *(1–3)*.

## Environmental fate

Chlorine dioxide rapidly decomposes into chlorite, chlorate, and chloride ions in treated water, chlorite being the predominant species. The reaction is favoured by alkaline conditions.

## 16.4.2 Analytical methods

Methods are available for the determination of chlorine dioxide, chlorite, and total available chlorine *(4, 5)*. The limits of detection for these methods are 8 µg/litre for chlorine dioxide, 4 µg/litre for total chlorine, and 10 µg/litre for chlorite and chlorate.

---

[1] Conversion factor in air: 1 ppm = 2.8 mg/m$^3$.

## 16.4.3 Environmental levels and human exposure

### *Water*

Chlorite occurs in drinking-water when chlorine dioxide is used for purification purposes. The levels of chlorite in water reported in one study ranged from 3.2 to 7.0 mg/litre (6).

### *Food*

Chlorine dioxide, chlorite, and chlorate may occur in foodstuffs as a result of their use in flour processing, as a decolorizing agent for carotenoids and other natural pigments (chlorine dioxide), as a bleaching agent in the preparation of modified food starch (sodium chlorite), as an indirect additive in paper and paperboard products used for food packaging (sodium chlorite), and as a defoliant, desiccant, and fungicide in agriculture (sodium chlorate) (7–9).

### *Estimated total exposure and relative contribution of drinking-water*

The major route of environmental exposure to chlorine dioxide, sodium chlorite, and sodium chlorate is through drinking-water.

## 16.4.4 Kinetics and metabolism in laboratory animals and humans

Chlorine dioxide is rapidly absorbed from the gastrointestinal tract. No particular organ appears to selectively concentrate the dose following exposure (10). Following oral ingestion by monkeys, chlorine dioxide was rapidly converted into chloride ion and, to a lesser extent, chlorite and chlorate (11). Excretion is mainly via the urine, smaller amounts being excreted in faeces (12).

Chlorite was readily absorbed when administered to rats, then randomly distributed throughout the tissues (12). It was transformed mainly into chloride in rats, smaller amounts appearing as unchanged chlorite. Excretion was mainly via the urine, followed by faeces (13).

Chlorate was readily absorbed and randomly distributed throughout the tissues of rats (12). It was excreted mainly in the form of chloride in the urine, smaller amounts appearing as chlorite and chlorate (13).

## 16.4.5 Effects on laboratory animals and *in vitro* test systems

### *Chlorine dioxide*

*Short-term exposure*
Drinking-water containing 0, 10, or 100 mg of chlorine dioxide per litre (equivalent to approximately 0, 1.5, or 15 mg/kg of body weight per day) was adminis-

tered to mice (10 per dose) for 30 days with no apparent effects on blood parameters. The NOAEL for this study was 15 mg/kg of body weight per day (*14*).

A total of 12 African green monkeys were exposed to water containing chlorine dioxide at concentrations of 0, 30, 100, or 200 mg/litre (corresponding to measured doses of 0, 3.5, 9.5, or 11 mg/kg of body weight per day) using a rising dose protocol. Each dose was maintained for 30–60 days. A slight suppression of thyroid function (decreased thyroxine) was observed in monkeys receiving the two highest doses. No other effects were noted. The NOAEL was 3.5 mg/kg of body weight per day (*11*).

Six monkeys were treated for 8 weeks with drinking-water containing chlorine dioxide at 100 mg/litre, corresponding to an average measured dose of about 4.6 mg/kg of body weight per day. Thyroxine level was reduced after 4 weeks of treatment but rebounded after a further 4 weeks. In the same study, drinking-water containing chlorine dioxide at 0, 100, or 200 mg/litre was administered to male rats (12 per dose) (equivalent to 0, 10, or 20 mg/kg of body weight per day). A dose-dependent decrease in thyroxine levels was observed after 8 weeks of treatment; there was no rebound. The exposure level of 100 mg/litre, equivalent to a dose of approximately 10 mg/kg of body weight per day, was the LOAEL in this study (*15*).

Sprague-Dawley rats (10 per sex per dose) were exposed to 0, 25, 50, 100, or 200 mg of chlorine dioxide per litre in drinking-water for 90 days (approximate dose levels of 0, 2, 4, 6, or 12 mg/kg of body weight per day for males and 0, 2, 5, 8, or 15 mg/kg of body weight per day for females). Water consumption was decreased in both sexes at the three highest dose levels, probably because of its reduced palatability. Food consumption was decreased in males receiving the highest dose. Goblet-cell hyperplasia was significantly increased in the nasal turbinates of females given 100 or 200 mg/litre and males at all doses. Inflammation of the nasal cavity was observed in males at 25 mg/litre and in both sexes at higher doses. The authors concluded that the lowest dose (2 mg/kg of body weight per day) was a LOAEL (*16*).

*Long-term exposure*

In a drinking-water study, chlorine dioxide was administered to rats (7 per sex per dose) at concentrations of 0, 0.5, 1, 5, 10, or 100 mg/litre (highest dose equivalent to about 13 mg/kg of body weight per day) for 2 years. At the highest dose level, survival rate was substantially decreased in both sexes, and mean life span was reduced compared with that for control animals. No correlation was observed between treatment and histopathological findings. In this study, a NOAEL of 10 mg/litre (1.3 mg/kg of body weight per day) was identified (*17*).

*Reproductive toxicity, embryotoxicity, and teratogenicity*

Female rats were exposed to 0, 1, 10, or 100 mg of chlorine dioxide per litre in drinking-water (equivalent to 0, 0.1, 1, or 10 mg/kg of body weight per day) for 2.5 months before mating and throughout gestation. At the highest dose, there was a slight reduction in the number of implants and live births per pregnancy. No effects were observed at 1 mg/kg of body weight per day, which was identified as the NOAEL (18).

Female Sprague-Dawley rats (13–16 per dose) were supplied with drinking-water containing 0, 2, 20, or 100 mg of chlorine dioxide per litre from 2 weeks before mating to gestation and lactation until pups were weaned on postnatal day 21. No significant effect on the body weight of either the dams or the pups was observed at any dose tested. At 100 mg/litre (14 mg/kg of body weight per day for the pregnant dam), a significant depression of serum thyroxine and an increase in serum triiodothyronine were observed in the pups at weaning, but not in the dams. Neurobehavioural exploratory and locomotor activities were decreased in pups born to dams exposed to 100 mg/litre but not to those exposed to 20 mg/litre (3 mg/kg of body weight per day), which was considered a NOAEL (19).

In a second experiment, rat pups were exposed directly (by gavage) to 14 mg of chlorine dioxide per kg of body weight per day (equivalent to the dose received by a pregnant dam drinking water containing 100 mg of chlorine dioxide per litre) on postnatal days 5–20. In this study, serum thyroxine levels were depressed, a somewhat greater and more consistent delay in the development of exploratory and locomotor activity was seen, and pup body weight gain was reduced. The decrease in serum triiodothyronine levels was not statistically significant. Based on decreased pup development and decreased thyroid hormone levels, a LOAEL of 14 mg/kg of body weight per day (the only dose tested) was identified (19).

Cell number was significantly depressed in the cerebellum of 21-day-old rat pups born to dams supplied during gestation and lactation with water containing 100 mg of chlorine dioxide per litre (about 14 mg/kg of body weight per day to the dam). A group of 12 rat pups dosed directly by gavage with 14 mg/kg of body weight per day had depressed cell numbers in both the cerebellum and forebrain at postnatal day 11 and displayed decreased voluntary running-wheel activity at postnatal days 50–60, despite the fact that chlorine dioxide treatments were terminated at 20 days of age. These data suggest that chlorine dioxide is capable of influencing brain development in neonatal rats. In this study, a LOAEL of 14 mg/kg of body weight per day, the only dose tested, was identified (20).

The developmental neurotoxic potential of chlorine dioxide was evaluated in a study in which it was administered to rat pups by oral intubation at 14 mg/kg of body weight per day on postnatal days 1–20. Forebrain cell proliferation was decreased on postnatal day 35, and there were decreases in forebrain weight and protein content on postnatal days 21 and 35. Cell proliferation in the cerebellum and olfactory bulbs was comparable to that in untreated controls, as were migration and aggregation of neuronal cells in the cerebral cortex. Histopathological examination of the forebrain, cerebellum, and brain stem did not reveal any lesions or changes in these tissues. In this study, a LOAEL of 14 mg/kg of body weight per day (the only dose tested) was identified (18).

*Mutagenicity and related end-points*
Chlorine dioxide was mutagenic in *Salmonella typhimurium* strain TA100 in the absence of a metabolic activation system (*21*). No sperm-head abnormalities were observed in male mice following chlorine dioxide gavage (*22*). No chromosomal abnormalities were seen in either the micronucleus test or a cytogenetic assay in mouse bone marrow cells following gavage dosing with chlorine dioxide (*22*).

## Carcinogenicity
Tumours were not observed in rats following 2-year exposures to chlorine dioxide in drinking-water (*17*).

## *Chlorite*

*Acute exposure*
An oral $LD_{50}$ of 105 mg/kg of body weight has been reported in rats (*23*). Quail were more resistant than rats; the $LD_{50}$ was 493 mg/kg of body weight (*24*).

*Short-term exposure*
Single doses of sodium chlorite administered orally to cats produced methaemoglobinaemia (*25*). A dose of 20 mg of chlorite per litre (equivalent to approximately 1.5 mg of chlorite per kg of body weight) caused up to 32% of the haemoglobin to be in the methaemoglobin state and was considered to be the LOAEL. A dose-dependent increase in methaemoglobinaemia and anaemia was observed in 12 African green monkeys treated with sodium chlorite at 0, 25, 50, 100, or 400 mg/litre in drinking-water using a rising dose protocol. Doses of chlorite were approximately 0, 3, 6, 13, and 50 mg/kg of body weight per day, and each dose level was maintained for 30–60 days (*11*).

Rats were exposed to chlorite ion at 0, 10, 50, 100, 250, or 500 mg/litre in drinking-water (equivalent to 0, 1, 5, 10, 25, or 50 mg/kg of body weight per day) for 30–90 days. Haematological parameters were monitored, and the three highest concentrations produced transient anaemia. At 90 days, red blood cell glutathione levels in the 100 mg/litre group were 40% below those of controls; there was at least a 20% reduction in the rats receiving 50 mg/litre. In this study, a NOAEL of 1 mg/kg of body weight per day was identified (*25*).

*Long-term exposure*
The effect of sodium chlorite in drinking-water at 0, 1, 2, 4, 8, 100, or 1000 mg/litre on the survival and postmortem pathology of albino rats (7 per sex per dose) was examined in a 2-year study. The life span of the animals was not significantly affected at any dose. No effects were observed in animals exposed to 8 mg/litre (0.7 mg/kg of body weight per day) or less. Animals exposed to 100 or 1000 mg/litre (9.3 or 81 mg/kg of body weight per day) exhibited treatment-related renal pathology; the author concluded that this was the result of a non-specific salt effect (*17*).

*Reproductive toxicity, embryotoxicity, and teratogenicity*
Female mice (10 per dose) were treated with sodium chlorite at 0 or 100 mg/litre in drinking-water (equivalent to 0 and 72 mg/kg of body weight per day) from day 1 of gestation and throughout lactation. Conception rates were 56% for controls and 39% for treated mice. The body weights of pups at weaning were reduced in treated mice relative to controls, so that 72 mg/kg of body weight per day is the LOAEL for this study (*14*).

In a series of experiments, sodium chlorite was administered to male rats (12 rats per dose) in drinking-water for 66–76 days at concentrations of 0, 1, 10, 100, or 500 mg/litre (equivalent to 0, 0.1, 1, 10, or 50 mg/kg of body weight per day). No compound-related abnormalities were observed on histopathological examination of the reproductive tract. Abnormal sperm morphology and decreased sperm motility were seen at the two highest dose levels, but no sperm effects were observed at 1 mg/kg of body weight per day, which can be identified as the NOAEL. In another part of the same study, male rats were bred with female rats treated at the same dose levels for 2 weeks before and throughout a 10-day breeding period. Females were exposed to sodium chlorite throughout gestation and lactation until the pups were weaned on day 21. There was no evidence of any adverse effects on conception rates, litter size, day of eye opening, or day of vaginal opening. Based on reproductive effects, a NOAEL of 10 mg/kg of body weight per day, the highest dose tested, was identified (*26*).

Treatment of maternal mice with 100 mg of sodium chlorite per litre in drinking-water (equivalent to 14 mg of chlorite per kg of body weight per day) throughout gestation and lactation resulted in pups with decreased body weights (14% below those of controls) at weaning. In this study, a LOAEL for developmental effects of 14 mg/kg of body weight per day was identified (*14*).

Fetuses from maternal rats exposed to chlorite ion via drinking-water at levels of up to 10 mg/litre (about 1 mg/kg of body weight per day) were examined. No compound-related skeletal or soft-tissue anomalies were observed. A NOAEL of 1 mg/kg of body weight per day was identified (*27*).

*Mutagenicity and related end-points*
No chromosomal abnormalities were seen in either the micronucleus test or a cytogenetic assay in mouse bone marrow cells following gavage dosing with chlorite (*22*).

*Carcinogenicity*
In a long-term study in which mice received sodium chlorite in drinking-water for 85 weeks, there was no significant increase in tumours as compared with controls at a dose of 250 mg/litre (about 36 mg of chlorite ion per kg of body weight per day). Although treated male mice exhibited an increased incidence of lung and liver tumours, tumour rates were within historical ranges for control mice, increases in liver tumours did not display a typical dose–response pattern, and

significant increases were seen only for benign tumours (*28*). Tumours were not observed in rats following 2-year exposures to sodium chlorite in drinking-water (*17*).

## Chlorate

*Acute exposure*
An acute oral dosing study in dogs demonstrated lethality at levels of sodium chlorate as low as 600 mg of chlorate ion per kg (*29*).

*Short-term exposure*
Beagle dogs (4 per sex per dose) were exposed by gavage to sodium chlorate at doses of 0, 10, 60, or 360 mg/kg of body weight per day for 3 months. There was no significant effect at any dose level on body weight, food consumption, clinical chemistry, organ weights, ophthalmic effects, gross necropsy, or tissue histopathology. Haematological changes were limited to a slight elevation in methaemoglobin level in the highest-dose animals, but this appeared to be within normal limits and was not judged to be treatment-related. In this study, a NOAEL of 360 mg/kg of body weight per day in dogs was identified (*30*).

Sprague-Dawley rats (14 per sex per dose) were exposed by gavage to sodium chlorate at doses of 0, 10, 100, or 1000 mg/kg of body weight per day for up to 3 months. No treatment-related effects were observed on mortality, physical appearance or behaviour, body weight, food consumption, clinical chemistry, gross necropsy, or organ histopathology. At the highest dose, haematological changes indicative of anaemia included decreases in erythrocyte count, haemoglobin concentration, and erythrocyte volume fraction (haematocrit). In this study, a NOAEL of 100 mg/kg of body weight per day was identified (*31*).

*Reproductive toxicity, embryotoxicity, and teratogenicity*
Sodium chlorate was administered to pregnant CD rats by gavage at doses of 0, 10, 100, or 1000 mg/kg of body weight per day on days 6–15 of gestation. There were no maternal deaths in treated animals or treatment-related effects on maternal body weight gain, food consumption, clinical observations, number of implantations, or gross necropsy. Examination of fetuses on day 20 revealed no effects on fetal weight or sex ratio, and no external, visceral, or skeletal abnormalities were detected. In this study, a developmental NOAEL of 1000 mg/kg of body weight per day in rats was identified (*32*).

*Mutagenicity and related end-points*
No chromosomal abnormalities were seen in either the micronucleus test or a cytogenetic assay in mouse bone marrow cells following gavage dosing with chlorate (*22*).

## 16.4.6 Effects on humans

### Chlorine dioxide

Six different doses of chlorine dioxide (0.1, 1, 5, 10, 18, or 24 mg/litre) in drinking-water were administered to each of 10 male volunteers using a rising dose protocol. Serum chemistry, blood count, and urinalysis parameters were monitored. A treatment-related change in group mean values for serum uric acid was observed, which the authors concluded was not physiologically detrimental. The highest dose tested, 24 mg/litre (about 0.34 mg/kg of body weight per day), can be identified as a single-dose NOAEL (33).

The same male volunteers drank 0.5 litres of water containing 5 mg of chlorine dioxide per litre each day for approximately 12 weeks, and were then kept under observation for 8 weeks. Serum chemistry, blood counts, and urinalysis revealed no abnormalities, except for a slight change in blood urea nitrogen, which the authors concluded was of doubtful physiological or toxicological significance. This exposure, equivalent to 36 µg/kg of body weight per day, can be considered a NOAEL (33).

In a prospective study of 197 persons, a portion of the population of a rural village exposed for 12 weeks to a chlorine dioxide-treated water supply (containing 0.25–1.1 mg of chlorine dioxide per litre and 0.45–0.91 mg of free chlorine per litre) experienced no significant changes in haematological parameters, serum creatinine, or total bilirubin (6).

### Chlorite

The effects of sodium chlorite on humans were evaluated in 10 male volunteers on a rising dose protocol. Single doses of 0.01, 0.1, 0.5, 1.0, 1.8, and 2.4 mg of chlorite ion in 1 litre of drinking-water were ingested by each subject. Changes in group mean values for serum urea nitrogen, creatinine, and urea nitrogen/creatinine ratio were observed, which the authors concluded were not adverse physiological effects. The highest dose tested, 2.4 mg/litre (0.034 mg/kg of body weight per day), can be identified as a single-dose NOAEL (33).

The same volunteers ingested 0.5 litres of water per day containing 5 mg of sodium chlorite per litre for approximately 12 weeks, and were then kept under observation for 8 weeks. Treatment was associated with a change in group mean corpuscular haemoglobin; however, as there was no trend over time for this change and values were within the normal ranges, the authors were reluctant to attach physiological significance to the observation. The dose tested, equivalent to 36 µg/kg of body weight per day, was identified as the NOAEL (33).

### Chlorate

Because of its use as a weed killer, a large number of cases of chlorate poisoning have been reported (3). Symptoms include methaemoglobinaemia, anuria, abdominal pain, and renal failure. For an adult human, the oral lethal dose is estimated to be as low as 20 g of sodium chlorate (230 mg of chlorate per kg of body weight) (*34*).

Ten male volunteers were given six separate doses of sodium chlorate following a rising dose protocol, single doses of 0.01, 0.1, 0.5, 1.0, 1.8, and 2.4 mg of chlorate ion in 1 litre of drinking-water being ingested by each volunteer. Very slight changes in group mean serum bilirubin, iron, and methaemoglobin were observed, but the authors concluded that they were not adverse physiological effects. The highest dose tested, 2.4 mg/litre (34 µg/kg of body weight per day), can be identified as a single-dose NOAEL (*33*).

The volunteers also ingested 0.5 litres of water per day containing 5 mg of sodium chlorate per litre (36 µg/kg of body weight per day) for approximately 12 weeks, and were then kept under observation for 8 weeks. Treatment was associated with slight changes in group mean serum urea nitrogen and mean corpuscular haemoglobin, but the authors concluded that these were not physiologically significant as values remained within the normal range for each parameter. The NOAEL was 36 µg/kg of body weight per day (*33*).

## 16.4.7 Guideline values

### Chlorine dioxide

Chlorine dioxide has been shown to impair neurobehavioural and neurological development in rats exposed perinatally. Significant depression of thyroid hormones has also been observed in rats and monkeys exposed to it in drinking-water studies.

A guideline value has not been established for chlorine dioxide because of its rapid breakdown and because the chlorite provisional guideline value (see below) is adequately protective for potential toxicity from chlorine dioxide. The taste and odour threshold for this compound is 0.4 mg/litre.

### Chlorite

Chlorite affects the red blood cells, resulting in methaemoglobin formation in cats and monkeys. IARC has concluded that chlorite is not classifiable as to its carcinogenicity to humans (Group 3) (*35*).

The TDI for chlorite is 10 µg/kg of body weight, based on the NOAEL of 1 mg/kg of body weight per day for decreased red blood cell glutathione levels in a 90-day study in rats exposed to chlorite in their drinking-water (*25*) and applying an uncertainty factor of 100 (to account for inter- and intraspecies variation). Owing to the acute nature of the response and the existence of a 2-year rat study, an additional uncertainty factor of 10 was not incorporated to account for the short duration of the key study. The TDI derived in this manner is consistent with the NOAEL (36 µg/kg of body weight per day) in a 12-week clinical study in a small number of human volunteers (*33*).

On the assumption that drinking-water contributes 80% of the total exposure, the provisional guideline value is 0.2 mg/litre (rounded figure). This guideline value is designated as provisional because use of chlorine dioxide as a disinfectant may result in the chlorite guideline value being exceeded, and difficulties in meeting the guideline value must never be a reason for compromising adequate disinfection.

## Chlorate

Available data on the effects of chlorate in humans and experimental animals are considered insufficient to permit the development of a guideline value. Data on accidental poisonings indicate that the lethal dose to humans is about 230 mg/kg of body weight per day. This is of the same order of magnitude as the NOAELs identified from studies in rats and dogs. Although no effects were observed in a 12-week clinical study in a small number of human volunteers ingesting 36 µg/kg of body weight per day, a guideline value was not derived from these results because no adverse effect level was determined.

Further research is needed to characterize the nonlethal effects of chlorate. Until data become available, it may be prudent to try to minimize chlorate levels. However, adequate disinfection should not be compromised.

## References

1. Budavari S, O'Neill M, Smith A, eds. *The Merck index. An encyclopedia of chemicals, drugs and biologicals,* 11th ed. Rahway, NJ, Merck, 1989.

2. Meister R, ed. *Farm chemicals handbook.* Willoughby, OH, Meister Publishing Co., 1989.

3. National Academy of Sciences. *Drinking water and health.* Vol. 7. Washington, DC, National Academy Press, 1987.

4. American Public Health Association. Method 4500, chlorine. In: *Standard methods for the examination of water and waste water,* 17th ed. Washington, DC, 1989:4.45-4.67.

5. American Public Health Association. Method 4500, chlorine dioxide. In: *Standard methods for the examination of water and waste water,* 17th ed. Washington, DC, 1989:4.75-4.83.

6. Michael GE et al. Chlorine dioxide water disinfection: a prospective epidemiology study. *Archives of environmental health,* 1981, 36:20-27.

7. Chemical Manufacturers Association. *A review of the uses, chemistry and health effects of chlorine dioxide and the chlorite ion.* Washington, DC, 1989.

8. US Food and Drug Administration. *Food and drugs*, Vol. 21, Parts 170-179. Washington, DC, Office of the Federal Register, 1990.

9. US Environmental Protection Agency. Sodium chlorate: exemption from the requirement of a tolerance. *Federal register*, 1983, 48:19028.

10. Abdel-Rahman MS. Pharmacokinetics of chlorine obtained from chlorine dioxide, chlorine, chloramine and chloride. In: Jolley RL et al., eds. *Water chlorination: environmental impact and health effects.* Vol. 5. Chelsea, MI, Lewis Publishers, 1985:281-293.

11. Bercz JP et al. Subchronic toxicity of chlorine dioxide and related compounds in drinking water in the nonhuman primate. *Environmental health perspectives,* 1982, 46:47-55.

12. Abdel-Rahman MS, Couri D, Bull RJ. Metabolism and pharmacokinetics of alternate drinking water disinfectants. *Environmental health perspectives,* 1982, 46:19-23.

13. Abdel-Rahman MS, Couri D, Bull RJ. The kinetics of chlorite and chlorate in rats. *Journal of environmental pathology, toxicology and oncology,* 1985, 6(1):97-103.

14. Moore GS, Calabrese EJ. Toxicological effects of chlorite in the mouse. *Environmental health perspectives,* 1982, 46:31-37.

15. Harrington RM, Shertzer HG, Bercz JP. Effects of chlorine dioxide on thyroid function in the African green monkey and the rat. *Journal of toxicology and environmental health,* 1986, 19:235-242.

16. Daniel FB et al. Comparative subchronic toxicity studies of three disinfectants. *Journal of the American Water Works Association,* 1990, 82:61-69.

17. Haag HB. *The effect on rats of chronic administration of sodium chlorite and chlorine dioxide in the drinking water.* Report to the Mathieson Alkali Works from the Medical College of Virginia, 1949.

18. Toth GP et al. Effects of chlorine dioxide on the developing rat brain. *Journal of toxicology and environmental health,* 1990, 31:29-44.

19. Orme J et al. Effects of chlorine dioxide on thyroid function in neonatal rats. *Journal of toxicology and environmental health,* 1985, 15:315-322.

20. Taylor DH, Pfohl RJ. Effects of chlorine dioxide on the neurobehavioral development of rats. In: Jolley RL et al., eds. *Water chlorination: environmental impact and health effects.* Vol. 5. Chelsea, MI, Lewis Publishers, 1985:355-364.

21. Ishidate M et al. Primary mutagenicity screening of food additives currently used in Japan. *Food chemistry and toxicology,* 1984, 22:623-636.

22. Meier JR et al. Evaluation of chemicals used for drinking water disinfection for production of chromosomal damage and sperm-head abnormalities in mice. *Environmental mutagenesis*, 1985, 7:201-211.

23. Musil J et al. Toxicologic aspects of chlorine dioxide application for the treatment of water containing phenols. *Technology of water*, 1964, 8:327-346.

24. Fletcher D. *Acute oral toxicity study with sodium chlorite in bobwhite quail.* Industrial Bio-Test Laboratory's report to Olin Corporation, 1973 (IBT No. J2119).

25. Heffernan WP, Guion C, Bull RJ. Oxidative damage to the erythrocyte induced by sodium chlorite, *in vivo. Journal of environmental pathology and toxicology*, 1979, 2:1487-1499.

26. Carlton BD et al. Sodium chlorite administration in Long-Evans rats: reproductive and endocrine effects. *Environmental research*, 1987, 42:238-245.

27. Suh DH, Abdel-Rahman MS, Bull RJ. Effect of chlorine dioxide and its metabolites in drinking water on fetal development in rats. *Journal of applied toxicology*, 1983, 3:75-79.

28. Kurokawa Y et al. Long-term *in vivo* carcinogenicity tests of potassium bromate, sodium hypochlorite and sodium chlorite conducted in Japan. *Environmental health perspectives*, 1986, 69:221-235.

29. Sheahan BJ, Pugh DM, Winstanley EW. Experimental sodium chlorate poisoning in dogs. *Research in veterinary science*, 1971, 12:387-389.

30. *A subchronic (3-month) oral toxicity study in the dog via gavage administration with sodium chlorate.* East Millston, NJ, Bio/dynamics, Inc., 1987 (unpublished report no. 86-3114, for Sodium Chlorate Task Force, Oklahoma City).

31. *A subchronic (3-month) oral toxicity study of sodium chlorate in the rat via gavage.* East Millston, NJ, Bio/dynamics, Inc., 1987 (unpublished report no. 86-3112, for Sodium Chlorate Task Force, Oklahoma City).

32. *A teratogenicity study in rats with sodium chlorate.* East Millston, NJ, Bio/dynamics, Inc., 1987 (unpublished report no. 86-3117, for Sodium Chlorate Task Force, Oklahoma City).

33. Lubbers JR, Chauhan S, Bianchine JR. Controlled clinical evaluations of chlorine dioxide, chlorite and chlorate in man. *Fundamental and applied toxicology*, 1981, 1:334-338.

34. National Academy of Sciences. *Drinking water and health.* Vol. 3. Washington, DC, National Academy Press, 1980.

35. International Agency for Research on Cancer. *Chlorinated drinking-water; chlorination by-products; some other halogenated compounds; cobalt and cobalt compounds.* Lyon, 1991:45-359 (IARC Monographs on the Evaluation of Carcinogenic Risks to Humans, Volume 52).

## 16.5 Iodine

### 16.5.1 General description

#### *Identity*

CAS no.:                7553-56-2
Molecular formula:      $I_2$

#### *Physicochemical properties* (1, 2)[1,2]

| Property | Value |
|---|---|
| Boiling point | 184.4 °C |
| Melting point | 113.5 °C |
| Density | 4.93 g/cm³ at 25 °C |
| Vapour pressure | 40 Pa at 25 °C |
| Water solubility | 0.34 g/litre at 25 °C |
| Log octanol–water partition coefficient | 2.49 |

#### *Organoleptic properties*

The taste and odour thresholds for iodine are 0.147–0.204 mg/litre in water and 9 mg/m³ in air (3).

#### *Major uses*

Iodine is used as an antiseptic for skin wounds, as a disinfecting agent in hospitals and laboratories, and for the emergency disinfection of drinking-water in the field. Iodide is used in pharmaceuticals and in photographic developing materials.

#### *Environmental fate*

Iodine occurs naturally in water in the form of iodide (I⁻), which is largely oxidized to iodine during water treatment.

---

[1] Also includes data from the Hazardous Substances Data Bank of the National Library of Medicine, Bethesda, MD.
[2] Conversion factor in air: 1 ppm = 10 mg/m³.

## 16.5.2 Analytical methods

Iodide in water is normally determined by a titrimetric procedure which can be used for solutions containing 2–20 mg of iodide per litre. A leuco crystal violet method may be used for the determination of iodide or molecular iodine in water. This photometric method is applicable to iodide concentrations of 50–6000 µg/litre; the detection limit for iodine is 10 µg/litre (*4, 5*).

## 16.5.3 Environmental levels and human exposure

### Water

The mean concentration of total iodine in drinking-water in the USA is 4 µg/litre, and the maximum concentration is 18 µg/litre (*2*). This is presumably predominantly iodide.

### Food

The main natural sources of dietary iodide are seafood (200–1000 µg/kg) and seaweed (0.1–0.2% iodide by weight). Iodide is also found in cow's milk (20–70 µg/litre) and may be added to table salt (100 µg of potassium iodide per gram of sodium chloride) to ensure an adequate intake of iodine (*2, 6*). The estimated dietary iodine requirement for adults ranges from 80 to 150 µg/day (*7*).

### Estimated total exposure

Exposure to iodine may occur through drinking-water, pharmaceuticals, and food. At a concentration of 4 µg/litre in drinking-water, adult human daily intake will be 8 µg of iodine, on the asssumption that 2 litres of drinking-water are consumed per day.

## 16.5.4 Kinetics and metabolism in laboratory animals and humans

Molecular iodine is rapidly converted into iodide following ingestion and this is efficiently absorbed throughout the gastrointestinal tract (*8*). Molecular iodine vapour is converted into iodide before absorption (*2*). The highest concentration of iodine in the human body is found in the thyroid, which contains 70–80% of the total iodine content (15–20 mg). Muscle and eyes also contain high iodide concentrations (*6, 8*).

Iodine is an essential element in the synthesis of the thyroid hormones thyroxine ($T_4$) and triiodothyronine ($T_3$) through the precursor protein thyroglobulin and the action of the enzyme thyroid peroxidase. Iodide is excreted primarily by the kidneys and is partially reabsorbed from the tubules following glomerular filtration (*8*). Smaller amounts of iodine are excreted in saliva, sweat, bile, and milk (*9*).

## 16.5.5 Effects on laboratory animals and *in vitro* test systems

### Acute exposure

The acute oral $LD_{50}$ for potassium iodide in rats was 4340 mg/kg of body weight (3320 mg of iodide per kg of body weight), and the lowest oral lethal dose in mice was 1862 mg/kg of body weight (1425 mg of iodide per kg of body weight) (*9*).

### Short-term exposure

The effects of iodide on autoimmune thyroiditis were investigated in two strains of chickens (CS and OS) known to be genetically susceptible to this disease. Administration of iodide in drinking-water (20 or 200 mg/litre, as potassium iodide) during the first 10 weeks of life increased the incidence of the disease, as determined by histological examination of the thyroid and measurement of $T_3$, $T_4$, and thyroglobulin antibodies. Excessive iodide consumption may increase the incidence of this disease in humans (*10*).

### Reproductive toxicity, embryotoxicity, and teratogenicity

No effects were observed on ovulation rate, implantation rate, or fetal development in female rats given doses of 0, 500, 1000, 1500, or 2000 mg of iodide (as potassium iodide) per kg of diet during gestation and lactation. The dose-related survival rate for pups ranged from 93% (controls) to 16% (2000 mg/kg). Milk secretion was absent or greatly diminished in females exposed to iodide and the high mortality in pups was attributed to the dams' lactational failure (*11*).

The effects of iodide on brain enzymes in rat pups born to females given 1.1 mg of iodide per day as potassium iodide (about 37 mg/kg of body weight per day) in drinking-water were studied. Transient increases in glutamate dehydrogenase and decreases in succinate dehydrogenase were observed. Increases in phosphofructokinase and malate enzymes were also noted, but no changes in hexokinase were reported. Serum $T_4$ levels did not differ significantly from control values (*12*).

Metabolism was severely disturbed in foals born to mares receiving excess iodine (48–432 mg of iodine per day) in the diet during pregnancy and lactation. The long bones of the legs of foals showed osteopetrosis (abnormally dense bones); phosphorus and alkaline phosphatase levels in the blood were elevated (*13*).

### Carcinogenicity

In a study on the tumorigenic effects of iodide on the thyroid, groups of 20 rats were fed diets containing 0 or 1000 mg of iodide per kg as potassium iodide (0 or 39 mg of iodide per kg of body weight per day) for 19 weeks. No tumours were found on histopathological examination of the thyroid in either the treated or untreated groups (*14*). The exposure period may have been too short for a carcinogenic effect to be detected.

## 16.5.6 Effects on humans

### Short-term exposure

Oral doses of 2000–3000 mg of iodine (about 30–40 mg/kg of body weight) are estimated to be lethal to humans, but survival has been reported after ingestion of 10 000 mg. Doses of 30–250 ml of tincture of iodine (about 16–130 mg of total iodine per kg of body weight) have been reported to be fatal. Acute oral toxicity is primarily due to irritation of the gastrointestinal tract, marked fluid loss and shock occurring in severe cases. Exposure to iodine vapour results in lung, eye, and skin irritation, while high concentrations rapidly lead to pulmonary oedema (*2*).

In rare instances, a hypersensitization reaction may occur immediately after or within several hours of oral or dermal exposure to iodide. The most striking symptoms are angio-oedema (acute, transitory swelling of the face, hands, feet, or viscera) and swelling of the larynx, which may cause suffocation (*8*). Iodide has been used in the past as an expectorant in the treatment of asthma and related conditions at a typical dose of 3.3 mg/kg of body weight (*2*).

### Long-term exposure

Chronic iodide exposure results in iodism; the symptoms resemble those of a sinus cold but may also include salivary gland swelling, gastrointestinal irritation, acneform skin, metallic or brassy taste, gingivitis, increased salivation, conjunctival irritation, and oedema of eyelids (*8*). Chronic ingestion of 2 mg of iodide per day (0.03 mg/kg of body weight per day) is considered by some authors to be excessive, but daily doses of 50–80 mg (0.8–1.3 mg/kg of body weight per day) are consumed by some Japanese without ill effect (*6*).

Chronic consumption of iodinated drinking-water has not been shown to cause adverse health effects in humans although some changes in thyroid status have been observed. In a 5-year study of prison inmates consuming water containing iodine at a concentration of 1 mg/litre (approximately 0.03 mg/kg of body weight per day), no cases of hyper- or hypothyroidism, urticaria, or iodism were seen. However, a small but statistically significant decrease in radioactive iodine uptake by the thyroid and an increase in protein-bound iodine concentrations were reported (*15*). No adverse health effects were reported in men who drank water providing iodide at doses of 0.17–0.27 mg/kg of body weight per day for 26 weeks (*16*).

In one study, the rate of radioactive iodide uptake by the thyroid was measured in 22 individuals with thyroid disease and 10 with normal thyroid function, before and after administration of 2.0 mg of iodide. Radioactive iodine uptake decreased by 54–99% in patients with thyroid disease but only by 8–54% in normal controls. These results suggest that iodide may aggravate certain pre-existing thyroid disease conditions (17).

Eight cases of congenital goitre and hypothyroidism in children were reported to be associated with maternal ingestion of iodide (18). Estimates of maternal iodide exposure ranged from 12 to 1650 mg/day (about 0.2–27 mg/kg of body weight per day) in individuals taking iodide as an expectorant in the treatment of asthma. No direct evidence of a cause-and-effect relationship between iodide exposure and health effects during pregnancy was reported.

Hypothyroidism has also been reported in infants of mothers receiving multiple topical applications of povidone–iodine (about 1% free iodine) during pregnancy and lactation (19).

## 16.5.7 Conclusions

In 1988, JECFA set a PMTDI for iodine of 1 mg/day (17 µg/kg of body weight per day) from all sources, based mainly on data on the effects of iodide (20). However, recent data from studies in rats indicate that the effects of iodine in drinking-water on thyroid hormone concentrations in the blood differ from those of iodide (21, 22).

Available data therefore suggest that derivation of a guideline value for iodine on the basis of information on the effects of iodide is inappropriate, and there are few relevant data on the effects of iodine. Because iodine is not recommended for long-term disinfection, lifetime exposure to iodine from water disinfection is unlikely. For these reasons, a guideline value for iodine has not been established at this time.

## References

1. Budavari S, O'Neill M, Smith A, eds. *The Merck index. An encyclopedia of chemicals, drugs, and biologicals*, 11th ed. Rahway, NJ, Merck, 1989.

2. National Academy of Sciences. *Drinking water and health*. Vol. 3. Washington, DC, National Academy Press, 1980.

3. Ruth JH. Odor thresholds and irritation levels of several chemical substances: a review. *Journal of the American Industrial Hygiene Association*, 1986, 47:A142-A151.

4. US Environmental Protection Agency. *Methods for chemical analysis of water and wastes*. Cincinnati, OH, 1983 (EPA-600/4-79-020).

5. American Public Health Association. *Standard methods for the examination of water and wastewater*, 17th ed. Washington, DC, 1989.

6.  Hetzel BS, Maberly GF. Iodine. In: Mertz W, ed., *Trace elements in human and animal nutrition*, 5th ed. New York, NY, Academic Press, 1986:139-208.

7.  National Research Council. *Recommended dietary allowances*. Washington, DC, National Academy Press, 1989:214.

8.  Welt LG, Blythe WB. Anions: phosphate, iodide, fluoride and other anions. In: Goodman LD, Gilman A, eds. *The pharmacological basis of therapeutics*, 4th ed. New York, Macmillan, 1970.

9.  Stokinger HE. The halogens and the nonmetals, boron and silicon. In: Clayton GD, Clayton FE, eds. *Patty's industrial hygiene and toxicology*, Vol. 2B, 3rd rev. ed. New York, NY, John Wiley, 1981:2937-3043.

10. Bagchi N et al. Induction of autoimmune thyroiditis in chickens by dietary iodine. *Science*, 1985, 230:325-327.

11. Ammerman CB et al. Reproduction and lactation in rats fed excessive iodine. *Journal of nutrition*, 1964, 84:107-112.

12. Morales de Villalobos LM, Campos G, Ryder E. Effect of chronic ingestion of iodide during pregnancy and lactation on rat pup brain enzymes. *Enzyme*, 1986, 35:96-101.

13. Silva CA et al. Consequence of excess iodine supply on a thoroughbred stud in southern Brazil. *Journal of reproduction and fertility*, 1987, 35(Suppl.):529-533.

14. Hiasa Y et al. Potassium perchlorate, potassium iodide, and propylthiouracil: promoting effect on the development of thyroid tumors in rats treated with $N$-bis(2-hydroxypropyl)-nitrosamine. *Japanese journal of cancer research*, 1987, 78:1335-1340.

15. Thomas WC et al. Iodine disinfection of water. *Archives of environmental health*, 1969, 19:124-128.

16. Morgan DP, Karpen RJ. Test of chronic toxicity of iodine as related to the purification of water. *U.S. Armed Forces medical journal*, 1953, 4:725-728.

17. Paris J et al. The effect of iodides on Hashimoto's thyroiditis. *Journal of clinical endocrinology and metabolism*, 1961, 21:1037-1043.

18. Carswell F, Kerr MM, Hutchinson JH. Congenital goiter and hypothyroidism produced by maternal ingestion of iodides. *Lancet*, 1970, i:1241–1243.

19. Danziger Y, Pertzelan A, Mimouni M. Transient congenital hypothyroidism after topical iodine in pregnancy and lactation. *Archives of disease in childhood*, 1987, 62:295-296.

20. Joint FAO/WHO Expert Committee on Food Additives. *Toxicological evaluation of certain food additives and contaminants.* Cambridge, Cambridge University Press, 1989 (WHO Food Additives Series, No. 24).

21. Thrall KD, Bull RJ. Differences in the distribution of iodine and iodide in the Sprague-Dawley rat. *Fundamental and applied toxicology*, 1990, 15:75-81.

22. Sherer TT, Thrall KD, Bull RJ. Comparison of toxicity induced by iodine and iodide in male and female rats. *Journal of toxicology and environmental health*, 1991, 32(1):89-101.

# Disinfectant by-products

## 16.6 Bromate

### 16.6.1 General description

**Identity**

| Compound | CAS no. | Molecular formula |
|---|---|---|
| Potassium bromate | 7758-01-2 | $KBrO_3$ |
| Sodium bromate | 7789-38-0 | $NaBrO_3$ |

The bromate ion ($BrO_3^-$) may exist in a number of salts, the most common of which are potassium and sodium bromate.

**Physicochemical properties** *(1)*

| Property | Sodium bromate | Potassium bromate |
|---|---|---|
| Boiling point (°C) | – | Decomposes at 370 °C |
| Melting point (°C) | 381 | 350 |
| Density at 20 °C (g/cm³) | 3.34 | 3.27 |
| Water solubility (g/litre) | 275 (8 °C) | 133 (40 °C) |
|  | 909 (100 °C) | 498 (100 °C) |

**Major uses**

Bromate is used in home permanent wave neutralizing solutions *(2)*. Small amounts may be added to flour as a maturing agent, to dough as a conditioner, and to fish paste. It may also be added to beer or cheese *(3)*.

**Environmental fate**

Its properties suggest that bromate will not volatilize and will be adsorbed only slightly on to soil or sediment. Because it is a strong oxidant, its commonest fate is probably reaction with organic matter, ultimately leading to the formation of bromide ion.

## 16.6.2 Analytical methods

Bromate may be determined by several different methods, including iodometric titration and high-performance liquid chromatography. Detection limits range from 0.05 to 1 mg/litre (3). Ion chromatography with conductivity detection has a detection limit of 5 µg/litre (US EPA draft method, available from Environmental Monitoring and Support Laboratory, Cincinnati, OH, USA).

## 16.6.3 Environmental levels and human exposure

### Water

Bromate is not normally present in water but may be formed from bromide during ozonation. Concentrations of 60–90 µg/litre have been reported in ozonated water (4, 5).

### Food

Small amounts of bromate may be added to flour or dough during the preparation of bread, but this is broken down to bromide during baking (3).

### Estimated total exposure and relative contribution of drinking-water

For most people, exposure to bromate is unlikely to be significant. If ozone is used to disinfect drinking-water, intake of bromate might range from 120 to 180 µg/day (5).

## 16.6.4 Kinetics and metabolism in laboratory animals and humans

Following oral administration, bromate is rapidly absorbed from the gastrointestinal tract (6). It was not detected in rat tissues following a single intragastric dose, but was significantly increased in plasma, red blood cells, pancreas, kidney, stomach, and small intestine (7).

Bromate may be converted into hydrobromic acid by hydrochloric acid in the stomach (6). Liver and kidney tissues may degrade bromate to bromide by a process involving glutathione (8), although only small amounts appear to be reduced in this way (6). Bromate is excreted mainly in the urine as bromate and bromide; some may also be eliminated in the faeces (7).

## 16.6.5 Effects on laboratory animals and in vitro test systems

### Acute exposure

Potassium bromate administered orally (9) and intraperitoneally (10) to mice gave $LD_{50}$s of 223–363 and 136 mg of bromate per kg of body weight, respectively. LD$_{50}$s of 280–495 mg/kg of body weight were obtained for rats, mice, and hamsters given potassium bromate by gavage (*11*).

## Short-term exposure

Potassium bromate was administered to groups of F344 rats (10 per sex per dose) in water at concentrations of 0, 150, 300, 600, 1250, 2500, 5000, or 10 000 mg/litre (approximately 16, 32, 63, 140, 270, 540, or 1080 mg of bromate per kg of body weight per day) for 13 weeks. All animals exposed to 2500 mg/litre or more died within 7 weeks. Observed signs of toxicity included significant inhibition of body weight gain in males at 600 mg/litre or above and significant increases in serum parameters in both sexes at 600 mg/litre (*11*).

## Long-term exposure

Male Wistar rats were exposed to 0.04% potassium bromate in drinking-water (approximately 30 mg of bromate per kg of body weight per day) for up to 15 months. Effects included markedly inhibited body weight gain in all exposed animals, karyopyknotic foci in tubules of the inner kidney medulla, increased blood urea nitrogen (BUN), and marked structural abnormalities of the cortical tubules. Based on body weight and renal effects, a LOAEL of 30 mg of bromate per kg of body weight per day was identified in this study (*12*).

## Reproductive toxicity, embryotoxicity, and teratogenicity

The reproductive effects of potassium bromate were evaluated in a study in which rats and mice were fed flour treated with 15 mg of potassium bromate per kg over five and eight generations, respectively. No effects on reproductive performance or survival were observed in either species (*11*).

## Mutagenicity and related end-points

Positive results were obtained for the mutagenicity of potassium bromate in *Salmonella typhimurium* strain TA100 using the Ames test and for chromosomal aberrations in cultured Chinese hamster fibroblast cells (*13*). Positive results were also obtained in an *in vivo* study of the acute cytogenetic effect of potassium bromate on rat bone marrow cells (*14*) and in the mouse micronucleus test (*9, 10*). Some evidence of DNA damage in rats given potassium bromate has been observed (*15*).

## Carcinogenicity

F344 rats (50 per sex per dose) were given drinking-water containing 0, 250, or 500 (reduced to 400 at week 60) mg of potassium bromate per litre (average doses 0, 9.6, and 21.3 mg of bromate per kg of body weight per day in males and

0, 9.6 or 19.6 mg of bromate per kg of body weight per day in females) for 110 weeks. The incidence of renal tumours in the three groups was 6%, 60%, and 88% in males and 0, 56%, and 80% in females. The incidence of peritoneal mesotheliomas in dosed males was also significantly elevated (11%, 33%, and 59%). The authors concluded that potassium bromate was carcinogenic in both male and female rats (16).

In a subsequent study, male F344 rats were given water containing potassium bromate at 0, 15, 30, 60, 125, 250, or 500 mg/litre (equivalent to 0, 0.7, 1.3, 2.5, 5.6, 12, or 33 mg of bromate per kg of body weight) for 104 weeks. The incidence of renal cell tumours in these dose groups was 0, 0, 0, 4%, 21%, 25%, and 45% and was significantly elevated at 12 mg/kg of body weight per day and above. The incidence of dysplastic foci (considered to be preneoplastic lesions) was 0, 5%, 25%, 25%, 50%, 95%, and 95% and was significantly elevated at 5.6 mg/kg of body weight per day and above (17).

The carcinogenic potential of potassium bromate was investigated in B6C3F$_1$ female mice (50 per dose) supplied with water containing 0, 500, or 1000 mg of potassium bromate per litre (average dose 0, 43.5, or 91.6 mg of bromate per kg of body weight per day) for 78 weeks. Based on the histological examination of tissues at week 104, no significant difference in tumour incidence as between exposed and control animals was apparent (16).

Male F344 rats were supplied with water containing 500 mg of potassium bromate per litre (average dose 32.3 mg of bromate per kg of body weight per day) for up to 104 weeks to assess the time-course of renal cell tumour induction. Dysplastic foci and renal adenomas were first observed after 26 weeks of treatment, but the incidence was not statistically significant. Renal dysplastic foci (62%) and adenomas (52% were significantly increased as compared with controls by 52 weeks of treatment. After 104 weeks, renal adenocarcinomas were observed in 3 of 20 rats (15%) and adenomas in 6 of 20 (30%). The combined incidence of follicular adenomas and adenocarcinomas of the thyroid (7/35) was significantly increased in rats receiving treatment for 104 weeks. The authors concluded that the minimum induction time for renal adenoma development was 26 weeks (18).

In a related study, the incidence of renal cell tumours was investigated in F344 rats exposed to water containing 500 mg of potassium bromate per litre (29.6–35.5 mg of bromate per kg of body weight per day) for up to 104 weeks. The incidence of renal dysplastic foci was 65% in animals exposed for 1–13 weeks and increased to 100% in animals exposed for 39–52 weeks (0% in controls). The combined incidence of adenomas and adenocarcinomas in rats exposed for 13–52 weeks ranged from 47% to 74%, which is similar to or higher than that in animals exposed continuously for 104 weeks (45%). The authors concluded that the minimum total cumulative dose necessary for the induction of renal adenomas and adenocarcinomas was 4 g of potassium bromate per kg (3.1 g of bromate per kg) and the minimum treatment period for the induction of these tumours was 13 weeks (18).

No significant differences were observed in the incidence of tumours in male or female newborn F344 rats or ICR mice when potassium bromate was administered subcutaneously (*19*).

## 16.6.6 Effects on humans

Most cases of human poisoning from bromate are due to the accidental or intentional ingestion of home permanent wave solutions, which can contain 2–10% bromate. In children, serious poisonings have been reported following ingestion of 60–120 ml of 2% potassium bromate (equivalent to 46–92 mg of bromate per kg of body weight per day for a 20-kg child). Lethal oral doses of potassium bromate are estimated to be 200–500 mg/kg of body weight (150–385 mg of bromate per kg of body weight) (*2*).

Toxic effects of bromate salts include nausea, vomiting, abdominal pain and diarrhoea, varying degrees of central nervous system depression, seizures, respiratory depression, and pulmonary oedema, most of which are reversible. Irreversible effects include renal failure and deafness, both of which have been observed following the ingestion of 240–500 mg of potassium bromate per kg of body weight (185–385 mg of bromate per kg of body weight) (*2*).

## 16.6.7 Provisional guideline value

JECFA evaluated bromate and recommended that there should be no residues in food when bromate is used in food processing (*20*). IARC has concluded that there is sufficient evidence for the carcinogenicity of potassium bromate in animals (*3*) and has classified it in Group 2B (possible human carcinogen). Bromate is mutagenic both *in vitro* and *in vivo*.

To estimate cancer risks, the linearized multistage model was applied to the incidence of renal tumours in male rats given potassium bromate in drinking-water (*16*), although it was noted that, if the mechanism of tumour induction is oxidative damage in the kidney, application of the low-dose cancer risk model may not be appropriate. The concentrations in drinking-water associated with excess lifetime cancer risks of $10^{-4}$, $10^{-5}$, and $10^{-6}$ are 30, 3, and 0.3 µg/litre, respectively.

Because of limitations in available analytical and treatment methods, a provisional guideline value of 25 µg/litre is recommended. This value is associated with a lifetime excess cancer risk of $7 \times 10^{-5}$.

## References

1. Weast RC, ed. *CRC handbook of chemistry and physics*. 67th ed. Boca Raton, FL, CRC Press, 1986.

2. Mack RB. Round up the usual suspects. Potassium bromate poisoning. *North Carolina medical journal*, 1988, 49:243-245.

3.  International Agency for Research on Cancer. *Some naturally occurring and synthetic food components, furocoumarins and ultraviolet radiation.* Lyon, 1986:207-220 (IARC Monographs on the Evaluation of the Carcinogenic Risk of Chemicals to Humans, Volume 40).

4.  Haag WR, Holgne J. Ozonation of bromide-containing waters: kinetics of formation of hypobromous acid and bromate. *Environmental science and technology,* 1983, 17:261-267.

5.  McGuire MJ, Krasner SW, Gramith JT. *Comments on bromide levels in state project water and impacts on control of disinfectant by-products.* Los Angeles, CA, Metropolitan Water District of Southern California, 1990.

6.  Kutom A et al. Bromate intoxication: hairdressers' anuria. *American journal of kidney disease,* 1990, 15:84-85.

7.  Fujie M et al. Metabolism of potassium bromate in rats. I. *In vivo* studies. *Chemosphere,* 1984, 13:1207-1212.

8.  Tanaka K et al. Metabolism of potassium bromate in rats. II. *In vitro* studies. *Chemosphere,* 1984, 13:1213-1219.

9.  Nakajima M et al. Effect of route of administration in the micronucleus test with potassium bromate. *Mutation research,* 1989, 223:399-402.

10. Hayashi M et al. Difference between intraperitoneal and oral gavage application in the micronucleus test: the 3rd collaborative study by CSGMT/JEMS·MMS. *Mutation research,* 1989, 223:329-344.

11. Kurokawa Y et al. Toxicity and carcinogenicity of potassium bromate—a new renal carcinogen. *Environmental health perspectives,* 1990, 87:309-335.

12. Nakano K et al. Renal changes induced by chronic oral administration of potassium bromate or ferric nitrilotriacetate in Wistar rats. *Japanese archives of internal medicine,* 1989, 36:41-47.

13. Ishidate M et al. Primary mutagenicity screening of food additives currently used in Japan. *Food chemistry and toxicology,* 1984, 22:623-636.

14. Fujie K et al. Acute cytogenetic effects of potassium bromate on rat bone marrow cells *in vivo. Mutation research,* 1988, 206:455-458.

15. Kasai H et al. Oral administration of the renal carcinogen, potassium bromate, specifically produces 8-hydroxy-deoxyguanosine in rat target organ DNA. *Carcinogenesis,* 1987, 8:1959-1961.

16. Kurokawa Y et al. Long-term *in vivo* carcinogenicity tests of potassium bromate, sodium hypochlorite and sodium chlorite conducted in Japan. *Environmental health perspectives,* 1986, 69:221-235.

17. Kurokawa Y et al. Dose-response studies on the carcinogenicity of potassium bromate in F344 rats after long-term oral administration. *Journal of the National Cancer Institute*, 1986, 77:977-982.

18. Kurokawa Y et al. Relationship between the duration of treatment and the incidence of renal cell tumors in male F344 rats administered potassium bromate. *Japanese journal of cancer research*, 1987, 78:358-364.

19. Matsushima Y et al. Lack of carcinogenicity of potassium bromate after subcutaneous injection to newborn mice and newborn rats. *Science reports of the Research Institutes, Tohoku University*, 1986, 33:22-26.

20. Joint FAO/WHO Expert Committee on Food Additives. *Toxicological evaluation of certain food additives and contaminants*. Cambridge, Cambridge University Press, 1989 (WHO Food Additives Series, No. 24).

## 16.7 Chlorophenols

### 16.7.1 General description

#### *Identity*

| Compound | CAS no. | Molecular formula |
|----------|---------|-------------------|
| 2-Chlorophenol | 95-57-8 | $ClC_6H_4OH$ |
| 2,4-Dichlorophenol | 120-83-2 | $Cl_2C_6H_3OH$ |
| 2,4,6-Trichlorophenol | 88-06-2 | $Cl_3C_6H_2OH$ |

A total of 19 possible chlorinated phenols exist, but only 2-chlorophenol (2-CP), 2,4-dichlorophenol (2,4-DCP), and 2,4,6-trichlorophenol (2,4,6-TCP) will be evaluated here, as these are the most likely to occur in drinking-water as possible by-products of disinfection.

#### *Physicochemical properties* (1–3)

| Property | 2-CP [1] | 2,4-DCP [2] | 2,4,6-TCP [3] |
|----------|----------|-------------|---------------|
| Boiling point (°C) | 175–176 | 210–211 | 246 |
| Melting point (°C) | 8.7 | 43–44 | 68 |
| Density (g/cm³) | 1.24 | 1.38 | 1.49 |
| Vapour pressure (kPa) | 0.133 (12.1 °C) | 0.133 (53 °C) | 0.133 (76 °C) |
| Water solubility (mg/litre) | 28 000 | 4500 | 900 |
| Log octanol–water partition coefficient | 2.15 | 3.06 | — |

[1] Conversion factor in air: 1 ppm = 5.26 mg/m³.
[2] Conversion factor in air: 1 ppm = 6.67 mg/m³.
[3] Conversion factor in air: 1 ppm = 8.08 mg/m³.

### Organoleptic properties

Chlorophenols generally have very low organoleptic thresholds. The taste thresholds in water for 2-CP, 2,4-DCP, and 2,4,6-TCP are 0.1, 0.3, and 2 µg/litre, respectively. Odour thresholds are 10, 40, and 300 µg/litre, respectively (2).

### Major uses

2-CP is used as a precursor in the production of higher chlorophenols and dyestuffs, and as a preservative. 2,4-DCP is used as a mothproofing agent, germicide and antiseptic, and in the production of the pesticide 2,4-D. 2,4,6-TCP is used in the production of 2,3,4,6-tetrachlorophenol and pentachlorophenol, and as a germicide, glue and wood preservative, and antimildew agent (4, 5).

## 16.7.2 Analytical methods

EPA methods 604 (6, 7), 525 (8), and 8270 (9) are used for the determination of chlorophenols. The most sensitive technique involves the formation of the pentafluorobenzyl ether derivatives (an option in method 604); the method has a detection limit of 0.5–5 µg/litre. Chlorophenols can also be determined by gas chromatography with an electron-capture detector. The detection limits are 1–10 µg/litre for monochlorophenols, 0.5 µg/litre for dichlorophenols, and 0.01 µg/litre for trichlorophenols (1).

## 16.7.3 Environmental levels and human exposure

### Water

Chlorophenols are present in drinking-water as a result of the chlorination of phenols during disinfection, as by-products of the reaction of hypochlorite with phenolic acids, as biocides, or as degradation products of phenoxy herbicides. Data from 40 Canadian treatment plants indicate that chlorophenol levels in drinking-water are generally quite low but vary considerably from one location to another (10). Chlorination increased the concentrations of 2-CP (maximum 65 ng/litre), 2,4-DCP (72 ng/litre), and 2,4,6-TCP (719 ng/litre). Drinking-water from the Ruhr area of Germany contained 2,4-DCP at 3–6 ng/litre and 2,4,6-TCP at 1 ng/litre (1). Several chlorophenols were present in Finnish tapwater at levels roughly one order of magnitude higher than those found in Germany (11).

## 16.7.4 Kinetics and metabolism in laboratory animals and humans

Chlorophenols are well absorbed after oral administration (12), and they readily penetrate the skin (13). They do not appear to accumulate in body tissues in rats but are rapidly metabolized and eliminated from the body (14–16). The major metabolite is the glucuronide conjugate of the parent chlorophenol. Less abundant metabolites include sulfate conjugates and possibly chloromethoxyphenol isomers of the parent compounds (*12, 14, 16, 17*). Chlorophenols are readily excreted as glucuronide conjugates in urine and, to a lesser extent, faeces (*12, 16, 18*).

## 16.7.5 Effects on laboratory animals and *in vitro* test systems

### *2-Chlorophenol*

*Acute exposure*
The oral $LD_{50}$ for 2-CP in mice was reported to be 670 mg/kg of body weight (*19*).

*Long-term exposure*
Immunological (e.g. humoral and cell-mediated immunity, macrophage function) and haematological (e.g. red and white blood cell count, haematocrit, haemoglobin) effects were assessed in groups of 12–20 weanling female Sprague-Dawley rats exposed to 0, 5, 50, or 500 mg of 2-CP per litre in drinking-water (0, 0.5, 5, or 50 mg/kg of body weight per day) in a reproductive study. Females were exposed from 3 weeks of age until breeding at 90 days, and throughout gestation to parturition. No treatment-related differences were found. A NOAEL of 50 mg/kg of body weight per day can be identified (*15, 20*).

*Reproductive toxicity, embryotoxicity, and teratogenicity*
Groups of 12–20 weanling female Sprague-Dawley rats were exposed to 0, 5, 50, or 500 mg of 2-CP per litre in drinking-water (0, 0.5, 5, or 50 mg/kg of body weight per day) for 10 weeks, then bred. Treatment was continued during breeding, gestation, and weaning. Parameters evaluated included percentage conception, litter size, birth weight, number of stillbirths, weanling weight, and haematology in weanling rats. A treatment-related increase in conception rate, an increase in the number of stillbirths, and a decrease in the size of the litters were observed at the highest dose (*15, 21*).

*Carcinogenicity*
In a 24-month experiment, female Sprague-Dawley rats (12–22 per dose) were given 2-CP in drinking-water at 0, 5, 50, or 500 mg/litre (0, 0.5, 5, or 50 mg/kg of body weight per day) for 10 weeks, then bred. Ethylurea and nitrite, precursors of the transplacental carcinogen nitrosoethylurea (NEU), were administered to females on days 14–21 of pregnancy. The effects on tumour incidence and latency were most evident in male progeny that received 2-CP with NEU, both pre- and postnatally. The lowest level of 2-CP appeared to exert the greatest effect. The authors suggested that 2-CP is a co-carcinogen (*21*).

## 2,4-Dichlorophenol

*Acute exposure*

The acute oral $LD_{50}$s for 2,4-DCP in rats ranged from 580 to 4000 mg/kg of body weight (*22, 23*). Acute oral $LD_{50}$s were 1276 and 1352 mg/kg of body weight for male and female CD-1 mice, respectively (*24*).

*Short-term exposure*

CD-1 mice (20 per sex per dose) were exposed to 2,4-DCP in drinking-water for 90 days at concentrations of 0.2, 0.6, or 2.0 g/litre (mean daily doses of 50, 143, and 491 mg/kg of body weight for females and 40, 114, and 383 mg/kg of body weight for males). There were no significant differences in body weight gain and no differences in terminal organ weights or organ weight ratios. Haematological differences, namely an increase in leukocytes (high dose) and in polymorpho-nuclear leukocytes (low dose), were observed only in males. Changes in clinical chemistry parameters, namely a decrease in creatinine (low dose), an increase in BUN/creatinine ratios (mid-dose), and an increase in alkaline phosphatase (high dose), were significant in females. These changes were not consistently dose-related, and a LOAEL cannot be established (*24*).

ICR mice of both sexes were fed 2,4-DCP in the diet at 0, 0.05%, 0.1%, or 0.2% (0, 45, 100, or 230 mg/kg of body weight per day) for 6 months. Hyper-plasia of hepatic cells was reported in one of seven animals receiving 0.2%. There were no other significant differences in histopathology, organ or body weight gains, red or white blood cell counts, or alanine aminotransferase and aspartate aminotransferase activities at any dose. The authors identified a NOAEL of 100 mg/kg of body weight per day (*23*).

Pre- and postnatal treatment of rats with 300 mg of 2,4-DCP per litre of drinking-water for 147 days significantly increased liver and spleen weights and enhanced humoral immune responsiveness. Cell-mediated immunity was depressed at 30 and 300 mg/litre. No histopathological changes were reported. Based on these findings, a NOAEL of 3 mg/litre (0.3 mg/kg of body weight per day) and a LOAEL of 30 mg/litre (3 mg/kg of body weight per day) can be identified (*25*).

*Long-term exposure*

Investigations of the effects of long-term exposure to 2,4-DCP have been designed primarily to test its carcinogenic properties and are described below.

*Reproductive toxicity, embryotoxicity, and teratogenicity*

Administration of 2,4-DCP (0, 50, 150, or 500 mg/kg of body weight per day) in drinking-water to male CD-1 mice for 90 days had no effect on sperm motility or ability to penetrate ova (*26*). Exposure of female rats to 0, 3, 30, or 300 mg of 2,4-DCP per litre in drinking-water from 3 weeks of age and throughout parturition and lactation had no significant effect on conception, litter size and weight, number of stillborn pups, or survival of weanlings continued on treatment for 5 weeks (*25*).

*Mutagenicity and related end-points*
2,4-DCP did not show mutagenic potential in *Salmonella typhimurium* strains TA98, TA100, TA1535, and TA1537 with and without metabolic activation (*27*). In eukaryotic test assays, 2,4-DCP was not mutagenic in primary hepatocyte cultures, as shown by the absence of unscheduled DNA synthesis (*28*).

*Carcinogenicity*
F344 rats and B6C3F$_1$ mice were given 2,4-DCP in feed for 2 years at dietary concentrations of 0, 5000, or 10 000 mg/kg (mice and male rats) and 0, 2500, or 5000 mg/kg (female rats) (male rats: 0, 210, or 440 mg/kg of body weight per day; female rats: 0, 210, or 250 mg/kg of body weight per day; male mice, 0, 800, or 1300 mg/kg of body weight per day; female mice, 0, 430, or 820 mg/kg of body weight per day). There was no evidence of carcinogenicity in either species. The maximum tolerated dose was probably reached, judging from the lower body weight in the treated animals, especially at the high dose. Survival was not affected in either species (*29*).

## 2,4,6-Trichlorophenol

*Acute exposure*
The oral LD$_{50}$ for 2,4,6-TCP has been reported as 820 mg/kg of body weight in rats (*30*).

*Short-term exposure*
2,4,6-TCP was mixed with corn oil and administered daily by gavage to Sprague-Dawley rats (10 per sex per dose) for 90 consecutive days at 0, 80, 240, or 720 mg/kg of body weight per day. At 240 mg/kg of body weight per day, liver weight increased in males and adrenal gland weight increased in females. At the highest dose, treatment-related effects included salivation, increased weights of the kidneys, liver, adrenal glands, and testes, and an increase in serum albumin, total protein, and serum alanine aminotransferase, as well as a decrease in urinary pH. No gross or histopathological changes were seen. In this study, a LOAEL of 240 mg/kg of body weight per day and a NOAEL of 80 mg/kg of body weight per day were identified (Bercz JP et al., unpublished data, 1989).

*Long-term exposure*
Female Sprague-Dawley rats (12–14 per dose) were exposed to 2,4,6-TCP in drinking-water at 0, 3, 30, or 300 mg/litre from 3 weeks of age and throughout breeding, gestation, parturition, and lactation. Ten pups from each dose group were weaned at 3 weeks and continued on treatment for 12–15 weeks. A dose-related increase in the liver weight of the pups reached statistical significance at

30 and 300 mg/litre. At 300 mg/litre, the spleen weight of the pups also increased significantly. No treatment-related changes in cell-mediated immunity, humoral immunity, or macrophage function were seen in the treated groups. In this study, a LOAEL of 30 mg/litre (3 mg/kg of body weight per day) and a NOAEL of 3 mg/litre (0.3 mg/kg of body weight per day) were identified (21).

F344 rats (50 per sex per dose) were given 2,4,6-TCP in their feed at 0, 5000, or 10 000 mg/kg (0, 250, or 500 mg/kg of body weight per day) for 106–107 weeks. Mean body weights of both dosed groups were lower than those of corresponding controls and were dose-related throughout the study. Other clinical signs were common to both the dosed and the control groups. There was no significant dose-related trend in mortality. In a similar experiment in B6C3F$_1$ mice, dose-related decreases in mean body weights were seen in male and female mice. Other clinical signs were common to both dosed and control groups. There was no statistically significant dose-related trend in mortality in either sex (30).

*Reproductive toxicity, embryotoxicity, and teratogenicity*
Sprague-Dawley rats were exposed to 2,4,6-TCP at 0, 30, or 300 mg/litre in drinking-water from 3 weeks of age to parturition. There were no statistically significant treatment-related effects on percentage conception, litter size, percentage stillborn, birth weight, and percentage survival to weaning (21).

Male Long-Evans hooded rats were given 2,4,6-TCP at 0 or 1000 mg/kg of body weight in corn oil by gavage, 5 days per week for 11 weeks (average 0 or 714 mg/kg of body weight per day), then bred with untreated females. No treatment-related effects were seen in copulatory behaviour, semen characteristics, organ weights, fertility, or fetal outcome. Female rats were given 0, 100, 500, or 1000 mg/kg of body weight by gavage, 5 days per week for 2 weeks prior to and during mating and up to day 21 of gestation. No treatment-related effects were reported in litter size or pup survival at the dose levels tested (31).

*Mutagenicity and related end-points*
Mutagenic activity was not detected in *S. typhimurium* strains TA98, TA100, TA1535, and TA1537 with and without metabolic activation (27). 2,4,6-TCP showed weak but significant mutagenic activity in the MP-1 strain *of Saccharomyces cerevisiae* (32). There was no effect on mitotic crossing-over or mitotic gene conversion. Pregnant mice injected with 2,4,6-TCP displayed a slightly increased frequency of spotted coat in the offspring, indicative of weak mutagenic activity (32).

*Carcinogenicity*
Administration of 2,4,6-TCP to mice at 100 mg/kg of body weight for 72 weeks led to increases in the incidences of hepatomas and reticulum-cell sarcomas. However, the incidences are not statistically significant if males and females are considered separately or if matched controls are considered (33).

F344 rats and B6C3F$_1$ mice were given 2,4,6-TCP (96–97% pure) in the feed for over 2 years. Rats and male mice received doses of 0, 5000, or 10 000 mg/kg of body weight and female mice received time-weighted average doses of 0, 5214, or 10 428 mg/kg of body weight. A statistically significant dose-related increase in the incidence of lymphomas or leukaemias was observed in male rats (3/20, 23/50, and 29/50 for the control, low-, and high-dose groups, respectively). In addition, the combined incidence of hepatocellular carcinomas and adenomas was significantly increased as compared with controls in both male and female mice (30). The 2,4,6-TCP may have been contaminated with 1,3,6,8-tetrachlorodibenzo-p-dioxin (1,3,6,8-TCDD), which might also be capable of inducing liver tumours in mice but is not expected to induce leukaemias in male rats, as the 2,3,7,8-TCDD isomer does not appear to do so (34).

## 16.7.6 Guideline values

### 2-Chlorophenol

Because of the limited database on the toxicity of 2-CP, no health-based guideline value has been derived.

### 2,4-Dichlorophenol

Because the database for the toxicity of 2,4-DCP is limited, no health-based guideline value has been derived.

### 2,4,6-Trichlorophenol

2,4,6-TCP has been reported to induce lymphomas and leukaemias in male rats and hepatic tumours in male and female mice. IARC has concluded that 2,4,6-TCP is possibly carcinogenic to humans (Group 2B) (35). The compound has not been shown to be mutagenic in the Ames test but has shown weak mutagenic activity in other in vitro and in vivo assays.

A guideline value can be derived for 2,4,6-TCP by applying the linearized multistage model to leukaemias in male rats observed in a 2-year feeding study (33). The hepatic tumours found in this study were not used for risk estimation, because of the possible role of contaminants in their induction. The concentrations of 2,4,6-TCP in drinking-water (and hence the guideline values) associated with $10^{-4}$, $10^{-5}$, and $10^{-6}$ excess lifetime cancer risks are 2000, 200, and 20 µg/litre, respectively.

The lowest reported taste threshold for 2,4,6-TCP is 2 µg/litre. If water containing this chlorophenol is free from taste, it is unlikely to present an undue risk to health.

# References

1.  Dietz F, Traud J. [Trace analysis of phenols, especially chlorophenols in water, by GC.] *Vom Wasser*, 1978, 51:235-237 (in German).

2.  Kozak VP et al. *Reviews of the environmental effects of pollutants: XI. Chlorophenols.* Washington, DC, US Environmental Protection Agency, 1979 (EPA 600/1-79-012).

3.  *Chlorophenols.* Geneva, World Health Organization, 1989 (Environmental Health Criteria, No. 93).

4.  Freiter ER. Chlorophenols. In: *Kirk-Othmer encyclopedia of chemical technology.* 3rd ed., Vol.5, New York, John Wiley, 1979:864-872.

5.  Doedens JD. Chlorophenols. In: *Kirk-Othmer encyclopedia of chemical technology.* 2nd ed. New York, John Wiley, 1963:325-338.

6.  US Environmental Protection Agency. *U.S. EPA Method 604—Phenols.* Washington, DC, 1985 (40 CFR, part 136).

7.  Kawahara FK. Analysis of mercaptans, phenols and organic acids in surface waters with use of pentafluorobenzyl derivatives. *Environmental science and technology,* 1971, 5:235-239.

8.  Environmental Monitoring and Support Labatory. *U.S. EPA Method 525—Detection of organic compounds in drinking water by liquid-solid extraction and capillary column gas chromatography. Revision 2.1.* Cincinnati, OH, US Environmental Protection Agency, 1988.

9.  Office of Solid Waste. *U.S. EPA Method 8270—Gas chromatography/mass spectrometry for semi-volatile organics, capillary column technique, test methods for evaluating solid waste,* 3rd ed. Washington, DC, US Environmental Protection Agency, 1986 (SW 846).

10. Sithole BB, Williams DT. Halogenated phenols in water at forty Canadian potable water treatment facilities. *Journal of the Association of Official Analytical Chemists,* 1986, 69(5):807-810.

11. Paasivirta J et al. Polychlorinated phenols, guaiacols and catechols in the environment. *Chemosphere,* 1985, 14(5):469-491.

12. Carpenter HM, Bender RC, Buhler DR. Absorption, metabolism and excretion of 2- and 4-chlorophenol in rats. *Toxicology,* 1985, 5:109 (abstract).

13. Roberts MS, Anderson RA, Swarbrick J. Permeability of human epidermis to phenolic compounds. *Journal of pharmacy and pharmacology,* 1977, 29:677-683.

14. Somani SM, Khalique A. Distribution and metabolism of 2,4-dichlorophenol in rats. *Journal of toxicology and environmental health*, 1982, 9:889-897.

15. Exon JH, Koller LD. Effects of transplacental exposure to chlorinated phenols. *Environmental health perspectives*, 1982, 46:137-140.

16. Bahig ME, Kraus A, Klein W. Excretion and metabolism of 2,4,6-trichlorophenol-$^{14}$C in rats. *Chemosphere*, 1981, 10(3):323-327.

17. Somani SM, Smart T, Khalique A. Metabolism of 2,4-dichlorophenol by isolated perfused rat liver. *Journal of toxicology and environmental health*, 1984, 13:787-798.

18. Korte F et al. Ecotoxicologic profile analysis. *Chemosphere*, 1978, 7(1):79-102.

19. Bubnov WD, Jafizov FN, Ogryzkov SE. [The toxic properties of activated *o*-chlorophenol for white mice and blue foxes]. *Trudy Vsesojuznogo Naučno-Issledovatel'skogo Instituta Veterinarnoj Sanitarij Ektoparazitologij*, 1969, 33:258-263 (in Russian) (cited in ref. 2).

20. Exon JH, Koller LD. Effects of chlorinated phenols on immunity in rats. *International journal of immunology and pharmacology*, 1983, 5(2):131-136.

21. Exon JH, Koller LD. Toxicity of 2-chlorophenol, 2,4-dichlorophenol and 2,4,6-trichlorophenol. In: Jolley RL et al., eds. *Water chlorination: chemistry, environmental impact and health effects*. Vol. 5. Chelsea, MI, Lewis Publishers, 1985:307-330.

22. Deichmann WB, Mergard EG. Comparative evaluation of methods employed to express the degree of toxicity of a compound. *Journal of industrial hygiene and toxicology*, 1948, 30:373.

23. Kobayashi S et al. [Chronic toxicity of 2,4-dichlorophenol in mice: a simple design for the toxicity of residual metabolites of pesticides.] *Toho University, Japan, journal of the Medical Society*, 1972, 19:356-362 (in Japanese).

24. Borzelleca JF et al. Acute and subchronic toxicity of 2,4-dichlorophenol in DC-1 mice. *Fundamental and applied toxicology*, 1985, 5:478-486.

25. Exon JH et al. Toxicologic, pathologic and immunotoxic effects of 2,4-dichlorophenol in rats. *Journal of toxicology and environmental health*, 1984, 14:723-730.

26. Seyler DE et al. The use of *in vitro* methods for assessing reproductive toxicity. Dichlorophenols. *Toxicology letters*, 1984, 20:309-315.

27. Rasanen L, Hattula ML, Arstila AU. The mutagenicity of MCPA and its soil metabolites, chlorinated phenols, catechols and some widely used slimicides in Finland. *Bulletin of environmental contamination and toxicology*, 1977, 18(5):565-571.

28. Probst GS et al. Chemically-induced unscheduled DNA synthesis in primary rat hepatocyte cultures: a comparison with bacterial mutagenicity using 218 compounds. *Environmental mutagenesis*, 1981, 3:11-32.

29. National Toxicology Program. *Toxicology and carcinogenesis studies of 2,4-dichlorophenol in F344/N rats and B6C3F₁ mice.* Research Triangle Park, NC, 1989 (NTP-TR-353).

30. National Cancer Institute. *Bioassay of 2,4,6-trichlorophenol for possible carcinogenicity.* Bethesda, MD, 1979 (NCI-CG-TR-155).

31. Blackburn K et al. Evaluation of the reproductive toxicology of 2,4,6-trichlorophenol in male and female rats. *Fundamental and applied toxicology*, 1986, 6:233-239.

32. Fahrig R, Nilsson CA, Rappe C. Genetic activity of chlorophenols and chlorophenol impurities. In: Rao KR, ed. *Pentachlorophenol: chemistry, pharmacology and environmental toxicology.* New York, NY, Plenum Press, 1978:325-338.

33. Bionetics Research Laboratories. *Evaluation of carcinogenic, teratogenic and mutagenic activities of selected pesticides and industrial chemicals.* Vol. 1. *Carcinogenic studies.* Bethesda, MD, National Cancer Institute, 1968.

34. Firestone D et al. Determination of polychlorodibenzo-*p*-dioxins and related compounds in commercial chlorophenols. *Journal of the Association of Official Analytical Chemists*, 1972, 55(1):85-92.

35. International Agency for Research on Cancer. *Overall evaluations of carcinogenicity: an updating of IARC Monographs volumes 1-42.* Lyon, 1987:154-156 (IARC Monographs on the Evaluation of Carcinogenic Risks to Humans, Suppl. 7).

# 16.8 Formaldehyde

## 16.8.1 General description

### Identity

CAS no.:              50-00-00
Molecular formula:    $CH_2O$

The IUPAC name for formaldehyde is methanal.

### *Physicochemical properties (1–4)*[1]

| Property | Value |
|---|---|
| Physical state | Colourless gas |
| Boiling point | -19.2 °C |
| Melting point | -118 °C |
| Relative density | 1.04 (air=1) |
| Vapour pressure | 52.6 kPa at -33 °C |
| Water solubility | Freely miscible at 25 °C |
| Log octanol–water partition coefficient | -1 |

### *Organoleptic properties*

Formaldehyde has a pungent, suffocating, hay- or straw-like odour. Taste and odour thresholds are 50 and 25 mg/litre, respectively (*3, 4*).

### *Major uses*

Formaldehyde's main industrial use is in the production of urea–formaldehyde, phenolic, melamine, pentaerythritol, and polyacetal resins. Its second largest use is in the industrial synthesis of a number of organic compounds. It is also used in cosmetics, fungicides, textiles, and embalming fluids (*1*).

## 16.8.2 Analytical methods

Formaldehyde in drinking-water is generally determined by a high-performance liquid chromatographic method following derivatization with 2,4-dinitrophenyl-hydrazine and liquid–solid extraction. The detection limit is 6.2 µg/litre (*5*).

## 16.8.3 Environmental levels and human exposure

### *Air*

Formaldehyde is emitted into air from plastics and resin glues. Low levels in air may also result from the photo-oxidation of hydrocarbons derived from fossil fuel. Typical levels in air are a few µg/m$^3$. Smokers are exposed to high levels of formaldehyde (*1, 6, 7*).

### *Water*

Formaldehyde in drinking-water is formed mainly by the oxidation of natural organic (humic) matter during ozonation (*8*) and chlorination (*9*). It also enters

---

[1] Conversion factor in air: 1 ppm = 1.2 mg/m$^3$ at 25 °C.

drinking-water via industrial effluents and leaching from polyacetal plastic fittings. Concentrations of up to 30 µg/litre have been found in ozonated drinking-water (*10, 11*).

## Food

Concentrations of formaldehyde ranging from 3 to 23 mg/kg have been reported in a variety of foods (*6*).

### Estimated total exposure and relative contribution of drinking-water

The general population is exposed to formaldehyde mainly by inhalation, smokers receiving about 0.38 mg/day by this route (*1, 7*). People are also exposed by ingesting contaminated drinking-water and food, and from the use of urea–formaldehyde foam in housing insulation, and of cosmetics containing formaldehyde.

## 16.8.4 Kinetics and metabolism in laboratory animals and humans

Ingested formaldehyde is readily absorbed by the gastrointestinal tract. In dermal studies, it was absorbed less readily in monkeys than in rats or guinea-pigs (*12*). It appears to be distributed mainly to muscle, lower levels being found in the intestines, liver, and other tissues (*13*).

Formaldehyde is rapidly oxidized to formic acid; the subsequent oxidation to carbon dioxide and water is slower in monkeys than in rats (*14*). Other metabolic products, such as *N,N'*-bis(hydroxymethyl)urea and *N*-(hydroxymethyl)urea, have been reported in rats (*15*). Metabolites are eliminated in the urine, faeces, and expired air, the relative amounts depending on the route of administration (*1, 16, 17*).

## 16.8.5 Effects on laboratory animals and *in vitro* test systems
### Acute exposure

Oral $LD_{50}$s of 800 and 260 mg/kg of body weight have been reported for the rat and guinea-pig, respectively (*18*).

### Short-term exposure

In a 4-week study, Wistar rats (10 per sex per dose) received formaldehyde in drinking-water at doses of 0, 5, 25, or 125 mg/kg of body weight per day. Rats receiving the highest dose showed lowered food and liquid intake, histopathological changes in the stomach (focal hyperkeratosis of the forestomach, moderate papillomatous hyperplasia) and, in males only, lowered total protein and albumin levels in plasma. The NOAEL was 25 mg/kg of body weight per day (*1, 19*).

Oral doses of 0, 50, 100, or 150 mg/kg of body weight per day in rats and 0, 50, 75, or 100 mg/kg of body weight per day in dogs for 91 days had no effect on haematology, clinical chemistry, urinalysis, or gross microscopic pathology. Depression in body weight gain was observed in both species at the highest dose levels and in male rats given 100 mg/kg of body weight per day (*20*).

### Long-term exposure

In a 2-year study, Wistar rats were exposed to formaldehyde in drinking-water at mean doses of 0, 1.2, 15, or 82 mg/kg of body weight per day for males and 0, 1.8, 21, or 109 mg/kg of body weight per day for females. Adverse effects were observed only in animals receiving the highest dose and included lower food and liquid intake, lower body weights, and pathological changes in the stomach, characterized by thickening of the mucosal wall. Relative kidney weights were increased in high-dose females, and an increased incidence of renal papillary necrosis was found in both sexes. Exposure did not appear to affect survival, haematology, or clinical chemistry. The NOAEL was 15 mg/kg of body weight per day (*21*).

In a similar study, Wistar rats were given formaldehyde in drinking-water at 10, 50, or 300 mg/kg of body weight per day. At the end of 12 months, rats of both sexes in the high-dose group were observed to have gastric erosions, ulcers, squamous cell hyperplasia, hyperkeratosis, and basal cell hyperplasia. Only one male and one female from the mid-dose group showed hyperkeratosis (*1, 22*).

### Reproductive toxicity, embryotoxicity, and teratogenicity

No teratogenic effects were reported in mice given formaldehyde at oral doses of 0, 74, 148, or 185 mg/kg of body weight per day on days 6–15 of gestation (*23*). Growth and viability of neonates from mice given oral doses of 540 mg/kg of body weight per day on days 8–12 of gestation were unaffected (*24*). No effects on reproductive performance or on the health of offspring were observed in beagle dogs fed 0, 3.1, or 9.4 mg of formaldehyde per kg of body weight per day in their diet on days 4–56 after mating (*25*). Sperm abnormalities were observed in male rats given single oral doses of 100–200 mg/kg of body weight (*26*). Intraperitoneal injection of formaldehyde at 8 or 16 mg/kg of body weight per day for 10 days resulted in degeneration of testicular tissue, inhibition of spermatogenesis, and lowered male reproductive organ weights in rats (*27*).

### Mutagenicity and related end-points

Formaldehyde has shown evidence of mutagenicity in prokaryotic and eukaryotic cells *in vitro*. It has also been shown to be genotoxic in *Drosophila melanogaster*. It binds readily to proteins, RNA, and single-stranded DNA to induce DNA–protein cross-links and breaks in single-stranded DNA. It reacts readily with macromolecules in cells, mainly at the point of exposure (*28*). *In vivo*, formaldehyde increases both DNA synthesis (*29*) and the number of micronuclei and nuclear anomalies in epithelial cells in rats (*30*).

### Carcinogenicity

There is little evidence that formaldehyde is carcinogenic by the oral route. In a 2-year study in which Wistar rats were exposed to formaldehyde in drinking water at mean doses of 0, 1.2, 15, or 82 mg/kg of body weight per day for males and 0, 1.8, 21, or 109 mg/kg of body weight per day for females, exposure did not appear to affect tumour incidence (*21*). In a 2-year study in which Sprague-Dawley rats were exposed to formaldehyde in drinking-water at dose levels of 0, 1, 5, 10, 50, 100, or 150 mg/kg of body weight per day, a dose-dependent increase in the incidence of leukaemia (mainly lymphoblastic) and lymphosarcoma was reported at dose levels of 5 mg/kg of body weight per day or greater. The increase in the incidence of gastrointestinal neoplasms was not dose-related. Tumours of this type were rare in historical controls and not detected in concurrent controls (*31*).

In a carcinogenicity study, a group of 10 rats was given drinking-water containing 0.5% formalin (0.2% formaldehyde) for 32 weeks. Histopathological changes were observed in the stomach, as well as neoplastic changes in the forestomach and papillomas. In addition, the authors reported evidence that formaldehyde had tumour-promoting activity. However, because of the presence of high levels of methanol in formalin, the usefulness of this information is limited (*32*). In another study, formaldehyde induced ornithine decarboxylase activity (an indication of tumour-promoting activity) in rats given a single oral formaldehyde dose of up to 100 mg/kg of body weight (*29*). There is no evidence that formaldehyde acts as a carcinogen or promoter when applied to mouse skin (*33*).

There is some evidence that inhalation exposure to formaldehyde causes cancer in rats and mice by irritating the nasal epithelium. Rats exposed to 17 mg of formaldehyde per m$^3$, 6 h per day, 5 days per week for 2 years, exhibited an increased incidence of squamous cell carcinoma of the nasal cavity. Tumours were also noted in mice at the same level of exposure, but this species was less sensitive than the rat (*34, 35*).

### 16.8.6 Effects on humans

Irritation and allergic contact dermatitis have been associated with exposure of the skin to formaldehyde at levels higher than those encountered in drinking-water (*36*). Its presence in some types of water filters has been associated with the occurrence of haemolytic anaemia in dialysis patients (*1, 37*).

There is some evidence that formaldehyde is a carcinogen in humans exposed by inhalation. Epidemiological investigations of the mortality of factory workers following prolonged occupational exposure to formaldehyde showed a slight excess of lung cancer that was not related to formaldehyde exposure (*2, 38*). An increase in the incidence of nasopharyngeal cancer was also noted but again did not appear to be related to formaldehyde (*39*).

## 16.8.7 Guideline value

Rats and mice exposed to formaldehyde by inhalation exhibited an increased incidence of carcinomas of the nasal cavity at doses that caused irritation of the nasal epithelium (*34, 35*). Ingestion of formaldehyde in drinking-water for 2 years caused stomach irritation in rats (*21, 22*). Papillomas of the stomach associated with severe tissue irritation were observed in one study (*32*).

On the basis of studies in which humans and experimental animals were exposed to formaldehyde by inhalation, IARC has classified formaldehyde in Group 2A (*40*). The weight of evidence indicates that formaldehyde is not carcinogenic by the oral route. A guideline value has been derived, therefore, on the basis of a TDI. A TDI of 150 µg/kg of body weight was calculated based on the NOAEL of 15 mg/kg of body weight per day in a 2-year study in rats (*21*), incorporating an uncertainty factor of 100 (for intra- and interspecies variation). No account was taken of potential carcinogenicity from the inhalation of formaldehyde from various indoor water uses, such as showering. With an allocation of 20% of the TDI to drinking-water, the guideline value is 900 µg/litre.

## References

1.  *Formaldehyde.* Geneva, World Health Organization, 1989 (Environmental Health Criteria, No. 89).

2.  Acheson ED et al. Formaldehyde process workers and lung cancer. *Lancet*, 1984, 1(8385):1066-1067 (letter).

3.  Bills D, Marking L, Chandler H Jr. *Investigation in fish control. 73. Formalin: Its toxicity to nontarget aquatic organisms, persistence and counteraction.* Washington, DC, US Department of the Interior, Fish and Wildlife Service, 1977:1-7.

4.  Verschueren K. *Handbook of environmental data on organic chemicals*, 2nd ed. New York, Van Nostrand Reinhold, 1983:678-679.

5.  Environmental Monitoring Systems Laboratory. *Method 554. Determination of carbonyl compounds in drinking water by DNPH derivatization and high performance liquid chromatography (HPLC).* Cincinnati, OH, US Environmental Protection Agency, 1991.

6.  International Agency for Research on Cancer. *Some industrial chemicals and dyestuffs.* Lyon, 1982:345-389 (IARC Monographs on the Evaluation of the Carcinogenic Risk of Chemicals to Humans, Volume 29).

7.  National Research Council. *Formaldehyde: an assessment of its health effects.* Washington, DC, National Academy of Sciences, 1980.

8.  Glaze WH, Koga M, Cancilla D. Ozonation by-products. 2. Improvement of an aqueous-phase derivatization method for the detection of formaldehyde and other carbonyl compounds formed by the ozonation of drinking water. *Environmental science and technology,* 1989, 23:838-847.

9.  Becher G, Ovrum NM, Christman RF. Novel chlorination by-products of aquatic humic substances. *Science of the total environment,* 1992, 117/118:509-520.

10. Tomkins BA et al. Liquid chromatographic determination of total formaldehyde in drinking water. *Journal of the Association of Official Analytical Chemists,* 1989, 72:835-839.

11. Krasner SW et al. The occurrence of disinfection by-products in US drinking water. *Journal of the American Water Works Association,* 1989, 81:41-53.

12. Jeffcoat AR. *Percutaneous penetration of formaldehyde. Final report (July 1981-July 1983).* Research Triangle Park, NC, Research Triangle Institute, 1983:59.

13. Bhatt HS, Lober SB, Combes B. Effect of glutathione depletion on aminopyrine and formaldehyde metabolism. *Biochemical pharmacology,* 1988, 37:1581-1589.

14. McMartin KE et al. Methanol poisoning. V. Role of formate metabolism in the monkey. *Journal of pharmacology and experimental therapeutics,* 1977, 201:564-572.

15. Mashford PM, Jones AR. Formaldehyde metabolism by the rat: a re-appraisal. *Xenobiotica,* 1982, 12:119-124.

16. Galli CL et al. Toxicological evaluation in rats and mice of the ingestion of a cheese made from milk with added formaldehyde. *Food chemistry and toxicology,* 1983, 21:313-317.

17. Upreti RK et al. Toxicokinetics and molecular interaction of [$^{14}$C]-formaldehyde in rats. *Archives of environmental contamination and toxicology,* 1987, 16:263-273.

18. Smyth HF Jr, Seaton J, Fischer L. The single dose toxicity of some glycols and derivatives. *Journal of industrial hygiene and toxicology,* 1941, 23:259-268.

19. Til HP et al. Evaluation of the oral toxicity of acetaldehyde and formaldehyde in a 4-week drinking-water study in rats. *Food chemistry and toxicology,* 1988, 26:447-452.

20. Johannsen FR, Levinskas GJ, Tegeris AS. Effects of formaldehyde in the rat and dog following oral exposure. *Toxicology letters,* 1986, 30:1-6.

21. Til HP et al. Two-year drinking-water study of formaldehyde in rats. *Food chemistry and toxicology,* 1989, 27:77-87.

22. Tobe M, Naito K, Kurokawa Y. Chronic toxicity study on formaldehyde administered orally to rats. *Toxicology*, 1989, 56:79-86.

23. Marks TA, Worthy WC, Staples RE. Influence of formaldehyde and Sonacide (potentiated acid glutaraldehyde) on embryo and fetal development in mice. *Teratology*, 1980, 22:51-58.

24. Seidenberg JM, Anderson DG, Becker RA. Validation of an *in vivo* developmental toxicity screen in the mouse. *Teratogenesis, carcinogenesis and mutagenesis*, 1987, 6:361-374.

25. Hurni H, Ohder H. Reproduction study with formaldehyde and hexamethylenetetramine in beagle dogs. *Food and cosmetics toxicology*, 1977, 11:459-462.

26. Cassidy SL, Dix KM, Jenkins T. Evaluation of a testicular sperm head counting technique using rats exposed to dimethoxyethyl phthalate (DMEP), glycerol alphamonochlorohydrin (GMCH), epichlorohydrin (ECH), formaldehyde (FA), or methyl methanesulphonate (MMS). *Archives of toxicology*, 1983, 53:71-78.

27. Shah BM et al. Formaldehyde-induced structural and functional changes in the testis of rats. *Journal of reproductive biology and comparative endocrinology*, 1987, 7:42-52.

28. Ma TH, Harris MM. Review of the genotoxicity of formaldehyde. *Mutation research*, 1988, 196:37-59.

29. Overman DO. Absence of embryotoxic effects of formaldehyde after percutaneous exposure in hamsters. *Toxicology letters*, 1985, 24:107-110.

30. Migliore L et al. Micronuclei and nuclear anomalies induced in the gastrointestinal epithelium of rats treated with formaldehyde. *Mutagenesis*, 1989, 4(5):327-334.

31. Soffritti M et al. Formaldehyde: an experimental multipotential carcinogen. *Toxicology and industrial health*, 1989, 5(5):699-730.

32. Takahashi M et al. Effects of ethanol, potassium metabisulfite, formaldehyde and hydrogen peroxide on gastric carcinogenesis in rats after initiation with *N*-methyl-*N¹*-nitro-*N*-nitrosoguanidine. *Japanese journal of cancer research (Gann)*, 1986, 77: 118-124.

33. Krivanek ND, Chromey NC, McAlack JW. Skin initiation-promotion study with formaldehyde in CD-1 mice. In: Clary JJ, Gibson JE, Waritz RS, eds. *Formaldehyde: toxicology, epidemiology, mechanisms*. New York, Marcel Dekker, 1983:159-171.

34. Swenberg JA et al. Induction of squamous cell carcinomas of the rat nasal cavity by inhalation exposure to formaldehyde vapor. *Cancer research*, 1980, 40:3398-3402.

35. Kerns WD et al. Carcinogenicity of formaldehyde in rats and mice after long-term inhalation exposure. *Cancer research*, 1983, 43:4382-4392.

36. Cosmetic, Toiletry and Fragrance Association. Final report on the safety assessment of formaldehyde. *Journal of the American College of Toxicologists*, 1984, 3:157-184.

37. Beall JR. Formaldehyde in dialysis patients. A review. In: Turosk V, ed. *Formaldehyde: analytical chemistry and toxicology*. Washington, DC, Chemical Society, 1985:275-287 (Advances in Chemistry Series, Vol. 210).

38. Acheson ED et al. Formaldehyde in the British chemical industry. An occupational cohort study. *Lancet*, 1984, 1(8377):611-616.

39. Collins JJ et al. Formaldehyde exposure and nasopharyngeal cancer: re-examination of the National Cancer Institute study and an update of one plant. *Journal of the National Cancer Institute*, 1988, 80:376-377.

40. International Agency for Research on Cancer. *Overall evaluations of carcinogenicity: an updating of IARC Monographs volumes 1-42*. Lyon, 1987:211-216 (IARC Monographs on the Evaluation of Carcinogenic Risks to Humans, Suppl. 7).

## 16.9 MX

### 16.9.1 General description

#### *Identity*

CAS no.:                77439-76-0
Molecular formula:      $C_5H_3Cl_3O_3$

MX is the common name for 3-chloro-4-dichloromethyl-5-hydroxy-2(5H)-furanone.

#### *Major uses*

MX does not have any commercial uses.

#### *Environmental fate*

In drinking-water at normal pH, MX exists in the open-ring form, i.e. as (Z)-2-chloro-3-(dichloromethyl)-4-oxobutenoic acid.

### 16.9.2 Analytical methods

MX in drinking-water can be determined by first concentrating organics using XAD resins, followed by high-pressure liquid chromatography, capillary-column gas chromatography, and mass spectroscopy (*1–3*).

## 16.9.3 Environmental levels and human exposure

### Water

MX is formed by the reaction of chlorine with complex organic matter in drinking-water and is present in the chlorinated effluents of pulp mills. It has been identified in chlorinated humic acid solutions and drinking-water in Finland, the United Kingdom and the USA, and was found to be present in 37 water sources at levels of 2–67 ng/litre (2, 4). Five drinking-water samples from different Japanese cities contained MX at concentrations ranging from <3 to 9 ng/litre (5).

## 16.9.4 Kinetics and metabolism in laboratory animals and humans

At least 40% of a dose of MX administered by gavage to rats was absorbed, about 5% of it being recovered in the liver, muscle, skin, kidneys, and blood (6). It has been demonstrated that MX is a substrate for direct conjugation with glutathione *in vitro* and that glutathione-*S*-transferase enhances the reaction (7). Cumulative excretion of label in 48 h by male rats given [14]C-labelled MX by gavage was about 34% in the urine and 47% in faeces (6). No parent compound was excreted in the urine from rats (8).

## 16.9.5 Effects on laboratory animals and *in vitro* test systems

### Acute exposure

An acute oral $LD_{50}$ of 128 mg/kg of body weight per day has been estimated for mice (9).

### Short-term exposure

MX in distilled water was administered to Swiss-Webster mice (5 per sex per dose) by gavage at 10, 20, 42, 88, or 184 mg/kg of body weight per day for 2 days. At 184 mg/kg of body weight per day, all animals died within 1 day following the second dose; enlarged stomachs and haemorrhagic areas of the forestomach were observed. At lower doses, no deaths occurred, no effects on body weight were noted during the 2-week observation period, and gross necropsy results were normal (9).

### Mutagenicity and related end-points

MX was reported to be an extremely potent mutagen in *Salmonella typhimurium* strain TA100 without metabolic activation by the S9 fraction of rat liver homogenate. The responses were also positive but not as strong in strains TA92, TA97,

TA98, TA102, and TA1535. No mutagenic response was found with TA1537. The addition of the S9 fraction dramatically decreased the responses of TA100, TA98, and TA1535 (*9, 10*).

MX has been examined for genotoxic activity in cultured mammalian cells. In Chinese hamster ovary cells (CHO-K1), it induced significant increases in structural chromosomal aberrations with and without metabolic activation (*9*). It also induced DNA strand breaks in suspensions of rat hepatocytes, rat testicular cells and V79 Chinese hamster cells (*11*), but not micronuclei in mouse bone marrow *in vivo*, despite its relatively high clastogenic activity in mammalian cells *in vitro* (*9*).

### Carcinogenicity

A skin tumour initiation–promotion assay was conducted in SENCAR mice (20–40 per dose). A single dose of MX was administered either topically in acetone or orally in distilled water at 5, 16, 28, or 50 mg/kg of body weight. Two weeks after treatment, 12-*O*-tetradecanoyl-phorbol-13-acetate (TPA) was applied topically three times per week for 30 weeks. At 24 weeks, no tumours were observed in animals receiving MX alone (topically or orally) without TPA promotion; results in topically treated animals with TPA promotion were similar to those in controls. In orally treated mice, both the tumour incidence and number of tumours per mouse were significantly elevated at 16 mg of MX per kg of body weight and above. Because of disparities in the tumour incidences for the topical and oral control groups, the data were reanalysed at 28 weeks, when tumour incidence was significantly higher than for controls only in the group receiving 16 mg/kg of body weight. The authors concluded that these results require confirmation before MX can be considered to possess tumour-initiating activity when administered orally (*4*).

### 16.9.6 Conclusions

There are very limited data on the toxicity of MX. $^{14}$C-labelled MX is rapidly absorbed, and most of the radioactivity is excreted in the urine within 24–48 h. It is unlikely to be absorbed as the parent compound because of its high reactivity. MX is an extremely potent mutagen in some strains of *Salmonella typhimurium*, but the addition of liver extract dramatically reduces the response. It is only weakly active or inactive in short-term tests for genotoxicity *in vivo*. Available data are inadequate to permit a guideline value for MX to be established.

### References

1. Munch JW et al. Determination of a chlorinated furanone (MX) in treated water. In: *Proceedings of the American Water Works Quality Technology Conference, Baltimore, MD, November 1987*. Denver, CO, American Water Works Association, 1987:933–942.

2.  Hemming J et al. Determination of the strong mutagen 3-chloro-4-(dichloro-methyl)-5-hydroxy-2(5H)-furanone in chlorinated drinking and humic waters. *Chemosphere*, 1986, 15:549-556.

3.  Kronberg L, Vartiainen T. Ames mutagenicity and concentration of the strong mutagen 3-chloro-4-(dichloromethyl)-5-hydroxy-2(5H)-furanone and of its geometric isomer (E)-2-chloro-3-(dichloromethyl)-4-oxobutenoic acid in chlorine-treated tapwater. *Mutation research*, 1988, 206:177-182.

4.  Meier JR et al. Genotoxic and carcinogenic properties of chlorinated furanones—important by-products of water chlorination. In: Waters MO et al., eds. *Genetic toxicology of complex mixtures: short-term bioassays in the analysis of complex environmental mixtures*. New York, Plenum Press, 1989:185-195.

5.  Suzuki N, Nakaniski J. The determination of strong mutagen, 3-chloro-4-(dichloromethyl)-5-hydroxy-2(5H)-furanone in drinking water in Japan. *Chemosphere*, 1990, 21:387-392.

6.  Ringhand HP et al. Synthesis of 3-$^{14}$C-3-chloro-4-(dichloromethyl)-5-hydroxy-2(5H)-furanone and its use in a tissue distribution study in the rat. *Chemosphere*, 1989, 18:2229-2236.

7.  Meier JR et al. Importance of glutathione in the *in vitro* detoxification of 3-chloro-4-(dichloromethyl)-5-hydroxy-2(5H)-furanone, an important mutagenic by-product of water chlorination. In: Jolley RL et al., eds. *Water chlorination: chemistry, environmental impact and health effects*. Chelsea, MI, Lewis Publishers, 1990.

8.  Komulainen H et al. Pharmacokinetics in rat of 3-chloro-4-(dichloromethyl)-5-hydroxy-2(5H)-furanone (MX), a drinking water mutagen, after a single dose. *Pharmacology and toxicology*, 1992, 70:424-428.

9.  Meier JR, Blazak WF, Knohl RB. Mutagenic and clastogenic properties of 3-chloro-4-(dichloromethyl)-5-hydroxy-2(5H)-furanone: a potent bacterial mutagen in drinking water. *Environmental molecular mutation*, 1987, 10:411-424.

10. Holmbom B et al. Fractionation, isolation, and characterization of Ames mutagenic compounds in kraft chlorination effluents. *Environmental science and technology*, 1984, 18(5):333-337.

11. Brunborg G et al. Genotoxic effects of the drinking water mutagen 3-chloro-4-(di-chloromethyl)-5-hydroxy-2[5H]-furanone (MX) in mammalian cells *in vitro* and rats *in vivo*. *Mutation research*, 1991, 260:55-64.

## 16.10 Trihalomethanes

### 16.10.1 General description

#### *Identity*

| Compound | CAS no. | Molecular formula |
|---|---|---|
| Bromoform | 75-25-2 | $CHBr_3$ |
| Dibromochloromethane (DBCM) | 124-48-1 | $CHBr_2Cl$ |
| Bromodichloromethane (BDCM) | 75-27-4 | $CHBrCl_2$ |
| Chloroform | 67-66-3 | $CHCl_3$ |

Trihalomethanes are halogen-substituted single-carbon compounds with the general formula $CHX_3$, where X may be fluorine, chlorine, bromine, or iodine, or a combination thereof. From the point of view of drinking-water contamination, only four members of the group are important, namely bromoform, DBCM, BDCM, and chloroform, the last of these being the one most commonly found. The IUPAC names of bromoform and chloroform are tribromomethane and trichloromethane, respectively.

#### *Physicochemical properties* (1–7)

| Property | Bromoform [1] | DBCM [2] | BDCM [3] | Chloroform [4] |
|---|---|---|---|---|
| Boiling point (°C) | 149–150 | 119 | 90 | 61–62 |
| Melting point (°C) | 8.3 | – | -57.1 | -63.5 |
| Density at 20 °C (g/cm³) | 2.90 | 2.38 | 1.98 | 1.48 |
| Vapour pressure (kPa) | 0.75 (25 °C) | 2.0 (10 °C) | 6.67 (20 °C) | 26.7 (25 °C) |
| Water solubility (mg/litre) | 3190 (30 °C) | 1050 (30 °C) | 3320 (30 °C) | 7220 (25 °C) |
| Log octanol–water partition coefficient | 2.38 | 2.08 | 1.88 | 1.97 |

#### *Organoleptic properties*

The odour threshold for bromoform in water is 0.3 mg/litre. Chloroform has a characteristic odour, with odour threshold values of 2.4 mg/litre in water and 420 mg/m³ in air (2, 7).

---

[1] Conversion factor in air: 1 ppm = 10.34 mg/m³.
[2] Conversion factor in air: 1 ppm = 8.52 mg/m³.
[3] Conversion factor in air: 1 ppm = 6.70 mg/m³.
[4] Conversion factor in air: 1 ppm = 4.96 mg/m³.

## Major uses

Brominated trihalomethanes have been used as laboratory reagents, as chemical intermediates for the synthesis of organic compounds, and as fluids for mineral ore separation. They were formerly used as solvents for fats, waxes, and resins and as flame retardants. Bromoform has been used as a sedative and cough suppressant (8).

Chloroform is used mainly as the starting material in the manufacture of the refrigerant fluorocarbon-22. It is an important extraction solvent for resins, gums, and other products. Chloroform was previously used as an anaesthetic, but it has been replaced by safer materials.

## Environmental fate

In air, brominated trihalomethanes may be degraded by photo-oxidative interaction with atmospheric hydroxyl radicals; their typical atmospheric half-life is about 2 months (1, 9). Chloroform can be photo-oxidized in air with a half-life of 26–260 days (10).

Volatilization is a major transport process for trihalomethanes. Estimated volatilization half-lives from rivers and streams are 1 h to 24 days for bromoform, 0.7 h to 16 days for DBCM, and 0.5–24 h for BDCM (11, 12). Volatilization half-lives for chloroform are 1–2 days for ponds and rivers and 9–10 days for lakes (13, 14).

Under anaerobic conditions, brominated trihalomethanes are readily biodegraded within days in the presence of methane-producing bacteria and under denitrifying and sulfate-reducing conditions (15, 16). Chloroform can be biodegraded in groundwater with a half-life ranging from weeks to years (13). Hydrolysis of brominated trihalomethanes in aqueous media is very slow; estimated half-lives are 1000, 274, and 686 years for BDCM, DBCM, and bromoform, respectively (17). Based on partition coefficients, bioaccumulation of trihalomethanes in aquatic organisms may occur, but only to a limited degree (8, 13).

Chloroform is not strongly absorbed by soil or sediments (13). Brominated trihalomethanes are expected to be mobile in soil, based on their partition coefficients and data from percolation studies (8). Studies in aqueous media suggest that anaerobic biodegradation could be a major removal process in soil if volatilization is restricted. Chloroform can be biodegraded in soil with a half-life of 4–24 weeks (13).

## 16.10.2 Analytical methods

The preferred technique for the determination of trihalomethanes is gas chromatography, with detection by flame ionization, electron capture, or mass spectroscopy (18). The purge-and-trap gas chromatographic procedure is well suited to biological and environmental samples that are soluble in water; it has a detection limit of approximately 0.5 µg/litre (*19*). The detection limit for chloroform in biological materials (e.g. blood, tissue, and food) when the purge-and-trap technique is used is in the range 0.1–1 µg/kg (*13*).

## 16.10.3 Environmental levels and human exposure

### Air

Ambient air concentrations at several urban locations in the USA averaged 37 ng/m$^3$ for bromoform, 32 ng/m$^3$ for DBCM, and 7.4 ng/m$^3$ for BDCM (highest values reported were 0.73, 0.23, and 1.3 µg/m$^3$, respectively). The maximum concentration of bromoform in the air sampled in Toronto (Canada) was 0.1 µg/m$^3$ (54 samples) (*20, 21*). Typical background levels of chloroform in outdoor air in rural/remote, urban/suburban, and source-dominated areas are 0.02–0.2, 0.2–3.4, and 0.2–13 µg/m$^3$, respectively (*13, 22–24*). Typical concentrations of chloroform in indoor air range from 0.07 to 3.6 µg/m$^3$ (*23, 25, 26*).

### Water

Trihalomethanes are generated principally as by-products of the chlorination of drinking-water. Hypochlorous acid oxidizes bromide ion to form hypobromous acid, which reacts with endogenous organic materials (e.g. humic or fulvic acids) to form brominated trihalomethanes (*1*). Chlorine reacts with the same organic substances in water to form chloroform. The amount of each trihalomethane formed depends on the temperature, pH, and chlorine and bromide ion concentrations (*27*). Trihalomethanes are rarely found in raw water but are often present in finished water (*28, 29*).

In a Canadian survey of the water supplies of 70 communities, the average concentrations of bromoform, DBCM, BDCM, and chloroform were 0.1, 0.4, 2.9, and 22.7 µg/litre, respectively (*30*). In a survey of 105 systems in the USA using surface water, bromoform was found in 14 supplies at <1.0–5.7 µg/litre (median 1.3 µg/litre), DBCM in 70 supplies at <0.5–45 µg/litre (median 3.2 µg/litre), and BDCM in 99 supplies at <0.5–62 µg/litre (median 8.2 µg/litre). In a survey of 315 systems using groundwater, bromoform was found in 81 supplies at <1.0–110 µg/litre (median 3.0 µg/litre), DBCM in 107 supplies at <0.5–32 µg/litre (median 4.1 µg/litre), and BDCM in 104 supplies at <0.5–51 µg/litre (median 3.5 µg/litre) (*31*). Chloroform was found in 99.5% of finished drinking-water samples in two surveys in the USA at concentrations ranging from the detection limit to 311 µg/litre; in most samples, concentrations were between 32 and 68 µg/litre (*32, 33*).

Trihalomethanes can be found in chlorinated swimming pools, total concentrations ranging from 120 to 660 µg/litre (*34*). BDCM concentrations were about the same in saltwater as in freshwater pools (13–34 µg/litre) (*35*).

## Food

BDCM is not a common food contaminant but has been found in trace amounts in some samples: 1.2 µg/kg in one dairy composite and 7 µg/kg in butter (*36*). Chloroform has been found in various foods, including seafood (3–180 µg/kg), dairy products (1–33 µg/kg), meat (1–4 µg/kg), oil and fat (2–10 µg/kg), beverages (0.4–18 µg/kg), fruit and vegetables (2–18 µg/kg), and bread (2 µg/kg) (*37*). Many drugs contain residual amounts of chloroform as a result of its use as a solvent or formation as a by-product in the manufacturing process (*38*).

## Estimated total exposure and relative contribution of drinking-water

The major routes of exposure to trihalomethanes are via drinking-water and inhalation. If it is assumed that the average human intake of air is 20 m$^3$/day, the average daily intake of chloroform by inhalation in urban areas can be estimated to be 4–68 µg. Indoor air contamination from such sources as volatilization from household uses of chlorinated water (e.g. showers, cleaning) probably contributes more to human exposure than outdoor air. It has been estimated that the ingestion of 2 litres of drinking-water per day by the average adult results in an exposure of 4–88 µg of chloroform (*13*).

## 16.10.4 Kinetics and metabolism in laboratory animals and humans

Available studies indicate that gastrointestinal absorption is high for all trihalomethanes, while chloroform is also rapidly and extensively absorbed through the lungs (*39–42*). Because of their high lipophilicity, accumulation is higher in tissues of high lipid content, including body fat, liver, and kidneys (*41, 42*).

In rats, trihalomethanes are oxidized by the hepatic cytochrome P-450 mixed-function oxidase system to trihalomethanols, which then decompose to yield highly reactive dihalocarbonyls (*43, 44*). The amount metabolized depends on the species, being higher in mice than in rats (*39, 42*). Under anaerobic conditions, chloroform is reduced by cytochrome P-450 to yield the dichloromethyl radical (*45*). As the reactive metabolites of trihalomethanes may be responsible for their toxicity or carcinogenicity (*14*), interspecies differences in metabolic patterns should be taken into account in the extrapolation of toxicity or carcinogenicity data from experimental animals to humans (*46*).

Excretion of unchanged compounds and carbon dioxide occurs primarily in exhaled air, only small amounts being excreted in urine (*39, 42*).

## 16.10.5 Effects on laboratory animals and *in vitro* test systems

### *Bromoform*

*Acute exposure*

The oral $LD_{50}$s for bromoform administered in an aqueous vehicle to male and female mice were 1400 and 1550 mg/kg of body weight, respectively (*47*). For male and female rats given bromoform in corn oil, $LD_{50}$s were 1388 and 1147 mg/kg of body weight, respectively (*48*).

*Short-term exposure*

Bromoform was administered in drinking-water at levels of 0, 5, 50, 500, or 2500 mg/litre (0, 0.6, 7, 52, or 250 mg/kg of body weight per day) to Sprague-Dawley rats (20 per sex per dose) for 90 days. Mild to moderate histological changes in the liver and thyroid and a significant increase in the severity of hepatic lesions were observed at the highest dose, and lactate dehydrogenase activity was significantly reduced. Based on the observed liver effect, the NOAEL was 52 mg/kg of body weight per day (*49*).

Young adult rats (10 per sex per dose) were given bromoform by gavage in corn oil at doses of 0, 12, 25, 50, 100, or 200 mg/kg of body weight per day, 5 days per week for 13 weeks. Male and female mice were given doses of 0, 25, 50, 100, 200, or 400 mg/kg of body weight per day. Growth was not affected except at the highest dose in male mice, in which it was slightly suppressed. Male mice at the two highest dose levels showed "minimal to moderate" hepatocellular vacuolation in a few cells. Male rats showed a dose-related increase in hepatocellular vacuolation, which became statistically significant at 50 mg/kg of body weight per day. The NOAELs for hepatocellular vacuolation were 25 and 100 mg/kg of body weight per day in male rats and male mice, respectively (*50*).

*Long-term exposure*

The effect of feeding bromoform (microencapsulated and mixed in the diet) was evaluated in Wistar SPF rats (40 per sex) dosed for 2 years at 0.04%, 0.16%, or 0.65% (18, 71, or 480 mg/kg of body weight per day for males and 30, 120, or 870 mg/kg of body weight per day for females). Animals given the highest dose exhibited body weight depression; decreases in serum triglycerides, nonesterified fatty acids, glucose, and cholinesterase activity; elevated γ-glutamyl transpeptidase activity; and yellowing and roughening of the liver surface. Similar but less severe effects were seen in the mid-dose groups. Based on body weight depression and serum enzyme changes, the authors considered the NOAELs to be 18 and 30 mg/kg of body weight per day for male and female rats, respectively (*51*).

Rats of both sexes and female mice (50 per dose) were given bromoform by gavage in corn oil at doses of 100 or 200 mg/kg of body weight per day, 5 days per week for 2 years. Male mice received 50 or 100 mg/kg of body weight per day. Survival was reduced relative to controls in male rats in the high-dose group.

A dose-related suppression of growth was also noted in male rats, but female rats showed an adverse effect on growth only at the high dose level. Male mice at the lower dose showed no effect on growth, but female mice showed a slight suppression that was not clearly related to dose. Rats of both sexes and female mice showed a dose-related increased incidence of fatty change (or vacuolation) in the liver. An increased incidence of mild fatty changes was noted in both low-dose and high-dose female mice but not in male mice. The LOAEL was 100 mg/kg of body weight per day for hepatocellular vacuolation and suppression of weight gain in rats and female mice (50).

*Reproductive toxicity, embryotoxicity, and teratogenicity*
The effect of bromoform on fertility and reproduction was investigated in Swiss CD-1 mice (20 pairs per dose) dosed for 105 days at 0, 50, 100, or 200 mg/kg of body weight per day in corn oil by gavage. No apparent effect on fertility or reproduction (e.g. litters per pair, live pups per litter, pup body weights) was reported in either the parental or the $F_1$ generation, and a reproductive NOAEL of 200 mg/kg of body weight per day was identified (52).

*Mutagenicity and related end-points*
Bromoform was positive in the Ames test in *Salmonella typhimurium* strain TA100 without activation (53, 54) and negative or equivocal in strains TA1535 or TA1937 with and without activation (50). Bromoform gave positive results in the following assays: chromosomal aberration in CHO cells with activation (54) and in mouse bone marrow cells *in vivo* (50), sister chromatid exchange in human lymphocytes (55), in CHO cells without activation (50), and in mouse bone marrow cells *in vivo* (50, 55), and gene mutation in mouse lymphoma cells (50). It was negative for sister chromatid exchange in CHO cells with activation (50), and results were equivocal in the micronucleus assay (50, 54).

*Carcinogenicity*
When bromoform (4, 48, or 100 mg/kg of body weight) was administered intraperitoneally to male strain A mice (20 per dose) 3 times per week for 8 weeks, and they were kept under observation for 16 additional weeks, an increased incidence of lung tumours was seen at the intermediate dose (56).

Groups of 50 male $B6C3F_1$ mice were given bromoform by gavage in corn oil at doses of 0, 50, or 100 mg/kg of body weight per day, 5 days per week for 105 weeks. Females received doses of 0, 100, or 200 mg/kg of body weight per day. No increase in tumours was reported in any tissue in any group. In a similar study, Fischer 344/N rats (50 per sex per dose) were also exposed to bromoform by gavage in corn oil at doses of 0, 100, or 200 mg/kg of body weight per day, 5 days per week for 105 weeks. Adenomatous polyps or adenocarcinoma (combined) of the large intestine (colon or rectum) were induced in three male rats given the highest dose and in eight female rats given the highest dose. The increase was considered to be significant, as these tumours are rare in control animals. On the basis of these data, it was concluded that there was "some evidence" of carcinogenic activity in male rats and "clear evidence" in female rats. There were no tumours in the control rats and one in a mid-dose female rat (*50*).

## Dibromochloromethane

### Acute exposure
The oral LD$_{50}$s for DBCM administered in an aqueous vehicle to male and female mice were 800 and 1200 mg/kg of body weight, respectively (*47*). LD$_{50}$s for male and female rats given the compound in corn oil were 1186 and 848 mg/kg of body weight, respectively (*48*).

### Short-term exposure
DBCM was administered in drinking-water at levels of 0, 5, 50, 500, or 2500 mg/litre (0, 0.6, 7, 52, or 250 mg/kg of body weight per day) to Sprague-Dawley rats (20 per sex per dose) for 90 days. Mild to moderate histological changes in the liver and thyroid and a significant increase in the severity of hepatic lesions were observed at the highest dose. Based on the observed liver effect, the NOAEL was 52 mg/kg of body weight per day (*49*).

Fischer 344/N rats and B6C3F$_1$ mice (10 per sex per dose) were given DBCM by gavage in corn oil at dose levels of 0, 15, 30, 60, 125, or 250 mg/kg of body weight per day, 5 days per week for 13 weeks. The final body weights of rats that received 250 mg/kg of body weight were depressed. A dose-dependent increase in hepatic vacuolation was observed in male rats. Based on this hepatic effect, the NOAEL in rats was 30 mg/kg of body weight per day. Kidney and liver toxicity were observed in male and female rats and male mice at 250 mg/kg of body weight per day. Survival rates for treated animals and corresponding controls were comparable except in high-dose rats. Clinical signs in the treated animals and controls were comparable. Based on the renal and hepatic lesions, a NOAEL of 125 mg/kg of body weight per day was identified in mice (*57*).

### Long-term exposure
The effect of feeding DBCM (microencapsulated and mixed in the diet) was evaluated in Wistar SPF rats (40 per sex) dosed for 2 years at 0.022%, 0.088%, or 0.35% (10, 39, or 210 mg/kg of body weight per day for males and 17, 66, or 350 mg/kg of body weight per day for females). Animals receiving the highest dose exhibited depressed body weight; decreases in serum triglycerides, nonesterified fatty acids, glucose, and cholinesterase activity; elevated γ-glutamyl transpeptidase activity; and yellowing and roughening of the liver surface. Similar but less severe findings were present in the mid-dose groups. Based on the body weight depression and serum enzyme changes, the authors considered the NOAELs to be 10 and 17 mg/kg of body weight per day for male and female rats, respectively (*51*).

Rats (50 per sex per dose) were given DBCM by gavage in corn oil at 0, 40, or 80 mg/kg of body weight, 5 days per week for 104 weeks, and mice (50 per sex per dose) received 0, 50, or 100 mg/kg of body weight by gavage for 105 weeks. Survival in rats and female mice was comparable in all dose groups, whereas it was decreased in high-dose male mice. An overdosing accident at week 58 killed 35 male mice in the low-dose group, so this group was not evaluated further. Mean body weights of high-dose male rats and high-dose mice of both sexes were lower than those of the vehicle controls. The incidence of fatty metamorphosis of the liver was increased in male and female rats and female mice at both low- and high-dose levels. Male mice showed liver effects at the high dose. There was an increased incidence of kidney nephrosis in female rats and in male mice but not in male rats or female mice. Follicular cell hyperplasia of the thyroid occurred at increased incidence in female mice but not in males. Based on the hepatic lesions, LOAELs of 50 and 40 mg/kg of body weight per day for mice and rats, respectively, were identified (57).

*Reproductive toxicity, embryotoxicity, and teratogenicity*
In a multigeneration reproductive study, groups of 10 male and 30 female ICR mice were treated with DBCM in emulphor at 0, 0.1, 1.0, or 4.0 g/litre (0, 17, 171, or 685 mg/kg of body weight per day) in drinking-water for 35 days, then mated; subsequent re-matings occurred 2 weeks after weaning. The $F_1$ mice were treated with the same test solution for 11 weeks after weaning and then mated; re-mating occurred 2 weeks after weaning. At 17 mg/kg of body weight per day, there was only a slight depression in the body weight of the newborn pups in the $F_{2b}$ generation. At 171 mg/kg of body weight per day, there was a significant decrease in female body weight and an increase in the occurrence of gross liver pathology of $F_0$ and $F_{1b}$ mice; the lesions varied in severity from fat accumulation to distinct masses on the liver surface. Although not occurring in every generation, there were significant decreases in litter size, pup viability, postnatal body weight, and lactation index. At 685 mg/kg of body weight per day, the effects were of the same types but more severe. Body weight gain was significantly reduced in both males and females at the highest dose (685 mg/kg of body weight per day) and in females at the middle dose (171 mg/kg of body weight per day). Animals in both these groups exhibited enlarged livers with gross morphological changes. In addition, the gestation index, fertility, and survival of the $F_1$ generation were significantly reduced. Based on maternal toxicity and fetotoxicity, a NOAEL of 17 mg/kg of body weight per day was identified (58).

*Mutagenicity and related end-points*
DBCM was positive in the Ames test with *S. typhimurium* strain TA100 without activation (53, 54) but negative in strains TA98, TA1535, and TA1537 with or without activation (58). It gave positive results for chromosomal aberration in CHO cells with activation (54) and for sister chromatid exchange in human lymphocytes and mouse bone marrow cells *in vivo* (55); it was negative in the micronucleus assay (54).

*Carcinogenicity*

DBCM was administered to rats and mice (50 per sex per dose) in corn oil by gavage at doses of 0, 40, or 80 mg/kg of body weight per day for rats and 0, 50, or 100 mg/kg of body weight per day for mice, 5 days per week for 104–105 weeks. An overdose killed 35 of the 50 low-dose male mice, so that this group could not be used for the study of carcinogenicity. DBCM significantly increased the incidence of hepatocellular adenomas and the combined incidence of hepato-cellular adenomas and carcinomas in high-dose female mice. The incidence of hepatocellular carcinomas was significantly increased in high-dose male mice; the combined incidence of hepatocellular adenomas and carcinomas was marginally significant by the life-table test but not by the incidental tumour test. DBCM did not produce an increased incidence of tumours in treated rats. There was "no evidence" of carcinogenic activity in male or female rats, "equivocal evidence" of carcinogenicity in male mice, and "some evidence" of carcinogenicity in female mice under the conditions of this study (*57*).

## Bromodichloromethane

*Acute exposure*

Oral $LD_{50}$s for BDCM administered in an aqueous vehicle to mice were 450 and 900 mg/kg of body weight for males and females, respectively (*47*). Male and fe-male rats given the compound in corn oil had $LD_{50}$s of 916 and 969 mg/kg of body weight, respectively (*48*).

*Short-term exposure*

BDCM was administered in drinking-water at levels of 0, 5, 50, 500, or 2500 mg/litre (0, 0.6, 7, 52, or 250 mg/kg of body weight per day) to Sprague-Dawley rats (20 per sex per dose) for 90 days. Mild to moderate histological changes in the liver and thyroid and a significant increase in the severity of hepatic lesions were observed at the highest dose. Based on the observed liver effect, the NOAEL was 52 mg/kg of body weight per day (*49*).

Fischer 344/N rats and B6C3F$_1$ mice were given BDCM by gavage in corn oil 5 days per week for 13 weeks. Rats (10 per sex per dose) were given 0, 19, 38, 75, 150, or 300 mg/kg of body weight per day. Male mice (10 per dose) were giv-en 0, 6.3, 12.5, 50, or 100 mg/kg of body weight per day, and female mice were given 0, 25, 50, 100, 200, or 400 mg/kg of body weight per day. Of the male and female rats that received the highest dose, 50% and 20% respectively died before the end of the study. None of the mice died. Body weights decreased significantly in male and female rats given BDCM at 150 and 300 mg/kg of body weight per day. Centrilobular degeneration of the liver was observed at 300 mg/kg of body weight per day in male and female rats and at 200 and 400 mg/kg of body weight per day in female mice. Degeneration and necrosis of the kidney were observed at 300 mg/kg of body weight per day in male rats and at 100 mg/kg of body weight per day in male mice. The NOAELs in rats were 75 and 150 mg/kg of body weight per day for body weight reduction and for hepatic and renal lesions, respectively. The NOAEL for renal lesions in mice was 50 mg/kg of body weight per day (*59*).

*Long-term exposure*

The effect of feeding BDCM (microencapsulated and mixed in the diet) was evaluated in Wistar SPF rats (40 per sex) dosed for 2 years at 0.014%, 0.055%, or 0.22% (6, 24, or 130 mg/kg of body weight per day for males and 11, 41, or 220 mg/kg of body weight per day for females). Animals receiving the highest dose exhibited depressed body weight; decreases in serum triglycerides, nonesterified fatty acids, glucose, and cholinesterase activity; elevated γ-glutamyl transpeptidase activity; and yellowing and roughening of the liver surface. Similar but less severe findings were present in the mid-dose groups. Based on the body weight depression and serum enzyme changes, the authors considered the NOAELs to be 6 and 11 mg/kg of body weight per day for male and female rats, respectively (*51*).

Groups of Fischer 344/N rats (50 per sex per dose) were given 0, 50, or 100 mg of BDCM per kg of body weight per day in corn oil by gavage 5 days per week for 102 weeks. Male B6C3F$_1$ mice (50 per dose) were given 0, 25, or 50 mg/kg of body weight per day, and female mice received 0, 75, or 150 mg/kg of body weight per day by gavage for 102 weeks. Renal cytomegaly was observed in male rats at 50 mg/kg of body weight per day and above and in male mice at 25 mg/kg of body weight per day and above. Fatty metamorphosis of the liver was observed in male and female rats at 50 mg/kg of body weight per day and above and in male mice at 25 mg/kg of body weight per day and above. Compound-related follicular cell hyperplasia of the thyroid was also observed in male and female mice. Survival was decreased in female mice only. Mean body weights were decreased at 100 mg/kg of body weight per day in rats and at 50 and 150 mg/kg of body weight per day in male and female mice, respectively. Based on the observed renal and liver effects, a LOAEL of 50 mg/kg of body weight per day was identified for rats. Based on the observed renal, liver, and thyroid effects in male mice and thyroid effects in female mice, a LOAEL of 25 mg/kg of body weight per day was identified for mice (*59*).

*Reproductive toxicity, embryotoxicity, and teratogenicity*

A dose-related increased incidence in sternebral anomalies was reported in fetuses from groups of 9–15 pregnant rats exposed to BDCM in corn oil by gavage at doses of 0, 50, 100, or 200 mg/kg of body weight per day on days 6–15 of gestation. The authors interpreted the sternebral anomalies as evidence of a fetotoxic (rather than a teratogenic) effect. The LOAEL based on this fetotoxic effect was 50 mg/kg of body weight per day (*60*).

*Mutagenicity and related end-points*
BDCM was positive in the Ames test with *S. typhimurium* strain TA100 without activation (*53, 54*) but negative in strains TA98, TA1535, and TA1537 with or without activation (*59*). It induced gene mutations in mouse lymphoma cells with, but not without, activation (*59*). BDCM gave conflicting results for chromosomal aberration in CHO cells with and without activation (*54, 59*), positive results for sister chromatid exchange in human lymphocytes and in mouse bone marrow cells *in vivo* (*55*), and negative results for the micronucleus assay (*54*) and sister chromatid exchange in CHO cells (*59*).

*Carcinogenicity*
When BDCM (20, 40, or 100 mg/kg of body weight) was administered intraperitoneally to male strain A mice (20 per dose) 3 times per week for 8 weeks, and they were kept under observation for 16 additional weeks, an increased incidence of lung tumours was seen at the highest dose (*56*).

Fischer 344/N rats (50 per sex per dose) were given BDCM in corn oil by gavage at 0, 50, or 100 mg/kg of body weight, 5 days per week for 102 weeks. Male B6C3F$_1$ mice (50 per dose) were given 0, 25, or 50 mg/kg of body weight per day by gavage, and females received 0, 75, or 150 mg/kg of body weight per day. BDCM caused a significant increase in tumours of the kidney in male mice, the liver in female mice, and the kidney and large intestine in male and female rats. In male mice, the incidences of tubular cell adenomas and the combined incidences of tubular-cell adenomas and adenocarcinomas of the kidneys were significantly increased at 50 mg/kg of body weight per day. In female mice, significant increases in hepatocellular adenomas occurred at 75 and 150 mg/kg of body weight per day, whereas hepatocellular carcinomas were significantly increased at 150 mg/kg of body weight per day. In male and female rats, the incidence of tubular cell adenomas, adenocarcinomas, and the combined incidence of adenomas and adenocarcinomas of the kidneys were significantly increased only at 100 mg/kg of body weight per day. Adenosarcomas of the large intestine were increased in male rats at both doses and in high-dose female rats. Adenomatous polyps were significantly increased in male rats in a dose-dependent manner but were present in females at the high dose only. Based on the data, it was concluded that, under the conditions of this study, there was "clear evidence" of carcinogenic activity for male and female mice and rats (*59*).

## Chloroform

*Acute exposure*
Oral LD$_{50}$s in rats and mice for chloroform range from 908 to 2000 mg/kg of body weight (*14*).

*Short-term exposure*
Six-week-old male Osborne-Mendel rats (30 per dose) were given chloroform in drinking-water at 0, 20, 38, 58, 81, or 160 mg/kg of body weight per day (based

on average weight and water intake) for 36, 60, or 90 days (*61*). A decrease in body weight was observed at the highest dose. No effects on percentage of kidney fat or serum biochemistry were observed, and gross and microscopic pathology findings were mild and not dose-related.

A similar study was conducted on B6C3F$_1$ female mice (30 per dose) given chloroform in drinking-water at approximately 0, 32, 64, 97, 145, 290, or 436 mg/kg of body weight per day (*61*). Histologically, centrilobular fatty changes in the liver appeared to be treatment-related. There was a statistically significant increase in the percentage of liver fat at the highest dose. Based on fatty changes in the liver, a NOAEL of 290 mg/kg of body weight per day and a LOAEL of 436 mg/kg of body weight per day were identified.

Chloroform was administered to weanling SD rats (20 per dose) in drinking-water at approximately 0, 0.7, 6, 50, or 180 mg/kg of body weight per day (based on average body weight and water intake) (*62*). Increased mortality, decreased growth rate, and decreased food intake were reported at the highest dose. Mild to moderate liver and thyroid lesions were observed in all groups. However, after a 90-day recovery period, these effects were not significantly different from controls, except for the thyroid lesions in the highest-dose males. No significant changes were observed in the serum biochemical or haematological parameters. A NOAEL of 50 mg/kg of body weight per day was established, based on thyroid lesions and decreased growth.

Chloroform was administered by gavage to B6C3F$_1$ mice (10 per sex per dose) at doses of 60, 130, or 270 mg/kg of body weight per day for 90 days, either in corn oil or in 2% emulphor (*63*). When chloroform was given in corn oil, there was a significant increase in aspartate aminotransferase levels in both male and female mice at 270 mg/kg of body weight per day, as well as a significant degree of diffuse parenchymal degeneration and mild to moderate early cirrhosis. Significant pathological lesions were not observed in the mice receiving chloroform in 2% emulphor. The data suggest that administration of chloroform by gavage in corn oil results in more marked hepatotoxicity than administration of chloroform in an aqueous suspension. The study identified 270 mg/kg of body weight per day as a LOAEL for serum enzyme elevation and diffuse liver pathology when chloroform is given in corn oil and the same level as a NOAEL when chloroform is given in an aqueous vehicle.

*Long-term exposure*
Male and female SD rats (50 per dose) were dosed by gavage with chloroform in a toothpaste-based vehicle at 0 or 60 mg/kg of body weight per day, 6 days per week for 80 weeks. There was a marginal but consistent and progressive retardation of weight gain in both sexes. A decrease in plasma cholinesterase activity and a significant decrease in relative liver weight were seen in treated female rats. No other significant effects on the liver or kidney were observed. In this study, a LOAEL of 60 mg/kg of body weight per day, based on decreases in body weight, liver weight, and plasma cholinesterase activity, was identified (*64*).

Drinking-water containing chloroform at 600 or 1800 mg/litre (86 or 258 mg/kg of body weight per day) was administered to B6C3F$_1$ mice (35 per dose) for 24 or 52 weeks. The animals in the high-dose group showed a statistically significant decrease in mean body weight. Focal areas of cellular necrosis were found in the kidneys and liver of treated mice, and focal areas of hepatic lipid accumulation were seen in the high-dose mice. A NOAEL was not identified (65).

Chloroform was administered to Osborne-Mendel rats (50–330 per dose) and B6C3F$_1$ mice (50–430 per dose) at concentrations of 0, 200, 400, 900, or 1800 mg/litre in drinking-water for 23 months. The time-weighted average doses were 0, 19, 38, 81, and 160 mg/kg of body weight per day for rats and 0, 34, 65, 130, and 263 mg/kg of body weight per day for mice. Although various blood chemistry and haematological parameters differed significantly from the control values at some time points, these parameters were not significantly different from those of matched controls with identical water consumption, and the authors concluded that the effects of chloroform were probably secondary to those of reduced water and food consumption. There was increased mortality in the two highest dose groups for mice. The percentage of fat in the mouse liver was significantly increased in the two highest dose groups at 6 months. A NOAEL was not established (66).

Chloroform was administered to beagle dogs (12–15 per dose) in a toothpaste base in gelatin capsules at dose levels of 15 or 30 mg/kg of body weight per day for 7.5 years. The most significant effect was the formation of hepatic "fatty cysts" and nodules of altered hepatocytes at both doses. There was also a moderate rise in serum enzyme (e.g. alanine aminotransferase) levels, which reached a peak in the sixth year of the study. Based on the increased alanine aminotransferase levels and increased frequency of fatty cysts, a LOAEL of 15 mg/kg of body weight per day was identified in this study (67).

*Reproductive toxicity, embryotoxicity, and teratogenicity*
Rats were given chloroform at doses of 0, 20, 50, or 126 mg/kg of body weight per day by gavage in corn oil on days 6–15 of gestation. Dams (25 per dose) receiving 50 or 126 mg/kg of body weight per day displayed signs of maternal toxicity (decreased weight gain, mild fatty changes in the liver). Reduced body weights were seen in the fetuses from dams dosed at the highest level. There was, however, no evidence of teratogenicity. The maternal and fetal NOAELs were 20 and 50 mg/kg of body weight per day, respectively (68).

In a similar study in rabbits, dams were dosed by gavage with chloroform at 0, 20, 35, or 50 mg/kg of body weight per day on days 6–18 of gestation. Maternal toxicity (decreased weight gain) was observed in dams given 50 mg/kg of body weight per day. Fetuses from dams (15 per dose) given 20 or 50 mg/kg of body weight per day had slightly reduced body weights. An increased incidence of incompletely ossified skull bones (usually parietals) was observed at 20 and 35 mg/kg of body weight per day. The authors did not consider these effects to be evidence of teratogenicity or fetotoxicity. The maternal NOAEL identified in this study was 35 mg/kg of body weight per day (*68*).

*Mutagenicity and related end-points*
Chloroform was not mutagenic in several Ames bacterial test systems with or without microsomal activation (*53, 69, 72*). However, positive responses were observed in a host-mediated assay in male mice (*71*), a sex-linked recessive lethal test in *Drosophila* (*70*), an assay utilizing yeast (*72*), and a sperm-head abnormality assay in mice (*73*).

*Carcinogenicity*
Osborne-Mendel rats (50 per sex per dose) were treated with chloroform in corn oil, 5 days per week for 78 weeks. Male rats received 90 or 180 mg/kg of body weight per day; females were treated with 125 or 250 mg/kg of body weight per day for 22 weeks and 90 or 180 mg/kg of body weight per day thereafter. Lower body weight gain and survival were observed in all treated groups. The most significant observation was a dose-related increase in renal epithelial tumours of tubular-cell origin in male rats. There was an increase in thyroid tumours in female rats, but this was not considered biologically significant by the authors (*74*).

B6C3F$_1$ mice (50 per sex per dose) were given chloroform in corn oil by gavage, 5 days per week for 78 weeks. For the first 18 weeks, dose levels were 100 or 200 mg/kg of body weight per day for males and 200 or 400 mg/kg of body weight per day for females; they were then raised to 150 or 300 mg/kg of body weight per day for males and 250 or 500 mg/kg of body weight per day for females for the rest of the study. Survival rate and weight gain were similar in all treated groups, except for an increase in lesions (including tumours) that tended to shorten the lives of the high-dose female mice. Statistically significant dose-related increases in hepatocellular carcinomas were observed in all treated groups. Nodular hyperplasia of the liver was observed in many male mice that had not developed hepatocellular carcinomas (*74*).

Male Osborne-Mendel rats (50–330 per dose) and female B6C3F$_1$ mice (50–430 per dose) were given chloroform in drinking-water at levels of 0, 200, 400, 900, or 1800 mg/litre (average dose 0, 19, 38, 81, or 160 mg/kg of body weight per day in rats and 0, 34, 65, 130, or 263 mg/kg of body weight per day in mice) for 104 weeks. The incidence of renal tubular adenomas and adenocarcinomas in male rats was increased in a dose-related manner (14% in the highest-dose group compared with 2% in the control group). In the female B6C3F$_1$ mice, there was no statistically significant increase in the incidence of hepatocellular carcinomas (*66*).

It is important to note that chloroform in corn oil at a dose of 250 mg/kg of body weight per day promoted the development of liver tumours in B6C3F$_1$ mice (*74*), whereas in drinking-water at 263 mg/kg of body weight per day it failed to induce such tumours in the same strain of mice (*66*). This may be due either to the toxicokinetic difference between the administration of chloroform as a bolus dose by gavage in corn oil as compared with continuous dosing in water or, alternatively, a synergistic interaction between chloroform and corn oil (74).

## 16.10.6 Effects on humans

In the past, orally administered bromoform was used as a sedative for children with whooping cough. Typical doses were around 180 mg, given 3-6 times per day. Deaths as a result of accidental overdose were occasionally reported. The clinical signs in fatal cases were central nervous system depression followed by respiratory failure (75, 76). Based on these clinical observations, the estimated lethal dose for a child weighing 10–20 kg is probably about 300 mg/kg of body weight, and the LOAEL for mild sedation is around 54 mg/kg of body weight per day.

Chloroform is a central nervous system depressant and can also affect liver and kidney function. Based on case reports, the mean lethal oral dose for humans was estimated at approximately 44 g (77), but a fatal dose may be as small as 211 mg/kg of body weight, death being caused by respiratory or cardiac arrest (14). Workers exposed to chloroform by inhalation at levels of 112–1158 mg/m$^3$ for one or more years complained of nausea, lassitude, dry mouth, flatulence, thirst, depression, irritability, and scalding urination (78). Workers inhaling chloroform at levels of 10-1000 mg/m$^3$ for 1–4 years had an increased incidence of viral hepatitis and enlarged liver (79).

In several epidemiological studies (80, 81), associations between the ingestion of chlorinated drinking-water (which typically contains trihalomethanes) and increased cancer mortality rates have been reported. In one study (82), there was an apparent association between bladder cancer and trihalomethanes, and a higher degree of correlation was noted with the brominated trihalomethanes than with chloroform. However, as chlorinated water contains many by-products, it is not possible from these epidemiological studies to conclude that brominated trihalomethanes are human carcinogens. In another study, no apparent association was found between chloroform ingested in drinking-water and risk of colorectal cancer (83).

## 16.10.7 Guideline values

The trihalomethanes may act as an indicator for the presence of other chlorination by-products. Control of the four most commonly occurring trihalomethanes in drinking-water should help to reduce levels of other uncharacterized chlorination by-products.

Because these four compounds usually occur together, it has been the practice to consider total trihalomethanes as a group, and a number of countries have set guidelines or standards on this basis. In the first edition of the *Guidelines for drinking-water quality,* a guideline value was established for chloroform only; few data existed for the remaining trihalomethanes and, for most water supplies, chloroform was the most commonly encountered member of the group. In this edition, no guideline value has been set for total trihalomethanes; however, guideline values have been established separately for all four trihalomethanes.

For authorities wishing to establish a total trihalomethane standard to account for additive toxicity, the following fractionation approach could be taken:

$$\frac{C_{bromoform}}{GV_{bromoform}} + \frac{C_{DBCM}}{GV_{DBCM}} + \frac{C_{BDCM}}{GV_{BDCM}} + \frac{C_{chloroform}}{GV_{chloroform}} \leq 1$$

where C = concentration and GV = guideline value.

Authorities wishing to use a guideline value for total trihalomethanes should not simply add up the guideline values for the individual compounds in order to arrive at a standard, because the four compounds are basically similar in toxicological action.

In controlling trihalomethanes, a multistep treatment system should be used to reduce organic trihalomethane precursors, and primary consideration should be given to ensuring that disinfection is never compromised.

### Bromoform

In a bioassay carried out by the National Toxicology Program (NTP) in the USA, bromoform induced a small increase in relatively rare tumours of the large intestine in rats of both sexes but did not induce tumours in mice. Data from a variety of assays on the genotoxicity of bromoform are equivocal. IARC has classified bromoform in Group 3.

A TDI was derived on the basis of a NOAEL of 25 mg/kg of body weight per day for the absence of histopathological lesions in the liver in a well-conducted and well-documented 90-day study in rats (*50*). This NOAEL is supported by the results of two long-term studies. The TDI is 17.9 µg/kg of body weight, correcting for exposure on 5 days per week and using an uncertainty factor of 1000 (100 for intra- and interspecies variation and 10 for possible carcinogenicity and the short duration of the study). With an allocation of 20% of the TDI to drinking-water, the guideline value is 100 µg/litre (rounded figure).

### Dibromochloromethane

In an NTP bioassay, DBCM induced hepatic tumours in female and possibly in male mice but not in rats. The genotoxicity of DBCM has been studied in a number of assays, but the available data are considered inconclusive. IARC has classified DBCM in Group 3.

A TDI was derived on the basis of a NOAEL of 30 mg/kg of body weight per day for the absence of histopathological effects in the liver in a well-conducted and well-documented 90-day study in rats (*57*). This NOAEL is supported by the results of long-term studies. The TDI is 21.4 μg/kg of body weight, correcting for exposure on 5 days per week and using an uncertainty factor of 1000 (100 for intra- and interspecies variation and 10 for the short duration of the study). An additional uncertainty factor for potential carcinogenicity was not applied because of the questions regarding mouse liver tumours from corn oil vehicles and inconclusive evidence of genotoxicity. With an allocation of 20% of the TDI to drinking-water, the guideline value is 100 μg/litre (rounded figure).

### Bromodichloromethane

In an NTP bioassay, BDCM induced renal adenomas and adenocarcinomas in both sexes of rats and male mice, rare tumours of the large intestine (adenomatous polyps and adenocarcinomas) in both sexes of rats, and hepatocellular adenomas and adenocarcinomas in female mice. BDCM has given both positive and negative results in a variety of *in vitro* and *in vivo* genotoxicity assays. IARC has classified bromodichloromethane in Group 2B (*84*).

Cancer risks have been estimated on the basis of increases in incidence of kidney tumours in male mice observed in the NTP bioassay (*59*), as these tumours yield the most protective value. Hepatic tumours in female mice were not considered owing to the possible role of the corn oil vehicle in their induction, although the estimated risks are within the same range. Using the linearized multistage model, the range of concentrations of BDCM in drinking-water associated with excess lifetime cancer risks of $10^{-4}$, $10^{-5}$, and $10^{-6}$ for kidney tumours are 600, 60, and 6 μg/litre, respectively. These values are supported by a recently published feeding study in rats that was not available for full evaluation.

### Chloroform

IARC has classified chloroform in Group 2B as a possible human carcinogen (*85*). In long-term studies, chloroform has been shown to induce hepatocellular carcinomas in mice when administered by gavage in oil-based vehicles but not in drinking-water; it has been reported to induce renal tubular adenomas and adenocarcinomas in male rats regardless of the carrier vehicle. Chloroform has been studied in a wide variety of genotoxicity assays and has been found to give both positive and negative results.

The guideline value is based on extrapolation of the observed increase in kidney tumours in male rats exposed to chloroform in drinking-water for 2 years (*66*), although it is recognized that chloroform may induce tumours through a non-genotoxic mechanism. Using the linearized multistage model, concentrations of chloroform in drinking-water of 2000, 200, and 20 μg/litre were calcu-

865

lated to correspond to excess lifetime cancer risks of $10^{-4}$, $10^{-5}$, and $10^{-6}$, respectively. The guideline value associated with an excess lifetime cancer risk of $10^{-5}$ is also supported by a 7.5-year study in dogs, in which a LOAEL of 15 mg/kg of body weight per day was observed for liver effects (applying an uncertainty factor of 1000 (100 for inter- and intraspecies variation and 10 for the use of a LOAEL) and allocating 50% of the TDI to drinking-water).

## References

1. Office of Water Regulations and Standards. *An exposure and risk assessment for trihalomethanes.* Washington, DC, US Environmental Protection Agency, 1980.

2. Budavari S, O'Neill M, Smith A, eds. *The Merck index. An encyclopedia of chemicals, drugs, and biologicals,* 11th ed. Rahway, NJ, Merck, 1989.

3. Verschueren K. *Handbook of environmental data on organic chemicals.* New York, Van Nostrand Reinhold, 1977.

4. Hawley GG. *The condensed chemical dictionary,* 10th ed. New York, Van Nostrand Reinhold, 1981:241.

5. Office of Research and Development. *Health assessment document for chloroform. Final report.* Research Triangle Park, NC, US Environmental Protection Agency, 1985 (EPA-600/8-84-004F).

6. Montgomery JH, Welkom LM. *Groundwater chemicals desk reference.* Chelsea, MI, Lewis Publishers, 1990.

7. Hansch C, Leo AJ. *Medchem Project Issue No. 26.* Claremont, CA, Pomona College, 1985.

8. Agency for Toxic Substances and Disease Registry. *Toxicological profile for bromoform and chlorodibromomethane.* Atlanta, GA, US Public Health Service, 1989.

9. Radding SB, Liu DH, Johnson HL. *Review of the environmental fate of selected chemicals.* Washington, DC, US Environmental Protection Agency, Office of Toxic Substances, 1977:69-72 (EPA 560/5-77-003).

10. Office of Toxic Substances and Environmental Criteria and Assessment Office. *Chemical fate rate constants for SARA Section 313 chemicals and Superfund health evaluation manual chemicals.* Washington, DC, US Environmental Protection Agency, 1989 (EPA-68-02-4254).

11. Kaczmar SW, D'Itri FM, Zabik MJ. Volatilization rates of selected haloforms from aqueous environments. *Environmental toxicology and chemistry,* 1985, 3(1):31-35 (cited in ref. 8).

12. Mackay DM et al. Vapor pressure corrections for low-volatility environmental chemicals. *Environmental science and technology*, 1982, 16:645-649.

13. Agency for Toxic Substances and Disease Registry. *Toxicological profile for chloroform*. Atlanta, GA, US Department of Health and Human Services, 1989.

14. Office of Research and Development. *Health assessment document for chloroform. Final report*. Research Triangle Park, NC, US Environmental Protection Agency, 1985 (EPA-600/8-84-004F).

15. Bouwer EJ, Rittman BE, McCarty PL. Anaerobic degradation of halogenated 1- and 2-carbon organic compounds. *Environmental science and technology*, 1981, 15(5): 596-599.

16. Bouwer EJ, McCarty PL. Transformation of halogenated organic compounds under denitrification conditions. *Applied environmental microbiology*, 1983, 45:1295-1299.

17. Mabey WR et al. *Aquatic fate process data for organic priority pollutants*. Washington, DC, US Environmental Protection Agency, Office of Water Regulation and Standards, 1982 (EPA 4014-81-PB87-16909).

18. Fishbein L. A survey of the analysis of halogenated alkanes and alkenes in biological samples. In: Fishbein L, O'Neil ID, eds. *Environmental carcinogens, selected methods of analysis*, Vol. 7. *Some volatile halogenated hydrocarbons*. Lyon, International Agency for Research on Cancer, 1985:141-168 (IARC Scientific Publications No. 68).

19. Environmental Monitoring and Support Laboratory. *Method 501.1. The analysis of trihalomethanes in finished waters by the purge and trap method*. Cincinnati, OH, US Environmental Protection Agency, 1979.

20. Environment Canada, Pollutant Management Division. *Ambient air concentrations of volatile compounds in Toronto and Montreal*. Ottawa, 1986.

21. Department of National Health and Welfare (Canada). *Draft review on trihalomethanes*. Ottawa, 1990.

22. Brodzinsky R, Singh HB. *Volatile organic chemicals in the atmosphere: an assessment of available data*. Menlo Park, CA, Atmospheric Science Center, SRI International, 1982 (Contract 68-02-3452).

23. Wallace LA. Personal exposure, indoor and outdoor air concentrations, and exhaled breath concentrations of selected volatile organic compounds measured for 600 residents of New Jersey, North Dakota, North Carolina, and California. *Toxicology and environmental chemistry*, 1986, 612:215-236.

24. Office of Research and Development. *The Total Exposure Assessment Methodology (TEAM) study: summary and analysis. I. Final report*. Washington, DC, US Environmental Protection Agency, 1986.

25. Andelman JB. Human exposures to volatile halogenated organic chemicals in indoor and outdoor air. *Environmental health perspectives*, 1985, 62:313-318.

26. Andelman JB. Inhalation exposure in the home to volatile organic contaminants of drinking water. *Science of the total environment*, 1985, 47:443-460.

27. Aizawa T, Magara Y, Musashi M. Effects of bromide ions on trihalomethane (THM) formation in water. *Aqua*, 1989, 38:165-175.

28. Boland PA. *National screening program for organics in drinking water*. Menlo Park, CA, SRI International, 1981 (report submitted to US Environmental Protection Agency, Office of Drinking Water, Washington, DC; contract no. 68-01-4666).

29. Rook JJ. Formation of haloforms during chlorination of natural waters. *Journal of the Society for Water Treatment and Examination*, 1974, 23:234-243.

30. Department of National Health and Welfare (Canada). *National survey for halo-methanes in drinking water*. Ottawa, 1977.

31. Brass HJ, Weisner MJ, Kingsley BA. *Community water supply survey: sampling and analysis for purgeable organics and total organic carbon*. Paper presented at the American Water Works Association Annual Meeting, Water Quality Division, 9 June 1981.

32. Brass HJ et al. The National Organic Monitoring Survey: sampling and analysis for purgeable organic compounds. In: Pojasek RB, ed. *Drinking water quality enhancement through source protection*. Ann Arbor, MI, Ann Arbor Science Publishers, 1977:393-416.

33. Symons JM, Bellar TA, Carswell JK. National Organic Reconnaissance Survey for halogenated organics. *Journal of the American Water Works Association*, 1975, 67:634-647.

34. Beech JA. Estimated worst case trihalomethane body burden of a child using a swimming pool. *Medical hypotheses*, 1980, 6:303-307.

35. Agency for Toxic Substances and Disease Registry. *Toxicological profile for bromo-dichloromethane. Draft for public comment*. Atlanta, GA, US Public Health Service, 1989.

36. Entz RC, Thomas KW, Diachenko EW. Residues of volatile halocarbons in foods using headspace gas chromatography. *Journal of agricultural chemistry*, 1982, 30:846-849.

37. McConnell G, Ferguson DM, Pearson CR. Chlorinated hydrocarbons and the environment. *Endeavour*, 1975, 34:13-18 (reviewed in ref. 14).

38. International Agency for Research on Cancer. *Some halogenated hydrocarbons. Chloroform.* Lyon, 1979:401-427 (IARC Monographs on the Evaluation of the Carcinogenic Risk of Chemicals to Humans, Volume 20).

39. Fry BJ, Taylor T, Hathway DE. Pulmonary elimination of chloroform and its metabolite in man. *Archives internationales de pharmacodynamie et de thérapie,* 1972, 196:98-111.

40. Lehman KB, Hasegawa O. Studies of the absorption of chlorinated hydrocarbons in animals and humans. *Archives of hygiene,* 1910, 72:327-342.

41. Brown DM et al. Metabolism of chloroform. I. The metabolism of $^{14}$C-chloroform by different species. *Xenobiotica,* 1974, 4:151-163 (reviewed in ref. 14).

42. Mink FL, Brown J, Rickabaugh J. Absorption, distribution and excretion of $^{14}$C-trihalomethanes in mice and rats. *Bulletin of environmental contamination and toxicology,* 1986, 37:752-758.

43. Ahmed AE, Kubic VL, Anders MW. Metabolism of haloforms to carbon monoxide. I. *In vitro* studies. *Drug metabolism and disposition,* 1977, 5:198-204.

44. Gopinath C, Ford EJ. The role of microsomal hydroxylases in the modification of chloroform hepatotoxicity in rats. *British journal of experimental pathology,* 1975, 56:412-522.

45. Wolf CR et al. The reduction of polyhalogenated methane by liver microsomal cytochrome P-450. *Molecular pharmacology,* 1977, 13:698-705.

46. Reitz RH, Gehring PJ, Park CN. Carcinogenic risk estimation for chloroform: an alternative to EPA's procedures. *Food and cosmetics toxicology,* 1978, 16:511-514.

47. Bowman FJ, Borzelleca JF, Munson AE. The toxicity of some halomethanes in mice. *Toxicology and applied pharmacology,* 1978, 44:213-215.

48. Chu I et al. The acute toxicity of four trihalomethanes in male and female rats. *Toxicology and applied pharmacology,* 1980, 52:351-353.

49. Chu I et al. Toxicity of trihalomethanes. I. The acute and subacute toxicity of chloroform, bromodichloromethane, chlorodibromomethane and bromoform in rats. *Journal of environmental science and health,* 1982, B17:205-224.

50. National Toxicology Program. *Toxicology and carcinogenesis studies of tribromomethane (bromoform) in F344/N rats and B6C3F1 mice (gavage studies).* Research Triangle Park, NC, US Department of Health and Human Services, 1989 (TR 350).

51. Tobe M et al. *Studies on the chronic oral toxicity of tribromomethane, dibromochloromethane and bromodichloromethane.* Tokyo, Tokyo Medical and Dental University, 1982 (unpublished interagency report to the National Institute of Hygienic Sciences).

52. National Toxicology Program. *Bromoform—reproduction and fertility assessment in Swiss CD-1 mice when administered by gavage.* Research Triangle Park, NC, National Institute of Environmental Health Sciences, 1989 (NTP-89-068).

53. Simmon VF, Kauhanen K, Tardiff RG. Mutagenic activity of chemicals identified in drinking water. *Developments in toxicology and environmental science*, 1977:249-258.

54. Ishidate M et al. *Studies on the mutagenicity of low boiling organohalogen compounds.* Tokyo, Tokyo Medical and Dental University, 1982 (unpublished interagency report to the National Institute of Hygienic Sciences).

55. Morimoto K, Koizumi A. Trihalomethanes induce sister chromatid exchanges in human lymphocytes *in vitro* and mouse bone marrow cells *in vivo*. *Environmental research*, 1983, 32(1):72-79.

56. Theiss JC et al. Test for carcinogenicity of organic contaminants of United States drinking waters by pulmonary tumor response in strain A mice. *Cancer research*, 1977, 37:2717-2720.

57. National Toxicology Program. *Toxicology and carcinogenesis studies of chlorodibromomethane in F344/N rats and B6C3F$_1$ mice (gavage studies).* Research Triangle Park, NC, US Department of Health and Human Services, 1985 (TR 282).

58. Borzelleca JF, Carchman RA. *Effects of selected organic drinking water contaminants on male reproduction.* Research Triangle Park, NC, US Environmental Protection Agency, 1982 (EPA 600/1-82-009; NTIS PB82-259847; Contract No. R804290).

59. National Toxicology Program. *Toxicology and carcinogenesis studies of bromodichloromethane in F344/N rats and B6C3F$_1$ mice (gavage studies).* Research Triangle Park, NC, US Department of Health and Human Services, 1987 (TR 321).

60. Ruddick JA, Villeneuve DC, Chu I. A teratological assessment of four trihalomethanes in rats. *Journal of environmental science and health*, 1983, B18:333-349.

61. Jorgenson TA, Rushbrook CJ. *Effects of chloroform in the drinking water of rats and mice: ninety-day subacute toxicity study.* Menlo Park, CA, SRI International, 1980 (prepared for US Environmental Protection Agency, contract no. 68-03-2626; publication no. EPA-600/1-80-030).

62. Chu I et al. Toxicity of trihalomethanes: II. Reversibility of toxicological changes produced by chloroform, bromodichloromethane, chlorodibromomethane and bromoform in rats. *Journal of environmental science and health*, 1982, B17:225-240.

63. Bull RJ et al. Enhancement of the hepatotoxicity of chloroform in B6C3F$_1$ mice by corn oil: implications for chloroform carcinogenesis. *Environmental health perspectives*, 1986, 69:9-58.

64. Palmer AK et al. Safety evaluation of toothpaste containing chloroform. II. Long-term studies in rats. *Journal of environmental pathology and toxicology*, 1979, 2:821-833.

65. Klaunig JE, Ruch RJ, Pereira MA. Carcinogenicity of chlorinated methane and ethane compounds administered in drinking water to mice. *Environmental health perspectives*, 1986, 69:89-95.

66. Jorgenson TA, Meierhenry EF, Rushbrook CJ. Carcinogenicity of chloroform in drinking water to male Osborne-Mendel rats and female B6C3F$_1$ mice. *Fundamental and applied toxicology*, 1985, 5:760-769.

67. Heywood R et al. Safety evaluation of toothpaste containing chloroform. III. Long-term study in beagle dogs. *Journal of environmental pathology and toxicology*, 1979, 2:835-851.

68. Thompson DJ, Warner SD, Robinson VB. Teratology studies on orally administered chloroform in the rat and rabbit. *Toxicology and applied pharmacology*, 1974, 29:348-357.

69. Uehleke H et al. Metabolic activation of haloalkanes and tests *in vitro* for mutagenicity. *Xenobiotica*, 1977, 7:393-400 (reviewed in ref. 14).

70. Gocke E et al. Mutagenicity of cosmetics ingredients licensed by the European communities. *Mutation research*, 1981, 90:91-109 (reviewed in ref. 14).

71. Agustin JS, Lim-Syliano CY. Mutagenic and clastogenic effects of chloroform. *Bulletin of the Philadelphia Biochemical Society*, 1978, 1:17-23.

72. Callen DF, Wolf CR, Philpot RM. Cytochrome P-450 mediated genetic activity and cytotoxicity of seven halogenated aliphatic hydrocarbons in *Saccharomyces cerevisiae*. *Mutation research*, 1980, 77:55-63.

73. Land PC, Owen EL, Linde HW. Morphologic changes in mouse spermatogen after exposure to inhalational anesthetics during early spermatogenesis. *Anesthesiology*, 1981, 54:53-56.

74. National Cancer Institute. *Report on carcinogenesis bioassay of chloroform.* Springfield, VA, 1976 (NTIS PB-264018).

75. Burton-Fanning FW. Poisoning by bromoform. *British medical journal*, 1901, May 18:1202-1203.

76. Dwelle EH. Fatal bromoform poisoning. *Journal of the American Medical Association*, 1903, 41:1540.

77. Gosselin RE et al. *Clinical toxicology of commercial products. Acute poisoning*, 4th ed. Baltimore, MD, Williams and Wilkins, 1976.

78. Challen P Jr, Hickish DE, Bedford J. Chronic chloroform intoxication. *British journal of industrial medicine*, 1958, 15:243-249.

79. Bomski H, Sobolewska A, Strakowski A. [Toxic damage of the liver by chloroform in chemical industry workers.] *Archiv für Gewerbepathologie und Gewerbehygiene*, 1967, 24:127-134 (in German).

80. Brenniman GR et al. Case-control study of cancer deaths in Illinois communities served by chlorinated or non-chlorinated water. In: Jolley R et al., eds. *Water chlorination: environmental impact and health effects*. Vol. 3. Ann Arbor, MI, Ann Arbor Science Publishers, 1980:1043-1057.

81. Cragle DL et al. A case-control study of colon cancer and water chlorination in North Carolina. In: Jolley RL et al., eds. *Water chlorination: chemistry, environmental impact and health effects*. Vol. 5. Chelsea, MI, Lewis Publishing, 1985:153-157.

82. US Environmental Protection Agency. *Preliminary assessment of suspected carcinogens in drinking water. Report to Congress*. Washington, DC, 1975 (EPA-56014-75-005, PB 260961).

83. Lawrence CE et al. Trihalomethanes in drinking water and human colorectal cancer. *Journal of the National Cancer Institute*, 1984, 72:563-568.

84. International Agency for Research on Cancer. *Chlorinated drinking-water; chlorination by-products; some other halogenated compounds; cobalt and cobalt compounds*. Lyon, 1991:45-359 (IARC Monographs on the Evaluation of Carcinogenic Risks to Humans, Volume 52).

85. International Agency for Research on Cancer. *Overall evaluations of carcinogenicity: an updating of IARC Monographs volumes 1-42*. Lyon, 1987:152-154 (IARC Monographs on the Evaluation of Carcinogenic Risks to Humans, Suppl. 7).

# Other chlorination by-products

A number of oxidation by-products are formed when chlorine reacts with organic materials, such as humic or fulvic acids, present in water as a result of the degradation of animal or plant matter. The following chlorination by-products are dealt with in this section: chlorinated acetic acids, trichloroacetaldehyde, chloroacetones, halogenated acetonitriles, cyanogen chloride, and chloropicrin.

# 16.11 Chlorinated acetic acids

## 16.11.1 General description

### Identity

| Compound | CAS no. | Molecular formula |
|---|---|---|
| Monochloroacetic acid | 79-11-8 | $ClCH_2COOH$ |
| Dichloroacetic acid | 79-43-6 | $Cl_2CHCOOH$ |
| Trichloroacetic acid | 76-03-9 | $Cl_3CCOOH$ |

The IUPAC names for these compounds are mono-, di- and trichloroethanoic acid, respectively.

### Physicochemical properties (1-3)

| Property | Monochloroacetic acid [1] | Dichloroacetic acid [2] | Trichloroacetic acid [3] |
|---|---|---|---|
| Boiling point (°C) | 187.8 | 194 | 197.5 |
| Melting point (°C) | 52.5 | 13.5 | — |
| Density (g/cm³) | 1.58 at 20 °C | 1.56 at 20 °C | 1.63 at 61°C |
| Vapour pressure (kPa) | 0.133 at 40 °C | 0.133 at 44 °C | 0.133 at 51 °C |
| Water solubility (g/litre) | Very soluble | 86.3 | 13 |
| Log octanol–water partition coefficient | — | 0.14 | 0.10 |

### Organoleptic properties

No information is available on the odour thresholds of chlorinated acetic acids in water.

### Major uses

Monochloroacetic acid is used as an intermediate or reagent in the synthesis of a variety of chemicals and as a pre-emergence herbicide. Dichloroacetic acid is used as a chemical intermediate in the synthesis of organic materials, as an ingredient in pharmaceuticals and medicines, as a topical astringent, and as a fungicide. Trichloroacetic acid is used as an intermediate in the synthesis of organic chemicals, and as a laboratory reagent, herbicide, soil sterilizer, and antiseptic (2–5).

---

[1] Conversion factor in air: 1 ppm = 3.87 mg/m³.
[2] Conversion factor in air: 1 ppm = 5.27 mg/m³.
[3] Conversion factor in air: 1 ppm = 6.68 mg/m³.

## 16.11.2 Analytical methods

The chloroacetic acids can be determined either by EPA Method 515.1 or draft EPA Method 552, which was developed for non-pesticidal haloacids and phenols, i.e. by capillary-column/electron-capture/gas chromatography. Data from a monitoring study of water supplies indicate that detection levels of 1 µg/litre are achievable.

## 16.11.3 Environmental levels and human exposure

### Water

Chlorinated acetic acids are formed from organic material during water chlorination (6); typical levels in finished drinking-water supplies range from 30 to 160 µg/litre (7). Limited data for drinking-water supplies in the USA indicate that monochloroacetic acid is generally present at concentrations of less than 1.2 µg/litre (8); it was detected in the finished water at six of 10 sites at levels below 10 µg/litre. Dichloroacetic acid was found in the distribution systems of six water-supply companies at concentrations ranging from 8 to 79 µg/litre; it was detected in the finished water of 10 of 10 companies surveyed and at levels of 10 µg/litre or higher at eight of them. Trichloroacetic acid was found in the distribution systems of six companies at concentrations ranging from 15 to 103 µg/litre; it was detected in finished water at six of 10 companies at concentrations of 10–100 µg/litre (four sites) and less than 10 µg/litre (two sites) (9).

## 16.11.4 Kinetics and metabolism in laboratory animals and humans

### Monochloroacetic acid

In rats given monochloroacetate subcutaneously, levels in liver and kidney were approximately the same and 4–5 times higher than those in plasma, brain, and heart. Approximately 50% of the dose was excreted in the urine within 17 h. Monochloroacetic acid is metabolized to oxalate and glycine. It can also be conjugated with glutathione, phospholipids, and cholesterol. The glutathione conjugate degrades to thiodiacetic acid (10, 11).

### Dichloroacetic acid

Plasma dichloroacetic acid concentrations peaked in rats 30 min after dosing by gavage, suggesting rapid intestinal absorption (12). Levels in liver and muscle increased following administration (13). In rats, dogs, and humans given sodium dichloroacetate intravenously, average half-lives of the parent compound in the plasma were 2.97, 20.8, and 0.43 h, respectively; the apparent dose dependence of plasma clearance suggests that metabolic transformation becomes rate-limiting at high doses (14). In the rat, dichloroacetate is rapidly metabolized by dechlorination to glyoxalate, which in turn is metabolized to oxalate (*15*). In humans, urinary excretion of unchanged dichloroacetate was negligible after 8 h, and cumulative excretion was less than 1% of the total dose in all subjects (*14*).

### Trichloroacetic acid

Trichloroacetic acid appears to be rapidly absorbed from the intestinal tract, metabolism occurring mainly in the liver. It can be converted into carbon dioxide and chloride ion or reduced to the aldehyde. A comparatively small proportion of trichloroacetic acid is metabolized, much of this compound being excreted unchanged in the urine (*16, 17*).

## 16.11.5 Effects on laboratory animals and *in vitro* test systems

### Monochloroacetic acid

*Acute exposure*
The acute oral $LD_{50}$s for monochloroacetic acid in mice, male rats, and male guinea-pigs were estimated to be 255, 76, and 80 mg/kg of body weight, respectively (*18*). In other studies, oral $LD_{50}$s in mice were found to be 165 mg/kg of body weight (*19*) and 260 mg/kg of body weight (*20*). In rats, an oral $LD_{50}$ of 2820 mg/kg of body weight in males and a dermal $LD_{50}$ of 8068 mg/kg of body weight were reported (*21*).

*Short-term exposure*
Mice (20 per sex per dose) received monochloroacetic acid by gavage at 0, 25, 50, 100, 150, or 200 mg/kg of body weight per day for 13 weeks. Mortality was increased at the highest dose, and females in this group experienced decreased weight gain and increased absolute and relative liver weights. Cholinesterase levels were decreased in females at 150 and 200 mg/kg of body weight per day. The NOAEL was 100 mg/kg of body weight per day for decreased cholinesterase levels (*22*).

In rats (20 per sex per dose) that received monochloroacetic acid by gavage at 0, 30, 60, 90, 120, or 150 mg/kg of body weight per day for 13 weeks, effects were seen at every dose level. At 90 mg/kg of body weight per day and above, they included accumulations of mononuclear inflammatory cells and myofibre degeneration, elevated blood levels of thyroxin and segmented neutrophils, and increased blood urea nitrogen levels in males. At 60 mg/kg of body weight per day and above, effects included decreased survival, decreased absolute and relative heart weights, degenerative and inflammatory changes (cardiomyopathy), elevated alanine and aspartate aminotransferases, increased actual liver weight and relative kidney weight in males, and increased blood urea nitrogen levels in females. At 30 mg/kg of body weight per day and above, effects included decreased lymphocyte counts and decreased relative heart weight in females. The LOAEL for this study was the lowest dose tested, 30 mg/kg of body weight per day (*22*).

*Long-term exposure*

F344/N rats (70 per sex per dose) received monochloroacetic acid by gavage at doses of 0, 15, or 30 mg/kg of body weight per day, 5 days per week for 2 years. No effects on body weight or clinical findings were observed. However, survival was significantly decreased in male rats at 30 mg/kg of body weight per day and in female rats in both dose groups. The incidence of uterine polyps was marginally (nonsignificantly) increased in females at both doses. The LOAEL for this study was 15 mg/kg of body weight per day for reduced survival (*22*).

In the same study, B6C3F$_1$ mice (60 per sex per dose) were dosed with monochloroacetic acid at 0, 50, or 100 mg/kg of body weight per day, 5 days per week for 2 years. Effects were seen only at the highest dose and included decreased survival in males, decreased mean body weight and metaplasia of the olfactory epithelium in females, and inflammation of the nasal mucosa and squamous hyperplasia of the forestomach in both sexes. The NOAEL for this study was 50 mg/kg of body weight per day (*22*).

*Mutagenicity and related end-points*

Monochloroacetic acid was positive in the mouse lymphoma cell forward mutation assay without metabolic activation (*23*). It was positive without, and negative with metabolic activation in the sister chromatid exchange assay in Chinese hamster ovary (CHO) cells. In the *in vitro* chromosomal aberration assay in CHO cells, monochloroacetic acid was negative both with and without metabolic activation (*24*).

*Carcinogenicity*

There was no evidence of carcinogenic activity in 2-year bioassays in F344/N rats and B6C3F$_1$ mice. Rats (70 per sex per dose) received monochloroacetic acid by gavage at 0, 15, or 30 mg/kg of body weight per day, and mice (60 per sex per dose) received 0, 50, or 100 mg/kg of body weight per day (*22*).

## Dichloroacetic acid

*Acute exposure*

LD$_{50}$s of 4480 and 5520 mg of dichloroacetic acid per kg of body weight have been reported in rats and mice, respectively (*18*).

*Short-term exposure*

In a study in which Sprague-Dawley rats (5 per sex per group) were given water containing 0, 30, 125, 500, or 1875 mg of dichloroacetate per litre (0, 2.4, 10, 40, or 150 mg/kg of body weight per day) for 14 days, none of the parameters monitored (e.g. body weight, lactate and pyruvate levels, blood glucose levels) was significantly altered. In this study, a NOAEL of 150 mg/kg of body weight per day was identified (*25*).

In a study in which sodium dichloroacetate was administered to Sprague-Dawley rats (10 per sex per dose) by gavage at dose levels of 0, 125, 500, or 2000 mg/kg of body weight per day for 3 months, body weight gain was significantly depressed in a dose-dependent manner at all dose levels. Minimal effects on haematological parameters were observed at the two highest doses. Mean relative weights of liver, kidneys, and adrenals were significantly increased in a dose-dependent fashion. Brain and testes were the principal target organs; brain lesions characterized by vacuolation of the myelinated white tracts resembling oedema were observed in the cerebrum and cerebellum of treated rats of both sexes in all dose groups. Based on effects on organ weights and brain lesions, a LOAEL of 125 mg/kg of body weight per day, the lowest dose tested, was identified in this study (26, 27).

Beagle dogs were given sodium dichloroacetate by capsule at 50, 75, or 100 mg/kg of body weight per day for 13 weeks. Both sexes exhibited dose-dependent weight losses. All dose levels were associated with a progressive depression in erythrocyte counts, erythrocyte volume fraction (haematocrit) and haemoglobin levels. Mean blood glucose, lactate, and pyruvate levels were significantly reduced in all treated animals. There was an increased incidence of lung consolidation among treated dogs. Histopathological examination indicated that all treated dogs suffered slight to moderate vacuolation of white myelinated tracts in the cerebrum and to a lesser extent in the cerebellum. There was an increased incidence of haemosiderin-laden Kupffer's cells in the liver and cystic mucosal hyperplasia in the gallbladder at all dose levels. A LOAEL of 50 mg/kg of body weight per day can be identified from this study (26, 27).

*Long-term exposure*
Male B6C3F$_1$ mice (50 per dose) received dichloroacetate in their drinking-water at 0, 0.05, 0.5, 3.5, or 5.0 g/litre (0, 7.6, 77, 410, or 486 mg/kg of body weight per day) for 60 weeks. Other groups of mice received dichloroacetate at 7.6 or 77 mg/kg of body weight per day for 75 weeks. In the highest-dose mice, water consumption was reduced to 60% of that of controls. Body weight was decreased at the two highest dose levels, and relative liver weight was increased at the three highest dose levels. An increase in kidney weight was seen only at 410 mg/kg of body weight per day. No effects were seen on testes or spleen weight. The NOAEL for the 60- and 75-week studies was 7.6 mg/kg of body weight per day (28).

*Mutagenicity and related end-points*
Dichloroacetic acid was reported to cause strand breaks in DNA when administered *in vivo* to rats and mice in one study (29) but not in a second study at higher doses (30).

*Carcinogenicity*

The carcinogenic potential of dichloroacetate was investigated in B6C3F$_1$ mice (50 males per dose) that received this compound in their drinking-water for 60 weeks at concentrations of 0, 0.05, 0.5, 3.5, or 5.0 g/litre (0, 7.6, 77, 410, or 486 mg/kg of body weight per day). Other groups of mice received dichloroacetate at 7.6 or 77 mg/kg of body weight per day for 75 weeks. Hyperplastic nodules were seen in 58% of the mice that received 410 mg/kg of body weight per day and in 83% of the mice that received 486 mg/kg of body weight per day. The incidences of hepatocellular adenomas were 100% and 80%, and those of hepatocellular carcinomas 67% and 83%, respectively. Incidences in the other dose groups were similar to those in controls (*28*).

The carcinogenic potential of dichloroacetic acid in mice was investigated in a complex regimen that included pretreatment with nitrosoethylurea (NEU) at various doses. Male B6C3F$_1$ mice were supplied with drinking-water containing 0, 2000, or 5000 mg of dichloroacetate per litre (0, 400, or 1000 mg/kg of body weight per day). Non-initiation protocols (without NEU) were used only at the high-dose level. The incidence of hepatocellular carcinomas was 0% in the control group (no NEU or dichloroacetic acid) and 81% at 1000 mg/kg of body weight per day (no NEU). With dichloroacetic acid and a low dose of NEU, the tumour incidences were 66–72% for the high and low doses. The authors concluded that dichloroacetic acid was carcinogenic at a dose of 1000 mg/kg of body weight per day without prior initiation (*31*).

Dichloroacetic acid exposure via drinking-water resulted in the induction of liver tumours in male B6C3F$_1$ mice. Groups of mice received dichloroacetic acid at 0, 1, or 2 g/litre (approximately 0, 137, or 295 mg/kg of body weight per day, based on the authors' calculations of total dose for each group) for 37 or 52 weeks. Hepatocellular carcinomas were seen only in 5 of 24 males (21%) that received the highest dose for 52 weeks (*32*).

## Trichloroacetic acid

*Acute exposure*

The LD$_{50}$ for trichloroacetic acid was 3320 mg/kg of body weight in rats and 4970 mg/kg of body weight in mice (*18*).

*Short-term exposure*

Groups of male Sprague-Dawley rats were exposed to trichloroacetate in drinking-water at a concentration of 5000 mg/litre (about 312 mg/kg of body weight per day) for 10, 20, or 30 days. No treatment-related changes in body weight, organ weight, gross necropsy, or histopathology were found, and a short-term NOAEL of 312 mg/kg of body weight per day can be identified (*33*).

Six male Fischer 344 [CDF (F-344)/CrlBR] rats and eight male B6C3F$_1$ mice were given trichloroacetic acid by gavage at 500 mg/kg of body weight per day for 10 days. The mean liver-to-body-weight ratios were significantly increased in both species, but there was no effect on the mean kidney-to-body-weight ratio. Cyanide-insensitive palmitoyl coenzyme (CoA) oxidation was increased in both species. The LOAEL for liver effects identified in this study was 500 mg/kg of body weight per day for both rats and mice (*34*).

Male Sprague-Dawley rats (10 per dose) received trichloroacetic acid in their drinking-water at 0, 50, 500, or 5000 mg/litre (0, 4.1, 36.5, or 355 mg/kg of body weight per day) for 90 days. No effects were seen on body weight or absolute weight of liver or kidneys. At the highest dose level, absolute spleen weight was reduced and relative liver and kidney weights were increased. Liver effects seen at the highest dose included increased hepatic peroxisomal beta-oxidation activity, focal hepatocellular enlargement, intracellular swelling, and glycogen accumulation. The NOAEL for this study was 36.5 mg/kg of body weight per day (*35*).

Dose-related increases in hepatic weight were associated with the administration of trichloroacetic acid in drinking-water at 0, 300, 1000, or 2000 mg/litre to male $B6C3F_1$ mice for 14 days. The effect was statistically significant at 1000 and 2000 mg/litre. The NOAEL was therefore 300 mg/litre or approximately 55 mg/kg of body weight per day (*36*) .

*Long-term exposure*
Male Sprague-Dawley rats were exposed to trichloroacetate in drinking-water at concentrations of 0, 50, 500, or 5000 mg/litre (0, 2.89, 29.6, and 277 mg/kg of body weight per day at 6 months) for up to 12 months. No significant changes were detected in body weight, organ weight, gross necropsy, or histopathology during the experiment. A NOAEL of 277 mg/kg of body weight per day was identified in this study (*33*).

In a study in which $B6C3F_1$ mice received trichloroacetate at 0, 1, or 2 g/litre in drinking-water for 37 or 52 weeks, both absolute liver weights and liver-to-body-weight ratios in male and female mice were significantly increased in a dose-related manner relative to controls. The LOAEL in this study was 1 g/litre, or 178 mg/kg of body weight per day, based on the authors' calculations of total dose for each group (*32*).

*Mutagenicity and related end-points*
Trichloroacetic acid was not mutagenic in *Salmonella typhimurium* strain TA100 without metabolic activation (*37*). It gave positive results in three *in vivo* chromosomal aberration assays in mice: the bone marrow assay, the micronucleus test, and the sperm-head abnormality assay (*38*).

*Carcinogenicity*
Male $B6C3F_1$ mice received trichloroacetic acid at 0, 1, or 2 g/litre (approximately 0, 178, or 319 mg/kg of body weight per day, based on the authors' calculations of total dose for each group) in drinking-water for 37 or 52 weeks. An increase in the incidence of hepatocellular carcinomas was seen in males in both treated groups, but none was seen in any of the females (*32*).

The carcinogenic potential of trichloroacetic acid in mice was investigated in a complex regimen that included pretreatment with NEU at various doses for 61 weeks. Male B6C3F$_1$ mice were supplied with drinking-water containing trichloroacetate at 0, 2000, or 5000 mg/litre (0, 400, or 1000 mg/kg of body weight per day). Non-initiation protocols (without NEU) were used at the high-dose level only. The incidence of hepatocellular carcinomas was 0% in the controls (no NEU or trichloroacetic acid) and 32% at the highest dose level (no NEU). In both groups given trichloroacetic acid with a low dose of NEU, the tumour incidence was 48%. The authors concluded that trichloroacetic acid was carcinogenic at a dose of 1000 mg/kg of body weight per day without prior initiation (31).

The results of two short-term tests conducted in rats—the hepatic enzyme-altered foci bioassay and stimulation of peroxisomal-dependent palmitoyl-CoA oxidation in liver—suggest that trichloroacetic acid may possess weak promoting activity in the rat liver (33, 39).

## 16.11.6 Effects on humans

Diabetic or hyperlipoproteinaemic patients received a daily oral dose of 3-4 g of dichloroacetate for 6–7 days. Some patients experienced mild sedation, but no other laboratory or clinical evidence of adverse effects was noted during or immediately after the treatment phase. Biochemical effects included significantly reduced fasting blood glucose levels, marked decreases in plasma lactate and alanine, significantly decreased plasma cholesterol levels, decreased triglyceride levels, elevated plasma ketone bodies, and elevated serum uric acid levels (40).

Daily oral doses of 50 mg of dichloroacetate per kg were administered to two young males to treat severe familial hypercholesterolaemia (41). In both patients, total serum cholesterol levels decreased significantly. No adverse clinical or laboratory signs were detected in one patient, but the second complained of tingling in his fingers and toes after 16 weeks. Physical examination revealed slight decreases in the strength of facial and finger muscles, diminished to absent deep tendon reflexes, and decreased strength in all muscle groups of the lower extremities. Electromyographic studies revealed denervation changes in foot and distal leg muscles. Mild slowing of conduction velocity was noted in both posterior tibial nerves, and no measurable response was obtained in the peroneal or sural nerves. Six months after discontinuation of the treatment the neuropathic effects had improved, although serum cholesterol returned to high levels (42).

## 16.11.7 Guideline values

### Monochloroacetic acid

No evidence of carcinogenicity was found in a recent 2-year bioassay in rats and mice (22). Available toxicity data are considered insufficient for deriving a guideline value.

## Dichloroacetic acid

In several bioassays, dichloroacetate has been shown to induce hepatic tumours in mice. No adequate data on genotoxicity are available. Because the evidence for the carcinogenicity of dichloroacetate is insufficient, a TDI of 7.6 µg/kg of body weight was calculated based on a study in which no effects were seen on the livers of mice exposed to dichloroacetate at 7.6 mg/kg of body weight per day for 75 weeks (*28*) and incorporating an uncertainty factor of 1000 (100 for intra- and interspecies variation and 10 for possible carcinogenicity). With an allocation of 20% of the TDI to drinking-water, the provisional guideline value is 50 µg/litre (rounded figure).

The guideline value is designated as provisional because the data are insufficient to ensure that the value is technically achievable. Difficulties in meeting a guideline value must never be a reason to compromise adequate disinfection.

## Trichloroacetic acid

Trichloroacetate has been shown to induce tumours in the liver of mice. It has not been found to be mutagenic in *in vitro* assays, but has been reported to cause chromosomal aberrations.

Because the evidence for the carcinogenicity of trichloroacetate is restricted to one species, a TDI of 17.8 µg/kg of body weight was calculated based on a LOAEL of 178 mg/kg of body weight per day from a study in which increased liver weight was seen in mice exposed to trichloroacetate in drinking-water for 52 weeks (*32*) and incorporating an uncertainty factor of 10 000 (100 for intra- and interspecies variation and 100 for the use of a slightly less-than-lifetime study, use of a LOAEL rather than a NOAEL, and possible carcinogenicity). The NOAEL in a 14-day study in mice for the same effect was one-third of the LOAEL in the 52-week study (*36*). Based on a 20% allocation of the TDI to drinking-water, the provisional guideline value is 100 µg/litre (rounded figure).

The guideline value is designated as provisional because of the limitations of the available toxicological database and because there are inadequate data to judge whether the guideline value is technically achievable. Difficulties in meeting the guideline value must never be a reason for compromising adequate disinfection.

## References

1.   Weast RC. *Handbook of chemistry and physics.* Cleveland, OH, CRC Press, 1988.

2.   Verschueren K. *Handbook of environmental data on organic chemicals.* New York, NY, Van Nostrand Reinhold, 1977.

3.   Budavari S, O'Neill M, Smith A, eds. *The Merck index. An encyclopedia of chemicals, drugs, and biologicals,* 11th ed. Rahway, NJ, Merck, 1989.

4. Hawley GG. *The condensed chemical dictionary*, 10th ed. New York, NY, Van Nostrand Reinhold, 1981:241.

5. Meister RT, ed. *Farm chemicals handbook*, 75th ed. Willoughby, OH, Meister Publishing Co., 1989.

6. Coleman WE et al. Identification of organic compounds in a mutagenic extract of a surface drinking water by a computerized gas chromatography/mass spectrometry system (GC/MS/COM). *Environmental science and technology*, 1980, 14:576-588.

7. Jolley RL. Basic issues in water chlorination: a chemical perspective. In: Jolley RL et al., eds. *Water chlorination: chemistry, environmental impact and health effects*, Vol. 5. Chelsea, MI, Lewis Publishers, 1985:19-38.

8. Bull RJ, Kopfler FC. Formation and occurrence of disinfectant by-products. In: *Health effects of disinfectants and disinfection by-products*. Denver, CO, American Water Works Association Research Foundation, 1991:55-103.

9. Stevens AA et al. By-products of chlorination at ten operating utilities. In: Jolley RL et al., eds. *Water chlorination: chemistry, environmental impact and health effects*, Vol. 6. Ann Arbor, MI, Ann Arbor Scientific Publishers, 1990:579-604.

10. Hayes FD, Short RD, Gibson JE. Differential toxicity of monochloroacetate, monofluoroacetate and monoiodoacetate in rats. *Toxicology and applied pharmacology*, 1973, 26:93-102.

11. Bhat HK, Ahmed AE, Ansari GAS. Toxicokinetics of monochloroacetic acid: a whole-body autoradiography study. *Toxicology*, 1990, 63:35-43.

12. Stacpoole PW et al. Dichloroacetate derivatives. Metabolic effects and pharmacodynamics in normal rats. *Life sciences*, 1987, 41:2167-2176.

13. Evans OB. Dichloroacetate tissue concentrations and its relationship to hypolactatemia and pyruvate dehydrogenase activation. *Biochemical pharmacology*, 1982, 31:3124-3126.

14. Lukas G et al. Biological disposition of sodium dichloroacetate in animals and humans after intravenous administration. *Journal of pharmaceutical science*, 1980, 69(4):419-421.

15. Crabb DW, Yount EA, Harris RA. The metabolic effects of dichloroacetate. *Metabolism*, 1981, 30:1024-1039.

16. Hobara T et al. Intestinal absorption of chloral hydrate, free trichloroethanol and trichloroacetic acid in dogs. *Pharmacology and toxicology*, 1988, 62:250-258.

17. Hobara T et al. Extra-hepatic metabolism of chloral hydrate, trichloroethanol and trichloroacetic acid in dogs. *Pharmacology and toxicology*, 1987, 61:58-62.

18. Woodard G et al. The acute oral toxicity of acetic, chloroacetic, dichloroacetic and trichloroacetic acids. *Journal of industrial hygiene and toxicology*, 1941, 23(2):78-82.

19. Morrison JL. Toxicity of certain halogen substituted aliphatic acids for white mice. *Journal of pharmacology and experimental therapeutics*, 1946, 86:336-338.

20. Berardi MR et al. Monochloroacetic acid toxicity in the mouse associated with blood-brain barrier damage. *Fundamental and applied toxicology*, 1987, 9:469-479.

21. Smyth HF, Carpenter CP, Weil CS. Range-finding toxicity data: list IV. *American Medical Association archives of industrial hygiene and occupational medicine*, 1951, 4:119-122.

22. National Toxicology Program. *NTP technical report on the toxicology and carcinogenesis studies of monochloroacetic acid in F344/N rats and B6C3F$_1$ mice (gavage studies)*. Research Triangle Park, NC, 1990 (NTP TR 396; NIH Publication No. 90-2851).

23. McGregor DB et al. Responses of the LS178Y tk$^+$/tk$^-$ mouse lymphoma cell forward mutation assay to coded chemicals. I: Results for nine compounds. *Environmental mutagenesis*, 1987, 9:143-160.

24. Galloway SM et al. Chromosome aberrations and sister chromatid exchanges in Chinese hamster ovary cells: evaluation of 108 chemicals. *Environmental and molecular mutagenesis*, 1987, 10(Suppl. 10):1-175.

25. Davis ME. Effect of chloroacetic acids on the kidneys. *Environmental health perspectives*, 1986, 69:209-214.

26. Katz R et al. *CGS 7927A (dichloroacetate): 90-day oral administration to rats.* Summit, NJ, Ciba-Geigy, 1978.

27. Katz R et al. Dichloroacetate, sodium: 3-month oral toxicity studies in rats and dogs. *Toxicology and applied pharmacology*, 1981, 57:273-287.

28. DeAngelo AB et al. The carcinogenicity of dichloroacetic acid in the male B6C3F$_1$ mouse. *Fundamental and applied toxicology*, 1991, 16:337-347.

29. Nelson MA, Bull RJ. Induction of strand breaks in DNA by trichloroethylene and metabolites in rat and mouse liver *in vivo*. *Toxicology and applied pharmacology*, 1988, 94:45-54.

30. Chang LW, Daniel FB, DeAngelo AB. Analysis of DNA strand breaks induced in rodent liver *in vivo*, hepatocytes in primary culture, and a human cell line by chloroacetic acids and chloroacetaldehydes. In: *Proceedings of the Annual Meeting of the Society of Toxicology, Atlanta, GA, 27 February – 3 March, 1989.* Research Triangle Park, NC, US Environmental Protection Agency, Health Effects Research Laboratory, 1989.

31. Herren-Freund SL, Pereira MA. Carcinogenicity of by-products of disinfection in mouse and rat liver. *Environmental health perspectives*, 1986, 69:59-65.

32. Bull RJ et al. Liver tumor induction in B6C3F$_1$ mice by dichloroacetate and trichloroacetate. *Toxicology*, 1990, 63:341-359.

33. Parnell MJ, Koller LD, Exon JH. Assessment of hepatic initiation-promotion properties of trichloroacetic acid. *Archives of environmental contamination and toxicology*, 1988, 17:429-436.

34. Goldsworthy TL, Popp JA. Chlorinated hydrocarbon-induced peroxisomal enzyme activity in relation to species and organ carcinogenicity. *Toxicology and applied pharmacology*, 1987, 88:225-233.

35. Mather GG, Exon JH, Koller LD. Subchronic 90-day toxicity of dichloroacetic and trichloroacetic acid in rats. *Toxicology*, 1990, 64:71-80.

36. Sanchez IM, Bull RJ. Early induction of reparative hyperplasia in the liver of B6C3F1 mice treated with dichloroacetate and trichloroacetate. *Toxicology*, 1990, 64:33-46.

37. Rapson WH, Nazar MA, Butsky VV. Mutagenicity produced by aqueous chlorination of organic compounds. *Bulletin of environmental contamination and toxicology*, 1980, 24:590-596.

38. Bhunya SP, Behera BC. Relative genotoxicity of trichloroacetic acid (TCA) as revealed by different cytogenetic assays: bone marrow chromosome aberration, micronucleus and sperm-head abnormality in the mouse. *Mutation research*, 1987, 188:215-221.

39. Parnell MJ et al. Trichloroacetic acid effects on rat liver peroxisomes and enzyme-altered foci. *Environmental health perspectives*, 1986, 69:73-79.

40. Stacpoole PW, Moore GW, Kornauser DM. Metabolic effects of dichloroacetate in patients with diabetes mellitus and hyperlipoproteinemia. *New England journal of medicine*, 1978, 298:526-530.

41. Moore GW et al. Reduction of serum cholesterol in two patients with homozygous familial hypercholesterolemia by dichloroacetate. *Atherosclerosis*, 1979, 33:285-293.

42. Stacpoole PW, Moore GW, Kornauser DM. Toxicity of chronic dichloroacetate. *New England journal of medicine*, 1979, 300:372 (letter).

## 16.12 Chloral hydrate (trichloroacetaldehyde)

### 16.12.1 General description

#### Identity

| Compound | CAS no. | Molecular formula |
|---|---|---|
| Trichloroacetaldehyde | 75-87-6 | $Cl_3CCHO$ |
| Chloral hydrate | 302-17-0 | $Cl_3CCH(OH)_2$ |

The IUPAC name for trichloroacetaldehyde is trichloroethanal.

#### Physicochemical properties (1–3)

| Property | Trichloroacetaldehyde [1] | Chloral hydrate [2] |
|---|---|---|
| Boiling point (°C) | 97.8 | 96.3 |
| Melting point (°C) | -57.5 | 57 |
| Density at 20 °C (g/cm³) | 1.512 | 1.908 |
| Water solubility (g/litre) | Freely soluble | 8300 at 25 °C |

#### Major uses

Hydrated trichloroacetaldehyde (chloral hydrate) is used as a sedative and hypnotic in human and veterinary medicine (3, 4).

### 16.12.2 Analytical methods

Trichloroacetaldehyde and chloral hydrate are determined by draft EPA Method 551, i.e. by capillary-column/electron-capture/gas chromatography. Monitoring data indicate that a quantification limit of 0.4 µg/litre is achievable for chloral hydrate.

### 16.12.3 Environmental levels and human exposure

#### Water

Trichloroacetaldehyde may enter water from industrial discharges or be formed as a by-product during the chlorination of water containing organic precursor molecules. Chloral hydrate is formed when trichloroacetaldehyde is dissolved in water; it was detected in six of 10 drinking-water supplies sampled, at concentrations ranging from 0.01 to 5 µg/litre (5). In another survey, chloral hydrate was detected in each of 10 drinking-water systems at concentrations ranging from 10 to 100 µg/litre (6).

---

[1] Conversion factor in air: 1 ppm = 6.03 mg/m³.
[2] Conversion factor in air: 1 ppm = 6.77 mg/m³.

885

## 16.12.4 Kinetics and metabolism in laboratory animals and humans

Chloral hydrate was rapidly absorbed in dogs and humans, most, if not all, being either oxidized to trichloroacetic acid or reduced to trichloroethanol. Most of the dose was excreted in the urine as trichloroethanol glucuronide, together with small amounts of free trichloroethanol. The remainder was excreted as trichloro-acetate (7, 8).

## 16.12.5 Effects on laboratory animals and *in vitro* test systems

### Acute exposure

The acute oral $LD_{50}$ for chloral hydrate in mice was 1265–1442 mg/kg of body weight (9). Rats are more sensitive than mice, acute oral $LD_{50}$s ranging from 285 mg/kg of body weight in newborn pups to 479 mg/kg of body weight in adults (10).

### Short-term exposure

Groups of male CD-1 mice were dosed with chloral hydrate by gavage at 14.4 or 144 mg/kg of body weight per day for 14 days. No significant effect on body weight was observed, but a dose-dependent increase in liver weight and decrease in spleen weight were observed. These changes were statistically significant at the higher dose. No effects on haematological or serum biochemical parameters were noted, except for an unusual decrease in lactate dehydrogenase at the higher dose. A NOAEL of 14.4 mg/kg of body weight per day was identified in this study (9).

Male and female CD-1 mice were supplied with chloral hydrate in drinking-water at 70 or 700 mg/litre (time-weighted average doses of approximately 16 or 160 mg/kg of body weight per day) for 90 days. The liver appeared to be the tissue most seriously affected. In males, dose-related hepatomegaly and microsomal proliferation were seen, accompanied by small changes in serum chemistry values for potassium, cholesterol, and glutathione, but no significant changes in serum enzyme levels. Females did not show hepatomegaly but did display changed hepatic microsomal parameters. No other significant toxicological changes were observed in either sex. Based on hepatomegaly, a LOAEL of 16 mg/kg of body weight per day (the lowest dose tested) was identified for chloral hydrate in this study (9).

### Long-term exposure

A chronic 2-year drinking-water study of chloral hydrate was conducted on groups of 40 male $B6C3F_1$ mice at dose levels of 0 and 1 g/litre (0 and 166 mg/kg of body weight per day). Lesions were primarily confined to the liver and included hepatocellular necrosis, inflammation, and cytomegaly. Organ weight changes were also evident, with increases in absolute and relative liver weights throughout the treatment period. Spleen, kidney, and testicular weights as well as pathological changes in these organs were comparable to those in controls (*11*).

## Reproductive toxicity, embryotoxicity, and teratogenicity

Female mice were exposed to chloral hydrate in drinking-water at concentrations corresponding to doses of 21.3 or 204.8 mg/kg of body weight per day from before breeding until weaning. No gross malformations were noted, and no significant effects were observed in gestational duration, number of pups delivered, pup weight, or number of stillborn pups. All pups showed the same rate of development and degree of performance on several neurobehavioural tests, except that pups from the high-dose group showed impaired retention in a passive avoidance learning task. A NOAEL of 21.3 mg/kg of body weight per day for developmental effects was identified in this study (*12*).

## Mutagenicity and related end-points

Chloral hydrate was reported to be mutagenic in *Salmonella typhimurium* strain TA98. Both chloral hydrate and trichloroacetaldehyde were reported to be mutagenic in *S. typhimurium* strain TA100, with and without metabolic activation. Mutagenic activity was also observed for chloral hydrate in *Streptomyces coelicolor* and *Aspergillus nidulans*. Neither chloral hydrate nor trichloroacetaldehyde was mutagenic in *S. typhimurium* strain TA1535 (*13, 14*).

Chloral hydrate administered to mice caused significant increases in the number of hyperhaploid cells, probably due to chromosome nondisjunction resulting from a disruptive effect of chloral hydrate on the mitotic spindle (*15*). Similar disruptive effects of chloral hydrate on chromosomal segregation have been observed in *A. nidulans* (*16*) and *Saccharomyces cerevisiae* (*17*). Chloral hydrate did not bind to DNA in mouse liver *in vivo* or form DNA–protein cross-links when incubated with rat liver nuclei *in vitro*, which suggests that it may have low genotoxic potential in animals (*18*).

## Carcinogenicity

The carcinogenic potential of chloral hydrate was investigated in male B6C3F$_1$ mice (40 per dose) that received the compound in their drinking-water at dose levels of 0 or 1 g/litre (0 or 166 mg/kg of body weight per day) for up to 104 weeks. The most prevalent lesions observed were hepatocellular carcinomas (46%) and hepatocellular adenomas (29%). Proliferative lesions were also observed in the untreated controls but at a lower incidence (2% and 1%, respectively). Hyperplastic nodules (4%) were observed in the treated group but not in untreated controls (*11*).

A single oral dose of chloral hydrate (10 mg/kg of body weight) administered to 15-day-old male mice resulted in a significant increase in liver tumours after 48–92 weeks (*19*).

## 16.12.6 Effects on humans

Chloral hydrate has been widely used as a sedative or hypnotic drug in humans at recommended oral doses of 0.25–1.0 g. Concentrated solutions are irritating to the gastrointestinal tract, and the ingestion of undiluted preparations causes nausea and vomiting. The acute oral toxic dose in humans is usually about 10 g, which causes severe respiratory depression and hypotension (*20*).

Adverse effects in patients given either 0.5 or 1.0 g of chloral hydrate included central nervous system depression, minor sensitivity reactions, gastrointestinal disturbances, and central nervous system excitement (*21*). Cardiac arrhythmias induced by chloral hydrate have been described (*22*).

The chronic use of chloral hydrate may result in the development of tolerance and physical dependence. Those physically dependent on it reportedly take as much as 12 g per day (*23*).

## 16.12.7 Provisional guideline value

Chloral hydrate causes liver tumours in mice. It has been shown to be mutagenic in short-term tests *in vitro*, but it does not bind to DNA. It has been shown to disrupt chromosome segregation in cell division. Because of the lack of adequate long-term studies, the guideline value for chloral hydrate is based on the LOAEL from a study in which liver effects were seen in mice that received chloral hydrate in drinking-water at 16 mg/kg of body weight per day for 90 days (*9*). A TDI of 1.6 µg/kg of body weight was calculated using this LOAEL and incorporating an uncertainty factor of 10 000 (100 for intra- and interspecies variation, 10 for the short duration of the study, and 10 for the use of a LOAEL instead of a NOAEL). With an allocation of 20% of the TDI to drinking-water, the provisional guideline value is 10 µg/litre (rounded figure). This guideline value is designated as provisional because of the limitations of the available database.

## References

1. Weast RC. *Handbook of chemistry and physics.* Cleveland, OH, CRC Press, 1988.

2. Verschueren K. *Handbook of environmental data on organic chemicals.* New York, NY, Van Nostrand Reinhold, 1977.

3. Budavari S, O'Neill M, Smith A, eds. *The Merck index. An encyclopedia of chemicals, drugs, and biologicals,* 11th ed. Rahway, NJ, Merck, 1989.

4. Hawley GG. *The condensed chemical dictionary*, 10th ed. New York, NY, Van Nostrand Reinhold, 1981:241.

5. Keith LH et al. Identification of organic compounds in drinking water from thirteen U.S. cities. In: Keith LH, ed. *Identification and analysis of organic pollutants in water*. Ann Arbor, MI, Ann Arbor Science Publishers, 1976:329-373.

6. Stevens AA et al. By-products of chlorination at ten operating utilities. In: Jolley RJ et al, eds. *Water chlorination: chemistry, environmental impact and health effects*. Vol. 6. Ann Arbor, MI, Ann Arbor Scientific Publishers, 1990:579-604.

7. Marshall EK, Owens AH. Absorption, excretion and metabolic fate of chloral hydrate and trichloroethanol. *Bulletin of the Johns Hopkins Hospital*, 1954, 95:1-18.

8. Butler TC. The metabolic fate of chloral hydrate. *Journal of pharmacology and experimental therapeutics*, 1948, 92:49-58.

9. Sanders VM et al. Toxicology of chloral hydrate in the mouse. *Environmental health perspectives*, 1982, 44:137-146.

10. Goldenthal EI. A compilation of $LD_{50}$ values in newborn and adult animals. *Toxicology and applied pharmacology*, 1971, 18:185-207.

11. Daniel FB et al. Hepatocarcinogenicity of chloral hydrate, 2-chloroacetaldehyde, and dichloroacetic acid in the male $B6C3F_1$ mouse. *Fundamental and applied toxicology*, 1992, 19(2):159-168.

12. Kallman MJ, Kaempf GL, Balster RL. Behavioral toxicity of chloral in mice: an approach to evaluation. *Neurobehavioral toxicology and teratology*, 1984, 6(2):137-146.

13. Bruce WR, Heddle JA. The mutagenic activity of 61 agents as determined by the micronucleus, *Salmonella*, and sperm abnormality assays. *Canadian journal of genetics and cytology*, 1979, 21:319-334.

14. Bignami M et al. Mutagenicity of halogenated aliphatic hydrocarbons in *Salmonella typhimurium, Streptomyces coelicolor* and *Aspergillus nidulans*. *Chemico-biological interactions*, 1980, 30:9-23.

15. Russo A, Pacchierotti F, Metalli P. Nondisjunction induced in mouse spermatogenesis by chloral hydrate, a metabolite of trichloroethylene. *Environmental mutagenesis*, 1984, 6(5):695-703.

16. Kafer E. Tests which distinguish induced crossing-over and aneuploidy from secondary segregation in *Aspergillus* treated with chloral hydrate or gamma rays. *Mutation research*, 1986, 164:145-166.

17. Sora S, Carbone ML. Chloral hydrate, methylmercury hydroxide and ethidium bromide affect chromosomal segregation during meiosis of *Saccharomyces cerevisiae*. *Mutation research*, 1987, 190:13-17.

18. Keller DA, Heck HD. Mechanistic studies on chloral toxicity: relationship to trichloroethylene carcinogenesis. *Toxicology letters*, 1988, 42:183-191.

19. Rijhsinghani KS et al. Induction of neoplastic lesions in the livers of $C_{57}BL$ x $C3HF_1$ mice by chloral hydrate. *Cancer detection and prevention*, 1986, 9:279-288.

20. Gilman AG et al., eds. Goodman and Gilman: *the pharmacological basis of therapeutics*, 7th ed. New York, NY, Macmillan Publishing, 1985:360-362.

21. Miller RR, Greenblatt DJ. Clinical effects of chloral hydrate in hospitalized medical patients. *Journal of clinical pharmacology*, 1979, 19:669-674.

22. Marshall AJ. Cardiac arrhythmias caused by chloral hydrate. *British medical journal*, 1977, 2:994.

23. Goodman LS, Gilman A. *The pharmacological basis of therapeutics*, 4th ed. New York, NY, Macmillan, 1970:123-125.

## 16.13 Chloroacetones

### 16.13.1 General description

**Identity**

| Compound | CAS no. | Molecular formula |
|----------|---------|-------------------|
| 1,1-Dichloroacetone | 513-88-2 | $Cl_2CHCOCH_3$ |
| 1,3-Dichloroacetone | 534-07-6 | $ClCH_2COCH_2Cl$ |

The IUPAC name for chloroacetone is chloropropanone.

**Physicochemical properties** (1–3)

| Property | 1,1-Dichloroacetone [1] | 1,3-Dichloroacetone [2] |
|----------|----------------------|----------------------|
| Boiling point (°C) | 120 | 173 |
| Melting point (°C) | - | 45 |
| Density at 20 °C (g/cm³) | 1.3 | 1.4 |
| Water solubility at 20 °C | Slightly soluble | Soluble |

---

[1] Conversion factor in air: 1 pmm = 5.19 mg/m³.
[2] Conversion factor in air: 1 pmm = 5.19 mg/m³.

### Major uses

Chlorinated acetones have been proposed for use in tear gas because they are lachrymators. Chloroacetone is used as a reagent in the synthesis of drugs, perfumes, insecticides, and vinyl compounds (3).

## 16.13.2 Analytical methods

Chloroacetones in water are usually determined by liquid–liquid extraction and gas chromatography with electron-capture detection. A detection limit of 13 ng/litre for 1,1,1-trichloroacetone has been achieved (4).

## 16.13.3 Environmental levels and human exposure

### Water

Dichloroacetones may be formed in water by the oxidation reaction between chlorine and large organic molecules. Concentrations in finished drinking-water are estimated at less than 10 µg/litre (5). Quarterly mean concentrations of 1,1-dichloroacetone ranged from 0.46 to 0.55 µg/litre in grab samples from 35 drinking-water treatment plants in the USA (6).

## 16.13.4 Effects on laboratory animals and *in vitro* test systems

### Acute exposure

Oral $LD_{50}$s of 250 mg/kg of body weight for 1,1-dichloroacetone and 25 mg/kg of body weight for 1,3-dichloroacetone have been reported in the mouse (7).

### Short-term exposure

The hepatotoxicity of 1,1- and 1,3-dichloroacetone was investigated in mice. Single oral doses of each compound were administered to CD-1 mice (5–12 per dose). A dose of 0.25 ml/kg of body weight (325 mg/kg of body weight) of 1,1-dichloroacetone caused significant increases in liver enzymes in serum, and histological examination showed evidence of periportal necrosis. These effects were not observed at doses of 130 mg/kg of body weight or lower. Liver glutathione levels were decreased at doses of 0.1 and 0.25 ml/kg of body weight but not at 0.05 ml/kg of body weight (65 mg/kg of body weight). Based on measurements of serum enzymes, liver glutathione, and histopathological examination, 1,3-dichloroacetone did not cause liver toxicity at doses of up to 20 mg/kg of body weight. NOAELs of 65 and 20 mg/kg of body weight for 1,1-dichloroacetone and 1,3-dichloroacetone, respectively, were identified in this study (7).

### Mutagenicity and related end-points

A number of chlorinated acetones, including 1,1-, 1,3-, 1,1,1-, 1,1,3,3-, and pentachloroacetone, were direct-acting mutagens in one or both of *Salmonella typhimurium* strains TA98 and TA100. Mutagenic activity decreased with increased chlorine substitutions at the C-1 and C-3 positions, although 1,1,1-trichloroacetone was 25 times as potent as 1,1-dichloroacetone (8).

### Carcinogenicity

The carcinogenic activity of 1,1-dichloroacetone and 1,1,1-trichloroacetone was studied in female SENCAR mice (60 per dose) that received a single oral (200 mg/kg) or topical (400 mg/kg) dose of 1,1-dichloroacetone or a single oral (50 mg/kg) or topical (400 mg/kg) dose of 1,1,1-trichloroacetone. The vehicle was 0.2 ml of dimethyl sulfoxide for oral exposure and 0.2 ml of ethanol for topical exposure. Two weeks after dosing, a tumour promotion schedule was begun with 1 µg of 12-*O*-tetradecanoyl-phorbol-13-acetate (TPA) three times per week for 20 weeks. However, 24 weeks after the start of the promotion schedule, there was no evidence of an increase in skin tumours attributable to either chemical (9).

The results of carcinogenicity studies with chlorinated acetones using the mouse skin assay have also been reported. Groups of 40 SENCAR mice received topical doses of 1,1-dichloroacetone at 400, 600, or 800 mg/kg; 1,3-dichloroacetone at 50, 75, or 100 mg/kg; or 1,1,3-trichloroacetone or 1,1,1-trichloroacetone at 50 mg/kg. Doses were applied six times over a 2-week period using 0.2 ml of ethanol as the vehicle. After 2 weeks, 1.0 µg of TPA in 0.2 ml of acetone was applied three times per week for 20 weeks. After 24 weeks, the percentages of animals with tumours in the respective dose groups were: 5% in controls; 0, 5%, and 5% for 1,1-dichloroacetone; 48%, 45%, and 30% for 1,3-dichloroacetone; 10%, 5%, and 0% for 1,1,1-trichloroacetone; and 10% for 1,1,3-trichloroacetone. The authors concluded that 1,3-dichloroacetone is a tumour initiator in mouse skin (10).

## 16.13.5 Conclusions

The toxicological data on the chloroacetones are very limited, although studies with single doses of 1,1-dichloroacetone indicate that it affects the liver. There are insufficient data at present to permit the proposal of guideline values for any of the chloroacetones.

## References

1.  Weast RC. *Handbook of chemistry and physics.* Cleveland, OH, CRC Press, 1988.

2.  Verschueren K. *Handbook of environmental data on organic chemicals.* New York, NY, Van Nostrand Reinhold, 1977.

3.   Budavari S, O'Neill M, Smith A, eds. *The Merck index. An encyclopedia of chemicals, drugs, and biologicals*, 11th ed. Rahway, NJ, Merck, 1989.

4.   Krasner SW et al. The occurrence of disinfection by-products in U.S. drinking water. *Journal of the American Water Works Association*, 1989, 81(8):41-53.

5.   Coleman WE et al. Identification of organic compounds in a mutagenic extract of a surface drinking water by a computerized gas chromatography/mass spectrometry system (GC/MS/COM). *Environmental science and technology*, 1980, 14:576-588.

6.   Bull RJ, Kopfler FC. Formation and occurrence of disinfectant by-products. In: *Health effects of disinfectants and disinfection by-products*. Denver, CO, American Water Works Association Research Foundation, 1991:55-103.

7.   Laurie RD et al. Studies of the toxic interactions of disinfection by-products. *Environmental health perspectives*, 1986, 69:203-207.

8.   Meier JR et al. Evaluation of chemicals used for drinking water disinfection for production of chromosomal damage and sperm-head abnormalities in mice. *Environmental mutagenesis*, 1985, 7:201-211.

9.   Bull RJ, Robinson M. Carcinogenic activity of haloacetonitrile and haloacetone derivatives in the mouse skin and lung. In: Jolley RL et al., eds. *Water chlorination: chemistry, environmental impact and health effects*, Vol. 5. Chelsea, MI, Lewis Publishers, 1985:221-227.

10.  Robinson J, Laurie RD, Bull RJ. Carcinogenic activity associated with halogenated acetones and acroleins in the mouse skin assay. *Cancer letter*, 1989, 48:197-203.

## 16.14 Halogenated acetonitriles

### 16.14.1 General description

#### *Identity*

| Compound | CAS no. | Molecular formula |
|----------|---------|-------------------|
| Dichloroacetonitrile | 3018-12-0 | $CHCl_2CN$ |
| Dibromoacetonitrile | 3252-43-5 | $CHBr_2CN$ |
| Bromochloroacetonitrile | 83463-62-1 | $CHBrClCN$ |
| Trichloroacetonitrile | 545-06-2 | $CCl_3CN$ |

The IUPAC name for acetonitrile is ethanenitrile.

### Physicochemical properties *(1–3)*

| Property | Dichloro-acetonitrile[1] | Dibromo-acetonitrile[2] | Bromochloro-acetonitrile[3] | Trichloro-acetonitrile [4] |
|---|---|---|---|---|
| Boiling point (°C) | 112.3 | 67–69 | 125–130 | 84.6 |
| Density at 20 °C (g/cm$^3$) | 1.37 | 2.30 | 1.68 | 1.44 |

### Major uses

Trichloroacetonitrile has been used as an insecticide *(3)*.

### Environmental fate

Halogenated acetonitriles are reported to undergo hydrolysis in water, yielding nonvolatile products *(4)*.

## 16.14.2 Analytical methods

Draft EPA Method 551 can be used for the determination of haloacetonitriles, by capillary-column/electron-capture/gas chromatography. Extremely low detection limits are achievable. Monitoring data indicate quantification limits of 0.4 µg/litre for dichloro-, dibromo-, bromochloro-, and trichloroacetonitrile.

## 16.14.3 Environmental levels and human exposure

### Water

Halogenated acetonitriles are formed from organic precursors during the chlorination of drinking-water. Dihalogenated acetonitriles are present in chlorinated water at concentrations ranging from 0.3 to 40 µg/litre *(5, 6)*; trichloroacetonitrile has been detected at a concentration of 0.1 µg/litre *(6)*.

## 16.14.4 Kinetics and metabolism in laboratory animals and humans

Dichloroacetonitrile is well absorbed from the gastrointestinal tract. Most is excreted in urine, smaller amounts being eliminated in expired air and faeces. Its metabolites are detected in highest concentrations in liver, blood, muscle, and skin. Differences in the pattern of label distribution in tissues and of label excre-

---

[1] Conversion factor in air: 1 ppm = 4.49 mg/m$^3$.
[2] Conversion factor in air: 1 ppm = 8.14 mg/m$^3$.
[3] Conversion factor in air: 1 ppm = 6.31 mg/m$^3$.
[4] Conversion factor in air: 1 ppm = 5.91 mg/m$^3$.

tion indicate that a substantial portion of dichloroacetonitrile is split into two one-carbon fragments that undergo different metabolic reactions (7).

Halogenated acetonitriles may be formed *in vivo* following the ingestion of chlorinated water. Dichloro- and dibromoacetonitrile were detected in the stomach contents of rats following the oral administration of sodium hypochlorite/potassium bromide, presumably formed by reaction with organic material in the stomach (8).

## 16.14.5 Effects on laboratory animals and *in vitro* test systems

### *Acute exposure*

Acute oral $LD_{50}$s for the halogenated acetonitriles in rodents range from 245 to 361 mg/kg of body weight (9–11).

### *Short-term exposure*

*Dichloroacetonitrile*
In a 14-day toxicity study, doses of 0, 12, 23, 45, or 90 mg/kg of body weight per day were administered to rats (10 per sex per dose). In males, a slight, nonsignificant depression in body weight gain was observed at the three highest doses, whereas decreased weight gain was noted only at the highest dose in females. No consistent treatment-related effects were observed in any of the haematological, serum chemistry, or urinary parameters measured. Absolute thymus weights in males given 23, 45, or 90 mg/kg of body weight per day were significantly decreased, but the thymus-to-body-weight ratio was decreased only at the highest dose. Based on decreased body weight as the most sensitive end-point, the NOAEL in this study was 45 mg/kg of body weight per day (11).

In a 90-day study, doses of 0, 8, 33, or 65 mg/kg of body weight per day were administered to groups of rats (20 per sex per dose). No consistent compound-related effects were observed in any of the haematological, urinary, or serum chemistry parameters measured. Body weight gain was significantly depressed in females at 65 mg/kg of body weight per day and in males at 33 mg/kg of body weight per day. The NOAEL in this study was 8 mg/kg of body weight per day (11).

*Dibromoacetonitrile*
The 14-day toxicity of dibromoacetonitrile was investigated in adult rats (10 per sex per dose) that received this compound by gavage at doses of 0, 23, 45, 90, or 180 mg/kg of body weight per day. There was increased mortality at 90 and 180 mg/kg of body weight per day (30% and 100%, respectively). No consistent compound-related effects were apparent in any of the serum chemistry, haematological, or urinary parameters measured. The authors concluded that decreased body weight was the most sensitive indicator of toxicity. In males, dose-dependent decreases occurred at 45 and 90 mg/kg of body weight per day. No effect on body

weight was noted in females. The authors concluded that the NOAEL was 45 mg/kg of body weight per day, but the body weight decrease in male rats exposed at this dose suggests that it should be 23 mg/kg of body weight per day (*11*).

In a 90-day study, dibromoacetonitrile doses of 0, 6, 23, or 45 mg/kg of body weight per day in corn oil were administered by gavage to rats (20 per sex per dose). Body weight gain was significantly depressed only in males at the highest dose tested. No compound-related deaths occurred, no consistent compound-related adverse effects were observed in the haematological, urinary, or serum chemistry parameters measured, and no remarkable findings were apparent at gross necropsy. The authors concluded that decreased body weight is the most sensitive end-point and identified a NOAEL of 23 mg/kg of body weight per day (*11*).

## Reproductive toxicity, embryotoxicity, and teratogenicity

*Dichloroacetonitrile*

Dichloroacetonitrile was administered to pregnant Long-Evans rats by gavage at doses of 0, 5, 15, 25, or 45 mg/kg of body weight per day on gestation days 6–18. At the two highest dose levels, fetal resorptions were significantly increased and fetal weight and size were decreased. Malformations of the cardiovascular, digestive, and urogenital systems were observed in fetuses from dams at the two highest dose levels. No effects were described at lower doses. This study indicated that 15 mg/kg of body weight per day is a developmental and teratogenic NOAEL for dichloroacetonitrile (*12*).

Pregnant Long-Evans rats were exposed via gavage to dichloroacetonitrile at 55 mg/kg of body weight per day on days 7–21 of gestation. Dichloroacetonitrile decreased the percentage of females delivering litters and increased the percentage of fetal resorptions. Mean birth weights were reduced, and postnatal survival was significantly reduced. A LOAEL of 55 mg/kg of body weight per day was identified in this study (*13, 14*).

Groups of 10 male B6C3F$_1$ mice were dosed with dichloroacetonitrile at 0, 12.5, 25, or 50 mg/kg of body weight by gavage for 5 consecutive days. No treatment-related effects were found on examination of sperm for abnormal sperm-head morphology (*9*).

*Dibromoacetonitrile*

Pregnant Long-Evans rats were exposed via gavage to dibromoacetonitrile at 50 mg/kg of body weight per day on gestation days 7–21. Maternal weight gain decreased during gestation, and mean birth weights were reduced. A LOAEL of 50 mg/kg of body weight per day was identified in this study (*13, 14*).

Groups of 10 male B6C3F$_1$ mice were dosed with dibromoacetonitrile at 0, 12.5, 25, or 50 mg/kg of body weight by gavage for 5 days. There were no treatment-related effects on sperm-head morphology (*9*).

*Bromochloroacetonitrile*

In a study in which pregnant Long-Evans rats were exposed via gavage to bromochloroacetonitrile at 55 mg/kg of body weight per day on days 7–21 of gestation, mean birth weights were reduced (*13, 14*). There were no treatment-related effects on sperm-head morphology when groups of 10 male B6C3F$_1$ mice were dosed with bromochloroacetonitrile at 0, 12.5, 25, or 50 mg/kg of body weight by gavage for 5 days (*9*).

*Trichloroacetonitrile*

Trichloroacetonitrile was administered to pregnant Long-Evans rats by gavage at doses of 0, 1, 7.5, 15, 35, or 55 mg/kg of body weight per day on gestation days 6–18. The highest dose was lethal in four of 19 dams, and there was 100% resorption in most survivors. Dose-related decreases in fetal weight and fetal viability were observed in animals exposed at all but the lowest dose. Numerous cardiovascular and urogenital malformations were seen in surviving fetuses. The frequency of soft-tissue malformations was dose-dependent, ranging from 18% at 7.5 mg/kg of body weight per day to 35% at 35 mg/kg of body weight per day. The malformation frequency at 1 mg/kg of body weight per day (8.4%) was not significantly different from that in controls (3.8%), but the authors expressed concern that this level of malformation could be of biological significance and suggested that a dose of 1 mg/kg of body weight per day might be the NOAEL or close to the LOAEL for teratogenic effects (*15*).

Pregnant Long-Evans rats were exposed via gavage to trichloroacetonitrile at 55 mg/kg of body weight per day on gestation days 7–21. Trichloroacetonitrile decreased the percentage of females delivering litters and increased the percentage of fetal resorptions, while mean birth weights were reduced, and postnatal survival was significantly reduced. A LOAEL of 55 mg/kg of body weight per day was identified in this study (*13, 14*).

Groups of 10 male B6C3F$_1$ mice were dosed with trichloroacetonitrile at 0, 12.5, 25, or 50 mg/kg of body weight by gavage for 5 days. Examination of sperm for abnormal sperm-head morphology revealed no treatment-related effects (*9*).

*Mutagenicity and related end-points*

No significant increase in the frequency of micronuclei was observed for any of the four halogenated acetonitriles in an *in vivo* assay in mice. All the halogenated acetonitriles induced sister chromatid exchanges in Chinese hamster ovary cells with metabolic activation and all except dichloroacetonitrile without it. Comparisons of potencies showed the order to be as follows: dibromoacetonitrile > bromochloroacetonitrile > trichloroacetonitrile > dichloroacetonitrile (*16*).

Results of the *Salmonella*/microsome assay, with and without metabolic activation by the S9 fraction of rat liver homogenate, suggested that dichloro- and bromochloroacetonitrile were direct-acting mutagens and that dibromo- and trichloroacetonitrile were nonmutagenic (*16*). Halogenated acetonitriles reportedly produced DNA strand breaks in cultured human lymphoblastic cells (*17*). The most potent initiator was trichloroacetonitrile, followed by bromochloro-, dibromo-, and dichloroacetonitrile. It was reported that dichloroacetonitrile formed a covalent adduct when incubated with calf thymus DNA (*18*).

### Carcinogenicity

Groups of 40 A/J female mice were given a single oral dose of dichloro-, dibromo-, bromochloro-, or trichloroacetonitrile of 10 mg/kg (4.3 mg/kg of body weight per day) three times per week for 8 weeks. The incidence of lung tumours (adenomas) was significantly increased in the groups given trichloro- and bromochloroacetonitrile, while dichloro- and dibromoacetonitrile produced marginal and nonsignificant increases in such tumours. The authors stated that the results should be interpreted with caution, as there is a relatively large variation in the background incidence of lung tumours in this strain of mice, and the dose level tested was considerably below the maximum tolerated dose (*19*).

The ability of the four halogenated acetonitriles to act as tumour initiators was studied in mouse skin. Six topical doses of 200, 400, or 800 mg/kg of body weight were applied to the shaved backs of female SENCAR mice (40 per dose) over a 2-week period to give total doses of 1200, 2400, and 4800 mg/kg of body weight. Two weeks after the last dose, a tumour promotion schedule involving the application of 1 µg of 12-*O*-tetradecanoyl-phorbol-13-acetate (TPA) three times per week was begun and continued for 20 weeks. After 1 year, the incidence of squamous cell carcinomas was significantly increased relative to the control group in mice treated with dibromo- and bromochloroacetonitrile. An increase in incidence with trichloroacetonitrile at 2400 mg/kg was not reproducible. No significant increases in carcinomas were observed with dichloroacetonitrile (*16*). Dichloro-, dibromo-, and trichloroacetonitrile were inactive as initiators in the rat liver γ-glutamyl transpeptidase foci assay (*20*).

## 16.14.6 Guideline values

IARC has concluded that dichloro-, dibromo-, bromochloro-, and trichloroacetonitriles are not classifiable as to their carcinogenicity to humans (Group 3) (*5*).

### Dichloroacetonitrile

A TDI of 15 µg/kg of body weight was calculated from the NOAEL of 15 mg/kg of body weight per day for fetal resorptions, decreases in fetal weight and size, and malformations of the cardiovascular, digestive, and urogenital systems in the offspring of rats exposed to this compound on gestation days 6–18 (*12*), incorporating an uncertainty factor of 1000 (100 for intra- and interspecies variation and 10 for the severity of the effects at doses above the NOAEL). This NOAEL is consistent with that observed for effects on body weight in a 90-day study in rats. The provisional guideline value is 90 µg/litre, allocating 20% of the TDI to drinking-water. This guideline value is designated as provisional because of the limitations of the database (i.e. lack of long-term toxicity and carcinogenicity bioassays).

### Dibromoacetonitrile

A TDI of 23 µg/kg of body weight was calculated based on a NOAEL of 23 mg/kg of body weight per day for effects on body weight in a 90-day study in rats (*11*), incorporating an uncertainty factor of 1000 (100 for intra- and interspecies variation and 10 for the short duration of the study). The provisional guideline value is 100 µg/litre (rounded figure), allocating 20% of the TDI to drinking-water. This guideline value is designated as provisional because of the limitations of the database (i.e. lack of long-term toxicity and carcinogenicity bioassays).

### Bromochloroacetonitrile

Available data are insufficient to serve as a basis for derivation of a guideline value for bromochloroacetonitrile.

### Trichloroacetonitrile

A TDI of 0.2 µg/kg of body weight was calculated from a NOAEL of 1 mg/kg of body weight per day for fetal resorption, decreased fetal weight and viability, and for numerous cardiovascular and urogenital malformations in a study in which rats were dosed on gestation days 6–18 (*15*), incorporating an uncertainty factor of 5000 (100 for intra- and interspecies variation, 10 for the severity of effects at doses above the NOAEL, and 5 for limitations of the database, i.e. lack of a 90-day study). The provisional guideline value is 1 µg/litre (rounded figure), assuming the allocation of 20% of the TDI to drinking-water. The guideline value is designated as provisional because of the limitations of the database (i.e. lack of long-term studies).

## References

1.  Weast RC. *Handbook of chemistry and physics.* Cleveland, OH, CRC Press, 1988.

2.  Verschueren K. *Handbook of environmental data on organic chemicals.* New York, NY, Van Nostrand Reinhold, 1977.

3.  Budavari S, O'Neill M, Smith A, eds. *The Merck index. An encyclopedia of chemicals, drugs, and biologicals,* 11th ed. Rahway, NJ, Merck, 1989.

4. Bieber TI, Trehy ML. Dihaloacetonitriles in chlorinated natural waters. In: Jolley RL et al., eds. *Water chlorination: environmental impact and health effects*, Vol. 4, Book 1. *Chemistry and water treatment*. Ann Arbor, MI, Ann Arbor Science Publishers, 1983:85-96.

5. International Agency for Research on Cancer. *Chlorinated drinking-water; chlorination by-products; some other halogenated compounds; cobalt and cobalt compounds*. Lyon, 1991:45-359 (IARC Monographs on the Evaluation of Carcinogenic Risks to Humans, Volume 52).

6. Bruchet A et al. Characterization of total halogenated compounds during various water treatment processes. In: Jolley RL et al., eds. *Water chlorination: chemistry, environmental impact and health effects*. Vol. 5. Chelsea, MI, Lewis Publishers, 1985:1165-1184.

7. Roby MR et al. Excretion and tissue disposition of dichloroacetonitrile in rats and mice. *Environmental health perspectives*, 1986, 69:215-220.

8. Mink FL et al. *In vivo* formation of halogenated reaction products following peroral sodium hypochlorite. *Bulletin of environmental contamination and toxicology*, 1983, 30:394-399.

9. Meier JR et al. Evaluation of chemicals used for drinking water disinfection for production of chromosomal damage and sperm-head abnormalities in mice. *Environmental mutagenesis*, 1985, 7:201-211.

10. Smyth HF et al. Range-finding toxicity data: list VI. *American Industrial Health Association journal*, 1962, 23:95-107.

11. Hayes JR, Condie LW, Borzelleca JF. Toxicology of haloacetonitriles. *Environmental health perspectives*, 1986, 69:183-202.

12. Smith MK et al. Developmental toxicity of dichloroacetonitrile, a by-product of drinking water disinfection. *Fundamental and applied toxicology*, 1989, 12:765-772.

13. Smith MK, Zenik H, George EL. Reproductive toxicology of disinfection by-products. *Environmental health perspectives*, 1986, 69:177-182.

14. Smith MK et al. Developmental toxicity of halogenated acetonitriles: drinking water by-products of chlorine disinfection. *Toxicology*, 1987, 46:83-93.

15. Smith MK et al. Teratogenic effects of trichloroacetonitrile in the Long-Evans rat. *Teratology*, 1988, 38:113-120.

16. Bull RJ et al. Evaluation of mutagenic and carcinogenic properties of brominated and chlorinated acetonitriles: by-products of chlorination. *Fundamental and applied toxicology*, 1985, 5:1065-1074.

17. Lin EL et al. Haloacetonitriles: metabolism, genotoxicity, and tumor-initiating activity. *Environmental health perspectives*, 1986, 69:67-71.

18. Daniel FB et al. Genotoxic properties of haloacetonitriles: drinking water by-products of chlorine disinfection. *Fundamental and applied toxicology*, 1986, 6:447-453.

19. Bull RJ, Robinson M. Carcinogenic activity of haloacetonitrile and haloacetone derivatives in the mouse skin and lung. In: Jolley RL et al., eds. *Water chlorination: chemistry, environmental impact and health effects*, Vol. 5. Chelsea, MI, Lewis Publishers, 1985:221-227.

20. Herren-Freund SL, Pereira MA. Carcinogenicity of by-products of disinfection in mouse and rat liver. *Environmental health perspectives*, 1986,69:59-65.

## 16.15 Cyanogen chloride

### 16.15.1 General description

**Identity**

CAS no.: 506-77-4
Molecular formula: CNCl

**Physicochemical properties** *(1–3)* [1]

Boiling point            12.7 °C
Melting point            -6 °C
Density                  1.186 g/cm$^3$ at 20 °C
Water solubility         Very soluble

**Major uses**

Cyanogen chloride is used in tear gas, in fumigant gases, and as a reagent in the synthesis of other compounds *(4)*.

### 16.15.2 Analytical methods

EPA Method 524.2, in which purge-and-trap gas chromatography is combined with mass spectroscopy, can be used for the determination of cyanogen chloride. This method has a practical quantification limit of 0.3 µg/litre.

---

[1] Conversion factor in air: 1 ppm = 2.5 mg/m$^3$.

## 16.15.3 Environmental levels and human exposure

### Water

Cyanogen chloride may be formed as a by-product of the chloramination or chlorination of water. It has been found in finished water supplies at concentrations below 10 µg/litre. The concentration in water when chlorination was used for disinfection was reported to be 0.4 µg/litre. The level was higher (1.6 µg/litre) in chloraminated water (6).

## 16.14.4 Kinetics and metabolism in laboratory animals and humans

In an *in vitro* study with rat blood, cyanogen chloride was metabolized to cyanide ion by haemoglobin and glutathione (7).

## 16.15.5 Effects on laboratory animals and *in vitro* test systems

### Acute exposure

Estimates of inhalation $LC_{50}$s range from 100 mg/m$^3$ in cats to 7536 mg/m$^3$ in rabbits (8). In other lethality tests, a concentration of 100 mg/m$^3$ was fatal to cats within 18 min, 120 mg/m$^3$ for 6 h was fatal to dogs, 5 mg/m$^3$ for 2 min was fatal to goats, and a subcutaneous dose of 20 mg/kg of body weight was fatal to rabbits (9). An $LD_{50}$ of 6 mg/kg of body weight was reported in rats following oral administration (10). Toxic signs included irritation of the respiratory tract, haemorrhagic exudate of the bronchi and trachea, and pulmonary oedema.

## 16.15.6 Effects on humans

On inhalation, a concentration of 2.5 mg/m$^3$ causes irritation. Cyanogen chloride was used as a war gas in the First World War. A concentration of 120 mg/m$^3$ was lethal (5).

## 16.15.7 Guideline value

Cyanogen chloride is rapidly metabolized to cyanide in the body. There are few data on the oral toxicity of cyanogen chloride, and the proposed guideline is therefore based on cyanide. A guideline value of 70 µg/litre for cyanide as total cyanogenic compounds is recommended (see Cyanide, p. 226).

## References

1. Weast RC. *Handbook of chemistry and physics.* Cleveland, OH, CRC Press, 1988.

2.  Verschueren K. *Handbook of environmental data on organic chemicals.* New York, NY, Van Nostrand Reinhold, 1977.

3.  Budavari S, O'Neill M, Smith A, eds. *The Merck index. An encyclopedia of chemicals, drugs, and biologicals,* 11th ed. Rahway, NJ, Merck, 1989.

4.  Hawley GG. *The condensed chemical dictionary,* 10th ed. New York, NY, Van Nostrand Reinhold, 1981:241.

5.  National Academy of Sciences. *Drinking water and health.* Washington, DC, 1977.

6.  Krasner SW et al. The occurrence of disinfection by-products in U.S. drinking water. *Journal of the American Water Works Association,* 1989, 81(8):41-53.

7.  Aldridge WN. The conversion of cyanogen chloride to cyanide in the presence of blood proteins and sulphydryl compounds. *Biochemical journal,* 1951, 48:271-276 (reviewed in ref. 5).

8.  Tatken RL, Lewis RJ Sr, eds. *Registry of toxic effects of chemical substances,* Vol. 2, 1981-82 ed. Cincinnati, OH, National Institute for Occupational Safety and Health, 1983 (DHHS (NIOSH) Publication No. 83-107).

9.  Flury F, Zernik F. *Schädliche Gase. [Harmful gases.]* Berlin, Springer, 1931 (reviewed in ref. 5).

10. Leitch JL, Bauer VE. *Oral toxicity of cyanogen chloride in water to rats.* Edgewood Arsenal, MD, US Chemical Warfare Service, 1945 (Medical Division Report No. 19) (reviewed in ref. 80).

## 16.16 Chloropicrin

### 16.16.1 General description

#### Identity

CAS no.:                   76-06-2
Molecular formula:         $CCl_3NO_2$

The IUPAC name for chloropicrin is trichloronitromethane.

#### *Physicochemical properties* (1–3)[1]

| Property | Value |
| --- | --- |
| Boiling point | 112 °C |
| Melting point | -64 °C |
| Density | 1.65 g/cm$^3$ at 20 °C |
| Vapour pressure | 2.27 kPa at 20 °C |

[1]  Conversion factor in air: 1 ppm = 6.68 mg/m$^3$.

## Major uses

Chloropicrin is used as a reagent in the synthesis of organic chemicals, in the manufacture of methyl violet, and as a fumigant for stored grain; it has also been used as a chemical warfare agent (*3, 5*).

## Environmental fate

Chloropicrin in water is reduced to chloroform when reducing agents are added to remove excess chlorine (*6*). In the presence of light, it is degraded to carbon dioxide, chloride ion, and nitrate ion (*7*).

## 16.16.2 Analytical methods

Draft EPA Method 551 can be used for the determination of chloropicrin, by capillary-column/electron-capture/gas chromatography. Extremely low detection limits can be achieved.

## 16.16.3 Environmental levels and human exposure

### Water

Chloropicrin is formed in water by the reaction of chlorine with humic acids, amino acids, and nitrophenols. The presence of nitrates increases the amount formed (*6*). Chloropicrin has been detected in drinking-water; however, in the presence of reducing agents, it is converted into chloroform (*6*). In one study, the mean chloropicrin concentration was 0.6 µg/litre; the highest concentration observed was 5.6 µg/litre in 36 water supplies expected to have high concentrations of chlorination by-products (*8*).

## 16.16.4 Effects on laboratory animals and *in vitro* test systems

### Acute exposure

An oral $LD_{50}$ of 250 mg/kg of body weight was reported in rats (*9*). An $LC_{50}$ of 66 mg/m$^3$ in mice was reported following a 4-h exposure to chloropicrin aerosol (*10*).

### Short-term exposure

In a 6-week range-finding test, Osborne-Mendel rats (5 per sex per group) were given chloropicrin by gavage at doses of 0, 16, 25, 40, 63, or 100 mg/kg of body weight per day, 5 days per week. Groups of B6C3F$_1$ mice were treated in the same manner with doses of 10, 16, 25, 40, or 63 mg/kg of body weight per day. In rats, chloropicrin produced no mortality at 40 mg/kg of body weight per day or less, except for one female at 25 mg/kg of body weight per day. At 40 and 63 mg/kg of body weight per day, mean body weight was depressed by 11% and

38% in males and by 17% and 30% in females, respectively. In mice, there was no mortality at any dose tested. At 40 and 63 mg/kg of body weight per day, mean body weight was depressed by 12% and 20% in males and by 3% and 6% in females, respectively. In both species, a NOAEL of 25 mg/kg of body weight per day was identified (*11*).

### Long-term exposure

The chronic toxicity of chloropicrin was investigated in a 78-week study on Osborne-Mendel rats and B6C3F$_1$ mice. Chloropicrin in corn oil was administered 5 days per week by gavage to animals (50 per sex per dose) at initial doses of 23 or 46 mg/kg of body weight per day for rats and 25 or 50 mg/kg of body weight per day for mice in a complex dosing regimen. Survival was decreased in both rats and mice. For rats, survival to the end of the study was 6% for high-dose males, 8% for low-dose males, 20% for high-dose females, and 22% for low-dose females. In both vehicle and untreated control groups, at least 50% of the animals survived past week 89. The associations between chloropicrin dose and accelerated mortality in mice were also significant when compared with the vehicle controls for both males and females (*11*).

### Mutagenicity and related end-points

The mutagenicity of chloropicrin in five strains of *Salmonella typhimurium* and one strain of *Escherichia coli* was studied. Chloropicrin was either negative or weakly positive in the absence of the S9 fraction of rat liver homogenate, but positive in one strain in its presence (*12*). Chloropicrin significantly increased the number of sister chromatid exchanges in cultured human lymphocytes *in vitro* in the absence of metabolic activation (*13*).

### Carcinogenicity

Osborne-Mendel rats (50 per sex per dose) and B6C3F$_1$ mice (50 per sex per dose) were given chloropicrin by gavage in corn oil 5 days per week for 78 weeks. A complex dosing regimen was employed in which varying doses were administered for varying periods; there were also periods during which no chloropicrin was given. The overall time-weighted average doses for the 78-week period were 25 or 26 mg/kg of body weight per day for male rats, 20 or 22 mg/kg of body weight per day for female rats, 66 mg/kg of body weight per day for male mice, and 33 mg/kg of body weight per day for female mice. Post-dosing observation periods were 32 weeks (rats) or 13 weeks (mice). In rats, the incidence of neoplasms in exposed animals was not higher than that in controls. However, mortality in exposed rats was high, and it is likely that most animals did not survive long enough to be at risk from tumours with long latency periods. A rapid decrease in survival after the first year of the study was also observed among the high-dose mice of both sexes. Although the mice did not exhibit any statistically significant incidence of tumours, two carcinomas and a papilloma of the squamous epithelium of the forestomach were reported, which were rare in historical controls. The authors concluded that the results of tests with rats did not permit an evaluation of carcinogenicity because of the short survival time of dosed animals, and that the results in mice did not demonstrate conclusive statistical evidence for carcinogenicity under the conditions of the study (11).

## 16.16.5 Effects on humans

Inhalation of chloropicrin at 2 mg/m$^3$ caused pulmonary effects following a 1-min exposure (9).

## 16.16.6 Conclusions

Because of the high mortality in the carcinogenesis bioassay and the limited number of end-points examined in the 78-week toxicity study, the available data are considered inadequate to support the establishment of a guideline value for chloropicrin.

## References

1.  Weast RC. *Handbook of chemistry and physics.* Cleveland, OH, CRC Press, 1988.

2.  Verschueren K. *Handbook of environmental data on organic chemicals.* New York, NY, Van Nostrand Reinhold, 1977.

3.  Budavari S, O'Neill M, Smith A, eds. *The Merck index. An encyclopedia of chemicals, drugs, and biologicals,* 11th ed. Rahway, NJ, Merck, 1989.

4.  Hawley GG. *The condensed chemical dictionary,* 10th ed. New York, NY, Van Nostrand Reinhold, 1981:241.

5.  Clayton GD, Clayton FE. *Patty's industrial hygiene and toxicology.* Vol. II, 2nd ed. New York, NY, Interscience, 1963:2082-2083.

6.  Sayato Y, Nakamuro K, Matsui S. [Studies on mechanism of volatile chlorinated organic compound formation. III. Mechanism of formation of chloroform and chloropicrin by chlorination of humic acid.] *Suishitsu odaku kenkyu,* 1982, 5:127-134 (in Japanese).

7.  Castro CE, Belser NO. Photohydrolysis of methyl bromide and chloropicrin. *Journal of agricultural and food chemistry,* 1981, 29:1005-1008.

8.  Bull RJ, Kopfler FC. Formation and occurrence of disinfectant by-products. In: *Health effects of disinfectants and disinfection by-products*. Denver, CO, American Water Works Association Research Foundation, 1991:55-103.

9.  Tatken RL, Lewis RJ Sr, eds. *Registry of toxic effects of chemical substances*, Vol. 2, 1981-82 ed. Cincinnati, OH, National Institute for Occupational Safety and Health, 1983 (DHHS (NIOSH) Publication No. 83-107).

10. Kawai M. [Inhalation toxicity of phosgene and trichloronitromethane (chloropicrin).] *Sangyo igaku*, 1973, 15:406-407 (abstract, in Japanese).

11. National Cancer Institute. *Carcinogenesis bioassay of chloropicrin*. Washington, DC, US Department of Health, Education, and Welfare, 1978 (Technical Report Series No. 65).

12. Moriya M et al. Further mutagenicity studies on pesticides in bacterial reversion assay systems. *Mutation research*, 1983, 116:185-216.

13. Garry VF, Nelson R, Markins M. Detection of genotoxicity of grain fumigants in human lymphocytes. *Environmental mutagenesis*, 1987, 9(Suppl. 8):38-39.

# 17.
# Radiological aspects

## 17.1 Introduction

The guideline levels for radioactivity in drinking-water recommended in the first edition of *Guidelines for drinking-water quality* in 1984 were based on the data available at that time on the risks of exposure to radiation sources. Since then, additional information has become available on the health consequences of exposure to radiation, risk estimates have been reviewed, and the recommendations of the International Commission on Radiological Protection (ICRP) have been revised. This new information (*1*) has been taken into account in the preparation of the recommendations in this chapter.

The purpose of these recommendations for radioactive substances in drinking-water is to guide the competent authorities in determining whether the water is of an appropriate quality for human consumption.

### 17.1.1 Environmental radiation exposure

Environmental radiation originates from a number of naturally occurring and man-made sources. The United Nations Scientific Committee on the Effects of Atomic Radiation (UNSCEAR) has estimated that exposure to natural sources contributes more than 98% of the radiation dose to the population (excluding medical exposure) (*2*). There is only a very small contribution from nuclear power production and nuclear weapons testing. The global average human exposure from natural sources is 2.4 mSv/year. There are large local variations in this exposure depending on a number of factors, such as height above sea level, the amount and type of radionuclides in the soil, and the amount taken into the body in air, food, and water. The contribution of drinking-water to the total exposure is very small and is due largely to naturally occurring radionuclides in the uranium and thorium decay series (*2*).

Levels of natural radionuclides in drinking-water may be increased by a number of human activities. Radionuclides from the nuclear fuel cycle and from medical and other uses of radioactive materials may enter drinking-water supplies; the contributions from these sources are normally limited by regulatory control of the source or practice, and it is through this regulatory mechanism that remedial action should be taken in the event that such sources cause concern by contaminating drinking-water.

## 17.1.2 Potential health consequences of radiation exposure

Exposure to ionizing radiation, whether natural or man-made, can cause two kinds of health effects. Effects for which the severity of the damage caused is proportional to the dose, and for which a threshold exists below which the effect does not occur, are called "deterministic" effects. Under normal conditions, the dose received from natural radioactivity and routine exposures from regulated practices is well below the threshold levels, and therefore deterministic effects are not relevant to these recommendations.

Effects for which the probability of the occurrence is proportional to dose are known as "stochastic" effects, and it is assumed that there is no threshold below which they do not occur. The main stochastic effect of concern is cancer.

Because different types of radiation have different biological effectiveness and different organs and tissues in the body have different sensitivities to radiation, the ICRP has introduced radiation and tissue-weighting factors to provide a measure of equal effect. The sum of the doubly weighted dose received by all the tissues and organs of the body gives a measure of the total harm and is referred to as the effective dose. Moreover, radionuclides taken into the body may persist and, in some cases, the resulting exposure may extend over many months or years. The committed effective dose is a measure of the total effective dose incurred over a lifetime following the intake of a radionuclide. It is this measure of exposure that is relevant to the present discussion; in what follows, the term "dose" refers to the committed effective dose, which is expressed in sieverts (Sv). The risk of adverse health consequences from radiation exposure is a function of the total dose received from all sources. A revised estimate of the risk (i.e., the mathematical expectation) of a lifetime fatal cancer for the general population has been estimated by the ICRP to be $5 \times 10^{-2}$ per sievert (1). (This does not include a small additional health risk from non-fatal cancers or hereditary effects.)

## 17.1.3 Recommendations

- The recommended reference level of committed effective dose is 0.1 mSv from 1 year's consumption of drinking-water. This reference level of dose represents less than 5% of the average effective dose attributable annually to natural background radiation.
- Below this reference level of dose, the drinking-water is acceptable for human consumption and action to reduce the radioactivity is not necessary.
- For practical purposes, the recommended guideline activity concentrations are 0.1 Bq/litre for gross alpha and 1 Bq/litre for gross beta activity.

The recommendations apply to routine operational conditions of existing or new water supplies. They do not apply to a water supply contaminated during an emergency involving the release of radionuclides into the environment. Guidelines covering emergencies are available elsewhere (3).

The recommendations do not differentiate between natural and man-made radionuclides.

## 17.2 Application of the reference level of dose

For practical purposes, the reference level of dose needs to be expressed as an activity concentration of radionuclides in drinking-water.

The dose to a human from radioactivity in drinking-water is dependent not only on intake but also on metabolic and dosimetric considerations. The guideline activity concentrations assume an intake of total radioactive material from the consumption of 2 litres of water per day for 1 year and are calculated on the basis of the metabolism of an adult. The influence of age on metabolism and variations in consumption of drinking-water do not require modification of the guideline activity concentrations, which are based on a lifetime exposure and provide an appropriate margin of safety. Metabolic and dosimetric considerations have been included in the development of dose conversion factors, expressed as sieverts per becquerel, which relate a dose expressed in sieverts to the quantity (in becquerels) of radioactive material ingested.

Examples of radionuclide concentrations (reference concentrations) corresponding to the reference level of dose, 0.1 mSv/year, are given in Table 17.1. These concentrations have been calculated using the dose conversion factors of the United Kingdom National Radiological Protection Board (4) from the formula:

reference concentration (Bq/litre)

$$= \frac{1 \times 10^{-4}\ (\mathrm{Sv/year})}{730\ (\mathrm{litre/year}) \times \text{dose conversion factor (Sv/Bq)}}$$

$$= \frac{1.4 \times 10^{-7}\ (\mathrm{Sv/litre})}{\text{dose conversion factor (Sv/Bq)}}$$

The previous guidelines recommended the use of an average gross alpha and gross beta activity concentration for routine screening. These were set at 0.1 Bq/litre and 1 Bq/litre, respectively. The doses associated with these levels of gross alpha and gross beta activity for selected radionuclides are shown in Table 17.2. For some radionuclides, such as $^{226}$Ra and $^{90}$Sr, the associated dose is much lower than 0.1 mSv per year. It can also be seen from this table that, if certain radionuclides, such as $^{232}$Th, $^{228}$Ra, or $^{210}$Pb, are singly responsible for 0.1 Bq/litre for gross alpha activity or 1 Bq/litre for gross beta activity, then the reference level of dose of 0.1 mSv per year would be exceeded. However, these radionuclides usually represent only a small fraction of the gross activity. In addition, an elevated activity concentration of these radionuclides would normally be associated with high activities from other radionuclides. This would elevate the gross

**Table 17.1 Activity concentration of various radionuclides in drinking-water corresponding to a dose of 0.1 mSv from 1 year's intake**

| Radionuclide[a] | Dose conversion factor (Sv/Bq)[b] | Calculated rounded value (Bq/litre) |
|---|---|---|
| $^3$H | $1.8 \times 10^{-11}$ | 7800 |
| $^{14}$C | $5.6 \times 10^{-10}$ | 250 |
| $^{60}$Co | $7.2 \times 10^{-9}$ | 20 |
| $^{89}$Sr | $3.8 \times 10^{-9}$ | 37 |
| $^{90}$Sr | $2.8 \times 10^{-8}$ | 5 |
| $^{129}$I | $1.1 \times 10^{-7}$ | 1 |
| $^{131}$I | $2.2 \times 10^{-8}$ | 6 |
| $^{134}$Cs | $1.9 \times 10^{-8}$ | 7 |
| $^{137}$Cs | $1.3 \times 10^{-8}$ | 10 |
| $^{210}$Pb | $1.3 \times 10^{-6}$ | 0.1 |
| $^{210}$Po | $6.2 \times 10^{-7}$ | 0.2 |
| $^{224}$Ra | $8.0 \times 10^{-8}$ | 2 |
| $^{226}$Ra | $2.2 \times 10^{-7}$ | 1 |
| $^{228}$Ra | $2.7 \times 10^{-7}$ | 1 |
| $^{232}$Th | $1.8 \times 10^{-6}$ | 0.1 |
| $^{234}$U | $3.9 \times 10^{-8}$ | 4 |
| $^{238}$U | $3.6 \times 10^{-8}$ | 4 |
| $^{239}$Pu | $5.6 \times 10^{-7}$ | 0.3 |

[a] For $^{40}$K, see below. For $^{222}$Rn, see section 17.2.3.
[b] Values from reference 4.

alpha or gross beta activity concentration above the investigation level and provoke specific radionuclide analysis. Therefore, the values of 0.1 Bq/litre for gross alpha activity and 1 Bq/litre for gross beta activity continue to be recommended as screening levels for drinking-water, below which no further action is required.

Radionuclides emitting low-energy beta particles such as $^3$H and $^{14}$C, and some gaseous or volatile radionuclides, such as $^{222}$Rn and $^{131}$I, will not be detected by standard methods of measurement. The values for average gross alpha and beta activities do not include such radionuclides, so that if their presence is suspected, special sampling techniques and measurements should be used.

It should not necessarily be assumed that the reference level of dose has been exceeded simply because the gross beta activity concentration approaches or exceeds 1 Bq/litre. This situation may well result from the presence of the naturally occurring radionuclide $^{40}$K, which makes up about 0.01% of natural potassium. The absorption of the essential element potassium is under homoeostatic control and takes place mainly from ingested food. Thus, the contribution to dose from the ingestion of $^{40}$K in drinking-water, with its relatively low dose conversion factor ($5 \times 10^{-9}$ Sv/Bq), will be much less than that of many other beta-emitting radionuclides. This situation will be clarified by the identification of the specific radionuclides in the sample.

***Table 17.2. Examples of the doses arising from 1 year's consumption of drinking-water containing any of the given alpha-emitting radionuclides at an activity concentration of 0.1 Bq/litre or of the given beta-emitting radionuclides at an activity concentration of 1 Bq/litre*** [a]

| Radionuclide | Dose (mSv) |
|---|---|
| Alpha emitters (0.1 Bq/litre) | |
| $^{210}$Po | 0.045 |
| $^{224}$Ra | 0.006 |
| $^{226}$Ra | 0.016 |
| $^{232}$Th | 0.130 |
| $^{234}$U | 0.003 |
| $^{238}$U | 0.003 |
| $^{239}$Pu | 0.04 |
| | |
| Beta emitters (1 Bq/litre) | |
| $^{60}$Co | 0.005 |
| $^{89}$Sr | 0.003 |
| $^{90}$Sr | 0.020 |
| $^{129}$I | 0.080 |
| $^{131}$I | 0.016 |
| $^{134}$Cs | 0.014 |
| $^{137}$Cs | 0.009 |
| $^{210}$Pb | 0.95 |
| $^{228}$Ra | 0.20 |

[a] Appropriate dose conversion factors taken from reference *4*.

## 17.2.1 Analytical methods

The International Organization for Standardization (ISO) has published standard methods for determining gross alpha (*5*) and gross beta (*6*) activity concentrations in water. Although the detection limits depend on the radionuclides present, the dissolved solids in the sample, and the counting conditions, the recommended levels for gross alpha and gross beta activity concentrations should be above the limits of detection. The ISO detection limit for gross alpha activity based on $^{239}$Pu is 0.04 Bq/litre, while that for gross beta activity based on $^{137}$Cs is between 0.04 and 0.1 Bq/litre.

For analyses of specific radionuclides in drinking-water, there are general compendium sources in addition to specific methods in the technical literature (*7–11*).

## 17.2.2 Strategy for assessing drinking-water

If either the gross alpha activity concentration of 0.1 Bq/litre or the gross beta activity concentration of 1 Bq/litre is exceeded, then the specific radionuclides should be identified and their individual activity concentrations measured. From these data, a dose estimate for each radionuclide should be made and the sum of

**Fig. 17.1. Application of recommendations on radionuclides in drinking-water based on an annual reference level of dose of 0.1 mSv**

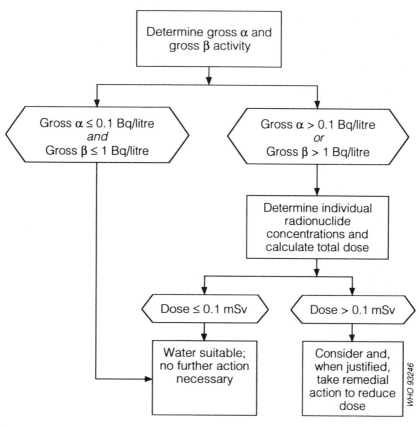

these doses determined. Where the following additive formula is satisfied, no further action is required:

$$\sum_i \frac{C_i}{RC_i} \leq 1$$

where $C_i$ is the measured activity concentration of radionuclide $i$ and $RC_i$ is the reference activity concentration of radionuclide $i$ that, at an intake of 2 litres per day for 1 year, will result in a committed effective dose of 0.1 mSv (see Table 17.1).

If alpha-emitting radionuclides with high dose conversion factors are suspected, this additive formula may also be invoked when the gross alpha and gross beta activity screening values of 0.1 Bq/litre and 1 Bq/litre are approached. Where the sum exceeds unity for a single sample, the reference level of dose of 0.1 mSv would be exceeded only if the exposure to the same measured concentrations were to continue for a full year. Hence, such a sample does not in itself imply that the water is unsuitable for consumption and should be regarded only as a level at which further investigation, including additional sampling, is needed.

The options available to the competent authority to reduce the dose should then be examined. Where remedial measures are contemplated, any strategy considered should first be justified (in the sense that it achieves a positive net benefit) and then optimized in accordance with the recommendations of ICRP (*1, 12*) in order to produce the maximum net benefit. The application of these recommendations is summarized in Fig. 17.1.

## 17.2.3 Radon

There are difficulties in applying the reference level of dose to derive activity concentrations of $^{222}$Rn in drinking-water (*2*). These difficulties arise from the ease with which radon is released from water during handling and the importance of the inhalation pathway. Stirring and transferring water from one container to another will liberate dissolved radon. Water that has been left to stand will have reduced radon activity, and boiling will remove radon completely. As a result, it is important that the form of water consumed is taken into account in assessing the dose from ingestion. Moreover, the use of water supplies for other domestic uses will increase the levels of radon in the air, thus increasing the dose from inhalation. This dose depends markedly on the form of domestic usage and housing construction (*13*). The form of water intake, the domestic use of water, and the construction of houses vary widely throughout the world. It is therefore not possible to derive an activity concentration for radon in drinking-water that is universally applicable.

The global average dose from inhalation of radon from all sources is about 1 mSv/year, which is roughly half of the total natural radiation exposure. In comparison, the global dose from ingestion of radon in drinking-water is relatively low. In a local situation, however, the risks from inhalation and from ingestion may be about equal. Because of this and because there may be other sources of radon gas entry to a house, ingestion cannot be considered in isolation from inhalation exposures.

All these factors should be assessed on a regional or national level by the appropriate authorities, in order to determine whether a reference level of dose of 0.1 mSv is appropriate for that region, and to determine an activity concentration that may be used to assess the suitability of the water supply. These judgements should be based not only on the ingestion and inhalation exposures resulting from the supply of water, but also on the inhalation doses from other radon sources in the home. In these circumstances, it would appear necessary to adopt an integrated approach and assess doses from all radon sources, especially to determine the optimum action to be undertaken where some sort of intervention is deemed necessary.

# References

1.  1990 Recommendations of the International Commission on Radiological Protection. *Annals of the ICRP*, 1990, 21 (1-3).

2.  United Nations Scientific Committee on the Effects of Atomic Radiation. *Sources, effects and risks of ionizing radiation.* New York, United Nations, 1988.

3.  World Health Organization. *Derived intervention levels for radionuclides in food.* Geneva, 1988.

4.  National Radiological Protection Board. *Committed equivalent organ doses and committed effective doses from intakes of radionuclides.* A report of the National Radiological Protection Board of the United Kingdom. Chilton, Didcot, 1991 (NRPB-R245).

5.  Association of Official Analytical Chemists. *Official methods of analysis of the Association of Official Analytical Chemists*, 15th ed. Washington, DC, 1990.

6.  Environmental Measurements Laboratory. *EML procedures manual.* New York, Department of Energy, 1990 (HASL-300).

7.  International Organization for Standardization. *Water quality — measurement of gross alpha activity in non-saline water — thick source method.* Geneva, 1990 (Draft International Standard 9696)

8.  International Organization for Standardization. *Water quality — measurement of gross beta activity in non-saline water.* Geneva, 1990 (Draft International Standard 9697).

9.  Suess MJ, ed. *Examination of water for pollution control.* 3 vols. Oxford, Pergamon Press, 1982.

10. United States Environmental Protection Agency. Eastern Environmental Radiation Facility. *Radiochemistry procedures manual.* Montgomery, AL, 1987 (EPA 520/5-84-006).

11. American Public Health Association. *Standard methods for the examination of water and wastewater*, 17th ed. Washington, DC, 1989.

12. Optimization and decision-making in radiological protection. *Annals of the ICRP*, 1989, 20(1).

13. National Council on Radiation Protection and Measurements. *Control of radon in houses. Recommendations of the National Council on Radiation Protection and Measurements.* Bethesda, MD, 1989 (NCRP Report No. 103)

# Annex 1

# List of participants in preparatory meetings

Consultation on Revision of WHO Guidelines for Drinking-Water Quality
(Rome, Italy, 17–19 October 1988)

## Members

L. Albanus, Head, Toxicology Laboratory, National Food Administration, Uppsala, Sweden

J. Alexander, Toxicological Department, National Institute of Public Health, Oslo, Norway

J.A. Cotruvo, Director, Criteria and Standards Division, United States Environmental Protection Agency, Washington, DC, USA

H. de Kruijf, Laboratory for Ecotoxicology, Environmental Chemistry and Drinking-Water, National Institute of Public Health and Environmental Protection, Bilthoven, Netherlands

H.H. Dieter, Director and Professor, Institute for Water, Soil and Air Hygiene of the Federal Office of Health, Berlin

J.K. Fawell, Principal Toxicologist, Water Research Centre, Medmenham, England (*Rapporteur*)

E. Funari, Department of Environmental Hygiene, Istituto Superiore di Sanità, Rome, Italy

J.R. Hickman, Acting Director-General, Environmental Health Directorate, Health and Welfare Canada, Ottawa, Canada

Y. Magara, Director, Department of Sanitary Engineering, Institute of Public Health, Tokyo, Japan

R.F. Packham, Chief Scientist, Water Research Centre, Medmenham, England

M. Waring, Department of Health and Social Security, London, England

G.A. Zapponi, Environmental Impact Assessment Section, Istituto Superiore di Sanità, Rome, Italy

## Observers

S. Blease, Administrator, Water Protection Division, Commission of European Communities, Brussels, Belgium

B. Julin, Regulatory Affairs Manager, International Group of National Associations of Manufacturers of Agrochemical Products, Wilmington, DE, USA

A. Pelfrène, International Group of National Associations of Manufacturers of Agrochemical Products, Paris, France

N. Sarti, Division of Water and Soil, Ministry of Health, Rome, Italy

### Secretariat

G. Burin, International Programme on Chemical Safety, Division of Environmental Health, World Health Organization, Geneva, Switzerland

R. Helmer, Prevention of Environmental Pollution, Division of Environmental Health, World Health Organization, Geneva, Switzerland

M. Mercier, Manager, International Programme on Chemical Safety, Division of Environmental Health, World Health Organization, Geneva, Switzerland

G. Ozolins, Manager, Prevention of Environmental Pollution, Division of Environmental Health, World Health Organization, Geneva, Switzerland (*Moderator*)

S. Tarkowski, Director, Environment and Health, WHO Regional Office for Europe, Copenhagen, Denmark

## Microbiology Consultation (London, England, 23 June 1989)

### Members

U. Blumental, London School of Hygiene and Tropical Medicine, London, England

S. Cairncross, London School of Hygiene and Tropical Medicine, London, England

A.H. Havelaar, National Institute of Public Health and Environmental Protection, Bilthoven, Netherlands

R.F. Packham, Marlow, England

W. Stelzer, Research Institute of Hygiene and Microbiology, Bad Elster, German Democratic Republic

H. Utkilen, Department of Sanitary Engineering and Environmental Protection, National Institute of Public Health, Oslo, Norway

R. Walter, Director, Institute for General and Community Hygiene, Dresden, German Democratic Republic

### Secretariat

J.K. Fawell, Principal Toxicologist, Water Research Centre, Medmenham, England

R. Helmer, Prevention of Environmental Pollution, Division of Environmental Health, World Health Organization, Geneva, Switzerland

B. Lloyd, Environmental Health Unit, Robens Institute of Industrial and Environmental Health and Safety, Guildford, England

E.B. Pike, Water Research Centre, Medmenham, England

## Coordination Consultation (Copenhagen, Denmark, 4–5 September 1989)

### Members

J.K. Fawell, Principal Toxicologist, Water Research Centre, Medmenham, England (*Co-Rapporteur*) '

E. Funari, Department of Environmental Hygiene, Istituto Superiore di Sanità, Rome, Italy

E.S. Jensen, Senior Technical Adviser on Water Supply and Sanitation Projects, Technical Advisory Division, Danish International Development Agency, Copenhagen, Denmark

A. Minderhoud, Laboratory for Ecotoxicology, Environmental Chemistry and Drinking Water, National Institute of Public Health and Environmental Protection, Bilthoven, Netherlands

B. Mintz, Chief, Health Effects Assessment Section, Criteria and Standards Division, Office of Drinking-Water, United States Environmental Protection Agency, Washington, DC, USA

P.A. Nielsen, Scientific Officer, Toxicologist, Institute of Toxicology, National Food Agency, Soborg, Denmark

E. Poulsen, Chief Adviser in Toxicology, Institute of Toxicology, National Food Agency, Soborg, Denmark

B. Schultz, Water Quality Institute, Horsholm, Denmark

### Secretariat

G. Burin, International Programme on Chemical Safety, Division of Environmental Health, World Health Organization, Geneva, Switzerland (*Co-Rapporteur*)

O. Espinoza, Regional Officer for International Water Decade, Environment and Health, WHO Regional Office for Europe, Copenhagen, Denmark

R. Helmer, Prevention of Environmental Pollution, Division of Environmental Health, World Health Organization, Geneva, Switzerland

D. Kello, Project Officer for Toxicology and Food Safety, Environment and Health, WHO Regional Office for Europe, Copenhagen, Denmark

S. Tarkowski, Director, Environment and Health, WHO Regional Office for Europe, Copenhagen, Denmark

## Coordination Group Meeting (Geneva, Switzerland, 13–14 March 1990)

### Members

J.K. Fawell, Principal Toxicologist, Water Research Centre, Medmenham, England

E. Funari, Department of Environmental Hygiene, Istituto Superiore di Sanità, Rome, Italy

J.R. Hickman, Acting Director-General, Environmental Health Directorate, Health and Welfare Canada, Ottawa, Canada

A. Minderhoud, Laboratory for Ecotoxicology, Environmental Chemistry and Drinking Water, National Institute of Public Health and Environmental Protection, Bilthoven, Netherlands

B. Mintz, Chief, Health Effects Assessment Section, Criteria and Standards Division, Office of Drinking-Water, United States Environmental Protection Agency, Washington, DC, USA

B. Schultz, Water Quality Institute, Horsholm, Denmark

### Secretariat

G. Burin, International Programme on Chemical Safety, Division of Environmental Health, World Health Organization, Geneva, Switzerland

O. Espinoza, Regional Officer for International Water Decade, Environment and Health, WHO Regional Office for Europe, Copenhagen, Denmark

R. Helmer, Prevention of Environmental Pollution, Division of Environmental Health, World Health Organization, Geneva, Switzerland

D. Kello, Project Officer for Toxicology and Food Safety, Environment and Health, WHO Regional Office for Europe, Copenhagen, Denmark

G. Ozolins, Manager, Prevention of Environmental Pollution, Division of Environmental Health, World Health Organization, Geneva, Switzerland

R. Plestina, International Programme on Chemical Safety, Division of Environmental Health, World Health Organization, Geneva, Switzerland

## First Review Group Meeting on Pesticides (Busto Garolfo, Italy, 25–30 June 1990)

### Members

H. Abouzaid, Chief, Water Quality Control Division, National Agency for Drinking-Water, Rabat-Chellah, Morocco

H. Atta-ur-Rahman, Director, H.E.J. Research Institute of Chemistry, Karachi, Pakistan

V. Benes, Chief, Toxicology and Reference Laboratory, Institute of Hygiene and Epidemiology, Prague, Czechoslovakia

J.F. Borzelleca, Pharmacology, Toxicology, Medical College of Virginia, Virginia Commonwealth University, Richmond, VA, USA

L. Brener, Chief, Department of Mineral Analysis, Research Laboratory, Société Lyonnaise des Eaux-Dumez, Paris, France

D. Calamari, Institute of Agricultural Entomology, Faculty of Agriculture, University of Milan, Italy

J. Du, Office of Drinking-Water, United States Environmental Protection Agency, Washington, DC, USA

J. K. Fawell, Principal Toxicologist, Water Research Centre, Medmenham, England (*Rapporteur*)

J. Forslund, National Agency of Environmental Protection, Copenhagen, Denmark

E. Funari, Department of Environmental Hygiene, Istituto Superiore di Sanità, Rome, Italy

A. Jaron, Commission of the European Communities, Brussels, Belgium

M. Maroni, Director, International Centre for Pesticide Safety, Busto Garolfo, Italy

Y. Patel, Health Effects Assessment, Office of Drinking-Water, United States Environmental Protection Agency, Washington, DC, USA

E. Poulsen, Chief Adviser in Toxicology, Institute of Toxicology, National Food Agency, Soborg, Denmark (*Chairman*)

J. Rueff, Department of Genetics, Faculty of Medical Science, Lisbon, Portugal

B. Schultz, Water Quality Institute, Horsholm, Denmark

J.A. Sokal, Head, Department of Toxicity Evaluation, Institute of Occupational Medicine, Lodz, Poland

M. Takeda, Director of Environmental Chemistry, National Institute of Hygienic Science, Tokyo, Japan

E.M. den Tonkelaar, National Institute of Public Health and Environmental Protection, Bilthoven, Netherlands

G. Wood, Acting Head, Criteria Section, Monitoring and Criteria Division, Environmental Health Directorate, Health and Welfare, Ottawa, Canada

## Observers

S. Behrendt, BASF AG, Limburgerhof, Federal Republic of Germany

S. Hahn, BASF AG, Limburgerhof, Federal Republic of Germany

H. Kieczka, BASF AG, Limburgerhof, Federal Republic of Germany

S. Kimura, Southern Fukuoka Prefecture, Water Spread Authority, Japan Water Works Association, Tokyo, Japan

F. Sarhan, CIBA-GEIGY Ltd, Basel, Switzerland

G.E. Veenstra, Shell International Petroleum, The Hague, Netherlands

### *Secretariat*

G. Burin, International Programme on Chemical Safety, Division of Environmental Health, World Health Organization, Geneva, Switzerland

D. Kello, Project Officer for Toxicology and Food Safety, Environment and Health, WHO Regional Office for Europe, Copenhagen, Denmark

R. Plestina, International Programme on Chemical Safety, Division of Environmental Health, World Health Organization, Geneva, Switzerland

## First Review Group Meeting on Organics (Copenhagen, Denmark, 6–10 November 1990)

### *Members*

C. Abernathy, Toxicologist, Health Effects Branch, Office of Drinking-Water, United States Environmental Protection Agency, Washingon, DC, USA

H.H. Dieter, Director and Professor, Institute for Water, Soil and Air Hygiene of the Federal Office of Health, Berlin, Germany

A.M. van Dijk-Looyaard, Drinking-Water Research Scientist, National Institute of Public Health and Environmental Protection, Bilthoven, Netherlands

J.K. Fawell, Principal Toxicologist, Water Research Centre, Medmenham, England (*Rapporteur*)

J. Forslund, National Agency of Environmental Protection, Copenhagen, Denmark

E. Funari, Department of Environmental Hygiene, Istituto Superiore di Sanità, Rome, Italy

K. Khanna, Pharmacologist, Health Effects Branch, Office of Drinking-Water, United States Environmental Protection Agency, Washington, DC, USA

R. van Leeuwen, Toxicologist, National Institute of Public Health and Environmental Protection, Bilthoven, Netherlands

U. Lund, Head, Department of Chemistry, Water Quality Institute, Horsholm, Denmark

M.E. Meek, Head, Priority Substances Section, Environmental Health Centre, Health and Welfare Canada, Ottawa, Canada

T. Ookubo, Head, Water Quality Examination Laboratory, Hachinohe Regional Water Supply Cooperation, Hachinohe, Japan

E. Sandberg, Toxicologist, National Food Administration, Uppsala, Sweden

U. Schlosser, Research Institute for Hygiene and Microbiology, Bad Elster, Germany

E.A. Simpson, Commission of the European Communities, Brussels, Belgium

J.A. Sokal, Head, Department of Toxicity Evaluation, Institute of Occupational Medicine, Lodz, Poland (*Chairman*)

M. Takeda, Director of Environmental Chemistry, National Institute of Hygienic Science, Tokyo, Japan

## Observer

A. Carlsen, Ministry of the Environment, National Agency of Environmental Protection, Miljöstyrelsen, Copenhagen, Denmark

## Secretariat

P. Bérubé, Programme Assistant, International Water Decade, Environment and Health, WHO Regional Office for Europe, Copenhagen, Denmark

O. Espinoza, Regional Officer for International Water Decade, Environment and Health, WHO Regional Office for Europe, Copenhagen, Denmark

D. Kello, Project Officer for Toxicology and Food Safety, Environment and Health, WHO Regional Office for Europe, Copenhagen, Denmark

D. Schutz, International Programme on Chemical Safety, Division of Environmental Health, World Health Organization, Geneva, Switzerland

S. Tarkowski, Director, Environment and Health, WHO Regional Office for Europe, Copenhagen, Denmark

J. Wilbourn, Unit of Carcinogen Identification and Evaluation, International Agency for Research on Cancer, Lyon, France

## First Review Group Meeting on Inorganics (Bilthoven, Netherlands, 18–22 March 1991)

### Members

E.A. Bababumni, Department of Biochemistry, University of Ibadan, Ibadan, Nigeria

K.L. Bailey, Health Effects Assessment Section, Criteria and Standards Division, Office of Drinking-Water, United States Environmental Protection Agency, Washington, DC, USA

G.F. Craun, Chief Epidemiologist, United States Environmental Protection Agency, Washington, DC, USA

A.M. van Dijk-Looyaard, Drinking-Water Research Scientist, National Institute of Public Health and Environmental Protection, Bilthoven, Netherlands

J.K. Fawell, Principal Toxicologist, Water Research Centre, Medmenham, England (*Rapporteur*)

R. van Leeuwen, Toxicologist, National Institute of Public Health and Environmental Protection, Bilthoven, Netherlands (*Chairman*)

M.E. Meek, Head, Priority Substances Section, Environmental Health Centre, Health and Welfare Canada, Ottawa, Canada

E. Poulsen, Chief Adviser in Toxicology, Institute of Toxicology, National Food Agency, Soborg, Denmark

Y.A. Rakhmanin, Head of Laboratory, Ministry of Health of the USSR Academy of Medical Sciences, A.N. Sysin Institute of General and Communal Hygiene, Moscow, USSR

V.R. Rao, Assistant Director and Head, Department of Toxicology, The Haffkine Institute, Parel, Bombay, India

F.G.R. Reyes, Professor of Food Toxicology, Department of Food Science, State University of Campinas, Brazil

F. Sartor, Institute of Hygiene and Epidemiology, Ministry of Public Health and the Family, Brussels, Belgium

J.A. Sokal, Head, Department of Toxicity Evaluation, Institute of Occupational Medicine, Lodz, Poland

M. Takeda, Director of Environmental Chemistry, National Institute of Hygienic Science, Tokyo, Japan

### Observers

J. Forslund, National Agency of Environmental Protection, Copenhagen, Denmark

I. Harimaya, Director of Water Quality Research, Kobe, Japan

M. Minowa, Director of Epidemiology, Institute of Public Health, Ministry of Health and Welfare, Tokyo, Japan

E.A. Simpson, Commission of the European Communities, Brussels, Belgium

J.F.M. Versteegh, National Institute of Public Health and Environmental Protection, Bilthoven, Netherlands

V. Vignier, Société Lyonnaise des Eaux Dumez, International Centre for Research on Water and the Environment (CIRSEE), Le Pecq, France

### Secretariat

B. Chen, International Programme on Chemical Safety, Division of Environmental Health, World Health Organization, Geneva, Switzerland

H. Galal-Gorchev, International Programme on Chemical Safety, Division of Environmental Health, World Health Organization, Geneva, Switzerland

## Second Review Group Meeting on Organics (Copenhagen, Denmark, 8–12 April 1991)

### Members

K. Bergman, Toxicologist, Medical Products Agency, Division of Pharmacology, Uppsala, Sweden

A. Carlsen, National Agency of Environmental Protection, Copenhagen, Denmark

H.H. Dieter, Director and Professor, Institute for Water, Soil and Air Hygiene of the Federal Office of Health, Berlin, Germany

P.M. Dudermel, Pasteur Institute, Lille, France

J.K. Fawell, Principal Toxicologist, Water Research Centre, Medmenham, England (*Rapporteur*)

J. Forslund, National Agency of Environmental Protection, Copenhagen, Denmark

R. Hasegawa, Section Chief, Division of Toxicology, National Institute of Hygienic Science, Tokyo, Japan

K. Hughes, Chemical Health Hazard Evaluator, Environmental Health Centre, Health and Welfare Canada, Ottawa, Canada

R. van Leeuwen, Toxicologist, National Institute of Public Health and Environmental Protection, Bilthoven, Netherlands

U. Lund, Head, Department of Chemistry, Water Quality Institute, Horsholm, Denmark

A. Patel, Toxicologist, Water Research Centre, Medmenham, England

Y. Richard, Chief, Department of Chemical Research, Société Degrémont, Rueil-Malmaison, France

E. Sandberg, Toxicologist, National Food Administration, Uppsala, Sweden

J.A. Sokal, Head, Department of Toxicity Evaluation, Institute of Occupational Medicine, Lodz, Poland (*Chairman*)

### Secretariat

X. Bonnefoy, Acting Regional Officer for Health Planning/Ecology, WHO Regional Office for Europe, Copenhagen, Denmark

H. Galal-Gorchev, International Programme on Chemical Safety, Division of Environmental Health, World Health Organization, Geneva, Switzerland

J. Gents, Secretary, International Water Decade, Environment and Health, WHO Regional Office for Europe, Copenhagen, Denmark

D. Kello, Project Officer for Toxicology and Food Safety, Environment and Health, WHO Regional Office for Europe, Copenhagen, Denmark

S. Tarkowski, Director, Environment and Health, WHO Regional Office for Europe, Copenhagen, Denmark

## Coordination Group Consultation (Geneva, Switzerland, 13–14 May 1991)

### Members

J. K. Fawell, Principal Toxicologist, Water Research Centre, Medmenham, England

J.R. Hickman, Director-General, Environmental Health Directorate, Health and Welfare Canada, Ottawa, Canada (*Moderator*)

U. Lund, Head, Department of Chemistry, Water Quality Institute, Horsholm, Denmark

B. Mintz, Chief, Health Effects Assessment Section, Criteria and Standards Division, Office of Drinking-Water, United States Environmental Protection Agency, Washington, DC, USA

E.B. Pike, Water Research Centre, Medmenham, England

### Secretariat

X. Bonnefoy, Acting Regional Officer for Health Planning/Ecology, WHO Regional Office for Europe, Copenhagen, Denmark (*Co-Rapporteur*)

H. Galal-Gorchev, International Programme on Chemical Safety, Division of Environmental Health, World Health Organization, Geneva, Switzerland (*Co-Rapporteur*)

R. Helmer, Prevention of Environmental Pollution, Division of Environmental Health, World Health Organization, Geneva, Switzerland

J. Kenny, Prevention of Environmental Pollution, Division of Environmental Health, World Health Organization, Geneva, Switzerland

M. Mercier, Manager, International Programme on Chemical Safety, Division of Environmental Health, World Health Organization, Geneva, Switzerland

G. Ozolins, Manager, Prevention of Environmental Pollution, Division of Environmental Health, World Health Organization, Geneva, Switzerland

P. Waight, Prevention of Environmental Pollution, Division of Environmental Health, World Health Organization, Geneva, Switzerland

## Review Group on Disinfectants and Disinfectant By-products (Bethesda, MD, USA, 10–14 June 1991)

### Members

H. Abouzaid, Chief, Water Quality Control Division, National Agency for Drinking-Water, Rabat-Chellah, Morocco

W. Almeida, Department of Preventive Medicine, State University of Campinas, Campinas, Brazil

M. Ando, National Institute of Hygienic Science, Division of Environmental Chemistry, Tokyo, Japan

R. Bull, Pharmacology/Toxicology Graduate Program, College of Pharmacy, Washington State University, Pullman, WA, USA

G. Burin, United States Environmental Protection Agency, Washington, DC, USA (*Vice-Chairman*)

J.K. Fawell, Principal Toxicologist, Water Research Centre, Medmenham, England (*Co-Rapporteur*)

B. Havlik, Institute of Hygiene and Epidemiology, Prague, Czechoslovakia

N. Mahabhol, Ministry of Public Health, Bangkok, Thailand

M.E. Meek, Head, Priority Substances Section, Environmental Health Centre, Health and Welfare Canada, Ottawa, Canada (*Co-Rapporteur*)

B. Mintz, Chief, Health Effects Assessment Section, Criteria and Standards Division, Office of Drinking-Water, United States Environmental Protection Agency, Washington, DC, USA (*Chairman*)

R. Packham, Marlow, England

J.F.M. Versteegh, National Institute of Public Health and Environmental Protection, Bilthoven, Netherlands

Z. Zholdakova, Academy of Medical Sciences, A.N. Sysin Institute of General and Communal Hygiene, Moscow, USSR

### Observers

J. Forslund, National Agency of Environmental Protection, Copenhagen, Denmark

E. Ohanian, Office of Science and Technology, United States Environmental Protection Agency, Washington, DC, USA

H. Sasaki, Water Quality Laboratory, Sapporro, Hokkaido, Japan

### Secretariat

R. Cantilli, United States Environmental Protection Agency, Washington, DC, USA

N. Chiu, United States Environmental Protection Agency, Washington, DC, USA

J. Du, United States Environmental Protection Agency, Washington, DC, USA

H. Galal-Gorchev, International Programme on Chemical Safety, Division of Environmental Health, World Health Organization, Geneva, Switzerland

J. Orme, Office of Science and Technology, United States Environmental Protection Agency, Washington, DC, USA

## Review Meeting on Pathogenic Agents and Volume 3 on Surveillance of Community Supplies (Harare, Zimbabwe, 24–28 June 1991)

### Members

H. Abouzaid, Chief, Water Quality Control Division, National Agency for Drinking-Water, Rabat-Chellah, Morocco

M.T. Boot, Programme Officer, IRC International Water and Sanitation Centre, The Hague, Netherlands

J.Z. Boutros, Consultant in Food and Water Control, Khartoum, Sudan (*Rapporteur*)

W. Fellows, Programme Officer, Water and Environmental Sanitation, UNICEF, Harare, Zimbabwe

F.J. Gumbo, Head of Water Laboratories, Operation, Maintenance and Water Laboratories Division, Ministry of Water (MAJI), Dar-es-Salaam, United Republic of Tanzania

A.H. Havelaar, National Institute of Public Health and Environmental Protection, Bilthoven, Netherlands

J. Hubley, Senior Lecturer in Health Education, Health Education Unit, Faculty of Health and Social Care, Leeds Polytechnic, Leeds, England

B. Jackson, Senior Engineering Advisor, British Development Division in East Africa, Nairobi, Kenya

E. Khaka, Ministry of Energy and Water Resources Development, Harare, Zimbabwe

S. Laver, Lecturer, Department of Community Medicine, University of Zimbabwe, Mount Pleasant, Harare, Zimbabwe

M.T. Martins, Associate Professor, Environmental Microbiology Laboratory, University of São Paulo, Brazil

P. Morgan, Advisor, Water and Sanitation, Ministry of Health, Blair Research Laboratory, Harare, Zimbabwe

S. Mtero, Principal Medical Research Officer, Ministry of Health, Blair Research Laboratory, Harare, Zimbabwe

S. Musingarabwi, Director, Environmental Health Services, Ministry of Health, Harare, Zimbabwe (*Vice-Chairman*)

F. Niang, Chief, Laboratory Service, Senegalese National Water Management Company, Dakar, Senegal

E.B. Pike, Water Research Centre, Medmenham, England

P.K. Ray, Director, Industrial Toxicology Research Centre, Lucknow, India

P. Taylor, Director, Training Centre for Water and Sanitation, Department of Civil Engineering, University of Zimbabwe, Harare, Zimbabwe (*Chairman*)

H. Utkilen, Scientist, National Institute of Public Health, Department of Environmental Medicine, Oslo, Norway

## Observers

M. Ellis, Primary Health Consultant, The Robens Institute of Health and Safety, University of Surrey, Guildford, England

D. Tolson, Aid Secretary, British High Commission, Harare, Zimbabwe

## Secretariat

J. Bartram, Manager, Overseas Development, The Robens Institute of Health and Safety, University of Surrey, Guildford, England

H. Galal-Gorchev, International Programme on Chemical Safety, Division of Environmental Health, World Health Organization, Geneva, Switzerland

R. Helmer, Prevention of Environmental Pollution, Division of Environmental Health, World Health Organization, Geneva, Switzerland

J. Kenny, Prevention of Environmental Pollution, Division of Environmental Health, World Health Organization, Geneva, Switzerland

V. Larby, The Robens Institute of Health and Safety, University of Surrey, Guildford, England

B. Lloyd, Head, Environmental Health, The Robens Institute of Health and Safety, University of Surrey, Guildford, England

K. Wedgwood, Research Officer, The Robens Institute of Health and Safety, University of Surrey, Guildford, England

F. Zawide, WHO Sanitary Engineer, Sub-region III, Harare, Zimbabwe

## Second Review Group Meeting on Pesticides (Rennes, France, 2–6 September 1991)

### Members

G. Burin, Toxicologist, United States Environmental Protection Agency, Washington, DC, USA (*Co-Rapporteur*)

A. Bruchet, Société Lyonnaise des Eaux Dumez, International Centre for Research on Water and the Environment (CIRSEE), Le Pecq, France

H.H. Dieter, Director and Professor, Institute for Water, Soil and Air Hygiene of the Federal Office of Health, Berlin, Germany

P.M. Dudermel, Pasteur Institute, Lille, France

J.K. Fawell, Principal Toxicologist, Water Research Centre, Medmenham, England (*Co-Rapporteur*)

J. Forslund, National Agency of Environmental Protection, Copenhagen, Denmark

E. Funari, Department of Environmental Hygiene, Istituto Superiore di Sanità, Rome, Italy

R. Halperin, Chief Engineer for Environmental Health, Ministry of Health, Jerusalem, Israel

K. Hughes, Chemical Health Hazard Evaluator, Priority Substances Section, Environmental Substances Division, Environmental Health Directorate, Environmental Health Centre, Ottawa, Canada

S. Kojima, Director of Environmental Chemistry, National Institute of Hygienic Science, Tokyo, Japan

A.M. Mahfouz, Senior Toxicologist and Pesticides Team Leader, Office of Science and Technology, United States Environmental Protection Agency, Washington, DC, USA

A. Montiel, Water Quality Control Officer, Water Management Company of Paris, Paris, France (*Chairman*)

E. Poulsen, Chief Adviser in Toxicology, Institute of Toxicology, National Food Agency, Soborg, Denmark

R. Seux, National School of Public Health, Rennes, France

E. Simpson, Commission of the European Communities, Brussels, Belgium

930

## Observers

M.J. Carroll, Area Registration Manager, Monsanto Services International, Brussels, Belgium

A. Hirata, Chief, Monitoring Section, Water Quality Management, Waterworks Bureau, Tokyo Metropolitan Government, Tokyo, Japan

H.P. Nigitz, Head, Regulatory Affairs, Agrolinz Agricultural Chemicals, Linz, Austria

E. Puri, Toxicologist, CIBA-GEIGY Ltd, Basel, Switzerland

G.A. Willis, Manager, Product Safety, ICI Agrochemicals, Fernhurst, Haslemere, Surrey, England

## Secretariat

X. Bonnefoy, Regional Adviser, Health Planning/Ecology, WHO Regional Office for Europe, Copenhagen, Denmark

H. Galal-Gorchev, International Programme on Chemical Safety, Division of Environmental Health, World Health Organization, Geneva, Switzerland

J. Gents, Programme Secretary, Environment and Health, WHO Regional Office for Europe, Copenhagen, Denmark

## Second Review Group Meeting on Inorganics (Brussels, Belgium, 14–18 October 1991)

## Members

Y. Aida, Senior Research Scientist, Division of Risk Assessment, National Institute of Hygienic Science, Kamiyoga, Setagayaku, Tokyo, Japan

J. Alexander, Deputy Director, Department of Environmental Medicine, National Institute of Public Health, Oslo, Norway

K.L. Bailey, Health Effects Assessment Section, Criteria and Standards Division, Office of Drinking-Water, United States Environmental Protection Agency, Washington, DC, USA

H.H. Dieter, Director and Professor, Toxicologist, Institute for Water, Soil and Air Hygiene of the Federal Office of Health, Berlin, Germany

J.K. Fawell, Principal Toxicologist, Water Research Centre, Medmenham, England (*Co-Rapporteur*)

A. Lafontaine, Honorary Director, Institute of Hygiene and Epidemiology, Brussels, Belgium

M.E. Meek, Head, Priority Substances Section, Environmental Health Centre, Health and Welfare Canada, Ottawa, Canada

B. Naima, Director, Water Quality Laboratory, National Agency for Drinking-Water, Rabat-Chellah, Morocco

G.D. Nielsen, Department of Environmental Medicine, Odense University, Odense, Denmark

R.F. Packham, Marlow, England

Y.A. Rakhmanin, Head of Laboratory, Ministry of Health of the USSR Academy of Medical Sciences, A.N. Sysin Institute of General and Communal Hygiene, Moscow, USSR

Tharwat Saleh, Project Manager, WHO Project EFY/CWS/002, Cairo, Egypt

R. Sarin, Assistant Director, Scientist and Head, Basic Research Division, National Environmental Engineering Research Institute (NEERI), Nehru Marg, Nagpur, India

F. Sartor, Institute of Hygiene and Epidemiology, Ministry of Public Health and the Family, Brussels, Belgium (*Chairman*)

J.F.M. Versteegh, National Institute of Public Health and Environmental Protection, Bilthoven, Netherlands

## *Observers*

J. Forslund, National Agency of Environmental Protection, Copenhagen, Denmark

E.A. Simpson, Commission of the European Communities, Brussels, Belgium

V. Vignier, Société Lyonnaise des Eaux Dumez, International Centre for Research on Water and the Environment (CIRSEE), Le Pecq, France

## *Secretariat*

X. Bonnefoy, Regional Adviser, Health Planning/Ecology, WHO Regional Office for Europe, Copenhagen, Denmark

H. Galal-Gorchev, International Programme on Chemical Safety, Division of Environmental Health, World Health Organization, Geneva, Switzerland (*Co-Rapporteur*)

C. Martin, Prevention of Environmental Pollution, Division of Environmental Health, World Health Organization, Geneva, Switzerland

## Radionuclides Meeting (Medmenham, England, 22–24 January 1992)

## *Members*

O. Hydes, Drinking-Water Inspectorate, Department of the Environment, London, England

D.P. Meyerhof, Bureau of Radiation and Medical Devices, Department of National Health and Welfare, Ottawa, Canada

J.-C. Nénot, Director of Research, Institute for Nuclear Protection and Safety, Fontenay-aux-Roses, France

K.C. Pillai, Health Physics Division, Bhabha Atomic Research Centre, Bombay, India

A. Randell, Senior Officer, Food Quality and Standards Service, Food and Agriculture Organization of the United Nations, Rome, Italy

C. Robinson, National Radiological Protection Board, Chilton, Didcot, England (*Co-Rapporteur*)

L.B. Sztanyik, Director, "Frédéric Joliot-Curie" National Research Institute for Radiobiology and Radiohygiene, Budapest, Hungary (*Chairman*)

E. Wirth, Institute for Radiation Hygiene, Federal Office for Radiation Protection, Neuerberg, Germany

### Secretariat

P.J. Waight, Prevention of Environmental Pollution, Division of Environmental Health, World Health Organization, Geneva, Switzerland (*Co-Rapporteur*)

## Analytical and Treatment Methods (Medmenham, England, 27–29 January 1992)

### Members

H. Abouzaid, Chief, Water Quality Control Division, National Agency for Drinking-Water, Rabat-Chellah, Morocco

S. Clark, Chief, Drinking Water Technology Branch, Office of Groundwater and Drinking Water, United States Environmental Protection Agency, Washington, DC, USA

A.M. van Dijk-Looyaard, Drinking-Water Research Scientist, National Institute of Public Health and Environmental Protection, Bilthoven, Netherlands

J. Forslund, National Agency of Environmental Protection, Copenhagen, Denmark

D. Green, Criteria Section, Environmental Health Centre, Department of National Health and Welfare, Ottawa, Canada (*Co-Rapporteur*)

I. Licsko, Research Centre for Water Resources Development (VITUKI), Budapest, Hungary

B. Lloyd, Head, Environmental Health, The Robens Institute of Health and Safety, University of Surrey, Guildford, England

D.P. Meyerhof, Bureau of Radiation and Medical Devices, Department of National Health and Welfare, Ottawa, Canada

A. Montiel, Water Quality Control Officer, Water Management Company of Paris, Paris, France (*Co-Rapporteur*)

R.F. Packham, Marlow, England (*Chairman*)

R. Sarin, Assistant Director, Scientist and Head, Basic Research Division, National Environmental Engineering Research Institute (NEERI), Nehru Marg, Nagpur, India

### Observers

T. Aizawa, Department of Sanitary Engineering, Institute of Public Health, Tokyo, Japan

R.A. Breach, Water Quality Manager, Severn Trent Water, Birmingham, England

O. Hydes, Drinking Water Inspectorate, Department of the Environment, London, England

M. Ichinohe, Bureau of Waterworks, Tokyo Metropolitan Government, Tokyo, Japan

E. Simpson, Commission of the European Communities, Brussels, Belgium

M. Tsuji, Ministry of Health and Welfare, Tokyo, Japan

### Secretariat

X. Bonnefoy, Regional Adviser, Health Planning/Ecology, WHO Regional Office for Europe, Copenhagen, Denmark

B. Crathorne, Water Research Centre, Medmenham, England

J.K. Fawell, Principal Toxicologist, Water Research Centre, Medmenham, England

H. Galal-Gorchev, International Programme on Chemical Safety, Division of Environmental Health, World Health Organization, Geneva, Switzerland

E.B. Pike, Water Research Centre, Medmenham, England

## WHO Consolidation Meeting on Organics and Pesticides (Medmenham, England, 30–31 January 1992)

### Members

J.K. Fawell, Principal Toxicologist, Water Research Centre, Medmenham, England

R. van Leeuwen, Toxicologist, National Institute of Public Health and Environmental Protection, Bilthoven, Netherlands (*Moderator*)

U. Lund, Head, Department of Chemistry, Water Quality Institute, Horsholm, Denmark

M. Sheffer, Scientific Editor, Orleans, Canada

### Secretariat

X. Bonnefoy, Regional Adviser, Health Planning/Ecology, WHO Regional Office for Europe, Copenhagen, Denmark (*Co-Rapporteur*)

H. Galal-Gorchev, International Programme on Chemical Safety, Division of Environmental Health, World Health Organization, Geneva, Switzerland (*Co-Rapporteur*)

## Final Drafts Preparation Meeting for Volumes 1 and 2 (Val David, Quebec, Canada, 19-22 May 1992)

### *Members*

K. Bentley, Director, Environmental Health, Health Advancement Division, Australian Department of Health, Housing and Community Services, Woden, Australia

J.K. Fawell, Principal Toxicologist, Water Research Centre, Medmenham, England

J.R. Hickman, Director-General, Environmental Health Directorate, Department of National Health and Welfare, Ottawa, Canada (*Chairman*)

U. Lund, Head, Department of Chemistry, Water Quality Institute, Horsholm, Denmark

M.E. Meek, Head, Priority Substances Section, Environmental Health Centre, Department of National Health and Welfare, Ottawa, Canada

B. Mintz, Chief, Health Effects Assessment Section, Criteria and Standards Division, Office of Drinking-Water, United States Environmental Protection Agency, Washington, DC, USA

R.F. Packham, Marlow, England

E.B. Pike, Water Research Centre, Medmenham, England

M. Sheffer, Scientific Editor, Orleans, Canada

P. Toft, Health Protection Branch, Environmental Health Directorate, Department of National Health and Welfare, Ottawa, Canada

G. Wood, Health Protection Branch, Environmental Health Directorate, Department of National Health and Welfare, Ottawa, Canada

### *Secretariat*

X. Bonnefoy, Regional Adviser, Health Planning/Ecology, WHO Regional Office for Europe, Copenhagen, Denmark (*Co-Rapporteur*)

H. Galal-Gorchev, International Programme on Chemical Safety, World Health Organization, Geneva, Switzerland (*Co-Rapporteur*)

G. Ozolins, Manager, Prevention of Environmental Pollution, Division of Environmental Health, World Health Organization, Geneva, Switzerland

## Final Task Group Meeting (Geneva, Switzerland, 21–25 September 1992)

### Members*

H. Abouzaid, Chief, Water Quality Control Division, National Agency for Drinking-Water, Rabat-Chellah, Morocco

M. Aguilar, Director of Basic Sanitation, Department of Environmental and Occupational Health and Basic Sanitation, Mexico City, Mexico

J. Alexander, Deputy Director, Department of Environmental Medicine, National Institute of Public Health, Oslo, Norway

V. Angjeli, Chief of Communal Hygiene Division, Research Institute of Hygiene and Epidemiology, Tirana, Albania

L. Anukam, Federal Environmental Protection Agency (FEPA), Department of Planning and Evaluation, Federal Secretariat Complex (Phase II), Ikoyi, Lagos, Nigeria

W.S. Assoy, Director, Environmental Health Service, Department of Health, Manila, Philippines

Changjie Chen, Director, Institute of Environmental Health Monitoring, Chinese Academy of Preventive Medicine, Beijing, China

M. Csanady, Department Leader, National Institute of Hygiene, Budapest, Hungary

H.H. Dieter, Director and Professor, Institute for Water, Soil and Air Hygiene of the Federal Office of Health, Berlin, Germany

F.K. El Jack, Head of Water Department, National Chemical Laboratories, Khartoum, Sudan

J. Forslund, National Agency of Environmental Protection, Copenhagen, Denmark (*Vice-Chairman*)

E. Funari, Department of Environmental Hygiene, Istituto Superiore di Sanità, Rome, Italy

E. Gonzalez, Chief, Department of Water Quality, Water Supply and Sewerage, San José, Costa Rica

F.J. Gumbo, Head of Water Laboratories, Operation, Maintenance and Water Laboratories Division, Ministry of Water (MAJI), Dar-es-Salaam, United Republic of Tanzania

B. Havlik, Head of Water Hygiene Branch, National Institute of Public Health, Prague, Czechoslovakia

H.M.S.S.D. Herath, Deputy Director General, Public Health Services, Ministry of Health, Colombo, Sri Lanka

---

* Invited but unable to attend: Director-General of Health, Islamabad, Pakistan; F. Sartor, Institute of Hygiene and Epidemiology, Ministry of Public Health and the Family, Brussels, Belgium.

L. Hiisvirta, Chief Engineer, Ministry of Social Affairs and Health, Helsinki, Finland

J. Kariuki, Senior Public Health Officer, Division of Environmental Health, Ministry of Health, Nairobi, Kenya

M. Kitenge, Director, Department of Local Production Control, Zaire Control Agency, Kinshasa, Zaire

F.X.R. van Leeuwen, Senior Toxicologist, National Institute of Public Health and Environmental Protection, Bilthoven, Netherlands

Y. Magara, Director, Department of Water Supply Engineering, Institute of Public Health, Tokyo, Japan

N.S. McDonald, Director, Water Branch, Department of Primary Industries and Energy, Canberra, Australia

B. Mintz, Chief, Exposure Assessment and Environmental Fate Section, Office of Science and Technology, United States Environmental Protection Agency, Washington, DC, USA

F. Niang, Chief, Laboratory Service, Senegalese National Water Management Company, Dakar, Senegal

R.F. Packham, Marlow, England

Y.A. Rakhmanin, Academician of Russian Academy of Natural Sciences, A.N. Sysin Research Institute of Human Ecology and Environmental Health, Moscow, Russian Federation

F.G.R. Reyes, Professor of Food Toxicology, Department of Food Science, State University of Campinas, Brazil (*Rapporteur*)

T. Saleh, WHO Regional Support Office, Cairo, Egypt

E. Sandberg, Senior Toxicologist, National Food Administration, Uppsala, Sweden

Nantana Santatiwut, Director, Environmental Health Division, Department of Health, Ministry of Public Health, Bangkok, Thailand

R. Sarin, Scientist, National Environmental Engineering Research Institute (NEERI), Nehru Marg, Nagpur, India

C. Shaw, Senior Advisor Scientist, Public Health Services, Department of Health, Wellington, New Zealand

J.A. Sokal, Director, Institute of Occupational Medicine and Environmental Health, Sosnowiec, Poland

P. Toft, Health Protection Branch, Environmental Health Directorate, Department of National Health and Welfare, Ottawa, Canada (*Chairman*)

D. Tricard, Sanitary Engineer, Ministry of Health and Humanitarian Action, Department of Health, Paris, France

## Observers

M.J. Crick, Radiation Safety Specialist, International Atomic Energy Agency, Vienna, Austria

A.M. van Dijk-Looyaard, Senior Scientist Drinking-Water Standards, KIWA N.V. Research and Consultancy, Nieuwegein, Netherlands

O. Hydes, Drinking Water Inspectorate, Department of the Environment, London, England

M. Rapinat, International Water Supply Association, Compagnie générale des Eaux, Paris, France

Y. Richard, Head Engineer, Société DEGREMONT-CIRSEE, Le Pecq, France

H. Rousseau, Division des Eaux de Consommation, Direction des Ecosystèmes urbains, Ministère de l'Environnement, Ste Foy, Québec, Canada

J.E. Samdal, Norwegian Institute for Water Research (NIVA), Oslo, Norway

F. Sarhan, CIBA-GEIGY Ltd, Basel, Switzerland (representing the International Group of National Associations of Manufacturers of Agrochemical Products)

E.A. Simpson, Commission of the European Communities, Brussels, Belgium

T. Yanagisawa, Director, Technical Management Section, Management and Planning Division, Bureau of Waterworks, Tokyo, Japan

## Secretariat

J. Bartram, Manager, Overseas Development, The Robens Institute of Health and Safety, University of Surrey, Guildford, England

X. Bonnefoy, Environmental Health Planning/Ecology, WHO Regional Office for Europe, Copenhagen, Denmark

A. Enevoldsen, Environmental Health Planning/Ecology, WHO Regional Office for Europe, Copenhagen, Denmark

J.K. Fawell, Principal Toxicologist, Water Research Centre, Medmenham, England

B.H. Fenger, Water and Waste Scientist, WHO European Office for Environment and Health, Rome, Italy

H. Galal-Gorchev, International Programme on Chemical Safety, World Health Organization, Geneva, Switzerland

R. Helmer, Prevention of Environmental Pollution, Division of Environmental Health, World Health Organization, Geneva, Switzerland

J. Kenny, Prevention of Environmental Pollution, Division of Environmental Health, World Health Organization, Geneva, Switzerland

U. Lund, Water Quality Institute, Horsholm, Denmark

M. Mercier, Director, International Programme on Chemical Safety, World Health Organization, Geneva, Switzerland

H. Moller, Scientist, Unit of Carcinogen Identification and Evaluation, International Agency for Research on Cancer, Lyon, France

G. Ozolins, Manager, Prevention of Environmental Pollution, Division of Environmental Health, World Health Organization, Geneva, Switzerland

E.B. Pike, Water Research Centre, Medmenham, England

M. Sheffer, Scientific Editor, Orleans, Canada

S. Tarkowski, Director, Environment and Health, WHO Regional Office for Europe, Copenhagen, Denmark

# Annex 2

# Tables of guideline values

The following tables present a summary of guideline values for microorganisms and chemicals in drinking-water. Individual values should not be used directly from the tables. The guideline values must be used and interpreted in conjunction with the information contained in the text.

## Table A2.1. *Bacteriological quality of drinking-water*[a]

| Organisms | Guideline value |
| --- | --- |
| **All water intended for drinking** | |
| *E. coli* or thermotolerant coliform bacteria[b,c] | Must not be detectable in any 100-ml sample |
| **Treated water entering the distribution system** | |
| *E. coli* or thermotolerant coliform bacteria[b] | Must not be detectable in any 100-ml sample |
| Total coliform bacteria | Must not be detectable in any 100-ml sample |
| **Treated water in the distribution system** | |
| *E. coli* or thermotolerant coliform bacteria[b] | Must not be detectable in any 100-ml sample |
| Total coliform bacteria | Must not be detectable in any 100-ml sample. In the case of large supplies, where sufficient samples are examined, must not be present in 95% of samples taken throughout any 12-month period |

[a] Immediate investigative action must be taken if either *E. coli* or total coliform bacteria are detected. The minimum action in the case of total coliform bacteria is repeat sampling; if these bacteria are detected in the repeat sample, the cause must be determined by immediate further investigation.

[b] Although *E. coli* is the more precise indicator of faecal pollution, the count of thermotolerant coliform bacteria is an acceptable alternative. If necessary, proper confirmatory tests must be carried out. Total coliform bacteria are not acceptable indicators of the sanitary quality of rural water supplies, particularly in tropical areas where many bacteria of no sanitary significance occur in almost all untreated supplies.

[c] It is recognized that, in the great majority of rural water supplies in developing countries, faecal contamination is widespread. Under these conditions, the national surveillance agency should set medium-term targets for the progressive improvement of water supplies, as recommended in Volume 3 of *Guidelines for drinking-water quality.*

## Table A2.2. Chemicals of health significance in drinking-water

### A. Inorganic constituents

| | Guideline value (mg/litre) | Remarks |
|---|---|---|
| antimony | 0.005 (P)[a] | |
| arsenic | 0.01[b](P) | For excess skin cancer risk of $6 \times 10^{-4}$ |
| barium | 0.7 | |
| beryllium | | NAD[c] |
| boron | 0.3 | |
| cadmium | 0.003 | |
| chromium | 0.05 (P) | |
| copper | 2 (P) | ATO[d] |
| cyanide | 0.07 | |
| fluoride | 1.5 | Climatic conditions, volume of water consumed, and intake from other sources should be considered when setting national standards |
| lead | 0.01 | It is recognized that not all water will meet the guideline value immediately; meanwhile, all other recommended measures to reduce the total exposure to lead should be implemented |
| manganese | 0.5 (P) | ATO |
| mercury (total) | 0.001 | |
| molybdenum | 0.07 | |
| nickel | 0.02 | |
| nitrate (as $NO_3^-$) | 50 | The sum of the ratio of the concentration of each to its respective guideline value should not exceed 1 |
| nitrite (as $NO_2^-$) | 3 (P) | |
| selenium | 0.01 | |
| uranium | | NAD |

## B. Organic constituents

| | Guideline value (µg/litre) | Remarks |
|---|---|---|
| *Chlorinated alkanes* | | |
| carbon tetrachloride | 2 | |
| dichloromethane | 20 | |
| 1,1-dichloroethane | | NAD |
| 1,2-dichloroethane | 30[b] | for excess risk of $10^{-5}$ |
| 1,1,1-trichloroethane | 2000 (P) | |
| *Chlorinated ethenes* | | |
| vinyl chloride | 5[b] | for excess risk of $10^{-5}$ |
| 1,1-dichloroethene | 30 | |
| 1,2-dichloroethene | 50 | |
| trichloroethene | 70 (P) | |
| tetrachloroethene | 40 | |
| *Aromatic hydrocarbons* | | |
| benzene | 10[b] | for excess risk of $10^{-5}$ |
| toluene | 700 | ATO |
| xylenes | 500 | ATO |
| ethylbenzene | 300 | ATO |
| styrene | 20 | ATO |
| benzo[a]pyrene | 0.7[b] | for excess risk of $10^{-5}$ |
| *Chlorinated benzenes* | | |
| monochlorobenzene | 300 | ATO |
| 1,2-dichlorobenzene | 1000 | ATO |
| 1,3-dichlorobenzene | | NAD |
| 1,4-dichlorobenzene | 300 | ATO |
| trichlorobenzenes (total) | 20 | ATO |
| *Miscellaneous* | | |
| di(2-ethylhexyl)adipate | 80 | |
| di(2-ethylhexyl)phthalate | 8 | |
| acrylamide | 0.5[b] | for excess risk of $10^{-5}$ |
| epichlorohydrin | 0.4 (P) | |
| hexachlorobutadiene | 0.6 | |
| edetic acid (EDTA) | 200 (P) | |
| nitrilotriacetic acid | 200 | |
| dialkyltins | | NAD |
| tributyltin oxide | 2 | |

## C. Pesticides

| | Guideline value (μg/litre) | Remarks |
|---|---|---|
| alachlor | 20[b] | for excess risk of $10^{-5}$ |
| aldicarb | 10 | |
| aldrin/dieldrin | 0.03 | |
| atrazine | 2 | |
| bentazone | 30 | |
| carbofuran | 5 | |
| chlordane | 0.2 | |
| chlorotoluron | 30 | |
| DDT | 2 | |
| 1,2-dibromo-3-chloropropane | 1[b] | for excess risk of $10^{-5}$ |
| 2,4-D | 30 | |
| 1,2-dichloropropane | 20 (P) | |
| 1,3-dichloropropane | | NAD |
| 1,3-dichloropropene | 20[b] | for excess risk of $10^{-5}$ |
| ethylene dibromide | | NAD |
| heptachlor and heptachlor epoxide | 0.03 | |
| hexachlorobenzene | 1[b] | for excess risk of $10^{-5}$ |
| isoproturon | 9 | |
| lindane | 2 | |
| MCPA | 2 | |
| methoxychlor | 20 | |
| metolachlor | 10 | |
| molinate | 6 | |
| pendimethalin | 20 | |
| pentachlorophenol | 9 (P) | |
| permethrin | 20 | |
| propanil | 20 | |
| pyridate | 100 | |
| simazine | 2 | |
| trifluralin | 20 | |
| chlorophenoxy herbicides other than 2,4-D and MCPA | | |
| 2,4-DB | 90 | |
| dichlorprop | 100 | |
| fenoprop | 9 | |
| MCPB | | NAD |
| mecoprop | 10 | |
| 2,4,5-T | 9 | |

## D. Disinfectants and disinfectant by-products

| Disinfectants | Guideline value (mg/litre) | Remarks |
|---|---|---|
| monochloramine | 3 | |
| di- and trichloramine | | NAD |
| chlorine | 5 | ATO. For effective disinfection there should be a residual concentration of free chlorine of $\geqslant 0.5$ mg/litre after at least 30 minutes contact time at pH $<8.0$ |
| chlorine dioxide | | A guideline value has not been established because of the rapid breakdown of chlorine dioxide and because the chlorite guideline value is adequately protective for potential toxicity from chlorine dioxide |
| iodine | | NAD |

| Disinfectant by-products | Guideline value ($\mu$g/litre) | Remarks |
|---|---|---|
| bromate | 25[b] (P) | for $7 \times 10^{-5}$ excess risk |
| chlorate | | NAD |
| chlorite | 200 (P) | |
| chlorophenols | | |
|   2-chlorophenol | | NAD |
|   2,4-dichlorophenol | | NAD |
|   2,4,6-trichlorophenol | 200[b] | for excess risk of $10^{-5}$, ATO |
| formaldehyde | 900 | |
| MX | | NAD |
| trihalomethanes | | The sum of the ratio of the concentration of each to its respective guideline value should not exceed 1 |
|   bromoform | 100 | |
|   dibromochloromethane | 100 | |
|   bromodichloromethane | 60[b] | for excess risk of $10^{-5}$ |
|   chloroform | 200[b] | for excess risk of $10^{-5}$ |
| chlorinated acetic acids | | |
|   monochloroacetic acid | | NAD |
|   dichloroacetic acid | 50 (P) | |
|   trichloroacetic acid | 100 (P) | |
| chloral hydrate | | |
|   (trichloroacetaldehyde) | 10 (P) | |
| chloroacetone | | NAD |

| Disinfectant by-products | Guideline value (µg/litre) | Remarks |
|---|---|---|
| halogenated acetonitriles | | |
| dichloroacetonitrile | 90 (P) | |
| dibromoacetonitrile | 100 (P) | |
| bromochloroacetonitrile | | NAD |
| trichloroacetonitrile | 1 (P) | |
| cyanogen chloride (as CN) | 70 | |
| chloropicrin | | NAD |

[a] (P) — Provisional guideline value. This term is used for constituents for which there is some evidence of a potential hazard but where the available information on health effects is limited; or where an uncertainty factor greater than 1000 has been used in the derivation of the tolerable daily intake (TDI). Provisional guideline values are also recommended: (1) for substances for which the calculated guideline value would be below the practical quantification level, or below the level that can be achieved through practical treatment methods; or (2) where disinfection is likely to result in the guideline value being exceeded.

[b] For substances that are considered to be carcinogenic, the guideline value is the concentration in drinking-water associated with an excess lifetime cancer risk of $10^{-5}$ (one additional cancer per 100 000 of the population ingesting drinking-water containing the substance at the guideline value for 70 years). Concentrations associated with estimated excess lifetime cancer risks of $10^{-4}$ and $10^{-6}$ can be calculated by multiplying and dividing, respectively, the guideline value by 10.

In cases in which the concentration associated with an excess lifetime cancer risk of $10^{-5}$ is not feasible as a result of inadequate analytical or treatment technology, a provisional guideline value is recommended at a practicable level and the estimated associated excess lifetime cancer risk presented.

It should be emphasized that the guideline values for carcinogenic substances have been computed from hypothetical mathematical models that cannot be verified experimentally and that the values should be interpreted differently than TDI-based values because of the lack of precision of the models. At best, these values must be regarded as rough estimates of cancer risk. However, the models used are conservative and probably err on the side of caution. Moderate short-term exposure to levels exceeding the guideline value for carcinogens does not significantly affect the risk.

[c] NAD— No adequate data to permit recommendation of a health-based guideline value.

[d] ATO— Concentrations of the substance at or below the health-based guideline value may affect the appearance, taste, or odour of the water.

*Table A2.3. Chemicals not of health significance at concentrations normally found in drinking-water*

| Chemical | Remarks |
|----------|---------|
| asbestos | U |
| silver | U |
| tin | U |

U — It is unnecessary to recommend a health-based guideline value for these compounds because they are not hazardous to human health at concentrations normally found in drinking-water.

*Table A2.4. Radioactive constituents of drinking-water*

| | Screening value (Bq/litre) | Remarks |
|---|---|---|
| gross alpha activity | 0.1 | If a screening value is exceeded, more detailed radionuclide analysis is necessary. Higher values do not necessarily imply that the water is unsuitable for human consumption |
| gross beta activity | 1 | |

### Table A2.5. Substances and parameters in drinking-water that may give rise to complaints from consumers

| | Levels likely to give rise to consumer complaints[a] | Reasons for consumer complaints |
|---|---|---|
| *Physical parameters* | | |
| colour | 15 TCU[b] | appearance |
| taste and odour | — | should be acceptable |
| temperature | — | should be acceptable |
| turbidity | 5 NTU[c] | appearance; for effective terminal disinfection, median turbidity ⩽1NTU, single sample ⩽5NTU |
| *Inorganic constituents* | | |
| aluminium | 0.2 mg/l | depositions, discoloration |
| ammonia | 1.5 mg/l | odour and taste |
| chloride | 250 mg/l | taste, corrosion |
| copper | 1 mg/l | staining of laundry and sanitary ware (health-based provisional guideline value 2 mg/litre) |
| hardness | — | high hardness: scale deposition, scum formation; low hardness: possible corrosion |
| hydrogen sulfide | 0.05 mg/l | odour and taste |
| iron | 0.3 mg/l | staining of laundry and sanitary ware |
| manganese | 0.1 mg/l | staining of laundry and sanitary ware (health-based provisional guideline value 0.5 mg/litre) |
| dissolved oxygen | — | indirect effects |
| pH | — | low pH: corrosion; high pH: taste, soapy feel; preferably <8.0 for effective disinfection with chlorine |
| sodium | 200 mg/l | taste |
| sulfate | 250 mg/l | taste, corrosion |
| total dissolved solids | 1000 mg/l | taste |
| zinc | 3 mg/l | appearance, taste |
| *Organic constituents* | | |
| toluene | 24–170 μg/l | odour, taste (health-based guideline value 700 μg/l) |
| xylene | 20–1800 μg/l | odour, taste (health-based guideline value 500 μg/l) |
| ethylbenzene | 2–200 μg/l | odour, taste (health-based guideline value 300 μg/l) |
| styrene | 4–2600 μg/l | odour, taste (health-based guideline value 20 μg/l) |

| | Levels likely to give rise to consumer complaints[a] | Reasons for consumer complaints |
|---|---|---|
| monochlorobenzene | 10–120 $\mu$g/l | odour, taste (health-based guideline value 300 $\mu$g/l) |
| 1,2-dichlorobenzene | 1–10 $\mu$g/l | odour, taste (health-based guideline value 1000 $\mu$g/l) |
| 1,4-dichlorobenzene | 0.3–30 $\mu$g/l | odour, taste (health-based guideline value 300 $\mu$g/l) |
| trichlorobenzenes (total) | 5–50 $\mu$g/l | odour, taste (health-based guideline value 20 $\mu$g/l) |
| synthetic detergents | — | foaming, taste, odour |
| *Disinfectants and disinfectant by-products* | | |
| chlorine | 600–1000 $\mu$g/l | taste and odour (health-based guideline value 5 mg/l) |
| chlorophenols | | |
| 2-chlorophenol | 0.1–10 $\mu$g/l | taste, odour |
| 2,4-dichlorophenol | 0.3–40 $\mu$g/l | taste, odour |
| 2,4,6-trichlorophenol | 2–300 $\mu$g/l | taste, odour (health-based guideline value 200 $\mu$g/l) |

[a] The levels indicated are not precise numbers. Problems may occur at lower or higher values according to local circumstances. A range of taste and odour threshold concentrations is given for organic constituents.

[b] TCU, true colour unit.

[c] NTU, nephelometric turbidity unit.

# Index

Page numbers in bold type indicate main discussions.

Aluminium **132–138**
  acceptable values 138, 948
  analytical methods 133
  animal toxicity studies 135–136
  coagulants 133
  effects on humans 136–138
  environmental levels/human exposure 133–134
  general description 132–133
  kinetics and metabolism 134
Aluminium sulfate (alum) 351
Alzheimer disease 137–138
δ-Aminolaevulinic acid dehydratase (δ-ALAD)
  260
Ammonia **142–146**
  acceptable level 948
  analytical methods 143
  animal toxicity studies 145
  effects on humans 146
  environmental levels/human exposure 143–144
  general description 142–143
  kinetics and metabolism 144–145
  mutagenicity 146
Ammonium cation *see* Ammonia
Amoebae
  free-living **60–62**
  *Legionella* growth inside 29, 62
Amoebic dysentery 59
Amoebic meningoencephalitis, primary 60, 62
Amyotrophic lateral sclerosis 136–137
*Anabaena* 75
Anaemia
  chlorite/chlorate-induced 808, 810
  haemolytic 701, 793
  lead-induced 260
  tin-induced 364
Anaerobic bacteria 83–84, 88
*Ancylostoma duodenale* 68, 73
Anencephaly 239
Angiosarcoma, liver 428, 429
Animals
  nuisance 78, 80–81, 106
  toxicity studies 122
Anthracene 498, 500
Antimony **147–152**
  analytical methods 148–149
  animal toxicity studies 150–151
  carcinogenicity 151, 152
  effects on humans 152
  environmental levels/human exposure 149
  general description 147–148
  guideline value, provisional 152, 942
  kinetics and metabolism 149–150
  mutagenicity 151
Aorta, coarctation of 161
*Aphanizomenon* 75

Aquifers *see* Groundwaters
Argyria 341
Arsenic **156–162**
  analytical methods 157
  animal toxicity studies 159
  carcinogenicity 159, 160–161, 162
  effects on humans 160–162
  environmental levels/human exposure 158
  general description 156–157
  guideline value, provisional 162, 942
  kinetics and metabolism 158–159
  mutagenicity 159
Asbestos **167–171**, 947
  analytical methods 168
  animal toxicity studies 170
  carcinogenicity 170–171
  effects on humans 170–171
  environmental levels/human exposure 168–169
  general description 167–168
  kinetics and metabolism 169
  mutagenicity 170
Asbestos/cement (A/C) pipes 169
*Ascaris lumbricoides* 68, 73
*Asellus aquaticus* 80, 81
Asthma, chlorinated water and 800
Astroviruses 43
Atrazine **608–612**
  analytical methods 609
  animal toxicity studies 610–611
  carcinogenicity 611
  effects on humans 611
  environmental levels/human exposure 609
  general description 608–609
  guideline value 612, 944
  kinetics and metabolism 609–610
  mutagenicity 611

Back-siphonage 117
Bacteria (*see also specific bacteria*)
  anaerobic 83–84, 88
  infective dose 14–15
  nuisance 78, 79–80
  pathogenic 10, 11, **18–36**
    excreted 18–27
    growing in supply systems 28–36
    methods of detection 89–90
    taste/odour problems 357–358
Bacteriological quality **94–96**
  guideline values 95, 941
Bacteriophages 82–83, **87–88**, 90
*Bacteroides fragilis* 83–84, 88
Balantidiasis 59
*Balantidium coli* 10, 52, **59**
Barium **173–180**
  analytical methods 175